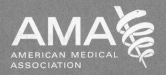

AMA
AMERICAN MEDICAL
ASSOCIATION

MW00836893

ICD-10-PCS 2023
The Complete Official Codebook

AMA publications fund initiatives that drive improvements in
patient health, practice innovation and medical education.

Notice

ICD-10-PCS: The Complete Official Codebook is designed to be an accurate and authoritative source regarding coding and every reasonable effort has been made to ensure accuracy and completeness of the content. However, the American Medical Association (AMA) makes no guarantee, warranty, or representation that this publication is accurate, complete, or without errors. It is understood that the AMA is not rendering any legal or other professional services or advice in this publication and that the AMA bears no liability for any results or consequences that may arise from the use of this book.

Our Commitment to Accuracy

The AMA is committed to producing accurate and reliable materials. To report corrections, please call the AMA Unified Service Center at (800) 621-8335. AMA product updates, errata, and addendum can be found at amaproductupdates.org.

To purchase additional copies, visit the AMA store at amastore.com. Refer to product number OP201123.

Copyright

Acknowledgments

Marianne Randall, CPC, *Product Manager*

Anita Schmidt, BS, RHIA, AHIMA-approved ICD-10-CM/PCS Trainer, *Subject Matter Expert*

LaJuana Green, RHIA, CCS, *Subject Matter Expert*

Stacy Perry, *Manager, Desktop Publishing*

Tracy Betzler, *Senior Desktop Publishing Specialist*

Hope M. Dunn, *Senior Desktop Publishing Specialist*

Katie Russell, *Desktop Publishing Specialist*

Kate Holden, *Editor*

Anita Schmidt, BS, RHIA, AHIMA-approved ICD-10-CM/PCS Trainer

Ms. Schmidt has expertise in ICD-10-CM/PCS, DRG, and CPT with more than 15 years' experience in coding in multiple settings, including inpatient, observation, and same-day surgery. Her experience includes analysis of medical record documentation, assignment of ICD-10-CM and PCS codes, and DRG validation. She has conducted training for ICD-10-CM/PCS and electronic health record. She has also collaborated with clinical documentation specialists to identify documentation needs and potential areas for physician education. Most recently she has been developing content for resource and educational products related to ICD-10-CM, ICD-10-PCS, DRG, and CPT. Ms. Schmidt is an AHIMA-approved ICD-10-CM/PCS trainer and is an active member of the American Health Information Management Association (AHIMA) and the Minnesota Health Information Management Association (MHIMA).

LaJuana Green, RHIA, CCS

Ms. Green is a registered health information administrator with over 35 years of experience in multiple areas of information management. She has proven expertise in the analysis of medical record documentation, assignment of ICD-10-CM and PCS codes, DRG validation, and CPT code assignment in ambulatory surgery units and the hospital outpatient setting. Her experience includes serving as a director of a health information management department, clinical technical editing, new technology research and writing, medical record management, utilization review activities, quality assurance, tumor registry, medical library services, and chargemaster maintenance. Ms. Green is an active member of the American Health Information Management Association (AHIMA).

Contents

Contents

What's New for 2023

The Centers for Medicare and Medicaid Services is the agency charged with maintaining and updating ICD-10-PCS. CMS released the most current revisions, a summary of which may be found on the CMS website at https://www.cms.gov/medicare/icd-10/2023-icd-10-pcs.

Due to the unique structure of ICD-10-PCS, a change in a character value may affect individual codes and several code tables.

Change Summary Table

2022 Total	New Codes	Revised Titles	Deleted Codes	2023 Total
78,229	331	0	64	78,496

ICD-10-PCS Code Totals, By Section

Medical and Surgical	68,024
Obstetrics	304
Placement	861
Administration	1,257
Measurement and Monitoring	422
Extracorporeal or Systemic Assistance and Performance	51
Extracorporeal or Systemic Therapies	46
Osteopathic	100
Other Procedures	78
Chiropractic	90
Imaging	2,978
Nuclear Medicine	463
Radiation Therapy	2,056
Physical Rehabilitation and Diagnostic Audiology	1,380
Mental Health	30
Substance Abuse Treatment	59
New Technology	297
Total	78,496

ICD-10-PCS Table Changes Highlights

- New qualifier Laser Interstitial Thermal Therapy (LITT) added to the root operation table, Destruction, in the following body systems:
  - Central Nervous System and Cranial Nerves
  - Respiratory System
  - Gastrointestinal System
  - Hepatobiliary System and Pancreas
  - Endocrine System
  - Skin and Breast
  - Male Reproductive System
- New qualifier Rapid Deployment Technique added to root operation table Replacement in the Heart and Great Vessels body system for the body part Aortic Valve and device value Zooplastic Tissue
- New qualifier values Prostatic Artery, Right and Prostatic Artery, Left, added to root operation table Occlusion in the Lower Arteries body system for body parts Internal Iliac Artery, Right, and Internal Iliac Artery, Left, respectively

- New qualifier values Bladder; Ureter, Right; Ureter, Left; and Ureters, Bilateral, added for body part Small Intestine and new qualifier value Bladder added for body part Large Intestine in the root operation table Transfer in the Gastrointestinal System body system
- New device value Infusion Device added for body part Skull in the root operation tables Removal and Revision in the Head and Facial Bones body system
- Approach values Via Natural or Artificial Opening and Via Natural or Artificial Opening Endoscopic added to body part Neck in the root operation table Drainage in the Anatomical Regions, General, body system
- New row added to root operation table Assistance, Physiological Systems, in the Extracorporeal or Systemic Assistance and Performance section to capture continuous supersaturated oxygenation of the Cardiac body system
- Qualifier value Supersaturated removed from Circulatory body system in the root operation table Assistance, Physiological Systems, in the Extracorporeal or Systemic Assistance and Performance section
- New row added to the root operation MRI, Respiratory System, in the Imaging section to capture the use of Hyperpolarized Xenon 129 (Xe-129) for the body part Lungs, Bilateral
- Modality qualifier value of Laser Interstitial Thermal Therapy removed from all root operation tables, Other Radiation, in the Radiation Therapy section
- Seven new tables added to the New Technology section:
  - X0H Nervous System, Insertion
  - X0Z Nervous System, Other Procedures
  - XF5 Hepatobiliary System and Pancreas, Destruction
  - XKU Muscles, Tendons, Bursae and Ligaments, Supplement
  - XNH Bones, Insertion
  - XRH Joints, Insertion
  - XRR Joints, Replacement
- One table deleted from the New Technology section:
  - XK0 Muscles, Tendons, Bursae and Ligaments, Introduction

New Definitions Addenda

Section 0 – Medical and Surgical
Body Part Definitions

ICD-10-PCS Value	Definition	
Internal Iliac Artery, Left	Add Add	Prostatic artery Superior vesical artery
Internal Iliac Artery, Right	Add Add	Prostatic artery Superior vesical artery
Add Peritoneal Cavity	Add	Abdominal cavity
Add Skin, Perineum	Add	Perianal skin
Superior Vena Cava	Add	Cavoatrial junction

Section 0 – Medical and Surgical Device Definitions

ICD-10-PCS Value	Definition	
Interbody Fusion Device in Lower Joints	Add	COALESCE® radiolucent interbody fusion device
	Add	COHERE® radiolucent interbody fusion device
	Add	nanoLOCK™ interbody fusion device
	Add	Titan Endoskeleton™
Interbody Fusion Device in Upper Joints	Add	COALESCE® radiolucent interbody fusion device
	Add	COHERE® radiolucent interbody fusion device
	Add	nanoLOCK™ interbody fusion device
	Add	Titan Endoskeleton™
Internal Fixation Device, Sustained Compression for Fusion in Lower Joints	Delete	DynaNail Mini®
	Delete	DynaNail®
	Add	DynaClip® (Forte)
	Add	DynaNail® (Hybrid)(Mini)
Internal Fixation Device, Sustained Compression for Fusion in Upper Joints	Delete	DynaNail Mini®
	Delete	DynaNail®
	Add	DynaClip® (Forte)
	Add	DynaNail® (Hybrid)(Mini)
Nonautologous Tissue Substitute	Add	MIRODERM™ Biologic Wound Matrix
Spinal Stabilization Device, Interspinous Process for Insertion in Lower Joints	Add	X-Spine Axle Cage
Spinal Stabilization Device, Interspinous Process for Insertion in Upper Joints	Add	X-Spine Axle Cage

Section 3 – Administration Substance Definitions

ICD-10-PCS Value	Definition	
Hematopoietic Stem/Progenitor Cells, Genetically Modified	Delete	OTL-103
	Delete	OTL-200
Add Other Substance	Add	CBMA (Concentrated Bone Marrow Aspirate)
	Add	Defitelio
	Add	MarrowStim™ PAD Kit for CBMA (concentrated bone marrow aspirate)

Section X – New Technology Root Operation Definitions

ICD-10-PCS Value	Definition	
Fusion	Delete	Explanation: The body part is joined together by fixation device, bone graft, or other means.
	Delete	Includes/Examples: Spinal fusion, ankle arthrodesis
Add Other Procedures	Add	Definition: Methodologies which attempt to remediate or cure a disorder or disease.
Replacement	Delete	Explanation: The body part may have been taken out or replaced, or may be taken out, physically eradicated, or rendered nonfunctional during the Replacement procedure. A Removal procedure is coded for taking out the device used in a previous replacement procedure.
	Delete	Includes/Examples: Total hip replacement, bone graft, free skin graft

Section X – New Technology Device/Substance/Technology Definitions

ICD-10-PCS Value	Definition	
Delete Bezlotoxumab Monoclonal Antibody	Delete	ZINPLAVA™
Add Afamitresgene Autoleucel Immunotherapy	Add	afami-cel
Add Betibeglogene Autotemcel	Add	beti-cel
Add Broad Consortium Microbiota-based Live Biotherapeutic Suspension	Add	REBYOTA®
Ciltacabtagene Autoleucel	Add	CARVYKTI™
Delete Concentrated Bone Marrow Aspirate	Delete	CBMA (concentrated bone marrow aspirate)
Delete Defibrotide Sodium Anticoagulant	Delete	Defitelio
Delete Interbody Fusion Device, Nanotextured Surface in New Technology	Delete	nanoLOCK™ interbody fusion device
Delete Interbody Fusion Device, Radiolucent Porous in New Technology	Delete	COALESCE® radiolucent interbody fusion device
	Delete	COHERE® radiolucent interbody fusion device
Delete Skin Substitute, Porcine Liver Derived in New Technology	Delete	MIRODERM™ Biologic Wound Matrix
Delete Zooplastic Tissue, Rapid Deployment Technique in New Technology	Delete	EDWARDS INTUITY Elite valve system
	Delete	INTUITY Elite valve system, EDWARDS
	Delete	Perceval sutureless valve
	Delete	Sutureless valve, Perceval
Add Daratumumab and Hyaluronidase-fihj	Add	Darzalex Faspro®
Add Engineered Allogeneic Thymus Tissue	Add	RETHYMIC®

ICD-10-PCS Value		Definition	
Add	Inebilizumab-cdon	Add	UPLIZNA®
Add	Internal Fixation Device with Tulip Connector in New Technology	Add	iFuse Bedrock™ Granite Implant System
Add	Maribavir Anti-infective	Add	LIVTENCITY™
Add	Neurostimulator Lead in New Technology	Add	Ischemic Stroke System (ISS500)
		Add	ISS500 (Ischemic Stroke System)
Add	Neurostimulator Lead with Paired Stimulation System in New Technology	Add	Vivistim® Paired VNS System Lead
Add	Posterior Spinal Motion Preservation Device in New Technology	Add	TOPS™ System
Add	Posterior Vertebral Tether in New Technology	Add	LigaPASS 2.0™ PJK Prevention System
Add	Synthetic Substitute, Lateral Meniscus in New Technology	Add	NUsurface® Meniscus Implant
Add	Synthetic Substitute, Medial Meniscus in New Technology	Add	NUsurface® Meniscus Implant
Add	Tabelecleucel Immunotherapy	Add	tab-cel®
Add	Taurolidine Anti-infective and Heparin Anticoagulant	Add	DefenCath™

List of Updated Files

2023 Official ICD-10-PCS Coding Guidelines
- New guideline B3.19 added and guidelines B4.1c and B6.1a revised in response to public comment and internal review.
- Downloadable PDF

2023 ICD-10-PCS Code Tables and Index (Zip file)
- Code tables for use beginning October 1, 2022.
- Downloadable PDF, file name is pcs_2023.pdf
- Downloadable xml files for developers, file names are icd10pcs_tables_2023.xml, icd10pcs_index_2023.xml, icd10pcs_definitions_2023.xml
- Accompanying schema for developers, file names are icd10pcs_tables.xsd, icd10pcs_index.xsd, icd10pcs_definitions.xsd

2023 ICD-10-PCS Codes File (Zip file)
- ICD-10-PCS Codes file is a simple format for nontechnical uses, containing the valid FY2023 ICD-10-PCS codes and their long titles.
- File is in text file format, file name is icd10pcs_codes_2023.txt
- Accompanying documentation for codes file, file name is icd10pcsCodesFile.pdf
- Codes file addenda in text format, file name is codes_addenda_2023.txt

2023 ICD-10-PCS Order File (Long and Abbreviated Titles) (Zip file)
- ICD-10-PCS order file is for developers, provides a unique five-digit "order number" for each ICD-10-PCS table and code, as well as a long and abbreviated code title.
- ICD-10-PCS order file name is icd10pcs_order_2023.txt
- Accompanying documentation for tabular order file, file name is icd10pcsOrderFile.pdf
- Tabular order file addenda in text format, file name is order_addenda_2023.txt

2023 ICD-10-PCS Final Addenda (Zip file)
- Addenda files in downloadable PDF, file names are tables_addenda_2023.pdf, index_addenda_2023.pdf, definitions_addenda_2023.pdf
- Addenda files also in machine readable text format for developers, file names are tables_addenda_2023.txt, index_addenda_2023.txt, definitions_addenda_2023.txt

2023 ICD-10-PCS Conversion Table (Zip file)
- ICD-10-PCS code conversion table is provided to assist users in data retrieval, in downloadable Excel spreadsheet, file name is icd10pcs_conversion_table_2023.xlsx
- Conversion table also in machine readable text format for developers, file name is icd10pcs_conversion_table_2023.txt
- Accompanying documentation for code conversion table, file name is icd10pcsConversionTable.pdf

Introduction

ICD-10-PCS: The Complete Official Code Set is your definitive coding resource for procedure coding in acute inpatient hospitals. In addition to the official ICD-10-PCS Coding System Files, revised and distributed by the Centers for Medicare and Medicaid Services (CMS), Optum's coding experts have incorporated Medicare-related coding edits and proprietary features, such as coding tools and appendixes, into a comprehensive and easy-to-use reference.

This manual provides the most current information that was available at the time of publication. For updates to official source documents that may have occurred after this manual was published, please refer to the following:

- **CMS International Classification of Disease, 10th Revision, Procedural Coding System (ICD-10-PCS):**

    https://www.cms.gov/medicare/icd-10/2023-icd-10-pcs

- **CMS Inpatient Prospective Payment System Proposed Rule, FY2023**

    https://www.cms.gov/medicare/acute-inpatient-pps/fy-2023-ipps-proposed-rule-home-page

- **CMS Inpatient Prospective Payment System Proposed Rule, FY 2023 - Proposed, version 40, MS-DRG Grouper software, Definitions Manual files and Medicare Code Editor (MCE) files**

    https://www.cms.gov/Medicare/Medicare-Fee-for-Service-Payment/AcuteInpatientPPS/MS-DRG-Classifications-and-Software

- **American Hospital Association (AHA) Coding Clinics**

    https://www.codingclinicadvisor.com/

ICD-10-PCS Code Structure

All codes in ICD-10-PCS are seven characters long. Each character in the seven-character code represents an aspect of the procedure, as shown in the following diagram of characters from the main section of ICD-10-PCS, called the Medical and Surgical section.

	Section	Body System	Root Operation	Body Part	Approach	Device	Qualifier
Characters:	1	2	3	4	5	6	7

One of 34 possible alphanumeric values—using the digits 0–9 and letters A–H, J–N, and P–Z—can be assigned to each character in a code. The letters O and I are not used so as to avoid confusion with the digits 0 and 1. A code is derived by choosing a specific value for each of the seven characters, based on details about the procedure performed. Because the definition of each character is a function of its physical position in the code, the same value placed in a different position means something different; the value 0 as the first character means something different from 0 as the second character or as the third character, and so on.

The first character always determines the broad procedure category, or section. The second through seventh characters have the same meaning within a specific section, but these meanings can change in a different section. For example, the sixth character means "device" in the Medical and Surgical section but "qualifier" in the Imaging section.

ICD-10-PCS Manual

Index

Codes may be found in the index based on the general type of procedure (e.g., resection, transfusion, fluoroscopy), or a more commonly used term (e.g., appendectomy). For example, the code for percutaneous intraluminal dilation of the coronary arteries with an intraluminal device can be found in the Index under *Dilation*, or a synonym of *Dilation* (e.g., angioplasty). The Index then specifies the first three or four values of the code or directs the user to see another term.

Example:

> **Dilation**
> > Artery
> > > Coronary
> > > > One Artery 0270

Based on the first three values of the code provided in the Index, the corresponding table can be located. In the example above, the first three values indicate table 027 is to be referenced for code completion.

The tables and characters are arranged first by number and then by letter for each character (tables for 00-, 01-, 02-, etc., are followed by those for 0B-, 0C-, 0D-, etc., followed by 0B1, 0B2, etc., followed by 0BB, 0BC, 0BD, etc.).

Note: The Tables section must be used to construct a complete and valid code by specifying the last three or four values.

Tables

The tables in ICD-10-PCS provide the valid combination of character values needed to build a unique procedure code. Each table is preceded by the first three characters of the code, along with their descriptions. In the Medical and Surgical section, for example, the first three characters contain the name of the section (character 1), the body system (character 2), and the root operation performed (character 3).

Listed underneath the first three characters is a table comprising four columns and one or more rows. The four columns in the table specify the last four characters needed to complete the ICD-10-PCS code. Depending on the section, the labels for each column may be different. In the Medical and Surgical section, they are labeled body part (character 4), approach (character 5), device (character 6), and qualifier (character 7). Each row in the table specifies the valid combination of values for characters 4 through 7.

Table 1: Row from table 027

Ø	Medical and Surgical	
2	Heart and Great Vessels	
7	Dilation	Definition: Expanding an orifice or the lumen of a tubular body part
		Explanation: The orifice can be a natural orifice or an artificially created orifice. Accomplished by stretching a tubular body part using intraluminal pressure or by cutting part of the orifice or wall of the tubular body part.

Body Part Character 4	Approach Character 5	Device Character 6	Qualifier Character 7
Ø Coronary Artery, One Artery 1 Coronary Artery, Two Arteries 2 Coronary Artery, Three Arteries 3 Coronary Artery, Four or More Arteries	Ø Open 3 Percutaneous 4 Percutaneous Endoscopic	4 Intraluminal Device, Drug-eluting 5 Intraluminal Device, Drug-eluting, Two 6 Intraluminal Device, Drug-eluting, Three 7 Intraluminal Device, Drug-eluting, Four or More D Intraluminal Device E Intraluminal Device, Two F Intraluminal Device, Three G Intraluminal Device, Four or More T Intraluminal Device, Radioactive Z No Device	6 Bifurcation Z No Qualifier

For instance, table 1 above shows the first row from table 027 in ICD-10-PCS. The values 027 specify the section *Medical and Surgical (Ø)*, the body system *Heart and Great Vessels (2)*, and the root operation *Dilation (7)*. As shown, the root operation (Dilation) is also accompanied by its corresponding definition and explanation. Note, a definition of the root operation is provided for every table in ICD-10-PCS; however, an explanation may not always be applicable.

In total, this single row can be used to construct 240 unique procedure codes. The valid codes shown in table 2 (below) are constructed using the body part (character 4) value of Ø, Coronary artery, one artery, combined with all valid approach (character 5) values, device (character 6) values, and a qualifier (character 7) value of Z, No Qualifier.

Table 2: Code titles for dilation of one coronary artery (Ø270)

027004Z	Dilation of Coronary Artery, One Artery with Drug-eluting Intraluminal Device, Open Approach
027005Z	Dilation of Coronary Artery, One Artery with Two Drug-eluting Intraluminal Devices, Open Approach
027006Z	Dilation of Coronary Artery, One Artery with Three Drug-eluting Intraluminal Devices, Open Approach
027007Z	Dilation of Coronary Artery, One Artery with Four or More Drug-eluting Intraluminal Devices, Open Approach
02700DZ	Dilation of Coronary Artery, One Artery with Intraluminal Device, Open Approach
02700EZ	Dilation of Coronary Artery, One Artery with Two Intraluminal Devices, Open Approach
02700FZ	Dilation of Coronary Artery, One Artery with Three Intraluminal Devices, Open Approach
02700GZ	Dilation of Coronary Artery, One Artery with Four or More Intraluminal Devices, Open Approach
02700TZ	Dilation of Coronary Artery, One Artery with Radioactive Intraluminal Device, Open Approach
02700ZZ	Dilation of Coronary Artery, One Artery, Open Approach
027034Z	Dilation of Coronary Artery, One Artery with Drug-eluting Intraluminal Device, Percutaneous Approach
027035Z	Dilation of Coronary Artery, One Artery with Two Drug-eluting Intraluminal Devices, Percutaneous Approach
027036Z	Dilation of Coronary Artery, One Artery with Three Drug-eluting Intraluminal Devices, Percutaneous Approach

027037Z	Dilation of Coronary Artery, One Artery with Four or More Drug-eluting Intraluminal Devices, Percutaneous Approach
02703DZ	Dilation of Coronary Artery, One Artery with Intraluminal Device, Percutaneous Approach
02703EZ	Dilation of Coronary Artery, One Artery with Two Intraluminal Devices, Percutaneous Approach
02703FZ	Dilation of Coronary Artery, One Artery with Three Intraluminal Devices, Percutaneous Approach
02703GZ	Dilation of Coronary Artery, One Artery with Four or More Intraluminal Devices, Percutaneous Approach
02703TZ	Dilation of Coronary Artery, One Artery with Radioactive Intraluminal Device, Percutaneous Approach
02703ZZ	Dilation of Coronary Artery, One Artery, Percutaneous Approach
027044Z	Dilation of Coronary Artery, One Artery with Drug-eluting Intraluminal Device, Percutaneous Endoscopic Approach
027045Z	Dilation of Coronary Artery, One Artery with Two Drug-eluting Intraluminal Devices, Percutaneous Endoscopic Approach
027046Z	Dilation of Coronary Artery, One Artery with Three Drug-eluting Intraluminal Devices, Percutaneous Endoscopic Approach
027047Z	Dilation of Coronary Artery, One Artery with Four or More Drug-eluting Intraluminal Devices, Percutaneous Endoscopic Approach
02704DZ	Dilation of Coronary Artery, One Artery with Intraluminal Device, Percutaneous Endoscopic Approach
02704EZ	Dilation of Coronary Artery, One Artery with Two Intraluminal Devices, Percutaneous Endoscopic Approach
02704FZ	Dilation of Coronary Artery, One Artery with Three Intraluminal Devices, Percutaneous Endoscopic Approach
02704GZ	Dilation of Coronary Artery, One Artery with Four or More Intraluminal Devices, Percutaneous Endoscopic Approach
02704TZ	Dilation of Coronary Artery, One Artery with Radioactive Intraluminal Device, Percutaneous Endoscopic Approach
02704ZZ	Dilation of Coronary Artery, One Artery, Percutaneous Endoscopic Approach

Table 3: Rows from table 00H

0	**Medical and Surgical**
0	**Central Nervous System and Cranial Nerves**
H	**Insertion**

Definition: Putting in a nonbiological appliance that monitors, assists, performs, or prevents a physiological function but does not physically take the place of a body part

Explanation: None

Body Part Character 4		Approach Character 5	Device Character 6	Qualifier Character 7

0 Brain
  Cerebrum
  Corpus callosum
  Encephalon
		0 Open	1 Radioactive Element
			2 Monitoring Device
			3 Infusion Device
			4 Radioactive Element, Cesium-131 Collagen Implant
			M Neurostimulator Lead
			Y Other Device
				Z No Qualifier

0 Brain
  Cerebrum
  Corpus callosum
  Encephalon
		3 Percutaneous
		4 Percutaneous Endoscopic
			1 Radioactive Element
			2 Monitoring Device
			3 Infusion Device
			M Neurostimulator Lead
			Y Other Device
				Z No Qualifier

6 Cerebral Ventricle
  Aqueduct of Sylvius
  Cerebral aqueduct (Sylvius)
  Choroid plexus
  Ependyma
  Foramen of Monro
    (intraventricular)
  Fourth ventricle
  Interventricular foramen
    (Monro)
  Left lateral ventricle
  Right lateral ventricle
  Third ventricle
	E Cranial Nerve
	U Spinal Canal
	  Epidural space, spinal
	  Extradural space, spinal
	  Subarachnoid space,
	    spinal
	  Subdural space, spinal
	  Vertebral canal
	V Spinal Cord
	  Dorsal root ganglion
		0 Open
		3 Percutaneous
		4 Percutaneous Endoscopic
			1 Radioactive Element
			2 Monitoring Device
			3 Infusion Device
			M Neurostimulator Lead
			Y Other Device
				Z No Qualifier

Table 3 is split into three rows; values of characters must all be selected from within the same row of the table. Rows 1 and 2 have the same body part (character 4) value of 0 Brain and the same qualifier value (character 7) of Z No Qualifier. However, the approach (character 5) values are not the same for these two rows, and there is one additional device (character 6) value in row 1 that is not included in row 2. As shown in row 1, body part value Brain (0) with device value Radioactive Element, Cesium-131 Collagen Implant (4) can only be used with approach value Open (0). In other words, code 00H034Z would be invalid as the approach value 3 is only applicable to row 2 and the device value 4 is only applicable to row 1. It would be inappropriate to build a code for body part 0 if all of the values are not contained in its own row.

Note: In this manual, there are instances in which some tables due to length must be continued on the next page. Each section must be used separately and value selection must be made within the same row of the table.

Character Meanings

In each section, each character has a specific meaning, and this character meaning remains constant within that section. Character meaning tables have been provided at the beginning of each body system in the Medical and Surgical section (0) and the Obstetric section (1) to help the user identify the character members available within that section. These tables have purple headers, unlike the official code tables that have green headers and **SHOULD NOT** be used to build a PCS code. Following is an excerpt of a character meaning table.

Table 4: Rows from Central Nervous System and Cranial Nerves - Character Meanings Table

Operation–Character 3	Body Part–Character 4	Approach–Character 5	Device–Character 6	Qualifier–Character 7
1 Bypass	0 Brain	0 Open	0 Drainage Device	0 Nasopharynx
2 Change	1 Cerebral Meninges	3 Percutaneous	1 Radioactive Element	1 Mastoid Sinus
5 Destruction	2 Dura Mater	4 Percutaneous Endoscopic	2 Monitoring Device	2 Atrium
7 Dilation	3 Epidural Space, Intracranial	X External	3 Infusion Device	3 Blood Vessel
8 Division	4 Subdural Space, Intracranial		4 Radioactive Element, Cesium-131 Collagen Implant	4 Pleural Cavity
9 Drainage	5 Subarachnoid Space, Intracranial		7 Autologous Tissue Substitute	5 Intestine
B Excision	6 Cerebral Ventricle		J Synthetic Substitute	6 Peritoneal Cavity
C Extirpation	7 Cerebral Hemisphere		K Nonautologous Tissue Substitute	7 Urinary Tract
D Extraction	8 Basal Ganglia		M Neurostimulator Lead	8 Bone Marrow
F Fragmentation	9 Thalamus		Y Other Device	9 Fallopian Tube
H Insertion	A Hypothalamus		Z No Device	A Subgaleal space
J Inspection	B Pons			B Cerebral Cisterns

Sections

The first character of the procedure code always specifies the section. There are 17 sections within the PCS manual, listed below.

Medical and Surgical Section

Ø   Medical and Surgical

Medical and Surgical-related Sections

1   Obstetrics

2   Placement

3   Administration

4   Measurement and Monitoring

5   Extracorporeal or Systemic Assistance and Performance

6   Extracorporeal or Systemic Therapies

7   Osteopathic

8   Other Procedures

9   Chiropractic

Ancillary Sections

B   Imaging

C   Nuclear Medicine

D   Radiation Therapy

F   Physical Rehabilitation and Diagnostic Audiology

G   Mental Health

H   Substance Abuse Treatment

New Technology Section

X   New Technology

Medical and Surgical Section (Ø)

The Medical and Surgical section contains codes for the vast majority of procedures typically reported in an inpatient setting.

Character Meaning

The seven characters for Medical and Surgical procedures have the following meaning:

Character	Meaning
1	Section
2	Body System
3	Root Operation
4	Body Part
5	Approach
6	Device
7	Qualifier

Section (Character 1)

Medical and Surgical procedure codes all have a first character value of Ø.

Body Systems (Character 2)

The second character represents the body system—the general physiological system or anatomical region where the procedure is being performed.

Body Systems

Ø   Central Nervous System and Cranial Nerves

1   Peripheral Nervous System

2   Heart and Great Vessels

3   Upper Arteries

4   Lower Arteries

5   Upper Veins

6   Lower Veins

7   Lymphatic and Hemic Systems

8   Eye

9   Ear, Nose, Sinus

B   Respiratory System

C   Mouth and Throat

D   Gastrointestinal System

F   Hepatobiliary System and Pancreas

G   Endocrine System

H   Skin and Breast

J   Subcutaneous Tissue and Fascia

K   Muscles

L   Tendons

M   Bursae and Ligaments

N   Head and Facial Bones

P   Upper Bones

Q   Lower Bones

R   Upper Joints

S   Lower Joints

T   Urinary System

U   Female Reproductive System

V   Male Reproductive System

W   Anatomical Regions, General

X   Anatomical Regions, Upper Extremities

Y   Anatomical Regions, Lower Extremities

Root Operations (Character 3)

The third character represents the root operation, or the primary objective, of the procedure. There are 31 different root operations in this section, each with its own precise definition.

- *Alteration:* Modifying the natural anatomic structure of a body part without affecting the function of the body part

- *Bypass:* Altering the route of passage of the contents of a tubular body part

- *Change:* Taking out or off a device from a body part and putting back an identical or similar device in or on the same body part without cutting or puncturing the skin or a mucous membrane

- *Control:* Stopping, or attempting to stop, postprocedural or other acute bleeding

- *Creation:* Putting in or on biological or synthetic material to form a new body part that to the extent possible replicates the anatomic structure or function of an absent body part

- *Destruction:* Physical eradication of all or a portion of a body part by the direct use of energy, force, or a destructive agent

- *Detachment:* Cutting off all or a portion of the upper or lower extremities
- *Dilation:* Expanding an orifice or the lumen of a tubular body part
- *Division:* Cutting into a body part without draining fluids and/or gases from the body part in order to separate or transect a body part
- *Drainage:* Taking or letting out fluids and/or gases from a body part
- *Excision:* Cutting out or off, without replacement, a portion of a body part
- *Extirpation:* Taking or cutting out solid matter from a body part
- *Extraction:* Pulling or stripping out or off all or a portion of a body part by the use of force
- *Fragmentation:* Breaking solid matter in a body part into pieces
- *Fusion:* Joining together portions of an articular body part rendering the articular body part immobile
- *Insertion:* Putting in a nonbiological appliance that monitors, assists, performs, or prevents a physiological function but does not physically take the place of a body part
- *Inspection:* Visually and/or manually exploring a body part
- *Map:* Locating the route of passage of electrical impulses and/or locating functional areas in a body part
- *Occlusion:* Completely closing an orifice or lumen of a tubular body part
- *Reattachment:* Putting back in or on all or a portion of a separated body part to its normal location or other suitable location
- *Release:* Freeing a body part from an abnormal physical constraint by cutting or by use of force
- *Removal:* Taking out or off a device from a body part
- *Repair:* Restoring, to the extent possible, a body part to its normal anatomic structure and function
- *Replacement:* Putting in or on biological or synthetic material that physically takes the place and/or function of all or a portion of a body part
- *Reposition:* Moving to its normal location or other suitable location all or a portion of a body part
- *Resection:* Cutting out or off, without replacement, all of a body part
- *Restriction:* Partially closing an orifice or lumen of a tubular body part
- *Revision:* Correcting, to the extent possible, a portion of a malfunctioning device or the position of a displaced device
- *Supplement:* Putting in or on biological or synthetic material that physically reinforces and/or augments the function of a portion of a body part
- *Transfer:* Moving, without taking out, all or a portion of a body part to another location to take over the function of all or a portion of a body part
- *Transplantation:* Putting in or on all or a portion of a living body part taken from another individual or animal to physically take the place and/or function of all or a portion of a similar body part

The standardized level of specificity designed into ICD-10-PCS restricts the use of broadly applicable "not otherwise specified (NOS)" or "unspecified code" options in the system. A minimal level of specificity is required to construct a valid code. "Not elsewhere classified (NEC)"

options are provided in ICD-10-PCS but only for specific, limited use. The root operation Repair in the Medical and Surgical section functions as a "not elsewhere classified" option. Repair is used only when the procedure performed is not one of the other specific root operations in the Medical and Surgical section.

Appendixes B and C provide additional subcategorization, explanations, and representative examples of the Medical and Surgical section root operations.

Body Part (Character 4)
The fourth character represents the body part, or specific anatomical site where the procedure was performed. The body system (second character) provides only a general indication of the procedure site. The body part and body system values, together, provide a precise description of the procedure site.

Approach (Character 5)
The fifth character represents the approach, or the technique used to reach the procedure site. There are seven different approach values in this section.

- *Open*: Cutting through the skin or mucous membrane and any other body layers necessary to expose the site of the procedure
- *Percutaneous*: Entry, by puncture or minor incision, of instrumentation through the skin or mucous membrane and any other body layers necessary to reach the site of the procedure
- *Percutaneous Endoscopic*: Entry, by puncture or minor incision, of instrumentation through the skin or mucous membrane and any other body layers necessary to reach and visualize the site of the procedure
- *Via Natural or Artificial Opening*: Entry of instrumentation through a natural or artificial external opening to reach the site of the procedure
- *Via Natural or Artificial Opening Endoscopic*: Entry of instrumentation through a natural or artificial external opening to reach and visualize the site of the procedure
- *Via Natural or Artificial Opening with Percutaneous Endoscopic Assistance:* Entry of instrumentation through a natural or artificial external opening and entry, by puncture or minor incision, of instrumentation through the skin or mucous membrane and any other body layers necessary to aid in the performance of the procedure
- *External*: Procedures performed directly on the skin or mucous membrane and procedures performed indirectly by the application of external force through the skin or mucous membrane

Appendix A provides definitions and comparisons of the components (access location, method, and type of instrumentation) for each approach and provides an example and illustration.

Device (Character 6)
The sixth character represents a device. Broad categories of devices found in this section include:

- Grafts (e.g., skin)
- Prostheses (e.g., hip joint)
- Implants (e.g., internal fixation device, mesh)
- Simple or Mechanical Appliances (e.g., drainage device, IUD)
- Electronic Appliances (e.g., pacemaker, monitoring device)

Depending on the procedure performed, there may or may not be a device left in place at the end of the procedure. For procedures that do not utilize a device, the value of *No Device* is available. For devices that cannot be categorized into one of the current values, many tables also have a device value of *Other Device*. This value is intended to be used temporarily until a more specific value can be added to the classification. No categories of medical or surgical devices are permanently classified to *Other Device*.

Instruments used to visualize the procedure site are specified in the fifth-character approach, not the sixth-character device value. Materials that are incidental to a procedure such as clips, ligatures, and sutures are not specified in the device character.

Appendix F compares the general device types and provides examples of each.

Appendix G provides an aggregation table that crosswalks specific device character values used for specific root operations to more general device character values used when the root operation represents an entire family of devices.

Qualifier (Character 7)
The seventh character is a qualifier that captures additional attributes of the procedure, where applicable.

Medical and Surgical Section Principles
In developing the Medical and Surgical procedure codes, several specific principles were followed.

Composite Terms Are Not Root Operations
Composite terms such as colonoscopy, sigmoidectomy, or appendectomy do not describe root operations, but they do specify multiple components of a specific root operation. In ICD-10-PCS, the components of a procedure are defined separately by the characters making up the complete code. The only component of a procedure specified in the root operation is the objective of the procedure. With each complete code the underlying objective of the procedure is specified by the root operation (third character), the precise part is specified by the body part (fourth character), and the method used to reach and visualize the procedure site is specified by the approach (fifth character). While colonoscopy, sigmoidectomy, and appendectomy are included in the Index, they do not constitute root operations in the Tables section. The objective of colonoscopy is the visualization of the colon and the root operation (character 3) is *Inspection*. Character 4 specifies the body part, which in this case is part of the colon. These composite terms, like colonoscopy or appendectomy, are included as cross-reference only. The index provides the correct root operation reference. Examples of other types of composite terms not representative of root operations are *partial* sigmoidectomy, *total* hysterectomy, and *partial* hip replacement. Always refer to the correct root operation in the Index and Tables section.

Root Operation Based on Objective of Procedure
The root operation is based on the objective of the procedure, such as *Resection* of transverse colon or *Dilation* of an artery. The assignment of the root operation is based on the procedure actually performed, which may or may not have been the intended procedure. If the intended procedure is modified or discontinued (e.g., excision instead of resection is performed), the root operation is determined by the procedure actually performed. If the desired result is not attained after completing the procedure (i.e., the artery does not remain expanded

after the dilation procedure), the root operation is still determined by the procedure actually performed.

Examples:

- Dilating the urethra is coded as *Dilation* since the objective of the procedure is to dilate the urethra. If dilation of the urethra includes putting in an intraluminal stent, the root operation remains *Dilation* and not *Insertion* of the intraluminal device because the underlying objective of the procedure is dilation of the urethra. The stent is identified by the intraluminal device value in the sixth character of the dilation procedure code.

- If the objective is solely to put a radioactive element in the urethra, then the procedure is coded to the root operation *Insertion*, with the radioactive element identified in the sixth character of the code.

- If the objective of the procedure is to correct a malfunctioning or displaced device, then the procedure is coded to the root operation *Revision*. In the root operation *Revision*, the original device being revised is identified in the device character. *Revision* is typically performed on mechanical appliances (e.g., pacemaker) or materials used in replacement procedures (e.g., synthetic substitute). Typical revision procedures include adjustment of pacemaker position and correction of malfunctioning knee prosthesis.

Combination Procedures Are Coded Separately
If multiple procedures as defined by distinct objectives are performed during an operative episode, then multiple codes are used. For example, obtaining the vein graft used for coronary bypass surgery is coded as a separate procedure from the bypass itself.

Redo of Procedures
The complete or partial redo of the original procedure is coded to the root operation that identifies the procedure performed rather than *Revision*.

Example:

A complete redo of a hip replacement procedure that requires putting in a new prosthesis is coded to the root operation *Replacement* rather than *Revision*.

The correction of complications arising from the original procedure, other than device complications, is coded to the procedure performed. Correction of a malfunctioning or displaced device would be coded to the root operation *Revision*.

Example:

A procedure to control hemorrhage arising from the original procedure is coded to *Control* rather than *Revision*.

Examples of Procedures Coded in the Medical Surgical Section
The following are examples of procedures from the Medical and Surgical section, coded in ICD-10-PCS.

- Suture of skin laceration, left lower arm: ØHQEXZZ

- Laparoscopic appendectomy: ØDTJ4ZZ

- Sigmoidoscopy with biopsy: ØDBN8ZX

- Tracheostomy with tracheostomy tube: ØB110F4

Obstetrics Section (1)

The Obstetrics section includes codes for procedures performed on the products of conception only. Procedures on pregnant females are coded in the Medical and Surgical section (e.g., episiotomy). The term "products of conception" refers to all physical components of a pregnancy, including the fetus, amnion, umbilical cord, and placenta. There is no differentiation of the products of conception based on gestational age. Thus, the diagnosis code, not the procedure code, specifies the products of conception as a zygote, embryo, or fetus, or of the trimester of the pregnancy.

Character Meanings

The seven characters in the Obstetrics section have the same meaning as in the Medical and Surgical section.

Character	Meaning
1	Section
2	Body System
3	Root Operation
4	Body Part
5	Approach
6	Device
7	Qualifier

Section (Character 1)

Obstetrics procedure codes have a first character value of *1*.

Body System (Character 2)

The second character represents the body system. There is only one value used in this section: *Pregnancy*.

Root Operation (Character 3)

The third character represents the root operation, or the primary objective, of the procedure. There are 12 values available in this section. Ten of these values specify root operations as defined in the Medical and Surgical section and include *Change, Drainage, Extraction, Insertion, Inspection, Removal, Repair, Reposition, Resection,* and *Transplantation.* The other two values are specific to this section only and are defined as follows:

- *Abortion*: Artificially terminating a pregnancy

- *Delivery*: Assisting the passage of the products of conception from the genital canal

A cesarean section is not a separate root operation because the underlying objective is *Extraction* (i.e., pulling out all or a portion of a body part).

Body Part (Character 4)

The fourth character represents the body part, which in this section is specific to the products of conception. The three values available are as follows:

- *Products of conception*
- *Products of conception, retained*
- *Products of conception, ectopic*

Approach (Character 5)

The fifth character represents the approach, as defined in the Medical and Surgical section.

Device (Character 6)

The sixth character represents a device used during the procedure, where applicable.

Qualifier (Character 7)

The seventh character is a qualifier that captures additional attributes of the procedure, where applicable.

Placement Section (2)

The Placement section includes codes for procedures that put a device in an orifice or on a body region, without making an incision or a puncture.

Character Meanings

The seven characters in the Placement section have the following meaning:

Character	Meaning
1	Section
2	Body System
3	Root Operation
4	Body Region
5	Approach
6	Device
7	Qualifier

Section (Character 1)

Placement procedure codes have a first character value of *2*.

Body System (Character 2)

The second character contains two values specifying either *Anatomical Regions* or *Anatomical Orifices*.

Root Operation (Character 3)

The third character represents the root operation, or the primary objective, of the procedure. There are seven values available in this section. Two of the values specify root operations as defined in the Medical and Surgical section and include *Change* and *Removal*. The other five values are specific to this section only and are defined as follows:

- *Compression*: Putting pressure on a body region

- *Dressing*: Putting material on a body region for protection

- *Immobilization*: Limiting or preventing motion of an external body region

- *Packing*: Putting material in a body region or orifice

- *Traction*: Exerting a pulling force on a body region in a distal direction

Body Region (Character 4)

The fourth character represents the specific body region or orifice. The body system (second character) provides only a general indication of the procedure site. The body region values and body system values, together, precisely describe the procedure site.

Approach (Character 5)

The fifth character represents the approach. Since all placement procedures are performed directly or indirectly on the skin or mucous membrane, the approach value is always *External*.

Device (Character 6)

The sixth character represents a device placed during the procedure, where applicable.

Except for devices used for fractures and dislocations, devices in this section are off the shelf and do not require any extensive design, fabrication, or fitting.

Qualifier (Character 7)

The seventh character is a qualifier. Because there are currently no specific qualifier values in this section, the value is always *No Qualifier*.

Administration Section (3)

The Administration section includes infusions, injections, and transfusions, as well as other related procedures, such as irrigation and tattooing. All codes in this section define procedures in which a diagnostic or therapeutic substance is given to the patient.

Character Meanings

The seven characters in the Administration section have the following meaning:

Character	Meaning
1	Section
2	Body System
3	Root Operation
4	Body System/Region
5	Approach
6	Substance
7	Qualifier

Section (Character 1)

Administration procedure codes have a first character value of *3*.

Body System (Character 2)

The second character can represent the general physiological system, anatomical region, or device to which a substance is being administered. The three values available in this section are *Indwelling Device, Physiological Systems and Anatomical Regions,* and *Circulatory System.*

Root Operation (Character 3)

The third character represents the root operation, or the primary objective, of the procedure. There are three values available in this section.

- *Introduction*: Putting in or on a therapeutic, diagnostic, nutritional, physiological, or prophylactic substance except blood or blood products

- *Irrigation*: Putting in or on a cleansing substance

- *Transfusion*: Putting in blood or blood products

Body/System Region (Character 4)

The fourth character represents the body system/region. The fourth character identifies the site where the substance is administered, not the site where the substance administered takes effect. Sites include *Skin and Mucous Membranes, Subcutaneous Tissue,* and *Muscle.* These differentiate intradermal, subcutaneous, and intramuscular injections, respectively. Other sites include *Eye, Respiratory Tract, Peritoneal Cavity,* and *Epidural Space.*

The body systems/regions for arteries and veins are *Peripheral Artery, Central Artery, Peripheral Vein,* and *Central Vein.* The *Peripheral Artery* or *Vein* is typically used when a substance is introduced locally into an artery or vein. For example, chemotherapy is the introduction of an antineoplastic substance into a peripheral artery or vein by a percutaneous approach. In general, the substance introduced into a peripheral artery or vein has a systemic effect.

The *Central Artery* or *Vein* is typically used when the site where the substance is introduced is distant from the point of entry into the artery or vein. For example, the introduction of a substance directly at the site of a clot within an artery or vein using a catheter is coded as an introduction of a thrombolytic substance into a central artery or vein by a percutaneous approach. In general, the substance introduced into a central artery or vein has a local effect.

Approach (Character 5)

The fifth character represents the approach, as defined in the Medical and Surgical section. The approach for intradermal, subcutaneous, and intramuscular introductions (i.e., injections) is *Percutaneous*. If a catheter is placed to introduce a substance into an internal site within the circulatory system, then the approach is also *Percutaneous*. For example, if a catheter is used to introduce contrast directly into the heart for angiography, then the procedure would be coded as a percutaneous introduction of contrast into the heart.

Substance (Character 6)

The sixth character represents the substance being introduced. Most of the values capture broad categories of substances to which several specific substances may be categorized.

Qualifier (Character 7)

The seventh character is a qualifier. The substance value (second character) provides the broad category to which a substance is classified. The qualifier and substance values, together, precisely describe the substance administered. Not every substance administered has its own unique qualifier.

Measurement and Monitoring Section (4)

The Measurement and Monitoring section represents procedures for determining the level of a physiological or physical function.

Character Meanings

The seven characters in the Measurement and Monitoring section have the following meaning:

Character	Meaning
1	Section
2	Body System
3	Root Operation
4	Body System
5	Approach
6	Function/Device
7	Qualifier

Section (Character 1)

Measurement and Monitoring procedure codes have a first character value of *4*.

Body System (Character 2)

The second character represents the body system or device being measured or monitored. There are two values available in this section, *Physiological Systems* and *Physiological Devices*.

Root Operation (Character 3)

The third character represents the root operation, or the primary objective, of the procedure. There are two values available in this section.

- *Measurement*: Determining the level of a physiological or physical function at a point in time
- *Monitoring*: Determining the level of a physiological or physical function repetitively over a period of time

Body System (Character 4)

The fourth character represents the specific body system measured or monitored.

Approach (Character 5)

The fifth character represents the approach, as defined in the Medical and Surgical section.

Function/Device (Character 6)

The sixth character represents the physiological or physical function, or the device function being measured or monitored.

Qualifier (Character 7)

The seventh character is a qualifier, which captures additional attributes of the procedure, where applicable.

Extracorporeal or Systemic Assistance and Performance Section (5)

The Extracorporeal or Systemic Assistance and Performance section describes procedures performed in a critical care setting, such as mechanical ventilation and cardioversion. It also includes other procedures, such as hemodialysis and hyperbaric oxygen treatment.

The procedures described in this section are meant to be temporary; that is, the equipment is used only for the duration of the procedure. The equipment resides primarily outside the body, though it may interface with the body via a tube or other means. Although parts of the equipment may be attached or inserted into the patient, such as lines or catheters, these are not coded as separate device insertion procedures.

Character Meanings

The seven characters in the Extracorporeal or Systemic Assistance and Performance section have the following meaning:

Character	Meaning
1	Section
2	Body System
3	Root Operation
4	Body System
5	Duration
6	Function
7	Qualifier

Section (Character 1)

Extracorporeal or Systemic Assistance and Performance procedure codes have a first character value of *5*.

Body System (Character 2)

The second character represents the body system. There is one value available in this section, *Physiological Systems*.

Root Operation (Character 3)

The third character represents the root operation, or the primary objective, of the procedure. There are three values available in this section.

- *Assistance*: Taking over a portion of a physiological function by extracorporeal means
- *Performance*: Completely taking over a physiological function by extracorporeal means
- *Restoration*: Returning, or attempting to return, a physiological function to its natural state by extracorporeal means

The root operation *Restoration* contains a single procedure code that identifies extracorporeal cardioversion.

Body System (Character 4)

The fourth character represents the body system for which support of a physiological function is required.

Duration (Character 5)

The fifth character specifies the duration of the procedure.

Function (Character 6)

The sixth character represents the physiological function assisted or performed (e.g., oxygenation, ventilation) during the procedure.

Qualifier (Character 7)

The seventh character is a qualifier, which captures additional attributes of the procedure, where applicable, such as the type of equipment used to support or assist a physiological function.

Extracorporeal or Systemic Therapies Section (6)

The Extracorporeal or Systemic Therapies section describes procedures in which equipment outside the body is used for a therapeutic purpose that does not involve the assistance or performance of a physiological function. For procedures such as hypothermia, for which the therapy is not applied to a specific body system but the entire body, a fourth character for *None* is used.

Character Meanings

The seven characters in the Extracorporeal or Systemic Therapies section have the following meaning:

Character	Meaning
1	Section
2	Body System
3	Root Operation
4	Body System
5	Duration
6	Qualifier
7	Qualifier

Section (Character 1)

Extracorporeal or Systemic Therapy procedure codes have a first character value of *6*.

Body System (Character 2)

The second character represents the body system. There is one value available in this section, *Physiological Systems*.

Root Operation (Character 3)

The third character represents the root operation, or the primary objective, of the procedure. There are 11 values available in this section.

- *Atmospheric Control*: Extracorporeal control of atmospheric pressure and composition

- *Decompression*: Extracorporeal elimination of undissolved gas from body fluids

  Decompression involves only one type of procedure: treatment for decompression sickness (the bends) in a hyperbaric chamber.

- *Electromagnetic Therapy*: Extracorporeal treatment by electromagnetic rays

- *Hyperthermia*: Extracorporeal raising of body temperature

  The term hyperthermia is used to describe both a temperature imbalance treatment and also as an adjunct radiation treatment for cancer. When treating the temperature imbalance, it is coded to this section; for the cancer treatment, it is coded in the Radiation Therapy section.

- *Hypothermia*: Extracorporeal lowering of body temperature

- *Perfusion*: Extracorporeal treatment by diffusion of therapeutic fluid

- *Pheresis*: Extracorporeal separation of blood products

  Pheresis may be used for two main purposes: to treat diseases when too much of a blood component is produced (e.g., leukemia) and to remove a blood product such as platelets from a donor, for transfusion into another patient.

- *Phototherapy*: Extracorporeal treatment by light rays

Phototherapy involves using a machine that exposes the blood to light rays outside the body, recirculates it, and then returns it to the body.

- *Shock Wave Therapy*: Extracorporeal treatment by shock waves

- *Ultrasound Therapy*: Extracorporeal treatment by ultrasound

- *Ultraviolet Light Therapy*: Extracorporeal treatment by ultraviolet light

Body System (Character 4)

The fourth character represents the body system on which the extracorporeal or systemic therapy is performed (e.g., skin, circulatory).

Duration (Character 5)

The fifth character specifies the duration of the procedure. There are two values available in this section, *Single* or *Multiple*.

Qualifier (Characters 6 and 7)

The sixth and seventh characters are qualifiers. The qualifier captures additional attributes of the procedure, where applicable.

Osteopathic Section (7)

Character Meanings

The seven characters in the Osteopathic section have the following meaning:

Character	Meaning
1	Section
2	Body System
3	Root Operation
4	Body Region
5	Approach
6	Method
7	Qualifier

Section (Character 1)

Osteopathic procedure codes have a first character value of *7*.

Body System (Character 2)

The second character represents the body system. There is one value available in this section, *Anatomical Regions*.

Root Operation (Character 3)

The third character represents the root operation, or the primary objective, of the procedure. There is one value available in this section.

- *Treatment*: Manual treatment to eliminate or alleviate somatic dysfunction and related disorders

Body Region (Character 4)

The fourth character represents the body region. The body system (second character) indicates only the anatomical region involved in the procedure. The body region values and body system value, together, precisely describe the procedure site.

Approach (Character 5)

The fifth character represents the approach. There is only one value available in this section, *External*.

Method (Character 6)

The sixth character represents the method used to carry out the osteopathic treatment.

Qualifier (Character 7)

The seventh character is a qualifier. Because there are currently no specific qualifier values in this section, the value is always *None*.

Other Procedures Section (8)

The Other Procedures section contains codes for procedures not included in the other medical and surgical-related sections, including computer- and robotic-assisted procedures.

Character Meanings

The seven characters in the Other Procedures section have the following meaning:

Character	Meaning
1	Section
2	Body System
3	Root Operation
4	Body Region
5	Approach
6	Method
7	Qualifier

Section (Character 1)

Other Procedures section codes have a first character value of *8*.

Body System (Character 2)

The second character represents the body system/region or a device. There are two values available in this section, *Physiological Systems and Anatomical Regions* and *Indwelling Device*.

Root Operation (Character 3)

The third character represents the root operation, or the primary objective, of the procedure. There is one value available in this section.

- *Other Procedures*: Methodologies that attempt to remediate or cure a disorder or disease.

Body Region (Character 4)

The fourth character contains specified body-region values, and also the body-region value *None*.

Approach (Character 5)

The fifth character represents the approach, as defined in the Medical and Surgical section.

Method (Character 6)

The sixth character specifies the method (e.g., *Acupuncture, Therapeutic Massage*).

Qualifier (Character 7)

The seventh character is a qualifier. The qualifier is used to capture additional attributes of the procedure, where applicable.

Chiropractic Section (9)

Character Meanings

The seven characters in the Chiropractic section have the following meaning:

Character	Meaning
1	Section
2	Body System
3	Root Operation
4	Body Region
5	Approach
6	Method
7	Qualifier

Section (Character 1)

Chiropractic section procedure codes have a first character value of *9*.

Body System (Character 2)

The second character represents the body region. There is one value available in this section, *Anatomical Regions*.

Root Operation (Character 3)

The third character represents the root operation, or the primary objective, of the procedure. There is one value available in this section.

- *Manipulation:* Manual procedure that involves a directed thrust to move a joint past the physiological range of motion, without exceeding the anatomical limit.

Body Region (Character 4)

The fourth character represents the body region on which the chiropractic manipulation is performed.

Approach (Character 5)

The fifth character represents the approach. There is only one value available in this section, *External*.

Method (Character 6)

The sixth character represents the method by which the manipulation is accomplished.

Qualifier (Character 7)

The seventh character is a qualifier. Because there are currently no specific qualifier values in this section, the value is always *None*.

Imaging Section (B)

The Imaging section contains codes for procedures such as plain radiography, fluoroscopy, CT, MRI, and ultrasound.

Procedures such as PET, uptakes, and scans are in the Nuclear Medicine section. Therapeutic radiation, for the treatment of cancer, is in the Radiation Therapy section.

Character Meanings

The seven characters in Imaging procedures have the following meaning:

Character	Meaning
1	Section
2	Body System
3	Root Type
4	Body Part
5	Contrast
6	Qualifier
7	Qualifier

Section (Character 1)

Imaging procedure codes have a first character value of *B*.

Body System (Character 2)

The second character represents the general body system where the imaging is being performed. The available values mimic those that are found in the Medical and Surgical section but may not be exact matches.

Root Type (Character 3)

The third character represents the root type. The section title, *Imaging,* essentially identifies the root operation, while the values for the third character describe the type of imaging being performed. There are six root types in this section.

- *Computerized Tomography (CT Scan)*: Computer reformatted digital display of multiplanar images developed from the capture of multiple exposures of external ionizing radiation

- *Fluoroscopy*: Single plane or bi-plane real time display of an image developed from the capture of external ionizing radiation on a fluorescent screen. The image may also be stored by either digital or analog means

- *Magnetic Resonance Imaging (MRI)*: Computer reformatted digital display of multiplanar images developed from the capture of radiofrequency signals emitted by nuclei in a body site excited within a magnetic field

- *Other Imaging:* Other specified modality for visualizing a body part

- *Plain Radiography*: Planar display of an image developed from the capture of external ionizing radiation on photographic or photoconductive plate

- *Ultrasonography*: Real time display of images of anatomy or flow information developed from the capture of reflected and attenuated high frequency sound waves

Body Part (Character 4)

The fourth character represents the body part, or specific anatomical site where the procedure was performed. The body system (second character) provides only a general indication of the procedure site. The body part and body system values, together, precisely describe the procedure site.

Contrast (Character 5)

The fifth character represents the type of contrast or enhancing material utilized to facilitate the procedure, when applicable.

Qualifier (Character 6)

The sixth character is a qualifier. The most common qualifier, *Unenhanced and Enhanced,* describes an image taken without contrast (unenhanced) followed by an image with contrast (enhanced). Other qualifier values describe other noncontrast material or technology used to facilitate the imaging.

Qualifier (Character 7)

The seventh character is a qualifier. The qualifier is used to capture additional attributes of the procedure, where applicable.

Nuclear Medicine Section (C)

The Nuclear Medicine section is organized like the Imaging section. Procedures captured in this section describe the introduction of radioactive material into the body to create an image, to diagnose or treat pathological conditions, or to assess metabolic functions.

The introduction of encapsulated radioactive material for the treatment of cancer is included in the Radiation Therapy section.

Character Meanings

The seven characters in the Nuclear Medicine section have the following meaning:

Character	Meaning
1	Section
2	Body System
3	Root Type
4	Body Part
5	Radionuclide
6	Qualifier
7	Qualifier

Section (Character 1)

Nuclear Medicine procedure codes have a first character value of *C*.

Body System (Character 2)

The second character represents the general body system or anatomical region to which the nuclear medicine procedure is performed.

Root Type (Character 3)

The third character represents the root type. The section title, *Nuclear Medicine*, essentially identifies the root operation, while the third character value describes the type of nuclear medicine being performed. There are seven root types available in this section.

- *Nonimaging Nuclear Medicine Assay:* Introduction of radioactive materials into the body for the study of body fluids and blood elements, by the detection of radioactive emissions

- *Nonimaging Nuclear Medicine Probe:* Introduction of radioactive materials into the body for the study of distribution and fate of certain substances by the detection of radioactive emissions; or alternatively, measurement of absorption of radioactive emissions from an external source

- *Nonimaging Nuclear Medicine Uptake:* Introduction of radioactive materials into the body for measurements of organ function, from the detection of radioactive emissions

- *Planar Nuclear Medicine Imaging*: Introduction of radioactive materials into the body for single-plane display of images developed from the capture of radioactive emissions
- *Positron Emission Tomography (PET) Imaging:* Introduction of radioactive materials into the body for three dimensional display of images developed from the simultaneous capture, 180 degrees apart, of radioactive emissions
- *Systemic Nuclear Medicine Therapy:* Introduction of unsealed radioactive materials into the body for treatment
- *Tomographic (Tomo) Nuclear Medicine Imaging*: Introduction of radioactive materials into the body for three dimensional display of images developed from the capture of radioactive emissions

Body Part (Character 4)
The fourth character represents the specific body part or region being studied, imaged, or treated. The body system (second character) provides only a general indication of the procedure site. The body part and body system values, together, provide a precise description of the procedure site.

Radionuclide (Character 5)
The fifth character represents the type of radioactive material utilized to facilitate the procedure, when applicable. The *Other Radionuclide* value is used for radioactive material that has been newly approved but does not yet have its own unique value in the coding system.

If more than one radioactive material is given to perform the procedure, more than one code is used.

Qualifier (Characters 6 and 7)
The sixth and seventh characters are qualifiers. Because there are currently no specific qualifier values in this section, the value is always *None*.

Radiation Therapy Section (D)
The Radiation Therapy section contains procedures performed for cancer treatment.

Character Meanings
The seven characters in the Radiation Therapy section have the following meaning:

Character	Meaning
1	Section
2	Body System
3	Modality
4	Treatment Site
5	Modality Qualifier
6	Isotope
7	Qualifier

Section (Character 1)
Radiation therapy procedure codes have a first character value of *D*.

Body System (Character 2)
The second character represents the general body system or anatomical region to which radiation therapy is being applied.

Modality (Character 3)
The third character represents the type of radiation, or modality, being used. There are four values available in this section.

- *Beam Radiation*
- *Brachytherapy*
- *Stereotactic Radiosurgery*
- *Other Radiation*

Treatment Site (Character 4)
The fourth character represents the specific body part or region being irradiated. The body system (second character) provides only a general indication of the procedure site. The treatment site and body system values, together, precisely describe the procedure site.

Modality Qualifier (Character 5)
The fifth character represents specific methods or materials unique to a particular type of radiation therapy. The modality (third character) and modality qualifier values, together, precisely describe the therapy performed.

Isotope (Character 6)
The sixth character represents the specific radioactive isotope introduced into the body, if applicable.

Qualifier (Character 7)
The seventh character is a qualifier. Besides the value of *None*, this section contains two other values, *Intraoperative* and *Unidirectional Source*.

Physical Rehabilitation and Diagnostic Audiology Section (F)

Character Meanings
The seven characters in the Physical Rehabilitation and Diagnostic Audiology section have the following meaning:

Character	Meaning
1	Section
2	Section Qualifier
3	Root Type
4	Body System/Region
5	Type Qualifier
6	Equipment
7	Qualifier

Section (Character 1)
Physical Rehabilitation and Diagnostic Audiology procedure codes have a first character value of *F*.

Section Qualifier (Character 2)
The second character qualifies which of the two services described in the section (character 1) is being represented. Therefore, only two values are available, *Rehabilitation* or *Diagnostic Audiology*.

Root Type (Character 3)
The third character represents the root type. The section qualifier (second character) identifies the root operation, while the third-character value describes the type of rehabilitation or diagnostic

audiology being performed. There are 14 root types available in this section, each classified into four general categories.

Assessment: Used to evaluate a patient's level of function to determine the type and timing of treatment required. Assessment procedures focus on the faculties of hearing and speech, on various aspects of body function, and on the patient's quality of life, such as muscle performance, neuromotor development, and reintegration skills.

There are six root type values available for assessment.

- *Speech Assessment:* Measurement of speech and related functions
- *Motor and/or Nerve Function Assessment:* Measurement of motor, nerve, and related functions
- *Activities of Daily Living Assessment:* Measurement of functional level for activities of daily living
- *Hearing Assessment:* Measurement of hearing and related functions
- *Hearing Aid Assessment:* Measurement of the appropriateness and/or effectiveness of a hearing device
- *Vestibular Assessment:* Measurement of the vestibular system and related functions

Treatment: Use of specific activities or methods to develop, improve, and/or restore the performance of necessary functions, compensate for dysfunction and/or minimize debilitation. Procedures include swallowing dysfunction exercises, bathing and showering techniques, wound management, gait training, and a host of activities typically associated with rehabilitation.

There are six root type values available for treatment.

- *Speech Treatment:* Application of techniques to improve, augment, or compensate for speech and related functional impairment
- *Motor Treatment:* Exercise or activities to increase or facilitate motor function
- *Activities of Daily Living Treatment:* Exercise or activities to facilitate functional competence for activities of daily living
- *Hearing Treatment:* Application of techniques to improve, augment, or compensate for hearing and related functional impairment
- *Cochlear Implant Treatment:* Application of techniques to improve the communication abilities of individuals with cochlear implant
- *Vestibular Treatment:* Application of techniques to improve, augment, or compensate for vestibular and related functional impairment

Caregiver Training: Educating a caregiver with the skills and knowledge needed to interact with and assist the patient.

There is only one root type value available for caregiver training.

- *Caregiver Training:* Training in activities to support patient's optimal level of function

Fitting(s): Design, fabrication, modification, selection, and/or application of splint, orthosis, prosthesis, hearing aids, and/or other rehabilitation device. The fifth character used in Device Fitting procedures describes the device being fitted rather than the method used to fit the device. Definitions of devices, when provided, are in the definitions portion of the ICD-10-PCS tables and index, under section F, character 5.

There is only one root type value available for fittings.

- *Device Fitting:* Fitting of a device designed to facilitate or support achievement of a higher level of function

Body System/Region (Character 4)
The fourth character represents the body system and body region, where applicable, that requires rehabilitation. For diagnostic audiology procedures, this value is always *None*.

Type Qualifier (Character 5)
The fifth character represents a type qualifier. The root type (third character) and type qualifier values, together, precisely describe the procedure performed.

Equipment (Character 6)
The sixth character represents any equipment used to facilitate the procedure. The values provided are broad categories that may capture several specific types of equipment.

Qualifier (Character 7)
The seventh character is a qualifier. As there are currently no specific qualifier values in this section, the value is always *None*.

Mental Health Section (G)

Character Meanings
The seven characters in the Mental Health section have the following meaning:

Character	Meaning
1	Section
2	Body System
3	Type
4	Qualifier
5	Qualifier
6	Qualifier
7	Qualifier

Section (Character 1)
Mental health procedure codes have a first character value of *G*.

Body System (Character 2)
The second character is always represented by the value of *None*. As mental health care manages the psychological aspects of a patient's health, there is no specific body system or region that can be represented in this section.

Type (Character 3)
The third character represents the type of procedure. There are 12 values available in this section.

- *Psychological Tests:* The administration and interpretation of standardized psychological tests and measurement instruments for the assessment of psychological function
- *Crisis Intervention:* Treatment of a traumatized, acutely disturbed, or distressed individual for the purpose of short-term stabilization
- *Medication Management:* Monitoring and adjusting the use of medications for the treatment of a mental health disorder

- *Individual Psychotherapy:* Treatment of an individual with a mental health disorder by behavioral, cognitive, psychoanalytic, psychodynamic, or psychophysiological means to improve functioning or well-being
- *Counseling:* The application of psychological methods to treat an individual with normal developmental issues and psychological problems in order to increase function, improve well-being, alleviate distress, maladjustment, or resolve crises
- *Family Psychotherapy:* Treatment that includes one or more family members of an individual with a mental health disorder by behavioral, cognitive, psychoanalytic, psychodynamic, or psychophysiological means to improve functioning or well-being
- *Electroconvulsive Therapy:* The application of controlled electrical voltages to treat a mental health disorder
- *Biofeedback:* Provision of information from the monitoring and regulating of physiological processes in conjunction with cognitive-behavioral techniques to improve patient functioning or well-being
- *Hypnosis:* Induction of a state of heightened suggestibility by auditory, visual, and tactile techniques to elicit an emotional or behavioral response
- *Narcosynthesis:* Administration of intravenous barbiturates in order to release suppressed or repressed thoughts
- *Group Psychotherapy:* Treatment of two or more individuals with a mental health disorder by behavioral, cognitive, psychoanalytic, psychodynamic, or psychophysiological means to improve functioning or well-being
- *Light Therapy:* Application of specialized light treatments to improve functioning or well-being

Qualifier (Character 4)

The fourth character is a qualifier. This value represents the specific technique used to evaluate or treat a patient's mental health. In conjunction with the type (third character), the qualifier value precisely describes the procedure.

Qualifier (Characters 5, 6, and 7)

The fifth, sixth, and seventh characters are qualifiers. As there are currently no specific qualifier values in this section, the value is always *None*.

Substance Abuse Treatment Section (H)

Character Meanings

The seven characters in the Substance Abuse Treatment section have the following meaning:

Character	Meaning
1	Section
2	Body System
3	Type
4	Qualifier
5	Qualifier
6	Qualifier
7	Qualifier

Section (Character 1)

Substance Abuse Treatment codes have a first character value of *H*.

Body System (Character 2)

The second character is always represented by the value of *None*. As the substance abuse treatment section describes management of the psychological aspects of a patient's health, there is no specific body system or region that can be represented in this section.

Type (Character 3)

The third character represents the specific type of treatment. There are seven values available in this section.

- *Detoxification Services:* Detoxification from alcohol and/or drugs
- *Individual Counseling:* The application of psychological methods to treat an individual with addictive behavior
- *Group Counseling:* The application of psychological methods to treat two or more individuals with addictive behavior
- *Individual Psychotherapy:* Treatment of an individual with addictive behavior by behavioral, cognitive, psychoanalytic, psychodynamic, or psychophysiological means
- *Family Counseling:* The application of psychological methods that includes one or more family members to treat an individual with addictive behavior
- *Medication Management:* Monitoring and adjusting the use of replacement medications for the treatment of addiction
- *Pharmacotherapy:* The use of replacement medications for the treatment of addiction

Qualifier (Character 4)

The fourth character is a qualifier. The qualifier value further characterizes the type (character 3) of treatment being rendered, where applicable.

Qualifier (Characters 5, 6, and 7)

The fifth, sixth, and seventh characters are qualifiers. As there are currently no specific qualifier values in this section, the value is always *None*.

New Technology Section (X)

General Information

Section X New Technology is a section added to ICD-10-PCS beginning October 1, 2015. The new section provides a place for codes that uniquely identify procedures requested via the New Technology Application Process or that capture other new technologies not currently classified in ICD-10-PCS.

Section X does not introduce any new coding concepts or unusual guidelines for correct coding. In fact, Section X codes maintain continuity with the other sections in ICD-10-PCS by using the same root operation and body part values as their closest counterparts in other sections of ICD-10-PCS. For example, the codes for the infusion of Sarilumab, use the same root operation (Introduction) and body part values (Central Vein and Peripheral Vein) in section X as the infusion codes in section 3 Administration, which are their closest counterparts in the other sections of ICD-10-PCS.

Character Meanings

The seven characters in the new technology section have the following meaning:

Character	Meaning
1	Section
2	Body System
3	Root Operation
4	Body Part
5	Approach
6	Device/Substance/Technology
7	Qualifier

Section (Character 1)

New technology procedure codes have a first character value of *X*.

Body System (Character 2)

The second character values for body system combine the uses of body system, body region, and physiological system as specified in other sections in ICD-10-PCS.

Root Operation (Character 3)

The third character utilizes the same root operation values as their counterparts in other sections of ICD-10-PCS.

Body Part (Character 4)

The fourth character represents the same body part values as their closest counterparts in other sections of ICD-10-PCS.

Approach (Character 5)

The fifth character represents the approach, as defined in the Medical and Surgical section.

Device/Substance/Technology (Character 6)

The sixth character represents the key feature of the new technology procedure. It may be specified as a new device, a new substance, or other new technology. Examples of sixth character values are *Robotic*

Waterjet Ablation, Interbody Fusion Device, Customizable, and *Nafamostat Anticoagulant.*

Qualifier (Character 7)

The seventh character qualifier is used exclusively to specify the new technology group, a number or letter that changes each year that new technology codes are added to the system. For example, Section X codes added for the first year have the seventh character value 1, *New Technology Group 1*, and the next year that Section X codes are added have the seventh character value 2, *New Technology Group 2*, and so on. Changing the seventh character value to a unique letter or number every year that there are new codes in the new technology section allows the ICD-10-PCS to "recycle" the values in the third, fourth, and sixth characters as needed.

New Technology Coding Instruction

Section X codes are standalone codes. They are not supplemental codes. Section X codes fully represent the specific procedure described in the code title, and do not require any additional codes from other sections of ICD-10-PCS. When section X contains a code title which describes a specific new technology procedure, only that X code is reported for the procedure. There is no need to report a broader, non-specific code in another section of ICD-10-PCS.

For example, code XW033G5 Introduction of Sarilumab into Peripheral Vein, Percutaneous Approach, New Technology Group 5, would be reported to indicate that Sarilumab was administered via peripheral vein. A separate code from table 3E0 in the Administration section of ICD-10-PCS would not be reported in addition to this code. The X section code fully identifies the administration of the sarilumab, and no additional code is needed.

The New Technology section codes are easily found by looking in the ICD-10-PCS Index or the Tables. In the Index, the name of the new technology device, substance or technology for a section X code is included as a main term. In addition, all codes in section X are listed under the main term New Technology. The new technology code index entry for sarilumab is shown below.

Sarilumab XW0

New Technology
   Sarilumab XW0

ICD-10-PCS Index and Tabular Format

The *ICD-10-PCS: The Complete Official Code Set* is based on the official version of the International Classification of Diseases, 10th Revision, Procedure Classification System, issued by the U.S. Department of Health and Human Services, Centers for Medicare and Medicaid Services. This book is consistent with the content of the government's version of ICD-10-PCS and follows their official format.

Index

The Alphabetic Index can be used to locate the appropriate table containing all the information necessary to construct a procedure code, however, the PCS tables should always be consulted to find the most appropriate valid code. Users may choose a valid code directly from the tables—he or she need not consult the index before proceeding to the tables to complete the code.

Main Terms

The Alphabetic Index reflects the structure of the tables. Therefore, the index is organized as an alphabetic listing. The index:

- Is based on the value of the third character
- Contains common procedure terms
- Lists anatomic sites
- Uses device terms

The main terms in the Alphabetic Index are root operations, root procedure types, or common procedure names. In addition, anatomic sites from the Body Part Key and device terms from the Device Key have been added for ease of use.

Examples:

> *Resection* (root operation)
>
> *Fluoroscopy* (root type)
>
> *Prostatectomy* (common procedure name)
>
> *Brachiocephalic artery* (body part)
>
> *Bard® Dulex™ mesh* (device)

The index provides at least the first three or four values of the code, and some entries may provide complete valid codes. However, the user should always consult the appropriate table to verify that the most appropriate valid code has been selected.

Root Operation and Procedure Type Main Terms

For the *Medical and Surgical* and related sections, the root operation values are used as main terms in the index. The subterms under the root operation main terms are body parts. For the Ancillary section of the tables, the main terms in the index are the general type of procedure performed.

Examples:

Biofeedback GZC9ZZZ
Destruction
  Acetabulum
    Left ØQ55
    Right ØQ54
  Adenoids ØC5Q
  Ampulla of Vater ØF5C
Planar Nuclear Medicine Imaging
  Abdomen CW1Ø

See Reference

The second type of term in the index uses common procedure names, such as "appendectomy" or "fundoplication." These common terms are listed as main terms with a "see" reference noting the PCS root operations that are possible valid code tables based on the objective of the procedure.

Examples:

Tendonectomy
  see Excision, Tendons ØLB
  see Resection, Tendons ØLT

Use Reference

The index also lists anatomic sites from the Body Part Key and device terms from the Device Key. These terms are listed with a "use" reference. The purpose of these references is to act as an additional reference to the terms located in the Appendix Keys. The term provided is the Body Part value or Device value to be selected when constructing a procedure code using the code tables. This type of index reference is not intended to direct the user to another term in the index, but to provide guidance regarding character value selection. Therefore, "use" references generally do not refer to specific valid code tables.

Examples:

CoAxia NeuroFlo catheter
  use Intraluminal Device
Epitrochlear lymph node
  use Lymphatic, Left Upper Extremity
  use Lymphatic, Right Upper Extremity
SynCardia Total Artificial Heart
  use Synthetic Substitute

Code Tables

ICD-10-PCS contains 17 sections of Code Tables organized by general type of procedure. The first three characters of a procedure code define each table. The tables consist of columns providing the possible last four characters of codes and rows providing valid values for each character. Within a PCS table, valid codes include all combinations of choices in characters 4 through 7 contained in the same row of the table. All seven characters must be specified to form a valid code.

There are three main sections of tables:

- Medical and Surgical section:
  - *Medical and Surgical* (Ø)
- Medical and Surgical-related sections:
  - *Obstetrics* (1)
  - *Placement* (2)
  - *Administration* (3)
  - *Measurement and Monitoring* (4)
  - *Extracorporeal or Systemic Assistance and Performance* (5)
  - *Extracorporeal or Systemic Therapies* (6)
  - *Osteopathic* (7)
  - *Other Procedures* (8)
  - *Chiropractic* (9)

- Ancillary sections:
  - *Imaging* (B)
  - *Nuclear Medicine* (C)
  - *Radiation Therapy* (D)
  - *Physical Rehabilitation and Diagnostic Audiology* (F)
  - *Mental Health* (G)
  - *Substance Abuse Treatment* (H)
- New Technology section:
  - *New Technology* (X)

The first three character values define each table. The root operation or root type designated for each table is accompanied by its official definition.

Example:

Table ØØF provides codes for procedures on the central nervous system that involve breaking up of solid matter into pieces:

Character 1, Section	Ø: Medical and Surgical
Character 2, Body System	Ø: Central Nervous System and Cranial Nerves
Character 3, Root Operation	F: Fragmentation: Breaking solid matter in a body part into pieces

Tables are arranged numerically, then alphabetically.

When reviewing tables, the user should keep in mind that:

- Some tables may cover multiple pages in the code book—to ensure maximum clarity about character choices, valid entries do not split rows between pages. For instance, the entire table of valid characters completing a code beginning with 4A1 is split between two pages, but the split is between, not within, rows. This means that all the valid sixth and seventh characters for, say, body system *Arterial* (3) and approach *External* (X) are contained on one page.
- Individual entries may be listed in several horizontal "selection" lines.
- When a table is continued onto another page, a note to this effect has been added in red.

Body Part Definitions:

An exclusive Optum feature in the tables is the incorporation of the body part definitions provided in appendix E into the Medical and Surgical section (Ø) tables under their appropriate body part characters in the first column (character 4). This provides the user a direct reference to all anatomical descriptions, terms, and sites that could be coded to that particular body part value.

Paired body parts typically have values for the right and left side and in some cases a value for bilateral. These paired body parts often have the same list of inclusive body part definitions. When there are paired body parts with the same body part definitions, the first listed body part (usually the right side) contains the list of body part definitions while the second listed body part (usually the left side) contains a *See* instruction. This *See* instruction references the body part value that contains the body part definitions. In the table below, body part value P – Upper Eyelid, Left is followed by a *See* instruction that states *See N Upper Eyelid, Right*. All body part descriptions under value N also apply to body part value P.

Example:

Ø   Medical and Surgical
8   Eye
M   Reattachment   Definition: Putting back in or on all or a portion of a separated body part to its normal location or other suitable location

Explanation: Vascular circulation and nervous pathways may or may not be reestablished

Body Part Character 4	Approach Character 5	Device Character 6	Qualifier Character 7
N Upper Eyelid, Right Lateral canthus Levator palpebrae superioris muscle Orbicularis oculi muscle Superior tarsal plate **P** Upper Eyelid, Left *See N Upper Eyelid, Right* **Q** Lower Eyelid, Right Inferior tarsal plate Medial canthus **R** Lower Eyelid, Left *See Q Lower Eyelid, Right*	**X** External	**Z** No Device	**Z** No Qualifier

ICD-10-PCS Additional Features

Use of Official Sources

Color-coding, symbol, and other annotations in this manual that identify coding and reimbursement issues are derived from various official federal government sources, including the *Federal Register*, volume 87, number 90, May 10, 2022 ("Hospital Inpatient Prospective Payment Systems for Acute Care Hospitals and the Long Term Care Hospital Prospective Payment System and Proposed Policy Changes and Fiscal Year 2023 Rates; Proposed Rule") and the proposed, version 40, MS-DRG Grouper software, Definitions Manual files and Medicare Code Editor (MCE) files published with the fiscal 2023 IPPS proposed rule. For the most current files related to IPPS, please refer to the following:

- FY2023 IPPS Final Rule
  https://www.cms.gov/Medicare/Medicare-Fee-for-Service-Payment/AcuteInpatientPPS/IPPS-Regulations-and-Notices

- FY2023 Final Version 40, MS-DRG Grouper software
  https://www.cms.gov/Medicare/Medicare-Fee-for-Service-Payment/AcuteInpatientPPS/MS-DRG-Classifications-and-Software

Table Notations

Many tables in ICD-10-PCS contain color or symbol annotations that may aid in code selection, provide clinical or coding information, or alert the coder to reimbursement issues affected by the PCS code assignment. These annotations may be displayed on or next to a character 4, character 6, or character 7 value. Please note that some values may have more than one annotation; this is true most often with the character 4 value.

Refer to the color/symbol legend at the bottom of each page in the tables section for an abridged description of each color and symbol.

Annotation Box

An annotation box has been appended to all tables that contain color-coding or symbol annotations. The color bar or symbol attached to a character value is provided in the box, as well as a list of the valid PCS code(s) to which that edit applies. The box may also list conditional criteria that must be met to satisfy the edit.

For example, see Table 00F. Four character 4 body part values have a gray color bar. In the annotation box below the table, the gray color bar is defined as "Non-OR," or a nonoperating room procedure edit. Following the Non-OR annotation are the PCS codes that are considered nonoperating room procedures from that row of Table 00F.

Bracketed Code Notation

The use of bracketed codes is an efficient convention to provide all valid character value alternatives for a specific set of circumstances. The character values in the brackets correspond to the valid values for the character in the position the bracket appears.

Examples:

In the annotation box for Table 00F the Noncovered Procedure edit (NC) applies to codes represented in the bracketed code 00F[3,4,5,6]XZZ.

00F[3,4,5,6]XZZ Fragmentation in (Central Nervous System and Cranial Nerves), External Approach

The valid fourth character values (body part) that may be selected for this specific circumstance are as follows:

3	Epidural Space, Intracranial
4	Subdural Space, Intracranial
5	Subarachnoid Space, Intracranial
6	Cerebral Ventricle

The fragmentation of matter in the spinal canal, Body Part value U, is not included in the noncovered procedure code edit.

Color-Coding/Symbols

New and Revised Text

Changes within the ICD-10-PCS tables, since the last published edition of this manual, are highlighted in two ways:

- **Red font** identifies new or revised text effective April 1, 2022.

- **Green font** identifies new or revised text effective October 1, 2022.

Medicare Code Edits

Medicare administrative contractors (MACs) and many payers use Medicare code edits to check the coding accuracy on claims. The coding edits provided in this manual include only those directly related to ICD-10-PCS codes used for acute care hospital inpatient admissions. These edits are based on the proposed, version 40, Medicare Code Editor (MCE) files published with the fiscal 2023 IPPS proposed rule.

The PCS related Medicare code edits are listed below:

- Invalid procedure code
- *Sex conflict
- *Questionable obstetric admission
- *Noncovered procedure
- *Limited coverage procedure

Starred edits above that are related to PCS issues are identified in this manual by symbols as described below.

Sex Edit Symbols

The sex edit symbols below are used to detect inconsistencies between the patient's sex and the procedure. The symbols below most often appear to the right of the body part (character 4) value but may also be found to the right of the qualifier (character 7) value:

♂ Male procedure only

♀ Female procedure only

Questionable Obstetric Admission

An inpatient admission is considered questionable when a vaginal or cesarean delivery code is assigned without a corresponding secondary diagnosis code describing the outcome of delivery. Both a delivery (ICD-10-PCS) code and an outcome-of-delivery (ICD-10-CM) code must be present to avoid errors in MS-DRG assignment. This symbol is found only in the Obstetrics Section, appearing to the right of the body part (character 4) value.

ɴᴄ Noncovered Procedure

Medicare does not cover all procedures. However, some noncovered procedures, due to the presence of certain diagnoses, are reimbursed.

ʟᴄ Limited Coverage

For certain procedures whose medical complexity and serious nature incur extraordinary associated costs, Medicare limits coverage to a portion of the cost. The limited coverage edit indicates the type of limited coverage.

ICD-10 MS-DRG Definitions Manual Edits

An MS-DRG is assigned based on specific patient attributes, such as principal diagnosis, secondary diagnoses, procedures, and discharge status. The attributes (edits) provided in this manual include only those directly related to ICD-10-PCS codes used for acute care hospital inpatient admissions. These edits are based on the proposed, version 40, MS-DRG Grouper software and Definitions Manual published with the fiscal 2023 IPPS proposed rule.

Non-Operating Room Procedures Not Affecting MS-DRG Assignment

In the Medical and Surgical section (001-0YW) and the Obstetric section (102-10Y) tables **only,** ICD-10-PCS procedures codes that DO NOT affect MS-DRG assignment are identified by a gray color bar over the body part (character 4) value and are considered non-operating room (non-OR) procedures.

NOTE: The majority of the ICD-10-PCS codes in the Medical and Surgical-Related, Ancillary and New Technology section tables are non-operating room procedures that do not typically affect MS-DRG assignment. Only the Valid Operating Room and DRG Non-Operating Room procedures are highlighted in these sections, *see* Non-Operating Room Procedures Affecting MS-DRG Assignment and Valid OR Procedure description below.

Non-Operating Room Procedures Affecting MS-DRG Assignment

Some ICD-10-PCS procedure codes, although considered non-operating room procedures, may still affect MS-DRG assignment. In all sections of the ICD-10-PCS book, these procedures are identified by a purple color bar over the body part (character 4) value.

Valid OR Procedure

In the Medical and Surgical-Related (2W0-9WB), Ancillary (B00-HZ9) and New Technology (X2A-XY0) section tables **only**, any codes that are considered a valid operating room procedure are identified with a blue color bar over the body part (character 4) value and will affect MS-DRG assignment. All codes without a color bar (blue or purple) are considered non-operating room procedures.

Hospital-Acquired Condition Related Procedures

Procedures associated with hospital-acquired conditions (HAC) are identified with the yellow color bar over the body part (character 4) value. Appendix K provides each specific HAC category and its associated ICD-10-CM and ICD-10-PCS codes.

Combination Only

Some ICD-10-PCS procedure codes that describe non-operating room procedures can group to a specific MS-DRG but only when used in combination with certain other ICD-10-PCS procedure codes. Such codes are designated by a red color bar over the body part (character 4) value.

⊞ Combination Member

A combination member, which can be either a valid operating room procedure or a non-operating room procedure, is an ICD-10-PCS procedure code that can influence MS-DRG assignment either on its own or in combination with other specific ICD-10-PCS procedure codes. Combination member codes are designated by a plus sign (⊞) to the right of the body part (character 4) value.

Note: In the few instances when a code is both a combination member and a non-operating room procedure affecting the MS-DRG assignment, the body part (character 4) value will have a purple color bar and the combination member icon.

See Appendix L for Procedure Combinations

Under certain circumstances, more than one procedure code is needed in order to group to a specific MS-DRG. When codes within a table have been identified as a Combination Only (red color bar) or Combination Member (⊞) code, there is also a footnote instructing the coder to *see Appendix L*. Appendix L contains tables that identify the other procedure codes needed in the combination and the title and number of the MS-DRG to which the combination will group.

Other Table Notations

AHA Coding Clinic:

Official citations from AHA's *Coding Clinic for ICD-10-CM/PCS* have been provided at the beginning of each section, when applicable. Each specific citation is listed below a header identifying the table to which that particular *Coding Clinic* citation applies. The citations appear in purple type with the year, quarter, and page of the reference as well as the title of the question as it appears in that *Coding Clinic's* table of contents. *Coding Clinic* citations included in this edition have been updated through second quarter 2022.

ɴᴛ New Technology Add-on Payment

This symbol identifies procedure codes that involve new technologies or medical services that have qualified for a new technology add-on payment (NTAP). CMS provides incremental payment, in addition to the DRG payment, for technologies that have received the NTAP designation. This symbol appears to the right of the sixth character value.

Note: Only specific brand or trade named devices, substances, or technologies receive NTAP approval. The sixth character value in the PCS table provides a generalized description that may be applicable to several brand or trade names. Unless otherwise specified in the annotation box, refer to appendix H or I to determine the specific brand or trade name of the device, substance, or technology that is applicable to the new technology add-on payment. New technology add-on payments are not exclusive to the New Technology (X) section.

Appendixes

The resources described below have been included as appendixes for *ICD-10-PCS The Complete Official Code Set*. These resources further instruct the coder on the appropriate application of the ICD-10-PCS code set.

Appendix A: Components of the Medical and Surgical Approach Definitions

This resource further defines the approach characters used in the Medical and Surgical (0) section. Complementing the detailed definition of the approach, additional information includes whether or not instrumentation is a part of the approach, the typical access location, the method used to initiate the approach, related procedural examples, and illustrations all of which will help the user determine the appropriate approach value.

Appendix B: Root Operation Definitions

This resource is a compilation of all root operations found in the Medical and Surgical-related sections (Ø-9) of this PCS manual. It provides a definition and in some cases a more detailed explanation of the root operation, to better reflect the purpose or objective. Examples of related procedure(s) may also be provided.

Appendix C: Comparison of Medical and Surgical Root Operations

The Medical and Surgical (Ø) section root operations are divided into groups that share similar attributes. These groups, and the root operations in each group, are listed in this resource along with information identifying the target of the root operation, the action used to perform the root operation, any clarification or further explanation on the objective of the root operation, and procedure examples.

Appendix D: Body Part Key

When an anatomical term or description is provided in the documentation but does not have a specific body part character within a table, the user can reference this resource to search for the anatomical description or site noted in the documentation to determine if there is a specific PCS body part character (character 4) to which the anatomical description or site could be coded.

Appendix E: Body Part Definitions

This resource is the reverse look-up of the Body Part Key. Each table in the Medical and Surgical section (Ø) of the PCS manual contains anatomical terms linked to a body part character or value, for example, in Table ØBB the Body Part (character 4) of 1 is Trachea. The body part Trachea may have anatomical structures or descriptions that may be used in procedure documentation instead of the term trachea. The Body Part Definitions list other anatomical structures or synonyms that are included in specific ICD-10-PCS body part values. According to the body part definitions, in the example above, cricoid cartilage is included in the Trachea (character 1) body part.

Appendix F: Device Classification

This resource provides an explanation of how a device is defined in the ICD-10-PCS classification along with two tables. The first table groups devices used in the ICD-10-PCS tables into general categories, including a definition of each device type and related examples. The second table provides definitions of transplant and grafting tissue types and associated terminology that may be found in the documentation.

Appendix G: Device Key and Aggregation Table

The Device Key helps users code the appropriate PCS sixth character for device. Devices are listed alphabetically by brand name or commonly used medical terminology and are translated to the appropriate PCS language or value. The key also reflects the body system where the device is located. For example, a SAPIEN valve used for transaortic valve replacement translates to Zooplastic Tissue in Heart and Great Vessels.

The following symbol **NT** has been placed next to those devices that have received an NTAP (new technology add-on payment) designation. When the code for this device is applied to an inpatient encounter, CMS provides incremental payment in addition to the DRG payment.

The Aggregation Table crosswalks specific device character value definitions for specific root operations in a specific body system to the more general device character value to be used when the root

operation covers a wide range of body parts and the device character represents an entire family of devices.

Appendix H: Device Definitions

This resource is a reverse look-up to the Device Key. The user may reference this resource to see all the specific devices that may be grouped to a particular device character (character 6).

Example:
The operative report states, "An internal fixation device was used to repair a fractured femur. Kirschner wire, bone screws and neutralization plate all used and left in the bone at the end of the procedure. "

Although PCS requires all devices left in the body to be coded and the operative report lists three different devices, a check in the device definitions shows that all of these devices are included in the PCS value "Internal Fixation Device" and require only one code.

The following symbol **NT** has been placed next to those devices that have received an NTAP (new technology add-on payment) designation. When the code for this device is applied to an inpatient encounter, CMS provides incremental payment in addition to the DRG payment.

Appendix I: Substance Key/Substance Definitions

The Substance Key lists substances by trade name or synonym and relates them to a PCS character in the Administration (3) or New Technology (X) section in the Substance (sixth character) or Qualifier (seventh character) column.

The Substance Definitions table is the reverse look-up of the substance key, relating all substance categories, the sixth- or seventh character values, to all trade name or synonyms that may be classified to that particular character.

The following symbol **NT** has been placed next to those substances/ technologies that have received an NTAP (new technology add-on payment) designation. When the code for this substance/technology is applied to an inpatient encounter, CMS provides incremental payment in addition to the DRG payment.

Appendix J: Sections B-H Character Definitions

In each ancillary section (B-H) the characters in a particular column may have different meanings depending on which section the user is working from. This resource provides the values for the characters in these sections as well as a definition of the character value.

Appendix K: Hospital Acquired Conditions

Hospital acquired conditions (HACs) are conditions that are considered reasonably preventable when occurring during the hospital admission and may prevent a case from grouping to a higher-paying MS-DRG. In certain instances the HACs are conditional, requiring a specific ICD-10-CM diagnosis code in combination with a specific ICD-10-PCS procedure code. This resource identifies these conditional HACs, listing the diagnosis and procedure codes that, in combination, may trigger a HAC edit. All codes, ICD-10-CM and ICD-10-PCS, are listed with their full descriptions.

Appendix L: Procedure Combination Tables

The procedure combination tables provided in this resource illustrate certain procedure combinations that must occur in order to assign a specific MS-DRG.

Appendix M: Coding Exercises and Answers

This resource provides the coding exercises with answers, and in some cases a brief explanation as to the reason that particular code was used.

ICD-10-PCS Official Guidelines for Coding and Reporting 2023

Narrative changes appear in **bold** text.

The Centers for Medicare and Medicaid Services (CMS) and the National Center for Health Statistics (NCHS), two departments within the U.S. Federal Government's Department of Health and Human Services (DHHS) provide the following guidelines for coding and reporting using the International Classification of Diseases, 10th Revision, Procedure Coding System (ICD-10-PCS). These guidelines should be used as a companion document to the official version of the ICD-10-PCS as published on the CMS website. The ICD-10-PCS is a procedure classification published by the United States for classifying procedures performed in hospital inpatient health care settings.

These guidelines have been approved by the four organizations that make up the Cooperating Parties for the ICD-10-PCS: the American Hospital Association (AHA), the American Health Information Management Association (AHIMA), CMS, and NCHS.

These guidelines are a set of rules that have been developed to accompany and complement the official conventions and instructions provided within the ICD-10-PCS itself. They are intended to provide direction that is applicable in most circumstances. However, there may be unique circumstances where exceptions are applied. The instructions and conventions of the classification take precedence over guidelines. These guidelines are based on the coding and sequencing instructions in the Tables, Index and Definitions of ICD-10-PCS, but provide additional instruction. Adherence to these guidelines when assigning ICD-10-PCS procedure codes is required under the Health Insurance Portability and Accountability Act (HIPAA). The procedure codes have been adopted under HIPAA for hospital inpatient healthcare settings. A joint effort between the healthcare provider and the coder is essential to achieve complete and accurate documentation, code assignment, and reporting of diagnoses and procedures. These guidelines have been developed to assist both the healthcare provider and the coder in identifying those procedures that are to be reported. The importance of consistent, complete documentation in the medical record cannot be overemphasized. Without such documentation accurate coding cannot be achieved.

Conventions

A1. ICD-10-PCS codes are composed of seven characters. Each character is an axis of classification that specifies information about the procedure performed. Within a defined code range, a character specifies the same type of information in that axis of classification.

Example:
The fifth axis of classification specifies the approach in sections Ø through 4 and 7 through 9 of the system.

A2. One of 34 possible values can be assigned to each axis of classification in the seven-character code: they are the numbers Ø through 9 and the alphabet (except I and O because they are easily confused with the numbers 1 and Ø). The number of unique values used in an axis of classification differs as needed.

Example:
Where the fifth axis of classification specifies the approach, seven different approach values are currently used to specify the approach.

A3. The valid values for an axis of classification can be added to as needed.

Example:
If a significantly distinct type of device is used in a new procedure, a new device value can be added to the system.

A4. As with words in their context, the meaning of any single value is a combination of its axis of classification and any preceding values on which it may be dependent.

Example:
The meaning of a body part value in the Medical and Surgical section is always dependent on the body system value. The body part value Ø in the Central Nervous body system specifies Brain and the body part value Ø in the Peripheral Nervous body system specifies Cervical Plexus.

A5. As the system is expanded to become increasingly detailed, over time more values will depend on preceding values for their meaning.

Example:
In the Lower Joints body system, the device value 3 in the root operation Insertion specifies Infusion Device and the device value 3 in the root operation Replacement specifies Ceramic Synthetic Substitute.

A6. The purpose of the alphabetic index is to locate the appropriate table that contains all information necessary to construct a procedure code. The PCS Tables should always be consulted to find the most appropriate valid code.

A7. It is not required to consult the index first before proceeding to the tables to complete the code. A valid code may be chosen directly from the tables.

A8. All seven characters must be specified to be a valid code. If the documentation is incomplete for coding purposes, the physician should be queried for the necessary information.

A9. Within a PCS table, valid codes include all combinations of choices in characters 4 through 7 contained in the same row of the table. In the example below, ØJHT3VZ is a valid code, and ØJHW3VZ is *not* a valid code.

Section:	Ø	Medical and Surgical	
Body System:	J	Subcutaneous Tissue and Fascia	
Operation:	H	Insertion	Putting in a nonbiological appliance that monitors, assists, performs, or prevents a physiological function but does not physically take the place of a body part

Body Part	Approach	Device	Qualifier
S Subcutaneous Tissue and Fascia, Head and Neck **V** Subcutaneous Tissue and Fascia, Upper Extremity **W** Subcutaneous Tissue and Fascia, Lower Extremity	**Ø** Open **3** Percutaneous	**1** Radioactive Element **3** Infusion Device **Y** Other Device	**Z** No Qualifier
T Subcutaneous Tissue and Fascia, Trunk	**Ø** Open **3** Percutaneous	**1** Radioactive Element **3** Infusion Device **V** Infusion Pump **Y** Other Device	**Z** No Qualifier

A10. "And," when used in a code description, means "and/or," except when used to describe a combination of multiple body parts for which separate values exist for each body part (e.g., Skin and Subcutaneous Tissue used as a qualifier, where there are separate body part values for "Skin" and "Subcutaneous Tissue").

Example:

Lower Arm and Wrist Muscle means lower arm and/or wrist muscle.

A11. Many of the terms used to construct PCS codes are defined within the system. It is the coder's responsibility to determine what the documentation in the medical record equates to in the PCS definitions. The physician is not expected to use the terms used in PCS code descriptions, nor is the coder required to query the physician when the correlation between the documentation and the defined PCS terms is clear.

Example:

When the physician documents "partial resection" the coder can independently correlate "partial resection" to the root operation Excision without querying the physician for clarification.

Medical and Surgical Section Guidelines (section Ø)

B2. Body System

General guidelines

B2.1a. The procedure codes in Anatomical Regions, General, Anatomical Regions, Upper Extremities and Anatomical Regions, Lower Extremities can be used when the procedure is performed on an anatomical region rather than a specific body part, or on the rare occasion when no information is available to support assignment of a code to a specific body part.

Examples:

Chest tube drainage of the pleural cavity is coded to the root operation Drainage found in the body system Anatomical Regions, General.

Suture repair of the abdominal wall is coded to the root operation Repair in the body system Anatomical Regions, General.

Amputation of the foot is coded to the root operation Detachment in the body system Anatomical Regions, Lower Extremities.

B2.1b. Where the general body part values "upper" and "lower" are provided as an option in the Upper Arteries, Lower Arteries, Upper Veins, Lower Veins, Muscles and Tendons body systems, "upper" or "lower" specifies body parts located above or below the diaphragm respectively.

Example:

Vein body parts above the diaphragm are found in the Upper Veins body system; vein body parts below the diaphragm are found in the Lower Veins body system.

B3. Root Operation

General guidelines

B3.1a. In order to determine the appropriate root operation, the full definition of the root operation as contained in the PCS Tables must be applied.

B3.1b. Components of a procedure specified in the root operation definition or explanation as integral to that root operation are not coded separately. Procedural steps necessary to reach the operative site and close the operative site, including anastomosis of a tubular body part, are also not coded separately.

Examples:

Resection of a joint as part of a joint replacement procedure is included in the root operation definition of Replacement and is not coded separately.

Laparotomy performed to reach the site of an open liver biopsy is not coded separately.

In a resection of sigmoid colon with anastomosis of descending colon to rectum, the anastomosis is not coded separately.

Multiple procedures

B3.2. During the same operative episode, multiple procedures are coded if:

a. The same root operation is performed on different body parts as defined by distinct values of the body part character.

Examples:

Diagnostic excision of liver and pancreas are coded separately.

Excision of lesion in the ascending colon and excision of lesion in the transverse colon are coded separately.

b. The same root operation is repeated in multiple body parts, and those body parts are separate and distinct body parts classified to a single ICD-10-PCS body part value.

Examples:

Excision of the sartorius muscle and excision of the gracilis muscle are both included in the upper leg muscle body part value, and multiple procedures are coded.

Extraction of multiple toenails are coded separately.

c. Multiple root operations with distinct objectives are performed on the same body part.

Example:

Destruction of sigmoid lesion and bypass of sigmoid colon are coded separately.

d. The intended root operation is attempted using one approach but is converted to a different approach.

Example:

Laparoscopic cholecystectomy converted to an open cholecystectomy is coded as percutaneous endoscopic Inspection and open Resection.

Discontinued or incomplete procedures

B3.3. If the intended procedure is discontinued or otherwise not completed, code the procedure to the root operation performed. If a procedure is discontinued before any other root operation is performed, code the root operation Inspection of the body part or anatomical region inspected.

Example:

A planned aortic valve replacement procedure is discontinued after the initial thoracotomy and before any incision is made in the heart muscle, when the patient becomes hemodynamically unstable. This procedure is coded as an open Inspection of the mediastinum.

Biopsy procedures

B3.4a. Biopsy procedures are coded using the root operations Excision, Extraction, or Drainage and the qualifier Diagnostic.

Examples:

Fine needle aspiration biopsy of fluid in the lung is coded to the root operation Drainage with the qualifier Diagnostic.

Biopsy of bone marrow is coded to the root operation Extraction with the qualifier Diagnostic.

Lymph node sampling for biopsy is coded to the root operation Excision with the qualifier Diagnostic.

Biopsy followed by more definitive treatment

B3.4b. If a diagnostic Excision, Extraction, or Drainage procedure (biopsy) is followed by a more definitive procedure, such as Destruction, Excision or Resection at the same procedure site, both the biopsy and the more definitive treatment are coded.

> *Example:*
> Biopsy of breast followed by partial mastectomy at the same procedure site, both the biopsy and the partial mastectomy procedure are coded.

Overlapping body layers

B3.5. If root operations such as Excision, Extraction, Repair or Inspection are performed on overlapping layers of the musculoskeletal system, the body part specifying the deepest layer is coded.

> *Example:*
> Excisional debridement that includes skin and subcutaneous tissue and muscle is coded to the muscle body part.

Bypass procedures

B3.6a. Bypass procedures are coded by identifying the body part bypassed "from" and the body part bypassed "to." The fourth character body part specifies the body part bypassed from, and the qualifier specifies the body part bypassed to.

> *Example:*
> Bypass from stomach to jejunum, stomach is the body part and jejunum is the qualifier.

B3.6b. Coronary artery bypass procedures are coded differently than other bypass procedures as described in the previous guideline. Rather than identifying the body part bypassed from, the body part identifies the number of coronary arteries bypassed to, and the qualifier specifies the vessel bypassed from.

> *Example:*
> Aortocoronary artery bypass of the left anterior descending coronary artery and the obtuse marginal coronary artery is classified in the body part axis of classification as two coronary arteries, and the qualifier specifies the aorta as the body part bypassed from.

B3.6c. If multiple coronary arteries are bypassed, a separate procedure is coded for each coronary artery that uses a different device and/or qualifier.

> *Example:*
> Aortocoronary artery bypass and internal mammary coronary artery bypass are coded separately.

Control vs. more specific root operations

B3.7. The root operation Control is defined as, "Stopping, or attempting to stop, postprocedural or other acute bleeding." Control is the root operation coded when the procedure performed to achieve hemostasis, beyond what would be considered integral to a procedure, utilizes techniques (e.g. cautery, application of substances or pressure, suturing or ligation or clipping of bleeding points at the site) that are not described by a more specific root operation definition, such as Bypass, Detachment, Excision, Extraction, Reposition, Replacement, or Resection. If a more specific root operation definition applies to the procedure performed, then the more specific root operation is coded instead of Control.

> *Example:*
> Silver nitrate cautery to treat acute nasal bleeding is coded to the root operation Control.

> *Example:*
> Liquid embolization of the right internal iliac artery to treat acute hematoma by stopping blood flow is coded to the root operation Occlusion.

> *Example:*
> Suctioning of residual blood to achieve hemostasis during a transbronchial cryobiopsy is considered integral to the cryobiopsy procedure and is not coded separately.

Excision vs. Resection

B3.8. PCS contains specific body parts for anatomical subdivisions of a body part, such as lobes of the lungs or liver and regions of the intestine. Resection of the specific body part is coded whenever all of the body part is cut out or off, rather than coding Excision of a less specific body part.

> *Example:*
> Left upper lung lobectomy is coded to Resection of Upper Lung Lobe, Left rather than Excision of Lung, Left.

Excision for graft

B3.9. If an autograft is obtained from a different procedure site in order to complete the objective of the procedure, a separate procedure is coded, except when the seventh character qualifier value in the ICD-10-PCS table fully specifies the site from which the autograft was obtained.

> *Examples:*
> Coronary bypass with excision of saphenous vein graft, excision of saphenous vein is coded separately.
>
> Replacement of breast with autologous deep inferior epigastric artery perforator (DIEP) flap, excision of the DIEP flap is not coded separately. The seventh character qualifier value Deep Inferior Epigastric Artery Perforator Flap in the Replacement table fully specifies the site of the autograft harvest.

Fusion procedures of the spine

B3.10a. The body part coded for a spinal vertebral joint(s) rendered immobile by a spinal fusion procedure is classified by the level of the spine (e.g. thoracic). There are distinct body part values for a single vertebral joint and for multiple vertebral joints at each spinal level.

> *Example:*
> Body part values specify Lumbar Vertebral Joint, Lumbar Vertebral Joints, 2 or More and Lumbosacral Vertebral Joint.

B3.10b. If multiple vertebral joints are fused, a separate procedure is coded for each vertebral joint that uses a different device and/or qualifier.

> *Example:*
> Fusion of lumbar vertebral joint, posterior approach, anterior column and fusion of lumbar vertebral joint, posterior approach, posterior column are coded separately.

B3.10c. Combinations of devices and materials are often used on a vertebral joint to render the joint immobile. When combinations of devices are used on the same vertebral joint, the device value coded for the procedure is as follows:

- If an interbody fusion device is used to render the joint immobile (containing bone graft or bone graft substitute), the procedure is coded with the device value Interbody Fusion Device

- If bone graft is the *only* device used to render the joint immobile, the procedure is coded with the device value Nonautologous Tissue Substitute or Autologous Tissue Substitute

- If a mixture of autologous and nonautologous bone graft (with or without biological or synthetic extenders or binders) is used to render the joint immobile, code the procedure with the device value Autologous Tissue Substitute

Examples:

Fusion of a vertebral joint using a cage style interbody fusion device containing morsellized bone graft is coded to the device Interbody Fusion Device.

Fusion of a vertebral joint using a bone dowel interbody fusion device made of cadaver bone and packed with a mixture of local morsellized bone and demineralized bone matrix is coded to the device Interbody Fusion Device.

Fusion of a vertebral joint using both autologous bone graft and bone bank bone graft is coded to the device Autologous Tissue Substitute.

Inspection procedures

B3.11a. Inspection of a body part(s) performed in order to achieve the objective of a procedure is not coded separately.

Example:

Fiberoptic bronchoscopy performed for irrigation of bronchus, only the irrigation procedure is coded.

B3.11b. If multiple tubular body parts are inspected, the most distal body part (the body part furthest from the starting point of the inspection) is coded. If multiple non-tubular body parts in a region are inspected, the body part that specifies the entire area inspected is coded.

Examples:

Cystoureteroscopy with inspection of bladder and ureters is coded to the ureter body part value.

Exploratory laparotomy with general inspection of abdominal contents is coded to the peritoneal cavity body part value.

B3.11c. When both an Inspection procedure and another procedure are performed on the same body part during the same episode, if the Inspection procedure is performed using a different approach than the other procedure, the Inspection procedure is coded separately.

Example:

Endoscopic Inspection of the duodenum is coded separately when open Excision of the duodenum is performed during the same procedural episode.

Occlusion vs. Restriction for vessel embolization procedures

B3.12. If the objective of an embolization procedure is to completely close a vessel, the root operation Occlusion is coded. If the objective of an embolization procedure is to narrow the lumen of a vessel, the root operation Restriction is coded.

Examples:

Tumor embolization is coded to the root operation Occlusion, because the objective of the procedure is to cut off the blood supply to the vessel.

Embolization of a cerebral aneurysm is coded to the root operation Restriction, because the objective of the procedure is not to close off the vessel entirely, but to narrow the lumen of the vessel at the site of the aneurysm where it is abnormally wide.

Release procedures

B3.13. In the root operation Release, the body part value coded is the body part being freed and not the tissue being manipulated or cut to free the body part.

Example:

Lysis of intestinal adhesions is coded to the specific intestine body part value.

Release vs. Division

B3.14. If the sole objective of the procedure is freeing a body part without cutting the body part, the root operation is Release. If the sole objective of the procedure is separating or transecting a body part, the root operation is Division.

Examples:

Freeing a nerve root from surrounding scar tissue to relieve pain is coded to the root operation Release.

Severing a nerve root to relieve pain is coded to the root operation Division.

Reposition for fracture treatment

B3.15. Reduction of a displaced fracture is coded to the root operation Reposition and the application of a cast or splint in conjunction with the Reposition procedure is not coded separately. Treatment of a nondisplaced fracture is coded to the procedure performed.

Examples:

Casting of a nondisplaced fracture is coded to the root operation Immobilization in the Placement section.

Putting a pin in a nondisplaced fracture is coded to the root operation Insertion.

Transplantation vs. Administration

B3.16. Putting in a mature and functioning living body part taken from another individual or animal is coded to the root operation Transplantation. Putting in autologous or nonautologous cells is coded to the Administration section.

Example:

Putting in autologous or nonautologous bone marrow, pancreatic islet cells or stem cells is coded to the Administration section.

Transfer procedures using multiple tissue layers

B3.17. The root operation Transfer contains qualifiers that can be used to specify when a transfer flap is composed of more than one tissue layer, such as a musculocutaneous flap. For procedures involving transfer of multiple tissue layers including skin, subcutaneous tissue, fascia or muscle, the procedure is coded to the body part value that describes the deepest tissue layer in the flap, and the qualifier can be used to describe the other tissue layer(s) in the transfer flap.

Example:

A musculocutaneous flap transfer is coded to the appropriate body part value in the body system Muscles, and the qualifier is used to describe the additional tissue layer(s) in the transfer flap.

Excision/Resection followed by replacement

B3.18. If an excision or resection of a body part is followed by a replacement procedure, code both procedures to identify each distinct objective, except when the excision or resection is considered integral and preparatory for the replacement procedure.

Examples:

Mastectomy followed by reconstruction, both resection and replacement of the breast are coded to fully capture the distinct objectives of the procedures performed.

Maxillectomy with obturator reconstruction, both excision and replacement of the maxilla are coded to fully capture the distinct objectives of the procedures performed.

Excisional debridement of tendon with skin graft, both the excision of the tendon and the replacement of the skin with a graft are coded to fully capture the distinct objectives of the procedures performed.

Esophagectomy followed by reconstruction with colonic interposition, both the resection and the transfer of the large intestine to function as the esophagus are coded to fully capture the distinct objectives of the procedures performed.

Examples:
Resection of a joint as part of a joint replacement procedure is considered integral and preparatory for the replacement of the joint and the resection is not coded separately.

Resection of a valve as part of a valve replacement procedure is considered integral and preparatory for the valve replacement and the resection is not coded separately.

Detachment procedures of extremities

B3.19. The root operation Detachment contains qualifiers that can be used to specify the level where the extremity was amputated. These qualifiers are dependent on the body part value in the "upper extremities" and "lower extremities" body systems. For procedures involving the detachment of all or part of the upper or lower extremities, the procedure is coded to the body part value that describes the site of the detachment.

> *Example:*
> An amputation at the proximal portion of the shaft of the tibia and fibula is coded to the Lower leg body part value in the body system Anatomical Regions, Lower Extremities, and the qualifier High is used to specify the level where the extremity was detached.

The following definitions were developed for the Detachment qualifiers

Body Part	Qualifier	Definition
Upper arm and upper leg	1	High: Amputation at the proximal portion of the shaft of the humerus or femur
	2	Mid: Amputation at the middle portion of the shaft of the humerus or femur
	3	Low: Amputation at the distal portion of the shaft of the humerus or femur
Lower arm and lower leg	1	High: Amputation at the proximal portion of the shaft of the radius/ulna or tibia/fibula
	2	Mid: Amputation at the middle portion of the shaft of the radius/ulna or tibia/fibula
	3	Low: Amputation at the distal portion of the shaft of the radius/ulna or tibia/fibula
Hand and Foot	0	Complete*
	4	Complete 1st Ray
	5	Complete 2nd Ray
	6	Complete 3rd Ray
	7	Complete 4th Ray
	8	Complete 5th Ray
	9	Partial 1st Ray
	B	Partial 2nd Ray
	C	Partial 3rd Ray
	D	Partial 4th Ray
	F	Partial 5th Ray

Body Part	Qualifier	Definition
Thumb, finger, or toe	0	Complete: Amputation at the metacarpophalangeal/metatarsal-phalangeal joint
	1	High: Amputation anywhere along the proximal phalanx
	2	Mid: Amputation through the proximal interphalangeal joint or anywhere along the middle phalanx
	3	Low: Amputation through the distal interphalangeal joint or anywhere along the distal phalanx

*When coding amputation of Hand and Foot, the following definitions are followed:

- **Complete:** Amputation through the carpometacarpal joint of the hand, or through the tarsal-metatarsal joint of the foot.
- **Partial:** Amputation anywhere along the shaft or head of the metacarpal bone of the hand, or of the metatarsal bone of the foot.

B4. Body Part

General guidelines

B4.1a. If a procedure is performed on a portion of a body part that does not have a separate body part value, code the body part value corresponding to the whole body part.

> *Example:*
> A procedure performed on the alveolar process of the mandible is coded to the mandible body part.

B4.1b. If the prefix "peri" is combined with a body part to identify the site of the procedure, and the site of the procedure is not further specified, then the procedure is coded to the body part named. This guideline applies only when a more specific body part value is not available.

> *Examples:*
> A procedure site identified as perirenal is coded to the kidney body part when the site of the procedure is not further specified.
>
> A procedure site described in the documentation as peri-urethral, and the documentation also indicates that it is the vulvar tissue and not the urethral tissue that is the site of the procedure, then the procedure is coded to the vulva body part.
>
> A procedure site documented as involving the periosteum is coded to the corresponding bone body part.

B4.1c. If a single vascular procedure is performed on a continuous section of an arterial or venous body part, code the body part value corresponding to the anatomically most proximal (closest to the heart) portion of the arterial or venous body part.

> *Example:*
> A procedure performed on a continuous section of artery from the femoral artery to the external iliac artery with the point of entry at the femoral artery is coded to the external iliac body part.
>
> A procedure performed on a continuous section of artery from the femoral artery to the external iliac artery with the point of entry at the external iliac artery is also coded to the external iliac artery body part.

Branches of body parts

B4.2. Where a specific branch of a body part does not have its own body part value in PCS, the body part is typically coded to the closest proximal branch that has a specific body part value. In the cardiovascular body systems, if a general body part is available in the correct root operation table, and coding to a proximal branch would require assigning a code in a different body system, the procedure is coded using the general body part value.

> *Examples:*
>
> A procedure performed on the mandibular branch of the trigeminal nerve is coded to the trigeminal nerve body part value.
>
> Occlusion of the bronchial artery is coded to the body part value Upper Artery in the body system Upper Arteries, and not to the body part value Thoracic Aorta, Descending in the body system Heart and Great Vessels.

Bilateral body part values

B4.3. Bilateral body part values are available for a limited number of body parts. If the identical procedure is performed on contralateral body parts, and a bilateral body part value exists for that body part, a single procedure is coded using the bilateral body part value. If no bilateral body part value exists, each procedure is coded separately using the appropriate body part value.

> *Examples:*
>
> The identical procedure performed on both fallopian tubes is coded once using the body part value Fallopian Tube, Bilateral.
>
> The identical procedure performed on both knee joints is coded twice using the body part values Knee Joint, Right and Knee Joint, Left.

Coronary arteries

B4.4. The coronary arteries are classified as a single body part that is further specified by number of arteries treated. One procedure code specifying multiple arteries is used when the same procedure is performed, including the same device and qualifier values.

> *Examples:*
>
> Angioplasty of two distinct coronary arteries with placement of two stents is coded as Dilation of Coronary Artery, Two Arteries with Two Intraluminal Devices.
>
> Angioplasty of two distinct coronary arteries, one with stent placed and one without, is coded separately as Dilation of Coronary Artery, One Artery with Intraluminal Device, and Dilation of Coronary Artery, One Artery with no device.

Tendons, ligaments, bursae and fascia near a joint

B4.5. Procedures performed on tendons, ligaments, bursae and fascia supporting a joint are coded to the body part in the respective body system that is the focus of the procedure. Procedures performed on joint structures themselves are coded to the body part in the joint body systems.

> *Examples:*
>
> Repair of the anterior cruciate ligament of the knee is coded to the knee bursa and ligament body part in the bursae and ligaments body system.
>
> Knee arthroscopy with shaving of articular cartilage is coded to the knee joint body part in the Lower Joints body system.

Skin, subcutaneous tissue and fascia overlying a joint

B4.6. If a procedure is performed on the skin, subcutaneous tissue or fascia overlying a joint, the procedure is coded to the following body part:

- Shoulder is coded to Upper Arm
- Elbow is coded to Lower Arm
- Wrist is coded to Lower Arm
- Hip is coded to Upper Leg
- Knee is coded to Lower Leg
- Ankle is coded to Foot

Fingers and toes

B4.7. If a body system does not contain a separate body part value for fingers, procedures performed on the fingers are coded to the body part value for the hand. If a body system does not contain a separate body part value for toes, procedures performed on the toes are coded to the body part value for the foot.

> *Example:*
>
> Excision of finger muscle is coded to one of the hand muscle body part values in the Muscles body system.

Upper and lower intestinal tract

B4.8. In the Gastrointestinal body system, the general body part values Upper Intestinal Tract and Lower Intestinal Tract are provided as an option for the root operations such as Change, Insertion, Inspection, Removal and Revision. Upper Intestinal Tract includes the portion of the gastrointestinal tract from the esophagus down to and including the duodenum, and Lower Intestinal Tract includes the portion of the gastrointestinal tract from the jejunum down to and including the rectum and anus.

> *Example:*
>
> In the root operation Change table, change of a device in the jejunum is coded using the body part Lower Intestinal Tract.

B5. Approach

Open approach with percutaneous endoscopic assistance

B5.2a. Procedures performed using the open approach with percutaneous endoscopic assistance are coded to the approach Open.

> *Example:*
>
> Laparoscopic-assisted sigmoidectomy is coded to the approach Open.

Percutaneous endoscopic approach with extension of incision

B5.2b. Procedures performed using the percutaneous endoscopic approach, with incision or extension of an incision to assist in the removal of all or a portion of a body part or to anastomose a tubular body part to complete the procedure, are coded to the approach value Percutaneous Endoscopic.

> *Examples:*
>
> Laparoscopic sigmoid colectomy with extension of stapling port for removal of specimen and direct anastomosis is coded to the approach value percutaneous endoscopic.
>
> Laparoscopic nephrectomy with midline incision for removing the resected kidney is coded to the approach value percutaneous endoscopic.
>
> Robotic-assisted laparoscopic prostatectomy with extension of incision for removal of the resected prostate is coded to the approach value percutaneous endoscopic.

External approach

B5.3a. Procedures performed within an orifice on structures that are visible without the aid of any instrumentation are coded to the approach External.

Example:
Resection of tonsils is coded to the approach External.

B5.3b. Procedures performed indirectly by the application of external force through the intervening body layers are coded to the approach External.

Example:
Closed reduction of fracture is coded to the approach External.

Percutaneous procedure via device

B5.4. Procedures performed percutaneously via a device placed for the procedure are coded to the approach Percutaneous.

Example:
Fragmentation of kidney stone performed via percutaneous nephrostomy is coded to the approach Percutaneous.

B6. Device

General guidelines

B6.1a. A device is coded only if a device remains after the procedure is completed. If no device remains, the device value No Device is coded. In limited root operations, the classification provides the qualifier values Temporary and Intraoperative, for specific procedures involving clinically significant devices, where the purpose of the device is to be utilized for a brief duration during the procedure or current inpatient stay. If a device that is intended to remain after the procedure is completed requires removal before the end of the operative episode in which it was inserted (for example, the device size is inadequate or **an event documented as a** complication occurs), both the insertion and removal of the device should be coded.

B6.1b. Materials such as sutures, ligatures, radiological markers and temporary post-operative wound drains are considered integral to the performance of a procedure and are not coded as devices.

B6.1c. Procedures performed on a device only and not on a body part are specified in the root operations Change, Irrigation, Removal and Revision, and are coded to the procedure performed.

Example:
Irrigation of percutaneous nephrostomy tube is coded to the root operation Irrigation of indwelling device in the Administration section.

Drainage device

B6.2. A separate procedure to put in a drainage device is coded to the root operation Drainage with the device value Drainage Device.

Obstetric Section Guidelines (section 1)

C. Obstetrics Section

Products of conception

C1. Procedures performed on the products of conception are coded to the Obstetrics section. Procedures performed on the pregnant female other than the products of conception are coded to the appropriate root operation in the Medical and Surgical section.

Examples:
Amniocentesis is coded to the products of conception body part in the Obstetrics section.

Repair of obstetric urethral laceration is coded to the urethra body part in the Medical and Surgical section.

Procedures following delivery or abortion

C2. Procedures performed following a delivery or abortion for curettage of the endometrium or evacuation of retained products of conception are all coded in the Obstetrics section, to the root operation Extraction and the body part Products of Conception, Retained.

Diagnostic or therapeutic dilation and curettage performed during times other than the postpartum or post-abortion period are all coded in the Medical and Surgical section, to the root operation Extraction and the body part Endometrium.

Radiation Therapy Section Guidelines (section D)

D. Radiation Therapy Section

Brachytherapy

D1.a. Brachytherapy is coded to the modality Brachytherapy in the Radiation Therapy section. When a radioactive brachytherapy source is left in the body at the end of the procedure, it is coded separately to the root operation Insertion with the device value Radioactive Element.

Example:
Brachytherapy with implantation of a low dose rate brachytherapy source left in the body at the end of the procedure is coded to the applicable treatment site in section D, Radiation Therapy, with the modality Brachytherapy, the modality qualifier value Low Dose Rate, and the applicable isotope value and qualifier value. The implantation of the brachytherapy source is coded separately to the device value Radioactive Element in the appropriate Insertion table of the Medical and Surgical section. The Radiation Therapy section code identifies the specific modality and isotope of the brachytherapy, and the root operation Insertion code identifies the implantation of the brachytherapy source that remains in the body at the end of the procedure.

Exception:
Implantation of Cesium-131 brachytherapy seeds embedded in a collagen matrix to the treatment site after resection of brain tumor is coded to the root operation Insertion with the device value Radioactive Element, Cesium-131 Collagen Implant. The procedure is coded to the root operation Insertion only, because the device value identifies both the implantation of the radioactive element and a specific brachytherapy isotope that is not included in the Radiation Therapy section tables.

D1.b. A separate procedure to place a temporary applicator for delivering the brachytherapy is coded to the root operation Insertion and the device value Other Device.

Examples:
Intrauterine brachytherapy applicator placed as a separate procedure from the brachytherapy procedure is coded to Insertion of Other Device, and the brachytherapy is coded separately using the modality Brachytherapy in the Radiation Therapy section.

Intrauterine brachytherapy applicator placed concomitantly with delivery of the brachytherapy dose is coded with a single code using the modality Brachytherapy in the Radiation Therapy section.

New Technology Section Guidelines (section X)

E. New Technology Section

General guidelines

E1.a. Section X codes fully represent the specific procedure described in the code title, and do not require additional codes from other sections of ICD-10-PCS. When section X contains a code title which fully describes a specific new technology procedure, and it is the only procedure performed, only the section X code is reported for the procedure. There is no need to report an additional code in another section of ICD-10-PCS.

Example:

XW043A6 Introduction of Cefiderocol Anti-infective into Central Vein, Percutaneous Approach, New Technology Group 6, can be coded to indicate that Cefiderocol Anti-infective was administered via a central vein. A separate code from table 3E0 in the Administration section of ICD-10-PCS is not coded in addition to this code.

E1.b. When multiple procedures are performed, New Technology section X codes are coded following the multiple procedures guideline.

Examples:

Dual filter cerebral embolic filtration used during transcatheter aortic valve replacement (TAVR), X2A5312 Cerebral Embolic Filtration, Dual Filter in Innominate Artery and Left Common Carotid Artery, Percutaneous Approach, New Technology Group 2, is coded for the cerebral embolic filtration, along with an ICD-10-PCS code for the TAVR procedure.

An extracorporeal flow reversal circuit for embolic neuroprotection placed during a transcarotid arterial revascularization procedure, a code from table X2A, Assistance of the Cardiovascular System is coded for the use of the extracorporeal flow reversal circuit, along with an ICD-10-PCS code for the transcarotid arterial revascularization procedure.

F. Selection of Principal Procedure

The following instructions should be applied in the selection of principal procedure and clarification on the importance of the relation to the principal diagnosis when more than one procedure is performed:

1. Procedure performed for definitive treatment of both principal diagnosis and secondary diagnosis

   a. Sequence procedure performed for definitive treatment most related to principal diagnosis as principal procedure.

2. Procedure performed for definitive treatment and diagnostic procedures performed for both principal diagnosis and secondary diagnosis.

   a. Sequence procedure performed for definitive treatment most related to principal diagnosis as principal procedure

3. A diagnostic procedure was performed for the principal diagnosis and a procedure is performed for definitive treatment of a secondary diagnosis.

   a. Sequence diagnostic procedure as principal procedure, since the procedure most related to the principal diagnosis takes precedence.

4. No procedures performed that are related to principal diagnosis; procedures performed for definitive treatment and diagnostic procedures were performed for secondary diagnosis

   a. Sequence procedure performed for definitive treatment of secondary diagnosis as principal procedure, since there are no procedures (definitive or nondefinitive treatment) related to principal diagnosis.

# #

3f (Aortic) Bioprosthesis valve *use* Zooplastic Tissue in Heart and Great Vessels

A

Abdominal aortic plexus *use* Abdominal Sympathetic Nerve
Abdominal cavity *use* Peritoneal Cavity
Abdominal esophagus *use* Esophagus, Lower
Abdominohysterectomy *see* Resection, Uterus ØUT9
Abdominoplasty
  see Alteration, Abdominal Wall ØWØF
  see Repair, Abdominal Wall ØWQF
  see Supplement, Abdominal Wall ØWUF
Abductor hallucis muscle
  use Foot Muscle, Left
  use Foot Muscle, Right
ABECMA® *use* Idecabtagene Vicleucel Immunotherapy
AbioCor® Total Replacement Heart *use* Synthetic Substitute
Ablation
  see Control bleeding in
  see Destruction
Abortion
  Abortifacient 10A07ZX
  Laminaria 10A07ZW
  Products of Conception 10A0
  Vacuum 10A07Z6
Abrasion *see* Extraction
Absolute Pro Vascular (OTW) Self-Expanding Stent System *use* Intraluminal Device
Accelerate PhenoTest™ BC XXE5XN6
Accessory cephalic vein
  use Cephalic Vein, Left
  use Cephalic Vein, Right
Accessory obturator nerve *use* Lumbar Plexus
Accessory phrenic nerve *use* Phrenic Nerve
Accessory spleen *use* Spleen
Acculink (RX) Carotid Stent System *use* Intraluminal Device
Acellular Hydrated Dermis *use* Nonautologous Tissue Substitute
Acetabular cup *use* Liner in Lower Joints
Acetabulectomy
  see Excision, Lower Bones ØQB
  see Resection, Lower Bones ØQT
Acetabulofemoral joint
  use Hip Joint, Left
  use Hip Joint, Right
Acetabuloplasty
  see Repair, Lower Bones ØQQ
  see Replacement, Lower Bones ØQR
  see Supplement, Lower Bones ØQU
Achilles tendon
  use Lower Leg Tendon, Left
  use Lower Leg Tendon, Right
Achillorrhaphy *see* Repair, Tendons ØLQ
Achillotenotomy, achillotomy
  see Division, Tendons ØL8
  see Drainage, Tendons ØL9
Acoustic Pulse Thrombolysis *see* Fragmentation, Artery
Acromioclavicular ligament
  use Shoulder Bursa and Ligament, Left
  use Shoulder Bursa and Ligament, Right
Acromion (process)
  use Scapula, Left
  use Scapula, Right
Acromionectomy
  see Excision, Upper Joints ØRB
  see Resection, Upper Joints ØRT
Acromioplasty
  see Repair, Upper Joints ØRQ
  see Replacement, Upper Joints ØRR
  see Supplement, Upper Joints ØRU
ACTEMRA® *use* Tocilizumab
Activa PC neurostimulator *use* Stimulator Generator, Multiple Array in ØJH
Activa RC neurostimulator *use* Stimulator Generator, Multiple Array Rechargeable in ØJH
Activa SC neurostimulator *use* Stimulator Generator, Single Array in ØJH
Activities of Daily Living Assessment FØ2

Activities of Daily Living Treatment FØ8
ACUITY™ Steerable Lead
  use Cardiac Lead, Defibrillator in Ø2H
  use Cardiac Lead, Pacemaker in Ø2H
Acupuncture
  Breast
    Anesthesia 8EØH3ØØ
    No Qualifier 8EØH3ØZ
  Integumentary System
    Anesthesia 8EØH3ØØ
    No Qualifier 8EØH3ØZ
Adductor brevis muscle
  use Upper Leg Muscle, Left
  use Upper Leg Muscle, Right
Adductor hallucis muscle
  use Foot Muscle, Left
  use Foot Muscle, Right
Adductor longus muscle
  use Upper Leg Muscle, Left
  use Upper Leg Muscle, Right
Adductor magnus muscle
  use Upper Leg Muscle, Left
  use Upper Leg Muscle, Right
Adenohypophysis *use* Pituitary Gland
Adenoidectomy
  see Excision, Adenoids ØCBQ
  see Resection, Adenoids ØCTQ
Adenoidotomy *see* Drainage, Adenoids ØC9Q
Adhesiolysis *see* Release
Administration
  Blood products *see* Transfusion
  Other substance *see* Introduction of substance in or on
Adrenalectomy
  see Excision, Endocrine System ØGB
  see Resection, Endocrine System ØGT
Adrenalorrhaphy *see* Repair, Endocrine System ØGQ
Adrenalotomy *see* Drainage, Endocrine System ØG9
Advancement
  see Reposition
  see Transfer
Advisa (MRI) *use* Pacemaker, Dual Chamber in ØJH
afami-cel *use* Afamitresgene Autoleucel Immunotherapy
Afamitresgene Autoleucel Immunotherapy XWØ
AFX® Endovascular AAA System *use* Intraluminal Device
Aidoc Briefcase for PE (pulmonary embolism) XXE3X27
AIGISRx Antibacterial Envelope *use* Anti-Infective Envelope
Alar ligament of axis *use* Head and Neck Bursa and Ligament
Alfapump® system *use* Other Device
Alfieri Stitch Valvuloplasty *see* Restriction, Valve, Mitral Ø2VG
Alimentation *see* Introduction of substance in or on
ALPPS (Associating liver partition and portal vein ligation)
  see Division, Hepatobiliary System and Pancreas ØF8
  see Resection, Hepatobiliary System and Pancreas ØFT
Alteration
  Abdominal Wall ØWØF
  Ankle Region
    Left ØYØL
    Right ØYØK
  Arm
    Lower
      Left ØXØF
      Right ØXØD
    Upper
      Left ØXØ9
      Right ØXØ8
  Axilla
    Left ØXØ5
    Right ØXØ4
  Back
    Lower ØWØL
    Upper ØWØK
  Breast
    Bilateral ØHØV
    Left ØHØU
    Right ØHØT
  Buttock
    Left ØYØ1

Alteration — *continued*
  Buttock — *continued*
    Right ØYØØ
  Chest Wall ØWØ8
  Ear
    Bilateral Ø9Ø2
    Left Ø9Ø1
    Right Ø9ØØ
  Elbow Region
    Left ØXØC
    Right ØXØB
  Extremity
    Lower
      Left ØYØB
      Right ØYØ9
    Upper
      Left ØXØ7
      Right ØXØ6
  Eyelid
    Lower
      Left Ø8ØR
      Right Ø8ØQ
    Upper
      Left Ø8ØP
      Right Ø8ØN
  Face ØWØ2
  Head ØWØØ
  Jaw
    Lower ØWØ5
    Upper ØWØ4
  Knee Region
    Left ØYØG
    Right ØYØF
  Leg
    Lower
      Left ØYØJ
      Right ØYØH
    Upper
      Left ØYØD
      Right ØYØC
  Lip
    Lower ØCØ1X
    Upper ØCØØX
  Nasal Mucosa and Soft Tissue Ø9ØK
  Neck ØWØ6
  Perineum
    Female ØWØN
    Male ØWØM
  Shoulder Region
    Left ØXØ3
    Right ØXØ2
  Subcutaneous Tissue and Fascia
    Abdomen ØJØ8
    Back ØJØ7
    Buttock ØJØ9
    Chest ØJØ6
    Face ØJØ1
    Lower Arm
      Left ØJØH
      Right ØJØG
    Lower Leg
      Left ØJØP
      Right ØJØN
    Neck
      Left ØJØ5
      Right ØJØ4
    Upper Arm
      Left ØJØF
      Right ØJØD
    Upper Leg
      Left ØJØM
      Right ØJØL
  Wrist Region
    Left ØXØH
    Right ØXØG
Alveolar process of mandible
  use Mandible, Left
  use Mandible, Right
Alveolar process of maxilla *use* Maxilla
Alveolectomy
  see Excision, Head and Facial Bones ØNB
  see Resection, Head and Facial Bones ØNT
Alveoloplasty
  see Repair, Head and Facial Bones ØNQ
  see Replacement, Head and Facial Bones ØNR
  see Supplement, Head and Facial Bones ØNU
Alveolotomy
  see Division, Head and Facial Bones ØN8

Alveolotomy — *continued*
see Drainage, Head and Facial Bones ØN9
Ambulatory cardiac monitoring 4A12X45
Amivantamab Monoclonal Antibody XWØ
Amniocentesis *see* Drainage, Products of Conception 1Ø9Ø
Amnioinfusion *see* Introduction of substance in or on, Products of Conception 3EØE
Amnioscopy 1ØJØ8ZZ
Amniotomy *see* Drainage, Products of Conception 1Ø9Ø
AMPLATZER® Muscular VSD Occluder *use* Synthetic Substitute
Amputation *see* Detachment
AMS 8ØØ® Urinary Control System *use* Artificial Sphincter in Urinary System
Anal orifice *use* Anus
Analog radiography *see* Plain Radiography
Analog radiology *see* Plain Radiography
Anastomosis *see* Bypass
Anatomical snuffbox
use Lower Arm and Wrist Muscle, Left
use Lower Arm and Wrist Muscle, Right
Andexanet Alfa, Factor Xa Inhibitor Reversal Agent *use* Coagulation Factor Xa, Inactivated
Andexxa *use* Coagulation Factor Xa, Inactivated
AneuRx® AAA Advantage® *use* Intraluminal Device
Angiectomy
see Excision, Heart and Great Vessels Ø2B
see Excision, Lower Arteries Ø4B
see Excision, Lower Veins Ø6B
see Excision, Upper Arteries Ø3B
see Excision, Upper Veins Ø5B
Angiocardiography
Combined right and left heart *see* Fluoroscopy, Heart, Right and Left B216
Left Heart *see* Fluoroscopy, Heart, Left B215
Right Heart *see* Fluoroscopy, Heart, Right B214
SPY system intravascular fluorescence *see* Monitoring, Physiological Systems 4A1
Angiography
see Computerized Tomography (CT Scan), Artery
see Fluoroscopy, Artery
see Magnetic Resonance Imaging (MRI), Artery
see Plain Radiography, Artery
Angioplasty
see Dilation, Heart and Great Vessels Ø27
see Dilation, Lower Arteries Ø47
see Dilation, Upper Arteries Ø37
see Repair, Heart and Great Vessels Ø2Q
see Repair, Lower Arteries Ø4Q
see Repair, Upper Arteries Ø3Q
see Replacement, Heart and Great Vessels Ø2R
see Replacement, Lower Arteries Ø4R
see Replacement, Upper Arteries Ø3R
see Supplement, Heart and Great Vessels Ø2U
see Supplement, Lower Arteries Ø4U
see Supplement, Upper Arteries Ø3U
Angiorrhaphy
see Repair, Heart and Great Vessels Ø2Q
see Repair, Lower Arteries Ø4Q
see Repair, Upper Arteries Ø3Q
Angioscopy Ø2JY4ZZ, Ø3JY4ZZ, Ø4JY4ZZ
Angiotensin II *use* Synthetic Human Angiotensin II
Angiotripsy
see Occlusion, Lower Arteries Ø4L
see Occlusion, Upper Arteries Ø3L
Angular artery *use* Face Artery
Angular vein
use Face Vein, Left
use Face Vein, Right
Annular ligament
use Elbow Bursa and Ligament, Left
use Elbow Bursa and Ligament, Right
Annuloplasty
see Repair, Heart and Great Vessels Ø2Q
see Supplement, Heart and Great Vessels Ø2U
Annuloplasty ring *use* Synthetic Substitute
Anoplasty
see Repair, Anus ØDQQ
see Supplement, Anus ØDUQ
Anorectal junction *use* Rectum
Anoscopy ØDJD8ZZ
Ansa cervicalis *use* Cervical Plexus
Antabuse therapy HZ93ZZZ

Antebrachial fascia
use Subcutaneous Tissue and Fascia, Left Lower Arm
use Subcutaneous Tissue and Fascia, Right Lower Arm
Anterior cerebral artery *use* Intracranial Artery
Anterior cerebral vein *use* Intracranial Vein
Anterior choroidal artery *use* Intracranial Artery
Anterior circumflex humeral artery
use Axillary Artery, Left
use Axillary Artery, Right
Anterior communicating artery *use* Intracranial Artery
Anterior cruciate ligament (ACL)
use Knee Bursa and Ligament, Left
use Knee Bursa and Ligament, Right
Anterior crural nerve *use* Femoral Nerve
Anterior facial vein
use Face Vein, Left
use Face Vein, Right
Anterior intercostal artery
use Internal Mammary Artery, Left
use Internal Mammary Artery, Right
Anterior interosseous nerve *use* Median Nerve
Anterior lateral malleolar artery
use Anterior Tibial Artery, Left
use Anterior Tibial Artery, Right
Anterior lingual gland *use* Minor Salivary Gland
Anterior (pectoral) lymph node
use Lymphatic, Left Axillary
use Lymphatic, Right Axillary
Anterior medial malleolar artery
use Anterior Tibial Artery, Left
use Anterior Tibial Artery, Right
Anterior spinal artery
use Vertebral Artery, Left
use Vertebral Artery, Right
Anterior tibial recurrent artery
use Anterior Tibial Artery, Left
use Anterior Tibial Artery, Right
Anterior ulnar recurrent artery
use Ulnar Artery, Left
use Ulnar Artery, Right
Anterior vagal trunk *use* Vagus Nerve
Anterior vertebral muscle
use Neck Muscle, Left
use Neck Muscle, Right
Antibacterial Envelope (TYRX) (AIGISRx) *use* Anti-Infective Envelope
Antibiotic-eluting Bone Void Filler XWØVØP7
Antigen-free air conditioning *see* Atmospheric Control, Physiological Systems 6AØ
Antihelix
use External Ear, Bilateral
use External Ear, Left
use External Ear, Right
Antimicrobial envelope *use* Anti-Infective Envelope
Anti-SARS-CoV-2 hyperimmune globulin *use* Hyperimmune Globulin
Antitragus
use External Ear, Bilateral
use External Ear, Left
use External Ear, Right
Antrostomy *see* Drainage, Ear, Nose, Sinus Ø99
Antrotomy *see* Drainage, Ear, Nose, Sinus Ø99
Antrum of Highmore
use Maxillary Sinus, Left
use Maxillary Sinus, Right
Aortic annulus *use* Aortic Valve
Aortic arch *use* Thoracic Aorta, Ascending/Arch
Aortic intercostal artery *use* Upper Artery
Aortography
see Fluoroscopy, Lower Arteries B41
see Fluoroscopy, Upper Arteries B31
see Plain Radiography, Lower Arteries B4Ø
see Plain Radiography, Upper Arteries B3Ø
Aortoplasty
see Repair, Aorta, Abdominal Ø4QØ
see Repair, Aorta, Thoracic, Ascending/Arch Ø2QX
see Repair, Aorta, Thoracic, Descending Ø2QW
see Replacement, Aorta, Abdominal Ø4RØ
see Replacement, Aorta, Thoracic, Ascending/Arch Ø2RX
see Replacement, Aorta, Thoracic, Descending Ø2RW
see Supplement, Aorta, Abdominal Ø4UØ

Aortoplasty — *continued*
see Supplement, Aorta, Thoracic, Ascending/Arch Ø2UX
see Supplement, Aorta, Thoracic, Descending Ø2UW
Apalutamide Antineoplastic XWØDXJ5
Apical (subclavicular) lymph node
use Lymphatic, Left Axillary
use Lymphatic, Right Axillary
ApiFix® Minimally Invasive Deformity Correction (MID-C) System *use* Posterior (Dynamic) Distraction Device in New Technology
Apneustic center *use* Pons
Appendectomy
see Excision, Appendix ØDBJ
see Resection, Appendix ØDTJ
Appendicolysis *see* Release, Appendix ØDNJ
Appendicotomy *see* Drainage, Appendix ØD9J
Application *see* Introduction of substance in or on
aprevo™ *use* Interbody Fusion Device, Customizable in New Technology
Aquablation therapy, prostate XV5Ø8A4
Aquapheresis 6A55ØZ3
Aqueduct of Sylvius *use* Cerebral Ventricle
Aqueous humour
use Anterior Chamber, Left
use Anterior Chamber, Right
Arachnoid mater, intracranial *use* Cerebral Meninges
Arachnoid mater, spinal *use* Spinal Meninges
Arcuate artery
use Foot Artery, Left
use Foot Artery, Right
Areola
use Nipple, Left
use Nipple, Right
AROM (artificial rupture of membranes) 1Ø9Ø7ZC
Arterial canal (duct) *use* Pulmonary Artery, Left
Arterial pulse tracing *see* Measurement, Arterial 4AØ3
Arteriectomy
see Excision, Heart and Great Vessels Ø2B
see Excision, Lower Arteries Ø4B
see Excision, Upper Arteries Ø3B
Arteriography
see Fluoroscopy, Heart B21
see Fluoroscopy, Lower Arteries B41
see Fluoroscopy, Upper Arteries B31
see Plain Radiography, Heart B2Ø
see Plain Radiography, Lower Arteries B4Ø
see Plain Radiography, Upper Arteries B3Ø
Arterioplasty
see Repair, Heart and Great Vessels Ø2Q
see Repair, Lower Arteries Ø4Q
see Repair, Upper Arteries Ø3Q
see Replacement, Heart and Great Vessels Ø2R
see Replacement, Lower Arteries Ø4R
see Replacement, Upper Arteries Ø3R
see Supplement, Heart and Great Vessels Ø2U
see Supplement, Lower Arteries Ø4U
see Supplement, Upper Arteries Ø3U
Arteriorrhaphy
see Repair, Heart and Great Vessels Ø2Q
see Repair, Lower Arteries Ø4Q
see Repair, Upper Arteries Ø3Q
Arterioscopy
see Inspection, Artery, Lower Ø4JY
see Inspection, Artery, Upper Ø3JY
see Inspection, Great Vessel Ø2JY
Arthrectomy
see Excision, Lower Joints ØSB
see Excision, Upper Joints ØRB
see Resection, Lower Joints ØST
see Resection, Upper Joints ØRT
Arthrocentesis
see Drainage, Lower Joints ØS9
see Drainage, Upper Joints ØR9
Arthrodesis
see Fusion, Lower Joints ØSG
see Fusion, Upper Joints ØRG
Arthrography
see Plain Radiography, Non-Axial Lower Bones BQØ
see Plain Radiography, Non-Axial Upper Bones BPØ
see Plain Radiography, Skull and Facial Bones BNØ
Arthrolysis
see Release, Lower Joints ØSN
see Release, Upper Joints ØRN

▽ **Subterms under main terms may continue to next column or page**

Arthropexy
　see Repair, Lower Joints ØSQ
　see Repair, Upper Joints ØRQ
　see Reposition, Lower Joints ØSS
　see Reposition, Upper Joints ØRS
Arthroplasty
　see Repair, Lower Joints ØSQ
　see Repair, Upper Joints ØRQ
　see Replacement, Lower Joints ØSR
　see Replacement, Upper Joints ØRR
　see Supplement, Lower Joints ØSU
　see Supplement, Upper Joints ØRU
Arthroplasty, radial head
　see Replacement, Radius, Left ØPRJ
　see Replacement, Radius, Right ØPRH
Arthroscopy
　see Inspection, Lower Joints ØSJ
　see Inspection, Upper Joints ØRJ
Arthrotomy
　see Drainage, Lower Joints ØS9
　see Drainage, Upper Joints ØR9
Articulating Spacer (Antibiotic) *use* Articulating
　Spacer in Lower Joints
Artificial anal sphincter (AAS) *use* Artificial Sphincter
　in Gastrointestinal System
Artificial bowel sphincter (neosphincter) *use* Artificial Sphincter in Gastrointestinal System
Artificial Sphincter
　Insertion of device in
　　Anus ØDHQ
　　Bladder ØTHB
　　Bladder Neck ØTHC
　　Urethra ØTHD
　Removal of device from
　　Anus ØDPQ
　　Bladder ØTPB
　　Urethra ØTPD
　Revision of device in
　　Anus ØDWQ
　　Bladder ØTWB
　　Urethra ØTWD
Artificial urinary sphincter (AUS) *use* Artificial
　Sphincter in Urinary System
Aryepiglottic fold *use* Larynx
Arytenoid cartilage *use* Larynx
Arytenoid muscle
　use Neck Muscle, Left
　use Neck Muscle, Right
Arytenoidectomy *see* Excision, Larynx ØCBS
Arytenoidopexy *see* Repair, Larynx ØCQS
Ascenda Intrathecal Catheter *use* Infusion Device
Ascending aorta *use* Thoracic Aorta, Ascending/Arch
Ascending palatine artery *use* Face Artery
Ascending pharyngeal artery
　use External Carotid Artery, Left
　use External Carotid Artery, Right
aScope™ Duodeno *see* New Technology, Hepatobiliary
　System and Pancreas XFJ
Aspiration, fine needle
　Fluid or gas *see* Drainage
　Tissue biopsy
　　see Excision
　　see Extraction
Assessment
　Activities of daily living *see* Activities of Daily Living
　　Assessment, Rehabilitation F02
　Hearing *see* Hearing Assessment, Diagnostic Audi-
　　ology F13
　Hearing aid *see* Hearing Aid Assessment, Diagnos-
　　tic Audiology F14
　Intravascular perfusion, using indocyanine green
　　(ICG) dye *see* Monitoring, Physiological Sys-
　　tems 4A1
　Motor function *see* Motor Function Assessment,
　　Rehabilitation F01
　Nerve function *see* Motor Function Assessment,
　　Rehabilitation F01
　Speech *see* Speech Assessment, Rehabilitation F00
　Vestibular *see* Vestibular Assessment, Diagnostic
　　Audiology F15
　Vocational *see* Activities of Daily Living Treatment,
　　Rehabilitation F08
Assistance
　Cardiac
　　Continuous
　　　Output
　　　　Balloon Pump 5AØ221Ø

Assistance — *continued*
　Cardiac — *continued*
　　Continuous — *continued*
　　　Output — *continued*
　　　　Impeller Pump 5AØ221D
　　　　Other Pump 5AØ2216
　　　　Pulsatile Compression 5AØ2215
　　　Oxygenation, Supersaturated 5AØ222C
　　Intermittent
　　　Balloon Pump 5AØ211Ø
　　　Impeller Pump 5AØ211D
　　　Other Pump 5AØ2116
　　　Pulsatile Compression 5AØ2115
　Circulatory
　　Continuous, Oxygenation, Hyperbaric
　　　5AØ5221
　　Intermittent, Oxygenation, Hyperbaric
　　　5AØ5121
　Respiratory
　　24-96 Consecutive Hours
　　　Continuous Negative Airway Pressure
　　　　5AØ9459
　　　Continuous Positive Airway Pressure
　　　　5AØ9457
　　　High Nasal Flow/Velocity 5AØ945A
　　　Intermittent Negative Airway Pressure
　　　　5AØ945B
　　　Intermittent Positive Airway Pressure
　　　　5AØ9458
　　　No Qualifier 5AØ945Z
　　Continuous, Filtration 5AØ920Z
　　Greater than 96 Consecutive Hours
　　　Continuous Negative Airway Pressure
　　　　5AØ9559
　　　Continuous Positive Airway Pressure
　　　　5AØ9557
　　　High Nasal Flow/Velocity 5AØ955A
　　　Intermittent Negative Airway Pressure
　　　　5AØ955B
　　　Intermittent Positive Airway Pressure
　　　　5AØ9558
　　　No Qualifier 5AØ955Z
　　Less than 24 Consecutive Hours
　　　Continuous Negative Airway Pressure
　　　　5AØ9359
　　　Continuous Positive Airway Pressure
　　　　5AØ9357
　　　High Nasal Flow/Velocity 5AØ935A
　　　Intermittent Negative Airway Pressure
　　　　5AØ935B
　　　Intermittent Positive Airway Pressure
　　　　5AØ9358
　　　No Qualifier 5AØ935Z
**Associating liver partition and portal vein ligation
　(ALPPS)**
　see Division, Hepatobiliary System and Pancreas
　　ØF8
　see Resection, Hepatobiliary System and Pancreas
　　ØFT
Assurant (Cobalt) stent *use* Intraluminal Device
Atezolizumab Antineoplastic XWØ
Atherectomy
　see Extirpation, Heart and Great Vessels Ø2C
　see Extirpation, Lower Arteries Ø4C
　see Extirpation, Upper Arteries Ø3C
Atlantoaxial joint *use* Cervical Vertebral Joint
Atmospheric Control 6AØZ
AtriClip LAA Exclusion System *use* Extraluminal De-
　vice
Atrioseptoplasty
　see Repair, Heart and Great Vessels Ø2Q
　see Replacement, Heart and Great Vessels Ø2R
　see Supplement, Heart and Great Vessels Ø2U
Atrioventricular node *use* Conduction Mechanism
Atrium dextrum cordis *use* Atrium, Right
Atrium pulmonale *use* Atrium, Left
Attain Ability® lead Ø2H
　use Cardiac Lead, Defibrillator in Ø2H
　use Cardiac Lead, Pacemaker in Ø2H
Attain Starfix® (OTW) lead
　use Cardiac Lead, Defibrillator in Ø2H
　use Cardiac Lead, Pacemaker in Ø2H
Audiology, diagnostic
　see Hearing Aid Assessment, Diagnostic Audiology
　　F14
　see Hearing Assessment, Diagnostic Audiology
　　F13

Audiology, diagnostic — *continued*
　see Vestibular Assessment, Diagnostic Audiology
　　F15
Audiometry *see* Hearing Assessment, Diagnostic Audi-
　ology F13
Auditory tube
　use Eustachian Tube, Left
　use Eustachian Tube, Right
Auerbach's (myenteric) plexus *use* Abdominal Sym-
　pathetic Nerve
Auricle
　use External Ear, Bilateral
　use External Ear, Left
　use External Ear, Right
Auricularis muscle *use* Head Muscle
Autograft *use* Autologous Tissue Substitute
AutoLITT® System *see* Destruction
Autologous artery graft
　use Autologous Arterial Tissue in Heart and Great
　　Vessels
　use Autologous Arterial Tissue in Lower Arteries
　use Autologous Arterial Tissue in Lower Veins
　use Autologous Arterial Tissue in Upper Arteries
　use Autologous Arterial Tissue in Upper Veins
Autologous vein graft
　use Autologous Venous Tissue in Heart and Great
　　Vessels
　use Autologous Venous Tissue in Lower Arteries
　use Autologous Venous Tissue in Lower Veins
　use Autologous Venous Tissue in Upper Arteries
　use Autologous Venous Tissue in Upper Veins
Automated Chest Compression (ACC) 5A1221J
AutoPulse® Resuscitation System 5A1221J
Autotransfusion *see* Transfusion
Autotransplant
　Adrenal tissue *see* Reposition, Endocrine System
　　ØGS
　Kidney *see* Reposition, Urinary System ØTS
　Pancreatic tissue *see* Reposition, Pancreas ØFSG
　Parathyroid tissue *see* Reposition, Endocrine Sys-
　　tem ØGS
　Thyroid tissue *see* Reposition, Endocrine System
　　ØGS
　Tooth *see* Reattachment, Mouth and Throat ØCM
Avulsion *see* Extraction
AVYCAZ® (ceftazidime-avibactam) *use* Other Anti-
　infective
Axial Lumbar Interbody Fusion System *use* Inter-
　body Fusion Device in Lower Joints
AxiaLIF® System *use* Interbody Fusion Device in Lower
　Joints
Axicabtagene Ciloleucel *use* Axicabtagene Ciloleucel
　Immunotherapy
Axicabtagene Ciloleucel Immunotherapy XWØ
Axillary fascia
　use Subcutaneous Tissue and Fascia, Left Upper
　　Arm
　use Subcutaneous Tissue and Fascia, Right Upper
　　Arm
Axillary nerve *use* Brachial Plexus
AZEDRA® *use* Iobenguane I-131 Antineoplastic

B

BAK/C® Interbody Cervical Fusion System *use* Inter-
　body Fusion Device in Upper Joints
BAL (bronchial alveolar lavage), diagnostic *see*
　Drainage, Respiratory System ØB9
Balanoplasty
　see Repair, Penis ØVQS
　see Supplement, Penis ØVUS
Balloon atrial septostomy (BAS) Ø2163Z7
Balloon Pump
　Continuous, Output 5AØ221Ø
　Intermittent, Output 5AØ211Ø
Bamlanivimab Monoclonal Antibody XWØ
Bandage, Elastic *see* Compression
Banding
　see Occlusion
　see Restriction
Banding, esophageal varices *see* Occlusion, Vein,
　Esophageal Ø6L3
Banding, laparoscopic (adjustable) gastric
　Initial procedure ØDV64CZ
　Surgical correction *see* Revision of device in,
　　Stomach ØDW6

Bard® Composix® Kugel® patch *use* Synthetic Substitute

Bard® Composix® (E/X) (LP) mesh *use* Synthetic Substitute

Bard® Dulex™ mesh *use* Synthetic Substitute

Bard® Ventralex™ hernia patch *use* Synthetic Substitute

Baricitinib XW0

Barium swallow *see* Fluoroscopy, Gastrointestinal System BD1

Baroreflex Activation Therapy® (BAT®)
 use Stimulator Generator in Subcutaneous Tissue and Fascia
 use Stimulator Lead in Upper Arteries

Barricaid® Annular Closure Device (ACD) *use* Synthetic Substitute

Bartholin's (greater vestibular) gland *use* Vestibular Gland

Basal (internal) cerebral vein *use* Intracranial Vein

Basal metabolic rate (BMR) *see* Measurement, Physiological Systems 4A0Z

Basal nuclei *use* Basal Ganglia

Base of Tongue *use* Pharynx

Basilar artery *use* Intracranial Artery

Basis pontis *use* Pons

Beam Radiation
 Abdomen DW03
  Intraoperative DW033Z0
 Adrenal Gland DG02
  Intraoperative DG023Z0
 Bile Ducts DF02
  Intraoperative DF023Z0
 Bladder DT02
  Intraoperative DT023Z0
 Bone
  Intraoperative DP0C3Z0
  Other DP0C
 Bone Marrow D700
  Intraoperative D7003Z0
 Brain D000
  Intraoperative D0003Z0
 Brain Stem D001
  Intraoperative D0013Z0
 Breast
  Left DM00
   Intraoperative DM003Z0
  Right DM01
   Intraoperative DM013Z0
 Bronchus DB01
  Intraoperative DB013Z0
 Cervix DU01
  Intraoperative DU013Z0
 Chest DW02
  Intraoperative DW023Z0
 Chest Wall DB07
  Intraoperative DB073Z0
 Colon DD05
  Intraoperative DD053Z0
 Diaphragm DB08
  Intraoperative DB083Z0
 Duodenum DD02
  Intraoperative DD023Z0
 Ear D900
  Intraoperative D9003Z0
 Esophagus DD00
  Intraoperative DD003Z0
 Eye D800
  Intraoperative D8003Z0
 Femur DP09
  Intraoperative DP093Z0
 Fibula DP0B
  Intraoperative DP0B3Z0
 Gallbladder DF01
  Intraoperative DF013Z0
 Gland
  Adrenal DG02
   Intraoperative DG023Z0
  Parathyroid DG04
   Intraoperative DG043Z0
  Pituitary DG00
   Intraoperative DG003Z0
  Thyroid DG05
   Intraoperative DG053Z0
 Glands
  Intraoperative D9063Z0
  Salivary D906
 Head and Neck DW01
  Intraoperative DW013Z0

Beam Radiation — *continued*
 Hemibody DW04
  Intraoperative DW043Z0
 Humerus DP06
  Intraoperative DP063Z0
 Hypopharynx D903
  Intraoperative D9033Z0
 Ileum DD04
  Intraoperative DD043Z0
 Jejunum DD03
  Intraoperative DD033Z0
 Kidney DT00
  Intraoperative DT003Z0
 Larynx D90B
  Intraoperative D90B3Z0
 Liver DF00
  Intraoperative DF003Z0
 Lung DB02
  Intraoperative DB023Z0
 Lymphatics
  Abdomen D706
   Intraoperative D7063Z0
  Axillary D704
   Intraoperative D7043Z0
  Inguinal D708
   Intraoperative D7083Z0
  Neck D703
   Intraoperative D7033Z0
  Pelvis D707
   Intraoperative D7073Z0
  Thorax D705
   Intraoperative D7053Z0
 Mandible DP03
  Intraoperative DP033Z0
 Maxilla DP02
  Intraoperative DP023Z0
 Mediastinum DB06
  Intraoperative DB063Z0
 Mouth D904
  Intraoperative D9043Z0
 Nasopharynx D90D
  Intraoperative D90D3Z0
 Neck and Head DW01
  Intraoperative DW013Z0
 Nerve
  Intraoperative D0073Z0
  Peripheral D007
 Nose D901
  Intraoperative D9013Z0
 Oropharynx D90F
  Intraoperative D90F3Z0
 Ovary DU00
  Intraoperative DU003Z0
 Palate
  Hard D908
   Intraoperative D9083Z0
  Soft D909
   Intraoperative D9093Z0
 Pancreas DF03
  Intraoperative DF033Z0
 Parathyroid Gland DG04
  Intraoperative DG043Z0
 Pelvic Bones DP08
  Intraoperative DP083Z0
 Pelvic Region DW06
  Intraoperative DW063Z0
 Pineal Body DG01
  Intraoperative DG013Z0
 Pituitary Gland DG00
  Intraoperative DG003Z0
 Pleura DB05
  Intraoperative DB053Z0
 Prostate DV00
  Intraoperative DV003Z0
 Radius DP07
  Intraoperative DP073Z0
 Rectum DD07
  Intraoperative DD073Z0
 Rib DP05
  Intraoperative DP053Z0
 Sinuses D907
  Intraoperative D9073Z0
 Skin
  Abdomen DH08
   Intraoperative DH083Z0
  Arm DH04
   Intraoperative DH043Z0
  Back DH07
   Intraoperative DH073Z0

Beam Radiation — *continued*
 Skin — *continued*
  Buttock DH09
   Intraoperative DH093Z0
  Chest DH06
   Intraoperative DH063Z0
  Face DH02
   Intraoperative DH023Z0
  Leg DH0B
   Intraoperative DH0B3Z0
  Neck DH03
   Intraoperative DH033Z0
 Skull DP00
  Intraoperative DP003Z0
 Spinal Cord D006
  Intraoperative D0063Z0
 Spleen D702
  Intraoperative D7023Z0
 Sternum DP04
  Intraoperative DP043Z0
 Stomach DD01
  Intraoperative DD013Z0
 Testis DV01
  Intraoperative DV013Z0
 Thymus D701
  Intraoperative D7013Z0
 Thyroid Gland DG05
  Intraoperative DG053Z0
 Tibia DP0B
  Intraoperative DP0B3Z0
 Tongue D905
  Intraoperative D9053Z0
 Trachea DB00
  Intraoperative DB003Z0
 Ulna DP07
  Intraoperative DP073Z0
 Ureter DT01
  Intraoperative DT013Z0
 Urethra DT03
  Intraoperative DT033Z0
 Uterus DU02
  Intraoperative DU023Z0
 Whole Body DW05
  Intraoperative DW053Z0

Bedside swallow F00ZJWZ

Berlin Heart Ventricular Assist Device *use* Implantable Heart Assist System in Heart and Great Vessels

Betibeglogene Autotemcel XW1

beti-cel *use* Betibeglogene Autotemcel

Bezlotoxumab infusion *see* Introduction with qualifier Other Therapeutic Monoclonal Antibody

Biceps brachii muscle
 use Upper Arm Muscle, Left
 use Upper Arm Muscle, Right

Biceps femoris muscle
 use Upper Leg Muscle, Left
 use Upper Leg Muscle, Right

Bicipital aponeurosis
 use Subcutaneous Tissue and Fascia, Left Lower Arm
 use Subcutaneous Tissue and Fascia, Right Lower Arm

Bicuspid valve *use* Mitral Valve

Bili light therapy *see* Phototherapy, Skin 6A60

Bioactive embolization coil(s) *use* Intraluminal Device, Bioactive in Upper Arteries

Bioengineered Allogeneic Construct, Skin XHRPXF7

Biofeedback GZC9ZZZ

BioFire® FilmArray® Pneumonia Panel XXEBXQ6

Biopsy
 see Drainage with qualifier Diagnostic
 see Excision with qualifier Diagnostic
 see Extraction with qualifier Diagnostic

BiPAP *see* Assistance, Respiratory 5A09

Bisection *see* Division

Biventricular external heart assist system *use* Short-term External Heart Assist System in Heart and Great Vessels

Blepharectomy
 see Excision, Eye 08B
 see Resection, Eye 08T

Blepharoplasty
 see Repair, Eye 08Q
 see Replacement, Eye 08R
 see Reposition, Eye 08S
 see Supplement, Eye 08U

Blepharorrhaphy *see* Repair, Eye 08Q

Blepharotomy see Drainage, Eye Ø89
Blinatumomab use Other Antineoplastic
BLINCYTO®(blinatumomab) use Other Antineoplastic
Block, Nerve, anesthetic injection 3EØT3BZ
Blood glucose monitoring system use Monitoring
   Device
Blood pressure see Measurement, Arterial 4AØ3
BMR (basal metabolic rate) see Measurement, Physi-
   ological Systems 4AØZ
Body of femur
   use Femoral Shaft, Left
   use Femoral Shaft, Right
Body of fibula
   use Fibula, Left
   use Fibula, Right
Bone anchored hearing device
   use Hearing Device, Bone Conduction in Ø9H
   use Hearing Device in Head and Facial Bones
Bone bank bone graft use Nonautologous Tissue
   Substitute
Bone Growth Stimulator
   Insertion of device in
      Bone
         Facial ØNHW
         Lower ØQHY
         Nasal ØNHB
         Upper ØPHY
         Skull ØNHØ
   Removal of device from
      Bone
         Facial ØNPW
         Lower ØQPY
         Nasal ØNPB
         Upper ØPPY
         Skull ØNPØ
   Revision of device in
      Bone
         Facial ØNWW
         Lower ØQWY
         Nasal ØNWB
         Upper ØPWY
         Skull ØNWØ
Bone marrow transplant see Transfusion, Circulatory
   3Ø2
Bone morphogenetic protein 2 (BMP 2) use Recombinant Bone Morphogenetic Protein
Bone screw (interlocking) (lag) (pedicle) (recessed)
   use Internal Fixation Device in Head and Facial
      Bones
   use Internal Fixation Device in Lower Bones
   use Internal Fixation Device in Upper Bones
Bony labyrinth
   use Inner Ear, Left
   use Inner Ear, Right
Bony orbit
   use Orbit, Left
   use Orbit, Right
Bony vestibule
   use Inner Ear, Left
   use Inner Ear, Right
Botallo's duct use Pulmonary Artery, Left
Bovine pericardial valve use Zooplastic Tissue in Heart
   and Great Vessels
Bovine pericardium graft use Zooplastic Tissue in
   Heart and Great Vessels
BP (blood pressure) see Measurement, Arterial 4AØ3
Brachial (lateral) lymph node
   use Lymphatic, Left Axillary
   use Lymphatic, Right Axillary
Brachialis muscle
   use Upper Arm Muscle, Left
   use Upper Arm Muscle, Right
Brachiocephalic artery use Innominate Artery
Brachiocephalic trunk use Innominate Artery
Brachiocephalic vein
   use Innominate Vein, Left
   use Innominate Vein, Right
Brachioradialis muscle
   use Lower Arm and Wrist Muscle, Left
   use Lower Arm and Wrist Muscle, Right
Brachytherapy
   Abdomen DW13
   Adrenal Gland DG12
   Back
      Lower DW1LBB
      Upper DW1KBB
   Bile Ducts DF12

Brachytherapy — continued
   Bladder DT12
   Bone Marrow D71Ø
   Brain DØ1Ø
   Brain Stem DØ11
   Breast
      Left DM1Ø
      Right DM11
   Bronchus DB11
   Cervix DU11
   Chest DW12
   Chest Wall DB17
   Colon DD15
   Cranial Cavity DW1ØBB
   Diaphragm DB18
   Duodenum DD12
   Ear D91Ø
   Esophagus DD1Ø
   Extremity
      Lower DW1YBB
      Upper DW1XBB
   Eye D81Ø
   Gallbladder DF11
   Gastrointestinal Tract DW1PBB
   Genitourinary Tract DW1RBB
   Gland
      Adrenal DG12
      Parathyroid DG14
      Pituitary DG1Ø
      Thyroid DG15
   Glands, Salivary D916
   Head and Neck DW11
   Hypopharynx D913
   Ileum DD14
   Jejunum DD13
   Kidney DT1Ø
   Larynx D91B
   Liver DF1Ø
   Lung DB12
   Lymphatics
      Abdomen D716
      Axillary D714
      Inguinal D718
      Neck D713
      Pelvis D717
      Thorax D715
   Mediastinum DB16
   Mouth D914
   Nasopharynx D91D
   Neck and Head DW11
   Nerve, Peripheral DØ17
   Nose D911
   Oropharynx D91F
   Ovary DU1Ø
   Palate
      Hard D918
      Soft D919
   Pancreas DF13
   Parathyroid Gland DG14
   Pelvic Region DW16
   Pineal Body DG11
   Pituitary Gland DG1Ø
   Pleura DB15
   Prostate DV1Ø
   Rectum DD17
   Respiratory Tract DW1QBB
   Sinuses D917
   Spinal Cord DØ16
   Spleen D712
   Stomach DD11
   Testis DV11
   Thymus D711
   Thyroid Gland DG15
   Tongue D915
   Trachea DB1Ø
   Ureter DT11
   Urethra DT13
   Uterus DU12
Brachytherapy, CivaSheet®
   see Brachytherapy with qualifier Unidirectional
      Source
   see Insertion with device Radioactive Element
Brachytherapy seeds use Radioactive Element
**Brain Electrical Activity, Computer-aided Semio-
   logic Analysis** XXEØX48
Breast procedures, skin only use Skin, Chest
Brexanolone XWØ

Brexucabtagene Autoleucel use Brexucabtagene
   Autoleucel Immunotherapy
Brexucabtagene Autoleucel Immunotherapy XWØ
Breyanzi® use Lisocabtagene Maraleucel Immunother-
   apy
**Broad Consortium Microbiota-based Live Biother-
   apeutic Suspension** XWØH7X8
Broad ligament use Uterine Supporting Structure
Bromelain-enriched Proteolytic Enzyme XWØ
Bronchial artery use Upper Artery
Bronchography
   see Fluoroscopy, Respiratory System BB1
   see Plain Radiography, Respiratory System BBØ
Bronchoplasty
   see Repair, Respiratory System ØBQ
   see Supplement, Respiratory System ØBU
Bronchorrhaphy see Repair, Respiratory System ØBQ
Bronchoscopy ØBJØ8ZZ
Bronchotomy see Drainage, Respiratory System ØB9
Bronchus Intermedius use Main Bronchus, Right
BRYAN® Cervical Disc System use Synthetic Substitute
Buccal gland use Buccal Mucosa
Buccinator lymph node use Lymphatic, Head
Buccinator muscle use Facial Muscle
Buckling, scleral with implant see Supplement, Eye
   Ø8U
Bulbospongiosus muscle use Perineum Muscle
Bulbourethral (Cowper's) gland use Urethra
Bundle of His use Conduction Mechanism
Bundle of Kent use Conduction Mechanism
Bunionectomy see Excision, Lower Bones ØQB
Bursectomy
   see Excision, Bursae and Ligaments ØMB
   see Resection, Bursae and Ligaments ØMT
Bursocentesis see Drainage, Bursae and Ligaments
   ØM9
Bursography
   see Plain Radiography, Non-Axial Lower Bones BQØ
   see Plain Radiography, Non-Axial Upper Bones BPØ
Bursotomy
   see Division, Bursae and Ligaments ØM8
   see Drainage, Bursae and Ligaments ØM9
BVS 5ØØØ Ventricular Assist Device use Short-term
   External Heart Assist System in Heart and Great
   Vessels
Bypass
   Anterior Chamber
      Left Ø8133
      Right Ø8123
   Aorta
      Abdominal Ø41Ø
      Thoracic
         Ascending/Arch Ø21X
         Descending Ø21W
   Artery
      Anterior Tibial
         Left Ø41Q
         Right Ø41P
      Axillary
         Left Ø316Ø
         Right Ø315Ø
      Brachial
         Left Ø318
         Right Ø317
      Common Carotid
         Left Ø31JØ
         Right Ø31HØ
      Common Iliac
         Left Ø41D
         Right Ø41C
      Coronary
         Four or More Arteries Ø213
         One Artery Ø21Ø
         Three Arteries Ø212
         Two Arteries Ø211
      External Carotid
         Left Ø31NØ
         Right Ø31MØ
      External Iliac
         Left Ø41J
         Right Ø41H
      Femoral
         Left Ø41L
         Right Ø41K
      Foot
         Left Ø41W
         Right Ø41V

Cardiolysis

Bypass

Bypass — *continued*
- Artery — *continued*
  - Hepatic 0413
  - Innominate 03120
  - Internal Carotid
    - Left 031L0
    - Right 031K0
  - Internal Iliac
    - Left 041F
    - Right 041E
  - Intracranial 031G0
  - Peroneal
    - Left 041U
    - Right 041T
  - Popliteal
    - Left 041N
    - Right 041M
  - Posterior Tibial
    - Left 041S
    - Right 041R
  - Pulmonary
    - Left 021R
    - Right 021Q
  - Pulmonary Trunk 021P
  - Radial
    - Left 031C
    - Right 031B
  - Splenic 0414
  - Subclavian
    - Left 03140
    - Right 03130
  - Temporal
    - Left 031T0
    - Right 031S0
  - Ulnar
    - Left 031A
    - Right 0319
- Atrium
  - Left 0217
  - Right 0216
- Bladder 0T1B
- Cavity, Cranial 0W110J
- Cecum 0D1H
- Cerebral Ventricle 0016
- Colon
  - Ascending 0D1K
  - Descending 0D1M
  - Sigmoid 0D1N
  - Transverse 0D1L
- Duct
  - Common Bile 0F19
  - Cystic 0F18
  - Hepatic
    - Common 0F17
    - Left 0F16
    - Right 0F15
  - Lacrimal
    - Left 081Y
    - Right 081X
  - Pancreatic 0F1D
    - Accessory 0F1F
- Duodenum 0D19
- Ear
  - Left 091E0
  - Right 091D0
- Esophagus 0D15
  - Lower 0D13
  - Middle 0D12
  - Upper 0D11
- Fallopian Tube
  - Left 0U16
  - Right 0U15
- Gallbladder 0F14
- Ileum 0D1B
- Intestine
  - Large 0D1E
  - Small 0D18
- Jejunum 0D1A
- Kidney Pelvis
  - Left 0T14
  - Right 0T13
- Pancreas 0F1G
- Pelvic Cavity 0W1J
- Peritoneal Cavity 0W1G
- Pleural Cavity
  - Left 0W1B
  - Right 0W19
- Spinal Canal 001U
- Stomach 0D16

Bypass — *continued*
- Trachea 0B11
- Ureter
  - Left 0T17
  - Right 0T16
- Ureters, Bilateral 0T18
- Vas Deferens
  - Bilateral 0V1Q
  - Left 0V1P
  - Right 0V1N
- Vein
  - Axillary
    - Left 0518
    - Right 0517
  - Azygos 0510
  - Basilic
    - Left 051C
    - Right 051B
  - Brachial
    - Left 051A
    - Right 0519
  - Cephalic
    - Left 051F
    - Right 051D
  - Colic 0617
  - Common Iliac
    - Left 061D
    - Right 061C
  - Esophageal 0613
  - External Iliac
    - Left 061G
    - Right 061F
  - External Jugular
    - Left 051Q
    - Right 051P
  - Face
    - Left 051V
    - Right 051T
  - Femoral
    - Left 061N
    - Right 061M
  - Foot
    - Left 061V
    - Right 061T
  - Gastric 0612
  - Hand
    - Left 051H
    - Right 051G
  - Hemiazygos 0511
  - Hepatic 0614
  - Hypogastric
    - Left 061J
    - Right 061H
  - Inferior Mesenteric 0616
  - Innominate
    - Left 0514
    - Right 0513
  - Internal Jugular
    - Left 051N
    - Right 051M
  - Intracranial 051L
  - Portal 0618
  - Renal
    - Left 061B
    - Right 0619
  - Saphenous
    - Left 061Q
    - Right 061P
  - Splenic 0611
  - Subclavian
    - Left 0516
    - Right 0515
  - Superior Mesenteric 0615
  - Vertebral
    - Left 051S
    - Right 051R
- Vena Cava
  - Inferior 0610
  - Superior 021V
- Ventricle
  - Left 021L
  - Right 021K

Bypass, cardiopulmonary 5A1221Z

C

Caesarean section *see* Extraction, Products of Conception 10D0

Calcaneocuboid joint
- *use* Tarsal Joint, Left
- *use* Tarsal Joint, Right

Calcaneocuboid ligament
- *use* Foot Bursa and Ligament, Left
- *use* Foot Bursa and Ligament, Right

Calcaneofibular ligament
- *use* Ankle Bursa and Ligament, Left
- *use* Ankle Bursa and Ligament, Right

Calcaneus
- *use* Tarsal, Left
- *use* Tarsal, Right

Cannulation
- *see* Bypass
- *see* Dilation
- *see* Drainage
- *see* Irrigation

Canthorrhaphy *see* Repair, Eye 08Q
Canthotomy *see* Release, Eye 08N
Capitate bone
- *use* Carpal, Left
- *use* Carpal, Right

Caplacizumab XW0
Capsulectomy, lens *see* Excision, Eye 08B
Capsulorrhaphy, joint
- *see* Repair, Lower Joints 0SQ
- *see* Repair, Upper Joints 0RQ

Caption Guidance system X2JAX47
Cardia *use* Esophagogastric Junction
Cardiac contractility modulation lead *use* Cardiac Lead in Heart and Great Vessels
Cardiac event recorder *use* Monitoring Device
Cardiac Lead
- Defibrillator
  - Atrium
    - Left 02H7
    - Right 02H6
  - Pericardium 02HN
  - Vein, Coronary 02H4
  - Ventricle
    - Left 02HL
    - Right 02HK
- Insertion of device in
  - Atrium
    - Left 02H7
    - Right 02H6
  - Pericardium 02HN
  - Vein, Coronary 02H4
  - Ventricle
    - Left 02HL
    - Right 02HK
- Pacemaker
  - Atrium
    - Left 02H7
    - Right 02H6
  - Pericardium 02HN
  - Vein, Coronary 02H4
  - Ventricle
    - Left 02HL
    - Right 02HK
- Removal of device from, Heart 02PA
- Revision of device in, Heart 02WA

Cardiac plexus *use* Thoracic Sympathetic Nerve
Cardiac Resynchronization Defibrillator Pulse Generator
- Abdomen 0JH8
- Chest 0JH6

Cardiac Resynchronization Pacemaker Pulse Generator
- Abdomen 0JH8
- Chest 0JH6

Cardiac resynchronization therapy (CRT) lead
- *use* Cardiac Lead, Defibrillator in 02H
- *use* Cardiac Lead, Pacemaker in 02H

Cardiac Rhythm Related Device
- Insertion of device in
  - Abdomen 0JH8
  - Chest 0JH6
- Removal of device from, Subcutaneous Tissue and Fascia, Trunk 0JPT
- Revision of device in, Subcutaneous Tissue and Fascia, Trunk 0JWT

Cardiocentesis *see* Drainage, Pericardial Cavity 0W9D
Cardioesophageal junction *use* Esophagogastric Junction
Cardiolysis *see* Release, Heart and Great Vessels 02N

CardioMEMS® pressure sensor *use* Monitoring Device, Pressure Sensor in 02H
Cardiomyotomy *see* Division, Esophagogastric Junction 0D84
Cardioplegia *see* Introduction of substance in or on, Heart 3E08
Cardiorrhaphy *see* Repair, Heart and Great Vessels 02Q
Cardioversion 5A2204Z
Caregiver Training F0FZ
Carmat total artificial heart (TAH) *use* Biologic with Synthetic Substitute, Autoregulated Electrohydraulic in 02R
Caroticotympanic artery
  use Internal Carotid Artery, Left
  use Internal Carotid Artery, Right
Carotid glomus
  use Carotid Bodies, Bilateral
  use Carotid Body, Left
  use Carotid Body, Right
Carotid sinus
  use Internal Carotid Artery, Left
  use Internal Carotid Artery, Right
Carotid (artery) sinus (baroreceptor) lead *use* Stimulator Lead in Upper Arteries
Carotid sinus nerve *use* Glossopharyngeal Nerve
Carotid WALLSTENT® Monorail® Endoprosthesis *use* Intraluminal Device
Carpectomy
  see Excision, Upper Bones 0PB
  see Resection, Upper Bones 0PT
Carpometacarpal ligament
  use Hand Bursa and Ligament, Left
  use Hand Bursa and Ligament, Right
CARVYKTI™ *use* Ciltacabtagene Autoleucel
Casirivimab (REGN10933) and Imdevimab (REGN10987) *use* REGN-COV2 Monoclonal Antibody
Casting *see* Immobilization
CAT scan *see* Computerized Tomography (CT Scan)
Catheterization
  see Dilation
  see Drainage
  see Insertion of device in
  see Irrigation
  Heart *see* Measurement, Cardiac 4A02
  Umbilical vein, for infusion 06H033T
Cauda equina *use* Lumbar Spinal Cord
Cauterization
  see Destruction
  see Repair
Cavernous plexus *use* Head and Neck Sympathetic Nerve
Cavoatrial junction *use* Superior Vena Cava
CBMA (Concentrated Bone Marrow Aspirate) *use* Other Substance
CBMA (Concentrated Bone Marrow Aspirate) injection *see* Introduction of substance in or on, Muscle 3E02
CD24Fc Immunomodulator XW0
Cecectomy
  see Excision, Cecum 0DBH
  see Resection, Cecum 0DTH
Cecocolostomy
  see Bypass, Gastrointestinal System 0D1
  see Drainage, Gastrointestinal System 0D9
Cecopexy
  see Repair, Cecum 0DQH
  see Reposition, Cecum 0DSH
Cecoplication *see* Restriction, Cecum 0DVH
Cecorrhaphy *see* Repair, Cecum 0DQH
Cecostomy
  see Bypass, Cecum 0D1H
  see Drainage, Cecum 0D9H
Cecotomy *see* Drainage, Cecum 0D9H
Cefiderocol Anti-infective XW0
Ceftazidime-avibactam *use* Other Anti-infective
Ceftolozane/Tazobactam Anti-infective XW0
Celiac ganglion *use* Abdominal Sympathetic Nerve
Celiac lymph node *use* Lymphatic, Aortic
Celiac (solar) plexus *use* Abdominal Sympathetic Nerve
Celiac trunk *use* Celiac Artery
Central axillary lymph node
  use Lymphatic, Left Axillary
  use Lymphatic, Right Axillary

Central venous pressure *see* Measurement, Venous 4A04
Centrimag® Blood Pump *use* Short-term External Heart Assist System in Heart and Great Vessels
Cephalogram BN00ZZZ
CERAMENT® G *use* Antibiotic-eluting Bone Void Filler
Ceramic on ceramic bearing surface *use* Synthetic Substitute, Ceramic in 0SR
Cerclage *see* Restriction
Cerebral aqueduct (Sylvius) *use* Cerebral Ventricle
Cerebral Embolic Filtration
  Dual Filter X2A5312
  Extracorporeal Flow Reversal Circuit X2A
  Single Deflection Filter X2A6325
Cerebrum *use* Brain
Cervical esophagus *use* Esophagus, Upper
Cervical facet joint
  use Cervical Vertebral Joint
  use Cervical Vertebral Joint, 2 or more
Cervical ganglion *use* Head and Neck Sympathetic Nerve
Cervical interspinous ligament *use* Head and Neck Bursa and Ligament
Cervical intertransverse ligament *use* Head and Neck Bursa and Ligament
Cervical Ligamentum Flavum *use* Head and Neck Bursa and Ligament
Cervical Lymph Node
  use Lymphatic, Left Neck
  use Lymphatic, Right Neck
Cervicectomy
  see Excision, Cervix 0UBC
  see Resection, Cervix 0UTC
Cervicothoracic facet joint *use* Cervicothoracic Vertebral Joint
Cesarean section *see* Extraction, Products of Conception 10D0
Cesium-131 Collagen Implant *use* Radioactive Element, Cesium-131 Collagen Implant in 00H
Change Device in
  Abdominal Wall 0W2FX
  Back
    Lower 0W2LX
    Upper 0W2KX
  Bladder 0T2BX
  Bone
    Facial 0N2WX
    Lower 0Q2YX
    Nasal 0N2BX
    Upper 0P2YX
  Bone Marrow 072TX
  Brain 0020X
  Breast
    Left 0H2UX
    Right 0H2TX
  Bursa and Ligament
    Lower 0M2YX
    Upper 0M2XX
  Cavity, Cranial 0W21X
  Chest Wall 0W28X
  Cisterna Chyli 072LX
  Diaphragm 0B2TX
  Duct
    Hepatobiliary 0F2BX
    Pancreatic 0F2DX
  Ear
    Left 092JX
    Right 092HX
  Epididymis and Spermatic Cord 0V2MX
  Extremity
    Lower
      Left 0Y2BX
      Right 0Y29X
    Upper
      Left 0X27X
      Right 0X26X
  Eye
    Left 0821X
    Right 0820X
  Face 0W22X
  Fallopian Tube 0U28X
  Gallbladder 0F24X
  Gland
    Adrenal 0G25X
    Endocrine 0G2SX
    Pituitary 0G20X
    Salivary 0C2AX
  Head 0W20X

Change Device in — *continued*
  Intestinal Tract
    Lower Intestinal Tract 0D2DXUZ
    Upper Intestinal Tract 0D20XUZ
  Jaw
    Lower 0W25X
    Upper 0W24X
  Joint
    Lower 0S2YX
    Upper 0R2YX
  Kidney 0T25X
  Larynx 0C2SX
  Liver 0F20X
  Lung
    Left 0B2LX
    Right 0B2KX
  Lymphatic 072NX
    Thoracic Duct 072KX
  Mediastinum 0W2CX
  Mesentery 0D2VX
  Mouth and Throat 0C2YX
  Muscle
    Lower 0K2YX
    Upper 0K2XX
  Nasal Mucosa and Soft Tissue 092KX
  Neck 0W26X
  Nerve
    Cranial 002EX
    Peripheral 012YX
  Omentum 0D2UX
  Ovary 0U23X
  Pancreas 0F2GX
  Parathyroid Gland 0G2RX
  Pelvic Cavity 0W2JX
  Penis 0V2SX
  Pericardial Cavity 0W2DX
  Perineum
    Female 0W2NX
    Male 0W2MX
  Peritoneal Cavity 0W2GX
  Peritoneum 0D2WX
  Pineal Body 0G21X
  Pleura 0B2QX
  Pleural Cavity
    Left 0W2BX
    Right 0W29X
  Products of Conception 10207
  Prostate and Seminal Vesicles 0V24X
  Retroperitoneum 0W2HX
  Scrotum and Tunica Vaginalis 0V28X
  Sinus 092YX
  Skin 0H2PX
  Skull 0N20X
  Spinal Canal 002UX
  Spleen 072PX
  Subcutaneous Tissue and Fascia
    Head and Neck 0J2SX
    Lower Extremity 0J2WX
    Trunk 0J2TX
    Upper Extremity 0J2VX
  Tendon
    Lower 0L2YX
    Upper 0L2XX
  Testis 0V2DX
  Thymus 072MX
  Thyroid Gland 0G2KX
  Trachea 0B21
  Tracheobronchial Tree 0B20X
  Ureter 0T29X
  Urethra 0T2DX
  Uterus and Cervix 0U2DXHZ
  Vagina and Cul-de-sac 0U2HXGZ
  Vas Deferens 0V2RX
  Vulva 0U2MX
Change Device in or on
  Abdominal Wall 2W03X
  Anorectal 2Y03X5Z
  Arm
    Lower
      Left 2W0DX
      Right 2W0CX
    Upper
      Left 2W0BX
      Right 2W0AX
  Back 2W05X
  Chest Wall 2W04X
  Ear 2Y02X5Z

Change Device in or on — *continued*
Extremity
  Lower
    Left 2W0MX
    Right 2W0LX
  Upper
    Left 2W09X
    Right 2W08X
Face 2W01X
Finger
  Left 2W0KX
  Right 2W0JX
Foot
  Left 2W0TX
  Right 2W0SX
Genital Tract, Female 2Y04X5Z
Hand
  Left 2W0FX
  Right 2W0EX
Head 2W00X
Inguinal Region
  Left 2W07X
  Right 2W06X
Leg
  Lower
    Left 2W0RX
    Right 2W0QX
  Upper
    Left 2W0PX
    Right 2W0NX
Mouth and Pharynx 2Y00X5Z
Nasal 2Y01X5Z
Neck 2W02X
Thumb
  Left 2W0HX
  Right 2W0GX
Toe
  Left 2W0VX
  Right 2W0UX
Urethra 2Y05X5Z
Chemoembolization *see* Introduction of substance in or on
Chemosurgery, Skin 3E00XTZ
Chemothalamectomy *see* Destruction, Thalamus 0059
Chemotherapy, Infusion for Cancer *see* Introduction of substance in or on
Chest compression (CPR), external
  Manual 5A12012
  Mechanical 5A1221J
Chest x-ray *see* Plain Radiography, Chest BW03
Chiropractic Manipulation
  Abdomen 9WB9X
  Cervical 9WB1X
  Extremities
    Lower 9WB6X
    Upper 9WB7X
  Head 9WB0X
  Lumbar 9WB3X
  Pelvis 9WB5X
  Rib Cage 9WB8X
  Sacrum 9WB4X
  Thoracic 9WB2X
Choana *use* Nasopharynx
Cholangiogram
  see Fluoroscopy, Hepatobiliary System and Pancreas BF1
  see Plain Radiography, Hepatobiliary System and Pancreas BF0
Cholecystectomy
  see Excision, Gallbladder 0FB4
  see Resection, Gallbladder 0FT4
Cholecystojejunostomy
  see Bypass, Hepatobiliary System and Pancreas 0F1
  see Drainage, Hepatobiliary System and Pancreas 0F9
Cholecystopexy
  see Repair, Gallbladder 0FQ4
  see Reposition, Gallbladder 0FS4
Cholecystoscopy 0FJ44ZZ
Cholecystostomy
  see Bypass, Gallbladder 0F14
  see Drainage, Gallbladder 0F94
Cholecystotomy *see* Drainage, Gallbladder 0F94
Choledochectomy
  see Excision, Hepatobiliary System and Pancreas 0FB

Choledochectomy — *continued*
  see Resection, Hepatobiliary System and Pancreas 0FT
Choledocholithotomy *see* Extirpation, Duct, Common Bile 0FC9
Choledochoplasty
  see Repair, Hepatobiliary System and Pancreas 0FQ
  see Replacement, Hepatobiliary System and Pancreas 0FR
  see Supplement, Hepatobiliary System and Pancreas 0FU
Choledochoscopy 0FJB8ZZ
Choledochotomy *see* Drainage, Hepatobiliary System and Pancreas 0F9
Cholelithotomy *see* Extirpation, Hepatobiliary System and Pancreas 0FC
Chondrectomy
  see Excision, Lower Joints 0SB
  see Excision, Upper Joints 0RB
  Knee *see* Excision, Lower Joints 0SB
  Semilunar cartilage *see* Excision, Lower Joints 0SB
Chondroglossus muscle *use* Tongue, Palate, Pharynx Muscle
Chorda tympani *use* Facial Nerve
Chordotomy *see* Division, Central Nervous System and Cranial Nerves 008
Choroid plexus *use* Cerebral Ventricle
Choroidectomy
  see Excision, Eye 08B
  see Resection, Eye 08T
Ciliary body
  use Eye, Left
  use Eye, Right
Ciliary ganglion *use* Head and Neck Sympathetic Nerve
Ciltacabtagene Autoleucel XW0
cilta-cel *use* Ciltacabtagene Autoleucel
Circle of Willis *use* Intracranial Artery
Circumcision 0VTTXZZ
Circumflex iliac artery
  use Femoral Artery, Left
  use Femoral Artery, Right
CivaSheet® *use* Radioactive Element
CivaSheet® Brachytherapy
  see Brachytherapy with qualifier Unidirectional Source
  see Insertion with device Radioactive Element
Clamp and rod internal fixation system (CRIF)
  use Internal Fixation Device in Lower Bones
  use Internal Fixation Device in Upper Bones
Clamping *see* Occlusion
Claustrum *use* Basal Ganglia
Claviculectomy
  see Excision, Upper Bones 0PB
  see Resection, Upper Bones 0PT
Claviculotomy
  see Division, Upper Bones 0P8
  see Drainage, Upper Bones 0P9
Clipping, aneurysm
  see Occlusion using Extraluminal Device
  see Restriction using Extraluminal Device
Clitorectomy, clitoridectomy
  see Excision, Clitoris 0UBJ
  see Resection, Clitoris 0UTJ
Clolar *use* Clofarabine
Closure
  see Occlusion
  see Repair
Clysis *see* Introduction of substance in or on
Coagulation *see* Destruction
Coagulation Factor Xa, Inactivated XW0
Coagulation Factor Xa, (Recombinant) Inactivated *use* Coagulation Factor Xa, Inactivated
COALESCE® radiolucent interbody fusion device
  use Interbody Fusion Device in Lower Joints
  use Interbody Fusion Device in Upper Joints
CoAxia NeuroFlo catheter *use* Intraluminal Device
Cobalt/chromium head and polyethylene socket *use* Synthetic Substitute, Metal on Polyethylene in 0SR
Cobalt/chromium head and socket *use* Synthetic Substitute, Metal in 0SR
Coccygeal body *use* Coccygeal Glomus
Coccygeus muscle
  use Trunk Muscle, Left
  use Trunk Muscle, Right

Cochlea
  use Inner Ear, Left
  use Inner Ear, Right
Cochlear implant (CI), multiple channel (electrode)
  use Hearing Device, Multiple Channel Cochlear Prosthesis in 09H
Cochlear implant (CI), single channel (electrode)
  use Hearing Device, Single Channel Cochlear Prosthesis in 09H
Cochlear Implant Treatment F0BZ0
Cochlear nerve *use* Acoustic Nerve
COGNIS® CRT-D *use* Cardiac Resynchronization Defibrillator Pulse Generator in 0JH
COHERE® radiolucent interbody fusion device
  use Interbody Fusion Device in Lower Joints
  use Interbody Fusion Device in Upper Joints
Colectomy
  see Excision, Gastrointestinal System 0DB
  see Resection, Gastrointestinal System 0DT
Collapse *see* Occlusion
Collection from
  Breast, Breast Milk 8E0HX62
  Indwelling Device
    Circulatory System
      Blood 8C02X6K
      Other Fluid 8C02X6L
    Nervous System
      Cerebrospinal Fluid 8C01X6J
      Other Fluid 8C01X6L
  Integumentary System, Breast Milk 8E0HX62
  Reproductive System, Male, Sperm 8E0VX63
Colocentesis *see* Drainage, Gastrointestinal System 0D9
Colofixation
  see Repair, Gastrointestinal System 0DQ
  see Reposition, Gastrointestinal System 0DS
Cololysis *see* Release, Gastrointestinal System 0DN
Colonic Z-Stent® *use* Intraluminal Device
Colonoscopy 0DJD8ZZ
Colopexy
  see Repair, Gastrointestinal System 0DQ
  see Reposition, Gastrointestinal System 0DS
Coloplication *see* Restriction, Gastrointestinal System 0DV
Coloproctectomy
  see Excision, Gastrointestinal System 0DB
  see Resection, Gastrointestinal System 0DT
Coloproctostomy
  see Bypass, Gastrointestinal System 0D1
  see Drainage, Gastrointestinal System 0D9
Colopuncture *see* Drainage, Gastrointestinal System 0D9
Colorrhaphy *see* Repair, Gastrointestinal System 0DQ
Colostomy
  see Bypass, Gastrointestinal System 0D1
  see Drainage, Gastrointestinal System 0D9
Colpectomy
  see Excision, Vagina 0UBG
  see Resection, Vagina 0UTG
Colpocentesis *see* Drainage, Vagina 0U9G
Colpopexy
  see Repair, Vagina 0UQG
  see Reposition, Vagina 0USG
Colpoplasty
  see Repair, Vagina 0UQG
  see Supplement, Vagina 0UUG
Colporrhaphy *see* Repair, Vagina 0UQG
Colposcopy 0UJH8ZZ
Columella *use* Nasal Mucosa and Soft Tissue
Common digital vein
  use Foot Vein, Left
  use Foot Vein, Right
Common facial vein
  use Face Vein, Left
  use Face Vein, Right
Common fibular nerve *use* Peroneal Nerve
Common hepatic artery *use* Hepatic Artery
Common iliac (subaortic) lymph node *use* Lymphatic, Pelvis
Common interosseous artery
  use Ulnar Artery, Left
  use Ulnar Artery, Right
Common peroneal nerve *use* Peroneal Nerve
Complete (SE) stent *use* Intraluminal Device
Compression
  see Restriction
  Abdominal Wall 2W13X

Compression — continued

Arm
  Lower
    Left 2W1DX
    Right 2W1CX
  Upper
    Left 2W1BX
    Right 2W1AX
Back 2W15X
Chest Wall 2W14X
Extremity
  Lower
    Left 2W1MX
    Right 2W1LX
  Upper
    Left 2W19X
    Right 2W18X
Face 2W11X
Finger
  Left 2W1KX
  Right 2W1JX
Foot
  Left 2W1TX
  Right 2W1SX
Hand
  Left 2W1FX
  Right 2W1EX
Head 2W10X
Inguinal Region
  Left 2W17X
  Right 2W16X
Leg
  Lower
    Left 2W1RX
    Right 2W1QX
  Upper
    Left 2W1PX
    Right 2W1NX
Neck 2W12X
Thumb
  Left 2W1HX
  Right 2W1GX
Toe
  Left 2W1VX
  Right 2W1UX

Computer Assisted Procedure

Extremity
  Lower
    No Qualifier 8E0YXBZ
    With Computerized Tomography
      8E0YXBG
    With Fluoroscopy 8E0YXBF
    With Magnetic Resonance Imaging
      8E0YXBH
  Upper
    No Qualifier 8E0XXBZ
    With Computerized Tomography
      8E0XXBG
    With Fluoroscopy 8E0XXBF
    With Magnetic Resonance Imaging
      8E0XXBH
Head and Neck Region
  No Qualifier 8E09XBZ
  With Computerized Tomography 8E09XBG
  With Fluoroscopy 8E09XBF
  With Magnetic Resonance Imaging 8E09XBH
Trunk Region
  No Qualifier 8E0WXBZ
  With Computerized Tomography 8E0WXBG
  With Fluoroscopy 8E0WXBF
  With Magnetic Resonance Imaging 8E0WXBH

Computer-aided Assessment, Intracranial Vascular Activity XXE0X07
Computer-aided Guidance, Transthoracic Echocardiography X2JAX47
Computer-aided Mechanical Aspiration X2C
Computer-aided Triage and Notification, Pulmonary Artery Flow XXE3X27
Computer-aided Valve Modeling and Notification, Coronary Artery Flow XXE3X68
Computer-assisted Intermittent Aspiration see New Technology, Cardiovascular System X2C
Computer-assisted Transcranial Magnetic Stimulation X0Z0X18
Computerized Tomography (CT Scan)
  Abdomen BW20
    Chest and Pelvis BW25
  Abdomen and Chest BW24

Computerized Tomography (CT Scan) — continued

Abdomen and Pelvis BW21
Airway, Trachea BB2F
Ankle
  Left BQ2H
  Right BQ2G
Aorta
  Abdominal B420
    Intravascular Optical Coherence
      B420Z2Z
  Thoracic B320
    Intravascular Optical Coherence
      B320Z2Z
Arm
  Left BP2F
  Right BP2E
Artery
  Celiac B421
    Intravascular Optical Coherence
      B421Z2Z
  Common Carotid
    Bilateral B325
    Intravascular Optical Coherence
      B325Z2Z
  Coronary
    Bypass Graft
      Intravascular Optical Coherence
        B223Z2Z
      Multiple B223
    Multiple B221
      Intravascular Optical Coherence
        B221Z2Z
  Internal Carotid
    Bilateral B328
    Intravascular Optical Coherence
      B328Z2Z
  Intracranial B32R
    Intravascular Optical Coherence
      B32RZ2Z
  Lower Extremity
    Bilateral B42H
      Intravascular Optical Coherence
        B42HZ2Z
    Left B42G
      Intravascular Optical Coherence
        B42GZ2Z
    Right B42F
      Intravascular Optical Coherence
        B42FZ2Z
  Pelvic B42C
    Intravascular Optical Coherence
      B42CZ2Z
  Pulmonary
    Left B32T
      Intravascular Optical Coherence
        B32TZ2Z
    Right B32S
      Intravascular Optical Coherence
        B32SZ2Z
  Renal
    Bilateral B428
      Intravascular Optical Coherence
        B428Z2Z
    Transplant B42M
      Intravascular Optical Coherence
        B42MZ2Z
  Superior Mesenteric B424
    Intravascular Optical Coherence
      B424Z2Z
  Vertebral
    Bilateral B32G
    Intravascular Optical Coherence
      B32GZ2Z
Bladder BT20
Bone
  Facial BN25
  Temporal BN2F
Brain B020
Calcaneus
  Left BQ2K
  Right BQ2J
Cerebral Ventricle B028
Chest, Abdomen and Pelvis BW25
Chest and Abdomen BW24
Cisterna B027
Clavicle
  Left BP25
  Right BP24
Coccyx BR2F

Computerized Tomography (CT Scan) — continued

Colon BD24
Ear B920
Elbow
  Left BP2H
  Right BP2G
Extremity
  Lower
    Left BQ2S
    Right BQ2R
  Upper
    Bilateral BP2V
    Left BP2U
    Right BP2T
Eye
  Bilateral B827
  Left B826
  Right B825
Femur
  Left BQ24
  Right BQ23
Fibula
  Left BQ2C
  Right BQ2B
Finger
  Left BP2S
  Right BP2R
Foot
  Left BQ2M
  Right BQ2L
Forearm
  Left BP2K
  Right BP2J
Gland
  Adrenal, Bilateral BG22
  Parathyroid BG23
  Parotid, Bilateral B926
  Salivary, Bilateral B92D
  Submandibular, Bilateral B929
  Thyroid BG24
Hand
  Left BP2P
  Right BP2N
Hands and Wrists, Bilateral BP2Q
Head BW28
Head and Neck BW29
Heart
  Intravascular Optical Coherence B226Z2Z
  Right and Left B226
Hepatobiliary System, All BF2C
Hip
  Left BQ21
  Right BQ20
Humerus
  Left BP2B
  Right BP2A
Intracranial Sinus B522
  Intravascular Optical Coherence B522Z2Z
Joint
  Acromioclavicular, Bilateral BP23
  Finger
    Left BP2DZZZ
    Right BP2CZZZ
  Foot
    Left BQ2Y
    Right BQ2X
  Hand
    Left BP2DZZZ
    Right BP2CZZZ
  Sacroiliac BR2D
  Sternoclavicular
    Bilateral BP22
    Left BP21
    Right BP20
  Temporomandibular, Bilateral BN29
  Toe
    Left BQ2Y
    Right BQ2X
Kidney
  Bilateral BT23
  Left BT22
  Right BT21
  Transplant BT29
Knee
  Left BQ28
  Right BQ27
Larynx B92J
Leg
  Left BQ2F

Computerized Tomography (CT Scan) — continued

Leg — *continued*
  Right BQ2D
Liver BF25
Liver and Spleen BF26
Lung, Bilateral BB24
Mandible BN26
Nasopharynx B92F
Neck BW2F
Neck and Head BW29
Orbit, Bilateral BN23
Oropharynx B92F
Pancreas BF27
Patella
  Left BQ2W
  Right BQ2V
Pelvic Region BW2G
Pelvis BR2C
  Chest and Abdomen BW25
Pelvis and Abdomen BW21
Pituitary Gland B029
Prostate BV23
Ribs
  Left BP2Y
  Right BP2X
Sacrum BR2F
Scapula
  Left BP27
  Right BP26
Sella Turcica B029
Shoulder
  Left BP29
  Right BP28
Sinus
  Intracranial B522
    Intravascular Optical Coherence B522Z2Z
  Paranasal B922
Skull BN20
Spinal Cord B02B
Spine
  Cervical BR20
  Lumbar BR29
  Thoracic BR27
Spleen and Liver BF26
Thorax BP2W
Tibia
  Left BQ2C
  Right BQ2B
Toe
  Left BQ2Q
  Right BQ2P
Trachea BB2F
Tracheobronchial Tree
  Bilateral BB29
  Left BB28
  Right BB27
Vein
  Pelvic (Iliac)
    Left B52G
      Intravascular Optical Coherence B52GZ2Z
    Right B52F
      Intravascular Optical Coherence B52FZ2Z
  Pelvic (Iliac) Bilateral B52H
    Intravascular Optical Coherence B52HZ2Z
  Portal B52T
    Intravascular Optical Coherence B52TZ2Z
  Pulmonary
    Bilateral B52S
      Intravascular Optical Coherence B52SZ2Z
    Left B52R
      Intravascular Optical Coherence B52RZ2Z
    Right B52Q
      Intravascular Optical Coherence B52QZ2Z
  Renal
    Bilateral B52L
      Intravascular Optical Coherence B52LZ2Z
    Left B52K
      Intravascular Optical Coherence B52KZ2Z
    Right B52J

Computerized Tomography (CT Scan) — continued

Vein — *continued*
  Renal — *continued*
    Right — *continued*
      Intravascular Optical Coherence B52JZ2Z
    Spanchnic B52T
      Intravascular Optical Coherence B52TZ2Z
  Vena Cava
    Inferior B529
      Intravascular Optical Coherence B529Z2Z
    Superior B528
      Intravascular Optical Coherence B528Z2Z
  Ventricle, Cerebral B028
  Wrist
    Left BP2M
    Right BP2L

Concerto II CRT-D *use* Cardiac Resynchronization Defibrillator Pulse Generator in 0JH
Condylectomy
  see Excision, Head and Facial Bones 0NB
  see Excision, Lower Bones 0QB
  see Excision, Upper Bones 0PB
Condyloid process
  use Mandible, Left
  use Mandible, Right
Condylotomy
  see Division, Head and Facial Bones 0N8
  see Division, Lower Bones 0Q8
  see Division, Upper Bones 0P8
  see Drainage, Head and Facial Bones 0N9
  see Drainage, Lower Bones 0Q9
  see Drainage, Upper Bones 0P9
Condylysis
  see Release, Head and Facial Bones 0NN
  see Release, Lower Bones 0QN
  see Release, Upper Bones 0PN
Conization, cervix *see* Excision, Cervix 0UBC
Conjunctivoplasty
  see Repair, Eye 08Q
  see Replacement, Eye 08R
CONSERVE® PLUS Total Resurfacing Hip System
  use Resurfacing Device in Lower Joints
Construction
  Auricle, ear *see* Replacement, Ear, Nose, Sinus 09R
  Ileal conduit *see* Bypass, Urinary System 0T1
Consulta CRT-D *use* Cardiac Resynchronization Defibrillator Pulse Generator in 0JH
Consulta CRT-P *use* Cardiac Resynchronization Pacemaker Pulse Generator in 0JH
Contact Radiation
  Abdomen DWY37ZZ
  Adrenal Gland DGY27ZZ
  Bile Ducts DFY27ZZ
  Bladder DTY27ZZ
  Bone, Other DPYC7ZZ
  Brain D0Y07ZZ
  Brain Stem D0Y17ZZ
  Breast
    Left DMY07ZZ
    Right DMY17ZZ
  Bronchus DBY17ZZ
  Cervix DUY07ZZ
  Chest DWY27ZZ
  Chest Wall DBY77ZZ
  Colon DDY57ZZ
  Diaphragm DBY87ZZ
  Duodenum DDY27ZZ
  Ear D9Y07ZZ
  Esophagus DDY07ZZ
  Eye D8Y07ZZ
  Femur DPY97ZZ
  Fibula DPYB7ZZ
  Gallbladder DFY17ZZ
  Gland
    Adrenal DGY27ZZ
    Parathyroid DGY47ZZ
    Pituitary DGY07ZZ
    Thyroid DGY57ZZ
  Glands, Salivary D9Y67ZZ
  Head and Neck DWY17ZZ
  Hemibody DWY47ZZ
  Humerus DPY67ZZ
  Hypopharynx D9Y37ZZ
  Ileum DDY47ZZ

Contact Radiation — continued

  Jejunum DDY37ZZ
  Kidney DTY07ZZ
  Larynx D9YB7ZZ
  Liver DFY07ZZ
  Lung DBY27ZZ
  Mandible DPY37ZZ
  Maxilla DPY27ZZ
  Mediastinum DBY67ZZ
  Mouth D9Y47ZZ
  Nasopharynx D9YD7ZZ
  Neck and Head DWY17ZZ
  Nerve, Peripheral D0Y77ZZ
  Nose D9Y17ZZ
  Oropharynx D9YF7ZZ
  Ovary DUY07ZZ
  Palate
    Hard D9Y87ZZ
    Soft D9Y97ZZ
  Pancreas DFY37ZZ
  Parathyroid Gland DGY47ZZ
  Pelvic Bones DPY87ZZ
  Pelvic Region DWY67ZZ
  Pineal Body DGY17ZZ
  Pituitary Gland DGY07ZZ
  Pleura DBY57ZZ
  Prostate DVY07ZZ
  Radius DPY77ZZ
  Rectum DDY77ZZ
  Rib DPY57ZZ
  Sinuses D9Y77ZZ
  Skin
    Abdomen DHY87ZZ
    Arm DHY47ZZ
    Back DHY77ZZ
    Buttock DHY97ZZ
    Chest DHY67ZZ
    Face DHY27ZZ
    Leg DHYB7ZZ
    Neck DHY37ZZ
  Skull DPY07ZZ
  Spinal Cord D0Y67ZZ
  Sternum DPY47ZZ
  Stomach DDY17ZZ
  Testis DVY17ZZ
  Thyroid Gland DGY57ZZ
  Tibia DPYB7ZZ
  Tongue D9Y57ZZ
  Trachea DBY07ZZ
  Ulna DPY77ZZ
  Ureter DTY17ZZ
  Urethra DTY37ZZ
  Uterus DUY27ZZ
  Whole Body DWY57ZZ
ContaCT software (Measurement of intracranial arterial flow) 4A03X5D
CONTAK RENEWAL® 3 RF (HE) CRT-D *use* Cardiac Resynchronization Defibrillator Pulse Generator in 0JH
Contegra Pulmonary Valved Conduit *use* Zooplastic Tissue in Heart and Great Vessels
CONTEPO™ *use* Fosfomycin Anti-Infective
Continent ileostomy *see* Bypass, Ileum 0D1B
Continuous Glucose Monitoring (CGM) device *use* Monitoring Device
Continuous Negative Airway Pressure
  24-96 Consecutive Hours, Ventilation 5A09459
  Greater than 96 Consecutive Hours, Ventilation 5A09559
  Less than 24 Consecutive Hours, Ventilation 5A09359
Continuous Positive Airway Pressure
  24-96 Consecutive Hours, Ventilation 5A09457
  Greater than 96 Consecutive Hours, Ventilation 5A09557
  Less than 24 Consecutive Hours, Ventilation 5A09357
Continuous renal replacement therapy (CRRT) 5A1D90Z
Contraceptive Device
  Change device in, Uterus and Cervix 0U2DXHZ
  Insertion of device in
    Cervix 0UHC
    Subcutaneous Tissue and Fascia
      Abdomen 0JH8
      Chest 0JH6
      Lower Arm
        Left 0JHH

Contraceptive Device — *continued*
  Insertion of device in — *continued*
    Subcutaneous Tissue and Fascia — *continued*
      Lower Arm — *continued*
        Right ØJHG
      Lower Leg
        Left ØJHP
        Right ØJHN
      Upper Arm
        Left ØJHF
        Right ØJHD
      Upper Leg
        Left ØJHM
        Right ØJHL
    Uterus ØUH9
  Removal of device from
    Subcutaneous Tissue and Fascia
      Lower Extremity ØJPW
      Trunk ØJPT
      Upper Extremity ØJPV
    Uterus and Cervix ØUPD
  Revision of device in
    Subcutaneous Tissue and Fascia
      Lower Extremity ØJWW
      Trunk ØJWT
      Upper Extremity ØJWV
    Uterus and Cervix ØUWD
Contractility Modulation Device
  Abdomen ØJH8
  Chest ØJH6
Control bleeding in
  Abdominal Wall ØW3F
  Ankle Region
    Left ØY3L
    Right ØY3K
  Arm
    Lower
      Left ØX3F
      Right ØX3D
    Upper
      Left ØX39
      Right ØX38
  Axilla
    Left ØX35
    Right ØX34
  Back
    Lower ØW3L
    Upper ØW3K
  Buttock
    Left ØY31
    Right ØY3Ø
  Cavity, Cranial ØW31
  Chest Wall ØW38
  Elbow Region
    Left ØX3C
    Right ØX3B
  Extremity
    Lower
      Left ØY3B
      Right ØY39
    Upper
      Left ØX37
      Right ØX36
  Face ØW32
  Femoral Region
    Left ØY38
    Right ØY37
  Foot
    Left ØY3N
    Right ØY3M
  Gastrointestinal Tract ØW3P
  Genitourinary Tract ØW3R
  Hand
    Left ØX3K
    Right ØX3J
  Head ØW3Ø
  Inguinal Region
    Left ØY36
    Right ØY35
  Jaw
    Lower ØW35
    Upper ØW34
  Knee Region
    Left ØY3G
    Right ØY3F
  Leg
    Lower
      Left ØY3J

Control bleeding in — *continued*
  Leg — *continued*
    Lower — *continued*
      Right ØY3H
    Upper
      Left ØY3D
      Right ØY3C
  Mediastinum ØW3C
  Nasal Mucosa and Soft Tissue Ø93K
  Neck ØW36
  Oral Cavity and Throat ØW33
  Pelvic Cavity ØW3J
  Pericardial Cavity ØW3D
  Perineum
    Female ØW3N
    Male ØW3M
  Peritoneal Cavity ØW3G
  Pleural Cavity
    Left ØW3B
    Right ØW39
  Respiratory Tract ØW3Q
  Retroperitoneum ØW3H
  Shoulder Region
    Left ØX33
    Right ØX32
  Wrist Region
    Left ØX3H
    Right ØX3G
Control bleeding using Tourniquet, External *see* Compression, Anatomical Regions 2W1
Control, Epistaxis *see* Control bleeding in, Nasal Mucosa and Soft Tissue Ø93K
Conus arteriosus *use* Ventricle, Right
Conus medullaris *use* Lumbar Spinal Cord
Convalescent Plasma (Nonautologous) *see* New Technology, Anatomical Regions XW1
Conversion
  Cardiac rhythm 5A22Ø4Z
  Gastrostomy to jejunostomy feeding device *see* Insertion of device in, Jejunum ØDHA
Cook Biodesign® Fistula Plug(s) *use* Nonautologous Tissue Substitute
Cook Biodesign® Hernia Graft(s) *use* Nonautologous Tissue Substitute
Cook Biodesign® Layered Graft(s) *use* Nonautologous Tissue Substitute
Cook Zenaprom™ Layered Graft(s) *use* Nonautologous Tissue Substitute
Cook Zenith AAA Endovascular Graft *use* Intraluminal Device
Cook Zenith® Fenestrated AAA Endovascular Graft
  use Intraluminal Device, Branched or Fenestrated, One or Two Arteries in Ø4V
  use Intraluminal Device, Branched or Fenestrated, Three or More Arteries in Ø4V
Coracoacromial ligament
  use Shoulder Bursa and Ligament, Left
  use Shoulder Bursa and Ligament, Right
Coracobrachialis muscle
  use Upper Arm Muscle, Left
  use Upper Arm Muscle, Right
Coracoclavicular ligament
  use Shoulder Bursa and Ligament, Left
  use Shoulder Bursa and Ligament, Right
Coracohumeral ligament
  use Shoulder Bursa and Ligament, Left
  use Shoulder Bursa and Ligament, Right
Coracoid process
  use Scapula, Left
  use Scapula, Right
Cordotomy *see* Division, Central Nervous System and Cranial Nerves ØØ8
Core needle biopsy *see* Excision with qualifier Diagnostic
CoreValve transcatheter aortic valve *use* Zooplastic Tissue in Heart and Great Vessels
Cormet Hip Resurfacing System *use* Resurfacing Device in Lower Joints
Corniculate cartilage *use* Larynx
CoRoent® XL *use* Interbody Fusion Device in Lower Joints
Coronary arteriography
  see Fluoroscopy, Heart B21
  see Plain Radiography, Heart B2Ø
Corox (OTW) Bipolar Lead
  use Cardiac Lead, Defibrillator in Ø2H
  use Cardiac Lead, Pacemaker in Ø2H

Corpus callosum *use* Brain
Corpus cavernosum *use* Penis
Corpus spongiosum *use* Penis
Corpus striatum *use* Basal Ganglia
Corrugator supercilii muscle *use* Facial Muscle
Cortical strip neurostimulator lead *use* Neurostimulator Lead in Central Nervous System and Cranial Nerves
Corvia IASD® *use* Synthetic Substitute
COSELA™ *use* Trilaciclib
Costatectomy
  see Excision, Upper Bones ØPB
  see Resection, Upper Bones ØPT
Costectomy
  see Excision, Upper Bones ØPB
  see Resection, Upper Bones ØPT
Costocervical trunk
  use Subclavian Artery, Left
  use Subclavian Artery, Right
Costochondrectomy
  see Excision, Upper Bones ØPB
  see Resection, Upper Bones ØPT
Costoclavicular ligament
  use Shoulder Bursa and Ligament, Left
  use Shoulder Bursa and Ligament, Right
Costosternoplasty
  see Repair, Upper Bones ØPQ
  see Replacement, Upper Bones ØPR
  see Supplement, Upper Bones ØPU
Costotomy
  see Division, Upper Bones ØP8
  see Drainage, Upper Bones ØP9
Costotransverse joint *use* Thoracic Vertebral Joint
Costotransverse ligament *use* Rib(s) Bursa and Ligament
Costovertebral joint *use* Thoracic Vertebral Joint
Costoxiphoid ligament *use* Sternum Bursa and Ligament
Counseling
  Family, for substance abuse, Other Family Counseling HZ63ZZZ
  Group
    12-Step HZ43ZZZ
    Behavioral HZ41ZZZ
    Cognitive HZ4ØZZZ
    Cognitive-Behavioral HZ42ZZZ
    Confrontational HZ48ZZZ
    Continuing Care HZ49ZZZ
    Infectious Disease
      Post-Test HZ4CZZZ
      Pre-Test HZ4CZZZ
    Interpersonal HZ44ZZZ
    Motivational Enhancement HZ47ZZZ
    Psychoeducation HZ46ZZZ
    Spiritual HZ4BZZZ
    Vocational HZ45ZZZ
  Individual
    12-Step HZ33ZZZ
    Behavioral HZ31ZZZ
    Cognitive HZ3ØZZZ
    Cognitive-Behavioral HZ32ZZZ
    Confrontational HZ38ZZZ
    Continuing Care HZ39ZZZ
    Infectious Disease
      Post-Test HZ3CZZZ
      Pre-Test HZ3CZZZ
    Interpersonal HZ34ZZZ
    Motivational Enhancement HZ37ZZZ
    Psychoeducation HZ36ZZZ
    Spiritual HZ3BZZZ
    Vocational HZ35ZZZ
  Mental Health Services
    Educational GZ6ØZZZ
    Other Counseling GZ63ZZZ
    Vocational GZ61ZZZ
Countershock, cardiac 5A22Ø4Z
COVID-19 Vaccine XWØ
COVID-19 Vaccine Booster XWØ
COVID-19 Vaccine Dose 1 XWØ
COVID-19 Vaccine Dose 2 XWØ
COVID-19 Vaccine Dose 3 XWØ
Cowper's (bulbourethral) gland *use* Urethra
CPAP (continuous positive airway pressure) *see* Assistance, Respiratory 5AØ9
Craniectomy
  see Excision, Head and Facial Bones ØNB
  see Resection, Head and Facial Bones ØNT

Cranioplasty
  see Repair, Head and Facial Bones ØNQ
  see Replacement, Head and Facial Bones ØNR
  see Supplement, Head and Facial Bones ØNU
Craniotomy
  see Division, Head and Facial Bones ØN8
  see Drainage, Central Nervous System and Cranial Nerves ØØ9
  see Drainage, Head and Facial Bones ØN9
Creation
  Perineum
    Female ØW4NØ
    Male ØW4MØ
  Valve
    Aortic Ø24FØ
    Mitral Ø24GØ
    Tricuspid Ø24JØ
Cremaster muscle *use* Perineum Muscle
CRESEMBA® (isavuconazonium sulfate) *use* Other Anti-infective
Cribriform plate
  use Ethmoid Bone, Left
  use Ethmoid Bone, Right
Cricoid cartilage *use* Trachea
Cricoidectomy *see* Excision, Larynx ØCBS
Cricothyroid artery
  use Thyroid Artery, Left
  use Thyroid Artery, Right
Cricothyroid muscle
  use Neck Muscle, Left
  use Neck Muscle, Right
Crisis Intervention GZ2ZZZZ
CRRT (Continuous renal replacement therapy) 5A1D9ØZ
Crural fascia
  use Subcutaneous Tissue and Fascia, Left Upper Leg
  use Subcutaneous Tissue and Fascia, Right Upper Leg
Crushing, nerve
  Cranial *see* Destruction, Central Nervous System and Cranial Nerves ØØ5
  Peripheral *see* Destruction, Peripheral Nervous System Ø15
Cryoablation *see* Destruction
Cryotherapy *see* Destruction
Cryptorchidectomy
  see Excision, Male Reproductive System ØVB
  see Resection, Male Reproductive System ØVT
Cryptorchiectomy
  see Excision, Male Reproductive System ØVB
  see Resection, Male Reproductive System ØVT
Cryptotomy
  see Division, Gastrointestinal System ØD8
  see Drainage, Gastrointestinal System ØD9
CT scan *see* Computerized Tomography (CT Scan)
CT sialogram *see* Computerized Tomography (CT Scan), Ear, Nose, Mouth and Throat B92
Cubital lymph node
  use Lymphatic, Left Upper Extremity
  use Lymphatic, Right Upper Extremity
Cubital nerve *use* Ulnar Nerve
Cuboid bone
  use Tarsal, Left
  use Tarsal, Right
Cuboideonavicular joint
  use Tarsal Joint, Left
  use Tarsal Joint, Right
Culdocentesis *see* Drainage, Cul-de-sac ØU9F
Culdoplasty
  see Repair, Cul-de-sac ØUQF
  see Supplement, Cul-de-sac ØUUF
Culdoscopy ØUJH8ZZ
Culdotomy *see* Drainage, Cul-de-sac ØU9F
Culmen *use* Cerebellum
Cultured epidermal cell autograft *use* Autologous Tissue Substitute
Cuneiform cartilage *use* Larynx
Cuneonavicular joint
  use Joint, Tarsal, Left
  use Joint, Tarsal, Right
Cuneonavicular ligament
  use Foot Bursa and Ligament, Left
  use Foot Bursa and Ligament, Right
Curettage
  see Excision
  see Extraction

Cutaneous (transverse) cervical nerve *use* Cervical Plexus
CVP (central venous pressure) *see* Measurement, Venous 4AØ4
Cyclodiathermy *see* Destruction, Eye Ø85
Cyclophotocoagulation *see* Destruction, Eye Ø85
CYPHER® Stent *use* Intraluminal Device, Drug-eluting in Heart and Great Vessels
Cystectomy
  see Excision, Bladder ØTBB
  see Resection, Bladder ØTTB
Cystocele repair *see* Repair, Subcutaneous Tissue and Fascia, Pelvic Region ØJQC
Cystography
  see Fluoroscopy, Urinary System BT1
  see Plain Radiography, Urinary System BTØ
Cystolithotomy *see* Extirpation, Bladder ØTCB
Cystopexy
  see Repair, Bladder ØTQB
  see Reposition, Bladder ØTSB
Cystoplasty
  see Repair, Bladder ØTQB
  see Replacement, Bladder ØTRB
  see Supplement, Bladder ØTUB
Cystorrhaphy *see* Repair, Bladder ØTQB
Cystoscopy ØTJB8ZZ
Cystostomy *see* Bypass, Bladder ØT1B
Cystostomy Tube *use* Drainage Device
Cystotomy *see* Drainage, Bladder ØT9B
Cystourethrography
  see Fluoroscopy, Urinary System BT1
  see Plain Radiography, Urinary System BTØ
Cystourethroplasty
  see Repair, Urinary System ØTQ
  see Replacement, Urinary System ØTR
  see Supplement, Urinary System ØTU
Cytarabine and Daunorubicin Liposome Antineoplastic XWØ

D

Daratumumab and Hyaluronidase-fihj XWØ1318
Darzalex Faspro® *use* Daratumumab and Hyaluronidase-fihj
DBS lead *use* Neurostimulator Lead in Central Nervous System and Cranial Nerves
DeBakey Left Ventricular Assist Device *use* Implantable Heart Assist System in Heart and Great Vessels
Debridement
  Excisional *see* Excision
  Non-excisional *see* Extraction
Decompression, Circulatory 6A15
Decortication, lung
  see Extirpation, Respiratory System ØBC
  see Release, Respiratory System ØBN
Deep brain neurostimulator lead *use* Neurostimulator Lead in Central Nervous System and Cranial Nerves
Deep cervical fascia
  use Subcutaneous Tissue and Fascia, Left Neck
  use Subcutaneous Tissue and Fascia, Right Neck
Deep cervical vein
  use Vertebral Vein, Left
  use Vertebral Vein, Right
Deep circumflex iliac artery
  use External Iliac Artery, Left
  use External Iliac Artery, Right
Deep facial vein
  use Face Vein, Left
  use Face Vein, Right
Deep femoral artery
  use Femoral Artery, Left
  use Femoral Artery, Right
Deep femoral (profunda femoris) vein
  use Femoral Vein, Left
  use Femoral Vein, Right
Deep Inferior Epigastric Artery Perforator Flap
  Replacement
    Bilateral ØHRVØ77
    Left ØHRUØ77
    Right ØHRTØ77
  Transfer
    Left ØKXG
    Right ØKXF

Deep palmar arch
  use Hand Artery, Left
  use Hand Artery, Right
Deep transverse perineal muscle *use* Perineum Muscle
DefenCath™ *use* Taurolidine Anti-infective and Heparin Anticoagulant
Deferential artery
  use Internal Iliac Artery, Left
  use Internal Iliac Artery, Right
Defibrillator Generator
  Abdomen ØJH8
  Chest ØJH6
Defibtech Automated Chest Compression (ACC) device 5A1221J
Defitelio *use* Other Substance
Defitelio® infusion *see* Introduction of substance in or on, Physiological Systems and Anatomical Regions 3EØ
Delivery
  Cesarean *see* Extraction, Products of Conception 1ØDØ
  Forceps *see* Extraction, Products of Conception 1ØDØ
  Manually assisted 1ØEØXZZ
  Products of Conception 1ØEØXZZ
  Vacuum assisted *see* Extraction, Products of Conception 1ØDØ
Delta frame external fixator
  use External Fixation Device, Hybrid in ØPH
  use External Fixation Device, Hybrid in ØPS
  use External Fixation Device, Hybrid in ØQH
  use External Fixation Device, Hybrid in ØQS
Delta III Reverse shoulder prosthesis *use* Synthetic Substitute, Reverse Ball and Socket in ØRR
Deltoid fascia
  use Subcutaneous Tissue and Fascia, Left Upper Arm
  use Subcutaneous Tissue and Fascia, Right Upper Arm
Deltoid ligament
  use Ankle Bursa and Ligament, Left
  use Ankle Bursa and Ligament, Right
Deltoid muscle
  use Shoulder Muscle, Left
  use Shoulder Muscle, Right
Deltopectoral (infraclavicular) lymph node
  use Lymphatic, Left Upper Extremity
  use Lymphatic, Right Upper Extremity
Denervation
  Cranial nerve *see* Destruction, Central Nervous System and Cranial Nerves ØØ5
  Peripheral nerve *see* Destruction, Peripheral Nervous System Ø15
Dens *use* Cervical Vertebra
Densitometry
  Plain Radiography
    Femur
      Left BQØ4ZZ1
      Right BQØ3ZZ1
    Hip
      Left BQØ1ZZ1
      Right BQØØZZ1
    Spine
      Cervical BRØØZZ1
      Lumbar BRØ9ZZ1
      Thoracic BRØ7ZZ1
      Whole BRØGZZ1
  Ultrasonography
    Elbow
      Left BP4HZZ1
      Right BP4GZZ1
    Hand
      Left BP4PZZ1
      Right BP4NZZ1
    Shoulder
      Left BP49ZZ1
      Right BP48ZZ1
    Wrist
      Left BP4MZZ1
      Right BP4LZZ1
Denticulate (dentate) ligament *use* Spinal Meninges
Depressor anguli oris muscle *use* Facial Muscle
Depressor labii inferioris muscle *use* Facial Muscle
Depressor septi nasi muscle *use* Facial Muscle
Depressor supercilii muscle *use* Facial Muscle
Dermabrasion *see* Extraction, Skin and Breast ØHD

Dermis use Skin
Descending genicular artery
  use Femoral Artery, Left
  use Femoral Artery, Right
Destruction
  Acetabulum
    Left 0Q55
    Right 0Q54
  Adenoids 0C5Q
  Ampulla of Vater 0F5C
  Anal Sphincter 0D5R
  Anterior Chamber
    Left 08533ZZ
    Right 08523ZZ
  Anus 0D5Q
  Aorta
    Abdominal
    Thoracic
      Ascending/Arch 025X
      Descending 025W
  Aortic Body 0G5D
  Appendix 0D5J
  Artery
    Anterior Tibial
      Left 045Q
      Right 045P
    Axillary
      Left 0356
      Right 0355
    Brachial
      Left 0358
      Right 0357
    Celiac 0451
    Colic
      Left 0457
      Middle 0458
      Right 0456
    Common Carotid
      Left 035J
      Right 035H
    Common Iliac
      Left 045D
      Right 045C
    External Carotid
      Left 035N
      Right 035M
    External Iliac
      Left 045J
      Right 045H
    Face 035R
    Femoral
      Left 045L
      Right 045K
    Foot
      Left 045W
      Right 045V
    Gastric 0452
    Hand
      Left 035F
      Right 035D
    Hepatic 0453
    Inferior Mesenteric 045B
    Innominate 0352
    Internal Carotid
      Left 035L
      Right 035K
    Internal Iliac
      Left 045F
      Right 045E
    Internal Mammary
      Left 0351
      Right 0350
    Intracranial 035G
    Lower 045Y
    Peroneal
      Left 045U
      Right 045T
    Popliteal
      Left 045N
      Right 045M
    Posterior Tibial
      Left 045S
      Right 045R
    Pulmonary
      Left 025R
      Right 025Q
    Pulmonary Trunk 025P
    Radial
      Left 035C

Destruction — *continued*
  Artery — *continued*
    Radial — *continued*
      Right 035B
    Renal
      Left 045A
      Right 0459
    Splenic 0454
    Subclavian
      Left 0354
      Right 0353
    Superior Mesenteric 0455
    Temporal
      Left 035T
      Right 035S
    Thyroid
      Left 035V
      Right 035U
    Ulnar
      Left 035A
      Right 0359
    Upper 035Y
    Vertebral
      Left 035Q
      Right 035P
  Atrium
    Left 0257
    Right 0256
  Auditory Ossicle
    Left 095A
    Right 0959
  Basal Ganglia 0058
  Bladder 0T5B
  Bladder Neck 0T5C
  Bone
    Ethmoid
      Left 0N5G
      Right 0N5F
    Frontal 0N51
    Hyoid 0N5X
    Lacrimal
      Left 0N5J
      Right 0N5H
    Nasal 0N5B
    Occipital 0N57
    Palatine
      Left 0N5L
      Right 0N5K
    Parietal
      Left 0N54
      Right 0N53
    Pelvic
      Left 0Q53
      Right 0Q52
    Sphenoid 0N5C
    Temporal
      Left 0N56
      Right 0N55
    Zygomatic
      Left 0N5N
      Right 0N5M
  Brain 0050
  Breast
    Bilateral 0H5V
    Left 0H5U
    Right 0H5T
  Bronchus
    Lingula 0B59
    Lower Lobe
      Left 0B5B
      Right 0B56
    Main
      Left 0B57
      Right 0B53
    Middle Lobe, Right 0B55
    Upper Lobe
      Left 0B58
      Right 0B54
  Buccal Mucosa 0C54
  Bursa and Ligament
    Abdomen
      Left 0M5J
      Right 0M5H
    Ankle
      Left 0M5R
      Right 0M5Q
    Elbow
      Left 0M54
      Right 0M53

Destruction — *continued*
  Bursa and Ligament — *continued*
    Foot
      Left 0M5T
      Right 0M5S
    Hand
      Left 0M58
      Right 0M57
    Head and Neck 0M50
    Hip
      Left 0M5M
      Right 0M5L
    Knee
      Left 0M5P
      Right 0M5N
    Lower Extremity
      Left 0M5W
      Right 0M5V
    Perineum 0M5K
    Rib(s) 0M5G
    Shoulder
      Left 0M52
      Right 0M51
    Spine
      Lower 0M5D
      Upper 0M5C
    Sternum 0M5F
    Upper Extremity
      Left 0M5B
      Right 0M59
    Wrist
      Left 0M56
      Right 0M55
  Carina 0B52
  Carotid Bodies, Bilateral 0G58
  Carotid Body
    Left 0G56
    Right 0G57
  Carpal
    Left 0P5N
    Right 0P5M
  Cecum 0D5H
  Cerebellum 005C
  Cerebral Hemisphere 0057
  Cerebral Meninges 0051
  Cerebral Ventricle 0056
  Cervix 0U5C
  Chordae Tendineae 0259
  Choroid
    Left 085B
    Right 085A
  Cisterna Chyli 075L
  Clavicle
    Left 0P5B
    Right 0P59
  Clitoris 0U5J
  Coccygeal Glomus 0G5B
  Coccyx 0Q5S
  Colon
    Ascending 0D5K
    Descending 0D5M
    Sigmoid 0D5N
    Transverse 0D5L
  Conduction Mechanism 0258
  Conjunctiva
    Left 085TXZZ
    Right 085SXZZ
  Cord
    Bilateral 0V5H
    Left 0V5G
    Right 0V5F
  Cornea
    Left 0859XZZ
    Right 0858XZZ
  Cul-de-sac 0U5F
  Diaphragm 0B5T
  Disc
    Cervical Vertebral 0R53
    Cervicothoracic Vertebral 0R55
    Lumbar Vertebral 0S52
    Lumbosacral 0S54
    Thoracic Vertebral 0R59
    Thoracolumbar Vertebral 0R5B
  Duct
    Common Bile 0F59
    Cystic 0F58
    Hepatic
      Common 0F57
      Left 0F56

Destruction — continued
- Duct — continued
  - Hepatic — continued
    - Right ØF55
  - Lacrimal
    - Left Ø85Y
    - Right Ø85X
  - Pancreatic ØF5D
    - Accessory ØF5F
  - Parotid
    - Left ØC5C
    - Right ØC5B
- Duodenum ØD59
- Dura Mater ØØ52
- Ear
  - External
    - Left Ø951
    - Right Ø950
  - External Auditory Canal
    - Left Ø954
    - Right Ø953
  - Inner
    - Left Ø95E
    - Right Ø95D
  - Middle
    - Left Ø956
    - Right Ø955
- Endometrium ØU5B
- Epididymis
  - Bilateral ØV5L
  - Left ØV5K
  - Right ØV5J
- Epiglottis ØC5R
- Esophagogastric Junction ØD54
- Esophagus ØD55
  - Lower ØD53
  - Middle ØD52
  - Upper ØD51
- Eustachian Tube
  - Left Ø95G
  - Right Ø95F
- Eye
  - Left Ø851XZZ
  - Right Ø850XZZ
- Eyelid
  - Lower
    - Left Ø85R
    - Right Ø85Q
  - Upper
    - Left Ø85P
    - Right Ø85N
- Fallopian Tube
  - Left ØU56
  - Right ØU55
- Fallopian Tubes, Bilateral ØU57
- Femoral Shaft
  - Left ØQ59
  - Right ØQ58
- Femur
  - Lower
    - Left ØQ5C
    - Right ØQ5B
  - Upper
    - Left ØQ57
    - Right ØQ56
- Fibula
  - Left ØQ5K
  - Right ØQ5J
- Finger Nail ØH5QXZZ
- Gallbladder ØF54
- Gingiva
  - Lower ØC56
  - Upper ØC55
- Gland
  - Adrenal
    - Bilateral ØG54
    - Left ØG52
    - Right ØG53
  - Lacrimal
    - Left Ø85W
    - Right Ø85V
  - Minor Salivary ØC5J
  - Parotid
    - Left ØC59
    - Right ØC58
  - Pituitary ØG5Ø
  - Sublingual
    - Left ØC5F
    - Right ØC5D

Destruction — continued
- Gland — continued
  - Submaxillary
    - Left ØC5H
    - Right ØC5G
  - Vestibular ØU5L
- Glenoid Cavity
  - Left ØP58
  - Right ØP57
- Glomus Jugulare ØG5C
- Humeral Head
  - Left ØP5D
  - Right ØP5C
- Humeral Shaft
  - Left ØP5G
  - Right ØP5F
- Hymen ØU5K
- Hypothalamus ØØ5A
- Ileocecal Valve ØD5C
- Ileum ØD5B
- Intestine
  - Large ØD5E
    - Left ØD5G
    - Right ØD5F
  - Small ØD58
- Iris
  - Left Ø85D3ZZ
  - Right Ø85C3ZZ
- Jejunum ØD5A
- Joint
  - Acromioclavicular
    - Left ØR5H
    - Right ØR5G
  - Ankle
    - Left ØS5G
    - Right ØS5F
  - Carpal
    - Left ØR5R
    - Right ØR5Q
  - Carpometacarpal
    - Left ØR5T
    - Right ØR5S
  - Cervical Vertebral ØR51
  - Cervicothoracic Vertebral ØR54
  - Coccygeal ØS56
  - Elbow
    - Left ØR5M
    - Right ØR5L
  - Finger Phalangeal
    - Left ØR5X
    - Right ØR5W
  - Hip
    - Left ØS5B
    - Right ØS59
  - Knee
    - Left ØS5D
    - Right ØS5C
  - Lumbar Vertebral ØS5Ø
  - Lumbosacral ØS53
  - Metacarpophalangeal
    - Left ØR5V
    - Right ØR5U
  - Metatarsal-Phalangeal
    - Left ØS5N
    - Right ØS5M
  - Occipital-cervical ØR5Ø
  - Sacrococcygeal ØS55
  - Sacroiliac
    - Left ØS58
    - Right ØS57
  - Shoulder
    - Left ØR5K
    - Right ØR5J
  - Sternoclavicular
    - Left ØR5F
    - Right ØR5E
  - Tarsal
    - Left ØS5J
    - Right ØS5H
  - Tarsometatarsal
    - Left ØS5L
    - Right ØS5K
  - Temporomandibular
    - Left ØR5D
    - Right ØR5C
  - Thoracic Vertebral ØR56
  - Thoracolumbar Vertebral ØR5A
  - Toe Phalangeal
    - Left ØS5Q

Destruction — continued
- Joint — continued
  - Toe Phalangeal — continued
    - Right ØS5P
  - Wrist
    - Left ØR5P
    - Right ØR5N
- Kidney
  - Left ØT51
  - Right ØT50
- Kidney Pelvis
  - Left ØT54
  - Right ØT53
- Larynx ØC5S
- Lens
  - Left Ø85K3ZZ
  - Right Ø85J3ZZ
- Lip
  - Lower ØC51
  - Upper ØC50
- Liver ØF50
  - Left Lobe ØF52
    - Ultrasound-guided Cavitation XF52X08
  - Right Lobe ØF51
    - Ultrasound-guided Cavitation XF51X08
  - Ultrasound-guided Cavitation XF50X08
- Lung
  - Bilateral ØB5M
  - Left ØB5L
  - Lower Lobe
    - Left ØB5J
    - Right ØB5F
  - Middle Lobe, Right ØB5D
  - Right ØB5K
  - Upper Lobe
    - Left ØB5G
    - Right ØB5C
- Lung Lingula ØB5H
- Lymphatic
  - Aortic Ø75D
  - Axillary
    - Left Ø756
    - Right Ø755
  - Head Ø750
  - Inguinal
    - Left Ø75J
    - Right Ø75H
  - Internal Mammary
    - Left Ø759
    - Right Ø758
  - Lower Extremity
    - Left Ø75G
    - Right Ø75F
  - Mesenteric Ø75B
  - Neck
    - Left Ø752
    - Right Ø751
  - Pelvis Ø75C
  - Thoracic Duct Ø75K
  - Thorax Ø757
  - Upper Extremity
    - Left Ø754
    - Right Ø753
- Mandible
  - Left ØN5V
  - Right ØN5T
- Maxilla ØN5R
- Medulla Oblongata ØØ5D
- Mesentery ØD5V
- Metacarpal
  - Left ØP5Q
  - Right ØP5P
- Metatarsal
  - Left ØQ5P
  - Right ØQ5N
- Muscle
  - Abdomen
    - Left ØK5L
    - Right ØK5K
  - Extraocular
    - Left Ø85M
    - Right Ø85L
  - Facial ØK51
  - Foot
    - Left ØK5W
    - Right ØK5V
  - Hand
    - Left ØK5D
    - Right ØK5C

▼ Subterms under main terms may continue to next column or page

Destruction — *continued*
  Muscle — *continued*
    Head 0K50
    Hip
      Left 0K5P
      Right 0K5N
    Lower Arm and Wrist
      Left 0K5B
      Right 0K59
    Lower Leg
      Left 0K5T
      Right 0K5S
    Neck
      Left 0K53
      Right 0K52
    Papillary 025D
    Perineum 0K5M
    Shoulder
      Left 0K56
      Right 0K55
    Thorax
      Left 0K5J
      Right 0K5H
    Tongue, Palate, Pharynx 0K54
    Trunk
      Left 0K5G
      Right 0K5F
    Upper Arm
      Left 0K58
      Right 0K57
    Upper Leg
      Left 0K5R
      Right 0K5Q
  Nasal Mucosa and Soft Tissue 095K
  Nasopharynx 095N
  Nerve
    Abdominal Sympathetic 015M
    Abducens 005L
    Accessory 005R
    Acoustic 005N
    Brachial Plexus 0153
    Cervical 0151
    Cervical Plexus 0150
    Facial 005M
    Femoral 015D
    Glossopharyngeal 005P
    Head and Neck Sympathetic 015K
    Hypoglossal 005S
    Lumbar 015B
    Lumbar Plexus 0159
    Lumbar Sympathetic 015N
    Lumbosacral Plexus 015A
    Median 0155
    Oculomotor 005H
    Olfactory 005F
    Optic 005G
    Peroneal 015H
    Phrenic 0152
    Pudendal 015C
    Radial 0156
    Sacral 015R
    Sacral Plexus 015Q
    Sacral Sympathetic 015P
    Sciatic 015F
    Thoracic 0158
    Thoracic Sympathetic 015L
    Tibial 015G
    Trigeminal 005K
    Trochlear 005J
    Ulnar 0154
    Vagus 005Q
  Nipple
    Left 0H5X
    Right 0H5W
  Omentum 0D5U
  Orbit
    Left 0N5Q
    Right 0N5P
  Ovary
    Bilateral 0U52
    Left 0U51
    Right 0U50
  Palate
    Hard 0C52
    Soft 0C53
  Pancreas 0F5G
  Para-aortic Body 0G59
  Paraganglion Extremity 0G5F
  Parathyroid Gland 0G5R

Destruction — *continued*
  Parathyroid Gland — *continued*
    Inferior
      Left 0G5P
      Right 0G5N
    Multiple 0G5Q
    Superior
      Left 0G5M
      Right 0G5L
  Patella
    Left 0Q5F
    Right 0Q5D
  Penis 0V5S
  Pericardium 025N
  Peritoneum 0D5W
  Phalanx
    Finger
      Left 0P5V
      Right 0P5T
    Thumb
      Left 0P5S
      Right 0P5R
    Toe
      Left 0Q5R
      Right 0Q5Q
  Pharynx 0C5M
  Pineal Body 0G51
  Pleura
    Left 0B5P
    Right 0B5N
  Pons 005B
  Prepuce 0V5T
  Prostate 0V50
    Robotic Waterjet Ablation XV508A4
  Radius
    Left 0P5J
    Right 0P5H
  Rectum 0D5P
  Retina
    Left 085F3ZZ
    Right 085E3ZZ
  Retinal Vessel
    Left 085H3ZZ
    Right 085G3ZZ
  Ribs
    1 to 2 0P51
    3 or More 0P52
  Sacrum 0Q51
  Scapula
    Left 0P56
    Right 0P55
  Sclera
    Left 0857XZZ
    Right 0856XZZ
  Scrotum 0V55
  Septum
    Atrial 0255
    Nasal 095M
    Ventricular 025M
  Sinus
    Accessory 095P
    Ethmoid
      Left 095V
      Right 095U
    Frontal
      Left 095T
      Right 095S
    Mastoid
      Left 095C
      Right 095B
    Maxillary
      Left 095R
      Right 095Q
    Sphenoid
      Left 095X
      Right 095W
  Skin
    Abdomen 0H57XZ
    Back 0H56XZ
    Buttock 0H58XZ
    Chest 0H55XZ
    Ear
      Left 0H53XZ
      Right 0H52XZ
    Face 0H51XZ
    Foot
      Left 0H5NXZ
      Right 0H5MXZ

Destruction — *continued*
  Skin — *continued*
    Hand
      Left 0H5GXZ
      Right 0H5FXZ
    Inguinal 0H5AXZ
    Lower Arm
      Left 0H5EXZ
      Right 0H5DXZ
    Lower Leg
      Left 0H5LXZ
      Right 0H5KXZ
    Neck 0H54XZ
    Perineum 0H59XZ
    Scalp 0H50XZ
    Upper Arm
      Left 0H5CXZ
      Right 0H5BXZ
    Upper Leg
      Left 0H5JXZ
      Right 0H5HXZ
  Skull 0N50
  Spinal Cord
    Cervical 005W
    Lumbar 005Y
    Thoracic 005X
  Spinal Meninges 005T
  Spleen 075P
  Sternum 0P50
  Stomach 0D56
    Pylorus 0D57
  Subcutaneous Tissue and Fascia
    Abdomen 0J58
    Back 0J57
    Buttock 0J59
    Chest 0J56
    Face 0J51
    Foot
      Left 0J5R
      Right 0J5Q
    Hand
      Left 0J5K
      Right 0J5J
    Lower Arm
      Left 0J5H
      Right 0J5G
    Lower Leg
      Left 0J5P
      Right 0J5N
    Neck
      Left 0J55
      Right 0J54
    Pelvic Region 0J5C
    Perineum 0J5B
    Scalp 0J50
    Upper Arm
      Left 0J5F
      Right 0J5D
    Upper Leg
      Left 0J5M
      Right 0J5L
  Tarsal
    Left 0Q5M
    Right 0Q5L
  Tendon
    Abdomen
      Left 0L5G
      Right 0L5F
    Ankle
      Left 0L5T
      Right 0L5S
    Foot
      Left 0L5W
      Right 0L5V
    Hand
      Left 0L58
      Right 0L57
    Head and Neck 0L50
    Hip
      Left 0L5K
      Right 0L5J
    Knee
      Left 0L5R
      Right 0L5Q
    Lower Arm and Wrist
      Left 0L56
      Right 0L55
    Lower Leg
      Left 0L5P

Subterms under main terms may continue to next column or page

Dilation — continued
Vein — continued
Axillary — continued
Right 0577
Azygos 0570
Basilic
Left 057C
Right 057B
Brachial
Left 057A
Right 0579
Cephalic
Left 057F
Right 057D
Colic 0677
Common Iliac
Left 067D
Right 067C
Esophageal 0673
External Iliac
Left 067G
Right 067F
External Jugular
Left 057Q
Right 057P
Face
Left 057V
Right 057T
Femoral
Left 067N
Right 067M
Foot
Left 067V
Right 067T
Gastric 0672
Hand
Left 057H
Right 057G
Hemiazygos 0571
Hepatic 0674
Hypogastric
Left 067J
Right 067H
Inferior Mesenteric 0676
Innominate
Left 0574
Right 0573
Internal Jugular
Left 057N
Right 057M
Intracranial 057L
Lower 067Y
Portal 0678
Pulmonary
Left 027T
Right 027S
Renal
Left 067B
Right 0679
Saphenous
Left 067Q
Right 067P
Splenic 0671
Subclavian
Left 0576
Right 0575
Superior Mesenteric 0675
Upper 057Y
Vertebral
Left 057S
Right 057R
Vena Cava
Inferior 0670
Superior 027V
Ventricle
Left 027L
Right 027K

Direct Lateral Interbody Fusion (DLIF) device *use* Interbody Fusion Device in Lower Joints
Disarticulation *see* Detachment
Discectomy, diskectomy
see Excision, Lower Joints 0SB
see Excision, Upper Joints 0RB
see Resection, Lower Joints 0ST
see Resection, Upper Joints 0RT
Discography
see Fluoroscopy, Axial Skeleton, Except Skull and Facial Bones BR1

Discography — continued
see Plain Radiography, Axial Skeleton, Except Skull and Facial Bones BR0
Dismembered pyeloplasty *see* Repair, Kidney Pelvis
Distal humerus
use Humeral Shaft, Left
use Humeral Shaft, Right
Distal humerus, involving joint
use Elbow Joint, Left
use Elbow Joint, Right
Distal radioulnar joint
use Wrist Joint, Left
use Wrist Joint, Right
Diversion *see* Bypass
Diverticulectomy *see* Excision, Gastrointestinal System 0DB
Division
Acetabulum
Left 0Q85
Right 0Q84
Anal Sphincter 0D8R
Basal Ganglia 0088
Bladder Neck 0T8C
Bone
Ethmoid
Left 0N8G
Right 0N8F
Frontal 0N81
Hyoid 0N8X
Lacrimal
Left 0N8J
Right 0N8H
Nasal 0N8B
Occipital 0N87
Palatine
Left 0N8L
Right 0N8K
Parietal
Left 0N84
Right 0N83
Pelvic
Left 0Q83
Right 0Q82
Sphenoid 0N8C
Temporal
Left 0N86
Right 0N85
Zygomatic
Left 0N8N
Right 0N8M
Brain 0080
Bursa and Ligament
Abdomen
Left 0M8J
Right 0M8H
Ankle
Left 0M8R
Right 0M8Q
Elbow
Left 0M84
Right 0M83
Foot
Left 0M8T
Right 0M8S
Hand
Left 0M88
Right 0M87
Head and Neck 0M80
Hip
Left 0M8M
Right 0M8L
Knee
Left 0M8P
Right 0M8N
Lower Extremity
Left 0M8W
Right 0M8V
Perineum 0M8K
Rib(s) 0M8G
Shoulder
Left 0M82
Right 0M81
Spine
Lower 0M8D
Upper 0M8C
Sternum 0M8F
Upper Extremity
Left 0M8B

Division — continued
Bursa and Ligament — continued
Upper Extremity — continued
Right 0M89
Wrist
Left 0M86
Right 0M85
Carpal
Left 0P8N
Right 0P8M
Cerebral Hemisphere 0087
Chordae Tendineae 0289
Clavicle
Left 0P8B
Right 0P89
Coccyx 0Q8S
Conduction Mechanism 0288
Esophagogastric Junction 0D84
Femoral Shaft
Left 0Q89
Right 0Q88
Femur
Lower
Left 0Q8C
Right 0Q8B
Upper
Left 0Q87
Right 0Q86
Fibula
Left 0Q8K
Right 0Q8J
Gland, Pituitary 0G80
Glenoid Cavity
Left 0P88
Right 0P87
Humeral Head
Left 0P8D
Right 0P8C
Humeral Shaft
Left 0P8G
Right 0P8F
Hymen 0U8K
Kidneys, Bilateral 0T82
Liver 0F80
Left Lobe 0F82
Right Lobe 0F81
Mandible
Left 0N8V
Right 0N8T
Maxilla 0N8R
Metacarpal
Left 0P8Q
Right 0P8P
Metatarsal
Left 0Q8P
Right 0Q8N
Muscle
Abdomen
Left 0K8L
Right 0K8K
Facial 0K81
Foot
Left 0K8W
Right 0K8V
Hand
Left 0K8D
Right 0K8C
Head 0K80
Hip
Left 0K8P
Right 0K8N
Lower Arm and Wrist
Left 0K8B
Right 0K89
Lower Leg
Left 0K8T
Right 0K8S
Neck
Left 0K83
Right 0K82
Papillary 028D
Perineum 0K8M
Shoulder
Left 0K86
Right 0K85
Thorax
Left 0K8J
Right 0K8H
Tongue, Palate, Pharynx 0K84

▽ **Subterms under main terms may continue to next column or page**

Division — *continued*
　Muscle — *continued*
　　Trunk
　　　Left 0K8G
　　　Right 0K8F
　　Upper Arm
　　　Left 0K88
　　　Right 0K87
　　Upper Leg
　　　Left 0K8R
　　　Right 0K8Q
　Nerve
　　Abdominal Sympathetic 018M
　　Abducens 008L
　　Accessory 008R
　　Acoustic 008N
　　Brachial Plexus 0183
　　Cervical 0181
　　Cervical Plexus 0180
　　Facial 008M
　　Femoral 018D
　　Glossopharyngeal 008P
　　Head and Neck Sympathetic 018K
　　Hypoglossal 008S
　　Lumbar 018B
　　Lumbar Plexus 0189
　　Lumbar Sympathetic 018N
　　Lumbosacral Plexus 018A
　　Median 0185
　　Oculomotor 008H
　　Olfactory 008F
　　Optic 008G
　　Peroneal 018H
　　Phrenic 0182
　　Pudendal 018C
　　Radial 0186
　　Sacral 018R
　　Sacral Plexus 018Q
　　Sacral Sympathetic 018P
　　Sciatic 018F
　　Thoracic 0188
　　Thoracic Sympathetic 018L
　　Tibial 018G
　　Trigeminal 008K
　　Trochlear 008J
　　Ulnar 0184
　　Vagus 008Q
　Orbit
　　Left 0N8Q
　　Right 0N8P
　Ovary
　　Bilateral 0U82
　　Left 0U81
　　Right 0U80
　Pancreas 0F8G
　Patella
　　Left 0Q8F
　　Right 0Q8D
　Perineum, Female 0W8NXZZ
　Phalanx
　　Finger
　　　Left 0P8V
　　　Right 0P8T
　　Thumb
　　　Left 0P8S
　　　Right 0P8R
　　Toe
　　　Left 0Q8R
　　　Right 0Q8Q
　Radius
　　Left 0P8J
　　Right 0P8H
　Ribs
　　1 to 2 0P81
　　3 or More 0P82
　Sacrum 0Q81
　Scapula
　　Left 0P86
　　Right 0P85
　Skin
　　Abdomen 0H87XZZ
　　Back 0H86XZZ
　　Buttock 0H88XZZ
　　Chest 0H85XZZ
　　Ear
　　　Left 0H83XZZ
　　　Right 0H82XZZ
　　Face 0H81XZZ

Division — *continued*
　Skin — *continued*
　　Foot
　　　Left 0H8NXZZ
　　　Right 0H8MXZZ
　　Hand
　　　Left 0H8GXZZ
　　　Right 0H8FXZZ
　　Inguinal 0H8AXZZ
　　Lower Arm
　　　Left 0H8EXZZ
　　　Right 0H8DXZZ
　　Lower Leg
　　　Left 0H8LXZZ
　　　Right 0H8KXZZ
　　Neck 0H84XZZ
　　Perineum 0H89XZZ
　　Scalp 0H80XZZ
　　Upper Arm
　　　Left 0H8CXZZ
　　　Right 0H8BXZZ
　　Upper Leg
　　　Left 0H8JXZZ
　　　Right 0H8HXZZ
　Skull 0N80
　Spinal Cord
　　Cervical 008W
　　Lumbar 008Y
　　Thoracic 008X
　Sternum 0P80
　Stomach, Pylorus 0D87
　Subcutaneous Tissue and Fascia
　　Abdomen 0J88
　　Back 0J87
　　Buttock 0J89
　　Chest 0J86
　　Face 0J81
　　Foot
　　　Left 0J8R
　　　Right 0J8Q
　　Hand
　　　Left 0J8K
　　　Right 0J8J
　　Head and Neck 0J8S
　　Lower Arm
　　　Left 0J8H
　　　Right 0J8G
　　Lower Extremity 0J8W
　　Lower Leg
　　　Left 0J8P
　　　Right 0J8N
　　Neck
　　　Left 0J85
　　　Right 0J84
　　Pelvic Region 0J8C
　　Perineum 0J8B
　　Scalp 0J80
　　Trunk 0J8T
　　Upper Arm
　　　Left 0J8F
　　　Right 0J8D
　　Upper Extremity 0J8V
　　Upper Leg
　　　Left 0J8M
　　　Right 0J8L
　Tarsal
　　Left 0Q8M
　　Right 0Q8L
　Tendon
　　Abdomen
　　　Left 0L8G
　　　Right 0L8F
　　Ankle
　　　Left 0L8T
　　　Right 0L8S
　　Foot
　　　Left 0L8W
　　　Right 0L8V
　　Hand
　　　Left 0L88
　　　Right 0L87
　　Head and Neck 0L80
　　Hip
　　　Left 0L8K
　　　Right 0L8J
　　Knee
　　　Left 0L8R
　　　Right 0L8Q

Division — *continued*
　Tendon — *continued*
　　Lower Arm and Wrist
　　　Left 0L86
　　　Right 0L85
　　Lower Leg
　　　Left 0L8P
　　　Right 0L8N
　　Perineum 0L8H
　　Shoulder
　　　Left 0L82
　　　Right 0L81
　　Thorax
　　　Left 0L8D
　　　Right 0L8C
　　Trunk
　　　Left 0L8B
　　　Right 0L89
　　Upper Arm
　　　Left 0L84
　　　Right 0L83
　　Upper Leg
　　　Left 0L8M
　　　Right 0L8L
　　Thyroid Gland Isthmus 0G8J
　　Tibia
　　　Left 0Q8H
　　　Right 0Q8G
　　Turbinate, Nasal 098L
　　Ulna
　　　Left 0P8L
　　　Right 0P8K
　　Uterine Supporting Structure 0U84
　　Vertebra
　　　Cervical 0P83
　　　Lumbar 0Q80
　　　Thoracic 0P84
Doppler study *see* Ultrasonography
Dorsal digital nerve *use* Radial Nerve
Dorsal metacarpal vein
　use Hand Vein, Left
　use Hand Vein, Right
Dorsal metatarsal artery
　use Foot Artery, Left
　use Foot Artery, Right
Dorsal metatarsal vein
　use Foot Vein, Left
　use Foot Vein, Right
Dorsal root ganglion
　use Cervical Spinal Cord
　use Lumbar Spinal Cord
　use Spinal Cord
　use Thoracic Spinal Cord
Dorsal scapular artery
　use Subclavian Artery, Left
　use Subclavian Artery, Right
Dorsal scapular nerve *use* Brachial Plexus
Dorsal venous arch
　use Foot Vein, Left
　use Foot Vein, Right
Dorsalis pedis artery
　use Anterior Tibial Artery, Left
　use Anterior Tibial Artery, Right
DownStream® System 5A0512C, 5A0522C
Drainage
　Abdominal Wall 0W9F
　Acetabulum
　　Left 0Q95
　　Right 0Q94
　Adenoids 0C9Q
　Ampulla of Vater 0F9C
　Anal Sphincter 0D9R
　Ankle Region
　　Left 0Y9L
　　Right 0Y9K
　Anterior Chamber
　　Left 0893
　　Right 0892
　Anus 0D9Q
　Aorta, Abdominal 0490
　Aortic Body 0G9D
　Appendix 0D9J
　Arm
　　Lower
　　　Left 0X9F
　　　Right 0X9D
　　Upper
　　　Left 0X99

Drainage — *continued*
  Arm — *continued*
    Upper — *continued*
      Right 0X98
  Artery
    Anterior Tibial
      Left 049Q
      Right 049P
    Axillary
      Left 0396
      Right 0395
    Brachial
      Left 0398
      Right 0397
    Celiac 0491
    Colic
      Left 0497
      Middle 0498
      Right 0496
    Common Carotid
      Left 039J
      Right 039H
    Common Iliac
      Left 049D
      Right 049C
    External Carotid
      Left 039N
      Right 039M
    External Iliac
      Left 049J
      Right 049H
    Face 039R
    Femoral
      Left 049L
      Right 049K
    Foot
      Left 049W
      Right 049V
    Gastric 0492
    Hand
      Left 039F
      Right 039D
    Hepatic 0493
    Inferior Mesenteric 049B
    Innominate 0392
    Internal Carotid
      Left 039L
      Right 039K
    Internal Iliac
      Left 049F
      Right 049E
    Internal Mammary
      Left 0391
      Right 0390
    Intracranial 039G
    Lower 049Y
    Peroneal
      Left 049U
      Right 049T
    Popliteal
      Left 049N
      Right 049M
    Posterior Tibial
      Left 049S
      Right 049R
    Radial
      Left 039C
      Right 039B
    Renal
      Left 049A
      Right 0499
    Splenic 0494
    Subclavian
      Left 0394
      Right 0393
    Superior Mesenteric 0495
    Temporal
      Left 039T
      Right 039S
    Thyroid
      Left 039V
      Right 039U
    Ulnar
      Left 039A
      Right 0399
    Upper 039Y
    Vertebral
      Left 039Q
      Right 039P

Drainage — *continued*
  Auditory Ossicle
    Left 099A
    Right 0999
  Axilla
    Left 0X95
    Right 0X94
  Back
    Lower 0W9L
    Upper 0W9K
  Basal Ganglia 0098
  Bladder 0T9B
  Bladder Neck 0T9C
  Bone
    Ethmoid
      Left 0N9G
      Right 0N9F
    Frontal 0N91
    Hyoid 0N9X
    Lacrimal
      Left 0N9J
      Right 0N9H
    Nasal 0N9B
    Occipital 0N97
    Palatine
      Left 0N9L
      Right 0N9K
    Parietal
      Left 0N94
      Right 0N93
    Pelvic
      Left 0Q93
      Right 0Q92
    Sphenoid 0N9C
    Temporal
      Left 0N96
      Right 0N95
    Zygomatic
      Left 0N9N
      Right 0N9M
  Bone Marrow 079T
  Brain 0090
  Breast
    Bilateral 0H9V
    Left 0H9U
    Right 0H9T
  Bronchus
    Lingula 0B99
    Lower Lobe
      Left 0B9B
      Right 0B96
    Main
      Left 0B97
      Right 0B93
    Middle Lobe, Right 0B95
    Upper Lobe
      Left 0B98
      Right 0B94
  Buccal Mucosa 0C94
  Bursa and Ligament
    Abdomen
      Left 0M9J
      Right 0M9H
    Ankle
      Left 0M9R
      Right 0M9Q
    Elbow
      Left 0M94
      Right 0M93
    Foot
      Left 0M9T
      Right 0M9S
    Hand
      Left 0M98
      Right 0M97
    Head and Neck 0M90
    Hip
      Left 0M9M
      Right 0M9L
    Knee
      Left 0M9P
      Right 0M9N
    Lower Extremity
      Left 0M9W
      Right 0M9V
    Perineum 0M9K
    Rib(s) 0M9G
    Shoulder
      Left 0M92

Drainage — *continued*
  Bursa and Ligament — *continued*
    Shoulder — *continued*
      Right 0M91
    Spine
      Lower 0M9D
      Upper 0M9C
    Sternum 0M9F
    Upper Extremity
      Left 0M9B
      Right 0M99
    Wrist
      Left 0M96
      Right 0M95
  Buttock
    Left 0Y91
    Right 0Y90
  Carina 0B92
  Carotid Bodies, Bilateral 0G98
  Carotid Body
    Left 0G96
    Right 0G97
  Carpal
    Left 0P9N
    Right 0P9M
  Cavity, Cranial 0W91
  Cecum 0D9H
  Cerebellum 009C
  Cerebral Hemisphere 0097
  Cerebral Meninges 0091
  Cerebral Ventricle 0096
  Cervix 0U9C
  Chest Wall 0W98
  Choroid
    Left 089B
    Right 089A
  Cisterna Chyli 079L
  Clavicle
    Left 0P9B
    Right 0P99
  Clitoris 0U9J
  Coccygeal Glomus 0G9B
  Coccyx 0Q9S
  Colon
    Ascending 0D9K
    Descending 0D9M
    Sigmoid 0D9N
    Transverse 0D9L
  Conjunctiva
    Left 089T
    Right 089S
  Cord
    Bilateral 0V9H
    Left 0V9G
    Right 0V9F
  Cornea
    Left 0899
    Right 0898
  Cul-de-sac 0U9F
  Diaphragm 0B9T
  Disc
    Cervical Vertebral 0R93
    Cervicothoracic Vertebral 0R95
    Lumbar Vertebral 0S92
    Lumbosacral 0S94
    Thoracic Vertebral 0R99
    Thoracolumbar Vertebral 0R9B
  Duct
    Common Bile 0F99
    Cystic 0F98
    Hepatic
      Common 0F97
      Left 0F96
      Right 0F95
    Lacrimal
      Left 089Y
      Right 089X
    Pancreatic 0F9D
      Accessory 0F9F
    Parotid
      Left 0C9C
      Right 0C9B
  Duodenum 0D99
  Dura Mater 0092
  Ear
    External
      Left 0991
      Right 0990

Drainage — *continued*
  Ear — *continued*
    External Auditory Canal
      Left 0994
      Right 0993
    Inner
      Left 099E
      Right 099D
    Middle
      Left 0996
      Right 0995
  Elbow Region
    Left 0X9C
    Right 0X9B
  Epididymis
    Bilateral 0V9L
    Left 0V9K
    Right 0V9J
  Epidural Space, Intracranial 0093
  Epiglottis 0C9R
  Esophagogastric Junction 0D94
  Esophagus 0D95
    Lower 0D93
    Middle 0D92
    Upper 0D91
  Eustachian Tube
    Left 099G
    Right 099F
  Extremity
    Lower
      Left 0Y9B
      Right 0Y99
    Upper
      Left 0X97
      Right 0X96
  Eye
    Left 0891
    Right 0890
  Eyelid
    Lower
      Left 089R
      Right 089Q
    Upper
      Left 089P
      Right 089N
  Face 0W92
  Fallopian Tube
    Left 0U96
    Right 0U95
  Fallopian Tubes, Bilateral 0U97
  Femoral Region
    Left 0Y98
    Right 0Y97
  Femoral Shaft
    Left 0Q99
    Right 0Q98
  Femur
    Lower
      Left 0Q9C
      Right 0Q9B
    Upper
      Left 0Q97
      Right 0Q96
  Fibula
    Left 0Q9K
    Right 0Q9J
  Finger Nail 0H9Q
  Foot
    Left 0Y9N
    Right 0Y9M
  Gallbladder 0F94
  Gingiva
    Lower 0C96
    Upper 0C95
  Gland
    Adrenal
      Bilateral 0G94
      Left 0G92
      Right 0G93
    Lacrimal
      Left 089W
      Right 089V
    Minor Salivary 0C9J
    Parotid
      Left 0C99
      Right 0C98
    Pituitary 0G90
    Sublingual
      Left 0C9F

Drainage — *continued*
  Gland — *continued*
    Sublingual — *continued*
      Right 0C9D
    Submaxillary
      Left 0C9H
      Right 0C9G
    Vestibular 0U9L
  Glenoid Cavity
    Left 0P98
    Right 0P97
  Glomus Jugulare 0G9C
  Hand
    Left 0X9K
    Right 0X9J
  Head 0W90
  Humeral Head
    Left 0P9D
    Right 0P9C
  Humeral Shaft
    Left 0P9G
    Right 0P9F
  Hymen 0U9K
  Hypothalamus 009A
  Ileocecal Valve 0D9C
  Ileum 0D9B
  Inguinal Region
    Left 0Y96
    Right 0Y95
  Intestine
    Large 0D9E
      Left 0D9G
      Right 0D9F
    Small 0D98
  Iris
    Left 089D
    Right 089C
  Jaw
    Lower 0W95
    Upper 0W94
  Jejunum 0D9A
  Joint
    Acromioclavicular
      Left 0R9H
      Right 0R9G
    Ankle
      Left 0S9G
      Right 0S9F
    Carpal
      Left 0R9R
      Right 0R9Q
    Carpometacarpal
      Left 0R9T
      Right 0R9S
    Cervical Vertebral 0R91
    Cervicothoracic Vertebral 0R94
    Coccygeal 0S96
    Elbow
      Left 0R9M
      Right 0R9L
    Finger Phalangeal
      Left 0R9X
      Right 0R9W
    Hip
      Left 0S9B
      Right 0S99
    Knee
      Left 0S9D
      Right 0S9C
    Lumbar Vertebral 0S90
    Lumbosacral 0S93
    Metacarpophalangeal
      Left 0R9V
      Right 0R9U
    Metatarsal-Phalangeal
      Left 0S9N
      Right 0S9M
    Occipital-cervical 0R90
    Sacrococcygeal 0S95
    Sacroiliac
      Left 0S98
      Right 0S97
    Shoulder
      Left 0R9K
      Right 0R9J
    Sternoclavicular
      Left 0R9F
      Right 0R9E

Drainage — *continued*
  Joint — *continued*
    Tarsal
      Left 0S9J
      Right 0S9H
    Tarsometatarsal
      Left 0S9L
      Right 0S9K
    Temporomandibular
      Left 0R9D
      Right 0R9C
    Thoracic Vertebral 0R96
    Thoracolumbar Vertebral 0R9A
    Toe Phalangeal
      Left 0S9Q
      Right 0S9P
    Wrist
      Left 0R9P
      Right 0R9N
  Kidney
    Left 0T91
    Right 0T90
  Kidney Pelvis
    Left 0T94
    Right 0T93
  Knee Region
    Left 0Y9G
    Right 0Y9F
  Larynx 0C9S
  Leg
    Lower
      Left 0Y9J
      Right 0Y9H
    Upper
      Left 0Y9D
      Right 0Y9C
  Lens
    Left 089K
    Right 089J
  Lip
    Lower 0C91
    Upper 0C90
  Liver 0F90
    Left Lobe 0F92
    Right Lobe 0F91
  Lung
    Bilateral 0B9M
    Left 0B9L
    Lower Lobe
      Left 0B9J
      Right 0B9F
    Middle Lobe, Right 0B9D
    Right 0B9K
    Upper Lobe
      Left 0B9G
      Right 0B9C
  Lung Lingula 0B9H
  Lymphatic
    Aortic 079D
    Axillary
      Left 0796
      Right 0795
    Head 0790
    Inguinal
      Left 079J
      Right 079H
    Internal Mammary
      Left 0799
      Right 0798
    Lower Extremity
      Left 079G
      Right 079F
    Mesenteric 079B
    Neck
      Left 0792
      Right 0791
    Pelvis 079C
    Thoracic Duct 079K
    Thorax 0797
    Upper Extremity
      Left 0794
      Right 0793
  Mandible
    Left 0N9V
    Right 0N9T
  Maxilla 0N9R
  Mediastinum 0W9C
  Medulla Oblongata 009D
  Mesentery 0D9V

Drainage — *continued*
- Metacarpal
  - Left 0P9Q
  - Right 0P9P
- Metatarsal
  - Left 0Q9P
  - Right 0Q9N
- Muscle
  - Abdomen
    - Left 0K9L
    - Right 0K9K
  - Extraocular
    - Left 089M
    - Right 089L
  - Facial 0K91
  - Foot
    - Left 0K9W
    - Right 0K9V
  - Hand
    - Left 0K9D
    - Right 0K9C
  - Head 0K90
  - Hip
    - Left 0K9P
    - Right 0K9N
  - Lower Arm and Wrist
    - Left 0K9B
    - Right 0K99
  - Lower Leg
    - Left 0K9T
    - Right 0K9S
  - Neck
    - Left 0K93
    - Right 0K92
  - Perineum 0K9M
  - Shoulder
    - Left 0K96
    - Right 0K95
  - Thorax
    - Left 0K9J
    - Right 0K9H
  - Tongue, Palate, Pharynx 0K94
  - Trunk
    - Left 0K9G
    - Right 0K9F
  - Upper Arm
    - Left 0K98
    - Right 0K97
  - Upper Leg
    - Left 0K9R
    - Right 0K9Q
- Nasal Mucosa and Soft Tissue 099K
- Nasopharynx 099N
- Neck 0W96
- Nerve
  - Abdominal Sympathetic 019M
  - Abducens 009L
  - Accessory 009R
  - Acoustic 009N
  - Brachial Plexus 0193
  - Cervical 0191
  - Cervical Plexus 0190
  - Facial 009M
  - Femoral 019D
  - Glossopharyngeal 009P
  - Head and Neck Sympathetic 019K
  - Hypoglossal 009S
  - Lumbar 019B
  - Lumbar Plexus 0199
  - Lumbar Sympathetic 019N
  - Lumbosacral Plexus 019A
  - Median 0195
  - Oculomotor 009H
  - Olfactory 009F
  - Optic 009G
  - Peroneal 019H
  - Phrenic 0192
  - Pudendal 019C
  - Radial 0196
  - Sacral 019R
  - Sacral Plexus 019Q
  - Sacral Sympathetic 019P
  - Sciatic 019F
  - Thoracic 0198
  - Thoracic Sympathetic 019L
  - Tibial 019G
  - Trigeminal 009K
  - Trochlear 009J
  - Ulnar 0194

Drainage — *continued*
- Nerve — *continued*
  - Vagus 009Q
- Nipple
  - Left 0H9X
  - Right 0H9W
- Omentum 0D9U
- Oral Cavity and Throat 0W93
- Orbit
  - Left 0N9Q
  - Right 0N9P
- Ovary
  - Bilateral 0U92
  - Left 0U91
  - Right 0U90
- Palate
  - Hard 0C92
  - Soft 0C93
- Pancreas 0F9G
- Para-aortic Body 0G9D
- Paraganglion Extremity 0G9F
- Parathyroid Gland 0G9R
  - Inferior
    - Left 0G9P
    - Right 0G9N
  - Multiple 0G9Q
  - Superior
    - Left 0G9M
    - Right 0G9L
- Patella
  - Left 0Q9F
  - Right 0Q9D
- Pelvic Cavity 0W9J
- Penis 0V9S
- Pericardial Cavity 0W9D
- Perineum
  - Female 0W9N
  - Male 0W9M
- Peritoneal Cavity 0W9G
- Peritoneum 0D9W
- Phalanx
  - Finger
    - Left 0P9V
    - Right 0P9T
  - Thumb
    - Left 0P9S
    - Right 0P9R
  - Toe
    - Left 0Q9R
    - Right 0Q9Q
- Pharynx 0C9M
- Pineal Body 0G91
- Pleura
  - Left 0B9P
  - Right 0B9N
- Pleural Cavity
  - Left 0W9B
  - Right 0W99
- Pons 009B
- Prepuce 0V9T
- Products of Conception
  - Amniotic Fluid
    - Diagnostic 1090
    - Therapeutic 1090
  - Fetal Blood 1090
  - Fetal Cerebrospinal Fluid 1090
  - Fetal Fluid, Other 1090
  - Fluid, Other 1090
- Prostate 0V90
- Radius
  - Left 0P9J
  - Right 0P9H
- Rectum 0D9P
- Retina
  - Left 089F
  - Right 089E
- Retinal Vessel
  - Left 089H
  - Right 089G
- Retroperitoneum 0W9H
- Ribs
  - 1 to 2 0P91
  - 3 or More 0P92
- Sacrum 0Q91
- Scapula
  - Left 0P96
  - Right 0P95
- Sclera
  - Left 0897

Drainage — *continued*
- Sclera — *continued*
  - Right 0896
- Scrotum 0V95
- Septum, Nasal 099M
- Shoulder Region
  - Left 0X93
  - Right 0X92
- Sinus
  - Accessory 099P
  - Ethmoid
    - Left 099V
    - Right 099U
  - Frontal
    - Left 099T
    - Right 099S
  - Mastoid
    - Left 099C
    - Right 099B
  - Maxillary
    - Left 099R
    - Right 099Q
  - Sphenoid
    - Left 099X
    - Right 099W
- Skin
  - Abdomen 0H97
  - Back 0H96
  - Buttock 0H98
  - Chest 0H95
  - Ear
    - Left 0H93
    - Right 0H92
  - Face 0H91
  - Foot
    - Left 0H9N
    - Right 0H9M
  - Hand
    - Left 0H9G
    - Right 0H9F
  - Inguinal 0H9A
  - Lower Arm
    - Left 0H9E
    - Right 0H9D
  - Lower Leg
    - Left 0H9L
    - Right 0H9K
  - Neck 0H94
  - Perineum 0H99
  - Scalp 0H90
  - Upper Arm
    - Left 0H9C
    - Right 0H9B
  - Upper Leg
    - Left 0H9J
    - Right 0H9H
- Skull 0N90
- Spinal Canal 009U
- Spinal Cord
  - Cervical 009W
  - Lumbar 009Y
  - Thoracic 009X
- Spinal Meninges 009T
- Spleen 079P
- Sternum 0P90
- Stomach 0D96
  - Pylorus 0D97
- Subarachnoid Space, Intracranial 0095
- Subcutaneous Tissue and Fascia
  - Abdomen 0J98
  - Back 0J97
  - Buttock 0J99
  - Chest 0J96
  - Face 0J91
  - Foot
    - Left 0J9R
    - Right 0J9Q
  - Hand
    - Left 0J9K
    - Right 0J9J
  - Lower Arm
    - Left 0J9H
    - Right 0J9G
  - Lower Leg
    - Left 0J9P
    - Right 0J9N
  - Neck
    - Left 0J95
    - Right 0J94

Drainage — *continued*
  Subcutaneous Tissue and Fascia — *continued*
    Pelvic Region ØJ9C
    Perineum ØJ9B
    Scalp ØJ9Ø
    Upper Arm
      Left ØJ9F
      Right ØJ9D
    Upper Leg
      Left ØJ9M
      Right ØJ9L
  Subdural Space, Intracranial ØØ94
  Tarsal
    Left ØQ9M
    Right ØQ9L
  Tendon
    Abdomen
      Left ØL9G
      Right ØL9F
    Ankle
      Left ØL9T
      Right ØL9S
    Foot
      Left ØL9W
      Right ØL9V
    Hand
      Left ØL98
      Right ØL97
    Head and Neck ØL9Ø
    Hip
      Left ØL9K
      Right ØL9J
    Knee
      Left ØL9R
      Right ØL9Q
    Lower Arm and Wrist
      Left ØL96
      Right ØL95
    Lower Leg
      Left ØL9P
      Right ØL9N
    Perineum ØL9H
    Shoulder
      Left ØL92
      Right ØL91
    Thorax
      Left ØL9D
      Right ØL9C
    Trunk
      Left ØL9B
      Right ØL99
    Upper Arm
      Left ØL94
      Right ØL93
    Upper Leg
      Left ØL9M
      Right ØL9L
  Testis
    Bilateral ØV9C
    Left ØV9B
    Right ØV99
  Thalamus ØØ99
  Thymus Ø79M
  Thyroid Gland ØG9K
    Left Lobe ØG9G
    Right Lobe ØG9H
  Tibia
    Left ØQ9H
    Right ØQ9G
  Toe Nail ØH9R
  Tongue ØC97
  Tonsils ØC9P
  Tooth
    Lower ØC9X
    Upper ØC9W
  Trachea ØB91
  Tunica Vaginalis
    Left ØV97
    Right ØV96
  Turbinate, Nasal Ø99L
  Tympanic Membrane
    Left Ø998
    Right Ø997
  Ulna
    Left ØP9L
    Right ØP9K
  Ureter
    Left ØT97
    Right ØT96

Drainage — *continued*
  Ureters, Bilateral ØT98
  Urethra ØT9D
  Uterine Supporting Structure ØU94
  Uterus ØU99
  Uvula ØC9N
  Vagina ØU9G
  Vas Deferens
    Bilateral ØV9Q
    Left ØV9P
    Right ØV9N
  Vein
    Axillary
      Left Ø598
      Right Ø597
    Azygos Ø59Ø
    Basilic
      Left Ø59C
      Right Ø59B
    Brachial
      Left Ø59A
      Right Ø599
    Cephalic
      Left Ø59F
      Right Ø59D
    Colic Ø697
    Common Iliac
      Left Ø69D
      Right Ø69C
    Esophageal Ø693
    External Iliac
      Left Ø69G
      Right Ø69F
    External Jugular
      Left Ø59Q
      Right Ø59P
    Face
      Left Ø59V
      Right Ø59T
    Femoral
      Left Ø69N
      Right Ø69M
    Foot
      Left Ø69V
      Right Ø69T
    Gastric Ø692
    Hand
      Left Ø59H
      Right Ø59G
    Hemiazygos Ø591
    Hepatic Ø694
    Hypogastric
      Left Ø69J
      Right Ø69H
    Inferior Mesenteric Ø696
    Innominate
      Left Ø594
      Right Ø593
    Internal Jugular
      Left Ø59N
      Right Ø59M
    Intracranial Ø59L
    Lower Ø69Y
    Portal Ø698
    Renal
      Left Ø69B
      Right Ø699
    Saphenous
      Left Ø69Q
      Right Ø69P
    Splenic Ø691
    Subclavian
      Left Ø596
      Right Ø595
    Superior Mesenteric Ø695
    Upper Ø59Y
    Vertebral
      Left Ø59S
      Right Ø59R
  Vena Cava, Inferior Ø69Ø
  Vertebra
    Cervical ØP93
    Lumbar ØQ9Ø
    Thoracic ØP94
  Vesicle
    Bilateral ØV93
    Left ØV92
    Right ØV91

Drainage — *continued*
  Vitreous
    Left Ø895
    Right Ø894
  Vocal Cord
    Left ØC9V
    Right ØC9T
  Vulva ØU9M
  Wrist Region
    Left ØX9H
    Right ØX9G
Dressing
  Abdominal Wall 2W23X4Z
  Arm
    Lower
      Left 2W2DX4Z
      Right 2W2CX4Z
    Upper
      Left 2W2BX4Z
      Right 2W2AX4Z
  Back 2W25X4Z
  Chest Wall 2W24X4Z
  Extremity
    Lower
      Left 2W2MX4Z
      Right 2W2LX4Z
    Upper
      Left 2W29X4Z
      Right 2W28X4Z
  Face 2W21X4Z
  Finger
    Left 2W2KX4Z
    Right 2W2JX4Z
  Foot
    Left 2W2TX4Z
    Right 2W2SX4Z
  Hand
    Left 2W2FX4Z
    Right 2W2EX4Z
  Head 2W2ØX4Z
  Inguinal Region
    Left 2W27X4Z
    Right 2W26X4Z
  Leg
    Lower
      Left 2W2RX4Z
      Right 2W2QX4Z
    Upper
      Left 2W2PX4Z
      Right 2W2NX4Z
  Neck 2W22X4Z
  Thumb
    Left 2W2HX4Z
    Right 2W2GX4Z
  Toe
    Left 2W2VX4Z
    Right 2W2UX4Z
Driver stent (RX) (OTW) *use* Intraluminal Device
Drotrecogin alfa, infusion *see* Introduction of Recombinant Human-activated Protein C
Duct of Santorini *use* Pancreatic Duct, Accessory
Duct of Wirsung *use* Pancreatic Duct
Ductogram, mammary *see* Plain Radiography, Skin, Subcutaneous Tissue and Breast BHØ
Ductography, mammary *see* Plain Radiography, Skin, Subcutaneous Tissue and Breast BHØ
Ductus deferens
  use Vas Deferens
  use Vas Deferens, Bilateral
  use Vas Deferens, Left
  use Vas Deferens, Right
Duodenal ampulla *use* Ampulla of Vater
Duodenectomy
  see Excision, Duodenum ØDB9
  see Resection, Duodenum ØDT9
Duodenocholedochotomy *see* Drainage, Gallbladder ØF94
Duodenocystostomy
  see Bypass, Gallbladder ØF14
  see Drainage, Gallbladder ØF94
Duodenoenterostomy
  see Bypass, Gastrointestinal System ØD1
  see Drainage, Gastrointestinal System ØD9
Duodenojejunal flexure *use* Jejunum
Duodenolysis *see* Release, Duodenum ØDN9
Duodenorrhaphy *see* Repair, Duodenum ØDQ9

Duodenoscopy, single-use (aScope™ Duodeno) (EXALT™ Model D) *see* New Technology, Hepatobiliary System and Pancreas XFJ
Duodenostomy
  see Bypass, Duodenum ØD19
  see Drainage, Duodenum ØD99
Duodenotomy *see* Drainage, Duodenum ØD99
Dura mater, intracranial *use* Dura Mater
Dura mater, spinal *use* Spinal Meninges
DuraGraft® Endothelial Damage Inhibitor *use* Endothelial Damage Inhibitor
DuraHeart Left Ventricular Assist System *use* Implantable Heart Assist System in Heart and Great Vessels
Dural venous sinus *use* Intracranial Vein
Durata® Defibrillation Lead *use* Cardiac Lead, Defibrillator in Ø2H
Durvalumab Antineoplastic XWØ
DynaClip® (Forte)
  use Internal Fixation Device, Sustained Compression in ØRG
  use Internal Fixation Device, Sustained Compression in ØSG
DynaNail® (Hybrid) (Mini)
  use Internal Fixation Device, Sustained Compression in ØRG
  use Internal Fixation Device, Sustained Compression in ØSG
Dynesys® Dynamic Stabilization System
  use Spinal Stabilization Device, Pedicle-Based in ØRH
  use Spinal Stabilization Device, Pedicle-Based in ØSH

E

Earlobe
  use Ear, External, Bilateral
  use Ear, External, Left
  use Ear, External, Right
ECCO2R (Extracorporeal Carbon Dioxide Removal) 5A0920Z
Echocardiogram *see* Ultrasonography, Heart B24
Echography *see* Ultrasonography
EchoTip® Insight™ Portosystemic Pressure Gradient Measurement System 4A044B2
ECMO *see* Performance, Circulatory 5A15
ECMO, intraoperative *see* Performance, Circulatory 5A15A
Eculizumab XWØ
EDWARDS INTUITY Elite valve system (rapid deployment technique) *see* Replacement, Valve, Aortic Ø2RF
EEG (electroencephalogram) *see* Measurement, Central Nervous 4A00
EGD (esophagogastroduodenoscopy) ØDJ08ZZ
Eighth cranial nerve *use* Acoustic Nerve
Ejaculatory duct
  use Vas Deferens
  use Vas Deferens, Bilateral
  use Vas Deferens, Left
  use Vas Deferens, Right
EKG (electrocardiogram) *see* Measurement, Cardiac 4A02
EKOS™ EkoSonic® Endovascular System *see* Fragmentation, Artery
Eladocagene exuparvovec XW0Q316
Electrical bone growth stimulator (EBGS)
  use Bone Growth Stimulator in Head and Facial Bones
  use Bone Growth Stimulator in Lower Bones
  use Bone Growth Stimulator in Upper Bones
Electrical muscle stimulation (EMS) lead *use* Stimulator Lead in Muscles
Electrocautery
  Destruction *see* Destruction
  Repair *see* Repair
Electroconvulsive Therapy
  Bilateral-Multiple Seizure GZB3ZZZ
  Bilateral-Single Seizure GZB2ZZZ
  Electroconvulsive Therapy, Other GZB4ZZZ
  Unilateral-Multiple Seizure GZB1ZZZ
  Unilateral-Single Seizure GZB0ZZZ
Electroencephalogram (EEG) *see* Measurement, Central Nervous 4A00

Electromagnetic Therapy
  Central Nervous 6A22
  Urinary 6A21
Electronic muscle stimulator lead *use* Stimulator Lead in Muscles
Electrophysiologic stimulation (EPS) *see* Measurement, Cardiac 4A02
Electroshock therapy *see* Electroconvulsive Therapy
Elevation, bone fragments, skull *see* Reposition, Head and Facial Bones ØNS
Eleventh cranial nerve *use* Accessory Nerve
Ellipsys® vascular access system *see* New Technology, Cardiovascular System X2K
E-Luminexx™ (Biliary) (Vascular) Stent *use* Intraluminal Device
Eluvia™ Drug-Eluting Vascular Stent System
  use Intraluminal Device, Sustained Release Drug-eluting in New Technology
  use Intraluminal Device, Sustained Release Drug-eluting, Two in New Technology
  use Intraluminal Device, Sustained Release Drug-eluting, Three in New Technology
  use Intraluminal Device, Sustained Release Drug-eluting, Four or More in New Technology
ELZONRIS™ *use* Tagraxofusp-erzs Antineoplastic
Embolectomy *see* Extirpation
Embolization
  see Occlusion
  see Restriction
Embolization coil(s) *use* Intraluminal Device
EMG (electromyogram) *see* Measurement, Musculoskeletal 4A0F
Encephalon *use* Brain
Endarterectomy
  see Extirpation, Lower Arteries Ø4C
  see Extirpation, Upper Arteries Ø3C
Endeavor® (III) (IV) (Sprint) Zotarolimus-eluting Coronary Stent System *use* Intraluminal Device, Drug-eluting in Heart and Great Vessels
EndoAVF procedure, using magnetic-guided radiofrequency *see* Bypass, Upper Arteries Ø31
EndoAVF procedure, using thermal resistance energy *see* New Technology, Cardiovascular System X2K
Endologix AFX® Endovascular AAA System *use* Intraluminal Device
EndoSure® sensor *use* Monitoring Device, Pressure Sensor in Ø2H
ENDOTAK RELIANCE® (G) Defibrillation Lead *use* Cardiac Lead, Defibrillator in Ø2H
Endothelial damage inhibitor, applied to vein graft XYØVX83
Endotracheal tube (cuffed) (double-lumen) *use* Intraluminal Device, Endotracheal Airway in Respiratory System
Endovascular fistula creation, using magnetic-guided radiofrequency *see* Bypass, Upper Arteries Ø31
Endovascular fistula creation, using thermal resistance energy *see* New Technology, Cardiovascular System X2K
Endurant® Endovascular Stent Graft *use* Intraluminal Device
Endurant® II AAA Stent Graft System *use* Intraluminal Device
Engineered Allogeneic Thymus Tissue XW020D8
Engineered Chimeric Antigen Receptor T-cell Immunotherapy
  Allogeneic XWØ
  Autologous XWØ
Enlargement
  see Dilation
  see Repair
EnRhythm *use* Pacemaker, Dual Chamber in ØJH
ENROUTE® Transcarotid Neuroprotection System *see* New Technology, Cardiovascular System X2A
ENSPRYNG™ *use* Satralizumab-mwge
Enterorrhaphy *see* Repair, Gastrointestinal System ØDQ
Enterra gastric neurostimulator *use* Stimulator Generator, Multiple Array in ØJH
Enucleation
  Eyeball *see* Resection, Eye Ø8T
  Eyeball with prosthetic implant *see* Replacement, Eye Ø8R
Ependyma *use* Cerebral Ventricle

Epicel® cultured epidermal autograft *use* Autologous Tissue Substitute
Epic™ Stented Tissue Valve (aortic) *use* Zooplastic Tissue in Heart and Great Vessels
Epidermis *use* Skin
Epididymectomy
  see Excision, Male Reproductive System ØVB
  see Resection, Male Reproductive System ØVT
Epididymoplasty
  see Repair, Male Reproductive System ØVQ
  see Supplement, Male Reproductive System ØVU
Epididymorrhaphy *see* Repair, Male Reproductive System ØVQ
Epididymotomy *see* Drainage, Male Reproductive System ØV9
Epidural space, spinal *use* Spinal Canal
Epiphysiodesis
  see Insertion of device in, Lower Bones ØQH
  see Insertion of device in, Upper Bones ØPH
  see Repair, Lower Bones ØQQ
  see Repair, Upper Bones ØPQ
Epiploic foramen *use* Peritoneum
Epiretinal Visual Prosthesis
  Left Ø8H105Z
  Right Ø8H005Z
Episiorrhaphy *see* Repair, Perineum, Female ØWQN
Episiotomy *see* Division, Perineum, Female ØW8N
Epithalamus *use* Thalamus
Epitrochlear lymph node
  use Lymphatic, Left Upper Extremity
  use Lymphatic, Right Upper Extremity
EPS (electrophysiologic stimulation) *see* Measurement, Cardiac 4A02
Eptifibatide, infusion *see* Introduction of Platelet Inhibitor
ERCP (endoscopic retrograde cholangiopancreatography) *see* Fluoroscopy, Hepatobiliary System and Pancreas BF1
Erdafitinib Antineoplastic XWØDXL5
Erector spinae muscle
  use Trunk Muscle, Left
  use Trunk Muscle, Right
ERLEADA™ *use* Apalutamide Antineoplastic
Esketamine Hydrochloride XW097M5
Esophageal artery *use* Upper Artery
Esophageal obturator airway (EOA) *use* Intraluminal Device, Airway in Gastrointestinal System
Esophageal plexus *use* Thoracic Sympathetic Nerve
Esophagectomy
  see Excision, Gastrointestinal System ØDB
  see Resection, Gastrointestinal System ØDT
Esophagocoloplasty
  see Repair, Gastrointestinal System ØDQ
  see Supplement, Gastrointestinal System ØDU
Esophagoenterostomy
  see Bypass, Gastrointestinal System ØD1
  see Drainage, Gastrointestinal System ØD9
Esophagoesophagostomy
  see Bypass, Gastrointestinal System ØD1
  see Drainage, Gastrointestinal System ØD9
Esophagogastrectomy
  see Excision, Gastrointestinal System ØDB
  see Resection, Gastrointestinal System ØDT
Esophagogastroduodenoscopy (EGD) ØDJ08ZZ
Esophagogastroplasty
  see Repair, Gastrointestinal System ØDQ
  see Supplement, Gastrointestinal System ØDU
Esophagogastroscopy ØDJ68ZZ
Esophagogastrostomy
  see Bypass, Gastrointestinal System ØD1
  see Drainage, Gastrointestinal System ØD9
Esophagojejunoplasty *see* Supplement, Gastrointestinal System ØDU
Esophagojejunostomy
  see Bypass, Gastrointestinal System ØD1
  see Drainage, Gastrointestinal System ØD9
Esophagomyotomy *see* Division, Esophagogastric Junction ØD84
Esophagoplasty
  see Repair, Gastrointestinal System ØDQ
  see Replacement, Esophagus ØDR5
  see Supplement, Gastrointestinal System ØDU
Esophagoplication *see* Restriction, Gastrointestinal System ØDV
Esophagorrhaphy *see* Repair, Gastrointestinal System ØDQ

Esophagoscopy ØDJØ8ZZ
Esophagotomy see Drainage, Gastrointestinal System ØD9
Esteem® implantable hearing system use Hearing Device in Ear, Nose, Sinus
ESWL (extracorporeal shock wave lithotripsy) see Fragmentation
Etesevimab Monoclonal Antibody XWØ
Ethmoidal air cell
  use Ethmoid Sinus, Left
  use Ethmoid Sinus, Right
Ethmoidectomy
  see Excision, Ear, Nose, Sinus Ø9B
  see Excision, Head and Facial Bones ØNB
  see Resection, Ear, Nose, Sinus Ø9T
  see Resection, Head and Facial Bones ØNT
Ethmoidotomy see Drainage, Ear, Nose, Sinus Ø99
Evacuation
  Hematoma *see* Extirpation
  Other Fluid *see* Drainage
Evera (XT) (S) (DR/VR) use Defibrillator Generator in ØJH
Everolimus-eluting coronary stent use Intraluminal Device, Drug-eluting in Heart and Great Vessels
Evisceration
  Eyeball *see* Resection, Eye Ø8T
  Eyeball with prosthetic implant *see* Replacement, Eye Ø8R
EVUSHELD™ use Tixagevimab and Cilgavimab Monoclonal Antibody
EXALT™ Model D Single-Use Duodenoscope see New Technology, Hepatobiliary System and Pancreas XFJ
Examination see Inspection
Exchange see Change device in
Excision
  Abdominal Wall ØWBF
  Acetabulum
    Left ØQB5
    Right ØQB4
  Adenoids ØCBQ
  Ampulla of Vater ØFBC
  Anal Sphincter ØDBR
  Ankle Region
    Left ØYBL
    Right ØYBK
  Anus ØDBQ
  Aorta
    Abdominal
    Thoracic
      Ascending/Arch Ø2BX
      Descending Ø2BW
  Aortic Body ØGBD
  Appendix ØDBJ
  Arm
    Lower
      Left ØXBF
      Right ØXBD
    Upper
      Left ØXB9
      Right ØXB8
  Artery
    Anterior Tibial
      Left Ø4BQ
      Right Ø4BP
    Axillary
      Left Ø3B6
      Right Ø3B5
    Brachial
      Left Ø3B8
      Right Ø3B7
    Celiac Ø4B1
    Colic
      Left Ø4B7
      Middle Ø4B8
      Right Ø4B6
    Common Carotid
      Left Ø3BJ
      Right Ø3BH
    Common Iliac
      Left Ø4BD
      Right Ø4BC
    External Carotid
      Left Ø3BN
      Right Ø3BM
    External Iliac
      Left Ø4BJ
      Right Ø4BH

Excision — *continued*
  Artery — *continued*
    Face Ø3BR
    Femoral
      Left Ø4BL
      Right Ø4BK
    Foot
      Left Ø4BW
      Right Ø4BV
    Gastric Ø4B2
    Hand
      Left Ø3BF
      Right Ø3BD
    Hepatic Ø4B3
    Inferior Mesenteric Ø4BB
    Innominate Ø3B2
    Internal Carotid
      Left Ø3BL
      Right Ø3BK
    Internal Iliac
      Left Ø4BF
      Right Ø4BE
    Internal Mammary
      Left Ø3B1
      Right Ø3BØ
    Intracranial Ø3BG
    Lower Ø4BY
    Peroneal
      Left Ø4BU
      Right Ø4BT
    Popliteal
      Left Ø4BN
      Right Ø4BM
    Posterior Tibial
      Left Ø4BS
      Right Ø4BR
    Pulmonary
      Left Ø2BR
      Right Ø2BQ
    Pulmonary Trunk Ø2BP
    Radial
      Left Ø3BC
      Right Ø3BB
    Renal
      Left Ø4BA
      Right Ø4B9
    Splenic Ø4B4
    Subclavian
      Left Ø3B4
      Right Ø3B3
    Superior Mesenteric Ø4B5
    Temporal
      Left Ø3BT
      Right Ø3BS
    Thyroid
      Left Ø3BV
      Right Ø3BU
    Ulnar
      Left Ø3BA
      Right Ø3B9
    Upper Ø3BY
    Vertebral
      Left Ø3BQ
      Right Ø3BP
  Atrium
    Left Ø2B7
    Right Ø2B6
  Auditory Ossicle
    Left Ø9BA
    Right Ø9B9
  Axilla
    Left ØXB5
    Right ØXB4
  Back
    Lower ØWBL
    Upper ØWBK
  Basal Ganglia ØØB8
  Bladder ØTBB
  Bladder Neck ØTBC
  Bone
    Ethmoid
      Left ØNBG
      Right ØNBF
    Frontal ØNB1
    Hyoid ØNBX
    Lacrimal
      Left ØNBJ
      Right ØNBH
    Nasal ØNBB

Excision — *continued*
  Bone — *continued*
    Occipital ØNB7
    Palatine
      Left ØNBL
      Right ØNBK
    Parietal
      Left ØNB4
      Right ØNB3
    Pelvic
      Left ØQB3
      Right ØQB2
    Sphenoid ØNBC
    Temporal
      Left ØNB6
      Right ØNB5
    Zygomatic
      Left ØNBN
      Right ØNBM
  Brain ØØBØ
  Breast
    Bilateral ØHBV
    Left ØHBU
    Right ØHBT
    Supernumerary ØHBY
  Bronchus
    Lingula ØBB9
    Lower Lobe
      Left ØBBB
      Right ØBB6
    Main
      Left ØBB7
      Right ØBB3
    Middle Lobe, Right ØBB5
    Upper Lobe
      Left ØBB8
      Right ØBB4
  Buccal Mucosa ØCB4
  Bursa and Ligament
    Abdomen
      Left ØMBJ
      Right ØMBH
    Ankle
      Left ØMBR
      Right ØMBQ
    Elbow
      Left ØMB4
      Right ØMB3
    Foot
      Left ØMBT
      Right ØMBS
    Hand
      Left ØMB8
      Right ØMB7
    Head and Neck ØMBØ
    Hip
      Left ØMBM
      Right ØMBL
    Knee
      Left ØMBP
      Right ØMBN
    Lower Extremity
      Left ØMBW
      Right ØMBV
    Perineum ØMBK
    Rib(s) ØMBG
    Shoulder
      Left ØMB2
      Right ØMB1
    Spine
      Lower ØMBD
      Upper ØMBC
    Sternum ØMBF
    Upper Extremity
      Left ØMBB
      Right ØMB9
    Wrist
      Left ØMB6
      Right ØMB5
  Buttock
    Left ØYB1
    Right ØYBØ
  Carina ØBB2
  Carotid Bodies, Bilateral ØGB8
  Carotid Body
    Left ØGB6
    Right ØGB7
  Carpal
    Left ØPBN

Excision — *continued*
  Skin — *continued*
    Foot — *continued*
      Right ØHBMXZ
    Hand
      Left ØHBGXZ
      Right ØHBFXZ
    Inguinal ØHBAXZ
    Lower Arm
      Left ØHBEXZ
      Right ØHBDXZ
    Lower Leg
      Left ØHBLXZ
      Right ØHBKXZ
    Neck ØHB4XZ
    Perineum ØHB9XZ
    Scalp ØHBØXZ
    Upper Arm
      Left ØHBCXZ
      Right ØHBBXZ
    Upper Leg
      Left ØHBJXZ
      Right ØHBHXZ
  Skull ØNBØ
  Spinal Cord
    Cervical ØØBW
    Lumbar ØØBY
    Thoracic ØØBX
  Spinal Meninges ØØBT
  Spleen Ø7BP
  Sternum ØPBØ
  Stomach ØDB6
    Pylorus ØDB7
  Subcutaneous Tissue and Fascia
    Abdomen ØJB8
    Back ØJB7
    Buttock ØJB9
    Chest ØJB6
    Face ØJB1
    Foot
      Left ØJBR
      Right ØJBQ
    Hand
      Left ØJBK
      Right ØJBJ
    Lower Arm
      Left ØJBH
      Right ØJBG
    Lower Leg
      Left ØJBP
      Right ØJBN
    Neck
      Left ØJB5
      Right ØJB4
    Pelvic Region ØJBC
    Perineum ØJBB
    Scalp ØJBØ
    Upper Arm
      Left ØJBF
      Right ØJBD
    Upper Leg
      Left ØJBM
      Right ØJBL
  Tarsal
    Left ØQBM
    Right ØQBL
  Tendon
    Abdomen
      Left ØLBG
      Right ØLBF
    Ankle
      Left ØLBT
      Right ØLBS
    Foot
      Left ØLBW
      Right ØLBV
    Hand
      Left ØLB8
      Right ØLB7
    Head and Neck ØLBØ
    Hip
      Left ØLBK
      Right ØLBJ
    Knee
      Left ØLBR
      Right ØLBQ
    Lower Arm and Wrist
      Left ØLB6
      Right ØLB5

Excision — *continued*
  Tendon — *continued*
    Lower Leg
      Left ØLBP
      Right ØLBN
    Perineum ØLBH
    Shoulder
      Left ØLB2
      Right ØLB1
    Thorax
      Left ØLBD
      Right ØLBC
    Trunk
      Left ØLBB
      Right ØLB9
    Upper Arm
      Left ØLB4
      Right ØLB3
    Upper Leg
      Left ØLBM
      Right ØLBL
  Testis
    Bilateral ØVBC
    Left ØVBB
    Right ØVB9
  Thalamus ØØB9
  Thymus Ø7BM
  Thyroid Gland
    Left Lobe ØGBG
    Right Lobe ØGBH
    Thyroid Gland Isthmus ØGBJ
  Tibia
    Left ØQBH
    Right ØQBG
  Toe Nail ØHBRXZ
  Tongue ØCB7
  Tonsils ØCBP
  Tooth
    Lower ØCBX
    Upper ØCBW
  Trachea ØBB1
  Tunica Vaginalis
    Left ØVB7
    Right ØVB6
  Turbinate, Nasal Ø9BL
  Tympanic Membrane
    Left Ø9B8
    Right Ø9B7
  Ulna
    Left ØPBL
    Right ØPBK
  Ureter
    Left ØTB7
    Right ØTB6
  Urethra ØTBD
  Uterine Supporting Structure ØUB4
  Uterus ØUB9
  Uvula ØCBN
  Vagina ØUBG
  Valve
    Aortic Ø2BF
    Mitral Ø2BG
    Pulmonary Ø2BH
    Tricuspid Ø2BJ
  Vas Deferens
    Bilateral ØVBQ
    Left ØVBP
    Right ØVBN
  Vein
    Axillary
      Left Ø5B8
      Right Ø5B7
    Azygos Ø5BØ
    Basilic
      Left Ø5BC
      Right Ø5BB
    Brachial
      Left Ø5BA
      Right Ø5B9
    Cephalic
      Left Ø5BF
      Right Ø5BD
    Colic Ø6B7
    Common Iliac
      Left Ø6BD
      Right Ø6BC
    Coronary Ø2B4
    Esophageal Ø6B3

Excision — *continued*
  Vein — *continued*
    External Iliac
      Left Ø6BG
      Right Ø6BF
    External Jugular
      Left Ø5BQ
      Right Ø5BP
    Face
      Left Ø5BV
      Right Ø5BT
    Femoral
      Left Ø6BN
      Right Ø6BM
    Foot
      Left Ø6BV
      Right Ø6BT
    Gastric Ø6B2
    Hand
      Left Ø5BH
      Right Ø5BG
    Hemiazygos Ø5B1
    Hepatic Ø6B4
    Hypogastric
      Left Ø6BJ
      Right Ø6BH
    Inferior Mesenteric Ø6B6
    Innominate
      Left Ø5B4
      Right Ø5B3
    Internal Jugular
      Left Ø5BN
      Right Ø5BM
    Intracranial Ø5BL
    Lower Ø6BY
    Portal Ø6B8
    Pulmonary
      Left Ø2BT
      Right Ø2BS
    Renal
      Left Ø6BB
      Right Ø6B9
    Saphenous
      Left Ø6BQ
      Right Ø6BP
    Splenic Ø6B1
    Subclavian
      Left Ø5B6
      Right Ø5B5
    Superior Mesenteric Ø6B5
    Upper Ø5BY
    Vertebral
      Left Ø5BS
      Right Ø5BR
  Vena Cava
    Inferior Ø6BØ
    Superior Ø2BV
  Ventricle
    Left Ø2BL
    Right Ø2BK
  Vertebra
    Cervical ØPB3
    Lumbar ØQBØ
    Thoracic ØPB4
  Vesicle
    Bilateral ØVB3
    Left ØVB2
    Right ØVB1
  Vitreous
    Left Ø8B53Z
    Right Ø8B43Z
  Vocal Cord
    Left ØCBV
    Right ØCBT
  Vulva ØUBM
  Wrist Region
    Left ØXBH
    Right ØXBG
EXCLUDER® AAA Endoprosthesis
  use Intraluminal Device
  use Intraluminal Device, Branched or Fenestrated, One or Two Arteries in Ø4V
  use Intraluminal Device, Branched or Fenestrated, Three or More Arteries in Ø4V
EXCLUDER® IBE Endoprosthesis *use* Intraluminal Device, Branched or Fenestrated, One or Two Arteries in Ø4V
Exclusion, Left atrial appendage (LAA) *see* Occlusion, Atrium, Left Ø2L7

Exercise, rehabilitation *see* Motor Treatment, Rehabilitation F07
Exploration *see* Inspection
Express® Biliary SD Monorail® Premounted Stent System *use* Intraluminal Device
Express® (LD) Premounted Stent System *use* Intraluminal Device
Express® SD Renal Monorail® Premounted Stent System *use* Intraluminal Device
Ex-PRESS™ mini glaucoma shunt *use* Synthetic Substitute
Extensor carpi radialis muscle
  use Lower Arm and Wrist Muscle, Left
  use Lower Arm and Wrist Muscle, Right
Extensor carpi ulnaris muscle
  use Lower Arm and Wrist Muscle, Left
  use Lower Arm and Wrist Muscle, Right
Extensor digitorum brevis muscle
  use Foot Muscle, Left
  use Foot Muscle, Right
Extensor digitorum longus muscle
  use Lower Leg Muscle, Left
  use Lower Leg Muscle, Right
Extensor hallucis brevis muscle
  use Foot Muscle, Left
  use Foot Muscle, Right
Extensor hallucis longus muscle
  use Lower Leg Muscle, Left
  use Lower Leg Muscle, Right
External anal sphincter *use* Anal Sphincter
External auditory meatus
  use External Auditory Canal, Left
  use External Auditory Canal, Right
External fixator
  use External Fixation Device in Head and Facial Bones
  use External Fixation Device in Lower Bones
  use External Fixation Device in Lower Joints
  use External Fixation Device in Upper Bones
  use External Fixation Device in Upper Joints
External maxillary artery *use* Face Artery
External naris *use* Nasal Mucosa and Soft Tissue
External oblique aponeurosis *use* Subcutaneous Tissue and Fascia, Trunk
External oblique muscle
  use Abdomen Muscle, Left
  use Abdomen Muscle, Right
External popliteal nerve *use* Peroneal Nerve
External pudendal artery
  use Femoral Artery, Left
  use Femoral Artery, Right
External pudendal vein
  use Saphenous Vein, Left
  use Saphenous Vein, Right
External urethral sphincter *use* Urethra
Extirpation
  Acetabulum
    Left 0QC5
    Right 0QC4
  Adenoids 0CCQ
  Ampulla of Vater 0FCC
  Anal Sphincter 0DCR
  Anterior Chamber
    Left 08C3
    Right 08C2
  Anus 0DCQ
  Aorta
    Abdominal 04C0
    Thoracic
      Ascending/Arch 02CX
      Descending 02CW
  Aortic Body 0GCD
  Appendix 0DCJ
  Artery
    Anterior Tibial
      Left 04CQ
      Right 04CP
    Axillary
      Left 03C6
      Right 03C5
    Brachial
      Left 03C8
      Right 03C7
    Celiac 04C1
    Colic
      Left 04C7
      Middle 04C8

Extirpation — *continued*
  Artery — *continued*
    Colic — *continued*
      Right 04C6
    Common Carotid
      Left 03CJ
      Right 03CH
    Common Iliac
      Left 04CD
      Right 04CC
    Coronary
      Four or More Arteries 02C3
      One Artery 02C0
      Three Arteries 02C2
      Two Arteries 02C1
    External Carotid
      Left 03CN
      Right 03CM
    External Iliac
      Left 04CJ
      Right 04CH
    Face 03CR
    Femoral
      Left 04CL
      Right 04CK
    Foot
      Left 04CW
      Right 04CV
    Gastric 04C2
    Hand
      Left 03CF
      Right 03CD
    Hepatic 04C3
    Inferior Mesenteric 04CB
    Innominate 03C2
    Internal Carotid
      Left 03CL
      Right 03CK
    Internal Iliac
      Left 04CF
      Right 04CE
    Internal Mammary
      Left 03C1
      Right 03C0
    Intracranial 03CG
    Lower 04CY
    Peroneal
      Left 04CU
      Right 04CT
    Popliteal
      Left 04CN
      Right 04CM
    Posterior Tibial
      Left 04CS
      Right 04CR
    Pulmonary
      Left 02CR
      Right 02CQ
    Pulmonary Trunk 02CP
    Radial
      Left 03CC
      Right 03CB
    Renal
      Left 04CA
      Right 04C9
    Splenic 04C4
    Subclavian
      Left 03C4
      Right 03C3
    Superior Mesenteric 04C5
    Temporal
      Left 03CT
      Right 03CS
    Thyroid
      Left 03CV
      Right 03CU
    Ulnar
      Left 03CA
      Right 03C9
    Upper 03CY
    Vertebral
      Left 03CQ
      Right 03CP
  Atrium
    Left 02C7
    Right 02C6
  Auditory Ossicle
    Left 09CA
    Right 09C9

Extirpation — *continued*
  Basal Ganglia 00C8
  Bladder 0TCB
  Bladder Neck 0TCC
  Bone
    Ethmoid
      Left 0NCG
      Right 0NCF
    Frontal 0NC1
    Hyoid 0NCX
    Lacrimal
      Left 0NCJ
      Right 0NCH
    Nasal 0NCB
    Occipital 0NC7
    Palatine
      Left 0NCL
      Right 0NCK
    Parietal
      Left 0NC4
      Right 0NC3
    Pelvic
      Left 0QC3
      Right 0QC2
    Sphenoid 0NCC
    Temporal
      Left 0NC6
      Right 0NC5
    Zygomatic
      Left 0NCN
      Right 0NCM
  Brain 00C0
  Breast
    Bilateral 0HCV
    Left 0HCU
    Right 0HCT
  Bronchus
    Lingula 0BC9
    Lower Lobe
      Left 0BCB
      Right 0BC6
    Main
      Left 0BC7
      Right 0BC3
    Middle Lobe, Right 0BC5
    Upper Lobe
      Left 0BC8
      Right 0BC4
  Buccal Mucosa 0CC4
  Bursa and Ligament
    Abdomen
      Left 0MCJ
      Right 0MCH
    Ankle
      Left 0MCR
      Right 0MCQ
    Elbow
      Left 0MC4
      Right 0MC3
    Foot
      Left 0MCT
      Right 0MCS
    Hand
      Left 0MC8
      Right 0MC7
    Head and Neck 0MC0
    Hip
      Left 0MCM
      Right 0MCL
    Knee
      Left 0MCP
      Right 0MCN
    Lower Extremity
      Left 0MCW
      Right 0MCV
    Perineum 0MCK
    Rib(s) 0MCG
    Shoulder
      Left 0MC2
      Right 0MC1
    Spine
      Lower 0MCD
      Upper 0MCC
    Sternum 0MCF
    Upper Extremity
      Left 0MCB
      Right 0MC9
    Wrist
      Left 0MC6

Extirpation — *continued*
  Bursa and Ligament — *continued*
    Wrist — *continued*
      Right ØMC5
  Carina ØBC2
  Carotid Bodies, Bilateral ØGC8
  Carotid Body
    Left ØGC6
    Right ØGC7
  Carpal
    Left ØPCN
    Right ØPCM
  Cavity, Cranial ØWC1
  Cecum ØDCH
  Cerebellum ØØCC
  Cerebral Hemisphere ØØC7
  Cerebral Meninges ØØC1
  Cerebral Ventricle ØØC6
  Cervix ØUCC
  Chordae Tendineae Ø2C9
  Choroid
    Left Ø8CB
    Right Ø8CA
  Cisterna Chyli Ø7CL
  Clavicle
    Left ØPCB
    Right ØPC9
  Clitoris ØUCJ
  Coccygeal Glomus ØGCB
  Coccyx ØQCS
  Colon
    Ascending ØDCK
    Descending ØDCM
    Sigmoid ØDCN
    Transverse ØDCL
  Computer-aided Mechanical Aspiration X2C
  Conduction Mechanism Ø2C8
  Conjunctiva
    Left Ø8CTXZZ
    Right Ø8CSXZZ
  Cord
    Bilateral ØVCH
    Left ØVCG
    Right ØVCF
  Cornea
    Left Ø8C9XZZ
    Right Ø8C8XZZ
  Cul-de-sac ØUCF
  Diaphragm ØBCT
  Disc
    Cervical Vertebral ØRC3
    Cervicothoracic Vertebral ØRC5
    Lumbar Vertebral ØSC2
    Lumbosacral ØSC4
    Thoracic Vertebral ØRC9
    Thoracolumbar Vertebral ØRCB
  Duct
    Common Bile ØFC9
    Cystic ØFC8
    Hepatic
      Common ØFC7
      Left ØFC6
      Right ØFC5
    Lacrimal
      Left Ø8CY
      Right Ø8CX
    Pancreatic ØFCD
      Accessory ØFCF
    Parotid
      Left ØCCC
      Right ØCCB
  Duodenum ØDC9
  Dura Mater ØØC2
  Ear
    External
      Left Ø9C1
      Right Ø9CØ
    External Auditory Canal
      Left Ø9C4
      Right Ø9C3
    Inner
      Left Ø9CE
      Right Ø9CD
    Middle
      Left Ø9C6
      Right Ø9C5
  Endometrium ØUCB
  Epididymis
    Bilateral ØVCL

Extirpation — *continued*
  Epididymis — *continued*
    Left ØVCK
    Right ØVCJ
  Epidural Space, Intracranial ØØC3
  Epiglottis ØCCR
  Esophagogastric Junction ØDC4
  Esophagus ØDC5
    Lower ØDC3
    Middle ØDC2
    Upper ØDC1
  Eustachian Tube
    Left Ø9CG
    Right Ø9CF
  Eye
    Left Ø8C1XZZ
    Right Ø8CØXZZ
  Eyelid
    Lower
      Left Ø8CR
      Right Ø8CQ
    Upper
      Left Ø8CP
      Right Ø8CN
  Fallopian Tube
    Left ØUC6
    Right ØUC5
  Fallopian Tubes, Bilateral ØUC7
  Femoral Shaft
    Left ØQC9
    Right ØQC8
  Femur
    Lower
      Left ØQCC
      Right ØQCB
    Upper
      Left ØQC7
      Right ØQC6
  Fibula
    Left ØQCK
    Right ØQCJ
  Finger Nail ØHCQXZZ
  Gallbladder ØFC4
  Gastrointestinal Tract ØWCP
  Genitourinary Tract ØWCR
  Gingiva
    Lower ØCC6
    Upper ØCC5
  Gland
    Adrenal
      Bilateral ØGC4
      Left ØGC2
      Right ØGC3
    Lacrimal
      Left Ø8CW
      Right Ø8CV
    Minor Salivary ØCCJ
    Parotid
      Left ØCC9
      Right ØCC8
    Pituitary ØGCØ
    Sublingual
      Left ØCCF
      Right ØCCD
    Submaxillary
      Left ØCCH
      Right ØCCG
    Vestibular ØUCL
  Glenoid Cavity
    Left ØPC8
    Right ØPC7
  Glomus Jugulare ØGCC
  Humeral Head
    Left ØPCD
    Right ØPCC
  Humeral Shaft
    Left ØPCG
    Right ØPCF
  Hymen ØUCK
  Hypothalamus ØØCA
  Ileocecal Valve ØDCC
  Ileum ØDCB
  Intestine
    Large ØDCE
      Left ØDCG
      Right ØDCF
    Small ØDC8
  Iris
    Left Ø8CD

Extirpation — *continued*
  Iris — *continued*
    Right Ø8CC
  Jaw
    Lower ØWC5
    Upper ØWC4
  Jejunum ØDCA
  Joint
    Acromioclavicular
      Left ØRCH
      Right ØRCG
    Ankle
      Left ØSCG
      Right ØSCF
    Carpal
      Left ØRCR
      Right ØRCQ
    Carpometacarpal
      Left ØRCT
      Right ØRCS
    Cervical Vertebral ØRC1
    Cervicothoracic Vertebral ØRC4
    Coccygeal ØSC6
    Elbow
      Left ØRCM
      Right ØRCL
    Finger Phalangeal
      Left ØRCX
      Right ØRCW
    Hip
      Left ØSCB
      Right ØSC9
    Knee
      Left ØSCD
      Right ØSCC
    Lumbar Vertebral ØSCØ
    Lumbosacral ØSC3
    Metacarpophalangeal
      Left ØRCV
      Right ØRCU
    Metatarsal-Phalangeal
      Left ØSCN
      Right ØSCM
    Occipital-cervical ØRCØ
    Sacrococcygeal ØSC5
    Sacroiliac
      Left ØSC8
      Right ØSC7
    Shoulder
      Left ØRCK
      Right ØRCJ
    Sternoclavicular
      Left ØRCF
      Right ØRCE
    Tarsal
      Left ØSCJ
      Right ØSCH
    Tarsometatarsal
      Left ØSCL
      Right ØSCK
    Temporomandibular
      Left ØRCD
      Right ØRCC
    Thoracic Vertebral ØRC6
    Thoracolumbar Vertebral ØRCA
    Toe Phalangeal
      Left ØSCQ
      Right ØSCP
    Wrist
      Left ØRCP
      Right ØRCN
  Kidney
    Left ØTC1
    Right ØTCØ
  Kidney Pelvis
    Left ØTC4
    Right ØTC3
  Larynx ØCCS
  Lens
    Left Ø8CK
    Right Ø8CJ
  Lip
    Lower ØCC1
    Upper ØCCØ
  Liver ØFCØ
    Left Lobe ØFC2
    Right Lobe ØFC1
  Lung
    Bilateral ØBCM

▽ **Subterms under main terms may continue to next column or page**

Extirpation — *continued*
Lung — *continued*
Left 0BCL
Lower Lobe
Left 0BCJ
Right 0BCF
Middle Lobe, Right 0BCD
Right 0BCK
Upper Lobe
Left 0BCG
Right 0BCC
Lung Lingula 0BCH
Lymphatic
Aortic 07CD
Axillary
Left 07C6
Right 07C5
Head 07C0
Inguinal
Left 07CJ
Right 07CH
Internal Mammary
Left 07C9
Right 07C8
Lower Extremity
Left 07CG
Right 07CF
Mesenteric 07CB
Neck
Left 07C2
Right 07C1
Pelvis 07CC
Thoracic Duct 07CK
Thorax 07C7
Upper Extremity
Left 07C4
Right 07C3
Mandible
Left 0NCV
Right 0NCT
Maxilla 0NCR
Mediastinum 0WCC
Medulla Oblongata 00CD
Mesentery 0DCV
Metacarpal
Left 0PCQ
Right 0PCP
Metatarsal
Left 0QCP
Right 0QCN
Muscle
Abdomen
Left 0KCL
Right 0KCK
Extraocular
Left 08CM
Right 08CL
Facial 0KC1
Foot
Left 0KCW
Right 0KCV
Hand
Left 0KCD
Right 0KCC
Head 0KC0
Hip
Left 0KCP
Right 0KCN
Lower Arm and Wrist
Left 0KCB
Right 0KC9
Lower Leg
Left 0KCT
Right 0KCS
Neck
Left 0KC3
Right 0KC2
Papillary 02CD
Perineum 0KCM
Shoulder
Left 0KC6
Right 0KC5
Thorax
Left 0KCJ
Right 0KCH
Tongue, Palate, Pharynx 0KC4
Trunk
Left 0KCG
Right 0KCF

Extirpation — *continued*
Muscle — *continued*
Upper Arm
Left 0KC8
Right 0KC7
Upper Leg
Left 0KCR
Right 0KCQ
Nasal Mucosa and Soft Tissue 09CK
Nasopharynx 09CN
Nerve
Abdominal Sympathetic 01CM
Abducens 00CL
Accessory 00CR
Acoustic 00CN
Brachial Plexus 01C3
Cervical 01C1
Cervical Plexus 01C0
Facial 00CM
Femoral 01CD
Glossopharyngeal 00CP
Head and Neck Sympathetic 01CK
Hypoglossal 00CS
Lumbar 01CB
Lumbar Plexus 01C9
Lumbar Sympathetic 01CN
Lumbosacral Plexus 01CA
Median 01C5
Oculomotor 00CH
Olfactory 00CF
Optic 00CG
Peroneal 01CH
Phrenic 01C2
Pudendal 01CC
Radial 01C6
Sacral 01CR
Sacral Plexus 01CQ
Sacral Sympathetic 01CP
Sciatic 01CF
Thoracic 01C8
Thoracic Sympathetic 01CL
Tibial 01CG
Trigeminal 00CK
Trochlear 00CJ
Ulnar 01C4
Vagus 00CQ
Nipple
Left 0HCX
Right 0HCW
Omentum 0DCU
Oral Cavity and Throat 0WC3
Orbit
Left 0NCQ
Right 0NCP
Orbital Atherectomy *see* Extirpation, Heart and
  Great Vessels 02C
Ovary
Bilateral 0UC2
Left 0UC1
Right 0UC0
Palate
Hard 0CC2
Soft 0CC3
Pancreas 0FCG
Para-aortic Body 0GC9
Paraganglion Extremity 0GCF
Parathyroid Gland 0GCR
Inferior
Left 0GCP
Right 0GCN
Multiple 0GCQ
Superior
Left 0GCM
Right 0GCL
Patella
Left 0QCF
Right 0QCD
Pelvic Cavity 0WCJ
Penis 0VCS
Pericardial Cavity 0WCD
Pericardium 02CN
Peritoneal Cavity 0WCG
Peritoneum 0DCW
Phalanx
Finger
Left 0PCV
Right 0PCT
Thumb
Left 0PCS

Extirpation — *continued*
Phalanx — *continued*
Thumb — *continued*
Right 0PCR
Toe
Left 0QCR
Right 0QCQ
Pharynx 0CCM
Pineal Body 0GC1
Pleura
Left 0BCP
Right 0BCN
Pleural Cavity
Left 0WCB
Right 0WC9
Pons 00CB
Prepuce 0VCT
Prostate 0VC0
Radius
Left 0PCJ
Right 0PCH
Rectum 0DCP
Respiratory Tract 0WCQ
Retina
Left 08CF
Right 08CE
Retinal Vessel
Left 08CH
Right 08CG
Retroperitoneum 0WCH
Ribs
1 to 2 0PC1
3 or More 0PC2
Sacrum 0QC1
Scapula
Left 0PC6
Right 0PC5
Sclera
Left 08C7XZZ
Right 08C6XZZ
Scrotum 0VC5
Septum
Atrial 02C5
Nasal 09CM
Ventricular 02CM
Sinus
Accessory 09CP
Ethmoid
Left 09CV
Right 09CU
Frontal
Left 09CT
Right 09CS
Mastoid
Left 09CC
Right 09CB
Maxillary
Left 09CR
Right 09CQ
Sphenoid
Left 09CX
Right 09CW
Skin
Abdomen 0HC7XZZ
Back 0HC6XZZ
Buttock 0HC8XZZ
Chest 0HC5XZZ
Ear
Left 0HC3XZZ
Right 0HC2XZZ
Face 0HC1XZZ
Foot
Left 0HCNXZZ
Right 0HCMXZZ
Hand
Left 0HCGXZZ
Right 0HCFXZZ
Inguinal 0HCAXZZ
Lower Arm
Left 0HCEXZZ
Right 0HCDXZZ
Lower Leg
Left 0HCLXZZ
Right 0HCKXZZ
Neck 0HC4XZZ
Perineum 0HC9XZZ
Scalp 0HC0XZZ
Upper Arm
Left 0HCCXZZ

Extirpation — *continued*
 Skin — *continued*
  Upper Arm — *continued*
   Right ØHCBXZZ
  Upper Leg
   Left ØHCJXZZ
   Right ØHCHXZZ
 Spinal Canal ØØCU
 Spinal Cord
  Cervical ØØCW
  Lumbar ØØCY
  Thoracic ØØCX
 Spinal Meninges ØØCT
 Spleen Ø7CP
 Sternum ØPCØ
 Stomach ØDC6
  Pylorus ØDC7
 Subarachnoid Space, Intracranial ØØC5
 Subcutaneous Tissue and Fascia
  Abdomen ØJC8
  Back ØJC7
  Buttock ØJC9
  Chest ØJC6
  Face ØJC1
  Foot
   Left ØJCR
   Right ØJCQ
  Hand
   Left ØJCK
   Right ØJCJ
  Lower Arm
   Left ØJCH
   Right ØJCG
  Lower Leg
   Left ØJCP
   Right ØJCN
  Neck
   Left ØJC5
   Right ØJC4
  Pelvic Region ØJCC
  Perineum ØJCB
  Scalp ØJCØ
  Upper Arm
   Left ØJCF
   Right ØJCD
  Upper Leg
   Left ØJCM
   Right ØJCL
 Subdural Space, Intracranial ØØC4
 Tarsal
  Left ØQCM
  Right ØQCL
 Tendon
  Abdomen
   Left ØLCG
   Right ØLCF
  Ankle
   Left ØLCT
   Right ØLCS
  Foot
   Left ØLCW
   Right ØLCV
  Hand
   Left ØLC8
   Right ØLC7
  Head and Neck ØLCØ
  Hip
   Left ØLCK
   Right ØLCJ
  Knee
   Left ØLCR
   Right ØLCQ
  Lower Arm and Wrist
   Left ØLC6
   Right ØLC5
  Lower Leg
   Left ØLCP
   Right ØLCN
  Perineum ØLCH
  Shoulder
   Left ØLC2
   Right ØLC1
  Thorax
   Left ØLCD
   Right ØLCC
  Trunk
   Left ØLCB
   Right ØLC9

Extirpation — *continued*
 Tendon — *continued*
  Upper Arm
   Left ØLC4
   Right ØLC3
  Upper Leg
   Left ØLCM
   Right ØLCL
 Testis
  Bilateral ØVCC
  Left ØVCB
  Right ØVC9
 Thalamus ØØC9
 Thymus Ø7CM
 Thyroid Gland ØGCK
  Left Lobe ØGCG
  Right Lobe ØGCH
 Tibia
  Left ØQCH
  Right ØQCG
 Toe Nail ØHCRXZZ
 Tongue ØCC7
 Tonsils ØCCP
 Tooth
  Lower ØCCX
  Upper ØCCW
 Trachea ØBC1
 Tunica Vaginalis
  Left ØVC7
  Right ØVC6
 Turbinate, Nasal Ø9CL
 Tympanic Membrane
  Left Ø9C8
  Right Ø9C7
 Ulna
  Left ØPCL
  Right ØPCK
 Ureter
  Left ØTC7
  Right ØTC6
 Urethra ØTCD
 Uterine Supporting Structure ØUC4
 Uterus ØUC9
 Uvula ØCCN
 Vagina ØUCG
 Valve
  Aortic Ø2CF
  Mitral Ø2CG
  Pulmonary Ø2CH
  Tricuspid Ø2CJ
 Vas Deferens
  Bilateral ØVCQ
  Left ØVCP
  Right ØVCN
 Vein
  Axillary
   Left Ø5C8
   Right Ø5C7
  Azygos Ø5CØ
  Basilic
   Left Ø5CC
   Right Ø5CB
  Brachial
   Left Ø5CA
   Right Ø5C9
  Cephalic
   Left Ø5CF
   Right Ø5CD
  Colic Ø6C7
  Common Iliac
   Left Ø6CD
   Right Ø6CC
  Coronary Ø2C4
  Esophageal Ø6C3
  External Iliac
   Left Ø6CG
   Right Ø6CF
  External Jugular
   Left Ø5CQ
   Right Ø5CP
  Face
   Left Ø5CV
   Right Ø5CT
  Femoral
   Left Ø6CN
   Right Ø6CM
  Foot
   Left Ø6CV
   Right Ø6CT

Extirpation — *continued*
 Vein — *continued*
  Gastric Ø6C2
  Hand
   Left Ø5CH
   Right Ø5CG
  Hemiazygos Ø5C1
  Hepatic Ø6C4
  Hypogastric
   Left Ø6CJ
   Right Ø6CH
  Inferior Mesenteric Ø6C6
  Innominate
   Left Ø5C4
   Right Ø5C3
  Internal Jugular
   Left Ø5CN
   Right Ø5CM
  Intracranial Ø5CL
  Lower Ø6CY
  Portal Ø6C8
  Pulmonary
   Left Ø2CT
   Right Ø2CS
  Renal
   Left Ø6CB
   Right Ø6C9
  Saphenous
   Left Ø6CQ
   Right Ø6CP
  Splenic Ø6C1
  Subclavian
   Left Ø5C6
   Right Ø5C5
  Superior Mesenteric Ø6C5
  Upper Ø5CY
  Vertebral
   Left Ø5CS
   Right Ø5CR
 Vena Cava
  Inferior Ø6CØ
  Superior Ø2CV
 Ventricle
  Left Ø2CL
  Right Ø2CK
 Vertebra
  Cervical ØPC3
  Lumbar ØQCØ
  Thoracic ØPC4
 Vesicle
  Bilateral ØVC3
  Left ØVC2
  Right ØVC1
 Vitreous
  Left Ø8C5
  Right Ø8C4
 Vocal Cord
  Left ØCCV
  Right ØCCT
 Vulva ØUCM
Extracorporeal Carbon Dioxide Removal (ECCO2R)
 5AØ92ØZ
Extracorporeal shock wave lithotripsy *see* Fragmentation
Extracranial-intracranial bypass (EC-IC) *see* Bypass, Upper Arteries Ø31
Extraction
 Acetabulum
  Left ØQD5ØZZ
  Right ØQD4ØZZ
 Ampulla of Vater ØFDC
 Anus ØDDQ
 Appendix ØDDJ
 Auditory Ossicle
  Left Ø9DAØZZ
  Right Ø9D9ØZZ
 Bone
  Ethmoid
   Left ØNDGØZZ
   Right ØNDFØZZ
  Frontal ØND1ØZZ
  Hyoid ØNDXØZZ
  Lacrimal
   Left ØNDJØZZ
   Right ØNDHØZZ
  Nasal ØNDBØZZ
  Occipital ØND7ØZZ
  Palatine
   Left ØNDLØZZ

Extraction — *continued*
- Bone — *continued*
  - Palatine — *continued*
    - Right 0NDK0ZZ
  - Parietal
    - Left 0ND40ZZ
    - Right 0ND30ZZ
  - Pelvic
    - Left 0QD30ZZ
    - Right 0QD20ZZ
  - Sphenoid 0NDC0ZZ
  - Temporal
    - Left 0ND60ZZ
    - Right 0ND50ZZ
  - Zygomatic
    - Left 0NDN0ZZ
    - Right 0NDM0ZZ
- Bone Marrow 07DT
  - Iliac 07DR
  - Sternum 07DQ
  - Vertebral 07DS
- Brain 00D0
- Breast
  - Bilateral 0HDV0ZZ
  - Left 0HDU0ZZ
  - Right 0HDT0ZZ
  - Supernumerary 0HDY0ZZ
- Bronchus
  - Lingula 0BD9
  - Lower Lobe
    - Left 0BDB
    - Right 0BD6
  - Main
    - Left 0BD7
    - Right 0BD3
  - Middle Lobe, Right 0BD5
  - Upper Lobe
    - Left 0BD8
    - Right 0BD4
- Bursa and Ligament
  - Abdomen
    - Left 0MDJ
    - Right 0MDH
  - Ankle
    - Left 0MDR
    - Right 0MDQ
  - Elbow
    - Left 0MD4
    - Right 0MD3
  - Foot
    - Left 0MDT
    - Right 0MDS
  - Hand
    - Left 0MD8
    - Right 0MD7
  - Head and Neck 0MD0
  - Hip
    - Left 0MDM
    - Right 0MDL
  - Knee
    - Left 0MDP
    - Right 0MDN
  - Lower Extremity
    - Left 0MDW
    - Right 0MDV
  - Perineum 0MDK
  - Rib(s) 0MDG
  - Shoulder
    - Left 0MD2
    - Right 0MD1
  - Spine
    - Lower 0MDD
    - Upper 0MDC
  - Sternum 0MDF
  - Upper Extremity
    - Left 0MDB
    - Right 0MD9
  - Wrist
    - Left 0MD6
    - Right 0MD5
- Carina 0BD2
- Carpal
  - Left 0PDN0ZZ
  - Right 0PDM0ZZ
- Cecum 0DDH
- Cerebellum 00DC
- Cerebral Hemisphere 00D7
- Cerebral Meninges 00D1
- Cisterna Chyli 07DL

Extraction — *continued*
- Clavicle
  - Left 0PDB0ZZ
  - Right 0PD90ZZ
- Coccyx 0QDS0ZZ
- Colon
  - Ascending 0DDK
  - Descending 0DDM
  - Sigmoid 0DDN
  - Transverse 0DDL
- Cornea
  - Left 08D9XZ
  - Right 08D8XZ
- Duct
  - Common Bile 0FD9
  - Cystic 0FD8
  - Hepatic
    - Common 0FD7
    - Left 0FD6
    - Right 0FD5
  - Pancreatic 0FDD
    - Accessory 0FDF
- Duodenum 0DD9
- Dura Mater 00D2
- Endometrium 0UDB
- Esophagogastric Junction 0DD4
- Esophagus 0DD5
  - Lower 0DD3
  - Middle 0DD2
  - Upper 0DD1
- Femoral Shaft
  - Left 0QD90ZZ
  - Right 0QD80ZZ
- Femur
  - Lower
    - Left 0QDC0ZZ
    - Right 0QDB0ZZ
  - Upper
    - Left 0QD70ZZ
    - Right 0QD60ZZ
- Fibula
  - Left 0QDK0ZZ
  - Right 0QDJ0ZZ
- Finger Nail 0HDQXZZ
- Gallbladder 0FD4
- Glenoid Cavity
  - Left 0PD80ZZ
  - Right 0PD70ZZ
- Hair 0HDSXZZ
- Humeral Head
  - Left 0PDD0ZZ
  - Right 0PDC0ZZ
- Humeral Shaft
  - Left 0PDG0ZZ
  - Right 0PDF0ZZ
- Ileocecal Valve 0DDC
- Ileum 0DDB
- Intestine
  - Large 0DDE
    - Left 0DDG
    - Right 0DDF
  - Small 0DD8
- Jejunum 0DDA
- Kidney
  - Left 0TD1
  - Right 0TD0
- Lens
  - Left 08DK3ZZ
  - Right 08DJ3ZZ
- Liver 0FD0
  - Left Lobe 0FD2
  - Right Lobe 0FD1
- Lung
  - Bilateral 0BDM
  - Left 0BDL
  - Lower Lobe
    - Left 0BDJ
    - Right 0BDF
  - Middle Lobe, Right 0BDD
  - Right 0BDK
  - Upper Lobe
    - Left 0BDG
    - Right 0BDC
- Lung Lingula 0BDH
- Lymphatic
  - Aortic 07DD
  - Axillary
    - Left 07D6
    - Right 07D5

Extraction — *continued*
- Lymphatic — *continued*
  - Head 07D0
  - Inguinal
    - Left 07DJ
    - Right 07DH
  - Internal Mammary
    - Left 07D9
    - Right 07D8
  - Lower Extremity
    - Left 07DG
    - Right 07DF
  - Mesenteric 07DB
  - Neck
    - Left 07D2
    - Right 07D1
  - Pelvis 07DC
  - Thoracic Duct 07DK
  - Thorax 07D7
  - Upper Extremity
    - Left 07D4
    - Right 07D3
- Mandible
  - Left 0NDV0ZZ
  - Right 0NDT0ZZ
- Maxilla 0NDR0ZZ
- Metacarpal
  - Left 0PDQ0ZZ
  - Right 0PDP0ZZ
- Metatarsal
  - Left 0QDP0ZZ
  - Right 0QDN0ZZ
- Muscle
  - Abdomen
    - Left 0KDL0ZZ
    - Right 0KDK0ZZ
  - Facial 0KD10ZZ
  - Foot
    - Left 0KDW0ZZ
    - Right 0KDV0ZZ
  - Hand
    - Left 0KDD0ZZ
    - Right 0KDC0ZZ
  - Head 0KD00ZZ
  - Hip
    - Left 0KDP0ZZ
    - Right 0KDN0ZZ
  - Lower Arm and Wrist
    - Left 0KDB0ZZ
    - Right 0KD90ZZ
  - Lower Leg
    - Left 0KDT0ZZ
    - Right 0KDS0ZZ
  - Neck
    - Left 0KD30ZZ
    - Right 0KD20ZZ
  - Perineum 0KDM0ZZ
  - Shoulder
    - Left 0KD60ZZ
    - Right 0KD50ZZ
  - Thorax
    - Left 0KDJ0ZZ
    - Right 0KDH0ZZ
  - Tongue, Palate, Pharynx 0KD40ZZ
  - Trunk
    - Left 0KDG0ZZ
    - Right 0KDF0ZZ
  - Upper Arm
    - Left 0KD80ZZ
    - Right 0KD70ZZ
  - Upper Leg
    - Left 0KDR0ZZ
    - Right 0KDQ0ZZ
- Nerve
  - Abdominal Sympathetic 01DM
  - Abducens 00DL
  - Accessory 00DR
  - Acoustic 00DN
  - Brachial Plexus 01D3
  - Cervical 01D1
  - Cervical Plexus 01D0
  - Facial 00DM
  - Femoral 01DD
  - Glossopharyngeal 00DP
  - Head and Neck Sympathetic 01DK
  - Hypoglossal 00DS
  - Lumbar 01DB
  - Lumbar Plexus 01D9
  - Lumbar Sympathetic 01DN

Extraction — *continued*
 Nerve — *continued*
  Lumbosacral Plexus 01DA
  Median 01D5
  Oculomotor 00DH
  Olfactory 00DF
  Optic 00DG
  Peroneal 01DH
  Phrenic 01D2
  Pudendal 01DC
  Radial 01D6
  Sacral 01DR
  Sacral Plexus 01DQ
  Sacral Sympathetic 01DP
  Sciatic 01DF
  Thoracic 01D8
  Thoracic Sympathetic 01DL
  Tibial 01DG
  Trigeminal 00DK
  Trochlear 00DJ
  Ulnar 01D4
  Vagus 00DQ
 Orbit
  Left 0NDQ0ZZ
  Right 0NDP0ZZ
 Ova 0UDN
 Pancreas 0FDG
 Patella
  Left 0QDF0ZZ
  Right 0QDD0ZZ
 Phalanx
  Finger
   Left 0PDV0ZZ
   Right 0PDT0ZZ
  Thumb
   Left 0PDS0ZZ
   Right 0PDR0ZZ
  Toe
   Left 0QDR0ZZ
   Right 0QDQ0ZZ
 Pleura
  Left 0BDP
  Right 0BDN
 Products of Conception
  Ectopic 10D2
  Extraperitoneal 10D00Z2
  High 10D00Z0
  High Forceps 10D07Z5
  Internal Version 10D07Z7
  Low 10D00Z1
  Low Forceps 10D07Z3
  Mid Forceps 10D07Z4
  Other 10D07Z8
  Retained 10D1
  Vacuum 10D07Z6
 Radius
  Left 0PDJ0ZZ
  Right 0PDH0ZZ
 Rectum 0DDP
 Ribs
  1 to 2 0PD10ZZ
  3 or More 0PD20ZZ
 Sacrum 0QD10ZZ
 Scapula
  Left 0PD60ZZ
  Right 0PD50ZZ
 Septum, Nasal 09DM
 Sinus
  Accessory 09DP
  Ethmoid
   Left 09DV
   Right 09DU
  Frontal
   Left 09DT
   Right 09DS
  Mastoid
   Left 09DC
   Right 09DB
  Maxillary
   Left 09DR
   Right 09DQ
  Sphenoid
   Left 09DX
   Right 09DW
 Skin
  Abdomen 0HD7XZZ
  Back 0HD6XZZ
  Buttock 0HD8XZZ
  Chest 0HD5XZZ

Extraction — *continued*
 Skin — *continued*
  Ear
   Left 0HD3XZZ
   Right 0HD2XZZ
  Face 0HD1XZZ
  Foot
   Left 0HDNXZZ
   Right 0HDMXZZ
  Hand
   Left 0HDGXZZ
   Right 0HDFXZZ
  Inguinal 0HDAXZZ
  Lower Arm
   Left 0HDEXZZ
   Right 0HDDXZZ
  Lower Leg
   Left 0HDLXZZ
   Right 0HDKXZZ
  Neck 0HD4XZZ
  Perineum 0HD9XZZ
  Scalp 0HD0XZZ
  Upper Arm
   Left 0HDCXZZ
   Right 0HDBXZZ
  Upper Leg
   Left 0HDJXZZ
   Right 0HDHXZZ
 Skull 0ND00ZZ
 Spinal Meninges 00DT
 Spleen 07DP
 Sternum 0PD00ZZ
 Stomach 0DD6
  Pylorus 0DD7
 Subcutaneous Tissue and Fascia
  Abdomen 0JD8
  Back 0JD7
  Buttock 0JD9
  Chest 0JD6
  Face 0JD1
  Foot
   Left 0JDR
   Right 0JDQ
  Hand
   Left 0JDK
   Right 0JDJ
  Lower Arm
   Left 0JDH
   Right 0JDG
  Lower Leg
   Left 0JDP
   Right 0JDN
  Neck
   Left 0JD5
   Right 0JD4
  Pelvic Region 0JDC
  Perineum 0JDB
  Scalp 0JD0
  Upper Arm
   Left 0JDF
   Right 0JDD
  Upper Leg
   Left 0JDM
   Right 0JDL
 Tarsal
  Left 0QDM0ZZ
  Right 0QDL0ZZ
 Tendon
  Abdomen
   Left 0LDG0ZZ
   Right 0LDF0ZZ
  Ankle
   Left 0LDT0ZZ
   Right 0LDS0ZZ
  Foot
   Left 0LDW0ZZ
   Right 0LDV0ZZ
  Hand
   Left 0LD80ZZ
   Right 0LD70ZZ
  Head and Neck 0LD00ZZ
  Hip
   Left 0LDK0ZZ
   Right 0LDJ0ZZ
  Knee
   Left 0LDR0ZZ
   Right 0LDQ0ZZ
  Lower Arm and Wrist
   Left 0LD60ZZ

Extraction — *continued*
 Tendon — *continued*
  Lower Arm and Wrist — *continued*
   Right 0LD50ZZ
  Lower Leg
   Left 0LDP0ZZ
   Right 0LDN0ZZ
  Perineum 0LDH0ZZ
  Shoulder
   Left 0LD20ZZ
   Right 0LD10ZZ
  Thorax
   Left 0LDD0ZZ
   Right 0LDC0ZZ
  Trunk
   Left 0LDB0ZZ
   Right 0LD90ZZ
  Upper Arm
   Left 0LD40ZZ
   Right 0LD30ZZ
  Upper Leg
   Left 0LDM0ZZ
   Right 0DLL0ZZ
 Thymus 07DM
 Tibia
  Left 0QDH0ZZ
  Right 0QDG0ZZ
 Toe Nail 0HDRXZZ
 Tooth
  Lower 0CDXXZ
  Upper 0CDWXZ
 Trachea 0BD1
 Turbinate, Nasal 09DL
 Tympanic Membrane
  Left 09D8
  Right 09D7
 Ulna
  Left 0PDL0ZZ
  Right 0PDK0ZZ
 Vein
  Basilic
   Left 05DC
   Right 05DB
  Brachial
   Left 05DA
   Right 05D9
  Cephalic
   Left 05DF
   Right 05DD
  Femoral
   Left 06DN
   Right 06DM
  Foot
   Left 06DV
   Right 06DT
  Hand
   Left 05DH
   Right 05DG
  Lower 06DY
  Saphenous
   Left 06DQ
   Right 06DP
  Upper 05DY
 Vertebra
  Cervical 0PD30ZZ
  Lumbar 0QD00ZZ
  Thoracic 0PD40ZZ
 Vocal Cord
  Left 0CDV
  Right 0CDT
Extradural space, intracranial *use* Epidural Space, Intracranial
Extradural space, spinal *use* Spinal Canal
EXtreme Lateral Interbody Fusion (XLIF) device *use* Interbody Fusion Device in Lower Joints

F

Face lift *see* Alteration, Face 0W02
Facet replacement spinal stabilization device
  use Spinal Stabilization Device, Facet Replacement in 0RH
  use Spinal Stabilization Device, Facet Replacement in 0SH
Facial artery *use* Face Artery
Factor Xa Inhibitor Reversal Agent, Andexanet Alfa *use* Coagulation Factor Xa, Inactivated
False vocal cord *use* Larynx

Falx cerebri *use* Dura Mater
Fascia lata
    use Subcutaneous Tissue and Fascia, Left Upper
        Leg
    use Subcutaneous Tissue and Fascia, Right Upper
        Leg
Fasciaplasty, fascioplasty
    see Repair, Subcutaneous Tissue and Fascia ØJQ
    see Replacement, Subcutaneous Tissue and Fascia
        ØJR
Fasciectomy *see* Excision, Subcutaneous Tissue and
    Fascia ØJB
Fasciorrhaphy *see* Repair, Subcutaneous Tissue and
    Fascia ØJQ
Fasciotomy
    see Division, Subcutaneous Tissue and Fascia ØJ8
    see Drainage, Subcutaneous Tissue and Fascia ØJ9
    see Release
Feeding Device
    Change device in
        Lower Intestinal Tract ØD2DXUZ
        Upper Intestinal Tract ØD20XUZ
    Insertion of device in
        Duodenum ØDH9
        Esophagus ØDH5
        Ileum ØDHB
        Intestine, Small ØDH8
        Jejunum ØDHA
        Stomach ØDH6
    Removal of device from
        Esophagus ØDP5
        Intestinal Tract
            Lower Intestinal Tract ØDPD
            Upper Intestinal Tract ØDPØ
        Stomach ØDP6
    Revision of device in
        Intestinal Tract
            Lower Intestinal Tract ØDWD
            Upper Intestinal Tract ØDWØ
        Stomach ØDW6
        Upper Intestinal Tract ØDWØ
Femoral head
    use Upper Femur, Left
    use Upper Femur, Right
Femoral lymph node
    use Lymphatic, Left Lower Extremity
    use Lymphatic, Right Lower Extremity
Femoropatellar joint
    use Knee Joint, Left
    use Knee Joint, Left, Tibial Surface
    use Knee Joint, Right
    use Knee Joint, Right, Femoral Surface
Femorotibial joint
    use Knee Joint, Left
    use Knee Joint, Left, Tibial Surface
    use Knee Joint, Right
    use Knee Joint, Right, Tibial Surface
FETROJA® *use* Cefiderocol Anti-infective
FGS (fluorescence-guided surgery) *see* Fluorescence
    Guided Procedure
Fibular artery
    use Peroneal Artery, Left
    use Peroneal Artery, Right
Fibular sesamoid
    use Metatarsal, Left
    use Metatarsal, Right
Fibularis brevis muscle
    use Lower Leg Muscle, Left
    use Lower Leg Muscle, Right
Fibularis longus muscle
    use Lower Leg Muscle, Left
    use Lower Leg Muscle, Right
Fifth cranial nerve *use* Trigeminal Nerve
Filum terminale *use* Spinal Meninges
Fimbriectomy
    see Excision, Female Reproductive System ØUB
    see Resection, Female Reproductive System ØUT
Fine needle aspiration
    Fluid or gas *see* Drainage
    Tissue biopsy
        see Excision
        see Extraction
First cranial nerve *use* Olfactory Nerve
First intercostal nerve *use* Brachial Plexus
Fistulization
    see Bypass
    see Drainage

Fistulization — *continued*
    see Repair
Fitting
    Arch bars, for fracture reduction *see* Reposition,
        Mouth and Throat ØCS
    Arch bars, for immobilization *see* Immobilization,
        Face 2W31
    Artificial limb *see* Device Fitting, Rehabilitation
        FØD
    Hearing aid *see* Device Fitting, Rehabilitation FØD
    Ocular prosthesis FØDZ8UZ
    Prosthesis, limb *see* Device Fitting, Rehabilitation
        FØD
    Prosthesis, ocular FØDZ8UZ
Fixation, bone
    External, with fracture reduction *see* Reposition
    External, without fracture reduction *see* Insertion
    Internal, with fracture reduction *see* Reposition
    Internal, without fracture reduction *see* Insertion
FLAIR® Endovascular Stent Graft *use* Intraluminal
    Device
Flexible Composite Mesh *use* Synthetic Substitute
Flexor carpi radialis muscle
    use Lower Arm and Wrist Muscle, Left
    use Lower Arm and Wrist Muscle, Right
Flexor carpi ulnaris muscle
    use Lower Arm and Wrist Muscle, Left
    use Lower Arm and Wrist Muscle, Right
Flexor digitorum brevis muscle
    use Foot Muscle, Left
    use Foot Muscle, Right
Flexor digitorum longus muscle
    use Lower Leg Muscle, Left
    use Lower Leg Muscle, Right
Flexor hallucis brevis muscle
    use Foot Muscle, Left
    use Foot Muscle, Right
Flexor hallucis longus muscle
    use Lower Leg Muscle, Left
    use Lower Leg Muscle, Right
Flexor pollicis longus muscle
    use Lower Arm and Wrist Muscle, Left
    use Lower Arm and Wrist Muscle, Right
Flow Diverter embolization device *use* Intraluminal
    Device, Flow Diverter in Ø3V
FlowSense Noninvasive Thermal Sensor 4B00XW0
Fluorescence Guided Procedure
    Extremity
        Lower 8E0Y
        Upper 8E0X
    Head and Neck Region 8E09
        Aminolevulinic Acid 8E090EM
        No Qualifier 8E090EZ
    Trunk Region 8E0W
Fluorescent Pyrazine, Kidney XT25XE5
Fluoroscopy
    Abdomen and Pelvis BW11
    Airway, Upper BB1DZZZ
    Ankle
        Left BQ1H
        Right BQ1G
    Aorta
        Abdominal B410
            Laser, Intraoperative B410
        Thoracic B310
            Laser, Intraoperative B310
        Thoraco-Abdominal B31P
            Laser, Intraoperative B31P
    Aorta and Bilateral Lower Extremity Arteries B41D
        Laser, Intraoperative B41D
    Arm
        Left BP1FZZZ
        Right BP1EZZZ
    Artery
        Brachiocephalic-Subclavian
            Laser, Intraoperative B311
            Right B311
         Bronchial B31L
            Laser, Intraoperative B31L
         Bypass Graft, Other B21F
         Cervico-Cerebral Arch B31Q
            Laser, Intraoperative B31Q
         Common Carotid
            Bilateral B315
                Laser, Intraoperative B315
            Left B314
                Laser, Intraoperative B314

Fluoroscopy — *continued*
    Artery — *continued*
        Common Carotid — *continued*
            Right B313
                Laser, Intraoperative B313
        Coronary
            Bypass Graft
                Multiple B213
                    Laser, Intraoperative B213
                Single B212
                    Laser, Intraoperative B212
            Multiple B211
                Laser, Intraoperative B211
            Single B210
                Laser, Intraoperative B210
        External Carotid
            Bilateral B31C
                Laser, Intraoperative B31C
            Left B31B
                Laser, Intraoperative B31B
            Right B319
                Laser, Intraoperative B319
        Hepatic B412
            Laser, Intraoperative B412
        Inferior Mesenteric B415
            Laser, Intraoperative B415
        Intercostal B31L
            Laser, Intraoperative B31L
        Internal Carotid
            Bilateral B318
                Laser, Intraoperative B318
            Left B317
                Laser, Intraoperative B317
            Right B316
                Laser, Intraoperative B316
        Internal Mammary Bypass Graft
            Left B218
            Right B217
        Intra-Abdominal
            Laser, Intraoperative B41B
            Other B41B
        Intracranial B31R
            Laser, Intraoperative B31R
        Lower
            Laser, Intraoperative B41J
            Other B41J
        Lower Extremity
            Bilateral and Aorta B41D
                Laser, Intraoperative B41D
            Left B41G
                Laser, Intraoperative B41G
            Right B41F
                Laser, Intraoperative B41F
        Lumbar B419
            Laser, Intraoperative B419
        Pelvic B41C
            Laser, Intraoperative B41C
        Pulmonary
            Left B31T
                Laser, Intraoperative B31T
            Right B31S
                Laser, Intraoperative B31S
        Pulmonary Trunk B31U
            Laser, Intraoperative B31U
        Renal
            Bilateral B418
                Laser, Intraoperative B418
            Left B417
                Laser, Intraoperative B417
            Right B416
                Laser, Intraoperative B416
        Spinal B31M
            Laser, Intraoperative B31M
        Splenic B413
            Laser, Intraoperative B413
        Subclavian
            Laser, Intraoperative B312
            Left B312
        Superior Mesenteric B414
            Laser, Intraoperative B414
        Upper
            Laser, Intraoperative B31N
            Other B31N
        Upper Extremity
            Bilateral B31K
                Laser, Intraoperative B31K
            Left B31J
                Laser, Intraoperative B31J
            Right B31H

Fluoroscopy — *continued*
  Artery — *continued*
    Upper Extremity — *continued*
      Right — *continued*
        Laser, Intraoperative B31H
      Vertebral
        Bilateral B31G
          Laser, Intraoperative B31G
        Left B31F
          Laser, Intraoperative B31F
        Right B31D
          Laser, Intraoperative B31D
  Bile Duct BF10
    Pancreatic Duct and Gallbladder BF14
  Bile Duct and Gallbladder BF13
  Biliary Duct BF11
  Bladder BT10
    Kidney and Ureter BT14
    Left BT1F
    Right BT1D
  Bladder and Urethra BT1B
  Bowel, Small BD1
  Calcaneus
    Left BQ1KZZZ
    Right BQ1JZZZ
  Clavicle
    Left BP15ZZZ
    Right BP14ZZZ
  Coccyx BR1F
  Colon BD14
  Corpora Cavernosa BV10
  Dialysis Fistula B51W
  Dialysis Shunt B51W
  Diaphragm BB16ZZZ
  Disc
    Cervical BR11
    Lumbar BR13
    Thoracic BR12
  Duodenum BD19
  Elbow
    Left BP1H
    Right BP1G
  Epiglottis B91G
  Esophagus BD11
  Extremity
    Lower BW1C
    Upper BW1J
  Facet Joint
    Cervical BR14
    Lumbar BR16
    Thoracic BR15
  Fallopian Tube
    Bilateral BU12
    Left BU11
    Right BU10
  Fallopian Tube and Uterus BU18
  Femur
    Left BQ14ZZZ
    Right BQ13ZZZ
  Finger
    Left BP1SZZZ
    Right BP1RZZZ
  Foot
    Left BQ1MZZZ
    Right BQ1LZZZ
  Forearm
    Left BP1KZZZ
    Right BP1JZZZ
  Gallbladder BF12
    Bile Duct and Pancreatic Duct BF14
  Gallbladder and Bile Duct BF13
  Gastrointestinal, Upper BD1
  Hand
    Left BP1PZZZ
    Right BP1NZZZ
  Head and Neck BW19
  Heart
    Left B215
    Right B214
    Right and Left B216
  Hip
    Left BQ11
    Right BQ10
  Humerus
    Left BP1BZZZ
    Right BP1AZZZ
  Ileal Diversion Loop BT1C
  Ileal Loop, Ureters and Kidney BT1G
  Intracranial Sinus B512

Fluoroscopy — *continued*
  Joint
    Acromioclavicular, Bilateral BP13ZZZ
    Finger
      Left BP1D
      Right BP1C
    Foot
      Left BQ1Y
      Right BQ1X
    Hand
      Left BP1D
      Right BP1C
    Lumbosacral BR1B
    Sacroiliac BR1D
    Sternoclavicular
      Bilateral BP12ZZZ
      Left BP11ZZZ
      Right BP10ZZZ
    Temporomandibular
      Bilateral BN19
      Left BN18
      Right BN17
    Thoracolumbar BR18
    Toe
      Left BQ1Y
      Right BQ1X
  Kidney
    Bilateral BT13
    Ileal Loop and Ureter BT1G
    Left BT12
    Right BT11
    Ureter and Bladder BT14
      Left BT1F
      Right BT1D
  Knee
    Left BQ18
    Right BQ17
  Larynx B91J
  Leg
    Left BQ1FZZZ
    Right BQ1DZZZ
  Liver BF15
  Lung
    Bilateral BB14ZZZ
    Left BB13ZZZ
    Right BB12ZZZ
  Mediastinum BB1CZZZ
  Mouth BD1B
  Neck and Head BW19
  Oropharynx BD1B
  Pancreatic Duct BF1
    Gallbladder and Bile Buct BF14
  Patella
    Left BQ1WZZZ
    Right BQ1VZZZ
  Pelvis BR1C
  Pelvis and Abdomen BW11
  Pharynix B91G
  Ribs
    Left BP1YZZZ
    Right BP1XZZZ
  Sacrum BR1F
  Scapula
    Left BP17ZZZ
    Right BP16ZZZ
  Shoulder
    Left BP19
    Right BP18
  Sinus, Intracranial B512
  Spinal Cord B01B
  Spine
    Cervical BR10
    Lumbar BR19
    Thoracic BR17
    Whole BR1G
  Sternum BR1H
  Stomach BD12
  Toe
    Left BQ1QZZZ
    Right BQ1PZZZ
  Tracheobronchial Tree
    Bilateral BB19YZZ
    Left BB18YZZ
    Right BB17YZZ
  Ureter
    Ileal Loop and Kidney BT1G
    Kidney and Bladder BT14
    Left BT1F
    Right BT1D

Fluoroscopy — *continued*
  Ureter — *continued*
    Left BT17
    Right BT16
  Urethra BT15
  Urethra and Bladder BT1B
  Uterus BU16
  Uterus and Fallopian Tube BU18
  Vagina BU19
  Vasa Vasorum BV18
  Vein
    Cerebellar B511
    Cerebral B511
    Epidural B510
    Jugular
      Bilateral B515
      Left B514
      Right B513
    Lower Extremity
      Bilateral B51D
      Left B51C
      Right B51B
    Other B51V
    Pelvic (Iliac)
      Left B51G
      Right B51F
    Pelvic (Iliac) Bilateral B51H
    Portal B51T
    Pulmonary
      Bilateral B51S
      Left B51R
      Right B51Q
    Renal
      Bilateral B51L
      Left B51K
      Right B51J
    Spanchnic B51T
    Subclavian
      Left B517
      Right B516
    Upper Extremity
      Bilateral B51P
      Left B51N
      Right B51M
  Vena Cava
    Inferior B519
    Superior B518
  Wrist
    Left BP1M
    Right BP1L
Fluoroscopy, laser intraoperative
  see Fluoroscopy, Heart B21
  see Fluoroscopy, Lower Arteries B41
  see Fluoroscopy, Upper Arteries B31
Flushing *see* Irrigation
Foley catheter *use* Drainage Device
Fontan completion procedure Stage II *see* Bypass, Vena Cava, Inferior 0610
Foramen magnum *use* Occipital Bone
Foramen of Monro (intraventricular) *use* Cerebral Ventricle
Foreskin *use* Prepuce
Formula™ Balloon-Expandable Renal Stent System *use* Intraluminal Device
Fosfomycin Anti-infective XW0
Fosfomycin injection *use* Fosfomycin Anti-infective
Fossa of Rosenmuller *use* Nasopharynx
Fostamatinib XW0
Fourth cranial nerve *use* Trochlear Nerve
Fourth ventricle *use* Cerebral Ventricle
Fovea
  use Retina, Left
  use Retina, Right
Fragmentation
  Ampulla of Vater 0FFC
  Anus 0DFQ
  Appendix 0DFJ
  Artery
    Anterior Tibial
      Left 04FQ3Z
      Right 04FP3Z
    Axillary
      Left 03F63Z
      Right 03F53Z
    Brachial
      Left 03F83Z
      Right 03F73Z

Fragmentation — *continued*
Artery — *continued*
 Common Iliac
  Left 04FD3Z
  Right 04FC3Z
 Coronary
  Four or More Arteries 02F33ZZ
  One Artery 02F03ZZ
  Three Arteries 02F23ZZ
  Two Arteries 02F13ZZ
 External Iliac
  Left 04FJ3Z
  Right 04FH3Z
 Femoral
  Left 04FL3Z
  Right 04FK3Z
 Innominate 03F23Z
 Internal Iliac
  Left 04FF3Z
  Right 04FE3Z
 Intracranial 03FG3Z
 Lower 04FY3Z
 Peroneal
  Left 04FU3Z
  Right 04FT3Z
 Popliteal
  Left 04FN3Z
  Right 04FM3Z
 Posterior Tibial
  Left 04FS3Z
  Right 04FR3Z
 Pulmonary
  Left 02FR3Z
  Right 02FQ3Z
 Pulmonary Trunk 02FP3Z
 Radial
  Left 03FC3Z
  Right 03FB3Z
 Subclavian
  Left 03F43Z
  Right 03F33Z
 Ulnar
  Left 03FA3Z
  Right 03F93Z
 Upper 03FY3Z
Bladder 0TFB
Bladder Neck 0TFC
Bronchus
 Lingula 0BF9
 Lower Lobe
  Left 0BFB
  Right 0BF6
 Main
  Left 0BF7
  Right 0BF3
 Middle Lobe, Right 0BF5
 Upper Lobe
  Left 0BF8
  Right 0BF4
Carina 0BF2
Cavity, Cranial 0WF1
Cecum 0DFH
Cerebral Ventricle 00F6
Colon
 Ascending 0DFK
 Descending 0DFM
 Sigmoid 0DFN
 Transverse 0DFL
Duct
 Common Bile 0FF9
 Cystic 0FF8
 Hepatic
  Common 0FF7
  Left 0FF6
  Right 0FF5
 Pancreatic 0FFD
  Accessory 0FFF
 Parotid
  Left 0CFC
  Right 0CFB
Duodenum 0DF9
Epidural Space, Intracranial 00F3
Esophagus 0DF5
Fallopian Tube
 Left 0UF6
 Right 0UF5
Fallopian Tubes, Bilateral 0UF7
Gallbladder 0FF4
Gastrointestinal Tract 0WFP

Fragmentation — *continued*
Genitourinary Tract 0WFR
Ileum 0DFB
Intestine
 Large 0DFE
  Left 0DFG
  Right 0DFF
 Small 0DF8
Jejunum 0DFA
Kidney Pelvis
 Left 0TF4
 Right 0TF3
Mediastinum 0WFC
Oral Cavity and Throat 0WF3
Pelvic Cavity 0WFJ
Pericardial Cavity 0WFD
Pericardium 02FN
Peritoneal Cavity 0WFG
Pleural Cavity
 Left 0WFB
 Right 0WF9
Rectum 0DFP
Respiratory Tract 0WFO
Spinal Canal 00FU
Stomach 0DF6
Subarachnoid Space, Intracranial 00F5
Subdural Space, Intracranial 00F4
Trachea 0BF1
Ureter
 Left 0TF7
 Right 0TF6
Urethra 0TFD
Uterus 0UF9
Vein
 Axillary
  Left 05F83Z
  Right 05F73Z
 Basilic
  Left 05FC3Z
  Right 05FB3Z
 Brachial
  Left 05FA3Z
  Right 05F93Z
 Cephalic
  Left 05FF3Z
  Right 05FD3Z
 Common Iliac
  Left 06FD3Z
  Right 06FC3Z
 External Iliac
  Left 06FG3Z
  Right 06FF3Z
 Femoral
  Left 06FN3Z
  Right 06FM3Z
 Hypogastric
  Left 06FJ3Z
  Right 06FH3Z
 Innominate
  Left 05F43Z
  Right 05F33Z
 Lower 06FY3Z
 Pulmonary
  Left 02FT3Z
  Right 02FS3Z
 Saphenous
  Left 06FQ3Z
  Right 06FP3Z
 Subclavian
  Left 05F63Z
  Right 05F53Z
 Upper 05FY3Z
Vitreous
 Left 08F5
 Right 08F4
Fragmentation, Ultrasonic *see* Fragmentation, Artery
Freestyle (Stentless) Aortic Root Bioprosthesis *use* Zooplastic Tissue in Heart and Great Vessels
Frenectomy
 see Excision, Mouth and Throat 0CB
 see Resection, Mouth and Throat 0CT
Frenoplasty, frenuloplasty
 see Repair, Mouth and Throat 0CQ
 see Replacement, Mouth and Throat 0CR
 see Supplement, Mouth and Throat 0CU
Frenotomy
 see Drainage, Mouth and Throat 0C9
 see Release, Mouth and Throat 0CN

Frenulotomy
 see Drainage, Mouth and Throat 0C9
 see Release, Mouth and Throat 0CN
Frenulum labii inferioris *use* Lower Lip
Frenulum labii superioris *use* Upper Lip
Frenulum linguae *use* Tongue
Frenulumectomy
 see Excision, Mouth and Throat 0CB
 see Resection, Mouth and Throat 0CT
Frontal lobe *use* Cerebral Hemisphere
Frontal vein
 use Face Vein, Left
 use Face Vein, Right
Frozen elephant trunk (FET) technique, aortic arch replacement
 see New Technology, Cardiovascular System X2R
 see Replacement, Heart and Great Vessels 02R
Frozen elephant trunk (FET) technique, thoracic aorta restriction
 see New Technology, Cardiovascular System X2V
 see Restriction, Heart and Great Vessels 02V
FUJIFILM EP-7000X System for Oxygen Saturation Endoscopic Imaging (OXEI) *see* New Technology, Gastrointestinal System XD2
Fulguration *see* Destruction
Fundoplication, gastroesophageal *see* Restriction, Esophagogastric Junction 0DV4
Fundus uteri *use* Uterus
Fusion
Acromioclavicular
 Left 0RGH
 Right 0RGG
Ankle
 Left 0SGG
 Right 0SGF
Carpal
 Left 0RGR
 Right 0RGQ
Carpometacarpal
 Left 0RGT
 Right 0RGS
Cervical Vertebral 0RG1
 2 or more 0RG2
Cervicothoracic Vertebral 0RG4
Coccygeal 0SG6
Elbow
 Left 0RGM
 Right 0RGL
Finger Phalangeal
 Left 0RGX
 Right 0RGW
Hip
 Left 0SGB
 Right 0SG9
Knee
 Left 0SGD
 Right 0SGC
Lumbar Vertebral 0SG0
 2 or more 0SG1
  Interbody Fusion Device, Customizable XRGC
  Interbody Fusion Device, Customizable XRGB
Lumbosacral 0SG3
 Interbody Fusion Device, Customizable XRGD
Metacarpophalangeal
 Left 0RGV
 Right 0RGU
Metatarsal-Phalangeal
 Left 0SGN
 Right 0SGM
Occipital-cervical 0RG0
Sacrococcygeal 0SG5
Sacroiliac
 Internal Fixation Device with Tulip Connector XRG
 Left 0SG8
 Right 0SG7
Shoulder
 Left 0RGK
 Right 0RGJ
Sternoclavicular
 Left 0RGF
 Right 0RGE
Tarsal
 Left 0SGJ
 Right 0SGH
Tarsometatarsal
 Left 0SGL

Fusion — *continued*
  Tarsometatarsal — *continued*
    Right ØSGK
  Temporomandibular
    Left ØRGD
    Right ØRGC
  Thoracic Vertebral ØRG6
    2 to 7 ØRG7
    8 or more ØRG8
  Thoracolumbar Vertebral ØRGA
    Interbody Fusion Device, Customizable XRGA
  Toe Phalangeal
    Left ØSGQ
    Right ØSGP
  Wrist
    Left ØRGP
    Right ØRGN
Fusion screw (compression) (lag) (locking)
  use Internal Fixation Device in Lower Joints
  use Internal Fixation Device in Upper Joints

G

Gait training *see* Motor Treatment, Rehabilitation FØ7
Galea aponeurotica *use* Subcutaneous Tissue and Fascia, Scalp
Gammaglobulin *use* Globulin
GammaTile™ *use* Radioactive Element, Cesium-131 Collagen Implant in ØØH
GAMUNEX-C, for COVID-19 treatment *use* High-Dose Intravenous Immune Globulin
Ganglion impar (ganglion of Walther) *use* Sacral Sympathetic Nerve
Ganglionectomy
  Destruction of lesion *see* Destruction
  Excision of lesion *see* Excision
Gasserian ganglion *use* Trigeminal Nerve
Gastrectomy
  Partial *see* Excision, Stomach ØDB6
  Total *see* Resection, Stomach ØDT6
  Vertical (sleeve) *see* Excision, Stomach ØDB6
Gastric electrical stimulation (GES) lead *use* Stimulator Lead in Gastrointestinal System
Gastric lymph node *use* Lymphatic, Aortic
Gastric pacemaker lead *use* Stimulator Lead in Gastrointestinal System
Gastric plexus *use* Abdominal Sympathetic Nerve
Gastrocnemius muscle
  use Lower Leg Muscle, Left
  use Lower Leg Muscle, Right
Gastrocolic ligament *use* Omentum
Gastrocolic omentum *use* Omentum
Gastrocolostomy
  see Bypass, Gastrointestinal System ØD1
  see Drainage, Gastrointestinal System ØD9
Gastroduodenal artery *use* Hepatic Artery
Gastroduodenectomy
  see Excision, Gastrointestinal System ØDB
  see Resection, Gastrointestinal System ØDT
Gastroduodenoscopy ØDJØ8ZZ
Gastroenteroplasty
  see Repair, Gastrointestinal System ØDQ
  see Supplement, Gastrointestinal System ØDU
Gastroenterostomy
  see Bypass, Gastrointestinal System ØD1
  see Drainage, Gastrointestinal System ØD9
Gastroesophageal (GE) junction *use* Esophagogastric Junction
Gastrogastrostomy
  see Bypass, Stomach ØD16
  see Drainage, Stomach ØD96
Gastrohepatic omentum *use* Omentum
Gastrojejunostomy
  see Bypass, Stomach ØD16
  see Drainage, Stomach ØD96
Gastrolysis *see* Release, Stomach ØDN6
Gastropexy
  see Repair, Stomach ØDQ6
  see Reposition, Stomach ØDS6
Gastrophrenic ligament *use* Omentum
Gastroplasty
  see Repair, Stomach ØDQ6
  see Supplement, Stomach ØDU6
Gastroplication *see* Restriction, Stomach ØDV6
Gastropylorectomy *see* Excision, Gastrointestinal System ØDB

Gastrorrhaphy *see* Repair, Stomach ØDQ6
Gastroscopy ØDJ68ZZ
Gastrosplenic ligament *use* Omentum
Gastrostomy
  see Bypass, Stomach ØD16
  see Drainage, Stomach ØD96
Gastrotomy *see* Drainage, Stomach ØD96
Gemellus muscle
  use Hip Muscle, Left
  use Hip Muscle, Right
Geniculate ganglion *use* Facial Nerve
Geniculate nucleus *use* Thalamus
Genioglossus muscle *use* Tongue, Palate, Pharynx Muscle
Genioplasty *see* Alteration, Jaw, Lower ØWØ5
Genitofemoral nerve *use* Lumbar Plexus
GIAPREZA™ *use* Synthetic Human Angiotensin II
Gilteritinib Antineoplastic XWØDXV5
Gingivectomy *see* Excision, Mouth and Throat ØCB
Gingivoplasty
  see Repair, Mouth and Throat ØCQ
  see Replacement, Mouth and Throat ØCR
  see Supplement, Mouth and Throat ØCU
Glans penis *use* Prepuce
Glenohumeral joint
  use Shoulder Joint, Left
  use Shoulder Joint, Right
Glenohumeral ligament
  use Shoulder Bursa and Ligament, Left
  use Shoulder Bursa and Ligament, Right
Glenoid fossa (of scapula)
  use Glenoid Cavity, Left
  use Glenoid Cavity, Right
Glenoid ligament (labrum)
  use Shoulder Joint, Left
  use Shoulder Joint, Right
Globus pallidus *use* Basal Ganglia
Glomectomy
  see Excision, Endocrine System ØGB
  see Resection, Endocrine System ØGT
Glossectomy
  see Excision, Tongue ØCB7
  see Resection, Tongue ØCT7
Glossoepiglottic fold *use* Epiglottis
Glossopexy
  see Repair, Tongue ØCQ7
  see Reposition, Tongue ØCS7
Glossoplasty
  see Repair, Tongue ØCQ7
  see Replacement, Tongue ØCR7
  see Supplement, Tongue ØCU7
Glossorrhaphy *see* Repair, Tongue ØCQ7
Glossotomy *see* Drainage, Tongue ØC97
Glottis *use* Larynx
Gluteal Artery Perforator Flap
  Replacement
    Bilateral ØHRVØ79
    Left ØHRUØ79
    Right ØHRTØ79
  Transfer
    Left ØKXG
    Right ØKXF
Gluteal lymph node *use* Lymphatic, Pelvis
Gluteal vein
  use Hypogastric Vein, Left
  use Hypogastric Vein, Right
Gluteus maximus muscle
  use Hip Muscle, Left
  use Hip Muscle, Right
Gluteus medius muscle
  use Hip Muscle, Left
  use Hip Muscle, Right
Gluteus minimus muscle
  use Hip Muscle, Left
  use Hip Muscle, Right
GORE EXCLUDER® AAA Endoprosthesis
  use Intraluminal Device
  use Intraluminal Device, Branched or Fenestrated, One or Two Arteries in Ø4V
  use Intraluminal Device, Branched or Fenestrated, Three or More Arteries in Ø4V
GORE EXCLUDER® IBE Endoprosthesis *use* Intraluminal Device, Branched or Fenestrated, One or Two Arteries in Ø4V
GORE TAG® Thoracic Endoprosthesis *use* Intraluminal Device

GORE® DUALMESH® *use* Synthetic Substitute
Gracilis muscle
  use Upper Leg Muscle, Left
  use Upper Leg Muscle, Right
Graft
  see Replacement
  see Supplement
Great auricular nerve *use* Cervical Plexus
Great cerebral vein *use* Intracranial Vein
Great(er) saphenous vein
  use Saphenous Vein, Left
  use Saphenous Vein, Right
Greater alar cartilage *use* Nasal Mucosa and Soft Tissue
Greater occipital nerve *use* Cervical Nerve
Greater Omentum *use* Omentum
Greater splanchnic nerve *use* Thoracic Sympathetic Nerve
Greater superficial petrosal nerve *use* Facial Nerve
Greater trochanter
  use Upper Femur, Left
  use Upper Femur, Right
Greater tuberosity
  use Humeral Head, Left
  use Humeral Head, Right
Greater vestibular (Bartholin's) gland *use* Vestibular Gland
Greater wing *use* Sphenoid Bone
GS-5734 *use* Remdesivir Anti-infective
Guedel airway *use* Intraluminal Device, Airway in Mouth and Throat
Guidance, catheter placement
  EKG *see* Measurement, Physiological Systems 4AØ
  Fluoroscopy *see* Fluoroscopy, Veins B51
  Ultrasound *see* Ultrasonography, Veins B54

H

Hallux
  use 1st Toe, Left
  use 1st Toe, Right
Hamate bone
  use Carpal, Left
  use Carpal, Right
Hancock Bioprosthesis (aortic) (mitral) valve *use* Zooplastic Tissue in Heart and Great Vessels
Hancock Bioprosthetic Valved Conduit *use* Zooplastic Tissue in Heart and Great Vessels
Harmony™ transcatheter pulmonary valve (TPV) placement Ø2RH38M
Harvesting, Stem Cells *see* Pheresis, Circulatory 6A55
hdIVIG (high-dose intravenous immunoglobulin), for COVID-19 treatment *use* High-Dose Intravenous Immune Globulin
Head of fibula
  use Fibula, Left
  use Fibula, Right
Hearing Aid Assessment F14Z
Hearing Assessment F13Z
Hearing Device
  Bone Conduction
    Left Ø9HE
    Right Ø9HD
  Insertion of device in
    Left ØNH6
    Right ØNH5
  Multiple Channel Cochlear Prosthesis
    Left Ø9HE
    Right Ø9HD
  Removal of device from, Skull ØNPØ
  Revision of device in, Skull ØNWØ
  Single Channel Cochlear Prosthesis
    Left Ø9HE
    Right Ø9HD
Hearing Treatment FØ9Z
Heart Assist System
  Implantable
    Insertion of device in, Heart Ø2HA
    Removal of device from, Heart Ø2PA
    Revision of device in, Heart Ø2WA
  Short-term External
    Insertion of device in, Heart Ø2HA
    Removal of device from, Heart Ø2PA
    Revision of device in, Heart Ø2WA
HeartMate 3™ LVAS *use* Implantable Heart Assist System in Heart and Great Vessels

HeartMate II® Left Ventricular Assist Device (LVAD)
    use Implantable Heart Assist System in Heart and Great Vessels
HeartMate XVE® Left Ventricular Assist Device (LVAD) *use* Implantable Heart Assist System in Heart and Great Vessels
HeartMate® implantable heart assist system *see* Insertion of device in, Heart 02HA
Helix
    use Ear, External, Bilateral
    use Ear, External, Left
    use Ear, External, Right
Hematopoietic cell transplant (HCT) *see* Transfusion, Circulatory 302
Hemicolectomy *see* Resection, Gastrointestinal System 0DT
Hemicystectomy *see* Excision, Urinary System 0TB
Hemigastrectomy *see* Excision, Gastrointestinal System 0DB
Hemiglossectomy *see* Excision, Mouth and Throat 0CB
Hemilaminectomy
    see Excision, Lower Bones 0QB
    see Excision, Upper Bones 0PB
Hemilaminotomy
    see Drainage, Lower Bones 0Q9
    see Drainage, Upper Bones 0P9
    see Excision, Lower Bones 0QB
    see Excision, Upper Bones 0PB
    see Release, Central Nervous System and Cranial Nerves 00N
    see Release, Lower Bones 0QN
    see Release, Peripheral Nervous System 01N
    see Release, Upper Bones 0PN
Hemilaryngectomy *see* Excision, Larynx 0CBS
Hemimandibulectomy *see* Excision, Head and Facial Bones 0NB
Hemimaxillectomy *see* Excision, Head and Facial Bones 0NB
Hemipylorectomy *see* Excision, Gastrointestinal System 0DB
Hemispherectomy
    see Excision, Central Nervous System and Cranial Nerves 00B
    see Resection, Central Nervous System and Cranial Nerves 00T
Hemithyroidectomy
    see Excision, Endocrine System 0GB
    see Resection, Endocrine System 0GT
Hemodialysis *see* Performance, Urinary 5A1D
Hemolung® Respiratory Assist System (RAS) 5A0920Z
Hemospray® Endoscopic Hemostat *use* Mineral-based Topical Hemostatic Agent
Hepatectomy
    see Excision, Hepatobiliary System and Pancreas 0FB
    see Resection, Hepatobiliary System and Pancreas 0FT
Hepatic artery proper *use* Hepatic Artery
Hepatic flexure *use* Transverse Colon
Hepatic lymph node *use* Lymphatic, Aortic
Hepatic plexus *use* Abdominal Sympathetic Nerve
Hepatic portal vein *use* Portal Vein
Hepaticoduodenostomy
    see Bypass, Hepatobiliary System and Pancreas 0F1
    see Drainage, Hepatobiliary System and Pancreas 0F9
Hepaticotomy *see* Drainage, Hepatobiliary System and Pancreas 0F9
Hepatocholedochostomy *see* Drainage, Duct, Common Bile 0F99
Hepatogastric ligament *use* Omentum
Hepatopancreatic ampulla *use* Ampulla of Vater
Hepatopexy
    see Repair, Hepatobiliary System and Pancreas 0FQ
    see Reposition, Hepatobiliary System and Pancreas 0FS
Hepatorrhaphy *see* Repair, Hepatobiliary System and Pancreas 0FQ
Hepatotomy *see* Drainage, Hepatobiliary System and Pancreas 0F9
Herculink (RX) Elite Renal Stent System *use* Intraluminal Device
Herniorrhaphy
    see Repair, Anatomical Regions, General 0WQ

Herniorrhaphy — *continued*
    see Repair, Anatomical Regions, Lower Extremities 0YQ
    With synthetic substitute
        see Supplement, Anatomical Regions, General 0WU
        see Supplement, Anatomical Regions, Lower Extremities 0YU
HIG (hyperimmune globulin), for COVID-19 treatment *use* Hyperimmune Globulin
High-Dose Intravenous Immune Globulin, for COVID-19 treatment XW1
High-dose intravenous immunoglobulin (hdIVIG), for COVID-19 treatment *use* High-Dose Intravenous Immune Globulin
Hip (joint) liner *use* Liner in Lower Joints
HIPEC (hyperthermic intraperitoneal chemotherapy) 3E0M30Y
HistoSonics® System *see* New Technology, Hepatobiliary System and Pancreas XF5
Histotripsy, liver *see* New Technology, Hepatobiliary System and Pancreas XF5
hIVIG (hyperimmune intravenous immunoglobulin), for COVID-19 treatment *use* Hyperimmune Globulin
Holter Monitoring 4A12X45
Holter valve ventricular shunt *use* Synthetic Substitute
Human angiotensin II, synthetic *use* Synthetic Human Angiotensin II
Humeroradial joint
    use Elbow Joint, Left
    use Elbow Joint, Right
Humeroulnar joint
    use Elbow Joint, Left
    use Elbow Joint, Right
Humerus, distal
    use Humeral Shaft, Left
    use Humeral Shaft, Right
Hydrocelectomy *see* Excision, Male Reproductive System 0VB
Hydrotherapy
    Assisted exercise in pool *see* Motor Treatment, Rehabilitation F07
    Whirlpool *see* Activities of Daily Living Treatment, Rehabilitation F08
Hymenectomy
    see Excision, Hymen 0UBK
    see Resection, Hymen 0UTK
Hymenoplasty
    see Repair, Hymen 0UQK
    see Supplement, Hymen 0UUK
Hymenorrhaphy *see* Repair, Hymen 0UQK
Hymenotomy
    see Division, Hymen 0U8K
    see Drainage, Hymen 0U9K
Hyoglossus muscle *use* Tongue, Palate, Pharynx Muscle
Hyoid artery
    use Thyroid Artery, Left
    use Thyroid Artery, Right
Hyperalimentation *see* Introduction of substance in or on
Hyperbaric oxygenation
    Decompression sickness treatment *see* Decompression, Circulatory 6A15
    Other treatment *see* Assistance, Circulatory 5A05
Hyperimmune globulin *use* Globulin
Hyperimmune Globulin, for COVID-19 treatment XW1
Hyperimmune intravenous immunoglobulin (hIVIG), for COVID-19 treatment *use* Hyperimmune Globulin
Hyperthermia
    Radiation Therapy
        Abdomen DWY38ZZ
        Adrenal Gland DGY28ZZ
        Bile Ducts DFY28ZZ
        Bladder DTY28ZZ
        Bone Marrow D7Y08ZZ
        Bone, Other DPYC8ZZ
        Brain D0Y08ZZ
        Brain Stem D0Y18ZZ
        Breast
            Left DMY08ZZ
            Right DMY18ZZ
        Bronchus DBY18ZZ

Hyperthermia — *continued*
    Radiation Therapy — *continued*
        Cervix DUY18ZZ
        Chest DWY28ZZ
        Chest Wall DBY78ZZ
        Colon DDY58ZZ
        Diaphragm DBY88ZZ
        Duodenum DDY28ZZ
        Ear D9Y08ZZ
        Esophagus DDY08ZZ
        Eye D8Y08ZZ
        Femur DPY98ZZ
        Fibula DPYB8ZZ
        Gallbladder DFY18ZZ
        Gland
            Adrenal DGY28ZZ
            Parathyroid DGY48ZZ
            Pituitary DGY08ZZ
            Thyroid DGY58ZZ
        Glands, Salivary D9Y68ZZ
        Head and Neck DWY18ZZ
        Hemibody DWY48ZZ
        Humerus DPY68ZZ
        Hypopharynx D9Y38ZZ
        Ileum DDY48ZZ
        Jejunum DDY38ZZ
        Kidney DTY08ZZ
        Larynx D9YB8ZZ
        Liver DFY08ZZ
        Lung DBY28ZZ
        Lymphatics
            Abdomen D7Y68ZZ
            Axillary D7Y48ZZ
            Inguinal D7Y88ZZ
            Neck D7Y38ZZ
            Pelvis D7Y78ZZ
            Thorax D7Y58ZZ
        Mandible DPY38ZZ
        Maxilla DPY28ZZ
        Mediastinum DBY68ZZ
        Mouth D9Y48ZZ
        Nasopharynx D9YD8ZZ
        Neck and Head DWY18ZZ
        Nerve, Peripheral D0Y78ZZ
        Nose D9Y18ZZ
        Oropharynx D9YF8ZZ
        Ovary DUY08ZZ
        Palate
            Hard D9Y88ZZ
            Soft D9Y98ZZ
        Pancreas DFY38ZZ
        Parathyroid Gland DGY48ZZ
        Pelvic Bones DPY88ZZ
        Pelvic Region DWY68ZZ
        Pineal Body DGY18ZZ
        Pituitary Gland DGY08ZZ
        Pleura DBY58ZZ
        Prostate DVY08ZZ
        Radius DPY78ZZ
        Rectum DDY78ZZ
        Rib DPY58ZZ
        Sinuses D9Y78ZZ
        Skin
            Abdomen DHY88ZZ
            Arm DHY48ZZ
            Back DHY78ZZ
            Buttock DHY98ZZ
            Chest DHY68ZZ
            Face DHY28ZZ
            Leg DHYB8ZZ
            Neck DHY38ZZ
        Skull DPY08ZZ
        Spinal Cord D0Y68ZZ
        Spleen D7Y28ZZ
        Sternum DPY48ZZ
        Stomach DDY18ZZ
        Testis DVY18ZZ
        Thymus D7Y18ZZ
        Thyroid Gland DGY58ZZ
        Tibia DPYB8ZZ
        Tongue D9Y58ZZ
        Trachea DBY08ZZ
        Ulna DPY78ZZ
        Ureter DTY18ZZ
        Urethra DTY38ZZ
        Uterus DUY28ZZ
        Whole Body DWY58ZZ
    Whole Body 6A3Z

Hyperthermic Intraperitoneal Chemotherapy (HIPEC) 3E0M30Y
Hypnosis GZFZZZZ
Hypogastric artery
  use Internal Iliac Artery, Left
  use Internal Iliac Artery, Right
Hypopharynx *use* Pharynx
Hypophysectomy
  see Excision, Gland, Pituitary 0GB0
  see Resection, Gland, Pituitary 0GT0
Hypophysis *use* Pituitary Gland
Hypothalamotomy *see* Destruction, Thalamus 0059
Hypothenar muscle
  use Hand Muscle, Left
  use Hand Muscle, Right
Hypothermia, Whole Body 6A4Z
Hysterectomy
  Supracervical *see* Resection, Uterus 0UT9
  Total *see* Resection, Uterus 0UT9
Hysterolysis *see* Release, Uterus 0UN9
Hysteropexy
  see Repair, Uterus 0UQ9
  see Reposition, Uterus 0US9
Hysteroplasty *see* Repair, Uterus 0UQ9
Hysterorrhaphy *see* Repair, Uterus 0UQ9
Hysteroscopy 0UJD8ZZ
Hysterotomy *see* Drainage, Uterus 0U99
Hysterotrachelectomy
  see Resection, Cervix 0UTC
  see Resection, Uterus 0UT9
Hysterotracheloplasty *see* Repair, Uterus 0UQ9
Hysterotrachelorrhaphy *see* Repair, Uterus 0UQ9

I

IABP (Intra-aortic balloon pump) *see* Assistance, Cardiac 5A02
IAEMT (Intraoperative anesthetic effect monitoring and titration) *see* Monitoring, Central Nervous 4A10
IASD® (InterAtrial Shunt Device), Corvia *use* Synthetic Substitute
Idarucizumab, Pradaxa® (dabigatran) reversal agent *use* Other Therapeutic Substance
Idecabtagene Vicleucel *use* Idecabtagene Vicleucel Immunotherapy
Idecabtagene Vicleucel Immunotherapy XW0
Ide-cel *use* Idecabtagene Vicleucel Immunotherapy
iFuse Bedrock™ Granite Implant System *use* Internal Fixation Device with Tulip Connector in New Technology
IGIV-C, for COVID-19 treatment *use* Hyperimmune Globulin
IHD (Intermittent hemodialysis) 5A1D70Z
Ileal artery *use* Superior Mesenteric Artery
Ileectomy
  see Excision, Ileum 0DBB
  see Resection, Ileum 0DTB
Ileocolic artery *use* Superior Mesenteric Artery
Ileocolic vein *use* Colic Vein
Ileopexy
  see Repair, Ileum 0DQB
  see Reposition, Ileum 0DSB
Ileorrhaphy *see* Repair, Ileum 0DQB
Ileoscopy 0DJD8ZZ
Ileostomy
  see Bypass, Ileum 0D1B
  see Drainage, Ileum 0D9B
Ileotomy *see* Drainage, Ileum 0D9B
Ileoureterostomy *see* Bypass, Urinary System 0T1
Iliac crest
  use Pelvic Bone, Left
  use Pelvic Bone, Right
Iliac fascia
  use Subcutaneous Tissue and Fascia, Left Upper Leg
  use Subcutaneous Tissue and Fascia, Right Upper Leg
Iliac lymph node *use* Lymphatic, Pelvis
Iliacus muscle
  use Hip Muscle, Left
  use Hip Muscle, Right
Iliofemoral ligament
  use Hip Bursa and Ligament, Left
  use Hip Bursa and Ligament, Right
Iliohypogastric nerve *use* Lumbar Plexus

Ilioinguinal nerve *use* Lumbar Plexus
Iliolumbar artery
  use Internal Iliac Artery, Left
  use Internal Iliac Artery, Right
Iliolumbar ligament *use* Lower Spine Bursa and Ligament
Iliotibial tract (band)
  use Subcutaneous Tissue and Fascia, Left Upper Leg
  use Subcutaneous Tissue and Fascia, Right Upper Leg
Ilium
  use Pelvic Bone, Left
  use Pelvic Bone, Right
Ilizarov external fixator
  use External Fixation Device, Ring in 0PH
  use External Fixation Device, Ring in 0PS
  use External Fixation Device, Ring in 0QH
  use External Fixation Device, Ring in 0QS
Ilizarov-Vecklich device
  use External Fixation Device, Limb Lengthening in 0PH
  use External Fixation Device, Limb Lengthening in 0QH
Imaging, diagnostic
  see Computerized Tomography (CT Scan)
  see Fluoroscopy
  see Magnetic Resonance Imaging (MRI)
  see Plain Radiography
  see Ultrasonography
Imdevimab (REGN10987) and Casirivimab (REGN10933) *use* REGN-COV2 Monoclonal Antibody
IMFINZI® *use* Durvalumab Antineoplastic
Imipenem-cilastatin-relebactam Anti-infective XW0
IMI/REL *use* Imipenem-cilastatin-relebactam Anti-infective
Immobilization
  Abdominal Wall 2W33X
  Arm
    Lower
      Left 2W3DX
      Right 2W3CX
    Upper
      Left 2W3BX
      Right 2W3AX
  Back 2W35X
  Chest Wall 2W34X
  Extremity
    Lower
      Left 2W3MX
      Right 2W3LX
    Upper
      Left 2W39X
      Right 2W38X
  Face 2W31X
  Finger
    Left 2W3KX
    Right 2W3JX
  Foot
    Left 2W3TX
    Right 2W3SX
  Hand
    Left 2W3FX
    Right 2W3EX
  Head 2W30X
  Inguinal Region
    Left 2W37X
    Right 2W36X
  Leg
    Lower
      Left 2W3RX
      Right 2W3QX
    Upper
      Left 2W3PX
      Right 2W3NX
  Neck 2W32X
  Thumb
    Left 2W3HX
    Right 2W3GX
  Toe
    Left 2W3VX
    Right 2W3UX
Immunization *see* Introduction of Serum, Toxoid, and Vaccine
Immunoglobulin *use* Globulin

Immunotherapy *see* Introduction of Immunotherapeutic Substance
Immunotherapy, antineoplastic
  Interferon *see* Introduction of Low-dose Interleukin-2
  Interleukin-2, high-dose *see* Introduction of High-dose Interleukin-2
  Interleukin-2, low-dose *see* Introduction of Low-dose Interleukin-2
  Monoclonal antibody *see* Introduction of Monoclonal Antibody
  Proleukin, high-dose *see* Introduction of High-dose Interleukin-2
  Proleukin, low-dose *see* Introduction of Low-dose Interleukin-2
Impella® heart pump *use* Short-term External Heart Assist System in Heart and Great Vessels
Impeller Pump
  Continuous, Output 5A0221D
  Intermittent, Output 5A0211D
Implantable cardioverter-defibrillator (ICD) *use* Defibrillator Generator in 0JH
Implantable drug infusion pump (anti-spasmodic) (chemotherapy) (pain) *use* Infusion Device, Pump in Subcutaneous Tissue and Fascia
Implantable glucose monitoring device *use* Monitoring Device
Implantable hemodynamic monitor (IHM) *use* Monitoring Device, Hemodynamic in 0JH
Implantable hemodynamic monitoring system (IHMS) *use* Monitoring Device, Hemodynamic in 0JH
Implantable Miniature Telescope™ (IMT) *use* Synthetic Substitute, Intraocular Telescope in 08R
Implantation
  see Insertion
  see Replacement
Implanted (venous)(access) port *use* Vascular Access Device, Totally Implantable in Subcutaneous Tissue and Fascia
IMV (intermittent mandatory ventilation) *see* Assistance, Respiratory 5A09
In Vitro Fertilization 8E0ZXY1
Incision, abscess *see* Drainage
Incudectomy
  see Excision, Ear, Nose, Sinus 09B
  see Resection, Ear, Nose, Sinus 09T
Incudopexy
  see Repair, Ear, Nose, Sinus 09Q
  see Reposition, Ear, Nose, Sinus 09S
Incus
  use Auditory Ossicle, Left
  use Auditory Ossicle, Right
Induction of labor
  Artificial rupture of membranes *see* Drainage, Pregnancy 109
  Oxytocin *see* Introduction of Hormone
InDura, intrathecal catheter (1P) (spinal) *use* Infusion Device
Inebilizumab-cdon XW0
Inferior cardiac nerve *use* Thoracic Sympathetic Nerve
Inferior cerebellar vein *use* Intracranial Vein
Inferior cerebral vein *use* Intracranial Vein
Inferior epigastric artery
  use External Iliac Artery, Left
  use External Iliac Artery, Right
Inferior epigastric lymph node *use* Lymphatic, Pelvis
Inferior genicular artery
  use Popliteal Artery, Left
  use Popliteal Artery, Right
Inferior gluteal artery
  use Internal Iliac Artery, Left
  use Internal Iliac Artery, Right
Inferior gluteal nerve *use* Sacral Plexus
Inferior hypogastric plexus *use* Abdominal Sympathetic Nerve
Inferior labial artery *use* Face Artery
Inferior longitudinal muscle *use* Tongue, Palate, Pharynx Muscle
Inferior mesenteric ganglion *use* Abdominal Sympathetic Nerve
Inferior mesenteric lymph node *use* Lymphatic, Mesenteric
Inferior mesenteric plexus *use* Abdominal Sympathetic Nerve
Inferior oblique muscle
  use Extraocular Muscle, Left

Inferior oblique muscle — *continued*
  use Extraocular Muscle, Right
Inferior pancreaticoduodenal artery *use* Superior
  Mesenteric Artery
Inferior phrenic artery *use* Abdominal Aorta
Inferior rectus muscle
  use Extraocular Muscle, Left
  use Extraocular Muscle, Right
Inferior suprarenal artery
  use Renal Artery, Left
  use Renal Artery, Right
Inferior tarsal plate
  use Lower Eyelid, Left
  use Lower Eyelid, Right
Inferior thyroid vein
  use Innominate Vein, Left
  use Innominate Vein, Right
Inferior tibiofibular joint
  use Ankle Joint, Left
  use Ankle Joint, Right
Inferior turbinate *use* Nasal Turbinate
Inferior ulnar collateral artery
  use Brachial Artery, Left
  use Brachial Artery, Right
Inferior vesical artery
  use Internal Iliac Artery, Left
  use Internal Iliac Artery, Right
Infraauricular lymph node *use* Lymphatic, Head
Infraclavicular (deltopectoral) lymph node
  use Lymphatic, Left Upper Extremity
  use Lymphatic, Right Upper Extremity
Infrahyoid muscle
  use Neck Muscle, Left
  use Neck Muscle, Right
Infraparotid lymph node *use* Lymphatic, Head
Infraspinatus fascia
  use Subcutaneous Tissue and Fascia, Left Upper
    Arm
  use Subcutaneous Tissue and Fascia, Right Upper
    Arm
Infraspinatus muscle
  use Shoulder Muscle, Left
  use Shoulder Muscle, Right
Infundibulopelvic ligament *use* Uterine Supporting
  Structure
Infusion *see* Introduction of substance in or on
Infusion Device, Pump
  Insertion of device in
    Abdomen ØJH8
    Back ØJH7
    Chest ØJH6
    Lower Arm
      Left ØJHH
      Right ØJHG
    Lower Leg
      Left ØJHP
      Right ØJHN
    Trunk ØJHT
    Upper Arm
      Left ØJHF
      Right ØJHD
    Upper Leg
      Left ØJHM
      Right ØJHL
  Removal of device from
    Lower Extremity ØJPW
    Trunk ØJPT
    Upper Extremity ØJPV
  Revision of device in
    Lower Extremity ØJWW
    Trunk ØJWT
    Upper Extremity ØJWV
Infusion, glucarpidase
  Central Vein 3E043GQ
  Peripheral Vein 3E033GQ
Inguinal canal
  use Inguinal Region, Bilateral
  use Inguinal Region, Left
  use Inguinal Region, Right
Inguinal triangle
  use Inguinal Region, Bilateral
  use Inguinal Region, Left
  use Inguinal Region, Right
Injection *see* Introduction of substance in or on
Injection reservoir, port *use* Vascular Access Device,
    Totally Implantable in Subcutaneous Tissue and
    Fascia

Injection reservoir, pump *use* Infusion Device, Pump
  in Subcutaneous Tissue and Fascia
Insemination, artificial 3E0P7LZ
Insertion
  Antimicrobial envelope *see* Introduction of Anti-
    infective
  Aqueous drainage shunt
    see Bypass, Eye 081
    see Drainage, Eye 089
  Bone, Pelvic, Internal Fixation Device with Tulip
    Connector XNH
  Joint
    Lumbar Vertebral, Posterior Spinal Motion
      Preservation Device XRHB018
    Lumbosacral, Posterior Spinal Motion
      Preservation Device XRHD018
  Neurostimulator Lead, Sphenopalatine Ganglion
    XØHK3Q8
  Neurostimulator Lead with Paired Stimulation
    System XØHQ3R8
  Products of Conception 10H0
  Spinal Stabilization Device
    see Insertion of device in, Lower Joints ØSH
    see Insertion of device in, Upper Joints ØRH
Insertion of device in
  Abdominal Wall ØWHF
  Acetabulum
    Left ØQH5
    Right ØQH4
  Anal Sphincter ØDHR
  Ankle Region
    Left ØYHL
    Right ØYHK
  Anus ØDHQ
  Aorta
    Abdominal 04H0
    Thoracic
      Ascending/Arch 02HX
      Descending 02HW
  Arm
    Lower
      Left ØXHF
      Right ØXHD
    Upper
      Left ØXH9
      Right ØXH8
  Artery
    Anterior Tibial
      Left 04HQ
      Right 04HP
    Axillary
      Left 03H6
      Right 03H5
    Brachial
      Left 03H8
      Right 03H7
    Celiac 04H1
    Colic
      Left 04H7
      Middle 04H8
      Right 04H6
    Common Carotid
      Left 03HJ
      Right 03HH
    Common Iliac
      Left 04HD
      Right 04HC
    Coronary
      Four or More Arteries 02H3
      One Artery 02H0
      Three Arteries 02H2
      Two Arteries 02H1
    External Carotid
      Left 03HN
      Right 03HM
    External Iliac
      Left 04HJ
      Right 04HH
    Face 03HR
    Femoral
      Left 04HL
      Right 04HK
    Foot
      Left 04HW
      Right 04HV
    Gastric 04H2
    Hand
      Left 03HF

Insertion of device in — *continued*
  Artery — *continued*
    Hand — *continued*
      Right 03HD
    Hepatic 04H3
    Inferior Mesenteric 04HB
    Innominate 03H2
    Internal Carotid
      Left 03HL
      Right 03HK
    Internal Iliac
      Left 04HF
      Right 04HE
    Internal Mammary
      Left 03H1
      Right 03H0
    Intracranial 03HG
    Lower 04HY
    Peroneal
      Left 04HU
      Right 04HT
    Popliteal
      Left 04HN
      Right 04HM
    Posterior Tibial
      Left 04HS
      Right 04HR
    Pulmonary
      Left 02HR
      Right 02HQ
    Pulmonary Trunk 02HP
    Radial
      Left 03HC
      Right 03HB
    Renal
      Left 04HA
      Right 04H9
    Splenic 04H4
    Subclavian
      Left 03H4
      Right 03H3
    Superior Mesenteric 04H5
    Temporal
      Left 03HT
      Right 03HS
    Thyroid
      Left 03HV
      Right 03HU
    Ulnar
      Left 03HA
      Right 03H9
    Upper 03HY
    Vertebral
      Left 03HQ
      Right 03HP
  Atrium
    Left 02H7
    Right 02H6
  Axilla
    Left ØXH5
    Right ØXH4
  Back
    Lower ØWHL
    Upper ØWHK
  Bladder ØTHB
  Bladder Neck ØTHC
  Bone
    Ethmoid
      Left ØNHG
      Right ØNHF
    Facial ØNHW
    Frontal ØNH1
    Hyoid ØNHX
    Lacrimal
      Left ØNHJ
      Right ØNHH
    Lower ØQHY
    Nasal ØNHB
    Occipital ØNH7
    Palatine
      Left ØNHL
      Right ØNHK
    Parietal
      Left ØNH4
      Right ØNH3
    Pelvic
      Left ØQH3
      Right ØQH2
    Sphenoid ØNHC

Insertion of device in — *continued*
- Bone — *continued*
  - Temporal
    - Left 0NH6
    - Right 0NH5
  - Upper 0PHY
  - Zygomatic
    - Left 0NHN
    - Right 0NHM
- Bone Marrow 07HT
- Brain 00H0
- Breast
  - Bilateral 0HHV
  - Left 0HHU
  - Right 0HHT
- Bronchus
  - Lingula 0BH9
  - Lower Lobe
    - Left 0BHB
    - Right 0BH6
  - Main
    - Left 0BH7
    - Right 0BH3
  - Middle Lobe, Right 0BH5
  - Upper Lobe
    - Left 0BH8
    - Right 0BH4
- Bursa and Ligament
  - Lower 0MHY
  - Upper 0MHX
- Buttock
  - Left 0YH1
  - Right 0YH0
- Carpal
  - Left 0PHN
  - Right 0PHM
- Cavity, Cranial 0WH1
- Cerebral Ventricle 00H6
- Cervix 0UHC
- Chest Wall 0WH8
- Cisterna Chyli 07HL
- Clavicle
  - Left 0PHB
  - Right 0PH9
- Coccyx 0QHS
- Cul-de-sac 0UHF
- Diaphragm 0BHT
- Disc
  - Cervical Vertebral 0RH3
  - Cervicothoracic Vertebral 0RH5
  - Lumbar Vertebral 0SH2
  - Lumbosacral 0SH4
  - Thoracic Vertebral 0RH9
  - Thoracolumbar Vertebral 0RHB
- Duct
  - Hepatobiliary 0FHB
  - Pancreatic 0FHD
- Duodenum 0DH9
- Ear
  - Inner
    - Left 09HE
    - Right 09HD
  - Left 09HJ
  - Right 09HH
- Elbow Region
  - Left 0XHC
  - Right 0XHB
- Epididymis and Spermatic Cord 0VHM
- Esophagus 0DH5
- Extremity
  - Lower
    - Left 0YHB
    - Right 0YH9
  - Upper
    - Left 0XH7
    - Right 0XH6
- Eye
  - Left 08H1
  - Right 08H0
- Face 0WH2
- Fallopian Tube 0UH8
- Femoral Region
  - Left 0YH8
  - Right 0YH7
- Femoral Shaft
  - Left 0QH9
  - Right 0QH8

Insertion of device in — *continued*
- Femur
  - Lower
    - Left 0QHC
    - Right 0QHB
  - Upper
    - Left 0QH7
    - Right 0QH6
- Fibula
  - Left 0QHK
  - Right 0QHJ
- Foot
  - Left 0YHN
  - Right 0YHM
- Gallbladder 0FH4
- Gastrointestinal Tract 0WHP
- Genitourinary Tract 0WHR
- Gland
  - Endocrine 0GHS
  - Salivary 0CHA
- Glenoid Cavity
  - Left 0PH8
  - Right 0PH7
- Hand
  - Left 0XHK
  - Right 0XHJ
- Head 0WH0
- Heart 02HA
- Humeral Head
  - Left 0PHD
  - Right 0PHC
- Humeral Shaft
  - Left 0PHG
  - Right 0PHF
- Ileum 0DHB
- Inguinal Region
  - Left 0YH6
  - Right 0YH5
- Intestinal Tract
  - Lower Intestinal Tract 0DHD
  - Upper Intestinal Tract 0DH0
- Intestine
  - Large 0DHE
  - Small 0DH8
- Jaw
  - Lower 0WH5
  - Upper 0WH4
- Jejunum 0DHA
- Joint
  - Acromioclavicular
    - Left 0RHH
    - Right 0RHG
  - Ankle
    - Left 0SHG
    - Right 0SHF
  - Carpal
    - Left 0RHR
    - Right 0RHQ
  - Carpometacarpal
    - Left 0RHT
    - Right 0RHS
  - Cervical Vertebral 0RH1
  - Cervicothoracic Vertebral 0RH4
  - Coccygeal 0SH6
  - Elbow
    - Left 0RHM
    - Right 0RHL
  - Finger Phalangeal
    - Left 0RHX
    - Right 0RHW
  - Hip
    - Left 0SHB
    - Right 0SH9
  - Knee
    - Left 0SHD
    - Right 0SHC
  - Lumbar Vertebral 0SH0
  - Lumbosacral 0SH3
  - Metacarpophalangeal
    - Left 0RHV
    - Right 0RHU
  - Metatarsal-Phalangeal
    - Left 0SHN
    - Right 0SHM
  - Occipital-cervical 0RH0
  - Sacrococcygeal 0SH5
  - Sacroiliac
    - Left 0SH8
    - Right 0SH7

Insertion of device in — *continued*
- Joint — *continued*
  - Shoulder
    - Left 0RHK
    - Right 0RHJ
  - Sternoclavicular
    - Left 0RHF
    - Right 0RHE
  - Tarsal
    - Left 0SHJ
    - Right 0SHH
  - Tarsometatarsal
    - Left 0SHL
    - Right 0SHK
  - Temporomandibular
    - Left 0RHD
    - Right 0RHC
  - Thoracic Vertebral 0RH6
  - Thoracolumbar Vertebral 0RHA
  - Toe Phalangeal
    - Left 0SHQ
    - Right 0SHP
  - Wrist
    - Left 0RHP
    - Right 0RHN
- Kidney 0TH5
- Knee Region
  - Left 0YHG
  - Right 0YHF
- Larynx 0CHS
- Leg
  - Lower
    - Left 0YHJ
    - Right 0YHH
  - Upper
    - Left 0YHD
    - Right 0YHC
- Liver 0FH0
  - Left Lobe 0FH2
  - Right Lobe 0FH1
- Lung
  - Left 0BHL
  - Right 0BHK
- Lymphatic 07HN
  - Thoracic Duct 07HK
- Mandible
  - Left 0NHV
  - Right 0NHT
- Maxilla 0NHR
- Mediastinum 0WHC
- Metacarpal
  - Left 0PHQ
  - Right 0PHP
- Metatarsal
  - Left 0QHP
  - Right 0QHN
- Mouth and Throat 0CHY
- Muscle
  - Lower 0KHY
  - Upper 0KHX
- Nasal Mucosa and Soft Tissue 09HK
- Nasopharynx 09HN
- Neck 0WH6
- Nerve
  - Cranial 00HE
  - Peripheral 01HY
- Nipple
  - Left 0HHX
  - Right 0HHW
- Oral Cavity and Throat 0WH3
- Orbit
  - Left 0NHQ
  - Right 0NHP
- Ovary 0UH3
- Pancreas 0FHG
- Patella
  - Left 0QHF
  - Right 0QHD
- Pelvic Cavity 0WHJ
- Penis 0VHS
- Pericardial Cavity 0WHD
- Pericardium 02HN
- Perineum
  - Female 0WHN
  - Male 0WHM
- Peritoneal Cavity 0WHG
- Phalanx
  - Finger
    - Left 0PHV

Insertion of device in — *continued*
  Phalanx — *continued*
    Finger — *continued*
      Right ØPHT
    Thumb
      Left ØPHS
      Right ØPHR
    Toe
      Left ØQHR
      Right ØQHQ
  Pleura ØBHQ
  Pleural Cavity
    Left ØWHB
    Right ØWH9
  Prostate ØVHØ
  Prostate and Seminal Vesicles ØVH4
  Radius
    Left ØPHJ
    Right ØPHH
  Rectum ØDHP
  Respiratory Tract ØWHQ
  Retroperitoneum ØWHH
  Ribs
    1 to 2 ØPH1
    3 or More ØPH2
  Sacrum ØQH1
  Scapula
    Left ØPH6
    Right ØPH5
  Scrotum and Tunica Vaginalis ØVH8
  Shoulder Region
    Left ØXH3
    Right ØXH2
  Sinus Ø9HY
  Skin ØHHPXYZ
  Skull ØNHØ
  Spinal Canal ØØHU
  Spinal Cord ØØHV
  Spleen Ø7HP
  Sternum ØPHØ
  Stomach ØDH6
  Subcutaneous Tissue and Fascia
    Abdomen ØJH8
    Back ØJH7
    Buttock ØJH9
    Chest ØJH6
    Face ØJH1
    Foot
      Left ØJHR
      Right ØJHQ
    Hand
      Left ØJHK
      Right ØJHJ
    Head and Neck ØJHS
    Lower Arm
      Left ØJHH
      Right ØJHG
    Lower Extremity ØJHW
    Lower Leg
      Left ØJHP
      Right ØJHN
    Neck
      Left ØJH5
      Right ØJH4
    Pelvic Region ØJHC
    Perineum ØJHB
    Scalp ØJHØ
    Trunk ØJHT
    Upper Arm
      Left ØJHF
      Right ØJHD
    Upper Extremity ØJHV
    Upper Leg
      Left ØJHM
      Right ØJHL
  Tarsal
    Left ØQHM
    Right ØQHL
  Tendon
    Lower ØLHY
    Upper ØLHX
  Testis ØVHD
  Thymus Ø7HM
  Tibia
    Left ØQHH
    Right ØQHG
  Tongue ØCH7
  Trachea ØBH1
  Tracheobronchial Tree ØBHØ

Insertion of device in — *continued*
  Ulna
    Left ØPHL
    Right ØPHK
  Ureter ØTH9
  Urethra ØTHD
  Uterus ØUH9
  Uterus and Cervix ØUHD
  Vagina ØUHG
  Vagina and Cul-de-sac ØUHH
  Vas Deferens ØVHR
  Vein
    Axillary
      Left Ø5H8
      Right Ø5H7
    Azygos Ø5HØ
    Basilic
      Left Ø5HC
      Right Ø5HB
    Brachial
      Left Ø5HA
      Right Ø5H9
    Cephalic
      Left Ø5HF
      Right Ø5HD
    Colic Ø6H7
    Common Iliac
      Left Ø6HD
      Right Ø6HC
    Coronary Ø2H4
    Esophageal Ø6H3
    External Iliac
      Left Ø6HG
      Right Ø6HF
    External Jugular
      Left Ø5HQ
      Right Ø5HP
    Face
      Left Ø5HV
      Right Ø5HT
    Femoral
      Left Ø6HN
      Right Ø6HM
    Foot
      Left Ø6HV
      Right Ø6HT
    Gastric Ø6H2
    Hand
      Left Ø5HH
      Right Ø5HG
    Hemiazygos Ø5H1
    Hepatic Ø6H4
    Hypogastric
      Left Ø6HJ
      Right Ø6HH
    Inferior Mesenteric Ø6H6
    Innominate
      Left Ø5H4
      Right Ø5H3
    Internal Jugular
      Left Ø5HN
      Right Ø5HM
    Intracranial Ø5HL
    Lower Ø6HY
    Portal Ø6H8
    Pulmonary
      Left Ø2HT
      Right Ø2HS
    Renal
      Left Ø6HB
      Right Ø6H9
    Saphenous
      Left Ø6HQ
      Right Ø6HP
    Splenic Ø6H1
    Subclavian
      Left Ø5H6
      Right Ø5H5
    Superior Mesenteric Ø6H5
    Upper Ø5HY
    Vertebral
      Left Ø5HS
      Right Ø5HR
  Vena Cava
    Inferior Ø6HØ
    Superior Ø2HV
  Ventricle
    Left Ø2HL
    Right Ø2HK

Insertion of device in — *continued*
  Vertebra
    Cervical ØPH3
    Lumbar ØQHØ
    Thoracic ØPH4
  Wrist Region
    Left ØXHH
    Right ØXHG

Inspection
  Abdominal Wall ØWJF
  Ankle Region
    Left ØYJL
    Right ØYJK
  Arm
    Lower
      Left ØXJF
      Right ØXJD
    Upper
      Left ØXJ9
      Right ØXJ8
  Artery
    Lower Ø4JY
    Upper Ø3JY
  Axilla
    Left ØXJ5
    Right ØXJ4
  Back
    Lower ØWJL
    Upper ØWJK
  Bladder ØTJB
  Bone
    Facial ØNJW
    Lower ØQJY
    Nasal ØNJB
    Upper ØPJY
  Bone Marrow Ø7JT
  Brain ØØJØ
  Breast
    Left ØHJU
    Right ØHJT
  Bursa and Ligament
    Lower ØMJY
    Upper ØMJX
  Buttock
    Left ØYJ1
    Right ØYJØ
  Cavity, Cranial ØWJ1
  Chest Wall ØWJ8
  Cisterna Chyli Ø7JL
  Diaphragm ØBJT
  Disc
    Cervical Vertebral ØRJ3
    Cervicothoracic Vertebral ØRJ5
    Lumbar Vertebral ØSJ2
    Lumbosacral ØSJ4
    Thoracic Vertebral ØRJ9
    Thoracolumbar Vertebral ØRJB
  Duct
    Hepatobiliary ØFJB
    Pancreatic ØFJD
  Ear
    Inner
      Left Ø9JE
      Right Ø9JD
    Left Ø9JJ
    Right Ø9JH
  Elbow Region
    Left ØXJC
    Right ØXJB
  Epididymis and Spermatic Cord ØVJM
  Extremity
    Lower
      Left ØYJB
      Right ØYJ9
    Upper
      Left ØXJ7
      Right ØXJ6
  Eye
    Left Ø8J1XZZ
    Right Ø8JØXZZ
  Face ØWJ2
  Fallopian Tube ØUJ8
  Femoral Region
    Bilateral ØYJE
    Left ØYJ8
    Right ØYJ7
  Finger Nail ØHJQXZZ
  Foot
    Left ØYJN

Inspection — continued

Foot — continued
Right ØYJM
Gallbladder ØFJ4
Gastrointestinal Tract ØWJP
Genitourinary Tract ØWJR
Gland
Adrenal ØGJ5
Endocrine ØGJS
Pituitary ØGJØ
Salivary ØCJA
Great Vessel Ø2JY
Hand
Left ØXJK
Right ØXJJ
Head ØWJØ
Heart Ø2JA
Inguinal Region
Bilateral ØYJA
Left ØYJ6
Right ØYJ5
Intestinal Tract
Lower Intestinal Tract ØDJD
Upper Intestinal Tract ØDJØ
Jaw
Lower ØWJ5
Upper ØWJ4
Joint
Acromioclavicular
Left ØRJH
Right ØRJG
Ankle
Left ØSJG
Right ØSJF
Carpal
Left ØRJR
Right ØRJQ
Carpometacarpal
Left ØRJT
Right ØRJS
Cervical Vertebral ØRJ1
Cervicothoracic Vertebral ØRJ4
Coccygeal ØSJ6
Elbow
Left ØRJM
Right ØRJL
Finger Phalangeal
Left ØRJX
Right ØRJW
Hip
Left ØSJB
Right ØSJ9
Knee
Left ØSJD
Right ØSJC
Lumbar Vertebral ØSJØ
Lumbosacral ØSJ3
Metacarpophalangeal
Left ØRJV
Right ØRJU
Metatarsal-Phalangeal
Left ØSJN
Right ØSJM
Occipital-cervical ØRJØ
Sacrococcygeal ØSJ5
Sacroiliac
Left ØSJ8
Right ØSJ7
Shoulder
Left ØRJK
Right ØRJJ
Sternoclavicular
Left ØRJF
Right ØRJE
Tarsal
Left ØSJJ
Right ØSJH
Tarsometatarsal
Left ØSJL
Right ØSJK
Temporomandibular
Left ØRJD
Right ØRJC
Thoracic Vertebral ØRJ6
Thoracolumbar Vertebral ØRJA
Toe Phalangeal
Left ØSJQ
Right ØSJP

Inspection — continued

Joint — continued
Wrist
Left ØRJP
Right ØRJN
Kidney ØTJ5
Knee Region
Left ØYJG
Right ØYJF
Larynx ØCJS
Leg
Lower
Left ØYJJ
Right ØYJH
Upper
Left ØYJD
Right ØYJC
Lens
Left Ø8JKXZZ
Right Ø8JJXZZ
Liver ØFJØ
Lung
Left ØBJL
Right ØBJK
Lymphatic Ø7JN
Thoracic Duct Ø7JK
Mediastinum ØWJC
Mesentery ØDJV
Mouth and Throat ØCJY
Muscle
Extraocular
Left Ø8JM
Right Ø8JL
Lower ØKJY
Upper ØKJX
Nasal Mucosa and Soft Tissue Ø9JK
Neck ØWJ6
Nerve
Cranial ØØJE
Peripheral Ø1JY
Omentum ØDJU
Oral Cavity and Throat ØWJ3
Ovary ØUJ3
Pancreas ØFJG
Parathyroid Gland ØGJR
Pelvic Cavity ØWJJ
Penis ØVJS
Pericardial Cavity ØWJD
Perineum
Female ØWJN
Male ØWJM
Peritoneal Cavity ØWJG
Peritoneum ØDJW
Pineal Body ØGJ1
Pleura ØBJQ
Pleural Cavity
Left ØWJB
Right ØWJ9
Products of Conception 1ØJØ
Ectopic 1ØJ2
Retained 1ØJ1
Prostate and Seminal Vesicles ØVJ4
Respiratory Tract ØWJQ
Retroperitoneum ØWJH
Scrotum and Tunica Vaginalis ØVJ8
Shoulder Region
Left ØXJ3
Right ØXJ2
Sinus Ø9JY
Skin ØHJPXZZ
Skull ØNJØ
Spinal Canal ØØJU
Spinal Cord ØØJV
Spleen Ø7JP
Stomach ØDJ6
Subcutaneous Tissue and Fascia
Head and Neck ØJJS
Lower Extremity ØJJW
Trunk ØJJT
Upper Extremity ØJJV
Tendon
Lower ØLJY
Upper ØLJX
Testis ØVJD
Thymus Ø7JM
Thyroid Gland ØGJK
Toe Nail ØHJRXZZ
Trachea ØBJ1
Tracheobronchial Tree ØBJØ

Inspection — continued

Tympanic Membrane
Left Ø9J8
Right Ø9J7
Ureter ØTJ9
Urethra ØTJD
Uterus and Cervix ØUJD
Vagina and Cul-de-sac ØUJH
Vas Deferens ØVJR
Vein
Lower Ø6JY
Upper Ø5JY
Vulva ØUJM
Wrist Region
Left ØXJH
Right ØXJG
Installation see Introduction of substance in or on
Insufflation see Introduction of substance in or on
Interatrial septum use Atrial Septum
InterAtrial Shunt Device IASD®, Corvia use Synthetic Substitute
Interbody fusion (spine) cage
use Interbody Fusion Device in Lower Joints
use Interbody Fusion Device in Upper Joints
Interbody Fusion Device, Customizable
Lumbar Vertebral XRGB
2 or more XRGC
Lumbosacral XRGD
Thoracolumbar Vertebral XRGA
Intercarpal joint
use Carpal Joint, Left
use Carpal Joint, Right
Intercarpal ligament
use Hand Bursa and Ligament, Left
use Hand Bursa and Ligament, Right
INTERCEPT Blood System for Plasma Pathogen Reduced Cryoprecipitated Fibrinogen Complex use Pathogen Reduced Cryoprecipitated Fibrinogen Complex
INTERCEPT Fibrinogen Complex use Pathogen Reduced Cryoprecipitated Fibrinogen Complex
Interclavicular ligament
use Shoulder Bursa and Ligament, Left
use Shoulder Bursa and Ligament, Right
Intercostal lymph node use Lymphatic, Thorax
Intercostal muscle
use Thorax Muscle, Left
use Thorax Muscle, Right
Intercostal nerve use Thoracic Nerve
Intercostobrachial nerve use Thoracic Nerve
Intercuneiform joint
use Tarsal Joint, Left
use Tarsal Joint, Right
Intercuneiform ligament
use Foot Bursa and Ligament, Left
use Foot Bursa and Ligament, Right
Intermediate bronchus use Main Bronchus, Right
Intermediate cuneiform bone
use Tarsal, Left
use Tarsal, Right
Intermittent Coronary Sinus Occlusion X2A7358
Intermittent hemodialysis (IHD) 5A1D7ØZ
Intermittent mandatory ventilation see Assistance, Respiratory 5AØ9
Intermittent Negative Airway Pressure
24-96 Consecutive Hours, Ventilation 5AØ945B
Greater than 96 Consecutive Hours, Ventilation 5AØ955B
Less than 24 Consecutive Hours, Ventilation 5AØ935B
Intermittent Positive Airway Pressure
24-96 Consecutive Hours, Ventilation 5AØ9458
Greater than 96 Consecutive Hours, Ventilation 5AØ9558
Less than 24 Consecutive Hours, Ventilation 5AØ9358
Intermittent positive pressure breathing see Assistance, Respiratory 5AØ9
Internal anal sphincter use Anal Sphincter
Internal carotid artery, intracranial portion use Intracranial Artery
Internal carotid plexus use Head and Neck Sympathetic Nerve
Internal (basal) cerebral vein use Intracranial Vein
Internal Fixation Device with Tulip Connector
Fusion, Joint, Sacroiliac XRG
Insertion, Bone, Pelvic XNH

Internal iliac vein
  use Hypogastric Vein, Left
  use Hypogastric Vein, Right
Internal maxillary artery
  use External Carotid Artery, Left
  use External Carotid Artery, Right
Internal naris *use* Nasal Mucosa and Soft Tissue
Internal oblique muscle
  use Abdomen Muscle, Left
  use Abdomen Muscle, Right
Internal pudendal artery
  use Internal Iliac Artery, Left
  use Internal Iliac Artery, Right
Internal pudendal vein
  use Hypogastric Vein, Left
  use Hypogastric Vein, Right
Internal thoracic artery
  use Internal Mammary Artery, Left
  use Internal Mammary Artery, Right
  use Subclavian Artery, Left
  use Subclavian Artery, Right
Internal urethral sphincter *use* Urethra
Interphalangeal (IP) joint
  use Finger Phalangeal Joint, Left
  use Finger Phalangeal Joint, Right
  use Toe Phalangeal Joint, Left
  use Toe Phalangeal Joint, Right
Interphalangeal ligament
  use Foot Bursa and Ligament, Left
  use Foot Bursa and Ligament, Right
  use Hand Bursa and Ligament, Left
  use Hand Bursa and Ligament, Right
Interrogation, cardiac rhythm related device
  Interrogation only *see* Measurement, Cardiac 4B02
  With cardiac function testing *see* Measurement, Cardiac 4A02
Interruption *see* Occlusion
Interspinalis muscle
  use Trunk Muscle, Left
  use Trunk Muscle, Right
Interspinous ligament, cervical *use* Head and Neck Bursa and Ligament
Interspinous ligament, lumbar *use* Lower Spine Bursa and Ligament
Interspinous ligament, thoracic *use* Upper Spine Bursa and Ligament
Interspinous process spinal stabilization device
  use Spinal Stabilization Device, Interspinous Process in 0RH
  use Spinal Stabilization Device, Interspinous Process in 0SH
InterStim® Therapy lead *use* Neurostimulator Lead in Peripheral Nervous System
InterStim™ II Therapy neurostimulator *use* Stimulator Generator, Single Array in 0JH
InterStim™ Micro Therapy neurostimulator *use* Stimulator Generator, Single Array Rechargeable in 0JH
Intertransversarius muscle
  use Trunk Muscle, Left
  use Trunk Muscle, Right
Intertransverse ligament, cervical *use* Head and Neck Bursa and Ligament
Intertransverse ligament, lumbar *use* Lower Spine Bursa and Ligament
Intertransverse ligament, thoracic *use* Upper Spine Bursa and Ligament
Interventricular foramen (Monro) *use* Cerebral Ventricle
Interventricular septum *use* Ventricular Septum
Intestinal lymphatic trunk *use* Cisterna Chyli
Intracranial Arterial Flow, Whole Blood mRNA XXE5XT7
Intraluminal Device
  Airway
    Esophagus 0DH5
    Mouth and Throat 0CHY
    Nasopharynx 09HN
  Bioactive
    Occlusion
      Common Carotid
        Left 03LJ
        Right 03LH
      External Carotid
        Left 03LN
        Right 03LM

Intraluminal Device — *continued*
  Bioactive — *continued*
    Occlusion — *continued*
      Internal Carotid
        Left 03LL
        Right 03LK
      Intracranial 03LG
      Vertebral
        Left 03LQ
        Right 03LP
    Restriction
      Common Carotid
        Left 03VJ
        Right 03VH
      External Carotid
        Left 03VN
        Right 03VM
      Internal Carotid
        Left 03VL
        Right 03VK
      Intracranial 03VG
      Vertebral
        Left 03VQ
        Right 03VP
  Endobronchial Valve
    Lingula 0BH9
    Lower Lobe
      Left 0BHB
      Right 0BH6
    Main
      Left 0BH7
      Right 0BH3
    Middle Lobe, Right 0BH5
    Upper Lobe
      Left 0BH8
      Right 0BH4
  Endotracheal Airway
    Change device in, Trachea 0B21XEZ
    Insertion of device in, Trachea 0BH1
  Pessary
    Change device in, Vagina and Cul-de-sac 0U2HXGZ
    Insertion of device in
      Cul-de-sac 0UHF
      Vagina 0UHG
Intramedullary (IM) rod (nail)
  use Internal Fixation Device, Intramedullary in Lower Bones
  use Internal Fixation Device, Intramedullary in Upper Bones
Intramedullary skeletal kinetic distractor (ISKD)
  use Internal Fixation Device, Intramedullary in Lower Bones
  use Internal Fixation Device, Intramedullary in Upper Bones
Intraocular Telescope
  Left 08RK30Z
  Right 08RJ30Z
Intraoperative Radiation Therapy (IORT)
  Anus DDY8CZZ
  Bile Ducts DFY2CZZ
  Bladder DTY2CZZ
  Brain D0Y0CZZ
  Brain Stem D0Y1CZZ
  Cervix DUY1CZZ
  Colon DDY5CZZ
  Duodenum DDY2CZZ
  Gallbladder DFY1CZZ
  Ileum DDY4CZZ
  Jejunum DDY3CZZ
  Kidney DTY0CZZ
  Larynx D9YBCZZ
  Liver DFY0CZZ
  Mouth D9Y4CZZ
  Nasopharynx D9YDCZZ
  Nerve, Peripheral D0Y7CZZ
  Ovary DUY0CZZ
  Pancreas DFY3CZZ
  Pharynx D9YCCZZ
  Prostate DVY0CZZ
  Rectum DDY7CZZ
  Spinal Cord D0Y6CZZ
  Stomach DDY1CZZ
  Ureter DTY1CZZ
  Urethra DTY3CZZ
  Uterus DUY2CZZ
Intra.OX 8E02XDZ

Intrauterine Device (IUD) *use* Contraceptive Device in Female Reproductive System
Intravascular fluorescence angiography (IFA) *see* Monitoring, Physiological Systems 4A1
Intravascular Lithotripsy (IVL) *see* Fragmentation
Intravascular ultrasound assisted thrombolysis *see* Fragmentation, Artery
Introduction of substance in or on
  Artery
    Central 3E06
      Analgesics 3E06
      Anesthetic, Intracirculatory 3E06
      Antiarrhythmic 3E06
      Anti-infective 3E06
      Anti-inflammatory 3E06
      Antineoplastic 3E06
      Destructive Agent 3E06
      Diagnostic Substance, Other 3E06
      Electrolytic Substance 3E06
      Hormone 3E06
      Hypnotics 3E06
      Immunotherapeutic 3E06
      Nutritional Substance 3E06
      Platelet Inhibitor 3E06
      Radioactive Substance 3E06
      Sedatives 3E06
      Serum 3E06
      Thrombolytic 3E06
      Toxoid 3E06
      Vaccine 3E06
      Vasopressor 3E06
      Water Balance Substance 3E06
    Coronary 3E07
      Diagnostic Substance, Other 3E07
      Platelet Inhibitor 3E07
      Thrombolytic 3E07
    Peripheral 3E05
      Analgesics 3E05
      Anesthetic, Intracirculatory 3E05
      Antiarrhythmic 3E05
      Anti-infective 3E05
      Anti-inflammatory 3E05
      Antineoplastic 3E05
      Destructive Agent 3E05
      Diagnostic Substance, Other 3E05
      Electrolytic Substance 3E05
      Hormone 3E05
      Hypnotics 3E05
      Immunotherapeutic 3E05
      Nutritional Substance 3E05
      Platelet Inhibitor 3E05
      Radioactive Substance 3E05
      Sedatives 3E05
      Serum 3E05
      Thrombolytic 3E05
      Toxoid 3E05
      Vaccine 3E05
      Vasopressor 3E05
      Water Balance Substance 3E05
  Biliary Tract 3E0J
    Analgesics 3E0J
    Anesthetic Agent 3E0J
    Anti-infective 3E0J
    Anti-inflammatory 3E0J
    Antineoplastic 3E0J
    Destructive Agent 3E0J
    Diagnostic Substance, Other 3E0J
    Electrolytic Substance 3E0J
    Gas 3E0J
    Hypnotics 3E0J
    Islet Cells, Pancreatic 3E0J
    Nutritional Substance 3E0J
    Radioactive Substance 3E0J
    Sedatives 3E0J
    Water Balance Substance 3E0J
  Bone 3E0V
    Analgesics 3E0V3NZ
    Anesthetic Agent 3E0V3BZ
    Anti-infective 3E0V32
    Anti-inflammatory 3E0V33Z
    Antineoplastic 3E0V30
    Destructive Agent 3E0V3TZ
    Diagnostic Substance, Other 3E0V3KZ
    Electrolytic Substance 3E0V37Z
    Hypnotics 3E0V3NZ
    Nutritional Substance 3E0V36Z
    Radioactive Substance 3E0V3HZ
    Sedatives 3E0V3NZ
    Water Balance Substance 3E0V37Z

Introduction of substance in or on — *continued*
Pericardial Cavity — *continued*
Water Balance Substance 3E0Y37Z
Peritoneal Cavity 3E0M
Adhesion Barrier 3E0M
Analgesics 3E0M3NZ
Anesthetic Agent 3E0M3BZ
Anti-infective 3E0M32
Anti-inflammatory 3E0M33Z
Antineoplastic 3E0M
Destructive Agent 3E0M3TZ
Diagnostic Substance, Other 3E0M3KZ
Electrolytic Substance 3E0M37Z
Gas 3E0M
Hypnotics 3E0M3NZ
Nutritional Substance 3E0M36Z
Radioactive Substance 3E0M3HZ
Sedatives 3E0M3NZ
Water Balance Substance 3E0M37Z
Pharynx 3E0D
Analgesics 3E0D
Anesthetic Agent 3E0D
Antiarrhythmic 3E0D
Anti-infective 3E0D
Anti-inflammatory 3E0D
Antineoplastic 3E0D
Destructive Agent 3E0D
Diagnostic Substance, Other 3E0D
Electrolytic Substance 3E0D
Hypnotics 3E0D
Nutritional Substance 3E0D
Radioactive Substance 3E0D
Sedatives 3E0D
Serum 3E0D
Toxoid 3E0D
Vaccine 3E0D
Water Balance Substance 3E0D
Pleural Cavity 3E0L
Adhesion Barrier 3E0L
Analgesics 3E0L3NZ
Anesthetic Agent 3E0L3BZ
Anti-infective 3E0L32
Anti-inflammatory 3E0L33Z
Antineoplastic 3E0L
Destructive Agent 3E0L3TZ
Diagnostic Substance, Other 3E0L3KZ
Electrolytic Substance 3E0L37Z
Gas 3E0L
Hypnotics 3E0L3NZ
Nutritional Substance 3E0L36Z
Radioactive Substance 3E0L3HZ
Sedatives 3E0L3NZ
Water Balance Substance 3E0L37Z
Products of Conception 3E0E
Analgesics 3E0E
Anesthetic Agent 3E0E
Anti-infective 3E0E
Anti-inflammatory 3E0E
Antineoplastic 3E0E
Destructive Agent 3E0E
Diagnostic Substance, Other 3E0E
Electrolytic Substance 3E0E
Gas 3E0E
Hypnotics 3E0E
Nutritional Substance 3E0E
Radioactive Substance 3E0E
Sedatives 3E0E
Water Balance Substance 3E0E
Reproductive
Female 3E0P
Adhesion Barrier 3E0P
Analgesics 3E0P
Anesthetic Agent 3E0P
Anti-infective 3E0P
Anti-inflammatory 3E0P
Antineoplastic 3E0P
Destructive Agent 3E0P
Diagnostic Substance, Other 3E0P
Electrolytic Substance 3E0P
Gas 3E0P
Hormone 3E0P
Hypnotics 3E0P
Nutritional Substance 3E0P
Ovum, Fertilized 3E0P
Radioactive Substance 3E0P
Sedatives 3E0P
Sperm 3E0P
Water Balance Substance 3E0P
Male 3E0N

Introduction of substance in or on — *continued*
Reproductive — *continued*
Male — *continued*
Analgesics 3E0N
Anesthetic Agent 3E0N
Anti-infective 3E0N
Anti-inflammatory 3E0N
Antineoplastic 3E0N
Destructive Agent 3E0N
Diagnostic Substance, Other 3E0N
Electrolytic Substance 3E0N
Gas 3E0N
Hypnotics 3E0N
Nutritional Substance 3E0N
Radioactive Substance 3E0N
Sedatives 3E0N
Water Balance Substance 3E0N
Respiratory Tract 3E0F
Analgesics 3E0F
Anesthetic Agent 3E0F
Anti-infective 3E0F
Anti-inflammatory 3E0F
Antineoplastic 3E0F
Destructive Agent 3E0F
Diagnostic Substance, Other 3E0F
Electrolytic Substance 3E0F
Gas 3E0F
Hypnotics 3E0F
Nutritional Substance 3E0F
Radioactive Substance 3E0F
Sedatives 3E0F
Water Balance Substance 3E0F
Skin 3E00XGC
Analgesics 3E00XNZ
Anesthetic Agent 3E00XBZ
Anti-infective 3E00X2
Anti-inflammatory 3E00X3Z
Antineoplastic 3E00X0
Destructive Agent 3E00XTZ
Diagnostic Substance, Other 3E00XKZ
Hypnotics 3E00XNZ
Pigment 3E00XMZ
Sedatives 3E00XNZ
Serum 3E00X4Z
Toxoid 3E00X4Z
Vaccine 3E00X4Z
Spinal Canal 3E0R3GC
Analgesics 3E0R3NZ
Anesthetic Agent 3E0R3BZ
Anti-infective 3E0R32
Anti-inflammatory 3E0R33Z
Antineoplastic 3E0R30
Destructive Agent 3E0R3TZ
Diagnostic Substance, Other 3E0R3KZ
Electrolytic Substance 3E0R37Z
Gas 3E0R
Hypnotics 3E0R3NZ
Nutritional Substance 3E0R36Z
Radioactive Substance 3E0R3HZ
Sedatives 3E0R3NZ
Stem Cells
Embryonic 3E0R
Somatic 3E0R
Water Balance Substance 3E0R37Z
Subcutaneous Tissue 3E013GC
Analgesics 3E013NZ
Anesthetic Agent 3E013BZ
Anti-infective 3E01
Anti-inflammatory 3E0133Z
Antineoplastic 3E0130
Destructive Agent 3E013TZ
Diagnostic Substance, Other 3E013KZ
Electrolytic Substance 3E0137Z
Hormone 3E013V
Hypnotics 3E013NZ
Nutritional Substance 3E0136Z
Radioactive Substance 3E013HZ
Sedatives 3E013NZ
Serum 3E0134Z
Toxoid 3E0134Z
Vaccine 3E0134Z
Water Balance Substance 3E0137Z
Vein
Central 3E04
Analgesics 3E04
Anesthetic, Intracirculatory 3E04
Antiarrhythmic 3E04
Anti-infective 3E04
Anti-inflammatory 3E04

Introduction of substance in or on — *continued*
Vein — *continued*
Central — *continued*
Antineoplastic 3E04
Destructive Agent 3E04
Diagnostic Substance, Other 3E04
Electrolytic Substance 3E04
Hormone 3E04
Hypnotics 3E04
Immunotherapeutic 3E04
Nutritional Substance 3E04
Platelet Inhibitor 3E04
Radioactive Substance 3E04
Sedatives 3E04
Serum 3E04
Thrombolytic 3E04
Toxoid 3E04
Vaccine 3E04
Vasopressor 3E04
Water Balance Substance 3E04
Peripheral 3E03
Analgesics 3E03
Anesthetic, Intracirculatory 3E03
Antiarrhythmic 3E03
Anti-Infective 3E03
Anti-inflammatory 3E03
Antineoplastic 3E03
Destructive Agent 3E03
Diagnostic Substance, Other 3E03
Electrolytic Substance 3E03
Hormone 3E03
Hypnotics 3E03
Immunotherapeutic 3E03
Islet Cells, Pancreatic 3E03
Nutritional Substance 3E03
Platelet Inhibitor 3E03
Radioactive Substance 3E03
Sedatives 3E03
Serum 3E03
Thrombolytic 3E03
Toxoid 3E03
Vaccine 3E03
Vasopressor 3E03
Water Balance Substance 3E03

Intubation
Airway
see Insertion of device in, Esophagus 0DH5
see Insertion of device in, Mouth and Throat 0CHY
see Insertion of device in, Trachea 0BH1
Drainage device *see* Drainage
Feeding Device *see* Insertion of device in, Gastrointestinal System 0DH
INTUITY Elite valve system, EDWARDS (rapid deployment technique) *see* Replacement, Valve, Aortic 02RF
Iobenguane I-131 Antineoplastic XW0
Iobenguane I-131, High Specific Activity (HSA) *use* Iobenguane I-131 Antineoplastic
IPPB (intermittent positive pressure breathing) *see* Assistance, Respiratory 5A09
IRE (Irreversible Electroporation) *see* Destruction, Hepatobiliary System and Pancreas 0F5
Iridectomy
see Excision, Eye 08B
see Resection, Eye 08T
Iridoplasty
see Repair, Eye 08Q
see Replacement, Eye 08R
see Supplement, Eye 08U
Iridotomy *see* Drainage, Eye 089
Irreversible Electroporation (IRE) *see* Destruction, Hepatobiliary System and Pancreas 0F5
Irrigation
Biliary Tract, Irrigating Substance 3E1J
Brain, Irrigating Substance 3E1Q38Z
Cranial Cavity, Irrigating Substance 3E1Q38Z
Ear, Irrigating Substance 3E1B
Epidural Space, Irrigating Substance 3E1S38Z
Eye, Irrigating Substance 3E1C
Gastrointestinal Tract
Lower, Irrigating Substance 3E1H
Upper, Irrigating Substance 3E1G
Genitourinary Tract, Irrigating Substance 3E1K
Irrigating Substance 3C1ZX8Z
Joint, Irrigating Substance 3E1U
Mucous Membrane, Irrigating Substance 3E10
Nose, Irrigating Substance 3E19

Irrigation — *continued*
  Pancreatic Tract, Irrigating Substance 3E1J
  Pericardial Cavity, Irrigating Substance 3E1Y38Z
  Peritoneal Cavity
    Dialysate 3E1M39Z
    Irrigating Substance 3E1M
  Pleural Cavity, Irrigating Substance 3E1L38Z
  Reproductive
    Female, Irrigating Substance 3E1P
    Male, Irrigating Substance 3E1N
  Respiratory Tract, Irrigating Substance 3E1F
  Skin, Irrigating Substance 3E10
  Spinal Canal, Irrigating Substance 3E1R38Z
Isavuconazole (isavuconazonium sulfate) *use* Other Anti-infective
Ischemic Stroke System (ISS500) *use* Neurostimulator Lead in New Technology
Ischiatic nerve *use* Sciatic Nerve
Ischiocavernosus muscle *use* Perineum Muscle
Ischiofemoral ligament
  use Hip Bursa and Ligament, Left
  use Hip Bursa and Ligament, Right
Ischium
  use Pelvic Bone, Left
  use Pelvic Bone, Right
ISC-REST kit
  ISCDx XXE5XT7
  QIAGEN Access Anti-SARS-CoV-2 Total Test XXE5XV7
  QIAstat-Dx Respiratory SARS-CoV-2 Panel XXE97U7
Isolation 8E0ZXY6
Isotope Administration, Other Radiation, Whole Body DWY5G
ISS500 (Ischemic Stroke System) *use* Neurostimulator Lead in New Technology
Itrel (3) (4) neurostimulator *use* Stimulator Generator, Single Array in 0JH

J

Jakafi® *use* Ruxolitinib
Jejunal artery *use* Superior Mesenteric Artery
Jejunectomy
  see Excision, Jejunum 0DBA
  see Resection, Jejunum 0DTA
Jejunocolostomy
  see Bypass, Gastrointestinal System 0D1
  see Drainage, Gastrointestinal System 0D9
Jejunopexy
  see Repair, Jejunum 0DQA
  see Reposition, Jejunum 0DSA
Jejunostomy
  see Bypass, Jejunum 0D1A
  see Drainage, Jejunum 0D9A
Jejunotomy *see* Drainage, Jejunum 0D9A
Joint fixation plate
  use Internal Fixation Device in Lower Joints
  use Internal Fixation Device in Upper Joints
Joint liner (insert) *use* Liner in Lower Joints
Joint spacer (antibiotic)
  use Spacer in Lower Joints
  use Spacer in Upper Joints
Jugular body *use* Glomus Jugulare
Jugular lymph node
  use Lymphatic, Left Neck
  use Lymphatic, Right Neck

K

Kappa *use* Pacemaker, Dual Chamber in 0JH
Kcentra *use* 4-Factor Prothrombin Complex Concentrate
Keratectomy, kerectomy
  see Excision, Eye 08B
  see Resection, Eye 08T
Keratocentesis *see* Drainage, Eye 089
Keratoplasty
  see Repair, Eye 08Q
  see Replacement, Eye 08R
  see Supplement, Eye 08U
Keratotomy
  see Drainage, Eye 089
  see Repair, Eye 08Q
KEVZARA® *use* Sarilumab

Keystone Heart TriGuard 3™ CEPD (cerebral embolic protection device) X2A6325
Kirschner wire (K-wire)
  use Internal Fixation Device in Head and Facial Bones
  use Internal Fixation Device in Lower Bones
  use Internal Fixation Device in Lower Joints
  use Internal Fixation Device in Upper Bones
  use Internal Fixation Device in Upper Joints
Knee (implant) insert *use* Liner in Lower Joints
KUB x-ray *see* Plain Radiography, Kidney, Ureter and Bladder BT04
Kuntscher nail
  use Internal Fixation Device, Intramedullary in Lower Bones
  use Internal Fixation Device, Intramedullary in Upper Bones
KYMRIAH® *use* Tisagenlecleucel Immunotherapy

L

Labia majora *use* Vulva
Labia minora *use* Vulva
Labial gland
  use Lower Lip
  use Upper Lip
Labiectomy
  see Excision, Female Reproductive System 0UB
  see Resection, Female Reproductive System 0UT
Lacrimal canaliculus
  use Lacrimal Duct, Left
  use Lacrimal Duct, Right
Lacrimal punctum
  use Lacrimal Duct, Left
  use Lacrimal Duct, Right
Lacrimal sac
  use Lacrimal Duct, Left
  use Lacrimal Duct, Right
LAGB (laparoscopic adjustable gastric banding)
  Initial procedure 0DV64CZ
  Surgical correction *see* Revision of device in, Stomach 0DW6
Laminectomy
  see Excision, Lower Bones 0QB
  see Excision, Upper Bones 0PB
  see Release, Central Nervous System and Cranial Nerves 00N
  see Release, Peripheral Nervous System 01N
Laminotomy
  see Drainage, Lower Bones 0Q9
  see Drainage, Upper Bones 0P9
  see Excision, Lower Bones 0QB
  see Excision, Upper Bones 0PB
  see Release, Central Nervous System and Cranial Nerves 00N
  see Release, Lower Bones 0QN
  see Release, Peripheral Nervous System 01N
  see Release, Upper Bones 0PN
Laparoscopic-assisted transanal pull-through
  see Excision, Gastrointestinal System 0DB
  see Resection, Gastrointestinal System 0DT
Laparoscopy *see* Inspection
Laparotomy
  Drainage *see* Drainage, Peritoneal Cavity 0W9G
  Exploratory *see* Inspection, Peritoneal Cavity 0WJG
LAP-BAND® adjustable gastric banding system *use* Extraluminal Device
Laryngectomy
  see Excision, Larynx 0CBS
  see Resection, Larynx 0CTS
Laryngocentesis *see* Drainage, Larynx 0C9S
Laryngogram *see* Fluoroscopy, Larynx B91J
Laryngopexy *see* Repair, Larynx 0CQS
Laryngopharynx *use* Pharynx
Laryngoplasty
  see Repair, Larynx 0CQS
  see Replacement, Larynx 0CRS
  see Supplement, Larynx 0CUS
Laryngorrhaphy *see* Repair, Larynx 0CQS
Laryngoscopy 0CJS8ZZ
Laryngotomy *see* Drainage, Larynx 0C9S
Laser Interstitial Thermal Therapy
  Ampulla of Vater 0F5C
  Anus 0D5Q
  Aortic Body 0G5D
  Appendix 0D5J

Laser Interstitial Thermal Therapy — *continued*
  Brain 0050
  Breast
    Bilateral 0H5V
    Left 0H5U
    Right 0H5T
  Carotid Bodies, Bilateral 0G58
  Carotid Body
    Left 0G56
    Right 0G57
  Cecum 0D5H
  Coccygeal Glomus 0G5B
  Colon
    Ascending 0D5K
    Descending 0D5M
    Sigmoid 0D5N
    Transverse 0D5L
  Duct
    Common Bile 0F59
    Cystic 0F58
    Hepatic
      Common 0F57
      Left 0F56
      Right 0F55
    Pancreatic 0F5D
      Accessory 0F5F
  Duodenum 0D59
  Esophagogastric Junction 0D54
  Esophagus 0D55
    Lower 0D53
    Middle 0D52
    Upper 0D51
  Gallbladder 0F54
  Gland
    Adrenal
      Bilateral 0G54
      Left 0G52
      Right 0G53
    Pituitary 0G50
  Glomus Jugulare 0G5C
  Ileocecal Valve 0D5C
  Ileum 0D5B
  Intestine
    Large 0D5E
      Left 0D5G
      Right 0D5F
    Small 0D58
  Jejunum 0D5A
  Liver 0F50
    Left Lobe 0F52
    Right Lobe 0F51
  Lung
    Bilateral 0B5M
    Left 0B5L
    Lower Lobe
      Left 0B5J
      Right 0B5F
    Middle Lobe, Right 0B5D
    Right 0B5K
    Upper Lobe
      Left 0B5G
      Right 0B5C
  Lung Lingula 0B5H
  Pancreas 0F5G
  Para-aortic Body 0G59
  Paraganglion Extremity 0G5F
  Parathyroid Gland 0G5R
    Inferior
      Left 0G5P
      Right 0G5N
    Multiple 0G5Q
    Superior
      Left 0G5M
      Right 0G5L
  Pineal Body 0G51
  Prostate 0V50
  Rectum 0D5P
  Spinal Cord
    Cervical 005W
    Lumbar 005Y
    Thoracic 005X
  Stomach 0D56
    Pylorus 0D57
  Thyroid Gland 0G5K
    Left Lobe 0G5G
    Right Lobe 0G5H
Lateral canthus
  use Upper Eyelid, Left
  use Upper Eyelid, Right

▽ **Subterms under main terms may continue to next column or page**

Lateral collateral ligament (LCL)
  use Knee Bursa and Ligament, Left
  use Knee Bursa and Ligament, Right
Lateral condyle of femur
  use Lower Femur, Left
  use Lower Femur, Right
Lateral condyle of tibia
  use Tibia, Left
  use Tibia, Right
Lateral cuneiform bone
  use Tarsal, Left
  use Tarsal, Right
Lateral epicondyle of femur
  use Lower Femur, Left
  use Lower Femur, Right
Lateral epicondyle of humerus
  use Humeral Shaft, Left
  use Humeral Shaft, Right
Lateral femoral cutaneous nerve *use* Lumbar Plexus
Lateral (brachial) lymph node
  use Lymphatic, Left Axillary
  use Lymphatic, Right Axillary
Lateral malleolus
  use Fibula, Left
  use Fibula, Right
Lateral meniscus
  use Knee Joint, Left
  use Knee Joint, Right
Lateral nasal cartilage *use* Nasal Mucosa and Soft
  Tissue
Lateral plantar artery
  use Foot Artery, Left
  use Foot Artery, Right
Lateral plantar nerve *use* Tibial Nerve
Lateral rectus muscle
  use Extraocular Muscle, Left
  use Extraocular Muscle, Right
Lateral sacral artery
  use Internal Iliac Artery, Left
  use Internal Iliac Artery, Right
Lateral sacral vein
  use Hypogastric Vein, Left
  use Hypogastric Vein, Right
Lateral sural cutaneous nerve *use* Peroneal Nerve
Lateral tarsal artery
  use Foot Artery, Left
  use Foot Artery, Right
Lateral temporomandibular ligament *use* Head and
  Neck Bursa and Ligament
Lateral thoracic artery
  use Axillary Artery, Left
  use Axillary Artery, Right
Latissimus dorsi muscle
  use Trunk Muscle, Left
  use Trunk Muscle, Right
Latissimus Dorsi Myocutaneous Flap
  Replacement
    Bilateral ØHRVØ75
    Left ØHRUØ75
    Right ØHRTØ75
  Transfer
    Left ØKXG
    Right ØKXF
Lavage
  see Irrigation
  Bronchial alveolar, diagnostic *see* Drainage, Respi-
    ratory System ØB9
Least splanchnic nerve *use* Thoracic Sympathetic
  Nerve
Lefamulin Anti-infective XWØ
Left ascending lumbar vein *use* Hemiazygos Vein
Left atrioventricular valve *use* Mitral Valve
Left auricular appendix *use* Atrium, Left
Left colic vein *use* Colic Vein
Left coronary sulcus *use* Heart, Left
Left gastric artery *use* Gastric Artery
Left gastroepiploic artery *use* Splenic Artery
Left gastroepiploic vein *use* Splenic Vein
Left inferior phrenic vein *use* Renal Vein, Left
Left inferior pulmonary vein *use* Pulmonary Vein,
  Left
Left jugular trunk *use* Thoracic Duct
Left lateral ventricle *use* Cerebral Ventricle
Left ovarian vein *use* Renal Vein, Left
Left second lumbar vein *use* Renal Vein, Left
Left subclavian trunk *use* Thoracic Duct

Left subcostal vein *use* Hemiazygos Vein
Left superior pulmonary vein *use* Pulmonary Vein,
  Left
Left suprarenal vein *use* Renal Vein, Left
Left testicular vein *use* Renal Vein, Left
Lengthening
  Bone, with device *see* Insertion of Limb Lengthen-
    ing Device
  Muscle, by incision *see* Division, Muscles ØK8
  Tendon, by incision *see* Division, Tendons ØL8
Leptomeninges, intracranial *use* Cerebral Meninges
Leptomeninges, spinal *use* Spinal Meninges
Leronlimab Monoclonal Antibody XWØ13K6
Lesser alar cartilage *use* Nasal Mucosa and Soft Tissue
Lesser occipital nerve *use* Cervical Plexus
Lesser Omentum *use* Omentum
Lesser saphenous vein
  use Saphenous Vein, Left
  use Saphenous Vein, Right
Lesser splanchnic nerve *use* Thoracic Sympathetic
  Nerve
Lesser trochanter
  use Upper Femur, Left
  use Upper Femur, Right
Lesser tuberosity
  use Humeral Head, Left
  use Humeral Head, Right
Lesser wing *use* Sphenoid Bone
Leukopheresis, therapeutic *see* Pheresis, Circulatory
  6A55
Levator anguli oris muscle *use* Facial Muscle
Levator ani muscle *use* Perineum Muscle
Levator labii superioris alaeque nasi muscle *use*
  Facial Muscle
Levator labii superioris muscle *use* Facial Muscle
Levator palpebrae superioris muscle
  use Upper Eyelid, Left
  use Upper Eyelid, Right
Levator scapulae muscle
  use Neck Muscle, Left
  use Neck Muscle, Right
Levator veli palatini muscle *use* Tongue, Palate,
  Pharynx Muscle
Levatores costarum muscle
  use Thorax Muscle, Left
  use Thorax Muscle, Right
**Lifeline ARM Automated Chest Compression (ACC)
  device** 5A1221J
LifeStent® (Flexstar) (XL) Vascular Stent System
  use Intraluminal Device
Lifileucel *use* Lifileucel Immunotherapy
Lifileucel Immunotherapy XWØ
Ligament of head of fibula
  use Knee Bursa and Ligament, Left
  use Knee Bursa and Ligament, Right
Ligament of the lateral malleolus
  use Ankle Bursa and Ligament, Left
  use Ankle Bursa and Ligament, Right
Ligamentum flavum, cervical *use* Head and Neck
  Bursa and Ligament
Ligamentum flavum, lumbar *use* Lower Spine Bursa
  and Ligament
Ligamentum flavum, thoracic *use* Upper Spine Bursa
  and Ligament
LigaPASS 2.Ø™ PJK Prevention System *use* Posterior
  Vertebral Tether in New Technology
Ligation *see* Occlusion
Ligation, hemorrhoid *see* Occlusion, Lower Veins,
  Hemorrhoidal Plexus
Light Therapy GZJZZZZ
Liner
  Removal of device from
    Hip
      Left ØSPBØ9Z
      Right ØSP9Ø9Z
    Knee
      Left ØSPDØ9Z
      Right ØSPCØ9Z
  Revision of device in
    Hip
      Left ØSWBØ9Z
      Right ØSW9Ø9Z
    Knee
      Left ØSWDØ9Z
      Right ØSWCØ9Z

Liner — *continued*
  Supplement
    Hip
      Left ØSUBØ9Z
        Acetabular Surface ØSUEØ9Z
        Femoral Surface ØSUSØ9Z
      Right ØSU9Ø9Z
        Acetabular Surface ØSUAØ9Z
        Femoral Surface ØSURØ9Z
    Knee
      Left ØSUDØ9
        Femoral Surface ØSUUØ9Z
        Tibial Surface ØSUWØ9Z
      Right ØSUCØ9
        Femoral Surface ØSUTØ9Z
        Tibial Surface ØSUVØ9Z
Lingual artery
  use External Carotid Artery, Left
  use External Carotid Artery, Right
Lingual tonsil *use* Pharynx
Lingulectomy, lung
  see Excision, Lung Lingula ØBBH
  see Resection, Lung Lingula ØBTH
Lisocabtagene Maraleucel *use* Lisocabtagene Mar-
  aleucel Immunotherapy
Lisocabtagene Maraleucel Immunotherapy XWØ
Lithoplasty *see* Fragmentation
Lithotripsy
  see Fragmentation
  With removal of fragments *see* Extirpation
LITT (laser interstitial thermal therapy)
  see Destruction
  see Laser Interstitial Thermal Therapy
LIVIAN™ CRT-D *use* Cardiac Resynchronization Defibrillator Pulse Generator in ØJH
LIVTENCITY™ *use* Maribavir Anti-infective
Lobectomy
  see Excision, Central Nervous System and Cranial
    Nerves ØØB
  see Excision, Endocrine System ØGB
  see Excision, Hepatobiliary System and Pancreas
    ØFB
  see Excision, Respiratory System ØBB
  see Resection, Endocrine System ØGT
  see Resection, Hepatobiliary System and Pancreas
    ØFT
  see Resection, Respiratory System ØBT
Lobotomy *see* Division, Brain ØØ8Ø
Localization
  see Imaging
  see Map
Locus ceruleus *use* Pons
Long thoracic nerve *use* Brachial Plexus
Loop ileostomy *see* Bypass, Ileum ØD1B
Loop recorder, implantable *use* Monitoring Device
Lower GI series *see* Fluoroscopy, Colon BD14
**Lower Respiratory Fluid Nucleic Acid-base Micro-
  bial Detection** XXEBXQ6
LTX Regional Anticoagulant *use* Nafamostat Antico-
  agulant
LUCAS® Chest Compression System 5A1221J
Lumbar artery *use* Abdominal Aorta
Lumbar facet joint *use* Lumbar Vertebral Joint
Lumbar ganglion *use* Lumbar Sympathetic Nerve
Lumbar lymph node *use* Lymphatic, Aortic
Lumbar lymphatic trunk *use* Cisterna Chyli
Lumbar splanchnic nerve *use* Lumbar Sympathetic
  Nerve
Lumbosacral facet joint *use* Lumbosacral Joint
Lumbosacral trunk *use* Lumbar Nerve
Lumpectomy *see* Excision
Lunate bone
  use Carpal, Left
  use Carpal, Right
Lunotriquetral ligament
  use Hand Bursa and Ligament, Left
  use Hand Bursa and Ligament, Right
Lurbinectedin XWØ
Lymphadenectomy
  see Excision, Lymphatic and Hemic Systems Ø7B
  see Resection, Lymphatic and Hemic Systems Ø7T
Lymphadenotomy *see* Drainage, Lymphatic and Hemic
  Systems Ø79
Lymphangiectomy
  see Excision, Lymphatic and Hemic Systems Ø7B
  see Resection, Lymphatic and Hemic Systems Ø7T

Lymphangiogram *see* Plain Radiography, Lymphatic System B70
Lymphangioplasty
   see Repair, Lymphatic and Hemic Systems 07Q
   see Supplement, Lymphatic and Hemic Systems 07U
Lymphangiorrhaphy *see* Repair, Lymphatic and Hemic Systems 07Q
Lymphangiotomy *see* Drainage, Lymphatic and Hemic Systems 079
Lysis *see* Release

M

Macula XXE5XR7
   use Retina, Left
   use Retina, Right
MAGEC® Spinal Bracing and Distraction System
   use Magnetically Controlled Growth Rod(s) in New Technology
Magnet extraction, ocular foreign body *see* Extirpation, Eye 08C
Magnetic Resonance Imaging (MRI)
  Abdomen BW30
  Ankle
    Left BQ3H
    Right BQ3G
  Aorta
    Abdominal B430
    Thoracic B330
  Arm
    Left BP3F
    Right BP3E
  Artery
    Celiac B431
    Cervico-Cerebral Arch B33Q
    Common Carotid, Bilateral B335
    Coronary
      Bypass Graft, Multiple B233
      Multiple B231
    Internal Carotid, Bilateral B338
    Intracranial B33R
    Lower Extremity
      Bilateral B43H
      Left B43G
      Right B43F
    Pelvic B43C
    Renal, Bilateral B438
    Spinal B33M
    Superior Mesenteric B434
    Upper Extremity
      Bilateral B33K
      Left B33J
      Right B33H
    Vertebral, Bilateral B33G
  Bladder BT30
  Brachial Plexus BW3P
  Brain B030
  Breast
    Bilateral BH32
    Left BH31
    Right BH30
  Calcaneus
    Left BQ3K
    Right BQ3J
  Chest BW33Y
  Coccyx BR3F
  Connective Tissue
    Lower Extremity BL31
    Upper Extremity BL30
  Corpora Cavernosa BV30
  Disc
    Cervical BR31
    Lumbar BR33
    Thoracic BR32
  Ear B930
  Elbow
    Left BP3H
    Right BP3G
  Eye
    Bilateral B837
    Left B836
    Right B835
  Femur
    Left BQ34
    Right BQ33
  Fetal Abdomen BY33

Magnetic Resonance Imaging (MRI) — *continued*
  Fetal Extremity BY35
  Fetal Head BY30
  Fetal Heart BY31
  Fetal Spine BY34
  Fetal Thorax BY32
  Fetus, Whole BY36
  Foot
    Left BQ3M
    Right BQ3L
  Forearm
    Left BP3K
    Right BP3J
  Gland
    Adrenal, Bilateral BG32
    Parathyroid BG33
    Parotid, Bilateral B936
    Salivary, Bilateral B93D
    Submandibular, Bilateral B939
    Thyroid BG34
  Head BW38
  Heart, Right and Left B236
  Hip
    Left BQ31
    Right BQ30
  Intracranial Sinus B532
  Joint
    Finger
      Left BP3D
      Right BP3C
    Hand
      Left BP3D
      Right BP3C
    Temporomandibular, Bilateral BN39
  Kidney
    Bilateral BT33
    Left BT32
    Right BT31
    Transplant BT39
  Knee
    Left BQ38
    Right BQ37
  Larynx B93J
  Leg
    Left BQ3F
    Right BQ3D
  Liver BF35
  Liver and Spleen BF36
  Lung Apices BB3G
  Lung, Bilateral, Hyperpolarized Xenon 129 (Xe-129) BB34Z3Z
  Nasopharynx B93F
  Neck BW3F
  Nerve
    Acoustic B03C
    Brachial Plexus BW3P
  Oropharynx B93F
  Ovary
    Bilateral BU35
    Left BU34
    Right BU33
  Ovary and Uterus BU3C
  Pancreas BF37
  Patella
    Left BQ3W
    Right BQ3V
  Pelvic Region BW3G
  Pelvis BR3C
  Pituitary Gland B039
  Plexus, Brachial BW3P
  Prostate BV33
  Retroperitoneum BW3H
  Sacrum BR3F
  Scrotum BV34
  Sella Turcica B039
  Shoulder
    Left BP39
    Right BP38
  Sinus
    Intracranial B532
    Paranasal B932
  Spinal Cord B03B
  Spine
    Cervical BR30
    Lumbar BR39
    Thoracic BR37
  Spleen and Liver BF36
  Subcutaneous Tissue
    Abdomen BH3H

Magnetic Resonance Imaging (MRI) — *continued*
  Subcutaneous Tissue — *continued*
    Extremity
      Lower BH3J
      Upper BH3F
    Head BH3D
    Neck BH3D
    Pelvis BH3H
    Thorax BH3G
  Tendon
    Lower Extremity BL33
    Upper Extremity BL32
  Testicle
    Bilateral BV37
    Left BV36
    Right BV35
  Toe
    Left BQ3Q
    Right BQ3P
  Uterus BU36
    Pregnant BU3B
  Uterus and Ovary BU3C
  Vagina BU39
  Vein
    Cerebellar B531
    Cerebral B531
    Jugular, Bilateral B535
    Lower Extremity
      Bilateral B53D
      Left B53C
      Right B53B
    Other B53V
    Pelvic (Iliac) Bilateral B53H
    Portal B53T
    Pulmonary, Bilateral B53S
    Renal, Bilateral B53L
    Spanchnic B53T
    Upper Extremity
      Bilateral B53P
      Left B53N
      Right B53M
  Vena Cava
    Inferior B539
    Superior B538
  Wrist
    Left BP3M
    Right BP3L
Magnetically Controlled Growth Rod(s)
  Cervical XNS3
  Lumbar XNS0
  Thoracic XNS4
Magnetic-guided radiofrequency endovascular fistula
  Radial Artery, Left 031C3ZF
  Radial Artery, Right 031B3ZF
  Ulnar Artery, Left 031A3ZF
  Ulnar Artery, Right 03193ZF
Magnus Neuromodulation System (MNS) X0Z0X18
Malleotomy *see* Drainage, Ear, Nose, Sinus 099
Malleus
  use Auditory Ossicle, Left
  use Auditory Ossicle, Right
Mammaplasty, mammoplasty
  see Alteration, Skin and Breast 0H0
  see Repair, Skin and Breast 0HQ
  see Replacement, Skin and Breast 0HR
  see Supplement, Skin and Breast 0HU
Mammary duct
  use Breast, Bilateral
  use Breast, Left
  use Breast, Right
Mammary gland
  use Breast, Bilateral
  use Breast, Left
  use Breast, Right
Mammectomy
  see Excision, Skin and Breast 0HB
  see Resection, Skin and Breast 0HT
Mammillary body *use* Hypothalamus
Mammography *see* Plain Radiography, Skin, Subcutaneous Tissue and Breast BH0
Mammotomy *see* Drainage, Skin and Breast 0H9
Mandibular nerve *use* Trigeminal Nerve
Mandibular notch
  use Mandible, Left
  use Mandible, Right
Mandibulectomy
  see Excision, Head and Facial Bones 0NB

Mandibulectomy — *continued*
see Resection, Head and Facial Bones ØNT
Manipulation
Adhesions *see* Release
Chiropractic *see* Chiropractic Manipulation
Manual removal, retained placenta *see* Extraction, Products of Conception, Retained 10D1
Manubrium *use* Sternum
Map
Basal Ganglia ØØK8
Brain ØØKØ
Cerebellum ØØKC
Cerebral Hemisphere ØØK7
Conduction Mechanism Ø2K8
Hypothalamus ØØKA
Medulla Oblongata ØØKD
Pons ØØKB
Thalamus ØØK9
Mapping
Doppler ultrasound *see* Ultrasonography
Electrocardiogram only *see* Measurement, Cardiac 4AØ2
Maribavir Anti-infective XWØ
Mark IV Breathing Pacemaker System *use* Stimulator Generator in Subcutaneous Tissue and Fascia
MarrowStim™ PAD Kit for CBMA (Concentrated Bone Marrow Aspirate) *use* Other Substance
MarrowStim™ PAD Kit, for injection of concentrated bone marrow aspirate *see* Introduction of substance in or on, Muscle 3EØ2
Marsupialization
see Drainage
see Excision
Massage, cardiac
External 5A12012
Open Ø2QAØZZ
Masseter muscle *use* Head Muscle
Masseteric fascia *use* Subcutaneous Tissue and Fascia, Face
Mastectomy
see Excision, Skin and Breast ØHB
see Resection, Skin and Breast ØHT
Mastoid air cells
use Mastoid Sinus, Left
use Mastoid Sinus, Right
Mastoid (postauricular) lymph node
use Lymphatic, Left Neck
use Lymphatic, Right Neck
Mastoid process
use Temporal Bone, Left
use Temporal Bone, Right
Mastoidectomy
see Excision, Ear, Nose, Sinus Ø9B
see Resection, Ear, Nose, Sinus Ø9T
Mastoidotomy *see* Drainage, Ear, Nose, Sinus Ø99
Mastopexy
see Repair, Skin and Breast ØHQ
see Reposition, Skin and Breast ØHS
Mastorrhaphy *see* Repair, Skin and Breast ØHQ
Mastotomy *see* Drainage, Skin and Breast ØH9
Maxillary artery
use External Carotid Artery, Left
use External Carotid Artery, Right
Maxillary nerve *use* Trigeminal Nerve
Maximo II DR (VR) *use* Defibrillator Generator in ØJH
Maximo II DR CRT-D *use* Cardiac Resynchronization Defibrillator Pulse Generator in ØJH
Measurement
Arterial
Flow
Coronary 4AØ3
Intracranial 4AØ3X5D
Peripheral 4AØ3
Pulmonary 4AØ3
Pressure
Coronary 4AØ3
Peripheral 4AØ3
Pulmonary 4AØ3
Thoracic, Other 4AØ3
Pulse
Coronary 4AØ3
Peripheral 4AØ3
Pulmonary 4AØ3
Saturation, Peripheral 4AØ3
Sound, Peripheral 4AØ3
Biliary
Flow 4AØC

Measurement — *continued*
Biliary — *continued*
Pressure 4AØC
Cardiac
Action Currents 4AØ2
Defibrillator 4BØ2XTZ
Electrical Activity 4AØ2
Guidance 4AØ2X4A
No Qualifier 4AØ2X4Z
Output 4AØ2
Pacemaker 4BØ2XSZ
Rate 4AØ2
Rhythm 4AØ2
Sampling and Pressure
Bilateral 4AØ2
Left Heart 4AØ2
Right Heart 4AØ2
Sound 4AØ2
Total Activity, Stress 4AØ2XM4
Central Nervous
Cerebrospinal Fluid Shunt, Wireless Sensor 4BØØXWØ
Conductivity 4AØØ
Electrical Activity 4AØØ
Pressure 4AØØØBZ
Intracranial 4AØØ
Saturation, Intracranial 4AØØ
Stimulator 4BØØXVZ
Temperature, Intracranial 4AØØ
Circulatory, Volume 4AØ5XLZ
Gastrointestinal
Motility 4AØB
Pressure 4AØB
Secretion 4AØB
Lower Respiratory Fluid Nucleic Acid-base Microbial Detection XXEBXQ6
Lymphatic
Flow 4AØ6
Pressure 4AØ6
Metabolism 4AØZ
Musculoskeletal
Contractility 4AØF
Pressure 4AØF3BE
Stimulator 4BØFXVZ
Olfactory, Acuity 4AØ8XØZ
Peripheral Nervous
Conductivity
Motor 4AØ1
Sensory 4AØ1
Electrical Activity 4AØ1
Stimulator 4BØ1XVZ
Positive Blood Culture Fluorescence Hybridization for Organism Identification, Concentration and Susceptibility XXE5XN6
Products of Conception
Cardiac
Electrical Activity 4AØH
Rate 4AØH
Rhythm 4AØH
Sound 4AØH
Nervous
Conductivity 4AØJ
Electrical Activity 4AØJ
Pressure 4AØJ
Respiratory
Capacity 4AØ9
Flow 4AØ9
Pacemaker 4BØ9XSZ
Rate 4AØ9
Resistance 4AØ9
Total Activity 4AØ9
Volume 4AØ9
Sleep 4AØZXQZ
Temperature 4AØZ
Urinary
Contractility 4AØD
Flow 4AØD
Pressure 4AØD
Resistance 4AØD
Volume 4AØD
Venous
Flow
Central 4AØ4
Peripheral 4AØ4
Portal 4AØ4
Pulmonary 4AØ4
Pressure
Central 4AØ4
Peripheral 4AØ4

Measurement — *continued*
Venous — *continued*
Pressure — *continued*
Portal 4AØ4
Pulmonary 4AØ4
Pulse
Central 4AØ4
Peripheral 4AØ4
Portal 4AØ4
Pulmonary 4AØ4
Saturation, Peripheral 4AØ4
Visual
Acuity 4AØ7XØZ
Mobility 4AØ7X7Z
Pressure 4AØ7XBZ
Whole Blood Nucleic Acid-base Microbial Detection XXE5XM5
Meatoplasty, urethra *see* Repair, Urethra ØTQD
Meatotomy *see* Drainage, Urinary System ØT9
Mechanical chest compression (mCPR) 5A1221J
Mechanical Initial Specimen Diversion Technique Using Active Negative Pressure (blood collection) XXE5XR7
Mechanical ventilation *see* Performance, Respiratory 5A19
Medial canthus
use Lower Eyelid, Left
use Lower Eyelid, Right
Medial collateral ligament (MCL)
use Knee Bursa and Ligament, Left
use Knee Bursa and Ligament, Right
Medial condyle of femur
use Lower Femur, Left
use Lower Femur, Right
Medial condyle of tibia
use Tibia, Left
use Tibia, Right
Medial cuneiform bone
use Tarsal, Left
use Tarsal, Right
Medial epicondyle of femur
use Lower Femur, Left
use Lower Femur, Right
Medial epicondyle of humerus
use Humeral Shaft, Left
use Humeral Shaft, Right
Medial malleolus
use Tibia, Left
use Tibia, Right
Medial meniscus
use Knee Joint, Left
use Knee Joint, Right
Medial plantar artery
use Foot Artery, Left
use Foot Artery, Right
Medial plantar nerve *use* Tibial Nerve
Medial popliteal nerve *use* Tibial Nerve
Medial rectus muscle
use Extraocular Muscle, Left
use Extraocular Muscle, Right
Medial sural cutaneous nerve *use* Tibial Nerve
Median antebrachial vein
use Basilic Vein, Left
use Basilic Vein, Right
Median cubital vein
use Basilic Vein, Left
use Basilic Vein, Right
Median sacral artery *use* Abdominal Aorta
Mediastinal cavity *use* Mediastinum
Mediastinal lymph node *use* Lymphatic, Thorax
Mediastinal space *use* Mediastinum
Mediastinoscopy ØWJC4ZZ
Medication Management GZ3ZZZZ
for substance abuse
Antabuse HZ83ZZZ
Bupropion HZ87ZZZ
Clonidine HZ86ZZZ
Levo-alpha-acetyl-methadol (LAAM) HZ82ZZZ
Methadone Maintenance HZ81ZZZ
Naloxone HZ85ZZZ
Naltrexone HZ84ZZZ
Nicotine Replacement HZ80ZZZ
Other Replacement Medication HZ89ZZZ
Psychiatric Medication HZ88ZZZ
Meditation 8EØZXY5

Medtronic Endurant® II AAA stent graft system *use* Intraluminal Device

Meissner's (submucous) plexus *use* Abdominal Sympathetic Nerve

Melody® transcatheter pulmonary valve *use* Zooplastic Tissue in Heart and Great Vessels

Membranous urethra *use* Urethra

Meningeorrhaphy
  see Repair, Cerebral Meninges 00Q1
  see Repair, Spinal Meninges 00QT

Meniscectomy, knee
  see Excision, Joint, Knee, Left 0SBD
  see Excision, Joint, Knee, Right 0SBC

Mental foramen
  use Mandible, Left
  use Mandible, Right

Mentalis muscle *use* Facial Muscle

Mentoplasty *see* Alteration, Jaw, Lower 0W05

Meropenem-vaborbactam Anti-infective XW0

Mesenterectomy *see* Excision, Mesentery 0DBV

Mesenteriorrhaphy, mesenterorrhaphy *see* Repair, Mesentery 0DQV

Mesenteriplication *see* Repair, Mesentery 0DQV

Mesoappendix *use* Mesentery

Mesocolon *use* Mesentery

Metacarpal ligament
  use Hand Bursa and Ligament, Left
  use Hand Bursa and Ligament, Right

Metacarpophalangeal ligament
  use Hand Bursa and Ligament, Left
  use Hand Bursa and Ligament, Right

Metal on metal bearing surface *use* Synthetic Substitute, Metal in 0SR

Metatarsal ligament
  use Foot Bursa and Ligament, Left
  use Foot Bursa and Ligament, Right

Metatarsectomy
  see Excision, Lower Bones 0QB
  see Resection, Lower Bones 0QT

Metatarsophalangeal (MTP) joint
  use Metatarsal-Phalangeal Joint, Left
  use Metatarsal-Phalangeal Joint, Right

Metatarsophalangeal ligament
  use Foot Bursa and Ligament, Left
  use Foot Bursa and Ligament, Right

Metathalamus *use* Thalamus

Micro-Driver stent (RX) (OTW) *use* Intraluminal Device

MicroMed HeartAssist *use* Implantable Heart Assist System in Heart and Great Vessels

Micrus CERECYTE Microcoil *use* Intraluminal Device, Bioactive in Upper Arteries

Midcarpal joint
  use Carpal Joint, Left
  use Carpal Joint, Right

Middle cardiac nerve *use* Thoracic Sympathetic Nerve

Middle cerebral artery *use* Intracranial Artery

Middle cerebral vein *use* Intracranial Vein

Middle colic vein *use* Colic Vein

Middle genicular artery
  use Popliteal Artery, Left
  use Popliteal Artery, Right

Middle hemorrhoidal vein
  use Hypogastric Vein, Left
  use Hypogastric Vein, Right

Middle rectal artery
  use Internal Iliac Artery, Left
  use Internal Iliac Artery, Right

Middle suprarenal artery *use* Abdominal Aorta

Middle temporal artery
  use Temporal Artery, Left
  use Temporal Artery, Right

Middle turbinate *use* Nasal Turbinate

Mineral-based Topical Hemostatic Agent XW0

MIRODERM™ Biologic Wound Matrix *use* Nonautologous Tissue Substitute

MIRODERM™ skin graft *see* Replacement, Skin and Breast 0HR

MitraClip valve repair system *use* Synthetic Substitute

Mitral annulus *use* Mitral Valve

Mitroflow® Aortic Pericardial Heart Valve *use* Zooplastic Tissue in Heart and Great Vessels

MNS (Magnus Neuromodulation System) X0Z0X18

Mobilization, adhesions *see* Release

Molar gland *use* Buccal Mucosa

MolecuLight i:X® wound imaging *see* Other Imaging, Anatomical Regions BW5

Monitoring
  Arterial
    Flow
      Coronary 4A13
      Peripheral 4A13
      Pulmonary 4A13
    Pressure
      Coronary 4A13
      Peripheral 4A13
      Pulmonary 4A13
    Pulse
      Coronary 4A13
      Peripheral 4A13
      Pulmonary 4A13
    Saturation, Peripheral 4A13
    Sound, Peripheral 4A13
  Cardiac
    Electrical Activity 4A12
      Ambulatory 4A12X45
      No Qualifier 4A12X4Z
    Output 4A12
    Rate 4A12
    Rhythm 4A12
    Sound 4A12
    Total Activity, Stress 4A12XM4
    Vascular Perfusion, Indocyanine Green Dye 4A12XSH
  Central Nervous
    Conductivity 4A10
    Electrical Activity
      Intraoperative 4A10
      No Qualifier 4A10
    Pressure 4A100BZ
      Intracranial 4A10
    Saturation, Intracranial 4A10
    Temperature, Intracranial 4A10
  Gastrointestinal
    Motility 4A1B
    Pressure 4A1B
    Secretion 4A1B
    Vascular Perfusion, Indocyanine Green Dye 4A1BXSH
  Kidney, Fluorescent Pyrazine XT25XE5
  Lymphatic
    Flow
      Indocyanine Green Dye 4A16
      No Qualifier 4A16
    Pressure 4A16
  Oxygen Saturation Endoscopic Imaging (OXEI) XD2
  Peripheral Nervous
    Conductivity
      Motor 4A11
      Sensory 4A11
    Electrical Activity
      Intraoperative 4A11
      No Qualifier 4A11
  Products of Conception
    Cardiac
      Electrical Activity 4A1H
      Rate 4A1H
      Rhythm 4A1H
      Sound 4A1H
    Nervous
      Conductivity 4A1J
      Electrical Activity 4A1J
      Pressure 4A1J
  Respiratory
    Capacity 4A19
    Flow 4A19
    Rate 4A19
    Resistance 4A19
    Volume 4A19
  Skin and Breast, Vascular Perfusion, Indocyanine Green Dye 4A1GXSH
  Sleep 4A1ZXQZ
  Temperature 4A1Z
  Urinary
    Contractility 4A1D
    Flow 4A1D
    Pressure 4A1D
    Resistance 4A1D
    Volume 4A1D
  Venous
    Flow
      Central 4A14
      Peripheral 4A14
      Portal 4A14

Monitoring — *continued*
  Venous — *continued*
    Flow — *continued*
      Pulmonary 4A14
    Pressure
      Central 4A14
      Peripheral 4A14
      Portal 4A14
      Pulmonary 4A14
    Pulse
      Central 4A14
      Peripheral 4A14
      Portal 4A14
      Pulmonary 4A14
    Saturation
      Central 4A14
      Portal 4A14
      Pulmonary 4A14

Monitoring Device, Hemodynamic
  Abdomen 0JH8
  Chest 0JH6

Mosaic Bioprosthesis (aortic) (mitral) valve *use* Zooplastic Tissue in Heart and Great Vessels

Mosunetuzumab Antineoplastic XW0

Motor Function Assessment F01

Motor Treatment F07

MR Angiography
  see Magnetic Resonance Imaging (MRI), Heart B23
  see Magnetic Resonance Imaging (MRI), Lower Arteries B43
  see Magnetic Resonance Imaging (MRI), Upper Arteries B33

MULTI-LINK (VISION) (MINI-VISION) (ULTRA) Coronary Stent System *use* Intraluminal Device

Multiple sleep latency test 4A0ZXQZ

Musculocutaneous nerve *use* Brachial Plexus

Musculopexy
  see Repair, Muscles 0KQ
  see Reposition, Muscles 0KS

Musculophrenic artery
  use Internal Mammary Artery, Left
  use Internal Mammary Artery, Right

Musculoplasty
  see Repair, Muscles 0KQ
  see Supplement, Muscles 0KU

Musculorrhaphy *see* Repair, Muscles 0KQ

Musculospiral nerve *use* Radial Nerve

Myectomy
  see Excision, Muscles 0KB
  see Resection, Muscles 0KT

Myelencephalon *use* Medulla Oblongata

Myelogram
  CT *see* Computerized Tomography (CT Scan), Central Nervous System B02
  MRI *see* Magnetic Resonance Imaging (MRI), Central Nervous System B03

Myenteric (Auerbach's) plexus *use* Abdominal Sympathetic Nerve

Myocardial Bridge Release *see* Release, Artery, Coronary

Myomectomy *see* Excision, Female Reproductive System 0UB

Myometrium *use* Uterus

Myopexy
  see Repair, Muscles 0KQ
  see Reposition, Muscles 0KS

Myoplasty
  see Repair, Muscles 0KQ
  see Supplement, Muscles 0KU

Myorrhaphy *see* Repair, Muscles 0KQ

Myoscopy *see* Inspection, Muscles 0KJ

Myotomy
  see Division, Muscles 0K8
  see Drainage, Muscles 0K9

Myringectomy
  see Excision, Ear, Nose, Sinus 09B
  see Resection, Ear, Nose, Sinus 09T

Myringoplasty
  see Repair, Ear, Nose, Sinus 09Q
  see Replacement, Ear, Nose, Sinus 09R
  see Supplement, Ear, Nose, Sinus 09U

Myringostomy *see* Drainage, Ear, Nose, Sinus 099

Myringotomy *see* Drainage, Ear, Nose, Sinus 099

N

NA-1 (Nerinitide) *use* Nerinitide
Nafamostat Anticoagulant XY0YX37
Nail bed
   use Finger Nail
   use Toe Nail
Nail plate
   use Finger Nail
   use Toe Nail
nanoLOCK™ interbody fusion device
   use Interbody Fusion Device in Lower Joints
   use Interbody Fusion Device in Upper Joints
Narcosynthesis GZGZZZZ
Narsoplimab Monoclonal Antibody XW0
Nasal cavity *use* Nasal Mucosa and Soft Tissue
Nasal concha *use* Nasal Turbinate
Nasalis muscle *use* Facial Muscle
Nasolacrimal duct
   use Lacrimal Duct, Left
   use Lacrimal Duct, Right
Nasopharyngeal airway (NPA) *use* Intraluminal Device, Airway in Ear, Nose, Sinus
Navicular bone
   use Tarsal, Left
   use Tarsal, Right
Near Infrared Spectroscopy, Circulatory System 8E02
Neck of femur
   use Upper Femur, Left
   use Upper Femur, Right
Neck of humerus (anatomical) (surgical)
   use Humeral Head, Left
   use Humeral Head, Right
Nelli® Seizure Monitoring System XXE0X48
Neovasc Reducer™ *use* Reduction Device in New Technology
Nephrectomy
   see Excision, Urinary System 0TB
   see Resection, Urinary System 0TT
Nephrolithotomy *see* Extirpation, Urinary System 0TC
Nephrolysis *see* Release, Urinary System 0TN
Nephropexy
   see Repair, Urinary System 0TQ
   see Reposition, Urinary System 0TS
Nephroplasty
   see Repair, Urinary System 0TQ
   see Supplement, Urinary System 0TU
Nephropyeloureterostomy
   see Bypass, Urinary System 0T1
   see Drainage, Urinary System 0T9
Nephrorrhaphy *see* Repair, Urinary System 0TQ
Nephroscopy, transurethral 0TJ58ZZ
Nephrostomy
   see Bypass, Urinary System 0T1
   see Drainage, Urinary System 0T9
Nephrotomography
   see Fluoroscopy, Urinary System BT1
   see Plain Radiography, Urinary System BT0
Nephrotomy
   see Division, Urinary System 0T8
   see Drainage, Urinary System 0T9
Nerinitide XW0
Nerve conduction study
   see Measurement, Central Nervous 4A00
   see Measurement, Peripheral Nervous 4A01
Nerve Function Assessment F01
Nerve to the stapedius *use* Facial Nerve
Nesiritide *use* Human B-Type Natriuretic Peptide
Neurectomy
   see Excision, Central Nervous System and Cranial Nerves 00B
   see Excision, Peripheral Nervous System 01B
Neurexeresis
   see Extraction, Central Nervous System and Cranial Nerves 00D
   see Extraction, Peripheral Nervous System 01D
NeuroBlate™ System *see* Destruction
Neurohypophysis *use* Pituitary Gland
Neurolysis
   see Release, Central Nervous System and Cranial Nerves 00N
   see Release, Peripheral Nervous System 01N
Neuromuscular electrical stimulation (NEMS) lead *use* Stimulator Lead in Muscles

Neurophysiologic monitoring *see* Monitoring, Central Nervous 4A10
Neuroplasty
   see Repair, Central Nervous System and Cranial Nerves 00Q
   see Repair, Peripheral Nervous System 01Q
   see Supplement, Central Nervous System and Cranial Nerves 00U
   see Supplement, Peripheral Nervous System 01U
Neurorrhaphy
   see Repair, Central Nervous System and Cranial Nerves 00Q
   see Repair, Peripheral Nervous System 01Q
Neurostimulator Generator
   Insertion of device in, Skull 0NH00NZ
   Removal of device from, Skull 0NP00NZ
   Revision of device in, Skull 0NW00NZ
Neurostimulator generator, multiple channel *use* Stimulator Generator, Multiple Array in 0JH
Neurostimulator generator, multiple channel rechargeable *use* Stimulator Generator, Multiple Array Rechargeable in 0JH
Neurostimulator generator, single channel *use* Stimulator Generator, Single Array in 0JH
Neurostimulator generator, single channel rechargeable *use* Stimulator Generator, Single Array Rechargeable in 0JH
Neurostimulator Lead
   Insertion of device in
     Brain 00H0
     Cerebral Ventricle 00H6
     Nerve
       Cranial 00HE
       Peripheral 01HY
     Spinal Canal 00HU
     Spinal Cord 00HV
     Vein
       Azygos 05H0
       Innominate
         Left 05H4
         Right 05H3
   Removal of device from
     Brain 00P0
     Cerebral Ventricle 00P6
     Nerve
       Cranial 00PE
       Peripheral 01PY
     Spinal Canal 00PU
     Spinal Cord 00PV
     Vein
       Azygos 05P0
       Innominate
         Left 05P4
         Right 05P3
   Revision of device in
     Brain 00W0
     Cerebral Ventricle 00W6
     Nerve
       Cranial 00WE
       Peripheral 01WY
     Spinal Canal 00WU
     Spinal Cord 00WV
     Vein
       Azygos 05W0
       Innominate
         Left 05W4
         Right 05W3
   Sphenopalatine Ganglion, Insertion X0HK3Q8
Neurostimulator Lead in Oropharynx XWHD7Q7
Neurostimulator Lead with Paired Stimulation System, Insertion X0HQ3R8
Neurotomy
   see Division, Central Nervous System and Cranial Nerves 008
   see Division, Peripheral Nervous System 018
Neurotripsy
   see Destruction, Central Nervous System and Cranial Nerves 005
   see Destruction, Peripheral Nervous System 015
Neutralization plate
   use Internal Fixation Device in Head and Facial Bones
   use Internal Fixation Device in Lower Bones
   use Internal Fixation Device in Upper Bones
New Technology
   Afamitresgene Autoleucel Immunotherapy XW0
   Amivantamab Monoclonal Antibody XW0
   Antibiotic-eluting Bone Void Filler XW0V0P7

New Technology — *continued*
   Aorta
     Thoracic Arch using Branched Synthetic Substitute with Intraluminal Device X2RX0N7
     Thoracic Descending using Branched Synthetic Substitute with Intraluminal Device X2VW0N7
   Apalutamide Antineoplastic XW0DXJ5
   Atezolizumab Antineoplastic XW0
   Axicabtagene Ciloleucel Immunotherapy XW0
   Bamlanivimab Monoclonal Antibody XW0
   Baricitinib XW0
   Betibeglogene Autotemcel XW1
   Bioengineered Allogeneic Construct, Skin XHRPXF7
   Brain Electrical Activity, Computer-aided Semiologic Analysis XXE0X48
   Brexanolone XW0
   Brexucabtagene Autoleucel Immunotherapy XW0
   Broad Consortium Microbiota-based Live Biotherapeutic Suspension XW0H7X8
   Bromelain-enriched Proteolytic Enzyme XW0
   Caplacizumab XW0
   CD24Fc Immunomodulator XW0
   Cefiderocol Anti-infective XW0
   Ceftolozane/Tazobactam Anti-infective XW0
   Cerebral Embolic Filtration
     Dual Filter X2A5312
     Extracorporeal Flow Reversal Circuit X2A
     Single Deflection Filter X2A6325
   Ciltacabtagene Autoleucel XW0
   Coagulation Factor Xa, Inactivated XW0
   Computer-aided Assessment, Intracranial Vascular Activity XXE0X07
   Computer-aided Guidance, Transthoracic Echocardiography X2JAX47
   Computer-aided Mechanical Aspiration X2C
   Computer-aided Triage and Notification, Pulmonary Artery Flow XXE3X27
   Computer-aided Valve Modeling and Notification, Coronary Artery Flow XXE3X68
   Computer-assisted Transcranial Magnetic Stimulation X0Z0X18
   Coronary Sinus, Reduction Device X2V73Q7
   COVID-19 Vaccine XW0
   COVID-19 Vaccine Booster XW0
   COVID-19 Vaccine Dose 1 XW0
   COVID-19 Vaccine Dose 2 XW0
   COVID-19 Vaccine Dose 3 XW0
   Cytarabine and Daunorubicin Liposome Antineoplastic XW0
   Daratumumab and Hyaluronidase-fihj XW01318
   Destruction
     Liver
       Left Lobe, Ultrasound-guided Cavitation XF52X08
       Right Lobe, Ultrasound-guided Cavitation XF51X08
       Ultrasound-guided Cavitation XF50X08
     Prostate, Robotic Waterjet Ablation XV508A4
   Dilation
     Anterior Tibial
       Left
         Sustained Release Drug-eluting Intraluminal Device X27Q385
         Four or More X27Q3C5
         Three X27Q3B5
         Two X27Q395
       Right
         Sustained Release Drug-eluting Intraluminal Device X27P385
         Four or More X27P3C5
         Three X27P3B5
         Two X27P395
     Femoral
       Left
         Sustained Release Drug-eluting Intraluminal Device X27J385
         Four or More X27J3C5
         Three X27J3B5
         Two X27J395
       Right
         Sustained Release Drug-eluting Intraluminal Device X27H385
         Four or More X27H3C5

New Technology — *continued*
  Dilation — *continued*
    Femoral — *continued*
      Right — *continued*
        Three X27H3B5
        Two X27H395
    Peroneal
      Left
        Sustained Release Drug-eluting Intraluminal Device X27U385
        Four or More X27U3C5
        Three X27U3B5
        Two X27U395
      Right
        Sustained Release Drug-eluting Intraluminal Device X27T385
        Four or More X27T3C5
        Three X27T3B5
        Two X27T395
    Popliteal
      Left Distal
        Sustained Release Drug-eluting Intraluminal Device X27N385
        Four or More X27N3C5
        Three X27N3B5
        Two X27N395
      Left Proximal
        Sustained Release Drug-eluting Intraluminal Device X27L385
        Four or More X27L3C5
        Three X27L3B5
        Two X27L395
      Right Distal
        Sustained Release Drug-eluting Intraluminal Device X27M385
        Four or More X27M3C5
        Three X27M3B5
        Two X27M395
      Right Proximal
        Sustained Release Drug-eluting Intraluminal Device X27K385
        Four or More X27K3C5
        Three X27K3B5
        Two X27K395
    Posterior Tibial
      Left
        Sustained Release Drug-eluting Intraluminal Device X27S385
        Four or More X27S3C5
        Three X27S3B5
        Two X27S395
      Right
        Sustained Release Drug-eluting Intraluminal Device X27R385
        Four or More X27R3C5
        Three X27R3B5
        Two X27R395
  Durvalumab Antineoplastic XW0
  Eculizumab XW0
  Eladocagene exuparvovec XW0Q316
  Endothelial Damage Inhibitor XY0VX83
  Engineered Allogeneic Thymus Tissue XW020D8
  Engineered Chimeric Antigen Receptor T-cell Immunotherapy
    Allogeneic XW0
    Autologous XW0
  Erdafitinib Antineoplastic XW0DXL5
  Esketamine Hydrochloride XW097M5
  Etesevimab Monoclonal Antibody XW0
  Fosfomycin Anti-infective XW0
  Fostamatinib XW0
  Fusion
    Lumbar Vertebral
      2 or more, Interbody Fusion Device, Customizable XRGC
      Interbody Fusion Device, Customizable XRGB
    Lumbosacral, Interbody Fusion Device, Customizable XRGD
    Sacroiliac, Internal Fixation Device with Tulip Connector XRG

New Technology — *continued*
  Fusion — *continued*
    Thoracolumbar Vertebral, Interbody Fusion Device, Customizable XRGA
  Gilteritinib Antineoplastic XW0DXV5
  High-Dose Intravenous Immune Globulin, for COVID-19 treatment XW1
  Hyperimmune Globulin, for COVID-19 treatment XW1
  Idecabtagene Vicleucel Immunotherapy XW0
  Imipenem-cilastatin-relebactam Anti-infective XW0
  Inebilizumab-cdon XW0
  Insertion
    Bone, Pelvic, Internal Fixation Device with Tulip Connector XNH
    Joint
      Lumbar Vertebral, Posterior Spinal Motion Preservation Device XRHB0I8
      Lumbosacral, Posterior Spinal Motion Preservation Device XRHD0I8
    Neurostimulator Lead, Sphenopalatine Ganglion X0HK3Q8
    Neurostimulator Lead with Paired Stimulation System X0HQ3R8
  Intermittent Coronary Sinus Occlusion X2A7358
  Intracranial Arterial Flow, Whole Blood mRNA XXE5XT7
  Iobenguane I-131 Antineoplastic XW0
  Kidney, Fluorescent Pyrazine XT25XE5
  Lefamulin Anti-infective XW0
  Leronlimab Monoclonal Antibody XW013K6
  Lifileucel Immunotherapy XW0
  Lisocabtagene Maraleucel Immunotherapy XW0
  Lower Respiratory Fluid Nucleic Acid-base Microbial Detection XXEBXQ6
  Lurbinectedin XW0
  Maribavir Anti-infective XW0
  Mechanical Initial Specimen Diversion Technique Using Active Negative Pressure (blood collection) XXE5XR7
  Meropenem-vaborbactam Anti-infective XW0
  Mineral-based Topical Hemostatic Agent XW0
  Mosunetuzumab Antineoplastic XW0
  Nafamostat Anticoagulant XY0YX37
  Narsoplimab Monoclonal Antibody XW0
  Nerinitide XW0
  Neurostimulator Lead in Oropharynx XWHD7Q7
  Omadacycline Anti-infective XW0
  Omidubicel XW1
  Other New Technology Monoclonal Antibody XW0
  Other New Technology Therapeutic Substance XW0
  OTL-103 XW1
  OTL-200 XW1
  Oxygen Saturation Endoscopic Imaging (OXEI) XD2
  Plasma, Convalescent (Nonautologous) XW1
  Plazomicin Anti-infective XW0
  Positive Blood Culture Fluorescence Hybridization for Organism Identification, Concentration and Susceptibility XXE5XN6
  Quantitative Flow Ratio Analysis, Coronary Artery Flow XXE3X58
  Radial artery arteriovenous fistula, using Thermal Resistance Energy X2K
  REGN-COV2 Monoclonal Antibody XW0
  Remdesivir Anti-infective XW0
  Replacement
    Lateral Meniscus Synthetic Substitute XRR
    Medial Meniscus Synthetic Substitute XRR
  Reposition
    Cervical, Magnetically Controlled Growth Rod(s) XNS3
    Lumbar
      Magnetically Controlled Growth Rod(s) XNS0
      Posterior (Dynamic) Distraction Device XNS0
    Thoracic
      Magnetically Controlled Growth Rod(s) XNS4
      Posterior (Dynamic) Distraction Device XNS4
  Ruxolitinib XW0DXT5
  Sarilumab XW0
  SARS-CoV-2 Antibody Detection, Serum/Plasma Nanoparticle Fluorescence XXE5XV7

New Technology — *continued*
  SARS-CoV-2 Polymerase Chain Reaction, Nasopharyngeal Fluid XXE97U7
  Satralizumab-mwge XW01397
  Single-use Duodenoscope XFJ
  Single-use Oversleeve with Intraoperative Colonic Irrigation XDPH8K7
  Spesolimab Monoclonal Antibody XW0
  Supplement
    Bursa and Ligament, Spine, Posterior Vertebral Tether XKU
    Vertebra
      Lumbar, Mechanically Expandable (Paired) Synthetic Substitute XNU0356
      Thoracic, Mechanically Expandable (Paired) Synthetic Substitute XNU4356
  Synthetic Human Angiotensin II XW0
  Tabelecleucel Immunotherapy XW0
  Tagraxofusp-erzs Antineoplastic XW0
  Taurolidine Anti-infective and Heparin Anticoagulant XY0YX28
  Teclistamab Antineoplastic XW01348
  Terlipressin XW0
  Tisagenlecleucel Immunotherapy XW0
  Tixagevimab and Cilgavimab Monoclonal Antibody XW023X7
  Tocilizumab XW0
  Treosulfan XW0
  Trilaciclib XW0
  Uridine Triacetate XW0DX82
  Venetoclax Antineoplastic XW0DXR5
  Whole Blood Nucleic Acid-base Microbial Detection XXE5XM5
  Whole Blood Reverse Transcription and Quantitative Real-time Polymerase Chain Reaction XXE5X38

NexoBrid™ *use* Bromelain-enriched Proteolytic Enzyme
Ninth cranial nerve *use* Glossopharyngeal Nerve
NIRS (Near Infrared Spectroscopy) *see* Physiological Systems and Anatomical Regions 8E0
Nitinol framed polymer mesh *use* Synthetic Substitute
Niyad™ *use* Nafamostat Anticoagulant
Nonimaging Nuclear Medicine Assay
  Bladder, Kidneys and Ureters CT63
  Blood C763
  Kidneys, Ureters and Bladder CT63
  Lymphatics and Hematologic System C76YYZZ
  Ureters, Kidneys and Bladder CT63
  Urinary System CT6YYZZ
Nonimaging Nuclear Medicine Probe
  Abdomen CW50
  Abdomen and Chest CW54
  Abdomen and Pelvis CW51
  Brain C050
  Central Nervous System C05YYZZ
  Chest CW53
  Chest and Abdomen CW54
  Chest and Neck CW56
  Extremity
    Lower CP5PZZZ
    Upper CP5NZZZ
  Head and Neck CW5B
  Heart C25YYZZ
    Right and Left C256
  Lymphatics
    Head C75J
    Head and Neck C755
    Lower Extremity C75P
    Neck C75K
    Pelvic C75D
    Trunk C75M
    Upper Chest C75L
    Upper Extremity C75N
  Lymphatics and Hematologic System C75YYZZ
  Musculoskeletal System, Other CP5YYZZ
  Neck and Chest CW56
  Neck and Head CW5B
  Pelvic Region CW5J
  Pelvis and Abdomen CW51
  Spine CP55ZZZ
Nonimaging Nuclear Medicine Uptake
  Endocrine System CG4YYZZ
  Gland, Thyroid CG42
Non-tunneled central venous catheter *use* Infusion Device

▽ Subterms under main terms may continue to next column or page

Nostril *use* Nasal Mucosa and Soft Tissue
Novacor Left Ventricular Assist Device *use* Implantable Heart Assist System in Heart and Great Vessels
Novation® Ceramic AHS® (Articulation Hip System) *use* Synthetic Substitute, Ceramic in ØSR
Nuclear medicine
　see Nonimaging Nuclear Medicine Assay
　see Nonimaging Nuclear Medicine Probe
　see Nonimaging Nuclear Medicine Uptake
　see Planar Nuclear Medicine Imaging
　see Positron Emission Tomographic (PET) Imaging
　see Systemic Nuclear Medicine Therapy
　see Tomographic (Tomo) Nuclear Medicine Imaging
Nuclear scintigraphy *see* Nuclear Medicine
NUsurface® Meniscus Implant
　use Synthetic Substitute, Lateral Meniscus in New Technology
　use Synthetic Substitute, Medial Meniscus in New Technology
Nutrition, concentrated substances
　Enteral infusion 3E0G36Z
　Parenteral (peripheral) infusion *see* Introduction of Nutritional Substance
NUZYRA™ *use* Omadacycline Anti-infective

O

Obliteration *see* Destruction
Obturator artery
　use Internal Iliac Artery, Left
　use Internal Iliac Artery, Right
Obturator lymph node *use* Lymphatic, Pelvis
Obturator muscle
　use Hip Muscle, Left
　use Hip Muscle, Right
Obturator nerve *use* Lumbar Plexus
Obturator vein
　use Hypogastric Vein, Left
　use Hypogastric Vein, Right
Obtuse margin *use* Heart, Left
Occipital artery
　use External Carotid Artery, Left
　use External Carotid Artery, Right
Occipital lobe *use* Cerebral Hemisphere
Occipital lymph node
　use Lymphatic, Left Neck
　use Lymphatic, Right Neck
Occipitofrontalis muscle *use* Facial Muscle
Occlusion
　Ampulla of Vater ØFLC
　Anus ØDLQ
　Aorta
　　Abdominal 04L0
　　Thoracic, Descending 02LW3DJ
　Artery
　　Anterior Tibial
　　　Left 04LQ
　　　Right 04LP
　　Axillary
　　　Left 03L6
　　　Right 03L5
　　Brachial
　　　Left 03L8
　　　Right 03L7
　　Celiac 04L1
　　Colic
　　　Left 04L7
　　　Middle 04L8
　　　Right 04L6
　　Common Carotid
　　　Left 03LJ
　　　Right 03LH
　　Common Iliac
　　　Left 04LD
　　　Right 04LC
　　External Carotid
　　　Left 03LN
　　　Right 03LM
　　External Iliac
　　　Left 04LJ
　　　Right 04LH
　　Face 03LR
　　Femoral
　　　Left 04LL
　　　Right 04LK

Occlusion — *continued*
　Artery — *continued*
　　Foot
　　　Left 04LW
　　　Right 04LV
　　Gastric 04L2
　　Hand
　　　Left 03LF
　　　Right 03LD
　　Hepatic 04L3
　　Inferior Mesenteric 04LB
　　Innominate 03L2
　　Internal Carotid
　　　Left 03LL
　　　Right 03LK
　　Internal Iliac
　　　Left 04LF
　　　Right 04LE
　　Internal Mammary
　　　Left 03L1
　　　Right 03L0
　　Intracranial 03LG
　　Lower 04LY
　　Peroneal
　　　Left 04LU
　　　Right 04LT
　　Popliteal
　　　Left 04LN
　　　Right 04LM
　　Posterior Tibial
　　　Left 04LS
　　　Right 04LR
　　Pulmonary
　　　Left 02LR
　　　Right 02LQ
　　Pulmonary Trunk 02LP
　　Radial
　　　Left 03LC
　　　Right 03LB
　　Renal
　　　Left 04LA
　　　Right 04L9
　　Splenic 04L4
　　Subclavian
　　　Left 03L4
　　　Right 03L3
　　Superior Mesenteric 04L5
　　Temporal
　　　Left 03LT
　　　Right 03LS
　　Thyroid
　　　Left 03LV
　　　Right 03LU
　　Ulnar
　　　Left 03LA
　　　Right 03L9
　　Upper 03LY
　　Vertebral
　　　Left 03LQ
　　　Right 03LP
　Atrium, Left 02L7
　Bladder ØTLB
　Bladder Neck ØTLC
　Bronchus
　　Lingula ØBL9
　　Lower Lobe
　　　Left ØBLB
　　　Right ØBL6
　　Main
　　　Left ØBL7
　　　Right ØBL3
　　Middle Lobe, Right ØBL5
　　Upper Lobe
　　　Left ØBL8
　　　Right ØBL4
　Carina ØBL2
　Cecum ØDLH
　Cisterna Chyli 07LL
　Colon
　　Ascending ØDLK
　　Descending ØDLM
　　Sigmoid ØDLN
　　Transverse ØDLL
　Cord
　　Bilateral ØVLH
　　Left ØVLG
　　Right ØVLF
　Cul-de-sac ØULF

Occlusion — *continued*
　Duct
　　Common Bile ØFL9
　　Cystic ØFL8
　　Hepatic
　　　Common ØFL7
　　　Left ØFL6
　　　Right ØFL5
　　Lacrimal
　　　Left Ø8LY
　　　Right Ø8LX
　　Pancreatic ØFLD
　　　Accessory ØFLF
　　Parotid
　　　Left ØCLC
　　　Right ØCLB
　Duodenum ØDL9
　Esophagogastric Junction ØDL4
　Esophagus ØDL5
　　Lower ØDL3
　　Middle ØDL2
　　Upper ØDL1
　Fallopian Tube
　　Left ØUL6
　　Right ØUL5
　Fallopian Tubes, Bilateral ØUL7
　Ileocecal Valve ØDLC
　Ileum ØDLB
　Intestine
　　Large ØDLE
　　　Left ØDLG
　　　Right ØDLF
　　Small ØDL8
　Jejunum ØDLA
　Kidney Pelvis
　　Left ØTL4
　　Right ØTL3
　Left atrial appendage (LAA) *see* Occlusion, Atrium, Left Ø2L7
　Lymphatic
　　Aortic 07LD
　　Axillary
　　　Left 07L6
　　　Right 07L5
　　Head 07L0
　　Inguinal
　　　Left 07LJ
　　　Right 07LH
　　Internal Mammary
　　　Left 07L9
　　　Right 07L8
　　Lower Extremity
　　　Left 07LG
　　　Right 07LF
　　Mesenteric 07LB
　　Neck
　　　Left 07L2
　　　Right 07L1
　　Pelvis 07LC
　　Thoracic Duct 07LK
　　Thorax 07L7
　　Upper Extremity
　　　Left 07L4
　　　Right 07L3
　Rectum ØDLP
　Stomach ØDL6
　　Pylorus ØDL7
　Trachea ØBL1
　Ureter
　　Left ØTL7
　　Right ØTL6
　Urethra ØTLD
　Vagina ØULG
　Valve, Pulmonary 02LH
　Vas Deferens
　　Bilateral ØVLQ
　　Left ØVLP
　　Right ØVLN
　Vein
　　Axillary
　　　Left Ø5L8
　　　Right Ø5L7
　　Azygos Ø5L0
　　Basilic
　　　Left Ø5LC
　　　Right Ø5LB
　　Brachial
　　　Left Ø5LA
　　　Right Ø5L9

Occlusion — *continued*
 Vein — *continued*
  Cephalic
   Left 05LF
   Right 05LD
  Colic 06L7
  Common Iliac
   Left 06LD
   Right 06LC
  Esophageal 06L3
  External Iliac
   Left 06LG
   Right 06LF
  External Jugular
   Left 05LQ
   Right 05LP
  Face
   Left 05LV
   Right 05LT
  Femoral
   Left 06LN
   Right 06LM
  Foot
   Left 06LV
   Right 06LT
  Gastric 06L2
  Hand
   Left 05LH
   Right 05LG
  Hemiazygos 05L1
  Hepatic 06L4
  Hypogastric
   Left 06LJ
   Right 06LH
  Inferior Mesenteric 06L6
  Innominate
   Left 05L4
   Right 05L3
  Internal Jugular
   Left 05LN
   Right 05LM
  Intracranial 05LL
  Lower 06LY
  Portal 06L8
  Pulmonary
   Left 02LT
   Right 02LS
  Renal
   Left 06LB
   Right 06L9
  Saphenous
   Left 06LQ
   Right 06LP
  Splenic 06L1
  Subclavian
   Left 05L6
   Right 05L5
  Superior Mesenteric 06L5
  Upper 05LY
  Vertebral
   Left 05LS
   Right 05LR
 Vena Cava
  Inferior 06L0
  Superior 02LV
Occlusion, REBOA (resuscitative endovascular balloon occlusion of the aorta)
 02LW3DJ
 04L03DJ
Occupational therapy *see* Activities of Daily Living Treatment, Rehabilitation F08
Octagam 10%, for COVID-19 treatment *use* High-Dose Intravenous Immune Globulin
Odentectomy
 see Excision, Mouth and Throat 0CB
 see Resection, Mouth and Throat 0CT
Odontoid process *use* Cervical Vertebra
Olecranon bursa
 use Elbow Bursa and Ligament, Left
 use Elbow Bursa and Ligament, Right
Olecranon process
 use Ulna, Left
 use Ulna, Right
Olfactory bulb *use* Olfactory Nerve
Olumiant® *use* Baricitinib
Omadacycline Anti-infective XW0
Omentectomy, omentumectomy
 see Excision, Gastrointestinal System 0DB

Omentectomy, omentumectomy — *continued*
 see Resection, Gastrointestinal System 0DT
Omentofixation *see* Repair, Gastrointestinal System 0DQ
Omentoplasty
 see Repair, Gastrointestinal System 0DQ
 see Replacement, Gastrointestinal System 0DR
 see Supplement, Gastrointestinal System 0DU
Omentorrhaphy *see* Repair, Gastrointestinal System 0DQ
Omentotomy *see* Drainage, Gastrointestinal System 0D9
Omidubicel XW1
Omnilink Elite Vascular Balloon Expandable Stent System *use* Intraluminal Device
Onychectomy
 see Excision, Skin and Breast 0HB
 see Resection, Skin and Breast 0HT
Onychoplasty
 see Repair, Skin and Breast 0HQ
 see Replacement, Skin and Breast 0HR
Onychotomy *see* Drainage, Skin and Breast 0H9
Oophorectomy
 see Excision, Female Reproductive System 0UB
 see Resection, Female Reproductive System 0UT
Oophoropexy
 see Repair, Female Reproductive System 0UQ
 see Reposition, Female Reproductive System 0US
Oophoroplasty
 see Repair, Female Reproductive System 0UQ
 see Supplement, Female Reproductive System 0UU
Oophororrhaphy *see* Repair, Female Reproductive System 0UQ
Oophorostomy *see* Drainage, Female Reproductive System 0U9
Oophorotomy
 see Division, Female Reproductive System 0U8
 see Drainage, Female Reproductive System 0U9
Oophorrhaphy *see* Repair, Female Reproductive System 0UQ
Open Pivot Aortic Valve Graft (AVG) *use* Synthetic Substitute
Open Pivot (mechanical) Valve *use* Synthetic Substitute
Ophthalmic artery *use* Intracranial Artery
Ophthalmic nerve *use* Trigeminal Nerve
Ophthalmic vein *use* Intracranial Vein
Opponensplasty
 Tendon replacement *see* Replacement, Tendons 0LR
 Tendon transfer *see* Transfer, Tendons 0LX
Optic chiasma *use* Optic Nerve
Optic disc
 use Retina, Left
 use Retina, Right
Optic foramen *use* Sphenoid Bone
Optical coherence tomography, intravascular *see* Computerized Tomography (CT Scan)
Optimizer™ III implantable pulse generator *use* Contractility Modulation Device in 0JH
Orbicularis oculi muscle
 use Upper Eyelid, Left
 use Upper Eyelid, Right
Orbicularis oris muscle *use* Facial Muscle
Orbital Atherectomy *see* Extirpation, Heart and Great Vessels 02C
Orbital fascia *use* Subcutaneous Tissue and Fascia, Face
Orbital portion of ethmoid bone
 use Orbit, Left
 use Orbit, Right
Orbital portion of frontal bone
 use Orbit, Left
 use Orbit, Right
Orbital portion of lacrimal bone
 use Orbit, Left
 use Orbit, Right
Orbital portion of maxilla
 use Orbit, Left
 use Orbit, Right
Orbital portion of palatine bone
 use Orbit, Left
 use Orbit, Right
Orbital portion of sphenoid bone
 use Orbit, Left
 use Orbit, Right

Orbital portion of zygomatic bone
 use Orbit, Left
 use Orbit, Right
Orchectomy, orchidectomy, orchiectomy
 see Excision, Male Reproductive System 0VB
 see Resection, Male Reproductive System 0VT
Orchidoplasty, orchioplasty
 see Repair, Male Reproductive System 0VQ
 see Replacement, Male Reproductive System 0VR
 see Supplement, Male Reproductive System 0VU
Orchidorrhaphy, orchiorrhaphy *see* Repair, Male Reproductive System 0VQ
Orchidotomy, orchiotomy, orchotomy *see* Drainage, Male Reproductive System 0V9
Orchiopexy
 see Repair, Male Reproductive System 0VQ
 see Reposition, Male Reproductive System 0VS
Oropharyngeal airway (OPA) *use* Intraluminal Device, Airway in Mouth and Throat
Oropharynx *use* Pharynx
Ossiculectomy
 see Excision, Ear, Nose, Sinus 09B
 see Resection, Ear, Nose, Sinus 09T
Ossiculotomy *see* Drainage, Ear, Nose, Sinus 099
Ostectomy
 see Excision, Head and Facial Bones 0NB
 see Excision, Lower Bones 0QB
 see Excision, Upper Bones 0PB
 see Resection, Head and Facial Bones 0NT
 see Resection, Lower Bones 0QT
 see Resection, Upper Bones 0PT
Osteoclasis
 see Division, Head and Facial Bones 0N8
 see Division, Lower Bones 0Q8
 see Division, Upper Bones 0P8
Osteolysis
 see Release, Head and Facial Bones 0NN
 see Release, Lower Bones 0QN
 see Release, Upper Bones 0PN
Osteopathic Treatment
 Abdomen 7W09X
 Cervical 7W01X
 Extremity
  Lower 7W06X
  Upper 7W07X
 Head 7W00X
 Lumbar 7W03X
 Pelvis 7W05X
 Rib Cage 7W08X
 Sacrum 7W04X
 Thoracic 7W02X
Osteopexy
 see Repair, Head and Facial Bones 0NQ
 see Repair, Lower Bones 0QQ
 see Repair, Upper Bones 0PQ
 see Reposition, Head and Facial Bones 0NS
 see Reposition, Lower Bones 0QS
 see Reposition, Upper Bones 0PS
Osteoplasty
 see Repair, Head and Facial Bones 0NQ
 see Repair, Lower Bones 0QQ
 see Repair, Upper Bones 0PQ
 see Replacement, Head and Facial Bones 0NR
 see Replacement, Lower Bones 0QR
 see Replacement, Upper Bones 0PR
 see Supplement, Head and Facial Bones 0NU
 see Supplement, Lower Bones 0QU
 see Supplement, Upper Bones 0PU
Osteorrhaphy
 see Repair, Head and Facial Bones 0NQ
 see Repair, Lower Bones 0QQ
 see Repair, Upper Bones 0PQ
Osteotomy, ostotomy
 see Division, Head and Facial Bones 0N8
 see Division, Lower Bones 0Q8
 see Division, Upper Bones 0P8
 see Drainage, Head and Facial Bones 0N9
 see Drainage, Lower Bones 0Q9
 see Drainage, Upper Bones 0P9
Other Imaging
 Bile Duct and Gallbladder, Indocyanine Green Dye, Intraoperative BF53200
 Bile Duct, Indocyanine Green Dye, Intraoperative BF50200
 Extremity
  Lower BW5CZ1Z
  Upper BW5JZ1Z

Other Imaging — *continued*

Gallbladder and Bile Duct, Indocyanine Green Dye, Intraoperative BF53200

Gallbladder, Indocyanine Green Dye, Intraoperative BF52200

Head and Neck BW59Z1Z

Hepatobiliary System, All, Indocyanine Green Dye, Intraoperative BF5C200

Liver and Spleen, Indocyanine Green Dye, Intraoperative BF56200

Liver, Indocyanine Green Dye, Intraoperative BF55200

Neck and Head BW59Z1Z

Pancreas, Indocyanine Green Dye, Intraoperative BF57200

Spleen and Liver, Indocyanine Green Dye, Intraoperative BF56200

Trunk BW52Z1Z

Other New Technology Monoclonal Antibody XW0

Other New Technology Therapeutic Substance XW0

Otic ganglion *use* Head and Neck Sympathetic Nerve

OTL-101 *use* Hematopoietic Stem/Progenitor Cells, Genetically Modified

OTL-103 XW1

OTL-200 XW1

Otoplasty

see Repair, Ear, Nose, Sinus 09Q

see Replacement, Ear, Nose, Sinus 09R

see Supplement, Ear, Nose, Sinus 09U

Otoscopy *see* Inspection, Ear, Nose, Sinus 09J

Oval window

use Middle Ear, Left

use Middle Ear, Right

Ovarian artery *use* Abdominal Aorta

Ovarian ligament *use* Uterine Supporting Structure

Ovariectomy

see Excision, Female Reproductive System 0UB

see Resection, Female Reproductive System 0UT

Ovariocentesis *see* Drainage, Female Reproductive System 0U9

Ovariopexy

see Repair, Female Reproductive System 0UQ

see Reposition, Female Reproductive System 0US

Ovariotomy

see Division, Female Reproductive System 0U8

see Drainage, Female Reproductive System 0U9

Ovatio™ CRT-D *use* Cardiac Resynchronization Defibrillator Pulse Generator in 0JH

Oversewing

Gastrointestinal ulcer *see* Repair, Gastrointestinal System 0DQ

Pleural bleb *see* Repair, Respiratory System 0BQ

Oviduct

use Fallopian Tube, Left

use Fallopian Tube, Right

Oximetry, Fetal pulse 10H073Z

OXINIUM *use* Synthetic Substitute, Oxidized Zirconium on Polyethylene in 0SR

Oxygen Saturation Endoscopic Imaging (OXEI) XD2

Oxygenation

Extracorporeal membrane (ECMO) *see* Performance, Circulatory 5A15

Hyperbaric *see* Assistance, Circulatory 5A05

Supersaturated *see* Assistance, Circulatory 5A05

P

Pacemaker

Dual Chamber

Abdomen 0JH8

Chest 0JH6

Intracardiac

Insertion of device in

Atrium

Left 02H7

Right 02H6

Vein, Coronary 02H4

Ventricle

Left 02HL

Right 02HK

Removal of device from, Heart 02PA

Revision of device in, Heart 02WA

Single Chamber

Abdomen 0JH8

Chest 0JH6

Pacemaker — *continued*

Single Chamber Rate Responsive

Abdomen 0JH8

Chest 0JH6

Packing

Abdominal Wall 2W43X5Z

Anorectal 2Y43X5Z

Arm

Lower

Left 2W4DX5Z

Right 2W4CX5Z

Upper

Left 2W4BX5Z

Right 2W4AX5Z

Back 2W45X5Z

Chest Wall 2W44X5Z

Ear 2Y42X5Z

Extremity

Lower

Left 2W4MX5Z

Right 2W4LX5Z

Upper

Left 2W49X5Z

Right 2W48X5Z

Face 2W41X5Z

Finger

Left 2W4KX5Z

Right 2W4JX5Z

Foot

Left 2W4TX5Z

Right 2W4SX5Z

Genital Tract, Female 2Y44X5Z

Hand

Left 2W4FX5Z

Right 2W4EX5Z

Head 2W40X5Z

Inguinal Region

Left 2W47X5Z

Right 2W46X5Z

Leg

Lower

Left 2W4RX5Z

Right 2W4QX5Z

Upper

Left 2W4PX5Z

Right 2W4NX5Z

Mouth and Pharynx 2Y40X5Z

Nasal 2Y41X5Z

Neck 2W42X5Z

Thumb

Left 2W4HX5Z

Right 2W4GX5Z

Toe

Left 2W4VX5Z

Right 2W4UX5Z

Urethra 2Y45X5Z

Paclitaxel-eluting coronary stent *use* Intraluminal Device, Drug-eluting in Heart and Great Vessels

Paclitaxel-eluting peripheral stent

use Intraluminal Device, Drug-eluting in Lower Arteries

use Intraluminal Device, Drug-eluting in Upper Arteries

Palatine gland *use* Buccal Mucosa

Palatine tonsil *use* Tonsils

Palatine uvula *use* Uvula

Palatoglossal muscle *use* Tongue, Palate, Pharynx Muscle

Palatopharyngeal muscle *use* Tongue, Palate, Pharynx Muscle

Palatoplasty

see Repair, Mouth and Throat 0CQ

see Replacement, Mouth and Throat 0CR

see Supplement, Mouth and Throat 0CU

Palatorrhaphy *see* Repair, Mouth and Throat 0CQ

Palmar cutaneous nerve

use Median Nerve

use Radial Nerve

Palmar (volar) digital vein

use Hand Vein, Left

use Hand Vein, Right

Palmar fascia (aponeurosis)

use Subcutaneous Tissue and Fascia, Left Hand

use Subcutaneous Tissue and Fascia, Right Hand

Palmar interosseous muscle

use Hand Muscle, Left

use Hand Muscle, Right

Palmar (volar) metacarpal vein

use Hand Vein, Left

use Hand Vein, Right

Palmar ulnocarpal ligament

use Wrist Bursa and Ligament, Left

use Wrist Bursa and Ligament, Right

Palmaris longus muscle

use Lower Arm and Wrist Muscle, Left

use Lower Arm and Wrist Muscle, Right

Pancreatectomy

see Excision, Pancreas 0FBG

see Resection, Pancreas 0FTG

Pancreatic artery *use* Splenic Artery

Pancreatic plexus *use* Abdominal Sympathetic Nerve

Pancreatic vein *use* Splenic Vein

Pancreaticoduodenostomy *see* Bypass, Hepatobiliary System and Pancreas 0F1

Pancreaticosplenic lymph node *use* Lymphatic, Aortic

Pancreatogram, endoscopic retrograde *see* Fluoroscopy, Pancreatic Duct BF18

Pancreatolithotomy *see* Extirpation, Pancreas 0FCG

Pancreatotomy

see Division, Pancreas 0F8G

see Drainage, Pancreas 0F9G

Panniculectomy

see Excision, Skin, Abdomen 0HB7

see Excision, Subcutaneous Tissue and Fascia, Abdomen 0JB8

Paraaortic lymph node *use* Lymphatic, Aortic

Paracentesis

Eye *see* Drainage, Eye 089

Peritoneal Cavity *see* Drainage, Peritoneal Cavity 0W9G

Tympanum *see* Drainage, Ear, Nose, Sinus 099

Parapharyngeal space *use* Neck

Pararectal lymph node *use* Lymphatic, Mesenteric

Parasternal lymph node *use* Lymphatic, Thorax

Parathyroidectomy

see Excision, Endocrine System 0GB

see Resection, Endocrine System 0GT

Paratracheal lymph node *use* Lymphatic, Thorax

Paraurethral (Skene's) gland *use* Vestibular Gland

Parenteral nutrition, total *see* Introduction of Nutritional Substance

Parietal lobe *use* Cerebral Hemisphere

Parotid lymph node *use* Lymphatic, Head

Parotid plexus *use* Facial Nerve

Parotidectomy

see Excision, Mouth and Throat 0CB

see Resection, Mouth and Throat 0CT

Pars flaccida

use Tympanic Membrane, Left

use Tympanic Membrane, Right

Partial joint replacement

Hip *see* Replacement, Lower Joints 0SR

Knee *see* Replacement, Lower Joints 0SR

Shoulder *see* Replacement, Upper Joints 0RR

Partially absorbable mesh *use* Synthetic Substitute

Patch, blood, spinal 3E0R3GC

Patellapexy

see Repair, Lower Bones 0QQ

see Reposition, Lower Bones 0QS

Patellaplasty

see Repair, Lower Bones 0QQ

see Replacement, Lower Bones 0QR

see Supplement, Lower Bones 0QU

Patellar ligament

use Knee Bursa and Ligament, Left

use Knee Bursa and Ligament, Right

Patellar tendon

use Knee Tendon, Left

use Knee Tendon, Right

Patellectomy

see Excision, Lower Bones 0QB

see Resection, Lower Bones 0QT

Patellofemoral joint

use Knee Joint, Left

use Knee Joint, Left, Femoral Surface

use Knee Joint, Right

use Knee Joint, Right, Femoral Surface

pAVF (percutaneous arteriovenous fistula), using magnetic-guided radiofrequency *see* Bypass, Upper Arteries 031

pAVF (percutaneous arteriovenous fistula), using thermal resistance energy *see* New Technology, Cardiovascular System X2K

Pectineus muscle
use Upper Leg Muscle, Left
use Upper Leg Muscle, Right

Pectoral fascia *use* Subcutaneous Tissue and Fascia, Chest

Pectoral (anterior) lymph node
use Lymphatic Left, Axillary
use Lymphatic Right, Axillary

Pectoralis major muscle
use Thorax Muscle, Left
use Thorax Muscle, Right

Pectoralis minor muscle
use Thorax Muscle, Left
use Thorax Muscle, Right

Pedicle-based dynamic stabilization device
use Spinal Stabilization Device, Pedicle-Based in ØSH
use Spinal Stabilization Device, Pedicle-Based in ØRH

PEEP (positive end expiratory pressure) *see* Assistance, Respiratory 5AØ9

PEG (percutaneous endoscopic gastrostomy) ØDH63UZ

PEJ (percutaneous endoscopic jejunostomy) ØDHA3UZ

Pelvic splanchnic nerve
use Abdominal Sympathetic Nerve
use Sacral Sympathetic Nerve

Penectomy
see Excision, Male Reproductive System ØVB
see Resection, Male Reproductive System ØVT

Penile urethra *use* Urethra

Penumbra Indigo® Aspiration System *see* New Technology, Cardiovascular System X2C

PERCEPT™ PC neurostimulator *use* Stimulator Generator, Multiple Array in ØJH

Perceval sutureless valve (rapid deployment technique) *see* Replacement, Valve, Aortic Ø2RF

Percutaneous endoscopic gastrojejunostomy (PEG/J) tube *use* Feeding Device in Gastrointestinal System

Percutaneous endoscopic gastrostomy (PEG) tube *use* Feeding Device in Gastrointestinal System

Percutaneous nephrostomy catheter *use* Drainage Device

Percutaneous transluminal coronary angioplasty (PTCA) *see* Dilation, Heart and Great Vessels Ø27

Performance
Biliary
Multiple, Filtration 5A1C6ØZ
Single, Filtration 5A1CØØZ
Cardiac
Continuous
Output 5A1221Z
Pacing 5A1223Z
Intermittent, Pacing 5A1213Z
Single, Output, Manual 5A12Ø12
Circulatory
Continuous
Central Membrane 5A1522F
Peripheral Veno-arterial Membrane 5A1522G
Peripheral Veno-venous Membrane 5A1522H
Intraoperative
Central Membrane 5A15A2F
Peripheral Veno-arterial Membrane 5A15A2G
Peripheral Veno-venous Membrane 5A15A2H
Respiratory
24-96 Consecutive Hours, Ventilation 5A1945Z
Greater than 96 Consecutive Hours, Ventilation 5A1955Z
Less than 24 Consecutive Hours, Ventilation 5A1935Z
Single, Ventilation, Nonmechanical 5A19Ø54
Urinary
Continuous, Greater than 18 hours per day, Filtration 5A1D9ØZ
Intermittent, Less than 6 Hours Per Day, Filtration 5A1D7ØZ

Performance — *continued*
Urinary — *continued*
Prolonged Intermittent, 6-18 hours per day, Filtration 5A1D8ØZ

Perfusion *see* Introduction of substance in or on

Perfusion, donor organ
Heart 6AB5ØBZ
Kidney(s) 6ABTØBZ
Liver 6ABFØBZ
Lung(s) 6ABBØBZ

Perianal skin *use* Skin, Perineum

Pericardiectomy
see Excision, Pericardium Ø2BN
see Resection, Pericardium Ø2TN

Pericardiocentesis *see* Drainage, Pericardial Cavity ØW9D

Pericardiolysis *see* Release, Pericardium Ø2NN

Pericardiophrenic artery
use Internal Mammary Artery, Left
use Internal Mammary Artery, Right

Pericardioplasty
see Repair, Pericardium Ø2QN
see Replacement, Pericardium Ø2RN
see Supplement, Pericardium Ø2UN

Pericardiorrhaphy *see* Repair, Pericardium Ø2QN

Pericardiostomy *see* Drainage, Pericardial Cavity ØW9D

Pericardiotomy *see* Drainage, Pericardial Cavity ØW9D

Perimetrium *use* Uterus

Peripheral Intravascular Lithotripsy (Peripheral IVL) *see* Fragmentation

Peripheral parenteral nutrition *see* Introduction of Nutritional Substance

Peripherally inserted central catheter (PICC) *use* Infusion Device

Peritoneal dialysis 3E1M39Z

Peritoneocentesis
see Drainage, Peritoneal Cavity ØW9G
see Drainage, Peritoneum ØD9W

Peritoneoplasty
see Repair, Peritoneum ØDQW
see Replacement, Peritoneum ØDRW
see Supplement, Peritoneum ØDUW

Peritoneoscopy ØDJW4ZZ

Peritoneotomy *see* Drainage, Peritoneum ØD9W

Peritoneumectomy *see* Excision, Peritoneum ØDBW

Peroneus brevis muscle
use Lower Leg Muscle, Left
use Lower Leg Muscle, Right

Peroneus longus muscle
use Lower Leg Muscle, Left
use Lower Leg Muscle, Right

Pessary ring *use* Intraluminal Device, Pessary in Female Reproductive System

PET scan *see* Positron Emission Tomographic (PET) Imaging

Petrous part of temporal bone
use Temporal Bone, Left
use Temporal Bone, Right

Phacoemulsification, lens
With IOL implant *see* Replacement, Eye Ø8R
Without IOL implant *see* Extraction, Eye Ø8D

Phagenyx® System XWHD7Q7

Phalangectomy
see Excision, Lower Bones ØQB
see Excision, Upper Bones ØPB
see Resection, Lower Bones ØQT
see Resection, Upper Bones ØPT

Phallectomy
see Excision, Penis ØVBS
see Resection, Penis ØVTS

Phalloplasty
see Repair, Penis ØVQS
see Supplement, Penis ØVUS

Phallotomy *see* Drainage, Penis ØV9S

Pharmacotherapy, for substance abuse
Antabuse HZ93ZZZ
Bupropion HZ97ZZZ
Clonidine HZ96ZZZ
Levo-alpha-acetyl-methadol (LAAM) HZ92ZZZ
Methadone Maintenance HZ91ZZZ
Naloxone HZ95ZZZ
Naltrexone HZ94ZZZ
Nicotine Replacement HZ9ØZZZ
Psychiatric Medication HZ98ZZZ
Replacement Medication, Other HZ99ZZZ

Pharyngeal constrictor muscle *use* Tongue, Palate, Pharynx Muscle

Pharyngeal plexus *use* Vagus Nerve
Pharyngeal recess *use* Nasopharynx
Pharyngeal tonsil *use* Adenoids
Pharyngogram *see* Fluoroscopy, Pharynix B91G

Pharyngoplasty
see Repair, Mouth and Throat ØCQ
see Replacement, Mouth and Throat ØCR
see Supplement, Mouth and Throat ØCU

Pharyngorrhaphy *see* Repair, Mouth and Throat ØCQ

Pharyngotomy *see* Drainage, Mouth and Throat ØC9

Pharyngotympanic tube
use Eustachian Tube, Left
use Eustachian Tube, Right

Pheresis
Erythrocytes 6A55
Leukocytes 6A55
Plasma 6A55
Platelets 6A55
Stem Cells
Cord Blood 6A55
Hematopoietic 6A55

Phlebectomy
see Excision, Lower Veins Ø6B
see Excision, Upper Veins Ø5B
see Extraction, Lower Veins Ø6D
see Extraction, Upper Veins Ø5D

Phlebography
see Plain Radiography, Veins B5Ø
Impedance 4AØ4X51

Phleborrhaphy
see Repair, Lower Veins Ø6Q
see Repair, Upper Veins Ø5Q

Phlebotomy
see Drainage, Lower Veins Ø69
see Drainage, Upper Veins Ø59

Photocoagulation
For Destruction *see* Destruction
For Repair *see* Repair

Photopheresis, therapeutic *see* Phototherapy, Circulatory 6A65

Phototherapy
Circulatory 6A65
Skin 6A6Ø
Ultraviolet light *see* Ultraviolet Light Therapy, Physiological Systems 6A8

Phrenectomy, phrenoneurectomy *see* Excision, Nerve, Phrenic Ø1B2

Phrenemphraxis *see* Destruction, Nerve, Phrenic Ø152

Phrenic nerve stimulator generator *use* Stimulator Generator in Subcutaneous Tissue and Fascia

Phrenic nerve stimulator lead *use* Diaphragmatic Pacemaker Lead in Respiratory System

Phreniclasis *see* Destruction, Nerve, Phrenic Ø152

Phrenicoexeresis *see* Extraction, Nerve, Phrenic Ø1D2

Phrenicotomy *see* Division, Nerve, Phrenic Ø182

Phrenicotripsy *see* Destruction, Nerve, Phrenic Ø152

Phrenoplasty
see Repair, Respiratory System ØBQ
see Supplement, Respiratory System ØBU

Phrenotomy *see* Drainage, Respiratory System ØB9

Physiatry *see* Motor Treatment, Rehabilitation FØ7

Physical medicine *see* Motor Treatment, Rehabilitation FØ7

Physical therapy *see* Motor Treatment, Rehabilitation FØ7

PHYSIOMESH™ Flexible Composite Mesh *use* Synthetic Substitute

Pia mater, intracranial *use* Cerebral Meninges
Pia mater, spinal *use* Spinal Meninges
PiCSO® Impulse System X2A7358

Pinealectomy
see Excision, Pineal Body ØGB1
see Resection, Pineal Body ØGT1

Pinealoscopy ØGJ14ZZ

Pinealotomy *see* Drainage, Pineal Body ØG91

Pinna
use External Ear, Bilateral
use External Ear, Left
use External Ear, Right

Pipeline™ (Flex) embolization device *use* Intraluminal Device, Flow Diverter in Ø3V

Piriform recess (sinus) *use* Pharynx

Piriformis muscle
use Hip Muscle, Left
use Hip Muscle, Right

PIRRT (Prolonged intermittent renal replacement therapy) 5A1D8ØZ

Subterms under main terms may continue to next column or page

Pisiform bone
  use Carpal, Left
  use Carpal, Right
Pisohamate ligament
  use Hand Bursa and Ligament, Left
  use Hand Bursa and Ligament, Right
Pisometacarpal ligament
  use Hand Bursa and Ligament, Left
  use Hand Bursa and Ligament, Right
Pituitectomy
  see Excision, Gland, Pituitary ØGBØ
  see Resection, Gland, Pituitary ØGTØ
Plain film radiology *see* Plain Radiography
Plain Radiography
  Abdomen BW00ZZZ
  Abdomen and Pelvis BW01ZZZ
  Abdominal Lymphatic
    Bilateral B701
    Unilateral B700
  Airway, Upper BB0DZZZ
  Ankle
    Left BQ0H
    Right BQ0G
  Aorta
    Abdominal B400
    Thoracic B300
    Thoraco-Abdominal B30P
  Aorta and Bilateral Lower Extremity Arteries B40D
  Arch
    Bilateral BN0DZZZ
    Left BN0CZZZ
    Right BN0BZZZ
  Arm
    Left BP0FZZZ
    Right BP0EZZZ
  Artery
    Brachiocephalic-Subclavian, Right B301
    Bronchial B30L
    Bypass Graft, Other B20F
    Cervico-Cerebral Arch B30Q
    Common Carotid
      Bilateral B305
      Left B304
      Right B303
    Coronary
      Bypass Graft
        Multiple B203
        Single B202
      Multiple B201
      Single B200
    External Carotid
      Bilateral B30C
      Left B30B
      Right B309
    Hepatic B402
    Inferior Mesenteric B405
    Intercostal B30L
    Internal Carotid
      Bilateral B308
      Left B307
      Right B306
    Internal Mammary Bypass Graft
      Left B208
      Right B207
    Intra-Abdominal, Other B40B
    Intracranial B30R
    Lower Extremity
      Bilateral and Aorta B40D
      Left B40G
      Right B40F
    Lower, Other B40J
    Lumbar B409
    Pelvic B40C
    Pulmonary
      Left B30T
      Right B30S
    Renal
      Bilateral B408
      Left B407
      Right B406
      Transplant B40M
    Spinal B30M
    Splenic B403
    Subclavian, Left B302
    Superior Mesenteric B404
    Upper Extremity
      Bilateral B30K
      Left B30J

Plain Radiography — *continued*
  Artery — *continued*
    Upper Extremity — *continued*
      Right B30H
      Upper, Other B30N
    Vertebral
      Bilateral B30G
      Left B30F
      Right B30D
  Bile Duct BF00
  Bile Duct and Gallbladder BF03
  Bladder BT00
    Kidney and Ureter BT04
  Bladder and Urethra BT0B
  Bone
    Facial BN05ZZZ
    Nasal BN04ZZZ
  Bones, Long, All BW0BZZZ
  Breast
    Bilateral BH02ZZZ
    Left BH01ZZZ
    Right BH00ZZZ
  Calcaneus
    Left BQ0KZZZ
    Right BQ0JZZZ
  Chest BW03ZZZ
  Clavicle
    Left BP05ZZZ
    Right BP04ZZZ
  Coccyx BR0FZZZ
  Corpora Cavernosa BV00
  Dialysis Fistula B50W
  Dialysis Shunt B50W
  Disc
    Cervical BR01
    Lumbar BR03
    Thoracic BR02
  Duct
    Lacrimal
      Bilateral B802
      Left B801
      Right B800
    Mammary
      Multiple
        Left BH06
        Right BH05
      Single
        Left BH04
        Right BH03
  Elbow
    Left BP0H
    Right BP0G
  Epididymis
    Left BV02
    Right BV01
  Extremity
    Lower BW0CZZZ
    Upper BW0JZZZ
  Eye
    Bilateral B807ZZZ
    Left B806ZZZ
    Right B805ZZZ
  Facet Joint
    Cervical BR04
    Lumbar BR06
    Thoracic BR05
  Fallopian Tube
    Bilateral BU02
    Left BU01
    Right BU00
  Fallopian Tube and Uterus BU08
  Femur
    Left, Densitometry BQ04ZZ1
    Right, Densitometry BQ03ZZ1
  Finger
    Left BP0SZZZ
    Right BP0RZZZ
  Foot
    Left BQ0MZZZ
    Right BQ0LZZZ
  Forearm
    Left BP0KZZZ
    Right BP0JZZZ
  Gallbladder and Bile Duct BF03
  Gland
    Parotid
      Bilateral B906
      Left B905
      Right B904

Plain Radiography — *continued*
  Gland — *continued*
    Salivary
      Bilateral B90D
      Left B90C
      Right B90B
    Submandibular
      Bilateral B909
      Left B908
      Right B907
  Hand
    Left BP0PZZZ
    Right BP0NZZZ
  Heart
    Left B205
    Right B204
    Right and Left B206
  Hepatobiliary System, All BF0C
  Hip
    Left BQ01
      Densitometry BQ01ZZ1
    Right BQ00
      Densitometry BQ00ZZ1
  Humerus
    Left BP0BZZZ
    Right BP0AZZZ
  Ileal Diversion Loop BT0C
  Intracranial Sinus B502
  Joint
    Acromioclavicular, Bilateral BP03ZZZ
    Finger
      Left BP0D
      Right BP0C
    Foot
      Left BQ0Y
      Right BQ0X
    Hand
      Left BP0D
      Right BP0C
    Lumbosacral BR0BZZZ
    Sacroiliac BR0D
    Sternoclavicular
      Bilateral BP02ZZZ
      Left BP01ZZZ
      Right BP00ZZZ
    Temporomandibular
      Bilateral BN09
      Left BN08
      Right BN07
    Thoracolumbar BR08ZZZ
    Toe
      Left BQ0Y
      Right BQ0X
  Kidney
    Bilateral BT03
    Left BT02
    Right BT01
    Ureter and Bladder BT04
  Knee
    Left BQ08
    Right BQ07
  Leg
    Left BQ0FZZZ
    Right BQ0DZZZ
  Lymphatic
    Head B704
    Lower Extremity
      Bilateral B70B
      Left B709
      Right B708
    Neck B704
    Pelvic B70C
    Upper Extremity
      Bilateral B707
      Left B706
      Right B705
  Mandible BN06ZZZ
  Mastoid B90HZZZ
  Nasopharynx B90FZZZ
  Optic Foramina
    Left B804ZZZ
    Right B803ZZZ
  Orbit
    Bilateral BN03ZZZ
    Left BN02ZZZ
    Right BN01ZZZ
  Oropharynx B90FZZZ
  Patella
    Left BQ0WZZZ

Plain Radiography — *continued*
Patella — *continued*
   Right BQ0VZZZ
Pelvis BR0CZZZ
Pelvis and Abdomen BW01ZZZ
Prostate BV03
Retroperitoneal Lymphatic
   Bilateral B701
   Unilateral B700
Ribs
   Left BP0YZZZ
   Right BP0XZZZ
Sacrum BR0FZZZ
Scapula
   Left BP07ZZZ
   Right BP06ZZZ
Shoulder
   Left BP09
   Right BP08
Sinus
   Intracranial B502
   Paranasal B902ZZZ
Skull BN00ZZZ
Spinal Cord B00B
Spine
   Cervical, Densitometry BR00ZZ1
   Lumbar, Densitometry BR09ZZ1
   Thoracic, Densitometry BR07ZZ1
   Whole, Densitometry BR0GZZ1
Sternum BR0HZZZ
Teeth
   All BN0JZZZ
   Multiple BN0HZZZ
Testicle
   Left BV06
   Right BV05
Toe
   Left BQ0QZZZ
   Right BQ0PZZZ
Tooth, Single BN0GZZZ
Tracheobronchial Tree
   Bilateral BB09YZZ
   Left BB08YZZ
   Right BB07YZZ
Ureter
   Bilateral BT08
   Kidney and Bladder BT04
   Left BT07
   Right BT06
Urethra BT05
Urethra and Bladder BT0B
Uterus BU06
Uterus and Fallopian Tube BU08
Vagina BU09
Vasa Vasorum BV08
Vein
   Cerebellar B501
   Cerebral B501
   Epidural B500
   Jugular
      Bilateral B505
      Left B504
      Right B503
   Lower Extremity
      Bilateral B50D
      Left B50C
      Right B50B
   Other B50V
   Pelvic (Iliac)
      Left B50G
      Right B50F
   Pelvic (Iliac) Bilateral B50H
   Portal B50T
   Pulmonary
      Bilateral B50S
      Left B50R
      Right B50Q
   Renal
      Bilateral B50L
      Left B50K
      Right B50J
   Spanchnic B50T
   Subclavian
      Left B507
      Right B506
   Upper Extremity
      Bilateral B50P
      Left B50N
      Right B50M

Plain Radiography — *continued*
Vena Cava
   Inferior B509
   Superior B508
Whole Body BW0KZZZ
   Infant BW0MZZZ
Whole Skeleton BW0LZZZ
Wrist
   Left BP0M
   Right BP0L
Planar Nuclear Medicine Imaging
Abdomen CW10
Abdomen and Chest CW14
Abdomen and Pelvis CW11
Anatomical Region, Other CW1ZZZZ
Anatomical Regions, Multiple CW1YYZZ
Bladder and Ureters CT1H
Bladder, Kidneys and Ureters CT13
Blood C713
Bone Marrow C710
Brain C010
Breast CH1YYZZ
   Bilateral CH12
   Left CH11
   Right CH10
Bronchi and Lungs CB12
Central Nervous System C01YYZZ
Cerebrospinal Fluid C015
Chest CW13
Chest and Abdomen CW14
Chest and Neck CW16
Digestive System CD1YYZZ
Ducts, Lacrimal, Bilateral C819
Ear, Nose, Mouth and Throat C91YYZZ
Endocrine System CG1YYZZ
Extremity
   Lower CW1D
      Bilateral CP1F
      Left CP1D
      Right CP1C
   Upper CW1M
      Bilateral CP1B
      Left CP19
      Right CP18
Eye C81YYZZ
Gallbladder CF14
Gastrointestinal Tract CD17
   Upper CD15
Gland
   Adrenal, Bilateral CG14
   Parathyroid CG11
   Thyroid CG12
Glands, Salivary, Bilateral C91B
Head and Neck CW1B
Heart C21YYZZ
   Right and Left C216
Hepatobiliary System, All CF1C
Hepatobiliary System and Pancreas CF1YYZZ
Kidneys, Ureters and Bladder CT13
Liver CF15
Liver and Spleen CF16
Lungs and Bronchi CB12
Lymphatics
   Head C71J
   Head and Neck C715
   Lower Extremity C71P
   Neck C71K
   Pelvic C71D
   Trunk C71M
   Upper Chest C71L
   Upper Extremity C71N
Lymphatics and Hematologic System C71YYZZ
Musculoskeletal System
   All CP1Z
   Other CP1YYZZ
Myocardium C21G
Neck and Chest CW16
Neck and Head CW1B
Pancreas and Hepatobiliary System CF1YYZZ
Pelvic Region CW1J
Pelvis CP16
Pelvis and Abdomen CW11
Pelvis and Spine CP17
Reproductive System, Male CV1YYZZ
Respiratory System CB1YYZZ
Skin CH1YYZZ
Skull CP11
Spine CP15
Spine and Pelvis CP17

Planar Nuclear Medicine Imaging — *continued*
Spleen C712
Spleen and Liver CF16
Subcutaneous Tissue CH1YYZZ
Testicles, Bilateral CV19
Thorax CP14
Ureters and Bladder CT1H
Ureters, Kidneys and Bladder CT13
Urinary System CT1YYZZ
Veins C51YYZZ
   Central C51R
   Lower Extremity
      Bilateral C51D
      Left C51C
      Right C51B
   Upper Extremity
      Bilateral C51Q
      Left C51P
      Right C51N
Whole Body CW1N
Plantar digital vein
   use Foot Vein, Left
   use Foot Vein, Right
Plantar fascia (aponeurosis)
   use Subcutaneous Tissue and Fascia, Left Foot
   use Subcutaneous Tissue and Fascia, Right Foot
Plantar metatarsal vein
   use Foot Vein, Left
   use Foot Vein, Right
Plantar venous arch
   use Foot Vein, Left
   use Foot Vein, Right
Plaque Radiation
Abdomen DWY3FZZ
Adrenal Gland DGY2FZZ
Anus DDY8FZZ
Bile Ducts DFY2FZZ
Bladder DTY2FZZ
Bone Marrow D7Y0FZZ
Bone, Other DPYCFZZ
Brain D0Y0FZZ
Brain Stem D0Y1FZZ
Breast
   Left DMY0FZZ
   Right DMY1FZZ
Bronchus DBY1FZZ
Cervix DUY1FZZ
Chest DWY2FZZ
Chest Wall DBY7FZZ
Colon DDY5FZZ
Diaphragm DBY8FZZ
Duodenum DDY2FZZ
Ear D9Y0FZZ
Esophagus DDY0FZZ
Eye D8Y0FZZ
Femur DPY9FZZ
Fibula DPYBFZZ
Gallbladder DFY1FZZ
Gland
   Adrenal DGY2FZZ
   Parathyroid DGY4FZZ
   Pituitary DGY0FZZ
   Thyroid DGY5FZZ
Glands, Salivary D9Y6FZZ
Head and Neck DWY1FZZ
Hemibody DWY4FZZ
Humerus DPY6FZZ
Ileum DDY4FZZ
Jejunum DDY3FZZ
Kidney DTY0FZZ
Larynx D9YBFZZ
Liver DFY0FZZ
Lung DBY2FZZ
Lymphatics
   Abdomen D7Y6FZZ
   Axillary D7Y4FZZ
   Inguinal D7Y8FZZ
   Neck D7Y3FZZ
   Pelvis D7Y7FZZ
   Thorax D7Y5FZZ
Mandible DPY3FZZ
Maxilla DPY2FZZ
Mediastinum DBY6FZZ
Mouth D9Y4FZZ
Nasopharynx D9YDFZZ
Neck and Head DWY1FZZ
Nerve, Peripheral D0Y7FZZ
Nose D9Y1FZZ

▽ **Subterms under main terms may continue to next column or page**

Plaque Radiation — *continued*
Ovary DUY0FZZ
Palate
    Hard D9Y8FZZ
    Soft D9Y9FZZ
Pancreas DFY3FZZ
Parathyroid Gland DGY4FZZ
Pelvic Bones DPY8FZZ
Pelvic Region DWY6FZZ
Pharynx D9YCFZZ
Pineal Body DGY1FZZ
Pituitary Gland DGY0FZZ
Pleura DBY5FZZ
Prostate DVY0FZZ
Radius DPY7FZZ
Rectum DDY7FZZ
Rib DPY5FZZ
Sinuses D9Y7FZZ
Skin
    Abdomen DHY8FZZ
    Arm DHY4FZZ
    Back DHY7FZZ
    Buttock DHY9FZZ
    Chest DHY6FZZ
    Face DHY2FZZ
    Foot DHYCFZZ
    Hand DHY5FZZ
    Leg DHYBFZZ
    Neck DHY3FZZ
Skull DPY0FZZ
Spinal Cord D0Y6FZZ
Spleen D7Y2FZZ
Sternum DPY4FZZ
Stomach DDY1FZZ
Testis DVY1FZZ
Thymus D7Y1FZZ
Thyroid Gland DGY5FZZ
Tibia DPYBFZZ
Tongue D9Y5FZZ
Trachea DBY0FZZ
Ulna DPY7FZZ
Ureter DTY1FZZ
Urethra DTY3FZZ
Uterus DUY2FZZ
Whole Body DWY5FZZ
Plasma, Convalescent (Nonautologous) XW1
Plasmapheresis, therapeutic *see* Pheresis, Physiological Systems 6A5
Plateletpheresis, therapeutic *see* Pheresis, Physiological Systems 6A5
Platysma muscle
use Neck Muscle, Left
use Neck Muscle, Right
Plazomicin Anti-infective XW0
Pleurectomy
see Excision, Respiratory System 0BB
see Resection, Respiratory System 0BT
Pleurocentesis *see* Drainage, Anatomical Regions, General 0W9
Pleurodesis, pleurosclerosis
    Chemical injection *see* Introduction of Substance in or on, Pleural Cavity 3E0L
    Surgical *see* Destruction, Respiratory System 0B5
Pleurolysis *see* Release, Respiratory System 0BN
Pleuroscopy 0BJQ4ZZ
Pleurotomy *see* Drainage, Respiratory System 0B9
Plica semilunaris
use Conjunctiva, Left
use Conjunctiva, Right
Plication *see* Restriction
Pneumectomy
see Excision, Respiratory System 0BB
see Resection, Respiratory System 0BT
Pneumocentesis *see* Drainage, Respiratory System 0B9
Pneumogastric nerve *use* Vagus Nerve
Pneumolysis *see* Release, Respiratory System 0BN
Pneumonectomy *see* Resection, Respiratory System 0BT
Pneumonolysis *see* Release, Respiratory System 0BN
Pneumonopexy
see Repair, Respiratory System 0BQ
see Reposition, Respiratory System 0BS
Pneumonorrhaphy *see* Repair, Respiratory System 0BQ
Pneumonotomy *see* Drainage, Respiratory System 0B9
Pneumotaxic center *use* Pons
Pneumotomy *see* Drainage, Respiratory System 0B9

Pollicization *see* Transfer, Anatomical Regions, Upper Extremities 0XX
Polyclonal hyperimmune globulin *use* Globulin
Polyethylene socket *use* Synthetic Substitute, Polyethylene in 0SR
Polymethylmethacrylate (PMMA) *use* Synthetic Substitute
Polypectomy, gastrointestinal *see* Excision, Gastrointestinal System 0DB
Polypropylene mesh *use* Synthetic Substitute
Polysomnogram 4A1ZXQZ
Pontine tegmentum *use* Pons
Popliteal ligament
use Knee Bursa and Ligament, Left
use Knee Bursa and Ligament, Right
Popliteal lymph node
use Lymphatic, Left Lower Extremity
use Lymphatic, Right Lower Extremity
Popliteal vein
use Femoral Vein, Left
use Femoral Vein, Right
Popliteus muscle
use Lower Leg Muscle, Left
use Lower Leg Muscle, Right
Porcine (bioprosthetic) valve *use* Zooplastic Tissue in Heart and Great Vessels
Positive Blood Culture Fluorescence Hybridization for Organism Identification, Concentration and Susceptibility XXE5XN6
Positive end expiratory pressure *see* Performance, Respiratory 5A19
Positron Emission Tomographic (PET) Imaging
    Brain C030
    Bronchi and Lungs CB32
    Central Nervous System C03YYZZ
    Heart C23YYZZ
    Lungs and Bronchi CB32
    Myocardium C23G
    Respiratory System CB3YYZZ
    Whole Body CW3NYZZ
Positron emission tomography *see* Positron Emission Tomographic (PET) Imaging
Postauricular (mastoid) lymph node
use Lymphatic, Left Neck
use Lymphatic, Right Neck
Postcava *use* Inferior Vena Cava
Posterior auricular artery
use External Carotid Artery, Left
use External Carotid Artery, Right
Posterior auricular nerve *use* Facial Nerve
Posterior auricular vein
use External Jugular Vein, Left
use External Jugular Vein, Right
Posterior cerebral artery *use* Intracranial Artery
Posterior chamber
use Eye, Left
use Eye, Right
Posterior circumflex humeral artery
use Axillary Artery, Left
use Axillary Artery, Right
Posterior communicating artery *use* Intracranial Artery
Posterior cruciate ligament (PCL)
use Knee Bursa and Ligament, Left
use Knee Bursa and Ligament, Right
Posterior (Dynamic) Distraction Device
    Lumbar XNS0
    Thoracic XNS4
Posterior facial (retromandibular) vein
use Face Vein, Left
use Face Vein, Right
Posterior femoral cutaneous nerve *use* Sacral Plexus
Posterior inferior cerebellar artery (PICA) *use* Intracranial Artery
Posterior interosseous nerve *use* Radial Nerve
Posterior labial nerve *use* Pudendal Nerve
Posterior (subscapular) lymph node
use Lymphatic, Left Axillary
use Lymphatic, Right Axillary
Posterior scrotal nerve *use* Pudendal Nerve
Posterior spinal artery
use Vertebral Artery, Left
use Vertebral Artery, Right
Posterior tibial recurrent artery
use Anterior Tibial Artery, Left
use Anterior Tibial Artery, Right

Posterior ulnar recurrent artery
use Ulnar Artery, Left
use Ulnar Artery, Right
Posterior vagal trunk *use* Vagus Nerve
PPN (peripheral parenteral nutrition) *see* Introduction of Nutritional Substance
Praxbind® (idarucizumab), Pradaxa® (dabigatran) reversal agent *use* Other Therapeutic Substance
Preauricular lymph node *use* Lymphatic, Head
Precava *use* Superior Vena Cava
PRECICE intramedullary limb lengthening system
use Internal Fixation Device, Intramedullary Limb Lengthening in 0PH
use Internal Fixation Device, Intramedullary Limb Lengthening in 0QH
Precision TAVI™ Coronary Obstruction Module XXE3X68
Prepatellar bursa
use Knee Bursa and Ligament, Left
use Knee Bursa and Ligament, Right
Preputiotomy *see* Drainage, Male Reproductive System 0V9
Pressure support ventilation *see* Performance, Respiratory 5A19
PRESTIGE® Cervical Disc *use* Synthetic Substitute
Pretracheal fascia
use Subcutaneous Tissue and Fascia, Left Neck
use Subcutaneous Tissue and Fascia, Right Neck
Prevertebral fascia
use Subcutaneous Tissue and Fascia, Left Neck
use Subcutaneous Tissue and Fascia, Right Neck
PrimeAdvanced neurostimulator (SureScan) (MRI Safe) *use* Stimulator Generator, Multiple Array in 0JH
Princeps pollicis artery
use Hand Artery, Left
use Hand Artery, Right
Probing, duct
    Diagnostic *see* Inspection
    Dilation *see* Dilation
PROCEED™ Ventral Patch *use* Synthetic Substitute
Procerus muscle *use* Facial Muscle
Proctectomy
see Excision, Rectum 0DBP
see Resection, Rectum 0DTP
Proctoclysis *see* Introduction of substance in or on, Gastrointestinal Tract, Lower 3E0H
Proctocolectomy
see Excision, Gastrointestinal System 0DB
see Resection, Gastrointestinal System 0DT
Proctocolpoplasty
see Repair, Gastrointestinal System 0DQ
see Supplement, Gastrointestinal System 0DU
Proctoperineoplasty
see Repair, Gastrointestinal System 0DQ
see Supplement, Gastrointestinal System 0DU
Proctoperineorrhaphy *see* Repair, Gastrointestinal System 0DQ
Proctopexy
see Repair, Rectum 0DQP
see Reposition, Rectum 0DSP
Proctoplasty
see Repair, Rectum 0DQP
see Supplement, Rectum 0DUP
Proctorrhaphy *see* Repair, Rectum 0DQP
Proctoscopy 0DJD8ZZ
Proctosigmoidectomy
see Excision, Gastrointestinal System 0DB
see Resection, Gastrointestinal System 0DT
Proctosigmoidoscopy 0DJD8ZZ
Proctostomy *see* Drainage, Rectum 0D9P
Proctotomy *see* Drainage, Rectum 0D9P
Prodisc-C *use* Synthetic Substitute
Prodisc-L *use* Synthetic Substitute
Production, atrial septal defect *see* Excision, Septum, Atrial 02B5
Profunda brachii
use Brachial Artery, Left
use Brachial Artery, Right
Profunda femoris (deep femoral) vein
use Femoral Vein, Left
use Femoral Vein, Right
PROLENE Polypropylene Hernia System (PHS) *use* Synthetic Substitute
Prolonged intermittent renal replacement therapy (PIRRT) 5A1D80Z

Pronator quadratus muscle
use Lower Arm and Wrist Muscle, Left
use Lower Arm and Wrist Muscle, Right
Pronator teres muscle
use Lower Arm and Wrist Muscle, Left
use Lower Arm and Wrist Muscle, Right
Prostatectomy
see Excision, Prostate ØVBØ
see Resection, Prostate ØVTØ
Prostatic artery
use Internal Iliac Artery, Left
use Internal Iliac Artery, Right
Prostatic urethra *use* Urethra
Prostatomy, prostatotomy *see* Drainage, Prostate ØV9Ø
Protecta XT CRT-D *use* Cardiac Resynchronization Defibrillator Pulse Generator in ØJH
Protecta XT DR (XT VR) *use* Defibrillator Generator in ØJH
Protege® RX Carotid Stent System *use* Intraluminal Device
Proximal radioulnar joint
use Elbow Joint, Left
use Elbow Joint, Right
Psoas muscle
use Hip Muscle, Left
use Hip Muscle, Right
PSV (pressure support ventilation) *see* Performance, Respiratory 5A19
Psychoanalysis GZ54ZZZ
Psychological Tests
Cognitive Status GZ14ZZZ
Developmental GZ10ZZZ
Intellectual and Psychoeducational GZ12ZZZ
Neurobehavioral Status GZ14ZZZ
Neuropsychological GZ13ZZZ
Personality and Behavioral GZ11ZZZ
Psychotherapy
Family, Mental Health Services GZ72ZZZ
Group GZHZZZZ
Mental Health Services GZHZZZZ
Individual
see Psychotherapy, Individual, Mental Health Services
for substance abuse
12-Step HZ53ZZZ
Behavioral HZ51ZZZ
Cognitive HZ50ZZZ
Cognitive-Behavioral HZ52ZZZ
Confrontational HZ58ZZZ
Interactive HZ55ZZZ
Interpersonal HZ54ZZZ
Motivational Enhancement HZ57ZZZ
Psychoanalysis HZ5BZZZ
Psychodynamic HZ5CZZZ
Psychoeducation HZ56ZZZ
Psychophysiological HZ5DZZZ
Supportive HZ59ZZZ
Mental Health Services
Behavioral GZ51ZZZ
Cognitive GZ52ZZZ
Cognitive-Behavioral GZ58ZZZ
Interactive GZ50ZZZ
Interpersonal GZ53ZZZ
Psychoanalysis GZ54ZZZ
Psychodynamic GZ55ZZZ
Psychophysiological GZ59ZZZ
Supportive GZ56ZZZ
PTCA (percutaneous transluminal coronary angioplasty) *see* Dilation, Heart and Great Vessels Ø27
Pterygoid muscle *use* Head Muscle
Pterygoid process *use* Sphenoid Bone
Pterygopalatine (sphenopalatine) ganglion *use* Head and Neck Sympathetic Nerve
Pubis
use Pelvic Bone, Left
use Pelvic Bone, Right
Pubofemoral ligament
use Hip Bursa and Ligament, Left
use Hip Bursa and Ligament, Right
Pudendal nerve *use* Sacral Plexus
Pull-through, laparoscopic-assisted transanal
see Excision, Gastrointestinal System ØDB
see Resection, Gastrointestinal System ØDT
Pull-through, rectal *see* Resection, Rectum ØDTP
Pulmoaortic canal *use* Pulmonary Artery, Left
Pulmonary annulus *use* Pulmonary Valve

Pulmonary artery wedge monitoring *see* Monitoring, Arterial 4A13
Pulmonary plexus
use Thoracic Sympathetic Nerve
use Vagus Nerve
Pulmonic valve *use* Pulmonary Valve
Pulpectomy *see* Excision, Mouth and Throat ØCB
Pulverization *see* Fragmentation
Pulvinar *use* Thalamus
Pump reservoir *use* Infusion Device, Pump in Subcutaneous Tissue and Fascia
Punch biopsy *see* Excision with qualifier Diagnostic
Puncture *see* Drainage
Puncture, lumbar *see* Drainage, Spinal Canal ØØ9U
Pure-Vu® System XDPH8K7
Pyelography
see Fluoroscopy, Urinary System BT1
see Plain Radiography, Urinary System BTØ
Pyeloileostomy, urinary diversion *see* Bypass, Urinary System ØT1
Pyeloplasty
see Repair, Urinary System ØTQ
see Replacement, Urinary System ØTR
see Supplement, Urinary System ØTU
Pyeloplasty, dismembered *see* Repair, Kidney Pelvis
Pyelorrhaphy *see* Repair, Urinary System ØTQ
Pyeloscopy ØTJ58ZZ
Pyelostomy
see Bypass, Urinary System ØT1
see Drainage, Urinary System ØT9
Pyelotomy *see* Drainage, Urinary System ØT9
Pylorectomy
see Excision, Stomach, Pylorus ØDB7
see Resection, Stomach, Pylorus ØDT7
Pyloric antrum *use* Stomach, Pylorus
Pyloric canal *use* Stomach, Pylorus
Pyloric sphincter *use* Stomach, Pylorus
Pylorodiosis *see* Dilation, Stomach, Pylorus ØD77
Pylorogastrectomy
see Excision, Gastrointestinal System ØDB
see Resection, Gastrointestinal System ØDT
Pyloroplasty
see Repair, Stomach, Pylorus ØDQ7
see Supplement, Stomach, Pylorus ØDU7
Pyloroscopy ØDJ68ZZ
Pylorotomy *see* Drainage, Stomach, Pylorus ØD97
Pyramidalis muscle
use Abdomen Muscle, Left
use Abdomen Muscle, Right

Q

QAngio XA® 3D XXE3X58
QFR® (Quantitative Flow Ratio) analysis of coronary angiography XXE3X58
Quadrangular cartilage *use* Nasal Septum
Quadrant resection of breast *see* Excision, Skin and Breast ØHB
Quadrate lobe *use* Liver
Quadratus femoris muscle
use Hip Muscle, Left
use Hip Muscle, Right
Quadratus lumborum muscle
use Trunk Muscle, Left
use Trunk Muscle, Right
Quadratus plantae muscle
use Foot Muscle, Left
use Foot Muscle, Right
Quadriceps (femoris)
use Upper Leg Muscle, Left
use Upper Leg Muscle, Right
Quantitative Flow Ratio Analysis, Coronary Artery Flow XXE3X58
Quarantine 8E0ZXY6

R

Radial artery arteriovenous fistula, using Thermal Resistance Energy X2K
Radial collateral carpal ligament
use Wrist Bursa and Ligament, Left
use Wrist Bursa and Ligament, Right
Radial collateral ligament
use Elbow Bursa and Ligament, Left
use Elbow Bursa and Ligament, Right

Radial notch
use Ulna, Left
use Ulna, Right
Radial recurrent artery
use Radial Artery, Left
use Radial Artery, Right
Radial vein
use Brachial Vein, Left
use Brachial Vein, Right
Radialis indicis
use Hand Artery, Left
use Hand Artery, Right
Radiation Therapy
see Beam Radiation
see Brachytherapy
see Other Radiation
see Stereotactic Radiosurgery
Radiation treatment *see* Radiation Therapy
Radiocarpal joint
use Wrist Joint, Left
use Wrist Joint, Right
Radiocarpal ligament
use Wrist Bursa and Ligament, Left
use Wrist Bursa and Ligament, Right
Radiography *see* Plain Radiography
Radiology, analog *see* Plain Radiography
Radiology, diagnostic *see* Imaging, Diagnostic
Radioulnar ligament
use Wrist Bursa and Ligament, Left
use Wrist Bursa and Ligament, Right
Range of motion testing *see* Motor Function Assessment, Rehabilitation FØ1
Rapid ASPECTS XXE0X07
REALIZE® Adjustable Gastric Band *use* Extraluminal Device
Reattachment
Abdominal Wall ØWMFØZZ
Ampulla of Vater ØFMC
Ankle Region
Left ØYMLØZZ
Right ØYMKØZZ
Arm
Lower
Left ØXMFØZZ
Right ØXMDØZZ
Upper
Left ØXM9ØZZ
Right ØXM8ØZZ
Axilla
Left ØXM5ØZZ
Right ØXM4ØZZ
Back
Lower ØWMLØZZ
Upper ØWMKØZZ
Bladder ØTMB
Bladder Neck ØTMC
Breast
Bilateral ØHMVXZZ
Left ØHMUXZZ
Right ØHMTXZZ
Bronchus
Lingula ØBM9ØZZ
Lower Lobe
Left ØBMBØZZ
Right ØBM6ØZZ
Main
Left ØBM7ØZZ
Right ØBM3ØZZ
Middle Lobe, Right ØBM5ØZZ
Upper Lobe
Left ØBM8ØZZ
Right ØBM4ØZZ
Bursa and Ligament
Abdomen
Left ØMMJ
Right ØMMH
Ankle
Left ØMMR
Right ØMMQ
Elbow
Left ØMM4
Right ØMM3
Foot
Left ØMMT
Right ØMMS
Hand
Left ØMM8
Right ØMM7

Release — *continued*
  Artery — *continued*
    Pulmonary — *continued*
      Right 02NQ
    Pulmonary Trunk 02NP
    Radial
      Left 03NC
      Right 03NB
    Renal
      Left 04NA
      Right 04N9
    Splenic 04N4
    Subclavian
      Left 03N4
      Right 03N3
    Superior Mesenteric 04N5
    Temporal
      Left 03NT
      Right 03NS
    Thyroid
      Left 03NV
      Right 03NU
    Ulnar
      Left 03NA
      Right 03N9
    Upper 03NY
    Vertebral
      Left 03NQ
      Right 03NP
  Atrium
    Left 02N7
    Right 02N6
  Auditory Ossicle
    Left 09NA
    Right 09N9
  Basal Ganglia 00N8
  Bladder 0TNB
  Bladder Neck 0TNC
  Bone
    Ethmoid
      Left 0NNG
      Right 0NNF
    Frontal 0NN1
    Hyoid 0NNX
    Lacrimal
      Left 0NNJ
      Right 0NNH
    Nasal 0NNB
    Occipital 0NN7
    Palatine
      Left 0NNL
      Right 0NNK
    Parietal
      Left 0NN4
      Right 0NN3
    Pelvic
      Left 0QN3
      Right 0QN2
    Sphenoid 0NNC
    Temporal
      Left 0NN6
      Right 0NN5
    Zygomatic
      Left 0NNN
      Right 0NNM
  Brain 00N0
  Breast
    Bilateral 0HNV
    Left 0HNU
    Right 0HNT
  Bronchus
    Lingula 0BN9
    Lower Lobe
      Left 0BNB
      Right 0BN6
    Main
      Left 0BN7
      Right 0BN3
    Middle Lobe, Right 0BN5
    Upper Lobe
      Left 0BN8
      Right 0BN4
  Buccal Mucosa 0CN4
  Bursa and Ligament
    Abdomen
      Left 0MNJ
      Right 0MNH
    Ankle
      Left 0MNR

Release — *continued*
  Bursa and Ligament — *continued*
    Ankle — *continued*
      Right 0MNQ
    Elbow
      Left 0MN4
      Right 0MN3
    Foot
      Left 0MNT
      Right 0MNS
    Hand
      Left 0MN8
      Right 0MN7
    Head and Neck 0MN0
    Hip
      Left 0MNM
      Right 0MNL
    Knee
      Left 0MNP
      Right 0MNN
    Lower Extremity
      Left 0MNW
      Right 0MNV
    Perineum 0MNK
    Rib(s) 0MNG
    Shoulder
      Left 0MN2
      Right 0MN1
    Spine
      Lower 0MND
      Upper 0MNC
    Sternum 0MNF
    Upper Extremity
      Left 0MNB
      Right 0MN9
    Wrist
      Left 0MN6
      Right 0MN5
  Carina 0BN2
  Carotid Bodies, Bilateral 0GN8
  Carotid Body
    Left 0GN6
    Right 0GN7
  Carpal
    Left 0PNN
    Right 0PNM
  Cecum 0DNH
  Cerebellum 00NC
  Cerebral Hemisphere 00N7
  Cerebral Meninges 00N1
  Cerebral Ventricle 00N6
  Cervix 0UNC
  Chordae Tendineae 02N9
  Choroid
    Left 08NB
    Right 08NA
  Cisterna Chyli 07NL
  Clavicle
    Left 0PNB
    Right 0PN9
  Clitoris 0UNJ
  Coccygeal Glomus 0GNB
  Coccyx 0QNS
  Colon
    Ascending 0DNK
    Descending 0DNM
    Sigmoid 0DNN
    Transverse 0DNL
  Conduction Mechanism 02N8
  Conjunctiva
    Left 08NTXZZ
    Right 08NSXZZ
  Cord
    Bilateral 0VNH
    Left 0VNG
    Right 0VNF
  Cornea
    Left 08N9XZZ
    Right 08N8XZZ
  Cul-de-sac 0UNF
  Diaphragm 0BNT
  Disc
    Cervical Vertebral 0RN3
    Cervicothoracic Vertebral 0RN5
    Lumbar Vertebral 0SN2
    Lumbosacral 0SN4
    Thoracic Vertebral 0RN9
    Thoracolumbar Vertebral 0RNB

Release — *continued*
  Duct
    Common Bile 0FN9
    Cystic 0FN8
    Hepatic
      Common 0FN7
      Left 0FN6
      Right 0FN5
    Lacrimal
      Left 08NY
      Right 08NX
    Pancreatic 0FND
      Accessory 0FNF
    Parotid
      Left 0CNC
      Right 0CNB
  Duodenum 0DN9
  Dura Mater 00N2
  Ear
    External
      Left 09N1
      Right 09N0
    External Auditory Canal
      Left 09N4
      Right 09N3
    Inner
      Left 09NE
      Right 09ND
    Middle
      Left 09N6
      Right 09N5
  Epididymis
    Bilateral 0VNL
    Left 0VNK
    Right 0VNJ
  Epiglottis 0CNR
  Esophagogastric Junction 0DN4
  Esophagus 0DN5
    Lower 0DN3
    Middle 0DN2
    Upper 0DN1
  Eustachian Tube
    Left 09NG
    Right 09NF
  Eye
    Left 08N1XZZ
    Right 08N0XZZ
  Eyelid
    Lower
      Left 08NR
      Right 08NQ
    Upper
      Left 08NP
      Right 08NN
  Fallopian Tube
    Left 0UN6
    Right 0UN5
  Fallopian Tubes, Bilateral 0UN7
  Femoral Shaft
    Left 0QN9
    Right 0QN8
  Femur
    Lower
      Left 0QNC
      Right 0QNB
    Upper
      Left 0QN7
      Right 0QN6
  Fibula
    Left 0QNK
    Right 0QNJ
  Finger Nail 0HNQXZZ
  Gallbladder 0FN4
  Gingiva
    Lower 0CN6
    Upper 0CN5
  Gland
    Adrenal
      Bilateral 0GN4
      Left 0GN2
      Right 0GN3
    Lacrimal
      Left 08NW
      Right 08NV
    Minor Salivary 0CNJ
    Parotid
      Left 0CN9
      Right 0CN8
    Pituitary 0GN0

Release — *continued*
　Gland — *continued*
　　Sublingual
　　　Left ØCNF
　　　Right ØCND
　　Submaxillary
　　　Left ØCNH
　　　Right ØCNG
　　Vestibular ØUNL
　Glenoid Cavity
　　Left ØPN8
　　Right ØPN7
　Glomus Jugulare ØGNC
　Humeral Head
　　Left ØPND
　　Right ØPNC
　Humeral Shaft
　　Left ØPNG
　　Right ØPNF
　Hymen ØUNK
　Hypothalamus ØØNA
　Ileocecal Valve ØDNC
　Ileum ØDNB
　Intestine
　　Large ØDNE
　　　Left ØDNG
　　　Right ØDNF
　　Small ØDN8
　Iris
　　Left Ø8ND3ZZ
　　Right Ø8NC3ZZ
　Jejunum ØDNA
　Joint
　　Acromioclavicular
　　　Left ØRNH
　　　Right ØRNG
　　Ankle
　　　Left ØSNG
　　　Right ØSNF
　　Carpal
　　　Left ØRNR
　　　Right ØRNQ
　　Carpometacarpal
　　　Left ØRNT
　　　Right ØRNS
　　Cervical Vertebral ØRN1
　　Cervicothoracic Vertebral ØRN4
　　Coccygeal ØSN6
　　Elbow
　　　Left ØRNM
　　　Right ØRNL
　　Finger Phalangeal
　　　Left ØRNX
　　　Right ØRNW
　　Hip
　　　Left ØSNB
　　　Right ØSN9
　　Knee
　　　Left ØSND
　　　Right ØSNC
　　Lumbar Vertebral ØSNØ
　　Lumbosacral ØSN3
　　Metacarpophalangeal
　　　Left ØRNV
　　　Right ØRNU
　　Metatarsal-Phalangeal
　　　Left ØSNN
　　　Right ØSNM
　　Occipital-cervical ØRNØ
　　Sacrococcygeal ØSN5
　　Sacroiliac
　　　Left ØSN8
　　　Right ØSN7
　　Shoulder
　　　Left ØRNK
　　　Right ØRNJ
　　Sternoclavicular
　　　Left ØRNF
　　　Right ØRNE
　　Tarsal
　　　Left ØSNJ
　　　Right ØSNH
　　Tarsometatarsal
　　　Left ØSNL
　　　Right ØSNK
　　Temporomandibular
　　　Left ØRND
　　　Right ØRNC
　　Thoracic Vertebral ØRN6

Release — *continued*
　Joint — *continued*
　　Thoracolumbar Vertebral ØRNA
　　Toe Phalangeal
　　　Left ØSNQ
　　　Right ØSNP
　　Wrist
　　　Left ØRNP
　　　Right ØRNN
　Kidney
　　Left ØTN1
　　Right ØTNØ
　Kidney Pelvis
　　Left ØTN4
　　Right ØTN3
　Larynx ØCNS
　Lens
　　Left Ø8NK3ZZ
　　Right Ø8NJ3ZZ
　Lip
　　Lower ØCN1
　　Upper ØCNØ
　Liver ØFNØ
　　Left Lobe ØFN2
　　Right Lobe ØFN1
　Lung
　　Bilateral ØBNM
　　Left ØBNL
　　Lower Lobe
　　　Left ØBNJ
　　　Right ØBNF
　　Middle Lobe, Right ØBND
　　Right ØBNK
　　Upper Lobe
　　　Left ØBNG
　　　Right ØBNC
　Lung Lingula ØBNH
　Lymphatic
　　Aortic Ø7ND
　　Axillary
　　　Left Ø7N6
　　　Right Ø7N5
　　Head Ø7NØ
　　Inguinal
　　　Left Ø7NJ
　　　Right Ø7NH
　　Internal Mammary
　　　Left Ø7N9
　　　Right Ø7N8
　　Lower Extremity
　　　Left Ø7NG
　　　Right Ø7NF
　　Mesenteric Ø7NB
　　Neck
　　　Left Ø7N2
　　　Right Ø7N1
　　Pelvis Ø7NC
　　Thoracic Duct Ø7NK
　　Thorax Ø7N7
　　Upper Extremity
　　　Left Ø7N4
　　　Right Ø7N3
　Mandible
　　Left ØNNV
　　Right ØNNT
　Maxilla ØNNR
　Medulla Oblongata ØØND
　Mesentery ØDNV
　Metacarpal
　　Left ØPNQ
　　Right ØPNP
　Metatarsal
　　Left ØQNP
　　Right ØQNN
　Muscle
　　Abdomen
　　　Left ØKNL
　　　Right ØKNK
　　Extraocular
　　　Left Ø8NM
　　　Right Ø8NL
　　Facial ØKN1
　　Foot
　　　Left ØKNW
　　　Right ØKNV
　　Hand
　　　Left ØKND
　　　Right ØKNC
　　Head ØKNØ

Release — *continued*
　Muscle — *continued*
　　Hip
　　　Left ØKNP
　　　Right ØKNN
　　Lower Arm and Wrist
　　　Left ØKNB
　　　Right ØKN9
　　Lower Leg
　　　Left ØKNT
　　　Right ØKNS
　　Neck
　　　Left ØKN3
　　　Right ØKN2
　　Papillary Ø2ND
　　Perineum ØKNM
　　Shoulder
　　　Left ØKN6
　　　Right ØKN5
　　Thorax
　　　Left ØKNJ
　　　Right ØKNH
　　Tongue, Palate, Pharynx ØKN4
　　Trunk
　　　Left ØKNG
　　　Right ØKNF
　　Upper Arm
　　　Left ØKN8
　　　Right ØKN7
　　Upper Leg
　　　Left ØKNR
　　　Right ØKNQ
　Myocardial Bridge *see* Release, Artery, Coronary
　Nasal Mucosa and Soft Tissue Ø9NK
　Nasopharynx Ø9NN
　Nerve
　　Abdominal Sympathetic Ø1NM
　　Abducens ØØNL
　　Accessory ØØNR
　　Acoustic ØØNN
　　Brachial Plexus Ø1N3
　　Cervical Ø1N1
　　Cervical Plexus Ø1NØ
　　Facial ØØNM
　　Femoral Ø1ND
　　Glossopharyngeal ØØNP
　　Head and Neck Sympathetic Ø1NK
　　Hypoglossal ØØNS
　　Lumbar Ø1NB
　　Lumbar Plexus Ø1N9
　　Lumbar Sympathetic Ø1NN
　　Lumbosacral Plexus Ø1NA
　　Median Ø1N5
　　Oculomotor ØØNH
　　Olfactory ØØNF
　　Optic ØØNG
　　Peroneal Ø1NH
　　Phrenic Ø1N2
　　Pudendal Ø1NC
　　Radial Ø1N6
　　Sacral Ø1NR
　　Sacral Plexus Ø1NQ
　　Sacral Sympathetic Ø1NP
　　Sciatic Ø1NF
　　Thoracic Ø1N8
　　Thoracic Sympathetic Ø1NL
　　Tibial Ø1NG
　　Trigeminal ØØNK
　　Trochlear ØØNJ
　　Ulnar Ø1N4
　　Vagus ØØNQ
　Nipple
　　Left ØHNX
　　Right ØHNW
　Omentum ØDNU
　Orbit
　　Left ØNNQ
　　Right ØNNP
　Ovary
　　Bilateral ØUN2
　　Left ØUN1
　　Right ØUNØ
　Palate
　　Hard ØCN2
　　Soft ØCN3
　Pancreas ØFNG
　Para-aortic Body ØGN9
　Paraganglion Extremity ØGNF
　Parathyroid Gland ØGNR

▽ Subterms under main terms may continue to next column or page

Release — *continued*
　Parathyroid Gland — *continued*
　　Inferior
　　　Left ØGNP
　　　Right ØGNN
　　Multiple ØGNQ
　　Superior
　　　Left ØGNM
　　　Right ØGNL
　Patella
　　Left ØQNF
　　Right ØQND
　Penis ØVNS
　Pericardium 02NN
　Peritoneum ØDNW
　Phalanx
　　Finger
　　　Left ØPNV
　　　Right ØPNT
　　Thumb
　　　Left ØPNS
　　　Right ØPNR
　　Toe
　　　Left ØQNR
　　　Right ØQNQ
　Pharynx ØCNM
　Pineal Body ØGN1
　Pleura
　　Left ØBNP
　　Right ØBNN
　Pons ØØNB
　Prepuce ØVNT
　Prostate ØVNØ
　Radius
　　Left ØPNJ
　　Right ØPNH
　Rectum ØDNP
　Retina
　　Left Ø8NF3ZZ
　　Right Ø8NE3ZZ
　Retinal Vessel
　　Left Ø8NH3ZZ
　　Right Ø8NG3ZZ
　Ribs
　　1 to 2 ØPN1
　　3 or More ØPN2
　Sacrum ØQN1
　Scapula
　　Left ØPN6
　　Right ØPN5
　Sclera
　　Left Ø8N7XZZ
　　Right Ø8N6XZZ
　Scrotum ØVN5
　Septum
　　Atrial 02N5
　　Nasal Ø9NM
　　Ventricular 02NM
　Sinus
　　Accessory Ø9NP
　　Ethmoid
　　　Left Ø9NV
　　　Right Ø9NU
　　Frontal
　　　Left Ø9NT
　　　Right Ø9NS
　　Mastoid
　　　Left Ø9NC
　　　Right Ø9NB
　　Maxillary
　　　Left Ø9NR
　　　Right Ø9NQ
　　Sphenoid
　　　Left Ø9NX
　　　Right Ø9NW
　Skin
　　Abdomen ØHN7XZZ
　　Back ØHN6XZZ
　　Buttock ØHN8XZZ
　　Chest ØHN5XZZ
　　Ear
　　　Left ØHN3XZZ
　　　Right ØHN2XZZ
　　Face ØHN1XZZ
　　Foot
　　　Left ØHNNXZZ
　　　Right ØHNMXZZ
　　Hand
　　　Left ØHNGXZZ

Release — *continued*
　Skin — *continued*
　　Hand — *continued*
　　　Right ØHNFXZZ
　　Inguinal ØHNAXZZ
　　Lower Arm
　　　Left ØHNEXZZ
　　　Right ØHNDXZZ
　　Lower Leg
　　　Left ØHNLXZZ
　　　Right ØHNKXZZ
　　Neck ØHN4XZZ
　　Perineum ØHN9XZZ
　　Scalp ØHNØXZZ
　　Upper Arm
　　　Left ØHNCXZZ
　　　Right ØHNBXZZ
　　Upper Leg
　　　Left ØHNJXZZ
　　　Right ØHNHXZZ
　Spinal Cord
　　Cervical ØØNW
　　Lumbar ØØNY
　　Thoracic ØØNX
　Spinal Meninges ØØNT
　Spleen 07NP
　Sternum ØPNØ
　Stomach ØDN6
　　Pylorus ØDN7
　Subcutaneous Tissue and Fascia
　　Abdomen ØJN8
　　Back ØJN7
　　Buttock ØJN9
　　Chest ØJN6
　　Face ØJN1
　　Foot
　　　Left ØJNR
　　　Right ØJNQ
　　Hand
　　　Left ØJNK
　　　Right ØJNJ
　　Lower Arm
　　　Left ØJNH
　　　Right ØJNG
　　Lower Leg
　　　Left ØJNP
　　　Right ØJNN
　　Neck
　　　Left ØJN5
　　　Right ØJN4
　　Pelvic Region ØJNC
　　Perineum ØJNB
　　Scalp ØJNØ
　　Upper Arm
　　　Left ØJNF
　　　Right ØJND
　　Upper Leg
　　　Left ØJNM
　　　Right ØJNL
　Tarsal
　　Left ØQNM
　　Right ØQNL
　Tendon
　　Abdomen
　　　Left ØLNG
　　　Right ØLNF
　　Ankle
　　　Left ØLNT
　　　Right ØLNS
　　Foot
　　　Left ØLNW
　　　Right ØLNV
　　Hand
　　　Left ØLN8
　　　Right ØLN7
　　Head and Neck ØLNØ
　　Hip
　　　Left ØLNK
　　　Right ØLNJ
　　Knee
　　　Left ØLNR
　　　Right ØLNQ
　　Lower Arm and Wrist
　　　Left ØLN6
　　　Right ØLN5
　　Lower Leg
　　　Left ØLNP
　　　Right ØLNN
　　Perineum ØLNH

Release — *continued*
　Tendon — *continued*
　　Shoulder
　　　Left ØLN2
　　　Right ØLN1
　　Thorax
　　　Left ØLND
　　　Right ØLNC
　　Trunk
　　　Left ØLNB
　　　Right ØLN9
　　Upper Arm
　　　Left ØLN4
　　　Right ØLN3
　　Upper Leg
　　　Left ØLNM
　　　Right ØLNL
　Testis
　　Bilateral ØVNC
　　Left ØVNB
　　Right ØVN9
　Thalamus ØØN9
　Thymus 07NM
　Thyroid Gland ØGNK
　　Left Lobe ØGNG
　　Right Lobe ØGNH
　Tibia
　　Left ØQNH
　　Right ØQNG
　Toe Nail ØHNRXZZ
　Tongue ØCN7
　Tonsils ØCNP
　Tooth
　　Lower ØCNX
　　Upper ØCNW
　Trachea ØBN1
　Tunica Vaginalis
　　Left ØVN7
　　Right ØVN6
　Turbinate, Nasal Ø9NL
　Tympanic Membrane
　　Left Ø9N8
　　Right Ø9N7
　Ulna
　　Left ØPNL
　　Right ØPNK
　Ureter
　　Left ØTN7
　　Right ØTN6
　Urethra ØTND
　Uterine Supporting Structure ØUN4
　Uterus ØUN9
　Uvula ØCNN
　Vagina ØUNG
　Valve
　　Aortic 02NF
　　Mitral 02NG
　　Pulmonary 02NH
　　Tricuspid 02NJ
　Vas Deferens
　　Bilateral ØVNQ
　　Left ØVNP
　　Right ØVNN
　Vein
　　Axillary
　　　Left Ø5N8
　　　Right Ø5N7
　　Azygos Ø5NØ
　　Basilic
　　　Left Ø5NC
　　　Right Ø5NB
　　Brachial
　　　Left Ø5NA
　　　Right Ø5N9
　　Cephalic
　　　Left Ø5NF
　　　Right Ø5ND
　　Colic 06N7
　　Common Iliac
　　　Left Ø6ND
　　　Right Ø6NC
　　Coronary 02N4
　　Esophageal Ø6N3
　　External Iliac
　　　Left Ø6NG
　　　Right Ø6NF
　　External Jugular
　　　Left Ø5NQ
　　　Right Ø5NP

Release — *continued*
- Vein — *continued*
  - Face
    - Left 05NV
    - Right 05NT
  - Femoral
    - Left 06NN
    - Right 06NM
  - Foot
    - Left 06NV
    - Right 06NT
  - Gastric 06N2
  - Hand
    - Left 05NH
    - Right 05NG
  - Hemiazygos 05N1
  - Hepatic 06N4
  - Hypogastric
    - Left 06NJ
    - Right 06NH
  - Inferior Mesenteric 06N6
  - Innominate
    - Left 05N4
    - Right 05N3
  - Internal Jugular
    - Left 05NN
    - Right 05NM
  - Intracranial 05NL
  - Lower 06NY
  - Portal 06N8
  - Pulmonary
    - Left 02NT
    - Right 02NS
  - Renal
    - Left 06NB
    - Right 06N9
  - Saphenous
    - Left 06NQ
    - Right 06NP
  - Splenic 06N1
  - Subclavian
    - Left 05N6
    - Right 05N5
  - Superior Mesenteric 06N5
  - Upper 05NY
  - Vertebral
    - Left 05NS
    - Right 05NR
- Vena Cava
  - Inferior 06N0
  - Superior 02NV
- Ventricle
  - Left 02NL
  - Right 02NK
- Vertebra
  - Cervical 0PN3
  - Lumbar 0QN0
  - Thoracic 0PN4
- Vesicle
  - Bilateral 0VN3
  - Left 0VN2
  - Right 0VN1
- Vitreous
  - Left 08N53ZZ
  - Right 08N43ZZ
- Vocal Cord
  - Left 0CNV
  - Right 0CNT
- Vulva 0UNM

Relocation *see* Reposition
Remdesivir Anti-infective XW0
Removal
- Abdominal Wall 2W53X
- Anorectal 2Y53X5Z
- Arm
  - Lower
    - Left 2W5DX
    - Right 2W5CX
  - Upper
    - Left 2W5BX
    - Right 2W5AX
- Back 2W55X
- Chest Wall 2W54X
- Ear 2Y52X5Z
- Extremity
  - Lower
    - Left 2W5MX
    - Right 2W5LX

Removal — *continued*
- Extremity — *continued*
  - Upper
    - Left 2W59X
    - Right 2W58X
- Face 2W51X
- Finger
  - Left 2W5KX
  - Right 2W5JX
- Foot
  - Left 2W5TX
  - Right 2W5SX
- Genital Tract, Female 2Y54X5Z
- Hand
  - Left 2W5FX
  - Right 2W5EX
- Head 2W50X
- Inguinal Region
  - Left 2W57X
  - Right 2W56X
- Leg
  - Lower
    - Left 2W5RX
    - Right 2W5QX
  - Upper
    - Left 2W5PX
    - Right 2W5NX
- Mouth and Pharynx 2Y50X5Z
- Nasal 2Y51X5Z
- Neck 2W52X
- Thumb
  - Left 2W5HX
  - Right 2W5GX
- Toe
  - Left 2W5VX
  - Right 2W5UX
- Urethra 2Y55X5Z
Removal of device from
- Abdominal Wall 0WPF
- Acetabulum
  - Left 0QP5
  - Right 0QP4
- Anal Sphincter 0DPR
- Anus 0DPQ
- Artery
  - Lower 04PY
  - Upper 03PY
- Back
  - Lower 0WPL
  - Upper 0WPK
- Bladder 0TPB
- Bone
  - Facial 0NPW
  - Lower 0QPY
  - Nasal 0NPB
  - Pelvic
    - Left 0QP3
    - Right 0QP2
  - Upper 0PPY
- Bone Marrow 07PT
- Brain 00P0
- Breast
  - Left 0HPU
  - Right 0HPT
- Bursa and Ligament
  - Lower 0MPY
  - Upper 0MPX
- Carpal
  - Left 0PPN
  - Right 0PPM
- Cavity, Cranial 0WP1
- Cerebral Ventricle 00P6
- Chest Wall 0WP8
- Cisterna Chyli 07PL
- Clavicle
  - Left 0PPB
  - Right 0PP9
- Coccyx 0QPS
- Diaphragm 0BPT
- Disc
  - Cervical Vertebral 0RP3
  - Cervicothoracic Vertebral 0RP5
  - Lumbar Vertebral 0SP2
  - Lumbosacral 0SP4
  - Thoracic Vertebral 0RP9
  - Thoracolumbar Vertebral 0RPB
- Duct
  - Hepatobiliary 0FPB
  - Pancreatic 0FPD

Removal of device from — *continued*
- Ear
  - Inner
    - Left 09PJ
    - Right 09PD
  - Left 09PJ
  - Right 09PH
- Epididymis and Spermatic Cord 0VPM
- Esophagus 0DP5
- Extremity
  - Lower
    - Left 0YPB
    - Right 0YP9
  - Upper
    - Left 0XP7
    - Right 0XP6
- Eye
  - Left 08P1
  - Right 08P0
- Face 0WP2
- Fallopian Tube 0UP8
- Femoral Shaft
  - Left 0QP9
  - Right 0QP8
- Femur
  - Lower
    - Left 0QPC
    - Right 0QPB
  - Upper
    - Left 0QP7
    - Right 0QP6
- Fibula
  - Left 0QPK
  - Right 0QPJ
- Finger Nail 0HPQX
- Gallbladder 0FP4
- Gastrointestinal Tract 0WPP
- Genitourinary Tract 0WPR
- Gland
  - Adrenal 0GP5
  - Endocrine 0GPS
  - Pituitary 0GP0
  - Salivary 0CPA
- Glenoid Cavity
  - Left 0PP8
  - Right 0PP7
- Great Vessel 02PY
- Hair 0HPSX
- Head 0WP0
- Heart 02PA
- Humeral Head
  - Left 0PPD
  - Right 0PPC
- Humeral Shaft
  - Left 0PPG
  - Right 0PPF
- Intestinal Tract
  - Lower Intestinal Tract 0DPD
  - Upper Intestinal Tract 0DP0
- Jaw
  - Lower 0WP5
  - Upper 0WP4
- Joint
  - Acromioclavicular
    - Left 0RPH
    - Right 0RPG
  - Ankle
    - Left 0SPG
    - Right 0SPF
  - Carpal
    - Left 0RPR
    - Right 0RPQ
  - Carpometacarpal
    - Left 0RPT
    - Right 0RPS
  - Cervical Vertebral 0RP1
  - Cervicothoracic Vertebral 0RP4
  - Coccygeal 0SP6
  - Elbow
    - Left 0RPM
    - Right 0RPL
  - Finger Phalangeal
    - Left 0RPX
    - Right 0RPW
  - Hip
    - Left 0SPB
      - Acetabular Surface 0SPE
      - Femoral Surface 0SPS
    - Right 0SP9

Removal of device from — *continued*
  Joint — *continued*
    Hip — *continued*
      Right — *continued*
        Acetabular Surface ØSPA
        Femoral Surface ØSPR
      Knee
        Left ØSPD
          Femoral Surface ØSPU
          Tibial Surface ØSPW
        Right ØSPC
          Femoral Surface ØSPT
          Tibial Surface ØSPV
    Lumbar Vertebral ØSPØ
    Lumbosacral ØSP3
    Metacarpophalangeal
      Left ØRPV
      Right ØRPU
    Metatarsal-Phalangeal
      Left ØSPN
      Right ØSPM
    Occipital-cervical ØRPØ
    Sacrococcygeal ØSP5
    Sacroiliac
      Left ØSP8
      Right ØSP7
    Shoulder
      Left ØRPK
      Right ØRPJ
    Sternoclavicular
      Left ØRPF
      Right ØRPE
    Tarsal
      Left ØSPJ
      Right ØSPH
    Tarsometatarsal
      Left ØSPL
      Right ØSPK
    Temporomandibular
      Left ØRPD
      Right ØRPC
    Thoracic Vertebral ØRP6
    Thoracolumbar Vertebral ØRPA
    Toe Phalangeal
      Left ØSPQ
      Right ØSPP
    Wrist
      Left ØRPP
      Right ØRPN
  Kidney ØTP5
  Larynx ØCPS
  Lens
    Left Ø8PK3
    Right Ø8PJ3
  Liver ØFPØ
  Lung
    Left ØBPL
    Right ØBPK
  Lymphatic Ø7PN
    Thoracic Duct Ø7PK
  Mediastinum ØWPC
  Mesentery ØDPV
  Metacarpal
    Left ØPPQ
    Right ØPPP
  Metatarsal
    Left ØQPP
    Right ØQPN
  Mouth and Throat ØCPY
  Muscle
    Extraocular
      Left Ø8PM
      Right Ø8PL
    Lower ØKPY
    Upper ØKPX
  Nasal Mucosa and Soft Tissue Ø9PK
  Neck ØWP6
  Nerve
    Cranial ØØPE
    Peripheral Ø1PY
  Omentum ØDPU
  Ovary ØUP3
  Pancreas ØFPG
  Parathyroid Gland ØGPR
  Patella
    Left ØQPF
    Right ØQPD
  Pelvic Cavity ØWPJ
  Penis ØVPS

Removal of device from — *continued*
  Pericardial Cavity ØWPD
  Perineum
    Female ØWPN
    Male ØWPM
  Peritoneal Cavity ØWPG
  Peritoneum ØDPW
  Phalanx
    Finger
      Left ØPPV
      Right ØPPT
    Thumb
      Left ØPPS
      Right ØPPR
    Toe
      Left ØQPR
      Right ØQPQ
  Pineal Body ØGP1
  Pleura ØBPQ
  Pleural Cavity
    Left ØWPB
    Right ØWP9
  Products of Conception 1ØPØ
  Prostate and Seminal Vesicles ØVP4
  Radius
    Left ØPPJ
    Right ØPPH
  Rectum ØDPP
  Respiratory Tract ØWPQ
  Retroperitoneum ØWPH
  Ribs
    1 to 2 ØPP1
    3 or More ØPP2
  Sacrum ØQP1
  Scapula
    Left ØPP6
    Right ØPP5
  Scrotum and Tunica Vaginalis ØVP8
  Sinus Ø9PY
  Skin ØHPPX
  Skull ØNPØ
  Spinal Canal ØØPU
  Spinal Cord ØØPV
  Spleen Ø7PP
  Sternum ØPPØ
  Stomach ØDP6
  Subcutaneous Tissue and Fascia
    Head and Neck ØJPS
    Lower Extremity ØJPW
    Trunk ØJPT
    Upper Extremity ØJPV
  Tarsal
    Left ØQPM
    Right ØQPL
  Tendon
    Lower ØLPY
    Upper ØLPX
  Testis ØVPD
  Thymus Ø7PM
  Thyroid Gland ØGPK
  Tibia
    Left ØQPH
    Right ØQPG
  Toe Nail ØHPRX
  Trachea ØBP1
  Tracheobronchial Tree ØBPØ
  Tympanic Membrane
    Left Ø9P8
    Right Ø9P7
  Ulna
    Left ØPPL
    Right ØPPK
  Ureter ØTP9
  Urethra ØTPD
  Uterus and Cervix ØUPD
  Vagina and Cul-de-sac ØUPH
  Vas Deferens ØVPR
  Vein
    Azygos Ø5PØ
    Innominate
      Left Ø5P4
      Right Ø5P3
    Lower Ø6PY
    Upper Ø5PY
  Vertebra
    Cervical ØPP3
    Lumbar ØQPØ
    Thoracic ØPP4
  Vulva ØUPM

Renal calyx
  use Kidney
  use Kidney, Left
  use Kidney, Right
  use Kidneys, Bilateral
Renal capsule
  use Kidney
  use Kidney, Left
  use Kidney, Right
  use Kidneys, Bilateral
Renal cortex
  use Kidney
  use Kidney, Left
  use Kidney, Right
  use Kidneys, Bilateral
Renal dialysis *see* Performance, Urinary 5A1D
Renal nerve *use* Abdominal Sympathetic Nerve
Renal plexus *use* Abdominal Sympathetic Nerve
Renal segment
  use Kidney
  use Kidney, Left
  use Kidney, Right
  use Kidneys, Bilateral
Renal segmental artery
  use Renal Artery, Left
  use Renal Artery, Right
Reopening, operative site
  Control of bleeding *see* Control bleeding in
  Inspection only *see* Inspection
Repair
  Abdominal Wall ØWQF
  Acetabulum
    Left ØQQ5
    Right ØQQ4
  Adenoids ØCQQ
  Ampulla of Vater ØFQC
  Anal Sphincter ØDQR
  Ankle Region
    Left ØYQL
    Right ØYQK
  Anterior Chamber
    Left Ø8Q33ZZ
    Right Ø8Q23ZZ
  Anus ØDQQ
  Aorta
    Abdominal Ø4QØ
    Thoracic
      Ascending/Arch Ø2QX
      Descending Ø2QW
  Aortic Body ØGQD
  Appendix ØDQJ
  Arm
    Lower
      Left ØXQF
      Right ØXQD
    Upper
      Left ØXQ9
      Right ØXQ8
  Artery
    Anterior Tibial
      Left Ø4QQ
      Right Ø4QP
    Axillary
      Left Ø3Q6
      Right Ø3Q5
    Brachial
      Left Ø3Q8
      Right Ø3Q7
    Celiac Ø4Q1
    Colic
      Left Ø4Q7
      Middle Ø4Q8
      Right Ø4Q6
    Common Carotid
      Left Ø3QJ
      Right Ø3QH
    Common Iliac
      Left Ø4QD
      Right Ø4QC
    Coronary
      Four or More Arteries Ø2Q3
      One Artery Ø2QØ
      Three Arteries Ø2Q2
      Two Arteries Ø2Q1
    External Carotid
      Left Ø3QN
      Right Ø3QM

⚄ **Subterms under main terms may continue to next column or page**

Repair — continued
  Artery — continued
    External Iliac
      Left 04QJ
      Right 04QH
    Face 03QR
    Femoral
      Left 04QL
      Right 04QK
    Foot
      Left 04QW
      Right 04QV
    Gastric 04Q2
    Hand
      Left 03QF
      Right 03QD
    Hepatic 04Q3
    Inferior Mesenteric 04QB
    Innominate 03Q2
    Internal Carotid
      Left 03QL
      Right 03QK
    Internal Iliac
      Left 04QF
      Right 04QE
    Internal Mammary
      Left 03Q1
      Right 03Q0
    Intracranial 03QG
    Lower 04QY
    Peroneal
      Left 04QU
      Right 04QT
    Popliteal
      Left 04QN
      Right 04QM
    Posterior Tibial
      Left 04QS
      Right 04QR
    Pulmonary
      Left 02QR
      Right 02QQ
    Pulmonary Trunk 02QP
    Radial
      Left 03QC
      Right 03QB
    Renal
      Left 04QA
      Right 04Q9
    Splenic 04Q4
    Subclavian
      Left 03Q4
      Right 03Q3
    Superior Mesenteric 04Q5
    Temporal
      Left 03QT
      Right 03QS
    Thyroid
      Left 03QV
      Right 03QU
    Ulnar
      Left 03QA
      Right 03Q9
    Upper 03QY
    Vertebral
      Left 03QQ
      Right 03QP
  Atrium
    Left 02Q7
    Right 02Q6
  Auditory Ossicle
    Left 09QA
    Right 09Q9
  Axilla
    Left 0XQ5
    Right 0XQ4
  Back
    Lower 0WQL
    Upper 0WQK
  Basal Ganglia 00Q8
  Bladder 0TQB
  Bladder Neck 0TQC
  Bone
    Ethmoid
      Left 0NQG
      Right 0NQF
    Frontal 0NQ1
    Hyoid 0NQX

Repair — continued
  Bone — continued
    Lacrimal
      Left 0NQJ
      Right 0NQH
    Nasal 0NQB
    Occipital 0NQ7
    Palatine
      Left 0NQL
      Right 0NQK
    Parietal
      Left 0NQ4
      Right 0NQ3
    Pelvic
      Left 0QQ3
      Right 0QQ2
    Sphenoid 0NQC
    Temporal
      Left 0NQ6
      Right 0NQ5
    Zygomatic
      Left 0NQN
      Right 0NQM
  Brain 00Q0
  Breast
    Bilateral 0HQV
    Left 0HQU
    Right 0HQT
    Supernumerary 0HQY
  Bronchus
    Lingula 0BQ9
    Lower Lobe
      Left 0BQB
      Right 0BQ6
    Main
      Left 0BQ7
      Right 0BQ3
    Middle Lobe, Right 0BQ5
    Upper Lobe
      Left 0BQ8
      Right 0BQ4
  Buccal Mucosa 0CQ4
  Bursa and Ligament
    Abdomen
      Left 0MQJ
      Right 0MQH
    Ankle
      Left 0MQR
      Right 0MQQ
    Elbow
      Left 0MQ4
      Right 0MQ3
    Foot
      Left 0MQT
      Right 0MQS
    Hand
      Left 0MQ8
      Right 0MQ7
    Head and Neck 0MQ0
    Hip
      Left 0MQM
      Right 0MQL
    Knee
      Left 0MQP
      Right 0MQN
    Lower Extremity
      Left 0MQW
      Right 0MQV
    Perineum 0MQK
    Rib(s) 0MQG
    Shoulder
      Left 0MQ2
      Right 0MQ1
    Spine
      Lower 0MQD
      Upper 0MQC
    Sternum 0MQF
    Upper Extremity
      Left 0MQB
      Right 0MQ9
    Wrist
      Left 0MQ6
      Right 0MQ5
  Buttock
    Left 0YQ1
    Right 0YQ0
  Carina 0BQ2
  Carotid Bodies, Bilateral 0GQ8

Repair — continued
  Carotid Body
    Left 0GQ6
    Right 0GQ7
  Carpal
    Left 0PQN
    Right 0PQM
  Cecum 0DQH
  Cerebellum 00QC
  Cerebral Hemisphere 00Q7
  Cerebral Meninges 00Q1
  Cerebral Ventricle 00Q6
  Cervix 0UQC
  Chest Wall 0WQ8
  Chordae Tendineae 02Q9
  Choroid
    Left 08QB
    Right 08QA
  Cisterna Chyli 07QL
  Clavicle
    Left 0PQB
    Right 0PQ9
  Clitoris 0UQJ
  Coccygeal Glomus 0GQB
  Coccyx 0QQS
  Colon
    Ascending 0DQK
    Descending 0DQM
    Sigmoid 0DQN
    Transverse 0DQL
  Conduction Mechanism 02Q8
  Conjunctiva
    Left 08QTXZZ
    Right 08QSXZZ
  Cord
    Bilateral 0VQH
    Left 0VQG
    Right 0VQF
  Cornea
    Left 08Q9XZZ
    Right 08Q8XZZ
  Cul-de-sac 0UQF
  Diaphragm 0BQT
  Disc
    Cervical Vertebral 0RQ3
    Cervicothoracic Vertebral 0RQ5
    Lumbar Vertebral 0SQ2
    Lumbosacral 0SQ4
    Thoracic Vertebral 0RQ9
    Thoracolumbar Vertebral 0RQB
  Duct
    Common Bile 0FQ9
    Cystic 0FQ8
    Hepatic
      Common 0FQ7
      Left 0FQ6
      Right 0FQ5
    Lacrimal
      Left 08QY
      Right 08QX
    Pancreatic 0FQD
      Accessory 0FQF
    Parotid
      Left 0CQC
      Right 0CQB
  Duodenum 0DQ9
  Dura Mater 00Q2
  Ear
    External
      Bilateral 09Q2
      Left 09Q1
      Right 09Q0
    External Auditory Canal
      Left 09Q4
      Right 09Q3
    Inner
      Left 09QE
      Right 09QD
    Middle
      Left 09Q6
      Right 09Q5
  Elbow Region
    Left 0XQC
    Right 0XQB
  Epididymis
    Bilateral 0VQL
    Left 0VQK
    Right 0VQJ
  Epiglottis 0CQR

Repair — *continued*
Esophagogastric Junction 0DQ4
Esophagus 0DQ5
  Lower 0DQ3
  Middle 0DQ2
  Upper 0DQ1
Eustachian Tube
  Left 09QG
  Right 09QF
Extremity
  Lower
    Left 0YQB
    Right 0YQ9
  Upper
    Left 0XQ7
    Right 0XQ6
Eye
  Left 08Q1XZZ
  Right 08Q0XZZ
Eyelid
  Lower
    Left 08QR
    Right 08QQ
  Upper
    Left 08QP
    Right 08QN
Face 0WQ2
Fallopian Tube
  Left 0UQ6
  Right 0UQ5
Fallopian Tubes, Bilateral 0UQ7
Femoral Region
  Bilateral 0YQE
  Left 0YQ8
  Right 0YQ7
Femoral Shaft
  Left 0QQ9
  Right 0QQ8
Femur
  Lower
    Left 0QQC
    Right 0QQB
  Upper
    Left 0QQ7
    Right 0QQ6
Fibula
  Left 0QQK
  Right 0QQJ
Finger
  Index
    Left 0XQP
    Right 0XQN
  Little
    Left 0XQW
    Right 0XQV
  Middle
    Left 0XQR
    Right 0XQQ
  Ring
    Left 0XQT
    Right 0XQS
Finger Nail 0HQQXZZ
Floor of mouth *see* Repair, Oral Cavity and Throat
  0WQ3
Foot
  Left 0YQN
  Right 0YQM
Gallbladder 0FQ4
Gingiva
  Lower 0CQ6
  Upper 0CQ5
Gland
  Adrenal
    Bilateral 0GQ4
    Left 0GQ2
    Right 0GQ3
  Lacrimal
    Left 08QW
    Right 08QV
  Minor Salivary 0CQJ
  Parotid
    Left 0CQ9
    Right 0CQ8
  Pituitary 0GQ0
  Sublingual
    Left 0CQF
    Right 0CQD
  Submaxillary
    Left 0CQH

Repair — *continued*
Gland — *continued*
  Submaxillary — *continued*
    Right 0CQG
  Vestibular 0UQL
Glenoid Cavity
  Left 0PQ8
  Right 0PQ7
Glomus Jugulare 0GQC
Hand
  Left 0XQK
  Right 0XQJ
Head 0WQ0
Heart 02QA
  Left 02QC
  Right 02QB
Humeral Head
  Left 0PQD
  Right 0PQC
Humeral Shaft
  Left 0PQG
  Right 0PQF
Hymen 0UQK
Hypothalamus 00QA
Ileocecal Valve 0DQC
Ileum 0DQB
Inguinal Region
  Bilateral 0YQA
  Left 0YQ6
  Right 0YQ5
Intestine
  Large 0DQE
    Left 0DQG
    Right 0DQF
  Small 0DQ8
Iris
  Left 08QD3ZZ
  Right 08QC3ZZ
Jaw
  Lower 0WQ5
  Upper 0WQ4
Jejunum 0DQA
Joint
  Acromioclavicular
    Left 0RQH
    Right 0RQG
  Ankle
    Left 0SQG
    Right 0SQF
  Carpal
    Left 0RQR
    Right 0RQQ
  Carpometacarpal
    Left 0RQT
    Right 0RQS
  Cervical Vertebral 0RQ1
  Cervicothoracic Vertebral 0RQ4
  Coccygeal 0SQ6
  Elbow
    Left 0RQM
    Right 0RQL
  Finger Phalangeal
    Left 0RQX
    Right 0RQW
  Hip
    Left 0SQB
    Right 0SQ9
  Knee
    Left 0SQD
    Right 0SQC
  Lumbar Vertebral 0SQ0
  Lumbosacral 0SQ3
  Metacarpophalangeal
    Left 0RQV
    Right 0RQU
  Metatarsal-Phalangeal
    Left 0SQN
    Right 0SQM
  Occipital-cervical 0RQ0
  Sacrococcygeal 0SQ5
  Sacroiliac
    Left 0SQ8
    Right 0SQ7
  Shoulder
    Left 0RQK
    Right 0RQJ
  Sternoclavicular
    Left 0RQF
    Right 0RQE

Repair — *continued*
Joint — *continued*
  Tarsal
    Left 0SQJ
    Right 0SQH
  Tarsometatarsal
    Left 0SQL
    Right 0SQK
  Temporomandibular
    Left 0RQD
    Right 0RQC
  Thoracic Vertebral 0RQ6
  Thoracolumbar Vertebral 0RQA
  Toe Phalangeal
    Left 0SQQ
    Right 0SQP
  Wrist
    Left 0RQP
    Right 0RQN
Kidney
  Left 0TQ1
  Right 0TQ0
Kidney Pelvis
  Left 0TQ4
  Right 0TQ3
Knee Region
  Left 0YQG
  Right 0YQF
Larynx 0CQS
Leg
  Lower
    Left 0YQJ
    Right 0YQH
  Upper
    Left 0YQD
    Right 0YQC
Lens
  Left 08QK3ZZ
  Right 08QJ3ZZ
Lip
  Lower 0CQ1
  Upper 0CQ0
Liver 0FQ0
  Left Lobe 0FQ2
  Right Lobe 0FQ1
Lung
  Bilateral 0BQM
  Left 0BQL
  Lower Lobe
    Left 0BQJ
    Right 0BQF
  Middle Lobe, Right 0BQD
  Right 0BQK
  Upper Lobe
    Left 0BQG
    Right 0BQC
Lung Lingula 0BQH
Lymphatic
  Aortic 07QD
  Axillary
    Left 07Q6
    Right 07Q5
  Head 07Q0
  Inguinal
    Left 07QJ
    Right 07QH
  Internal Mammary
    Left 07Q9
    Right 07Q8
  Lower Extremity
    Left 07QG
    Right 07QF
  Mesenteric 07QB
  Neck
    Left 07Q2
    Right 07Q1
  Pelvis 07QC
  Thoracic Duct 07QK
  Thorax 07Q7
  Upper Extremity
    Left 07Q4
    Right 07Q3
Mandible
  Left 0NQV
  Right 0NQT
Maxilla 0NQR
Mediastinum 0WQC
Medulla Oblongata 00QD
Mesentery 0DQV

Repair — continued

Metacarpal
  Left ØPQQ
  Right ØPQP
Metatarsal
  Left ØQQP
  Right ØQQN
Muscle
  Abdomen
    Left ØKQL
    Right ØKQK
  Extraocular
    Left Ø8QM
    Right Ø8QL
  Facial ØKQ1
  Foot
    Left ØKQW
    Right ØKQV
  Hand
    Left ØKQD
    Right ØKQC
  Head ØKQ0
  Hip
    Left ØKQP
    Right ØKQN
  Lower Arm and Wrist
    Left ØKQB
    Right ØKQ9
  Lower Leg
    Left ØKQT
    Right ØKQS
  Neck
    Left ØKQ3
    Right ØKQ2
  Papillary Ø2QD
  Perineum ØKQM
  Shoulder
    Left ØKQ6
    Right ØKQ5
  Thorax
    Left ØKQJ
    Right ØKQH
  Tongue, Palate, Pharynx ØKQ4
  Trunk
    Left ØKQG
    Right ØKQF
  Upper Arm
    Left ØKQ8
    Right ØKQ7
  Upper Leg
    Left ØKQR
    Right ØKQQ
Nasal Mucosa and Soft Tissue Ø9QK
Nasopharynx Ø9QN
Neck ØWQ6
Nerve
  Abdominal Sympathetic Ø1QM
  Abducens ØØQL
  Accessory ØØQR
  Acoustic ØØQN
  Brachial Plexus Ø1Q3
  Cervical Ø1Q1
  Cervical Plexus Ø1Q0
  Facial ØØQM
  Femoral Ø1QD
  Glossopharyngeal ØØQP
  Head and Neck Sympathetic Ø1QK
  Hypoglossal ØØQS
  Lumbar Ø1QB
  Lumbar Plexus Ø1Q9
  Lumbar Sympathetic Ø1QN
  Lumbosacral Plexus Ø1QA
  Median Ø1Q5
  Oculomotor ØØQH
  Olfactory ØØQF
  Optic ØØQG
  Peroneal Ø1QH
  Phrenic Ø1Q2
  Pudendal Ø1QC
  Radial Ø1Q6
  Sacral Ø1QR
  Sacral Plexus Ø1QQ
  Sacral Sympathetic Ø1QP
  Sciatic Ø1QF
  Thoracic Ø1Q8
  Thoracic Sympathetic Ø1QL
  Tibial Ø1QG
  Trigeminal ØØQK
  Trochlear ØØQJ

Repair — continued

Nerve — continued
  Ulnar Ø1Q4
  Vagus ØØQQ
Nipple
  Left ØHQX
  Right ØHQW
Omentum ØDQU
Oral Cavity and Throat ØWQ3
Orbit
  Left ØNQQ
  Right ØNQP
Ovary
  Bilateral ØUQ2
  Left ØUQ1
  Right ØUQ0
Palate
  Hard ØCQ2
  Soft ØCQ3
Pancreas ØFQG
Para-aortic Body ØGQ9
Paraganglion Extremity ØGQF
Parathyroid Gland ØGQR
  Inferior
    Left ØGQP
    Right ØGQN
  Multiple ØGQQ
  Superior
    Left ØGQM
    Right ØGQL
Patella
  Left ØQQF
  Right ØQQD
Penis ØVQS
Pericardium Ø2QN
Perineum
  Female ØWQN
  Male ØWQM
Peritoneum ØDQW
Phalanx
  Finger
    Left ØPQV
    Right ØPQT
  Thumb
    Left ØPQS
    Right ØPQR
  Toe
    Left ØQQR
    Right ØQQQ
Pharynx ØCQM
Pineal Body ØGQ1
Pleura
  Left ØBQP
  Right ØBQN
Pons ØØQB
Prepuce ØVQT
Products of Conception 10Q0
Prostate ØVQ0
Radius
  Left ØPQJ
  Right ØPQH
Rectum ØDQP
Retina
  Left Ø8QF3ZZ
  Right Ø8QE3ZZ
Retinal Vessel
  Left Ø8QH3ZZ
  Right Ø8QG3ZZ
Ribs
  1 to 2 ØPQ1
  3 or More ØPQ2
Sacrum ØQQ1
Scapula
  Left ØPQ6
  Right ØPQ5
Sclera
  Left Ø8Q7XZZ
  Right Ø8Q6XZZ
Scrotum ØVQ5
Septum
  Atrial Ø2Q5
  Nasal Ø9QM
  Ventricular Ø2QM
Shoulder Region
  Left ØXQ3
  Right ØXQ2
Sinus
  Accessory Ø9QP

Repair — continued

Sinus — continued
  Ethmoid
    Left Ø9QV
    Right Ø9QU
  Frontal
    Left Ø9QT
    Right Ø9QS
  Mastoid
    Left Ø9QC
    Right Ø9QB
  Maxillary
    Left Ø9QR
    Right Ø9QQ
  Sphenoid
    Left Ø9QX
    Right Ø9QW
Skin
  Abdomen ØHQ7XZZ
  Back ØHQ6XZZ
  Buttock ØHQ8XZZ
  Chest ØHQ5XZZ
  Ear
    Left ØHQ3XZZ
    Right ØHQ2XZZ
  Face ØHQ1XZZ
  Foot
    Left ØHQNXZZ
    Right ØHQMXZZ
  Hand
    Left ØHQGXZZ
    Right ØHQFXZZ
  Inguinal ØHQAXZZ
  Lower Arm
    Left ØHQEXZZ
    Right ØHQDXZZ
  Lower Leg
    Left ØHQLXZZ
    Right ØHQKXZZ
  Neck ØHQ4XZZ
  Perineum ØHQ9XZZ
  Scalp ØHQ0XZZ
  Upper Arm
    Left ØHQCXZZ
    Right ØHQBXZZ
  Upper Leg
    Left ØHQJXZZ
    Right ØHQHXZZ
Skull ØNQ0
Spinal Cord
  Cervical ØØQW
  Lumbar ØØQY
  Thoracic ØØQX
Spinal Meninges ØØQT
Spleen Ø7QP
Sternum ØPQ0
Stomach ØDQ6
  Pylorus ØDQ7
Subcutaneous Tissue and Fascia
  Abdomen ØJQ8
  Back ØJQ7
  Buttock ØJQ9
  Chest ØJQ6
  Face ØJQ1
  Foot
    Left ØJQR
    Right ØJQQ
  Hand
    Left ØJQK
    Right ØJQJ
  Lower Arm
    Left ØJQH
    Right ØJQG
  Lower Leg
    Left ØJQP
    Right ØJQN
  Neck
    Left ØJQ5
    Right ØJQ4
  Pelvic Region ØJQC
  Perineum ØJQB
  Scalp ØJQ0
  Upper Arm
    Left ØJQF
    Right ØJQD
  Upper Leg
    Left ØJQM
    Right ØJQL

Subterms under main terms may continue to next column or page

Repair — *continued*
- Tarsal
  - Left ØQQM
  - Right ØQQL
- Tendon
  - Abdomen
    - Left ØLQG
    - Right ØLQF
  - Ankle
    - Left ØLQT
    - Right ØLQS
  - Foot
    - Left ØLQW
    - Right ØLQV
  - Hand
    - Left ØLQ8
    - Right ØLQ7
  - Head and Neck ØLQ0
  - Hip
    - Left ØLQK
    - Right ØLQJ
  - Knee
    - Left ØLQR
    - Right ØLQQ
  - Lower Arm and Wrist
    - Left ØLQ6
    - Right ØLQ5
  - Lower Leg
    - Left ØLQP
    - Right ØLQN
  - Perineum ØLQH
  - Shoulder
    - Left ØLQ2
    - Right ØLQ1
  - Thorax
    - Left ØLQD
    - Right ØLQC
  - Trunk
    - Left ØLQB
    - Right ØLQ9
  - Upper Arm
    - Left ØLQ4
    - Right ØLQ3
  - Upper Leg
    - Left ØLQM
    - Right ØLQL
- Testis
  - Bilateral ØVQC
  - Left ØVQB
  - Right ØVQ9
- Thalamus 00Q9
- Thumb
  - Left ØXQM
  - Right ØXQL
- Thymus 07QM
- Thyroid Gland ØGQK
  - Left Lobe ØGQG
  - Right Lobe ØGQH
- Thyroid Gland Isthmus ØGQJ
- Tibia
  - Left ØQQH
  - Right ØQQG
- Toe
  - 1st
    - Left ØYQQ
    - Right ØYQP
  - 2nd
    - Left ØYQS
    - Right ØYQR
  - 3rd
    - Left ØYQU
    - Right ØYQT
  - 4th
    - Left ØYQW
    - Right ØYQV
  - 5th
    - Left ØYQY
    - Right ØYQX
- Toe Nail ØHQRXZZ
- Tongue ØCQ7
- Tonsils ØCQP
- Tooth
  - Lower ØCQX
  - Upper ØCQW
- Trachea ØBQ1
- Tunica Vaginalis
  - Left ØVQ7
  - Right ØVQ6
- Turbinate, Nasal 09QL

Repair — *continued*
- Tympanic Membrane
  - Left 09Q8
  - Right 09Q7
- Ulna
  - Left ØPQL
  - Right ØPQK
- Ureter
  - Left ØTQ7
  - Right ØTQ6
- Urethra ØTQD
- Uterine Supporting Structure ØUQ4
- Uterus ØUQ9
- Uvula ØCQN
- Vagina ØUQG
- Valve
  - Aortic 02QF
  - Mitral 02QG
  - Pulmonary 02QH
  - Tricuspid 02QJ
- Vas Deferens
  - Bilateral ØVQQ
  - Left ØVQP
  - Right ØVQN
- Vein
  - Axillary
    - Left 05Q8
    - Right 05Q7
  - Azygos 05Q0
  - Basilic
    - Left 05QC
    - Right 05QB
  - Brachial
    - Left 05QA
    - Right 05Q9
  - Cephalic
    - Left 05QF
    - Right 05QD
  - Colic 06Q7
  - Common Iliac
    - Left 06QD
    - Right 06QC
  - Coronary 02Q4
  - Esophageal 06Q3
  - External Iliac
    - Left 06QG
    - Right 06QF
  - External Jugular
    - Left 05QQ
    - Right 05QP
  - Face
    - Left 05QV
    - Right 05QT
  - Femoral
    - Left 06QN
    - Right 06QM
  - Foot
    - Left 06QV
    - Right 06QT
  - Gastric 06Q2
  - Hand
    - Left 05QH
    - Right 05QG
  - Hemiazygos 05Q1
  - Hepatic 06Q4
  - Hypogastric
    - Left 06QJ
    - Right 06QH
  - Inferior Mesenteric 06Q6
  - Innominate
    - Left 05Q4
    - Right 05Q3
  - Internal Jugular
    - Left 05QN
    - Right 05QM
  - Intracranial 05QL
  - Lower 06QY
  - Portal 06Q8
  - Pulmonary
    - Left 02QT
    - Right 02QS
  - Renal
    - Left 06QB
    - Right 06Q9
  - Saphenous
    - Left 06QQ
    - Right 06QP
  - Splenic 06Q1

Repair — *continued*
- Vein — *continued*
  - Subclavian
    - Left 05Q6
    - Right 05Q5
  - Superior Mesenteric 06Q5
  - Upper 05QY
  - Vertebral
    - Left 05QS
    - Right 05QR
- Vena Cava
  - Inferior 06Q0
  - Superior 02QV
- Ventricle
  - Left 02QL
  - Right 02QK
- Vertebra
  - Cervical ØPQ3
  - Lumbar ØQQ0
  - Thoracic ØPQ4
- Vesicle
  - Bilateral ØVQ3
  - Left ØVQ2
  - Right ØVQ1
- Vitreous
  - Left 08Q53ZZ
  - Right 08Q43ZZ
- Vocal Cord
  - Left ØCQV
  - Right ØCQT
- Vulva ØUQM
- Wrist Region
  - Left ØXQH
  - Right ØXQG

Repair, obstetric laceration, periurethral ØUQMXZZ

Replacement
- Acetabulum
  - Left ØQR5
  - Right ØQR4
- Ampulla of Vater ØFRC
- Anal Sphincter ØDRR
- Aorta
  - Abdominal 04R0
  - Thoracic
    - Ascending/Arch 02RX
    - Descending 02RW
- Artery
  - Anterior Tibial
    - Left 04RQ
    - Right 04RP
  - Axillary
    - Left 03R6
    - Right 03R5
  - Brachial
    - Left 03R8
    - Right 03R7
  - Celiac 04R1
  - Colic
    - Left 04R7
    - Middle 04R8
    - Right 04R6
  - Common Carotid
    - Left 03RJ
    - Right 03RH
  - Common Iliac
    - Left 04RD
    - Right 04RC
  - External Carotid
    - Left 03RN
    - Right 03RM
  - External Iliac
    - Left 04RJ
    - Right 04RH
  - Face 03RR
  - Femoral
    - Left 04RL
    - Right 04RK
  - Foot
    - Left 04RW
    - Right 04RV
  - Gastric 04R2
  - Hand
    - Left 03RF
    - Right 03RD
  - Hepatic 04R3
  - Inferior Mesenteric 04RB
  - Innominate 03R2
  - Internal Carotid
    - Left 03RL

Replacement — continued
Joint — continued
  Hip
    Left ØSRB
      Acetabular Surface ØSRE
      Femoral Surface ØSRS
    Right ØSR9
      Acetabular Surface ØSRA
      Femoral Surface ØSRR
  Knee
    Left ØSRD
      Femoral Surface ØSRU
      Tibial Surface ØSRW
    Right ØSRC
      Femoral Surface ØSRT
      Tibial Surface ØSRV
  Lumbar Vertebral ØSR00
  Lumbosacral ØSR30
  Metacarpophalangeal
    Left ØRRV0
    Right ØRRU0
  Metatarsal-Phalangeal
    Left ØSRN0
    Right ØSRM0
  Occipital-cervical ØRR00
  Sacrococcygeal ØSR50
  Sacroiliac
    Left ØSR80
    Right ØSR70
  Shoulder
    Left ØRRK
    Right ØRRJ
  Sternoclavicular
    Left ØRRF0
    Right ØRRE0
  Tarsal
    Left ØSRJ0
    Right ØSRH0
  Tarsometatarsal
    Left ØSRL0
    Right ØSRK0
  Temporomandibular
    Left ØRRD0
    Right ØRRC0
  Thoracic Vertebral ØRR60
  Thoracolumbar Vertebral ØRRA0
  Toe Phalangeal
    Left ØSRQ0
    Right ØSRP0
  Wrist
    Left ØRRP0
    Right ØRRN0
Kidney Pelvis
  Left ØTR4
  Right ØTR3
Larynx ØCRS
Lens
  Left Ø8RK30Z
  Right Ø8RJ30Z
Lip
  Lower ØCR1
  Upper ØCR0
Mandible
  Left ØNRV
  Right ØNRT
Maxilla ØNRR
Mesentery ØDRV
Metacarpal
  Left ØPRQ
  Right ØPRP
Metatarsal
  Left ØQRP
  Right ØQRN
Muscle
  Abdomen
    Left ØKRL
    Right ØKRK
  Facial ØKR1
  Foot
    Left ØKRW
    Right ØKRV
  Hand
    Left ØKRD
    Right ØKRC
  Head ØKR0
  Hip
    Left ØKRP
    Right ØKRN

Replacement — continued
Muscle — continued
  Lower Arm and Wrist
    Left ØKRB
    Right ØKR9
  Lower Leg
    Left ØKRT
    Right ØKRS
  Neck
    Left ØKR3
    Right ØKR2
  Papillary Ø2RD
  Perineum ØKRM
  Shoulder
    Left ØKR6
    Right ØKR5
  Thorax
    Left ØKRJ
    Right ØKRH
  Tongue, Palate, Pharynx ØKR4
  Trunk
    Left ØKRG
    Right ØKRF
  Upper Arm
    Left ØKR8
    Right ØKR7
  Upper Leg
    Left ØKRR
    Right ØKRQ
Nasal Mucosa and Soft Tissue Ø9RK
Nasopharynx Ø9RN
Nerve
  Abducens ØØRL
  Accessory ØØRR
  Acoustic ØØRN
  Cervical Ø1R1
  Facial ØØRM
  Femoral Ø1RD
  Glossopharyngeal ØØRP
  Hypoglossal ØØRS
  Lumbar Ø1RB
  Median Ø1R5
  Oculomotor ØØRH
  Olfactory ØØRF
  Optic ØØRG
  Peroneal Ø1RH
  Phrenic Ø1R2
  Pudendal Ø1RC
  Radial Ø1R6
  Sacral Ø1RR
  Sciatic Ø1RF
  Thoracic Ø1R8
  Tibial Ø1RG
  Trigeminal ØØRK
  Trochlear ØØRJ
  Ulnar Ø1R4
  Vagus ØØRQ
Nipple
  Left ØHRX
  Right ØHRW
Omentum ØDRU
Orbit
  Left ØNRQ
  Right ØNRP
Palate
  Hard ØCR2
  Soft ØCR3
Patella
  Left ØQRF
  Right ØQRD
Pericardium Ø2RN
Peritoneum ØDRW
Phalanx
  Finger
    Left ØPRV
    Right ØPRT
  Thumb
    Left ØPRS
    Right ØPRR
  Toe
    Left ØQRR
    Right ØQRQ
Pharynx ØCRM
Radius
  Left ØPRJ
  Right ØPRH
Retinal Vessel
  Left Ø8RH3
  Right Ø8RG3

Replacement — continued
Ribs
  1 to 2 ØPR1
  3 or More ØPR2
Sacrum ØQR1
Scapula
  Left ØPR6
  Right ØPR5
Sclera
  Left Ø8R7X
  Right Ø8R6X
Septum
  Atrial Ø2R5
  Nasal Ø9RM
  Ventricular Ø2RM
Skin
  Abdomen ØHR7
  Back ØHR6
  Buttock ØHR8
  Chest ØHR5
  Ear
    Left ØHR3
    Right ØHR2
  Face ØHR1
  Foot
    Left ØHRN
    Right ØHRM
  Hand
    Left ØHRG
    Right ØHRF
  Inguinal ØHRA
  Lower Arm
    Left ØHRE
    Right ØHRD
  Lower Leg
    Left ØHRL
    Right ØHRK
  Neck ØHR4
  Perineum ØHR9
  Scalp ØHR0
  Upper Arm
    Left ØHRC
    Right ØHRB
  Upper Leg
    Left ØHRJ
    Right ØHRH
Skull ØNR0
Spinal Meninges ØØRT
Sternum ØPR0
Subcutaneous Tissue and Fascia
  Abdomen ØJR8
  Back ØJR7
  Buttock ØJR9
  Chest ØJR6
  Face ØJR1
  Foot
    Left ØJRR
    Right ØJRQ
  Hand
    Left ØJRK
    Right ØJRJ
  Lower Arm
    Left ØJRH
    Right ØJRG
  Lower Leg
    Left ØJRP
    Right ØJRN
  Neck
    Left ØJR5
    Right ØJR4
  Pelvic Region ØJRC
  Perineum ØJRB
  Scalp ØJR0
  Upper Arm
    Left ØJRF
    Right ØJRD
  Upper Leg
    Left ØJRM
    Right ØJRL
Tarsal
  Left ØQRM
  Right ØQRL
Tendon
  Abdomen
    Left ØLRG
    Right ØLRF
  Ankle
    Left ØLRT
    Right ØLRS

Replacement — *continued*
  Tendon — *continued*
    Foot
      Left ØLRW
      Right ØLRV
    Hand
      Left ØLR8
      Right ØLR7
    Head and Neck ØLRØ
    Hip
      Left ØLRK
      Right ØLRJ
    Knee
      Left ØLRR
      Right ØLRQ
    Lower Arm and Wrist
      Left ØLR6
      Right ØLR5
    Lower Leg
      Left ØLRP
      Right ØLRN
    Perineum ØLRH
    Shoulder
      Left ØLR2
      Right ØLR1
    Thorax
      Left ØLRD
      Right ØLRC
    Trunk
      Left ØLRB
      Right ØLR9
    Upper Arm
      Left ØLR4
      Right ØLR3
    Upper Leg
      Left ØLRM
      Right ØLRL
  Testis
    Bilateral ØVRCØJZ
    Left ØVRBØJZ
    Right ØVR9ØJZ
  Thumb
    Left ØXRM
    Right ØXRL
  Tibia
    Left ØQRH
    Right ØQRG
  Toe Nail ØHRRX
  Tongue ØCR7
  Tooth
    Lower ØCRX
    Upper ØCRW
  Trachea ØBR1
  Turbinate, Nasal Ø9RL
  Tympanic Membrane
    Left Ø9R8
    Right Ø9R7
  Ulna
    Left ØPRL
    Right ØPRK
  Ureter
    Left ØTR7
    Right ØTR6
  Urethra ØTRD
  Uvula ØCRN
  Valve
    Aortic Ø2RF
    Mitral Ø2RG
    Pulmonary Ø2RH
    Tricuspid Ø2RJ
  Vein
    Axillary
      Left Ø5R8
      Right Ø5R7
    Azygos Ø5RØ
    Basilic
      Left Ø5RC
      Right Ø5RB
    Brachial
      Left Ø5RA
      Right Ø5R9
    Cephalic
      Left Ø5RF
      Right Ø5RD
    Colic Ø6R7
    Common Iliac
      Left Ø6RD
      Right Ø6RC
    Esophageal Ø6R3

Replacement — *continued*
  Vein — *continued*
    External Iliac
      Left Ø6RG
      Right Ø6RF
    External Jugular
      Left Ø5RQ
      Right Ø5RP
    Face
      Left Ø5RV
      Right Ø5RT
    Femoral
      Left Ø6RN
      Right Ø6RM
    Foot
      Left Ø6RV
      Right Ø6RT
    Gastric Ø6R2
    Hand
      Left Ø5RH
      Right Ø5RG
    Hemiazygos Ø5R1
    Hepatic Ø6R4
    Hypogastric
      Left Ø6RJ
      Right Ø6RH
    Inferior Mesenteric Ø6R6
    Innominate
      Left Ø5R4
      Right Ø5R3
    Internal Jugular
      Left Ø5RN
      Right Ø5RM
    Intracranial Ø5RL
    Lower Ø6RY
    Portal Ø6R8
    Pulmonary
      Left Ø2RT
      Right Ø2RS
    Renal
      Left Ø6RB
      Right Ø6R9
    Saphenous
      Left Ø6RQ
      Right Ø6RP
    Splenic Ø6R1
    Subclavian
      Left Ø5R6
      Right Ø5R5
    Superior Mesenteric Ø6R5
    Upper Ø5RY
    Vertebral
      Left Ø5RS
      Right Ø5RR
  Vena Cava
    Inferior Ø6RØ
    Superior Ø2RV
  Ventricle
    Left Ø2RL
    Right Ø2RK
  Vertebra
    Cervical ØPR3
    Lumbar ØQRØ
    Thoracic ØPR4
  Vitreous
    Left Ø8R53
    Right Ø8R43
  Vocal Cord
    Left ØCRV
    Right ØCRT
Replacement, hip
  Partial or total *see* Replacement, Lower Joints ØSR
  Resurfacing only *see* Supplement, Lower Joints ØSU
Replacement, knee
  Meniscus implant only *see* New Technology, Joints XRR
  Partial or total *see* Replacement, Lower Joints ØSR
Replantation *see* Reposition
Replantation, scalp *see* Reattachment, Skin, Scalp ØHMØ
Reposition
  Acetabulum
    Left ØQS5
    Right ØQS4
  Ampulla of Vater ØFSC
  Anus ØDSQ

Reposition — *continued*
  Aorta
    Abdominal Ø4SØ
    Thoracic
      Ascending/Arch Ø2SXØZZ
      Descending Ø2SWØZZ
  Artery
    Anterior Tibial
      Left Ø4SQ
      Right Ø4SP
    Axillary
      Left Ø3S6
      Right Ø3S5
    Brachial
      Left Ø3S8
      Right Ø3S7
    Celiac Ø4S1
    Colic
      Left Ø4S7
      Middle Ø4S8
      Right Ø4S6
    Common Carotid
      Left Ø3SJ
      Right Ø3SH
    Common Iliac
      Left Ø4SD
      Right Ø4SC
    Coronary
      One Artery Ø2SØØZZ
      Two Arteries Ø2S1ØZZ
    External Carotid
      Left Ø3SN
      Right Ø3SM
    External Iliac
      Left Ø4SJ
      Right Ø4SH
    Face Ø3SR
    Femoral
      Left Ø4SL
      Right Ø4SK
    Foot
      Left Ø4SW
      Right Ø4SV
    Gastric Ø4S2
    Hand
      Left Ø3SF
      Right Ø3SD
    Hepatic Ø4S3
    Inferior Mesenteric Ø4SB
    Innominate Ø3S2
    Internal Carotid
      Left Ø3SL
      Right Ø3SK
    Internal Iliac
      Left Ø4SF
      Right Ø4SE
    Internal Mammary
      Left Ø3S1
      Right Ø3SØ
    Intracranial Ø3SG
    Lower Ø4SY
    Peroneal
      Left Ø4SU
      Right Ø4ST
    Popliteal
      Left Ø4SN
      Right Ø4SM
    Posterior Tibial
      Left Ø4SS
      Right Ø4SR
    Pulmonary
      Left Ø2SRØZZ
      Right Ø2SQØZZ
    Pulmonary Trunk Ø2SPØZZ
    Radial
      Left Ø3SC
      Right Ø3SB
    Renal
      Left Ø4SA
      Right Ø4S9
    Splenic Ø4S4
    Subclavian
      Left Ø3S4
      Right Ø3S3
    Superior Mesenteric Ø4S5
    Temporal
      Left Ø3ST
      Right Ø3SS

Reposition — *continued*
Artery — *continued*
Thyroid
Left 03SV
Right 03SU
Ulnar
Left 03SA
Right 03S9
Upper 03SY
Vertebral
Left 03SQ
Right 03SP
Auditory Ossicle
Left 09SA
Right 09S9
Bladder 0TSB
Bladder Neck 0TSC
Bone
Ethmoid
Left 0NSG
Right 0NSF
Frontal 0NS1
Hyoid 0NSX
Lacrimal
Left 0NSJ
Right 0NSH
Nasal 0NSB
Occipital 0NS7
Palatine
Left 0NSL
Right 0NSK
Parietal
Left 0NS4
Right 0NS3
Pelvic
Left 0QS3
Right 0QS2
Sphenoid 0NSC
Temporal
Left 0NS6
Right 0NS5
Zygomatic
Left 0NSN
Right 0NSM
Breast
Bilateral 0HSV0ZZ
Left 0HSU0ZZ
Right 0HST0ZZ
Bronchus
Lingula 0BS90ZZ
Lower Lobe
Left 0BSB0ZZ
Right 0BS60ZZ
Main
Left 0BS70ZZ
Right 0BS30ZZ
Middle Lobe, Right 0BS50ZZ
Upper Lobe
Left 0BS80ZZ
Right 0BS40ZZ
Bursa and Ligament
Abdomen
Left 0MSJ
Right 0MSH
Ankle
Left 0MSR
Right 0MSQ
Elbow
Left 0MS4
Right 0MS3
Foot
Left 0MST
Right 0MSS
Hand
Left 0MS8
Right 0MS7
Head and Neck 0MS0
Hip
Left 0MSM
Right 0MSL
Knee
Left 0MSP
Right 0MSN
Lower Extremity
Left 0MSW
Right 0MSV
Perineum 0MSK
Rib(s) 0MSG

Reposition — *continued*
Bursa and Ligament — *continued*
Shoulder
Left 0MS2
Right 0MS1
Spine
Lower 0MSD
Upper 0MSC
Sternum 0MSF
Upper Extremity
Left 0MSB
Right 0MS9
Wrist
Left 0MS6
Right 0MS5
Carina 0BS20ZZ
Carpal
Left 0PSN
Right 0PSM
Cecum 0DSH
Cervix 0USC
Clavicle
Left 0PSB
Right 0PS9
Coccyx 0QSS
Colon
Ascending 0DSK
Descending 0DSM
Sigmoid 0DSN
Transverse 0DSL
Cord
Bilateral 0VSH
Left 0VSG
Right 0VSF
Cul-de-sac 0USF
Diaphragm 0BST0ZZ
Duct
Common Bile 0FS9
Cystic 0FS8
Hepatic
Common 0FS7
Left 0FS6
Right 0FS5
Lacrimal
Left 08SY
Right 08SX
Pancreatic 0FSD
Accessory 0FSF
Parotid
Left 0CSC
Right 0CSB
Duodenum 0DS9
Ear
Bilateral 09S2
Left 09S1
Right 09S0
Epiglottis 0CSR
Esophagus 0DS5
Eustachian Tube
Left 09SG
Right 09SF
Eyelid
Lower
Left 08SR
Right 08SQ
Upper
Left 08SP
Right 08SN
Fallopian Tube
Left 0US6
Right 0US5
Fallopian Tubes, Bilateral 0US7
Femoral Shaft
Left 0QS9
Right 0QS8
Femur
Lower
Left 0QSC
Right 0QSB
Upper
Left 0QS7
Right 0QS6
Fibula
Left 0QSK
Right 0QSJ
Gallbladder 0FS4
Gland
Adrenal
Left 0GS2

Reposition — *continued*
Gland — *continued*
Adrenal — *continued*
Right 0GS3
Lacrimal
Left 08SW
Right 08SV
Glenoid Cavity
Left 0PS8
Right 0PS7
Hair 0HSSXZZ
Humeral Head
Left 0PSD
Right 0PSC
Humeral Shaft
Left 0PSG
Right 0PSF
Ileum 0DSB
Intestine
Large 0DSE
Small 0DS8
Iris
Left 08SD3ZZ
Right 08SC3ZZ
Jejunum 0DSA
Joint
Acromioclavicular
Left 0RSH
Right 0RSG
Ankle
Left 0SSG
Right 0SSF
Carpal
Left 0RSR
Right 0RSQ
Carpometacarpal
Left 0RST
Right 0RSS
Cervical Vertebral 0RS1
Cervicothoracic Vertebral 0RS4
Coccygeal 0SS6
Elbow
Left 0RSM
Right 0RSL
Finger Phalangeal
Left 0RSX
Right 0RSW
Hip
Left 0SSB
Right 0SS9
Knee
Left 0SSD
Right 0SSC
Lumbar Vertebral 0SS0
Lumbosacral 0SS3
Metacarpophalangeal
Left 0RSV
Right 0RSU
Metatarsal-Phalangeal
Left 0SSN
Right 0SSM
Occipital-cervical 0RS0
Sacrococcygeal 0SS5
Sacroiliac
Left 0SS8
Right 0SS7
Shoulder
Left 0RSK
Right 0RSJ
Sternoclavicular
Left 0RSF
Right 0RSE
Tarsal
Left 0SSJ
Right 0SSH
Tarsometatarsal
Left 0SSL
Right 0SSK
Temporomandibular
Left 0RSD
Right 0RSC
Thoracic Vertebral 0RS6
Thoracolumbar Vertebral 0RSA
Toe Phalangeal
Left 0SSQ
Right 0SSP
Wrist
Left 0RSP
Right 0RSN

Reposition — *continued*
Kidney
  Left 0TS1
  Right 0TS0
Kidney Pelvis
  Left 0TS4
  Right 0TS3
Kidneys, Bilateral 0TS2
Lens
  Left 08SK3ZZ
  Right 08SJ3ZZ
Lip
  Lower 0CS1
  Upper 0CS0
Liver 0FS0
Lung
  Left 0BSL0ZZ
  Lower Lobe
    Left 0BSJ0ZZ
    Right 0BSF0ZZ
  Middle Lobe, Right 0BSD0ZZ
  Right 0BSK0ZZ
  Upper Lobe
    Left 0BSG0ZZ
    Right 0BSC0ZZ
Lung Lingula 0BSH0ZZ
Mandible
  Left 0NSV
  Right 0NST
Maxilla 0NSR
Metacarpal
  Left 0PSQ
  Right 0PSP
Metatarsal
  Left 0QSP
  Right 0QSN
Muscle
  Abdomen
    Left 0KSL
    Right 0KSK
  Extraocular
    Left 08SM
    Right 08SL
  Facial 0KS1
  Foot
    Left 0KSW
    Right 0KSV
  Hand
    Left 0KSD
    Right 0KSC
  Head 0KS0
  Hip
    Left 0KSP
    Right 0KSN
  Lower Arm and Wrist
    Left 0KSB
    Right 0KS9
  Lower Leg
    Left 0KST
    Right 0KSS
  Neck
    Left 0KS3
    Right 0KS2
  Perineum 0KSM
  Shoulder
    Left 0KS6
    Right 0KS5
  Thorax
    Left 0KSJ
    Right 0KSH
  Tongue, Palate, Pharynx 0KS4
  Trunk
    Left 0KSG
    Right 0KSF
  Upper Arm
    Left 0KS8
    Right 0KS7
  Upper Leg
    Left 0KSR
    Right 0KSQ
Nasal Mucosa and Soft Tissue 09SK
Nerve
  Abducens 00SL
  Accessory 00SR
  Acoustic 00SN
  Brachial Plexus 01S3
  Cervical 01S1
  Cervical Plexus 01S0
  Facial 00SM

Reposition — *continued*
Nerve — *continued*
  Femoral 01SD
  Glossopharyngeal 00SP
  Hypoglossal 00SS
  Lumbar 01SB
  Lumbar Plexus 01S9
  Lumbosacral Plexus 01SA
  Median 01S5
  Oculomotor 00SH
  Olfactory 00SF
  Optic 00SG
  Peroneal 01SH
  Phrenic 01S2
  Pudendal 01SC
  Radial 01S6
  Sacral 01S5
  Sacral Plexus 01SQ
  Sciatic 01SF
  Thoracic 01S8
  Tibial 01SG
  Trigeminal 00SK
  Trochlear 00SJ
  Ulnar 01S4
  Vagus 00SQ
Nipple
  Left 0HSXXZZ
  Right 0HSWXZZ
Orbit
  Left 0NSQ
  Right 0NSP
Ovary
  Bilateral 0US2
  Left 0US1
  Right 0US0
Palate
  Hard 0CS2
  Soft 0CS3
Pancreas 0FSG
Parathyroid Gland 0GSR
  Inferior
    Left 0GSP
    Right 0GSN
  Multiple 0GSQ
  Superior
    Left 0GSM
    Right 0GSL
Patella
  Left 0QSF
  Right 0QSD
Phalanx
  Finger
    Left 0PSV
    Right 0PST
  Thumb
    Left 0PSS
    Right 0PSR
  Toe
    Left 0QSR
    Right 0QSQ
Products of Conception 10S0
  Ectopic 10S2
Radius
  Left 0PSJ
  Right 0PSH
Rectum 0DSP
Retinal Vessel
  Left 08SH3ZZ
  Right 08SG3ZZ
Ribs
  1 to 2 0PS1
  3 or More 0PS2
Sacrum 0QS1
Scapula
  Left 0PS6
  Right 0PS5
Septum, Nasal 09SM
Sesamoid Bone(s) 1st Toe
  see Reposition, Metatarsal, Left 0QSP
  see Reposition, Metatarsal, Right 0QSN
Skull 0NS0
Spinal Cord
  Cervical 00SW
  Lumbar 00SY
  Thoracic 00SX
Spleen 07SP0ZZ
Sternum 0PS0
Stomach 0DS6

Reposition — *continued*
Tarsal
  Left 0QSM
  Right 0QSL
Tendon
  Abdomen
    Left 0LSG
    Right 0LSF
  Ankle
    Left 0LST
    Right 0LSS
  Foot
    Left 0LSW
    Right 0LSV
  Hand
    Left 0LS8
    Right 0LS7
  Head and Neck 0LS0
  Hip
    Left 0LSK
    Right 0LSJ
  Knee
    Left 0LSR
    Right 0LSQ
  Lower Arm and Wrist
    Left 0LS6
    Right 0LS5
  Lower Leg
    Left 0LSP
    Right 0LSN
  Perineum 0LSH
  Shoulder
    Left 0LS2
    Right 0LS1
  Thorax
    Left 0LSD
    Right 0LSC
  Trunk
    Left 0LSB
    Right 0LS9
  Upper Arm
    Left 0LS4
    Right 0LS3
  Upper Leg
    Left 0LSM
    Right 0LSL
Testis
  Bilateral 0VSC
  Left 0VSB
  Right 0VS9
Thymus 07SM0ZZ
Thyroid Gland
  Left Lobe 0GSG
  Right Lobe 0GSH
Tibia
  Left 0QSH
  Right 0QSG
Tongue 0CS7
Tooth
  Lower 0CSX
  Upper 0CSW
Trachea 0BS10ZZ
Turbinate, Nasal 09SL
Tympanic Membrane
  Left 09S8
  Right 09S7
Ulna
  Left 0PSL
  Right 0PSK
Ureter
  Left 0TS7
  Right 0TS6
Ureters, Bilateral 0TS8
Urethra 0TSD
Uterine Supporting Structure 0US4
Uterus 0US9
Uvula 0CSN
Vagina 0USG
Vein
  Axillary
    Left 05S8
    Right 05S7
  Azygos 05S0
  Basilic
    Left 05SC
    Right 05SB
  Brachial
    Left 05SA
    Right 05S9

Reposition — *continued*

   Vein — *continued*

      Cephalic
         Left 05SF
         Right 05SD
      Colic 06S7
      Common Iliac
         Left 06SD
         Right 06SC
      Esophageal 06S3
      External Iliac
         Left 06SG
         Right 06SF
      External Jugular
         Left 05SQ
         Right 05SP
      Face
         Left 05SV
         Right 05ST
      Femoral
         Left 06SN
         Right 06SM
      Foot
         Left 06SV
         Right 06ST
      Gastric 06S2
      Hand
         Left 05SH
         Right 05SG
      Hemiazygos 05S1
      Hepatic 06S4
      Hypogastric
         Left 06SJ
         Right 06SH
      Inferior Mesenteric 06S6
      Innominate
         Left 05S4
         Right 05S3
      Internal Jugular
         Left 05SN
         Right 05SM
      Intracranial 05SL
      Lower 06SY
      Portal 06S8
      Pulmonary
         Left 02ST0ZZ
         Right 02SS0ZZ
      Renal
         Left 06SB
         Right 06S9
      Saphenous
         Left 06SQ
         Right 06SP
      Splenic 06S1
      Subclavian
         Left 05S6
         Right 05S5
      Superior Mesenteric 06S5
      Upper 05SY
      Vertebral
         Left 05SS
         Right 05SR
   Vena Cava
      Inferior 06S0
      Superior 02SV0ZZ
   Vertebra
      Cervical 0PS3
         Magnetically Controlled Growth Rod(s)
           XNS3
      Lumbar 0QS0
         Magnetically Controlled Growth Rod(s)
           XNS0
         Posterior (Dynamic) Distraction Device
           XNS0
      Thoracic 0PS4
         Magnetically Controlled Growth Rod(s)
           XNS4
         Posterior (Dynamic) Distraction Device
           XNS4
   Vocal Cord
      Left 0CSV
      Right 0CST

Resection

   Acetabulum
      Left 0QT50ZZ
      Right 0QT40ZZ
   Adenoids 0CTQ
   Ampulla of Vater 0FTC
   Anal Sphincter 0DTR

Resection — *continued*

   Anus 0DTQ
   Aortic Body 0GTD
   Appendix 0DTJ
   Auditory Ossicle
      Left 09TA
      Right 09T9
   Bladder 0TTB
   Bladder Neck 0TTC
   Bone
      Ethmoid
         Left 0NTG0ZZ
         Right 0NTF0ZZ
      Frontal 0NT10ZZ
      Hyoid 0NTX0ZZ
      Lacrimal
         Left 0NTJ0ZZ
         Right 0NTH0ZZ
      Nasal 0NTB0ZZ
      Occipital 0NT70ZZ
      Palatine
         Left 0NTL0ZZ
         Right 0NTK0ZZ
      Parietal
         Left 0NT40ZZ
         Right 0NT30ZZ
      Pelvic
         Left 0QT30ZZ
         Right 0QT20ZZ
      Sphenoid 0NTC0ZZ
      Temporal
         Left 0NT60ZZ
         Right 0NT50ZZ
      Zygomatic
         Left 0NTN0ZZ
         Right 0NTM0ZZ
   Breast
      Bilateral 0HTV0ZZ
      Left 0HTU0ZZ
      Right 0HTT0ZZ
      Supernumerary 0HTY0ZZ
   Bronchus
      Lingula 0BT9
      Lower Lobe
         Left 0BTB
         Right 0BT6
      Main
         Left 0BT7
         Right 0BT3
      Middle Lobe, Right 0BT5
      Upper Lobe
         Left 0BT8
         Right 0BT4
   Bursa and Ligament
      Abdomen
         Left 0MTJ
         Right 0MTH
      Ankle
         Left 0MTR
         Right 0MTQ
      Elbow
         Left 0MT4
         Right 0MT3
      Foot
         Left 0MTT
         Right 0MTS
      Hand
         Left 0MT8
         Right 0MT7
      Head and Neck 0MT0
      Hip
         Left 0MTM
         Right 0MTL
      Knee
         Left 0MTP
         Right 0MTN
      Lower Extremity
         Left 0MTW
         Right 0MTV
      Perineum 0MTK
      Rib(s) 0MTG
      Shoulder
         Left 0MT2
         Right 0MT1
      Spine
         Lower 0MTD
         Upper 0MTC
      Sternum 0MTF

Resection — *continued*

   Bursa and Ligament — *continued*
      Upper Extremity
         Left 0MTB
         Right 0MT9
      Wrist
         Left 0MT6
         Right 0MT5
   Carina 0BT2
   Carotid Bodies, Bilateral 0GT8
   Carotid Body
      Left 0GT6
      Right 0GT7
   Carpal
      Left 0PTN0ZZ
      Right 0PTM0ZZ
   Cecum 0DTH
   Cerebral Hemisphere 00T7
   Cervix 0UTC
   Chordae Tendineae 02T9
   Cisterna Chyli 07TL
   Clavicle
      Left 0PTB0ZZ
      Right 0PT90ZZ
   Clitoris 0UTJ
   Coccygeal Glomus 0GTB
   Coccyx 0QTS0ZZ
   Colon
      Ascending 0DTK
      Descending 0DTM
      Sigmoid 0DTN
      Transverse 0DTL
   Conduction Mechanism 02T8
   Cord
      Bilateral 0VTH
      Left 0VTG
      Right 0VTF
   Cornea
      Left 08T9XZZ
      Right 08T8XZZ
   Cul-de-sac 0UTF
   Diaphragm 0BTT
   Disc
      Cervical Vertebral 0RT30ZZ
      Cervicothoracic Vertebral 0RT50ZZ
      Lumbar Vertebral 0ST20ZZ
      Lumbosacral 0ST40ZZ
      Thoracic Vertebral 0RT90ZZ
      Thoracolumbar Vertebral 0RTB0ZZ
   Duct
      Common Bile 0FT9
      Cystic 0FT8
      Hepatic
         Common 0FT7
         Left 0FT6
         Right 0FT5
      Lacrimal
         Left 08TY
         Right 08TX
      Pancreatic 0FTD
         Accessory 0FTF
      Parotid
         Left 0CTC0ZZ
         Right 0CTB0ZZ
   Duodenum 0DT9
   Ear
      External
         Left 09T1
         Right 09T0
      Inner
         Left 09TE
         Right 09TD
      Middle
         Left 09T6
         Right 09T5
   Epididymis
      Bilateral 0VTL
      Left 0VTK
      Right 0VTJ
   Epiglottis 0CTR
   Esophagogastric Junction 0DT4
   Esophagus 0DT5
      Lower 0DT3
      Middle 0DT2
      Upper 0DT1
   Eustachian Tube
      Left 09TG
      Right 09TF

▽ **Subterms under main terms may continue to next column or page**

Resection — *continued*
  Parathyroid Gland — *continued*
    Multiple ØGTQ
    Superior
      Left ØGTM
      Right ØGTL
  Patella
    Left ØQTFØZZ
    Right ØQTDØZZ
  Penis ØVTS
  Pericardium Ø2TN
  Phalanx
    Finger
      Left ØPTVØZZ
      Right ØPTTØZZ
    Thumb
      Left ØPTSØZZ
      Right ØPTRØZZ
    Toe
      Left ØQTRØZZ
      Right ØQTQØZZ
  Pharynx ØCTM
  Pineal Body ØGT1
  Prepuce ØVTT
  Products of Conception, Ectopic 1ØT2
  Prostate ØVTØ
  Radius
    Left ØPTJØZZ
    Right ØPTHØZZ
  Rectum ØDTP
  Ribs
    1 to 2 ØPT1ØZZ
    3 or More ØPT2ØZZ
  Scapula
    Left ØPT6ØZZ
    Right ØPT5ØZZ
  Scrotum ØVT5
  Septum
    Atrial Ø2T5
    Nasal Ø9TM
    Ventricular Ø2TM
  Sinus
    Accessory Ø9TP
    Ethmoid
      Left Ø9TV
      Right Ø9TU
    Frontal
      Left Ø9TT
      Right Ø9TS
    Mastoid
      Left Ø9TC
      Right Ø9TB
    Maxillary
      Left Ø9TR
      Right Ø9TQ
    Sphenoid
      Left Ø9TX
      Right Ø9TW
  Spleen Ø7TP
  Sternum ØPTØØZZ
  Stomach ØDT6
    Pylorus ØDT7
  Tarsal
    Left ØQTMØZZ
    Right ØQTLØZZ
  Tendon
    Abdomen
      Left ØLTG
      Right ØLTF
    Ankle
      Left ØLTT
      Right ØLTS
    Foot
      Left ØLTW
      Right ØLTV
    Hand
      Left ØLT8
      Right ØLT7
    Head and Neck ØLTØ
    Hip
      Left ØLTK
      Right ØLTJ
    Knee
      Left ØLTR
      Right ØLTQ
    Lower Arm and Wrist
      Left ØLT6
      Right ØLT5

Resection — *continued*
  Tendon — *continued*
    Lower Leg
      Left ØLTP
      Right ØLTN
    Perineum ØLTH
    Shoulder
      Left ØLT2
      Right ØLT1
    Thorax
      Left ØLTD
      Right ØLTC
    Trunk
      Left ØLTB
      Right ØLT9
    Upper Arm
      Left ØLT4
      Right ØLT3
    Upper Leg
      Left ØLTM
      Right ØLTL
  Testis
    Bilateral ØVTC
    Left ØVTB
    Right ØVT9
  Thymus Ø7TM
  Thyroid Gland ØGTK
    Left Lobe ØGTG
    Right Lobe ØGTH
  Thyroid Gland Isthmus ØGTJ
  Tibia
    Left ØQTHØZZ
    Right ØQTGØZZ
  Toe Nail ØHTRXZZ
  Tongue ØCT7
  Tonsils ØCTP
  Tooth
    Lower ØCTXØZ
    Upper ØCTWØZ
  Trachea ØBT1
  Tunica Vaginalis
    Left ØVT7
    Right ØVT6
  Turbinate, Nasal Ø9TL
  Tympanic Membrane
    Left Ø9T8
    Right Ø9T7
  Ulna
    Left ØPTLØZZ
    Right ØPTKØZZ
  Ureter
    Left ØTT7
    Right ØTT6
  Urethra ØTTD
  Uterine Supporting Structure ØUT4
  Uterus ØUT9
  Uvula ØCTN
  Vagina ØUTG
  Valve, Pulmonary Ø2TH
  Vas Deferens
    Bilateral ØVTQ
    Left ØVTP
    Right ØVTN
  Vesicle
    Bilateral ØVT3
    Left ØVT2
    Right ØVT1
  Vitreous
    Left Ø8T53ZZ
    Right Ø8T43ZZ
  Vocal Cord
    Left ØCTV
    Right ØCTT
  Vulva ØUTM
Resection, Left ventricular outflow tract obstruction (LVOT) *see* Dilation, Ventricle, Left Ø27L
Resection, Subaortic membrane (Left ventricular outflow tract obstruction) *see* Dilation, Ventricle, Left Ø27L
Restoration, Cardiac, Single, Rhythm 5A22Ø4Z
RestoreAdvanced neurostimulator (SureScan) (MRI Safe) *use* Stimulator Generator, Multiple Array Rechargeable in ØJH
RestoreSensor neurostimulator (SureScan) (MRI Safe) *use* Stimulator Generator, Multiple Array Rechargeable in ØJH

RestoreUltra neurostimulator (SureScan) (MRI Safe) *use* Stimulator Generator, Multiple Array Rechargeable in ØJH
Restriction
  Ampulla of Vater ØFVC
  Anus ØDVQ
  Aorta
    Abdominal Ø4VØ
      Intraluminal Device, Branched or Fenestrated Ø4VØ
    Thoracic
      Ascending/Arch, Intraluminal Device, Branched or Fenestrated Ø2VX
      Descending, Intraluminal Device, Branched or Fenestrated Ø2VW
  Artery
    Anterior Tibial
      Left Ø4VQ
      Right Ø4VP
    Axillary
      Left Ø3V6
      Right Ø3V5
    Brachial
      Left Ø3V8
      Right Ø3V7
    Celiac Ø4V1
    Colic
      Left Ø4V7
      Middle Ø4V8
      Right Ø4V6
    Common Carotid
      Left Ø3VJ
      Right Ø3VH
    Common Iliac
      Left Ø4VD
      Right Ø4VC
    External Carotid
      Left Ø3VN
      Right Ø3VM
    External Iliac
      Left Ø4VJ
      Right Ø4VH
    Face Ø3VR
    Femoral
      Left Ø4VL
      Right Ø4VK
    Foot
      Left Ø4VW
      Right Ø4VV
    Gastric Ø4V2
    Hand
      Left Ø3VF
      Right Ø3VD
    Hepatic Ø4V3
    Inferior Mesenteric Ø4VB
    Innominate Ø3V2
    Internal Carotid
      Left Ø3VL
      Right Ø3VK
    Internal Iliac
      Left Ø4VF
      Right Ø4VE
    Internal Mammary
      Left Ø3V1
      Right Ø3VØ
    Intracranial Ø3VG
    Lower Ø4VY
    Peroneal
      Left Ø4VU
      Right Ø4VT
    Popliteal
      Left Ø4VN
      Right Ø4VM
    Posterior Tibial
      Left Ø4VS
      Right Ø4VR
    Pulmonary
      Left Ø2VR
      Right Ø2VQ
    Pulmonary Trunk Ø2VP
    Radial
      Left Ø3VC
      Right Ø3VB
    Renal
      Left Ø4VA
      Right Ø4V9
    Splenic Ø4V4
    Subclavian
      Left Ø3V4

Restriction — *continued*
  Artery — *continued*
    Subclavian — *continued*
      Right 03V3
    Superior Mesenteric 04V5
    Temporal
      Left 03VT
      Right 03VS
    Thyroid
      Left 03VV
      Right 03VU
    Ulnar
      Left 03VA
      Right 03V9
    Upper 03VY
    Vertebral
      Left 03VQ
      Right 03VP
  Bladder 0TVB
  Bladder Neck 0TVC
  Bronchus
    Lingula 0BV9
    Lower Lobe
      Left 0BVB
      Right 0BV6
    Main
      Left 0BV7
      Right 0BV3
    Middle Lobe, Right 0BV5
    Upper Lobe
      Left 0BV8
      Right 0BV4
  Carina 0BV2
  Cecum 0DVH
  Cervix 0UVC
  Cisterna Chyli 07VL
  Colon
    Ascending 0DVK
    Descending 0DVM
    Sigmoid 0DVN
    Transverse 0DVL
  Duct
    Common Bile 0FV9
    Cystic 0FV8
    Hepatic
      Common 0FV7
      Left 0FV6
      Right 0FV5
    Lacrimal
      Left 08VY
      Right 08VX
    Pancreatic 0FVD
      Accessory 0FVF
    Parotid
      Left 0CVC
      Right 0CVB
  Duodenum 0DV9
  Esophagogastric Junction 0DV4
  Esophagus 0DV5
    Lower 0DV3
    Middle 0DV2
    Upper 0DV1
  Heart 02VA
  Ileocecal Valve 0DVC
  Ileum 0DVB
  Intestine
    Large 0DVE
      Left 0DVG
      Right 0DVF
    Small 0DV8
  Jejunum 0DVA
  Kidney Pelvis
    Left 0TV4
    Right 0TV3
  Lymphatic
    Aortic 07VD
    Axillary
      Left 07V6
      Right 07V5
    Head 07V0
    Inguinal
      Left 07VJ
      Right 07VH
    Internal Mammary
      Left 07V9
      Right 07V8
    Lower Extremity
      Left 07VG
      Right 07VF

Restriction — *continued*
  Lymphatic — *continued*
    Mesenteric 07VB
    Neck
      Left 07V2
      Right 07V1
    Pelvis 07VC
    Thoracic Duct 07VK
    Thorax 07V7
    Upper Extremity
      Left 07V4
      Right 07V3
  Rectum 0DVP
  Stomach 0DV6
    Pylorus 0DV7
  Trachea 0BV1
  Ureter
    Left 0TV7
    Right 0TV6
  Urethra 0TVD
  Valve, Mitral 02VG
  Vein
    Axillary
      Left 05V8
      Right 05V7
    Azygos 05V0
    Basilic
      Left 05VC
      Right 05VB
    Brachial
      Left 05VA
      Right 05V9
    Cephalic
      Left 05VF
      Right 05VD
    Colic 06V7
    Common Iliac
      Left 06VD
      Right 06VC
    Esophageal 06V3
    External Iliac
      Left 06VG
      Right 06VF
    External Jugular
      Left 05VQ
      Right 05VP
    Face
      Left 05VV
      Right 05VT
    Femoral
      Left 06VN
      Right 06VM
    Foot
      Left 06VV
      Right 06VT
    Gastric 06V2
    Hand
      Left 05VH
      Right 05VG
    Hemiazygos 05V1
    Hepatic 06V4
    Hypogastric
      Left 06VJ
      Right 06VH
    Inferior Mesenteric 06V6
    Innominate
      Left 05V4
      Right 05V3
    Internal Jugular
      Left 05VN
      Right 05VM
    Intracranial 05VL
    Lower 06VY
    Portal 06V8
    Pulmonary
      Left 02VT
      Right 02VS
    Renal
      Left 06VB
      Right 06V9
    Saphenous
      Left 06VQ
      Right 06VP
    Splenic 06V1
    Subclavian
      Left 05V6
      Right 05V5
    Superior Mesenteric 06V5
    Upper 05VY

Restriction — *continued*
  Vein — *continued*
    Vertebral
      Left 05VS
      Right 05VR
    Vena Cava
      Inferior 06V0
      Superior 02VV
    Ventricle, Left 02VL
Resurfacing Device
  Removal of device from
    Left 0SPB0BZ
    Right 0SP90BZ
  Revision of device in
    Left 0SWB0BZ
    Right 0SW90BZ
  Supplement
    Left 0SUB0BZ
      Acetabular Surface 0SUE0BZ
      Femoral Surface 0SUS0BZ
    Right 0SU90BZ
      Acetabular Surface 0SUA0BZ
      Femoral Surface 0SUR0BZ
Resuscitation
  Cardiopulmonary *see* Assistance, Cardiac 5A02
  Cardioversion 5A2204Z
  Defibrillation 5A2204Z
  Endotracheal intubation *see* Insertion of device in, Trachea 0BH1
  External chest compression, manual 5A12012
  External chest compression, mechanical 5A1221J
  Pulmonary 5A19054
Resuscitative endovascular balloon occlusion of the aorta (REBOA)
  02LW3DJ
  04L03DJ
Resuture, Heart valve prosthesis *see* Revision of device in, Heart and Great Vessels 02W
Retained placenta, manual removal *see* Extraction, Products of Conception, Retained 10D1
RETHYMIC® *use* Engineered Allogeneic Thymus Tissue
Retraining
  Cardiac *see* Motor Treatment, Rehabilitation F07
  Vocational *see* Activities of Daily Living Treatment, Rehabilitation F08
Retrogasserian rhizotomy *see* Division, Nerve, Trigeminal 008K
Retroperitoneal cavity *use* Retroperitoneum
Retroperitoneal lymph node *use* Lymphatic, Aortic
Retroperitoneal space *use* Retroperitoneum
Retropharyngeal lymph node
  use Lymphatic, Left Neck
  use Lymphatic, Right Neck
Retropharyngeal space *use* Neck
Retropubic space *use* Pelvic Cavity
Reveal (LINQ) (DX) (XT) *use* Monitoring Device
Reverse total shoulder replacement *see* Replacement, Upper Joints 0RR
Reverse® Shoulder Prosthesis *use* Synthetic Substitute, Reverse Ball and Socket in 0RR
Revision
  Correcting a portion of existing device *see* Revision of device in
  Removal of device without replacement *see* Removal of device from
  Replacement of existing device
    see Removal of device from
    see Root operation to place new device, e.g., Insertion, Replacement, Supplement
Revision of device in
  Abdominal Wall 0WWF
  Acetabulum
    Left 0QW5
    Right 0QW4
  Anal Sphincter 0DWR
  Anus 0DWQ
  Artery
    Lower 04WY
    Upper 03WY
  Auditory Ossicle
    Left 09WA
    Right 09W9
  Back
    Lower 0WWL
    Upper 0WWK
  Bladder 0TWB
  Bone
    Facial 0NWW

Revision of device in — continued
Bone — continued
 Lower 0QWY
 Nasal 0NWB
 Pelvic
  Left 0QW3
  Right 0QW2
 Upper 0PWY
Bone Marrow 07WT
Brain 00W0
Breast
 Left 0HWU
 Right 0HWT
Bursa and Ligament
 Lower 0MWY
 Upper 0MWX
Carpal
 Left 0PWN
 Right 0PWM
Cavity, Cranial 0WW1
Cerebral Ventricle 00W6
Chest Wall 0WW8
Cisterna Chyli 07WL
Clavicle
 Left 0PWB
 Right 0PW9
Coccyx 0QWS
Diaphragm 0BWT
Disc
 Cervical Vertebral 0RW3
 Cervicothoracic Vertebral 0RW5
 Lumbar Vertebral 0SW2
 Lumbosacral 0SW4
 Thoracic Vertebral 0RW9
 Thoracolumbar Vertebral 0RWB
Duct
 Hepatobiliary 0FWB
 Pancreatic 0FWD
Ear
 Inner
  Left 09WE
  Right 09WD
 Left 09WJ
 Right 09WH
Epididymis and Spermatic Cord 0VWM
Esophagus 0DW5
Extremity
 Lower
  Left 0YWB
  Right 0YW9
 Upper
  Left 0XW7
  Right 0XW6
Eye
 Left 08W1
 Right 08W0
Face 0WW2
Fallopian Tube 0UW8
Femoral Shaft
 Left 0QW9
 Right 0QW8
Femur
 Lower
  Left 0QWC
  Right 0QWB
 Upper
  Left 0QW7
  Right 0QW6
Fibula
 Left 0QWK
 Right 0QWJ
Finger Nail 0HWQX
Gallbladder 0FW4
Gastrointestinal Tract 0WWP
Genitourinary Tract 0WWR
Gland
 Adrenal 0GW5
 Endocrine 0GWS
 Pituitary 0GW0
 Salivary 0CWA
Glenoid Cavity
 Left 0PW8
 Right 0PW7
Great Vessel 02WY
Hair 0HWSX
Head 0WW0
Heart 02WA
Humeral Head
 Left 0PWD

Revision of device in — continued
Humeral Head — continued
 Right 0PWC
Humeral Shaft
 Left 0PWG
 Right 0PWF
Intestinal Tract
 Lower Intestinal Tract 0DWD
 Upper Intestinal Tract 0DW0
Intestine
 Large 0DWE
 Small 0DW8
Jaw
 Lower 0WW5
 Upper 0WW4
Joint
 Acromioclavicular
  Left 0RWH
  Right 0RWG
 Ankle
  Left 0SWG
  Right 0SWF
 Carpal
  Left 0RWR
  Right 0RWQ
 Carpometacarpal
  Left 0RWT
  Right 0RWS
 Cervical Vertebral 0RW1
 Cervicothoracic Vertebral 0RW4
 Coccygeal 0SW6
 Elbow
  Left 0RWM
  Right 0RWL
 Finger Phalangeal
  Left 0RWX
  Right 0RWW
 Hip
  Left 0SWB
   Acetabular Surface 0SWE
   Femoral Surface 0SWS
  Right 0SW9
   Acetabular Surface 0SWA
   Femoral Surface 0SWR
 Knee
  Left 0SWD
   Femoral Surface 0SWU
   Tibial Surface 0SWW
  Right 0SWC
   Femoral Surface 0SWT
   Tibial Surface 0SWV
 Lumbar Vertebral 0SW0
 Lumbosacral 0SW3
 Metacarpophalangeal
  Left 0RWV
  Right 0RWU
 Metatarsal-Phalangeal
  Left 0SWN
  Right 0SWM
 Occipital-cervical 0RW0
 Sacrococcygeal 0SW5
 Sacroiliac
  Left 0SW8
  Right 0SW7
 Shoulder
  Left 0RWK
  Right 0RWJ
 Sternoclavicular
  Left 0RWF
  Right 0RWE
 Tarsal
  Left 0SWJ
  Right 0SWH
 Tarsometatarsal
  Left 0SWL
  Right 0SWK
 Temporomandibular
  Left 0RWD
  Right 0RWC
 Thoracic Vertebral 0RW6
 Thoracolumbar Vertebral 0RWA
 Toe Phalangeal
  Left 0SWQ
  Right 0SWP
 Wrist
  Left 0RWP
  Right 0RWN
Kidney 0TW5
Larynx 0CWS

Revision of device in — continued
Lens
 Left 08WK
 Right 08WJ
Liver 0FW0
Lung
 Left 0BWL
 Right 0BWK
Lymphatic 07WN
 Thoracic Duct 07WK
Mediastinum 0WWC
Mesentery 0DWV
Metacarpal
 Left 0PWQ
 Right 0PWP
Metatarsal
 Left 0QWP
 Right 0QWN
Mouth and Throat 0CWY
Muscle
 Extraocular
  Left 08WM
  Right 08WL
 Lower 0KWY
 Upper 0KWX
Nasal Mucosa and Soft Tissue 09WK
Neck 0WW6
Nerve
 Cranial 00WE
 Peripheral 01WY
Omentum 0DWU
Ovary 0UW3
Pancreas 0FWG
Parathyroid Gland 0GWR
Patella
 Left 0QWF
 Right 0QWD
Pelvic Cavity 0WWJ
Penis 0VWS
Pericardial Cavity 0WWD
Perineum
 Female 0WWN
 Male 0WWM
Peritoneal Cavity 0WWG
Peritoneum 0DWW
Phalanx
 Finger
  Left 0PWV
  Right 0PWT
 Thumb
  Left 0PWS
  Right 0PWR
 Toe
  Left 0QWR
  Right 0QWQ
Pineal Body 0GW1
Pleura 0BWQ
Pleural Cavity
 Left 0WWB
 Right 0WW9
Prostate and Seminal Vesicles 0VW4
Radius
 Left 0PWJ
 Right 0PWH
Respiratory Tract 0WWQ
Retroperitoneum 0WWH
Ribs
 1 to 2 0PW1
 3 or More 0PW2
Sacrum 0QW1
Scapula
 Left 0PW6
 Right 0PW5
Scrotum and Tunica Vaginalis 0VW8
Septum
 Atrial 02W5
 Ventricular 02WM
Sinus 09WY
Skin 0HWPX
Skull 0NW0
Spinal Canal 00WU
Spinal Cord 00WV
Spleen 07WP
Sternum 0PW0
Stomach 0DW6
Subcutaneous Tissue and Fascia
 Head and Neck 0JWS
 Lower Extremity 0JWW
 Trunk 0JWT

Revision of device in — *continued*
  Subcutaneous Tissue and Fascia — *continued*
    Upper Extremity ØJWV
  Tarsal
    Left ØQWM
    Right ØQWL
  Tendon
    Lower ØLWY
    Upper ØLWX
  Testis ØVWD
  Thymus Ø7WM
  Thyroid Gland ØGWK
  Tibia
    Left ØQWH
    Right ØQWG
  Toe Nail ØHWRX
  Trachea ØBW1
  Tracheobronchial Tree ØBWØ
  Tympanic Membrane
    Left Ø9W8
    Right Ø9W7
  Ulna
    Left ØPWL
    Right ØPWK
  Ureter ØTW9
  Urethra ØTWD
  Uterus and Cervix ØUWD
  Vagina and Cul-de-sac ØUWH
  Valve
    Aortic Ø2WF
    Mitral Ø2WG
    Pulmonary Ø2WH
    Tricuspid Ø2WJ
  Vas Deferens ØVWR
  Vein
    Azygos Ø5WØ
    Innominate
      Left Ø5W4
      Right Ø5W3
    Lower Ø6WY
    Upper Ø5WY
  Vertebra
    Cervical ØPW3
    Lumbar ØQWØ
    Thoracic ØPW4
  Vulva ØUWM
Revo MRI™ SureScan® pacemaker *use* Pacemaker, Dual Chamber in ØJH
rhBMP-2 *use* Recombinant Bone Morphogenetic Protein
Rheos® System device *use* Stimulator Generator in Subcutaneous Tissue and Fascia
Rheos® System lead *use* Stimulator Lead in Upper Arteries
Rhinopharynx *use* Nasopharynx
Rhinoplasty
  see Alteration, Nasal Mucosa and Soft Tissue Ø9ØK
  see Repair, Nasal Mucosa and Soft Tissue Ø9QK
  see Replacement, Nasal Mucosa and Soft Tissue Ø9RK
  see Supplement, Nasal Mucosa and Soft Tissue Ø9UK
Rhinorrhaphy *see* Repair, Nasal Mucosa and Soft Tissue Ø9QK
Rhinoscopy Ø9JKXZZ
Rhizotomy
  see Division, Central Nervous System and Cranial Nerves ØØ8
  see Division, Peripheral Nervous System Ø18
Rhomboid major muscle
  use Trunk Muscle, Left
  use Trunk Muscle, Right
Rhomboid minor muscle
  use Trunk Muscle, Left
  use Trunk Muscle, Right
Rhythm electrocardiogram *see* Measurement, Cardiac 4AØ2
Rhytidectomy *see* Alteration, Face ØWØ2
Right ascending lumbar vein *use* Azygos Vein
Right atrioventricular valve *use* Tricuspid Valve
Right auricular appendix *use* Atrium, Right
Right colic vein *use* Colic Vein
Right coronary sulcus *use* Heart, Right
Right gastric artery *use* Gastric Artery
Right gastroepiploic vein *use* Superior Mesenteric Vein
Right inferior phrenic vein *use* Inferior Vena Cava

Right inferior pulmonary vein *use* Pulmonary Vein, Right
Right jugular trunk *use* Lymphatic, Right Neck
Right lateral ventricle *use* Cerebral Ventricle
Right lymphatic duct *use* Lymphatic, Right Neck
Right ovarian vein *use* Inferior Vena Cava
Right second lumbar vein *use* Inferior Vena Cava
Right subclavian trunk *use* Lymphatic, Right Neck
Right subcostal vein *use* Azygos Vein
Right superior pulmonary vein *use* Pulmonary Vein, Right
Right suprarenal vein *use* Inferior Vena Cava
Right testicular vein *use* Inferior Vena Cava
Rima glottidis *use* Larynx
Risorius muscle *use* Facial Muscle
RNS System lead *use* Neurostimulator Lead in Central Nervous System and Cranial Nerves
RNS system neurostimulator generator *use* Neurostimulator Generator in Head and Facial Bones
Robotic Assisted Procedure
  Extremity
    Lower 8EØY
    Upper 8EØX
  Head and Neck Region 8EØ9
  Trunk Region 8EØW
Robotic Waterjet Ablation, Destruction, Prostate XV5Ø8A4
Rotation of fetal head
  Forceps 1ØSØ7ZZ
  Manual 1ØSØXZZ
Round ligament of uterus *use* Uterine Supporting Structure
Round window
  use Inner Ear, Left
  use Inner Ear, Right
Roux-en-Y operation
  see Bypass, Gastrointestinal System ØD1
  see Bypass, Hepatobiliary System and Pancreas ØF1
Rupture
  Adhesions *see* Release
  Fluid collection *see* Drainage
Ruxolitinib XWØDXT5
RYBREVANT™ *use* Amivantamab Monoclonal Antibody

S

Sacral ganglion *use* Sacral Sympathetic Nerve
Sacral lymph node *use* Lymphatic, Pelvis
Sacral nerve modulation (SNM) lead *use* Stimulator Lead in Urinary System
Sacral neuromodulation lead *use* Stimulator Lead in Urinary System
Sacral splanchnic nerve *use* Sacral Sympathetic Nerve
Sacrectomy *see* Excision, Lower Bones ØQB
Sacrococcygeal ligament *use* Lower Spine Bursa and Ligament
Sacrococcygeal symphysis *use* Sacrococcygeal Joint
Sacroiliac ligament *use* Lower Spine Bursa and Ligament
Sacrospinous ligament *use* Lower Spine Bursa and Ligament
Sacrotuberous ligament *use* Lower Spine Bursa and Ligament
Salpingectomy
  see Excision, Female Reproductive System ØUB
  see Resection, Female Reproductive System ØUT
Salpingolysis *see* Release, Female Reproductive System ØUN
Salpingopexy
  see Repair, Female Reproductive System ØUQ
  see Reposition, Female Reproductive System ØUS
Salpingopharyngeus muscle *use* Tongue, Palate, Pharynx Muscle
Salpingoplasty
  see Repair, Female Reproductive System ØUQ
  see Supplement, Female Reproductive System ØUU
Salpingorrhaphy *see* Repair, Female Reproductive System ØUQ
Salpingoscopy ØUJ88ZZ
Salpingostomy *see* Drainage, Female Reproductive System ØU9
Salpingotomy *see* Drainage, Female Reproductive System ØU9
Salpinx
  use Fallopian Tube, Left

Salpinx — *continued*
  use Fallopian Tube, Right
Saphenous nerve *use* Femoral Nerve
SAPIEN transcatheter aortic valve *use* Zooplastic Tissue in Heart and Great Vessels
Sarilumab XWØ
SARS-CoV-2 Antibody Detection, Serum/Plasma Nanoparticle Fluorescence XXE5XV7
SARS-CoV-2 Polymerase Chain Reaction, Nasopharyngeal Fluid XXE97U7
Sartorius muscle
  use Upper Leg Muscle, Left
  use Upper Leg Muscle, Right
Satralizumab-mwge XWØ1397
SAVAL below-the-knee (BTK) drug-eluting stent system
  use Intraluminal Device, Sustained Release Drug-eluting in New Technology
  use Intraluminal Device, Sustained Release Drug-eluting, Two in New Technology
  use Intraluminal Device, Sustained Release Drug-eluting, Three in New Technology
  use Intraluminal Device, Sustained Release Drug-eluting, Four or More in New Technology
Scalene muscle
  use Neck Muscle, Left
  use Neck Muscle, Right
Scan
  Computerized Tomography (CT) *see* Computerized Tomography (CT Scan)
  Radioisotope *see* Planar Nuclear Medicine Imaging
Scaphoid bone
  use Carpal, Left
  use Carpal, Right
Scapholunate ligament
  use Wrist Bursa and Ligament, Left
  use Wrist Bursa and Ligament, Right
Scaphotrapezium ligament
  use Hand Bursa and Ligament, Left
  use Hand Bursa and Ligament, Right
Scapulectomy
  see Excision, Upper Bones ØPB
  see Resection, Upper Bones ØPT
Scapulopexy
  see Repair, Upper Bones ØPQ
  see Reposition, Upper Bones ØPS
Scarpa's (vestibular) ganglion *use* Acoustic Nerve
Sclerectomy *see* Excision, Eye Ø8B
Sclerotherapy, mechanical *see* Destruction
Sclerotherapy, via injection of sclerosing agent
  see Introduction, Destructive Agent
Sclerotomy *see* Drainage, Eye Ø89
Scrotectomy
  see Excision, Male Reproductive System ØVB
  see Resection, Male Reproductive System ØVT
Scrotoplasty
  see Repair, Male Reproductive System ØVQ
  see Supplement, Male Reproductive System ØVU
Scrotorrhaphy *see* Repair, Male Reproductive System ØVQ
Scrototomy *see* Drainage, Male Reproductive System ØV9
Sebaceous gland *use* Skin
Second cranial nerve *use* Optic Nerve
Section, cesarean *see* Extraction, Pregnancy 1ØD
Secura (DR) (VR) *use* Defibrillator Generator in ØJH
Sella turcica *use* Sphenoid Bone
Semicircular canal
  use Inner Ear, Left
  use Inner Ear, Right
Semimembranosus muscle
  use Upper Leg Muscle, Left
  use Upper Leg Muscle, Right
Semitendinosus muscle
  use Upper Leg Muscle, Left
  use Upper Leg Muscle, Right
Sentinel™ Cerebral Protection System (CPS) X2A5312
Seprafilm *use* Adhesion Barrier
Septal cartilage *use* Nasal Septum
Septectomy
  see Excision, Ear, Nose, Sinus Ø9B
  see Excision, Heart and Great Vessels Ø2B
  see Resection, Ear, Nose, Sinus Ø9T
  see Resection, Heart and Great Vessels Ø2T
SeptiCyte® RAPID XXE5X38

Septoplasty
 see Repair, Ear, Nose, Sinus Ø9Q
 see Repair, Heart and Great Vessels Ø2Q
 see Replacement, Ear, Nose, Sinus Ø9R
 see Replacement, Heart and Great Vessels Ø2R
 see Reposition, Ear, Nose, Sinus Ø9S
 see Supplement, Ear, Nose, Sinus Ø9U
 see Supplement, Heart and Great Vessels Ø2U
Septostomy, balloon atrial Ø2163Z7
Septotomy *see* Drainage, Ear, Nose, Sinus Ø99
Sequestrectomy, bone *see* Extirpation
Serratus anterior muscle
 use Thorax Muscle, Left
 use Thorax Muscle, Right
Serratus posterior muscle
 use Trunk Muscle, Left
 use Trunk Muscle, Right
Seventh cranial nerve *use* Facial Nerve
Shapshot_NIR 8E02XDZ
Sheffield hybrid external fixator
 use External Fixation Device, Hybrid in ØPH
 use External Fixation Device, Hybrid in ØPS
 use External Fixation Device, Hybrid in ØQH
 use External Fixation Device, Hybrid in ØQS
Sheffield ring external fixator
 use External Fixation Device, Ring in ØPH
 use External Fixation Device, Ring in ØPS
 use External Fixation Device, Ring in ØQH
 use External Fixation Device, Ring in ØQS
Shirodkar cervical cerclage ØUVC7ZZ
Shock Wave Therapy, Musculoskeletal 6A93
Shockwave Intravascular Lithotripsy (Shockwave IVL) *see* Fragmentation
Short gastric artery *use* Splenic Artery
Shortening
 see Excision
 see Repair
 see Reposition
Shunt creation *see* Bypass
Sialoadenectomy
 Complete *see* Resection, Mouth and Throat ØCT
 Partial *see* Excision, Mouth and Throat ØCB
Sialodochoplasty
 see Repair, Mouth and Throat ØCQ
 see Replacement, Mouth and Throat ØCR
 see Supplement, Mouth and Throat ØCU
Sialoectomy
 see Excision, Mouth and Throat ØCB
 see Resection, Mouth and Throat ØCT
Sialography *see* Plain Radiography, Ear, Nose, Mouth and Throat B90
Sialolithotomy *see* Extirpation, Mouth and Throat ØCC
S-ICD™ lead *use* Subcutaneous Defibrillator Lead in Subcutaneous Tissue and Fascia
Sigmoid artery *use* Inferior Mesenteric Artery
Sigmoid flexure *use* Sigmoid Colon
Sigmoid vein *use* Inferior Mesenteric Vein
Sigmoidectomy
 see Excision, Gastrointestinal System ØDB
 see Resection, Gastrointestinal System ØDT
Sigmoidorrhaphy *see* Repair, Gastrointestinal System ØDQ
Sigmoidoscopy ØDJD8ZZ
Sigmoidotomy *see* Drainage, Gastrointestinal System ØD9
Single lead pacemaker (atrium) (ventricle) *use* Pacemaker, Single Chamber in ØJH
Single lead rate responsive pacemaker (atrium) (ventricle) *use* Pacemaker, Single Chamber Rate Responsive in ØJH
Single-use Duodenoscope XFJ
Single-use Oversleeve with Intraoperative Colonic Irrigation XDPH8K7
Sinoatrial node *use* Conduction Mechanism
Sinogram
 Abdominal Wall *see* Fluoroscopy, Abdomen and Pelvis BW11
 Chest Wall *see* Plain Radiography, Chest BWØ3
 Retroperitoneum *see* Fluoroscopy, Abdomen and Pelvis BW11
Sinus venosus *use* Atrium, Right
Sinusectomy
 see Excision, Ear, Nose, Sinus Ø9B
 see Resection, Ear, Nose, Sinus Ø9T
Sinusoscopy Ø9JY4ZZ
Sinusotomy *see* Drainage, Ear, Nose, Sinus Ø99

Sirolimus-eluting coronary stent *use* Intraluminal Device, Drug-eluting in Heart and Great Vessels
Sixth cranial nerve *use* Abducens Nerve
Size reduction, breast *see* Excision, Skin and Breast ØHB
SJM Biocor® Stented Valve System *use* Zooplastic Tissue in Heart and Great Vessels
Skene's (paraurethral) gland *use* Vestibular Gland
Sling
 Fascial, orbicularis muscle (mouth) *see* Supplement, Muscle, Facial ØKU1
 Levator muscle, for urethral suspension *see* Reposition, Bladder Neck ØTSC
 Pubococcygeal, for urethral suspension *see* Reposition, Bladder Neck ØTSC
 Rectum *see* Reposition, Rectum ØDSP
Small bowel series *see* Fluoroscopy, Bowel, Small BD13
Small saphenous vein
 use Saphenous Vein, Left
 use Saphenous Vein, Right
Snapshot_NIR 8E02XDZ
Snaring, polyp, colon *see* Excision, Gastrointestinal System ØDB
Solar (celiac) plexus *use* Abdominal Sympathetic Nerve
Soleus muscle
 use Lower Leg Muscle, Left
 use Lower Leg Muscle, Right
Soliris® *use* Eculizumab
Spacer
 Insertion of device in
  Disc
   Lumbar Vertebral ØSH2
   Lumbosacral ØSH4
  Joint
   Acromioclavicular
    Left ØRHH
    Right ØRHG
   Ankle
    Left ØSHG
    Right ØSHF
   Carpal
    Left ØRHR
    Right ØRHQ
   Carpometacarpal
    Left ØRHT
    Right ØRHS
   Cervical Vertebral ØRH1
   Cervicothoracic Vertebral ØRH4
   Coccygeal ØSH6
   Elbow
    Left ØRHM
    Right ØRHL
   Finger Phalangeal
    Left ØRHX
    Right ØRHW
   Hip
    Left ØSHB
    Right ØSH9
   Knee
    Left ØSHD
    Right ØSHC
   Lumbar Vertebral ØSHØ
   Lumbosacral ØSH3
   Metacarpophalangeal
    Left ØRHV
    Right ØRHU
   Metatarsal-Phalangeal
    Left ØSHN
    Right ØSHM
   Occipital-cervical ØRHØ
   Sacrococcygeal ØSH5
   Sacroiliac
    Left ØSH8
    Right ØSH7
   Shoulder
    Left ØRHK
    Right ØRHJ
   Sternoclavicular
    Left ØRHF
    Right ØRHE
   Tarsal
    Left ØSHJ
    Right ØSHH
   Tarsometatarsal
    Left ØSHL
    Right ØSHK

Spacer — *continued*
 Insertion of device in — *continued*
  Joint — *continued*
   Temporomandibular
    Left ØRHD
    Right ØRHC
   Thoracic Vertebral ØRH6
   Thoracolumbar Vertebral ØRHA
   Toe Phalangeal
    Left ØSHQ
    Right ØSHP
   Wrist
    Left ØRHP
    Right ØRHN
 Removal of device from
  Acromioclavicular
   Left ØRPH
   Right ØRPG
  Ankle
   Left ØSPG
   Right ØSPF
  Carpal
   Left ØRPR
   Right ØRPQ
  Carpometacarpal
   Left ØRPT
   Right ØRPS
  Cervical Vertebral ØRP1
  Cervicothoracic Vertebral ØRP4
  Coccygeal ØSP6
  Elbow
   Left ØRPM
   Right ØRPL
  Finger Phalangeal
   Left ØRPX
   Right ØRPW
  Hip
   Left ØSPB
   Right ØSP9
  Knee
   Left ØSPD
   Right ØSPC
  Lumbar Vertebral ØSPØ
  Lumbosacral ØSP3
  Metacarpophalangeal
   Left ØRPV
   Right ØRPU
  Metatarsal-Phalangeal
   Left ØSPN
   Right ØSPM
  Occipital-cervical ØRPØ
  Sacrococcygeal ØSP5
  Sacroiliac
   Left ØSP8
   Right ØSP7
  Shoulder
   Left ØRPK
   Right ØRPJ
  Sternoclavicular
   Left ØRPF
   Right ØRPE
  Tarsal
   Left ØSPJ
   Right ØSPH
  Tarsometatarsal
   Left ØSPL
   Right ØSPK
  Temporomandibular
   Left ØRPD
   Right ØRPC
  Thoracic Vertebral ØRP6
  Thoracolumbar Vertebral ØRPA
  Toe Phalangeal
   Left ØSPQ
   Right ØSPP
  Wrist
   Left ØRPP
   Right ØRPN
 Revision of device in
  Acromioclavicular
   Left ØRWH
   Right ØRWG
  Ankle
   Left ØSWG
   Right ØSWF
  Carpal
   Left ØRWR
   Right ØRWQ

Spacer — *continued*
  Revision of device in — *continued*
    Carpometacarpal
      Left ØRWT
      Right ØRWS
    Cervical Vertebral ØRW1
    Cervicothoracic Vertebral ØRW4
    Coccygeal ØSW6
    Elbow
      Left ØRWM
      Right ØRWL
    Finger Phalangeal
      Left ØRWX
      Right ØRWW
    Hip
      Left ØSWB
      Right ØSW9
    Knee
      Left ØSWD
      Right ØSWC
    Lumbar Vertebral ØSWØ
    Lumbosacral ØSW3
    Metacarpophalangeal
      Left ØRWV
      Right ØRWU
    Metatarsal-Phalangeal
      Left ØSWN
      Right ØSWM
    Occipital-cervical ØRWØ
    Sacrococcygeal ØSW5
    Sacroiliac
      Left ØSW8
      Right ØSW7
    Shoulder
      Left ØRWK
      Right ØRWJ
    Sternoclavicular
      Left ØRWF
      Right ØRWE
    Tarsal
      Left ØSWJ
      Right ØSWH
    Tarsometatarsal
      Left ØSWL
      Right ØSWK
    Temporomandibular
      Left ØRWD
      Right ØRWC
    Thoracic Vertebral ØRW6
    Thoracolumbar Vertebral ØRWA
    Toe Phalangeal
      Left ØSWQ
      Right ØSWP
    Wrist
      Left ØRWP
      Right ØRWN
Spacer, Articulating (Antibiotic) *use* Articulating Spacer in Lower Joints
Spacer, Static (Antibiotic) *use* Spacer in Lower Joints
Spectroscopy
  Intravascular Near Infrared 8E023DZ
  Near Infrared *see* Physiological Systems and Anatomical Regions 8E0
Speech Assessment F00
Speech therapy *see* Speech Treatment, Rehabilitation F06
Speech Treatment F06
Spesolimab Monoclonal Antibody XW0
Sphenoidectomy
  see Excision, Ear, Nose, Sinus 09B
  see Excision, Head and Facial Bones ØNB
  see Resection, Ear, Nose, Sinus 09T
  see Resection, Head and Facial Bones ØNT
Sphenoidotomy *see* Drainage, Ear, Nose, Sinus 099
Sphenomandibular ligament *use* Head and Neck Bursa and Ligament
Sphenopalatine (pterygopalatine) ganglion *use* Head and Neck Sympathetic Nerve
Sphincterorrhaphy, anal *see* Repair, Anal Sphincter ØDQR
Sphincterotomy, anal
  see Division, Anal Sphincter ØD8R
  see Drainage, Anal Sphincter ØD9R
Spinal cord neurostimulator lead *use* Neurostimulator Lead in Central Nervous System and Cranial Nerves

Spinal growth rods, magnetically controlled *use* Magnetically Controlled Growth Rod(s) in New Technology
Spinal nerve, cervical *use* Cervical Nerve
Spinal nerve, lumbar *use* Lumbar Nerve
Spinal nerve, sacral *use* Sacral Nerve
Spinal nerve, thoracic *use* Thoracic Nerve
Spinal Stabilization Device
  Facet Replacement
    Cervical Vertebral ØRH1
    Cervicothoracic Vertebral ØRH4
    Lumbar Vertebral ØSHØ
    Lumbosacral ØSH3
    Occipital-cervical ØRHØ
    Thoracic Vertebral ØRH6
    Thoracolumbar Vertebral ØRHA
  Interspinous Process
    Cervical Vertebral ØRH1
    Cervicothoracic Vertebral ØRH4
    Lumbar Vertebral ØSHØ
    Lumbosacral ØSH3
    Occipital-cervical ØRHØ
    Thoracic Vertebral ØRH6
    Thoracolumbar Vertebral ØRHA
  Pedicle-Based
    Cervical Vertebral ØRH1
    Cervicothoracic Vertebral ØRH4
    Lumbar Vertebral ØSHØ
    Lumbosacral ØSH3
    Occipital-cervical ØRHØ
    Thoracic Vertebral ØRH6
    Thoracolumbar Vertebral ØRHA
SpineJack® system *use* Synthetic Substitute, Mechanically Expandable (Paired) in New Technology
Spinous process
  use Cervical Vertebra
  use Lumbar Vertebra
  use Thoracic Vertebra
Spiral ganglion *use* Acoustic Nerve
Spiration IBV™ Valve System *use* Intraluminal Device, Endobronchial Valve in Respiratory System
Splenectomy
  see Excision, Lymphatic and Hemic Systems 07B
  see Resection, Lymphatic and Hemic Systems 07T
Splenic flexure *use* Transverse Colon
Splenic plexus *use* Abdominal Sympathetic Nerve
Splenius capitis muscle *use* Head Muscle
Splenius cervicis muscle
  use Neck Muscle, Left
  use Neck Muscle, Right
Splenolysis *see* Release, Lymphatic and Hemic Systems 07N
Splenopexy
  see Repair, Lymphatic and Hemic Systems 07Q
  see Reposition, Lymphatic and Hemic Systems 07S
Splenoplasty *see* Repair, Lymphatic and Hemic Systems 07Q
Splenorrhaphy *see* Repair, Lymphatic and Hemic Systems 07Q
Splenotomy *see* Drainage, Lymphatic and Hemic Systems 079
Splinting, musculoskeletal *see* Immobilization, Anatomical Regions 2W3
SPRAVATO™ *use* Esketamine Hydrochloride
SPY PINPOINT fluorescence imaging system
  see Monitoring, Physiological Systems 4A1
  see Other Imaging, Hepatobiliary System and Pancreas BF5
SPY system intraoperative fluorescence cholangiography *see* Other Imaging, Hepatobiliary System and Pancreas BF5
SPY system intravascular fluorescence angiography *see* Monitoring, Physiological Systems 4A1
SSO2 (Supersaturated Oxygen) therapy, cardiac intra-arterial 5A0222C
Staged hepatectomy
  see Division, Hepatobiliary System and Pancreas ØF8
  see Resection, Hepatobiliary System and Pancreas ØFT
Stapedectomy
  see Excision, Ear, Nose, Sinus 09B
  see Resection, Ear, Nose, Sinus 09T
Stapediolysis *see* Release, Ear, Nose, Sinus 09N
Stapedioplasty
  see Repair, Ear, Nose, Sinus 09Q
  see Replacement, Ear, Nose, Sinus 09R

Stapedioplasty — *continued*
  see Supplement, Ear, Nose, Sinus 09U
Stapedotomy *see* Drainage, Ear, Nose, Sinus 099
Stapes
  use Auditory Ossicle, Left
  use Auditory Ossicle, Right
Static Spacer (Antibiotic) *use* Spacer in Lower Joints
STELARA® *use* Other New Technology Therapeutic Substance
Stellate ganglion *use* Head and Neck Sympathetic Nerve
Stem cell transplant *see* Transfusion, Circulatory 302
Stensen's duct
  use Parotid Duct, Left
  use Parotid Duct, Right
Stent, intraluminal (cardiovascular) (gastrointestinal) (hepatobiliary) (urinary) *use* Intraluminal Device
Stent retriever thrombectomy *see* Extirpation, Upper Arteries 03C
Stented tissue valve *use* Zooplastic Tissue in Heart and Great Vessels
Stereotactic Radiosurgery
  Abdomen DW23
  Adrenal Gland DG22
  Bile Ducts DF22
  Bladder DT22
  Bone Marrow D720
  Brain D020
  Brain Stem D021
  Breast
    Left DM20
    Right DM21
  Bronchus DB21
  Cervix DU21
  Chest DW22
  Chest Wall DB27
  Colon DD25
  Diaphragm DB28
  Duodenum DD22
  Ear D920
  Esophagus DD20
  Eye D820
  Gallbladder DF21
  Gamma Beam
    Abdomen DW23JZZ
    Adrenal Gland DG22JZZ
    Bile Ducts DF22JZZ
    Bladder DT22JZZ
    Bone Marrow D720JZZ
    Brain D020JZZ
    Brain Stem D021JZZ
    Breast
      Left DM20JZZ
      Right DM21JZZ
    Bronchus DB21JZZ
    Cervix DU21JZZ
    Chest DW22JZZ
    Chest Wall DB27JZZ
    Colon DD25JZZ
    Diaphragm DB28JZZ
    Duodenum DD22JZZ
    Ear D920JZZ
    Esophagus DD20JZZ
    Eye D820JZZ
    Gallbladder DF21JZZ
    Gland
      Adrenal DG22JZZ
      Parathyroid DG24JZZ
      Pituitary DG20JZZ
      Thyroid DG25JZZ
    Glands, Salivary D926JZZ
    Head and Neck DW21JZZ
    Ileum DD24JZZ
    Jejunum DD23JZZ
    Kidney DT20JZZ
    Larynx D92BJZZ
    Liver DF20JZZ
    Lung DB22JZZ
    Lymphatics
      Abdomen D726JZZ
      Axillary D724JZZ
      Inguinal D728JZZ
      Neck D723JZZ
      Pelvis D727JZZ
      Thorax D725JZZ
    Mediastinum DB26JZZ
    Mouth D924JZZ

▼ **Subterms under main terms may continue to next column or page**

Stereotactic Radiosurgery — *continued*
Gamma Beam — *continued*
Nasopharynx D92DJZZ
Neck and Head DW21JZZ
Nerve, Peripheral D027JZZ
Nose D921JZZ
Ovary DU20JZZ
Palate
Hard D928JZZ
Soft D929JZZ
Pancreas DF23JZZ
Parathyroid Gland DG24JZZ
Pelvic Region DW26JZZ
Pharynx D92CJZZ
Pineal Body DG21JZZ
Pituitary Gland DG20JZZ
Pleura DB25JZZ
Prostate DV20JZZ
Rectum DD27JZZ
Sinuses D927JZZ
Spinal Cord D026JZZ
Spleen D722JZZ
Stomach DD21JZZ
Testis DV21JZZ
Thymus D721JZZ
Thyroid Gland DG25JZZ
Tongue D925JZZ
Trachea DB20JZZ
Ureter DT21JZZ
Urethra DT23JZZ
Uterus DU22JZZ
Gland
Adrenal DG22
Parathyroid DG24
Pituitary DG20
Thyroid DG25
Glands, Salivary D926
Head and Neck DW21
Ileum DD24
Jejunum DD23
Kidney DT20
Larynx D92B
Liver DF20
Lung DB22
Lymphatics
Abdomen D726
Axillary D724
Inguinal D728
Neck D723
Pelvis D727
Thorax D725
Mediastinum DB26
Mouth D924
Nasopharynx D92D
Neck and Head DW21
Nerve, Peripheral D027
Nose D921
Other Photon
Abdomen DW23DZZ
Adrenal Gland DG22DZZ
Bile Ducts DF22DZZ
Bladder DT22DZZ
Bone Marrow D720DZZ
Brain D020DZZ
Brain Stem D021DZZ
Breast
Left DM20DZZ
Right DM21DZZ
Bronchus DB21DZZ
Cervix DU21DZZ
Chest DW22DZZ
Chest Wall DB27DZZ
Colon DD25DZZ
Diaphragm DB28DZZ
Duodenum DD22DZZ
Ear D920DZZ
Esophagus DD20DZZ
Eye D820DZZ
Gallbladder DF21DZZ
Gland
Adrenal DG22DZZ
Parathyroid DG24DZZ
Pituitary DG20DZZ
Thyroid DG25DZZ
Glands, Salivary D926DZZ
Head and Neck DW21DZZ
Ileum DD24DZZ
Jejunum DD23DZZ
Kidney DT20DZZ

Stereotactic Radiosurgery — *continued*
Other Photon — *continued*
Larynx D92BDZZ
Liver DF20DZZ
Lung DB22DZZ
Lymphatics
Abdomen D726DZZ
Axillary D724DZZ
Inguinal D728DZZ
Neck D723DZZ
Pelvis D727DZZ
Thorax D725DZZ
Mediastinum DB26DZZ
Mouth D924DZZ
Nasopharynx D92DDZZ
Neck and Head DW21DZZ
Nerve, Peripheral D027DZZ
Nose D921DZZ
Ovary DU20DZZ
Palate
Hard D928DZZ
Soft D929DZZ
Pancreas DF23DZZ
Parathyroid Gland DG24DZZ
Pelvic Region DW26DZZ
Pharynx D92CDZZ
Pineal Body DG21DZZ
Pituitary Gland DG20DZZ
Pleura DB25DZZ
Prostate DV20DZZ
Rectum DD27DZZ
Sinuses D927DZZ
Spinal Cord D026DZZ
Spleen D722DZZ
Stomach DD21DZZ
Testis DV21DZZ
Thymus D721DZZ
Thyroid Gland DG25DZZ
Tongue D925DZZ
Trachea DB20DZZ
Ureter DT21DZZ
Urethra DT23DZZ
Uterus DU22DZZ
Ovary DU20
Palate
Hard D928
Soft D929
Pancreas DF23
Parathyroid Gland DG24
Particulate
Abdomen DW23HZZ
Adrenal Gland DG22HZZ
Bile Ducts DF22HZZ
Bladder DT22HZZ
Bone Marrow D720HZZ
Brain D020HZZ
Brain Stem D021HZZ
Breast
Left DM20HZZ
Right DM21HZZ
Bronchus DB21HZZ
Cervix DU21HZZ
Chest DW22HZZ
Chest Wall DB27HZZ
Colon DD25HZZ
Diaphragm DB28HZZ
Duodenum DD22HZZ
Ear D920HZZ
Esophagus DD20HZZ
Eye D820HZZ
Gallbladder DF21HZZ
Gland
Adrenal DG22HZZ
Parathyroid DG24HZZ
Pituitary DG20HZZ
Thyroid DG25HZZ
Glands, Salivary D926HZZ
Head and Neck DW21HZZ
Ileum DD24HZZ
Jejunum DD23HZZ
Kidney DT20HZZ
Larynx D92BHZZ
Liver DF20HZZ
Lung DB22HZZ
Lymphatics
Abdomen D726HZZ
Axillary D724HZZ
Inguinal D728HZZ
Neck D723HZZ

Stereotactic Radiosurgery — *continued*
Particulate — *continued*
Lymphatics — *continued*
Pelvis D727HZZ
Thorax D725HZZ
Mediastinum DB26HZZ
Mouth D924HZZ
Nasopharynx D92DHZZ
Neck and Head DW21HZZ
Nerve, Peripheral D027HZZ
Nose D921HZZ
Ovary DU20HZZ
Palate
Hard D928HZZ
Soft D929HZZ
Pancreas DF23HZZ
Parathyroid Gland DG24HZZ
Pelvic Region DW26HZZ
Pharynx D92CHZZ
Pineal Body DG21HZZ
Pituitary Gland DG20HZZ
Pleura DB25HZZ
Prostate DV20HZZ
Rectum DD27HZZ
Sinuses D927HZZ
Spinal Cord D026HZZ
Spleen D722HZZ
Stomach DD21HZZ
Testis DV21HZZ
Thymus D721HZZ
Thyroid Gland DG25HZZ
Tongue D925HZZ
Trachea DB20HZZ
Ureter DT21HZZ
Urethra DT23HZZ
Uterus DU22HZZ
Pelvic Region DW26
Pharynx D92C
Pineal Body DG21
Pituitary Gland DG20
Pleura DB25
Prostate DV20
Rectum DD27
Sinuses D927
Spinal Cord D026
Spleen D722
Stomach DD21
Testis DV21
Thymus D721
Thyroid Gland DG25
Tongue D925
Trachea DB20
Ureter DT21
Urethra DT23
Uterus DU22
Steripath® Micro™ Blood Collection System
XXE5XR7
Sternoclavicular ligament
use Shoulder Bursa and Ligament, Left
use Shoulder Bursa and Ligament, Right
Sternocleidomastoid artery
use Thyroid Artery, Left
use Thyroid Artery, Right
Sternocleidomastoid muscle
use Neck Muscle, Left
use Neck Muscle, Right
Sternocostal ligament *use* Sternum Bursa and Ligament
Sternotomy
see Division, Sternum 0P80
see Drainage, Sternum 0P90
Stimulation, cardiac
Cardioversion 5A2204Z
Electrophysiologic testing *see* Measurement, Cardiac 4A02
Stimulator Generator
Insertion of device in
Abdomen 0JH8
Back 0JH7
Chest 0JH6
Multiple Array
Abdomen 0JH8
Back 0JH7
Chest 0JH6
Multiple Array Rechargeable
Abdomen 0JH8
Back 0JH7
Chest 0JH6

Stimulator Generator — *continued*
  Removal of device from, Subcutaneous Tissue and
    Fascia, Trunk ØJPT
  Revision of device in, Subcutaneous Tissue and
    Fascia, Trunk ØJWT
  Single Array
    Abdomen ØJH8
    Back ØJH7
    Chest ØJH6
  Single Array Rechargeable
    Abdomen ØJH8
    Back ØJH7
    Chest ØJH6
Stimulator Lead
  Insertion of device in
    Anal Sphincter ØDHR
    Artery
      Left Ø3HL
      Right Ø3HK
    Bladder ØTHB
    Muscle
      Lower ØKHY
      Upper ØKHX
    Stomach ØDH6
    Ureter ØTH9
  Removal of device from
    Anal Sphincter ØDPR
    Artery, Upper Ø3PY
    Bladder ØTPB
    Muscle
      Lower ØKPY
      Upper ØKPX
    Stomach ØDP6
    Ureter ØTP9
  Revision of device in
    Anal Sphincter ØDWR
    Artery, Upper Ø3WY
    Bladder ØTWB
    Muscle
      Lower ØKWY
      Upper ØKWX
    Stomach ØDW6
    Ureter ØTW9
Stoma
  Excision
    Abdomen Wall ØWBFXZ2
    Neck ØWB6XZ2
  Repair
    Abdomen Wall ØWQFXZ2
    Neck ØWQ6XZ2
Stomatoplasty
  see Repair, Mouth and Throat ØCQ
  see Replacement, Mouth and Throat ØCR
  see Supplement, Mouth and Throat ØCU
Stomatorrhaphy *see* Repair, Mouth and Throat ØCQ
StrataGraft® *use* Bioengineered Allogeneic Construct
Stratos LV *use* Cardiac Resynchronization Pacemaker
  Pulse Generator in ØJH
Stress test 4AØ2XM4, 4A12XM4
Stripping *see* Extraction
Study
  Electrophysiologic stimulation, cardiac *see* Mea-
    surement, Cardiac 4AØ2
  Ocular motility 4AØ7X7Z
  Pulmonary airway flow measurement *see* Measure-
    ment, Respiratory 4AØ9
  Visual acuity 4AØ7XØZ
Styloglossus muscle *use* Tongue, Palate, Pharynx
  Muscle
Stylomandibular ligament *use* Head and Neck Bursa
  and Ligament
Stylopharyngeus muscle *use* Tongue, Palate, Pharynx
  Muscle
Subacromial bursa
  use Shoulder Bursa and Ligament, Left
  use Shoulder Bursa and Ligament, Right
Subaortic (common iliac) lymph node *use* Lymphat-
  ic, Pelvis
Subarachnoid space, spinal *use* Spinal Canal
Subclavicular (apical) lymph node
  use Lymphatic, Left Axillary
  use Lymphatic, Right Axillary
Subclavius muscle
  use Thorax Muscle, Left
  use Thorax Muscle, Right
Subclavius nerve *use* Brachial Plexus
Subcostal artery *use* Upper Artery

Subcostal muscle
  use Thorax Muscle, Left
  use Thorax Muscle, Right
Subcostal nerve *use* Thoracic Nerve
Subcutaneous Defibrillator Lead
  Insertion of device in, Subcutaneous Tissue and
    Fascia, Chest ØJH6
  Removal of device from, Subcutaneous Tissue and
    Fascia, Trunk ØJPT
  Revision of device in, Subcutaneous Tissue and
    Fascia, Trunk ØJWT
Subcutaneous injection reservoir, port *use* Vascular
  Access Device, Totally Implantable in Subcuta-
  neous Tissue and Fascia
Subcutaneous injection reservoir, pump *use* Infu-
  sion Device, Pump in Subcutaneous Tissue and
  Fascia
Subdermal progesterone implant *use* Contraceptive
  Device in Subcutaneous Tissue and Fascia
Subdural space, spinal *use* Spinal Canal
Submandibular ganglion
  use Facial Nerve
  use Head and Neck Sympathetic Nerve
Submandibular gland
  use Submaxillary Gland, Left
  use Submaxillary Gland, Right
Submandibular lymph node *use* Lymphatic, Head
Submandibular space *use* Subcutaneous Tissue and
  Fascia, Face
Submaxillary ganglion *use* Head and Neck Sympa-
  thetic Nerve
Submaxillary lymph node *use* Lymphatic, Head
Submental artery *use* Face Artery
Submental lymph node *use* Lymphatic, Head
Submucous (Meissner's) plexus *use* Abdominal
  Sympathetic Nerve
Suboccipital nerve *use* Cervical Nerve
Suboccipital venous plexus
  use Vertebral Vein, Left
  use Vertebral Vein, Right
Subparotid lymph node *use* Lymphatic, Head
Subscapular aponeurosis
  use Subcutaneous Tissue and Fascia, Left Upper
    Arm
  use Subcutaneous Tissue and Fascia, Right Upper
    Arm
Subscapular artery
  use Axillary Artery, Left
  use Axillary Artery, Right
Subscapular (posterior) lymph node
  use Lymphatic, Axillary, Left
  use Lymphatic, Axillary, Right
Subscapularis muscle
  use Shoulder Muscle, Left
  use Shoulder Muscle, Right
Substance Abuse Treatment
  Counseling
    Family, for substance abuse, Other Family
      Counseling HZ63ZZZ
    Group
      12-Step HZ43ZZZ
      Behavioral HZ41ZZZ
      Cognitive HZ40ZZZ
      Cognitive-Behavioral HZ42ZZZ
      Confrontational HZ48ZZZ
      Continuing Care HZ49ZZZ
      Infectious Disease
        Post-Test HZ4CZZZ
        Pre-Test HZ4CZZZ
      Interpersonal HZ44ZZZ
      Motivational Enhancement HZ47ZZZ
      Psychoeducation HZ46ZZZ
      Spiritual HZ4BZZZ
      Vocational HZ45ZZZ
    Individual
      12-Step HZ33ZZZ
      Behavioral HZ31ZZZ
      Cognitive HZ30ZZZ
      Cognitive-Behavioral HZ32ZZZ
      Confrontational HZ38ZZZ
      Continuing Care HZ39ZZZ
      Infectious Disease
        Post-Test HZ3CZZZ
        Pre-Test HZ3CZZZ
      Interpersonal HZ34ZZZ
      Motivational Enhancement HZ37ZZZ
      Psychoeducation HZ36ZZZ

Substance Abuse Treatment — *continued*
  Counseling — *continued*
    Individual — *continued*
      Spiritual HZ3BZZZ
      Vocational HZ35ZZZ
  Detoxification Services, for substance abuse
    HZ2ZZZZ
  Medication Management
    Antabuse HZ83ZZZ
    Bupropion HZ87ZZZ
    Clonidine HZ86ZZZ
    Levo-alpha-acetyl-methadol (LAAM)
      HZ82ZZZ
    Methadone Maintenance HZ81ZZZ
    Naloxone HZ85ZZZ
    Naltrexone HZ84ZZZ
    Nicotine Replacement HZ80ZZZ
    Other Replacement Medication HZ89ZZZ
    Psychiatric Medication HZ88ZZZ
  Pharmacotherapy
    Antabuse HZ93ZZZ
    Bupropion HZ97ZZZ
    Clonidine HZ96ZZZ
    Levo-alpha-acetyl-methadol (LAAM)
      HZ92ZZZ
    Methadone Maintenance HZ91ZZZ
    Naloxone HZ95ZZZ
    Naltrexone HZ94ZZZ
    Nicotine Replacement HZ90ZZZ
    Psychiatric Medication HZ98ZZZ
    Replacement Medication, Other HZ99ZZZ
  Psychotherapy
    12-Step HZ53ZZZ
    Behavioral HZ51ZZZ
    Cognitive HZ50ZZZ
    Cognitive-Behavioral HZ52ZZZ
    Confrontational HZ58ZZZ
    Interactive HZ55ZZZ
    Interpersonal HZ54ZZZ
    Motivational Enhancement HZ57ZZZ
    Psychoanalysis HZ5BZZZ
    Psychodynamic HZ5CZZZ
    Psychoeducation HZ56ZZZ
    Psychophysiological HZ5DZZZ
    Supportive HZ59ZZZ
Substantia nigra *use* Basal Ganglia
Subtalar (talocalcaneal) joint
  use Tarsal Joint, Left
  use Tarsal Joint, Right
Subtalar ligament
  use Foot Bursa and Ligament, Left
  use Foot Bursa and Ligament, Right
Subthalamic nucleus *use* Basal Ganglia
Suction curettage (D&C), nonobstetric *see* Extraction, Endometrium ØUDB
Suction curettage, obstetric post-delivery *see* Ex-
  traction, Products of Conception, Retained 10D1
Superficial circumflex iliac vein
  use Saphenous Vein, Left
  use Saphenous Vein, Right
Superficial epigastric artery
  use Femoral Artery, Left
  use Femoral Artery, Right
Superficial epigastric vein
  use Saphenous Vein, Left
  use Saphenous Vein, Right
Superficial Inferior Epigastric Artery Flap
  Replacement
    Bilateral ØHRV078
    Left ØHRU078
    Right ØHRT078
  Transfer
    Left ØKXG
    Right ØKXF
Superficial palmar arch
  use Hand Artery, Left
  use Hand Artery, Right
Superficial palmar venous arch
  use Hand Vein, Left
  use Hand Vein, Right
Superficial temporal artery
  use Temporal Artery, Left
  use Temporal Artery, Right
Superficial transverse perineal muscle *use* Perineum
  Muscle
Superior cardiac nerve *use* Thoracic Sympathetic
  Nerve
Superior cerebellar vein *use* Intracranial Vein

Superior cerebral vein *use* Intracranial Vein	**Supplement** — *continued*	**Supplement** — *continued*
Superior clunic (cluneal) nerve *use* Lumbar Nerve	Artery — *continued*	Atrium
Superior epigastric artery	Brachial	Left 02U7
use Internal Mammary Artery, Left	Left 03U8	Right 02U6
use Internal Mammary Artery, Right	Right 03U7	Auditory Ossicle
Superior genicular artery	Celiac 04U1	Left 09UA
use Popliteal Artery, Left	Colic	Right 09U9
use Popliteal Artery, Right	Left 04U7	Axilla
Superior gluteal artery	Middle 04U8	Left 0XU5
use Internal Iliac Artery, Left	Right 04U6	Right 0XU4
use Internal Iliac Artery, Right	Common Carotid	Back
Superior gluteal nerve *use* Lumbar Plexus	Left 03UJ	Lower 0WUL
Superior hypogastric plexus *use* Abdominal Sympathetic Nerve	Right 03UH	Upper 0WUK
Superior labial artery *use* Face Artery	Common Iliac	Bladder 0TUB
Superior laryngeal artery	Left 04UD	Bladder Neck 0TUC
use Thyroid Artery, Left	Right 04UC	Bone
use Thyroid Artery, Right	Coronary	Ethmoid
Superior laryngeal nerve *use* Vagus Nerve	Four or More Arteries 02U3	Left 0NUG
Superior longitudinal muscle *use* Tongue, Palate, Pharynx Muscle	One Artery 02U0	Right 0NUF
	Three Arteries 02U2	Frontal 0NU1
Superior mesenteric ganglion *use* Abdominal Sympathetic Nerve	Two Arteries 02U1	Hyoid 0NUX
	External Carotid	Lacrimal
Superior mesenteric lymph node *use* Lymphatic, Mesenteric	Left 03UN	Left 0NUJ
	Right 03UM	Right 0NUH
Superior mesenteric plexus *use* Abdominal Sympathetic Nerve	External Iliac	Nasal 0NUB
	Left 04UJ	Occipital 0NU7
Superior oblique muscle	Right 04UH	Palatine
use Extraocular Muscle, Left	Face 03UR	Left 0NUL
use Extraocular Muscle, Right	Femoral	Right 0NUK
Superior olivary nucleus *use* Pons	Left 04UL	Parietal
Superior rectal artery *use* Inferior Mesenteric Artery	Right 04UK	Left 0NU4
Superior rectal vein *use* Inferior Mesenteric Vein	Foot	Right 0NU3
Superior rectus muscle	Left 04UW	Pelvic
use Extraocular Muscle, Left	Right 04UV	Left 0QU3
use Extraocular Muscle, Right	Gastric 04U2	Right 0QU2
Superior tarsal plate	Hand	Sphenoid 0NUC
use Upper Eyelid, Left	Left 03UF	Temporal
use Upper Eyelid, Right	Right 03UD	Left 0NU6
Superior thoracic artery	Hepatic 04U3	Right 0NU5
use Axillary Artery, Left	Inferior Mesenteric 04UB	Zygomatic
use Axillary Artery, Right	Innominate 03U2	Left 0NUN
Superior thyroid artery	Internal Carotid	Right 0NUM
use External Carotid Artery, Left	Left 03UL	Breast
use External Carotid Artery, Right	Right 03UK	Bilateral 0HUV
use Thyroid Artery, Left	Internal Iliac	Left 0HUU
use Thyroid Artery, Right	Left 04UF	Right 0HUT
Superior turbinate *use* Nasal Turbinate	Right 04UE	Bronchus
Superior ulnar collateral artery	Internal Mammary	Lingula 0BU9
use Brachial Artery, Left	Left 03U1	Lower Lobe
use Brachial Artery, Right	Right 03U0	Left 0BUB
Superior vesical artery	Intracranial 03UG	Right 0BU6
use Internal Iliac Artery, Left	Lower 04UY	Main
use Internal Iliac Artery, Right	Peroneal	Left 0BU7
Supersaturated Oxygen therapy 5A0512C, 5A0522C	Left 04UU	Right 0BU3
Supersaturated Oxygen (SSO2) therapy, cardiac intra-arterial 5A0222C	Right 04UT	Middle Lobe, Right 0BU5
	Popliteal	Upper Lobe
Supplement	Left 04UN	Left 0BU8
Abdominal Wall 0WUF	Right 04UM	Right 0BU4
Acetabulum	Posterior Tibial	Buccal Mucosa 0CU4
Left 0QU5	Left 04US	Bursa and Ligament
Right 0QU4	Right 04UR	Abdomen
Ampulla of Vater 0FUC	Pulmonary	Left 0MUJ
Anal Sphincter 0DUR	Left 02UR	Right 0MUH
Ankle Region	Right 02UQ	Ankle
Left 0YUL	Pulmonary Trunk 02UP	Left 0MUR
Right 0YUK	Radial	Right 0MUQ
Anus 0DUQ	Left 03UC	Elbow
Aorta	Right 03UB	Left 0MU4
Abdominal 04U0	Renal	Right 0MU3
Thoracic	Left 04UA	Foot
Ascending/Arch 02UX	Right 04U9	Left 0MUT
Descending 02UW	Splenic 04U4	Right 0MUS
Arm	Subclavian	Hand
Lower	Left 03U4	Left 0MU8
Left 0XUF	Right 03U3	Right 0MU7
Right 0XUD	Superior Mesenteric 04U5	Head and Neck 0MU0
Upper	Temporal	Hip
Left 0XU9	Left 03UT	Left 0MUM
Right 0XU8	Right 03US	Right 0MUL
Artery	Thyroid	Knee
Anterior Tibial	Left 03UV	Left 0MUP
Left 04UQ	Right 03UU	Right 0MUN
Right 04UP	Ulnar	Lower Extremity
Axillary	Left 03UA	Left 0MUW
Left 03U6	Right 03U9	Right 0MUV
Right 03U5	Upper 03UY	Perineum 0MUK
	Vertebral	Rib(s) 0MUG
	Left 03UQ	Shoulder
	Right 03UP	Left 0MU2

Supplement — *continued*
Bursa and Ligament — *continued*
Shoulder — *continued*
Right ØMU1
Spine
Lower ØMUD
Posterior Vertebral Tether XKU
Upper ØMUC
Sternum ØMUF
Upper Extremity
Left ØMUB
Right ØMU9
Wrist
Left ØMU6
Right ØMU5
Buttock
Left ØYU1
Right ØYUØ
Carina ØBU2
Carpal
Left ØPUN
Right ØPUM
Cecum ØDUH
Cerebral Meninges ØØU1
Cerebral Ventricle ØØU6
Chest Wall ØWU8
Chordae Tendineae Ø2U9
Cisterna Chyli Ø7UL
Clavicle
Left ØPUB
Right ØPU9
Clitoris ØUUJ
Coccyx ØQUS
Colon
Ascending ØDUK
Descending ØDUM
Sigmoid ØDUN
Transverse ØDUL
Cord
Bilateral ØVUH
Left ØVUG
Right ØVUF
Cornea
Left Ø8U9
Right Ø8U8
Cul-de-sac ØUUF
Diaphragm ØBUT
Disc
Cervical Vertebral ØRU3
Cervicothoracic Vertebral ØRU5
Lumbar Vertebral ØSU2
Lumbosacral ØSU4
Thoracic Vertebral ØRU9
Thoracolumbar Vertebral ØRUB
Duct
Common Bile ØFU9
Cystic ØFU8
Hepatic
Common ØFU7
Left ØFU6
Right ØFU5
Lacrimal
Left Ø8UY
Right Ø8UX
Pancreatic ØFUD
Accessory ØFUF
Duodenum ØDU9
Dura Mater ØØU2
Ear
External
Bilateral Ø9U2
Left Ø9U1
Right Ø9UØ
Inner
Left Ø9UE
Right Ø9UD
Middle
Left Ø9U6
Right Ø9U5
Elbow Region
Left ØXUC
Right ØXUB
Epididymis
Bilateral ØVUL
Left ØVUK
Right ØVUJ
Epiglottis ØCUR
Esophagogastric Junction ØDU4
Esophagus ØDU5

Supplement — *continued*
Esophagus — *continued*
Lower ØDU3
Middle ØDU2
Upper ØDU1
Extremity
Lower
Left ØYUB
Right ØYU9
Upper
Left ØXU7
Right ØXU6
Eye
Left Ø8U1
Right Ø8UØ
Eyelid
Lower
Left Ø8UR
Right Ø8UQ
Upper
Left Ø8UP
Right Ø8UN
Face ØWU2
Fallopian Tube
Left ØUU6
Right ØUU5
Fallopian Tubes, Bilateral ØUU7
Femoral Region
Bilateral ØYUE
Left ØYU8
Right ØYU7
Femoral Shaft
Left ØQU9
Right ØQU8
Femur
Lower
Left ØQUC
Right ØQUB
Upper
Left ØQU7
Right ØQU6
Fibula
Left ØQUK
Right ØQUJ
Finger
Index
Left ØXUP
Right ØXUN
Little
Left ØXUW
Right ØXUV
Middle
Left ØXUR
Right ØXUQ
Ring
Left ØXUT
Right ØXUS
Foot
Left ØYUN
Right ØYUM
Gingiva
Lower ØCU6
Upper ØCU5
Glenoid Cavity
Left ØPU8
Right ØPU7
Hand
Left ØXUK
Right ØXUJ
Head ØWUØ
Heart Ø2UA
Humeral Head
Left ØPUD
Right ØPUC
Humeral Shaft
Left ØPUG
Right ØPUF
Hymen ØUUK
Ileocecal Valve ØDUC
Ileum ØDUB
Inguinal Region
Bilateral ØYUA
Left ØYU6
Right ØYU5
Intestine
Large ØDUE
Left ØDUG
Right ØDUF
Small ØDU8

Supplement — *continued*
Iris
Left Ø8UD
Right Ø8UC
Jaw
Lower ØWU5
Upper ØWU4
Jejunum ØDUA
Joint
Acromioclavicular
Left ØRUH
Right ØRUG
Ankle
Left ØSUG
Right ØSUF
Carpal
Left ØRUR
Right ØRUQ
Carpometacarpal
Left ØRUT
Right ØRUS
Cervical Vertebral ØRU1
Cervicothoracic Vertebral ØRU4
Coccygeal ØSU6
Elbow
Left ØRUM
Right ØRUL
Finger Phalangeal
Left ØRUX
Right ØRUW
Hip
Left ØSUB
Acetabular Surface ØSUE
Femoral Surface ØSUS
Right ØSU9
Acetabular Surface ØSUA
Femoral Surface ØSUR
Knee
Left ØSUD
Femoral Surface ØSUUØ9Z
Tibial Surface ØSUWØ9Z
Right ØSUC
Femoral Surface ØSUTØ9Z
Tibial Surface ØSUVØ9Z
Lumbar Vertebral ØSUØ
Lumbosacral ØSU3
Metacarpophalangeal
Left ØRUV
Right ØRUU
Metatarsal-Phalangeal
Left ØSUN
Right ØSUM
Occipital-cervical ØRUØ
Sacrococcygeal ØSU5
Sacroiliac
Left ØSU8
Right ØSU7
Shoulder
Left ØRUK
Right ØRUJ
Sternoclavicular
Left ØRUF
Right ØRUE
Tarsal
Left ØSUJ
Right ØSUH
Tarsometatarsal
Left ØSUL
Right ØSUK
Temporomandibular
Left ØRUD
Right ØRUC
Thoracic Vertebral ØRU6
Thoracolumbar Vertebral ØRUA
Toe Phalangeal
Left ØSUQ
Right ØSUP
Wrist
Left ØRUP
Right ØRUN
Kidney Pelvis
Left ØTU4
Right ØTU3
Knee Region
Left ØYUG
Right ØYUF
Larynx ØCUS

Subterms under main terms may continue to next column or page

Supplement — *continued*
- Tendon — *continued*
  - Thorax
    - Left ØLUD
    - Right ØLUC
  - Trunk
    - Left ØLUB
    - Right ØLU9
  - Upper Arm
    - Left ØLU4
    - Right ØLU3
  - Upper Leg
    - Left ØLUM
    - Right ØLUL
- Testis
  - Bilateral ØVUCØ
  - Left ØVUBØ
  - Right ØVU9Ø
- Thumb
  - Left ØXUM
  - Right ØXUL
- Tibia
  - Left ØQUH
  - Right ØQUG
- Toe
  - 1st
    - Left ØYUQ
    - Right ØYUP
  - 2nd
    - Left ØYUS
    - Right ØYUR
  - 3rd
    - Left ØYUU
    - Right ØYUT
  - 4th
    - Left ØYUW
    - Right ØYUV
  - 5th
    - Left ØYUY
    - Right ØYUX
- Tongue ØCU7
- Trachea ØBU1
- Tunica Vaginalis
  - Left ØVU7
  - Right ØVU6
- Turbinate, Nasal Ø9UL
- Tympanic Membrane
  - Left Ø9U8
  - Right Ø9U7
- Ulna
  - Left ØPUL
  - Right ØPUK
- Ureter
  - Left ØTU7
  - Right ØTU6
- Urethra ØTUD
- Uterine Supporting Structure ØUU4
- Uvula ØCUN
- Vagina ØUUG
- Valve
  - Aortic Ø2UF
  - Mitral Ø2UG
  - Pulmonary Ø2UH
  - Tricuspid Ø2UJ
- Vas Deferens
  - Bilateral ØVUQ
  - Left ØVUP
  - Right ØVUN
- Vein
  - Axillary
    - Left Ø5U8
    - Right Ø5U7
  - Azygos Ø5UØ
  - Basilic
    - Left Ø5UC
    - Right Ø5UB
  - Brachial
    - Left Ø5UA
    - Right Ø5U9
  - Cephalic
    - Left Ø5UF
    - Right Ø5UD
  - Colic Ø6U7
  - Common Iliac
    - Left Ø6UD
    - Right Ø6UC
  - Esophageal Ø6U3
  - External Iliac
    - Left Ø6UG

Supplement — *continued*
- Vein — *continued*
  - External Iliac — *continued*
    - Right Ø6UF
  - External Jugular
    - Left Ø5UQ
    - Right Ø5UP
  - Face
    - Left Ø5UV
    - Right Ø5UT
  - Femoral
    - Left Ø6UN
    - Right Ø6UM
  - Foot
    - Left Ø6UV
    - Right Ø6UT
  - Gastric Ø6U2
  - Hand
    - Left Ø5UH
    - Right Ø5UG
  - Hemiazygos Ø5U1
  - Hepatic Ø6U4
  - Hypogastric
    - Left Ø6UJ
    - Right Ø6UH
  - Inferior Mesenteric Ø6U6
  - Innominate
    - Left Ø5U4
    - Right Ø5U3
  - Internal Jugular
    - Left Ø5UN
    - Right Ø5UM
  - Intracranial Ø5UL
  - Lower Ø6UY
  - Portal Ø6U8
  - Pulmonary
    - Left Ø2UT
    - Right Ø2US
  - Renal
    - Left Ø6UB
    - Right Ø6U9
  - Saphenous
    - Left Ø6UQ
    - Right Ø6UP
  - Splenic Ø6U1
  - Subclavian
    - Left Ø5U6
    - Right Ø5U5
  - Superior Mesenteric Ø6U5
  - Upper Ø5UY
  - Vertebral
    - Left Ø5US
    - Right Ø5UR
- Vena Cava
  - Inferior Ø6UØ
  - Superior Ø2UV
- Ventricle
  - Left Ø2UL
  - Right Ø2UK
- Vertebra
  - Cervical ØPU3
  - Lumbar ØQUØ
    - Mechanically Expandable (Paired) Synthetic Substitute XNUØ356
  - Thoracic ØPU4
    - Mechanically Expandable (Paired) Synthetic Substitute XNU4356
- Vesicle
  - Bilateral ØVU3
  - Left ØVU2
  - Right ØVU1
- Vocal Cord
  - Left ØCUV
  - Right ØCUT
- Vulva ØUUM
- Wrist Region
  - Left ØXUH
  - Right ØXUG

Supraclavicular (Virchow's) lymph node
- *use* Lymphatic, Left Neck
- *use* Lymphatic, Right Neck

Supraclavicular nerve *use* Cervical Plexus
Suprahyoid lymph node *use* Lymphatic, Head
Suprahyoid muscle
- *use* Neck Muscle, Left
- *use* Neck Muscle, Right

Suprainguinal lymph node *use* Lymphatic, Pelvis

Supraorbital vein
- *use* Face Vein, Left
- *use* Face Vein, Right

Suprarenal gland
- *use* Adrenal Gland
- *use* Adrenal Gland, Bilateral
- *use* Adrenal Gland, Left
- *use* Adrenal Gland, Right

Suprarenal plexus *use* Abdominal Sympathetic Nerve
Suprascapular nerve *use* Brachial Plexus
Supraspinatus fascia
- *use* Subcutaneous Tissue and Fascia, Left Upper Arm
- *use* Subcutaneous Tissue and Fascia, Right Upper Arm

Supraspinatus muscle
- *use* Shoulder Muscle, Left
- *use* Shoulder Muscle, Right

Supraspinous ligament
- *use* Lower Spine Bursa and Ligament
- *use* Upper Spine Bursa and Ligament

Suprasternal notch *use* Sternum
Supratrochlear lymph node
- *use* Lymphatic, Left Upper Extremity
- *use* Lymphatic, Right Upper Extremity

Sural artery
- *use* Popliteal Artery, Left
- *use* Popliteal Artery, Right

Surpass Streamline™ Flow Diverter *use* Intraluminal Device, Flow Diverter in Ø3V

Suspension
- Bladder Neck *see* Reposition, Bladder Neck ØTSC
- Kidney *see* Reposition, Urinary System ØTS
- Urethra *see* Reposition, Urinary System ØTS
- Urethrovesical *see* Reposition, Bladder Neck ØTSC
- Uterus *see* Reposition, Uterus ØUS9
- Vagina *see* Reposition, Vagina ØUSG

Sustained Release Drug-eluting Intraluminal Device
- Dilation
  - Anterior Tibial
    - Left X27Q385
    - Right X27P385
  - Femoral
    - Left X27J385
    - Right X27H385
  - Peroneal
    - Left X27U385
    - Right X27T385
  - Popliteal
    - Left Distal X27N385
    - Left Proximal X27L385
    - Right Distal X27M385
    - Right Proximal X27K385
  - Posterior Tibial
    - Left X27S385
    - Right X27R385
- Four or More
  - Anterior Tibial
    - Left X27Q3C5
    - Right X27P3C5
  - Femoral
    - Left X27J3C5
    - Right X27H3C5
  - Peroneal
    - Left X27U3C5
    - Right X27T3C5
  - Popliteal
    - Left Distal X27N3C5
    - Left Proximal X27L3C5
    - Right Distal X27M3C5
    - Right Proximal X27K3C5
  - Posterior Tibial
    - Left X27S3C5
    - Right X27R3C5
- Three
  - Anterior Tibial
    - Left X27Q3B5
    - Right X27P3B5
  - Femoral
    - Left X27J3B5
    - Right X27H3B5
  - Peroneal
    - Left X27U3B5
    - Right X27T3B5
  - Popliteal
    - Left Distal X27N3B5
    - Left Proximal X27L3B5

Subterms under main terms may continue to next column or page

Sustained Release Drug-eluting Intraluminal Device
— *continued*
Three — *continued*
Popliteal — *continued*
Right Distal X27M3B5
Right Proximal X27K3B5
Posterior Tibial
Left X27S3B5
Right X27R3B5
Two
Anterior Tibial
Left X27Q395
Right X27P395
Femoral
Left X27J395
Right X27H395
Peroneal
Left X27U395
Right X27T395
Popliteal
Left Distal X27N395
Left Proximal X27L395
Right Distal X27M395
Right Proximal X27K395
Posterior Tibial
Left X27S395
Right X27R395
Suture
Laceration repair *see* Repair
Ligation *see* Occlusion
Suture Removal
Extremity
Lower 8E0YXY8
Upper 8E0XXY8
Head and Neck Region 8E09XY8
Trunk Region 8E0WXY8
Sutureless valve, Perceval (rapid deployment technique) *see* Replacement, Valve, Aortic 02RF
Sweat gland *use* Skin
Sympathectomy *see* Excision, Peripheral Nervous System 01B
SynCardia (temporary) total artificial heart (TAH) *use* Synthetic Substitute, Pneumatic in 02R
SynCardia Total Artificial Heart *use* Synthetic Substitute
Synchra CRT-P *use* Cardiac Resynchronization Pacemaker Pulse Generator in 0JH
SynchroMed pump *use* Infusion Device, Pump in Subcutaneous Tissue and Fascia
Synechiotomy, iris *see* Release, Eye 08N
Synovectomy
Lower joint *see* Excision, Lower Joints 0SB
Upper joint *see* Excision, Upper Joints 0RB
Synthetic Human Angiotensin II XW0
Systemic Nuclear Medicine Therapy
Abdomen CW70
Anatomical Regions, Multiple CW7YYZZ
Chest CW73
Thyroid CW7G
Whole Body CW7N

T

tab-cel® *use* Tabelecleucel Immunotherapy
Tabelecleucel Immunotherapy XW0
Tagraxofusp-erzs Antineoplastic XW0
Takedown
Arteriovenous shunt *see* Removal of device from, Upper Arteries 03P
Arteriovenous shunt, with creation of new shunt *see* Bypass, Upper Arteries 031
Stoma
see Excision
see Reposition
Talent® Converter *use* Intraluminal Device
Talent® Occluder *use* Intraluminal Device
Talent® Stent Graft (abdominal) (thoracic) *use* Intraluminal Device
Talocalcaneal (subtalar) joint
use Tarsal Joint, Left
use Tarsal Joint, Right
Talocalcaneal ligament
use Foot Bursa and Ligament, Left
use Foot Bursa and Ligament, Right
Talocalcaneonavicular joint
use Tarsal Joint, Left
use Tarsal Joint, Right

Talocalcaneonavicular ligament
use Foot Bursa and Ligament, Left
use Foot Bursa and Ligament, Right
Talocrural joint
use Ankle Joint, Left
use Joint, Ankle, Right
Talofibular ligament
use Ankle Bursa and Ligament, Left
use Ankle Bursa and Ligament, Right
Talus bone
use Tarsal, Left
use Tarsal, Right
TandemHeart® System *use* Short-term External Heart Assist System in Heart and Great Vessels
Tarsectomy
see Excision, Lower Bones 0QB
see Resection, Lower Bones 0QT
Tarsometatarsal ligament
use Foot Bursa and Ligament, Left
use Foot Bursa and Ligament, Right
Tarsorrhaphy *see* Repair, Eye 08Q
Tattooing
Cornea 3E0CXMZ
Skin *see* Introduction of substance in or on, Skin 3E00
Taurolidine Anti-infective and Heparin Anticoagulant XY0YX28
TAXUS® Liberte® Paclitaxel-eluting Coronary Stent System *use* Intraluminal Device, Drug-eluting in Heart and Great Vessels
TBNA (transbronchial needle aspiration)
Fluid or gas *see* Drainage, Respiratory System 0B9
Tissue biopsy *see* Extraction, Respiratory System 0BD
Tecartus™ *use* Brexucabtagene Autoleucel Immunotherapy
TECENTRIQ® *use* Atezolizumab Antineoplastic
Teclistamab Antineoplastic XW01348
Telemetry 4A12X4Z
Ambulatory 4A12X45
Temperature gradient study 4A0ZXKZ
Temporal lobe *use* Cerebral Hemisphere
Temporalis muscle *use* Head Muscle
Temporoparietalis muscle *use* Head Muscle
Tendolysis *see* Release, Tendons 0LN
Tendonectomy
see Excision, Tendons 0LB
see Resection, Tendons 0LT
Tendonoplasty, tenoplasty
see Repair, Tendons 0LQ
see Replacement, Tendons 0LR
see Supplement, Tendons 0LU
Tendorrhaphy *see* Repair, Tendons 0LQ
Tendototomy
see Division, Tendons 0L8
see Drainage, Tendons 0L9
Tenectomy, tenonectomy
see Excision, Tendons 0LB
see Resection, Tendons 0LT
Tenolysis *see* Release, Tendons 0LN
Tenontorrhaphy *see* Repair, Tendons 0LQ
Tenontotomy
see Division, Tendons 0L8
see Drainage, Tendons 0L9
Tenorrhaphy *see* Repair, Tendons 0LQ
Tenosynovectomy
see Excision, Tendons 0LB
see Resection, Tendons 0LT
Tenotomy
see Division, Tendons 0L8
see Drainage, Tendons 0L9
Tensor fasciae latae muscle
use Hip Muscle, Left
use Hip Muscle, Right
Tensor veli palatini muscle *use* Tongue, Palate, Pharynx Muscle
Tenth cranial nerve *use* Vagus Nerve
Tentorium cerebelli *use* Dura Mater
Teres major muscle
use Shoulder Muscle, Left
use Shoulder Muscle, Right
Teres minor muscle
use Shoulder Muscle, Left
use Shoulder Muscle, Right
Terlipressin XW0
TERLIVAZ® *use* Terlipressin

Termination of pregnancy
Aspiration curettage 10A07ZZ
Dilation and curettage 10A07ZZ
Hysterotomy 10A00ZZ
Intra-amniotic injection 10A03ZZ
Laminaria 10A07ZW
Vacuum 10A07Z6
Testectomy
see Excision, Male Reproductive System 0VB
see Resection, Male Reproductive System 0VT
Testicular artery *use* Abdominal Aorta
Testing
Glaucoma 4A07XBZ
Hearing *see* Hearing Assessment, Diagnostic Audiology F13
Mental health *see* Psychological Tests
Muscle function, electromyography (EMG) *see* Measurement, Musculoskeletal 4A0F
Muscle function, manual *see* Motor Function Assessment, Rehabilitation F01
Neurophysiologic monitoring, intra-operative *see* Monitoring, Physiological Systems 4A1
Range of motion *see* Motor Function Assessment, Rehabilitation F01
Vestibular function *see* Vestibular Assessment, Diagnostic Audiology F15
Thalamectomy *see* Excision, Thalamus 00B9
Thalamotomy *see* Drainage, Thalamus 0099
Thenar muscle
use Hand Muscle, Left
use Hand Muscle, Right
Therapeutic Massage
Musculoskeletal System 8E0KX1Z
Reproductive System
Prostate 8E0VX1C
Rectum 8E0VX1D
Therapeutic occlusion coil(s) *use* Intraluminal Device
Thermography 4A0ZXKZ
Thermotherapy, prostate *see* Destruction, Prostate 0V50
Third cranial nerve *use* Oculomotor Nerve
Third occipital nerve *use* Cervical Nerve
Third ventricle *use* Cerebral Ventricle
Thoracectomy *see* Excision, Anatomical Regions, General 0WB
Thoracentesis *see* Drainage, Anatomical Regions, General 0W9
Thoracic aortic plexus *use* Thoracic Sympathetic Nerve
Thoracic esophagus *use* Esophagus, Middle
Thoracic facet joint *use* Thoracic Vertebral Joint
Thoracic ganglion *use* Thoracic Sympathetic Nerve
Thoracoacromial artery
use Axillary Artery, Left
use Axillary Artery, Right
Thoracocentesis *see* Drainage, Anatomical Regions, General 0W9
Thoracolumbar facet joint *use* Thoracolumbar Vertebral Joint
Thoracoplasty
see Repair, Anatomical Regions, General 0WQ
see Supplement, Anatomical Regions, General 0WU
Thoracostomy, for lung collapse *see* Drainage, Respiratory System 0B9
Thoracostomy tube *use* Drainage Device
Thoracotomy *see* Drainage, Anatomical Regions, General 0W9
Thoraflex™ Hybrid device *use* Branched Synthetic Substitute with Intraluminal Device in New Technology
Thoratec IVAD (Implantable Ventricular Assist Device) *use* Implantable Heart Assist System in Heart and Great Vessels
Thoratec Paracorporeal Ventricular Assist Device *use* Short-term External Heart Assist System in Heart and Great Vessels
Thrombectomy *see* Extirpation
Thrombolysis, Ultrasound assisted *see* Fragmentation, Artery
Thymectomy
see Excision, Lymphatic and Hemic Systems 07B
see Resection, Lymphatic and Hemic Systems 07T
Thymopexy
see Repair, Lymphatic and Hemic Systems 07Q
see Reposition, Lymphatic and Hemic Systems 07S
Thymus gland *use* Thymus
Thyroarytenoid muscle
use Neck Muscle, Left

Traction — *continued*
- Thumb
  - Left 2W6HX
  - Right 2W6GX
- Toe
  - Left 2W6VX
  - Right 2W6UX

Tractotomy *see* Division, Central Nervous System and Cranial Nerves 008

Tragus
- *use* External Ear, Bilateral
- *use* External Ear, Left
- *use* External Ear, Right

Training, caregiver *see* Caregiver Training

TRAM (transverse rectus abdominis myocuta-neous) flap reconstruction
- Free *see* Replacement, Skin and Breast 0HR
- Pedicled *see* Transfer, Muscles 0KX

Transcatheter Pulmonary Valve (TPV) placement
- In conduit 02RH38L
- Native site 02RH38M

Transdermal Glomerular Filtration Rate (GFR) Measurement System XT25XE5

Transection *see* Division

Transfer
- Buccal Mucosa 0CX4
- Bursa and Ligament
  - Abdomen
    - Left 0MXJ
    - Right 0MXH
  - Ankle
    - Left 0MXR
    - Right 0MXQ
  - Elbow
    - Left 0MX4
    - Right 0MX3
  - Foot
    - Left 0MXT
    - Right 0MXS
  - Hand
    - Left 0MX8
    - Right 0MX7
  - Head and Neck 0MX0
  - Hip
    - Left 0MXM
    - Right 0MXL
  - Knee
    - Left 0MXP
    - Right 0MXN
  - Lower Extremity
    - Left 0MXW
    - Right 0MXV
  - Perineum 0MXK
  - Rib(s) 0MXG
  - Shoulder
    - Left 0MX2
    - Right 0MX1
  - Spine
    - Lower 0MXD
    - Upper 0MXC
  - Sternum 0MXF
  - Upper Extremity
    - Left 0MXB
    - Right 0MX9
  - Wrist
    - Left 0MX6
    - Right 0MX5
- Finger
  - Left 0XXP0ZM
  - Right 0XXN0ZL
- Gingiva
  - Lower 0CX6
  - Upper 0CX5
- Intestine
  - Large 0DXE
  - Small 0DX8
- Lip
  - Lower 0CX1
  - Upper 0CX0
- Muscle
  - Abdomen
    - Left 0KXL
    - Right 0KXK
  - Extraocular
    - Left 08XM
    - Right 08XL
  - Facial 0KX1

Transfer — *continued*
- Muscle — *continued*
  - Foot
    - Left 0KXW
    - Right 0KXV
  - Hand
    - Left 0KXD
    - Right 0KXC
  - Head 0KX0
  - Hip
    - Left 0KXP
    - Right 0KXN
  - Lower Arm and Wrist
    - Left 0KXB
    - Right 0KX9
  - Lower Leg
    - Left 0KXT
    - Right 0KXS
  - Neck
    - Left 0KX3
    - Right 0KX2
  - Perineum 0KXM
  - Shoulder
    - Left 0KX6
    - Right 0KX5
  - Thorax
    - Left 0KXJ
    - Right 0KXH
  - Tongue, Palate, Pharynx 0KX4
  - Trunk
    - Left 0KXG
    - Right 0KXF
  - Upper Arm
    - Left 0KX8
    - Right 0KX7
  - Upper Leg
    - Left 0KXR
    - Right 0KXQ
- Nerve
  - Abducens 00XL
  - Accessory 00XR
  - Acoustic 00XN
  - Cervical 01X1
  - Facial 00XM
  - Femoral 01XD
  - Glossopharyngeal 00XP
  - Hypoglossal 00XS
  - Lumbar 01XB
  - Median 01X5
  - Oculomotor 00XH
  - Olfactory 00XF
  - Optic 00XG
  - Peroneal 01XH
  - Phrenic 01X2
  - Pudendal 01XC
  - Radial 01X6
  - Sciatic 01XF
  - Thoracic 01X8
  - Tibial 01XG
  - Trigeminal 00XK
  - Trochlear 00XJ
  - Ulnar 01X4
  - Vagus 00XQ
- Palate, Soft 0CX3
- Prepuce 0VXT
- Skin
  - Abdomen 0HX7XZZ
  - Back 0HX6XZZ
  - Buttock 0HX8XZZ
  - Chest 0HX5XZZ
  - Ear
    - Left 0HX3XZZ
    - Right 0HX2XZZ
  - Face 0HX1XZZ
  - Foot
    - Left 0HXNXZZ
    - Right 0HXMXZZ
  - Hand
    - Left 0HXGXZZ
    - Right 0HXFXZZ
  - Inguinal 0HXAXZZ
  - Lower Arm
    - Left 0HXEXZZ
    - Right 0HXDXZZ
  - Lower Leg
    - Left 0HXLXZZ
    - Right 0HXKXZZ
  - Neck 0HX4XZZ
  - Perineum 0HX9XZZ

Transfer — *continued*
- Skin — *continued*
  - Scalp 0HX0XZZ
  - Upper Arm
    - Left 0HXCXZZ
    - Right 0HXBXZZ
  - Upper Leg
    - Left 0HXJXZZ
    - Right 0HXHXZZ
- Stomach 0DX6
- Subcutaneous Tissue and Fascia
  - Abdomen 0JX8
  - Back 0JX7
  - Buttock 0JX9
  - Chest 0JX6
  - Face 0JX1
  - Foot
    - Left 0JXR
    - Right 0JXQ
  - Hand
    - Left 0JXK
    - Right 0JXJ
  - Lower Arm
    - Left 0JXH
    - Right 0JXG
  - Lower Leg
    - Left 0JXP
    - Right 0JXN
  - Neck
    - Left 0JX5
    - Right 0JX4
  - Pelvic Region 0JXC
  - Perineum 0JXB
  - Scalp 0JX0
  - Upper Arm
    - Left 0JXF
    - Right 0JXD
  - Upper Leg
    - Left 0JXM
    - Right 0JXL
- Tendon
  - Abdomen
    - Left 0LXG
    - Right 0LXF
  - Ankle
    - Left 0LXT
    - Right 0LXS
  - Foot
    - Left 0LXW
    - Right 0LXV
  - Hand
    - Left 0LX8
    - Right 0LX7
  - Head and Neck 0LX0
  - Hip
    - Left 0LXK
    - Right 0LXJ
  - Knee
    - Left 0LXR
    - Right 0LXQ
  - Lower Arm and Wrist
    - Left 0LX6
    - Right 0LX5
  - Lower Leg
    - Left 0LXP
    - Right 0LXN
  - Perineum 0LXH
  - Shoulder
    - Left 0LX2
    - Right 0LX1
  - Thorax
    - Left 0LXD
    - Right 0LXC
  - Trunk
    - Left 0LX9
    - Right 0LX9
  - Upper Arm
    - Left 0LX4
    - Right 0LX3
  - Upper Leg
    - Left 0LXM
    - Right 0LXL
- Tongue 0CX7

Transfusion
- Immunotherapy *see* New Technology, Anatomical Regions XW2
- Products of Conception
  - Antihemophilic Factors 3027

Transfusion — *continued*
  Products of Conception — *continued*
    Blood
      Platelets 3027
      Red Cells 3027
        Frozen 3027
      White Cells 3027
      Whole 3027
    Factor IX 3027
    Fibrinogen 3027
    Globulin 3027
    Plasma
      Fresh 3027
      Frozen 3027
    Plasma Cryoprecipitate 3027
    Serum Albumin 3027
  Vein
    4-Factor Prothrombin Complex Concentrate 30283B1
    Central
      Antihemophilic Factors 30243V
      Blood
        Platelets 30243R
        Red Cells 30243N
          Frozen 30243P
        White Cells 30243Q
        Whole 30243H
      Bone Marrow 30243G
      Factor IX 30243W
      Fibrinogen 30243T
      Globulin 30243S
      Hematopoietic Stem/Progenitor Cells (HSPC), Genetically Modified 30243C0
      Pathogen Reduced Cryoprecipitated Fibrinogen Complex 30243D1
      Plasma
        Fresh 30243L
        Frozen 30243K
      Plasma Cryoprecipitate 30243M
      Serum Albumin 30243J
      Stem Cells
        Cord Blood 30243X
        Embryonic 30243AZ
        Hematopoietic 30243Y
        T-cell Depleted Hematopoietic 30243U
    Peripheral
      Antihemophilic Factors 30233V
      Blood
        Platelets 30233R
        Red Cells 30233N
          Frozen 30233P
        White Cells 30233Q
        Whole 30233H
      Bone Marrow 30233G
      Factor IX 30233W
      Fibrinogen 30233T
      Globulin 30233S
      Hematopoietic Stem/Progenitor Cells (HSPC), Genetically Modified 30233C0
      Pathogen Reduced Cryoprecipitated Fibrinogen Complex 30233D1
      Plasma
        Fresh 30233L
        Frozen 30233K
      Plasma Cryoprecipitate 30233M
      Serum Albumin 30233J
      Stem Cells
        Cord Blood 30233X
        Embryonic 30233AZ
        Hematopoietic 30233Y
        T-cell Depleted Hematopoietic 30233U
Transplant *see* Transplantation
Transplantation
  Bone marrow *see* Transfusion, Circulatory 302
  Esophagus 0DY50Z
  Face 0WY20Z
  Hand
    Left 0XYK0Z
    Right 0XYJ0Z
  Heart 02YA0Z
  Hematopoietic cell *see* Transfusion, Circulatory 302
  Intestine
    Large 0DYE0Z
    Small 0DY80Z

Transplantation — *continued*
  Kidney
    Left 0TY10Z
    Right 0TY00Z
  Liver 0FY00Z
  Lung
    Bilateral 0BYM0Z
    Left 0BYL0Z
    Lower Lobe
      Left 0BYJ0Z
      Right 0BYF0Z
    Middle Lobe, Right 0BYD0Z
    Right 0BYK0Z
    Upper Lobe
      Left 0BYG0Z
      Right 0BYC0Z
  Lung Lingula 0BYH0Z
  Ovary
    Left 0UY10Z
    Right 0UY00Z
  Pancreas 0FYG0Z
  Penis 0VYS0Z
  Products of Conception 10Y0
  Scrotum 0VY50Z
  Spleen 07YP0Z
  Stem cell *see* Transfusion, Circulatory 302
  Stomach 0DY60Z
  Thymus 07YM0Z
  Uterus 0UY90Z
Transposition
  see Bypass
  see Reposition
  see Transfer
Transversalis fascia *use* Subcutaneous Tissue and Fascia, Trunk
Transverse acetabular ligament
  use Hip Bursa and Ligament, Left
  use Hip Bursa and Ligament, Right
Transverse (cutaneous) cervical nerve *use* Cervical Plexus
Transverse facial artery
  use Temporal Artery, Left
  use Temporal Artery, Right
Transverse foramen *use* Cervical Vertebra
Transverse humeral ligament
  use Shoulder Bursa and Ligament, Left
  use Shoulder Bursa and Ligament, Right
Transverse ligament of atlas *use* Head and Neck Bursa and Ligament
Transverse process
  use Cervical Vertebra
  use Lumbar Vertebra
  use Thoracic Vertebra
Transverse Rectus Abdominis Myocutaneous Flap
  Replacement
    Bilateral 0HRV076
    Left 0HRU076
    Right 0HRT076
  Transfer
    Left 0KXL
    Right 0KXK
Transverse scapular ligament
  use Shoulder Bursa and Ligament, Left
  use Shoulder Bursa and Ligament, Right
Transverse thoracis muscle
  use Thorax Muscle, Left
  use Thorax Muscle, Right
Transversospinalis muscle
  use Trunk Muscle, Left
  use Trunk Muscle, Right
Transversus abdominis muscle
  use Abdomen Muscle, Left
  use Abdomen Muscle, Right
Trapezium bone
  use Carpal, Left
  use Carpal, Right
Trapezius muscle
  use Trunk Muscle, Left
  use Trunk Muscle, Right
Trapezoid bone
  use Carpal, Left
  use Carpal, Right
Treosulfan XW0
Triceps brachii muscle
  use Upper Arm Muscle, Left
  use Upper Arm Muscle, Right
Tricuspid annulus *use* Tricuspid Valve

Trifacial nerve *use* Trigeminal Nerve
Trifecta™ Valve (aortic) *use* Zooplastic Tissue in Heart and Great Vessels
Trigone of bladder *use* Bladder
TriGuard 3™ CEPD (cerebral embolic protection device) X2A6325
Trilaciclib XW0
Trimming, excisional *see* Excision
Triquetral bone
  use Carpal, Left
  use Carpal, Right
Trochanteric bursa
  use Hip Bursa and Ligament, Left
  use Hip Bursa and Ligament, Right
TUMT (transurethral microwave thermotherapy of prostate) 0V507ZZ
TUNA (transurethral needle ablation of prostate) 0V507ZZ
Tunneled central venous catheter *use* Vascular Access Device, Tunneled in Subcutaneous Tissue and Fascia
Tunneled spinal (intrathecal) catheter *use* Infusion Device
Turbinectomy
  see Excision, Ear, Nose, Sinus 09B
  see Resection, Ear, Nose, Sinus 09T
Turbinoplasty
  see Repair, Ear, Nose, Sinus 09Q
  see Replacement, Ear, Nose, Sinus 09R
  see Supplement, Ear, Nose, Sinus 09U
Turbinotomy
  see Division, Ear, Nose, Sinus 098
  see Drainage, Ear, Nose, Sinus 099
TURP (transurethral resection of prostate) 0VB07ZZ
  see Excision, Prostate 0VB0
  see Resection, Prostate 0VT0
Twelfth cranial nerve *use* Hypoglossal Nerve
Two lead pacemaker *use* Pacemaker, Dual Chamber in 0JH
Tympanic cavity
  use Middle Ear, Left
  use Middle Ear, Right
Tympanic nerve *use* Glossopharyngeal Nerve
Tympanic part of temoporal bone
  use Temporal Bone, Left
  use Temporal Bone, Right
Tympanogram *see* Hearing Assessment, Diagnostic Audiology F13
Tympanoplasty
  see Repair, Ear, Nose, Sinus 09Q
  see Replacement, Ear, Nose, Sinus 09R
  see Supplement, Ear, Nose, Sinus 09U
Tympanosympathectomy *see* Excision, Nerve, Head and Neck Sympathetic 01BK
Tympanotomy *see* Drainage, Ear, Nose, Sinus 099
TYRX Antibacterial Envelope *use* Anti-Infective Envelope

U

Ulnar collateral carpal ligament
  use Wrist Bursa and Ligament, Left
  use Wrist Bursa and Ligament, Right
Ulnar collateral ligament
  use Elbow Bursa and Ligament, Left
  use Elbow Bursa and Ligament, Right
Ulnar notch
  use Radius, Left
  use Radius, Right
Ulnar vein
  use Brachial Vein, Left
  use Brachial Vein, Right
Ultrafiltration
  Hemodialysis *see* Performance, Urinary 5A1D
  Therapeutic plasmapheresis *see* Pheresis, Circulatory 6A55
Ultraflex™ Precision Colonic Stent System *use* Intraluminal Device
ULTRAPRO Hernia System (UHS) *use* Synthetic Substitute
ULTRAPRO Partially Absorbable Lightweight Mesh *use* Synthetic Substitute
ULTRAPRO Plug *use* Synthetic Substitute
Ultrasonic osteogenic stimulator
  use Bone Growth Stimulator in Head and Facial Bones

Ultrasonic osteogenic stimulator — *continued*
  use Bone Growth Stimulator in Lower Bones
  use Bone Growth Stimulator in Upper Bones
Ultrasonography
  Abdomen BW40ZZZ
  Abdomen and Pelvis BW41ZZZ
  Abdominal Wall BH49ZZZ
  Aorta
    Abdominal, Intravascular B440ZZ3
    Thoracic, Intravascular B340ZZ3
  Appendix BD48ZZZ
  Artery
    Brachiocephalic-Subclavian, Right, Intravascular B341ZZ3
    Celiac and Mesenteric, Intravascular B44KZZ3
    Common Carotid
      Bilateral, Intravascular B345ZZ3
      Left, Intravascular B344ZZ3
      Right, Intravascular B343ZZ3
    Coronary
      Multiple B241YZZ
        Intravascular B241ZZ3
        Transesophageal B241ZZ4
      Single B240YZZ
        Intravascular B240ZZ3
        Transesophageal B240ZZ4
    Femoral, Intravascular B44LZZ3
    Inferior Mesenteric, Intravascular B445ZZ3
    Internal Carotid
      Bilateral, Intravascular B348ZZ3
      Left, Intravascular B347ZZ3
      Right, Intravascular B346ZZ3
    Intra-Abdominal, Other, Intravascular B44BZZ3
    Intracranial, Intravascular B34RZZ3
    Lower Extremity
      Bilateral, Intravascular B44HZZ3
      Left, Intravascular B44GZZ3
      Right, Intravascular B44FZZ3
    Mesenteric and Celiac, Intravascular B44KZZ3
    Ophthalmic, Intravascular B34VZZ3
    Penile, Intravascular B44NZZ3
    Pulmonary
      Left, Intravascular B34TZZ3
      Right, Intravascular B34SZZ3
    Renal
      Bilateral, Intravascular B448ZZ3
      Left, Intravascular B447ZZ3
      Right, Intravascular B446ZZ3
    Subclavian, Left, Intravascular B342ZZ3
    Superior Mesenteric, Intravascular B444ZZ3
    Upper Extremity
      Bilateral, Intravascular B34KZZ3
      Left, Intravascular B34JZZ3
      Right, Intravascular B34HZZ3
  Bile Duct BF40ZZZ
  Bile Duct and Gallbladder BF43ZZZ
  Bladder BT40ZZZ
    and Kidney BT4JZZZ
  Brain B040ZZZ
  Breast
    Bilateral BH42ZZZ
    Left BH41ZZZ
    Right BH40ZZZ
  Chest Wall BH4BZZZ
  Coccyx BR4FZZZ
  Connective Tissue
    Lower Extremity BL41ZZZ
    Upper Extremity BL40ZZZ
  Duodenum BD49ZZZ
  Elbow
    Left, Densitometry BP4HZZ1
    Right, Densitometry BP4GZZ1
  Esophagus BD41ZZZ
  Extremity
    Lower BH48ZZZ
    Upper BH47ZZZ
  Eye
    Bilateral B847ZZZ
    Left B846ZZZ
    Right B845ZZZ
  Fallopian Tube
    Bilateral BU42
    Left BU41
    Right BU40
  Fetal Umbilical Cord BY47ZZZ
  Fetus
    First Trimester, Multiple Gestation BY4BZZZ

Ultrasonography — *continued*
  Fetus — *continued*
    Second Trimester, Multiple Gestation BY4DZZZ
    Single
      First Trimester BY49ZZZ
      Second Trimester BY4CZZZ
      Third Trimester BY4FZZZ
    Third Trimester, Multiple Gestation BY4GZZZ
  Gallbladder BF42ZZZ
  Gallbladder and Bile Duct BF43ZZZ
  Gastrointestinal Tract BD47ZZZ
  Gland
    Adrenal
      Bilateral BG42ZZZ
      Left BG41ZZZ
      Right BG40ZZZ
    Parathyroid BG43ZZZ
    Thyroid BG44ZZZ
  Hand
    Left, Densitometry BP4PZZ1
    Right, Densitometry BP4NZZ1
  Head and Neck BH4C7ZZ
  Heart
    Left B245YZZ
      Intravascular B245ZZ3
      Transesophageal B245ZZ4
    Pediatric B24DYZZ
      Intravascular B24DZZ3
      Transesophageal B24DZZ4
    Right B244YZZ
      Intravascular B244ZZ3
      Transesophageal B244ZZ4
    Right and Left B246YZZ
      Intravascular B246ZZ3
      Transesophageal B246ZZ4
  Heart with Aorta B24BYZZ
    Intravascular B24BZZ3
    Transesophageal B24BZZ4
  Hepatobiliary System, All BF4CZZZ
  Hip
    Bilateral BQ42ZZZ
    Left BQ41ZZZ
    Right BQ40ZZZ
  Kidney
    and Bladder BT4JZZZ
    Bilateral BT43ZZZ
    Left BT42ZZZ
    Right BT41ZZZ
    Transplant BT49ZZZ
  Knee
    Bilateral BQ49ZZZ
    Left BQ48ZZZ
    Right BQ47ZZZ
  Liver BF45ZZZ
  Liver and Spleen BF46ZZZ
  Mediastinum BB4CZZZ
  Neck BW4FZZZ
  Ovary
    Bilateral BU45
    Left BU44
    Right BU43
  Ovary and Uterus BU4C
  Pancreas BF47ZZZ
  Pelvic Region BW4GZZZ
  Pelvis and Abdomen BW41ZZZ
  Penis BV4BZZZ
  Pericardium B24CYZZ
    Intravascular B24CZZ3
    Transesophageal B24CZZ4
  Placenta BY48ZZZ
  Pleura BB4BZZZ
  Prostate and Seminal Vesicle BV49ZZZ
  Rectum BD4CZZZ
  Sacrum BR4FZZZ
  Scrotum BV44ZZZ
  Seminal Vesicle and Prostate BV49ZZZ
  Shoulder
    Left, Densitometry BP49ZZ1
    Right, Densitometry BP48ZZ1
  Spinal Cord B04BZZZ
  Spine
    Cervical BR40ZZZ
    Lumbar BR49ZZZ
    Thoracic BR47ZZZ
  Spleen and Liver BF46ZZZ
  Stomach BD42ZZZ
  Tendon
    Lower Extremity BL43ZZZ

Ultrasonography — *continued*
  Tendon — *continued*
    Upper Extremity BL42ZZZ
  Ureter
    Bilateral BT48ZZZ
    Left BT47ZZZ
    Right BT46ZZZ
  Urethra BT45ZZZ
  Uterus BU46
  Uterus and Ovary BU4C
  Vein
    Jugular
      Left, Intravascular B544ZZ3
      Right, Intravascular B543ZZ3
    Lower Extremity
      Bilateral, Intravascular B54DZZ3
      Left, Intravascular B54CZZ3
      Right, Intravascular B54BZZ3
    Portal, Intravascular B54TZZ3
    Renal
      Bilateral, Intravascular B54LZZ3
      Left, Intravascular B54KZZ3
      Right, Intravascular B54JZZ3
    Spanchnic, Intravascular B541ZZ3
    Subclavian
      Left, Intravascular B547ZZ3
      Right, Intravascular B546ZZ3
    Upper Extremity
      Bilateral, Intravascular B54PZZ3
      Left, Intravascular B54NZZ3
      Right, Intravascular B54MZZ3
  Vena Cava
    Inferior, Intravascular B549ZZ3
    Superior, Intravascular B548ZZ3
  Wrist
    Left, Densitometry BP4MZZ1
    Right, Densitometry BP4LZZ1
Ultrasound bone healing system
  use Bone Growth Stimulator in Head and Facial Bones
  use Bone Growth Stimulator in Lower Bones
  use Bone Growth Stimulator in Upper Bones
Ultrasound Therapy
  Heart 6A75
  No Qualifier 6A75
  Vessels
    Head and Neck 6A75
    Other 6A75
    Peripheral 6A75
Ultraviolet Light Therapy, Skin 6A80
Umbilical artery
  use Internal Iliac Artery, Left
  use Internal Iliac Artery, Right
  use Lower Artery
Uniplanar external fixator
  use External Fixation Device, Monoplanar in 0PH
  use External Fixation Device, Monoplanar in 0PS
  use External Fixation Device, Monoplanar in 0QH
  use External Fixation Device, Monoplanar in 0QS
UPLIZNA® *use* Inebilizumab-cdon
Upper GI series *see* Fluoroscopy, Gastrointestinal, Upper BD15
Ureteral orifice
  use Ureter
  use Ureter, Left
  use Ureter, Right
  use Ureters, Bilateral
Ureterectomy
  see Excision, Urinary System 0TB
  see Resection, Urinary System 0TT
Ureterocolostomy *see* Bypass, Urinary System 0T1
Ureterocystostomy *see* Bypass, Urinary System 0T1
Ureteroenterostomy *see* Bypass, Urinary System 0T1
Ureteroileostomy *see* Bypass, Urinary System 0T1
Ureterolithotomy *see* Extirpation, Urinary System 0TC
Ureterolysis *see* Release, Urinary System 0TN
Ureteroneocystostomy
  see Bypass, Urinary System 0T1
  see Reposition, Urinary System 0TS
Ureteropelvic junction (UPJ)
  use Kidney Pelvis, Left
  use Kidney Pelvis, Right
Ureteropexy
  see Repair, Urinary System 0TQ
  see Reposition, Urinary System 0TS
Ureteroplasty
  see Repair, Urinary System 0TQ

Ureteroplasty — *continued*
see Replacement, Urinary System ØTR
see Supplement, Urinary System ØTU
Ureteroplication see Restriction, Urinary System ØTV
Ureteropyelography see Fluoroscopy, Urinary System BT1
Ureterorrhaphy see Repair, Urinary System ØTQ
Ureteroscopy ØTJ98ZZ
Ureterostomy
see Bypass, Urinary System ØT1
see Drainage, Urinary System ØT9
Ureterotomy see Drainage, Urinary System ØT9
Ureteroureterostomy see Bypass, Urinary System ØT1
Ureterovesical orifice
use Ureter
use Ureter, Left
use Ureter, Right
use Ureters, Bilateral
Urethral catheterization, indwelling ØT9B7ØZ
Urethrectomy
see Excision, Urethra ØTBD
see Resection, Urethra ØTTD
Urethrolithotomy see Extirpation, Urethra ØTCD
Urethrolysis see Release, Urethra ØTND
Urethropexy
see Repair, Urethra ØTQD
see Reposition, Urethra ØTSD
Urethroplasty
see Repair, Urethra ØTQD
see Replacement, Urethra ØTRD
see Supplement, Urethra ØTUD
Urethrorrhaphy see Repair, Urethra ØTQD
Urethroscopy ØTJD8ZZ
Urethrotomy see Drainage, Urethra ØT9D
Uridine Triacetate XWØDX82
Urinary incontinence stimulator lead use Stimulator Lead in Urinary System
Urography see Fluoroscopy, Urinary System BT1
Ustekinumab use Other New Technology Therapeutic Substance
Uterine Artery
use Internal Iliac Artery, Left
use Internal Iliac Artery, Right
Uterine artery embolization (UAE) see Occlusion, Lower Arteries Ø4L
Uterine cornu use Uterus
Uterine tube
use Fallopian Tube, Left
use Fallopian Tube, Right
Uterine vein
use Hypogastric Vein, Left
use Hypogastric Vein, Right
Uvulectomy
see Excision, Uvula ØCBN
see Resection, Uvula ØCTN
Uvulorrhaphy see Repair, Uvula ØCQN
Uvulotomy see Drainage, Uvula ØC9N

V

Vabomere™ use Meropenem-vaborbactam Anti-infective
Vaccination see Introduction of Serum, Toxoid, and Vaccine
Vacuum extraction, obstetric 10D07Z6
Vaginal artery
use Internal Iliac Artery, Left
use Internal Iliac Artery, Right
Vaginal pessary use Intraluminal Device, Pessary in Female Reproductive System
Vaginal vein
use Hypogastric Vein, Left
use Hypogastric Vein, Right
Vaginectomy
see Excision, Vagina ØUBG
see Resection, Vagina ØUTG
Vaginofixation
see Repair, Vagina ØUQG
see Reposition, Vagina ØUSG
Vaginoplasty
see Repair, Vagina ØUQG
see Supplement, Vagina ØUUG
Vaginorrhaphy see Repair, Vagina ØUQG
Vaginoscopy ØUJH8ZZ
Vaginotomy see Drainage, Female Reproductive System ØU9

Vagotomy see Division, Nerve, Vagus 008Q
Valiant Thoracic Stent Graft use Intraluminal Device
Valvotomy, valvulotomy
see Division, Heart and Great Vessels 028
see Release, Heart and Great Vessels 02N
Valvuloplasty
see Repair, Heart and Great Vessels 02Q
see Replacement, Heart and Great Vessels 02R
see Supplement, Heart and Great Vessels 02U
Valvuloplasty, Alfieri Stitch see Restriction, Valve, Mitral 02VG
Vascular Access Device
Totally Implantable
Insertion of device in
Abdomen ØJH8
Chest ØJH6
Lower Arm
Left ØJHH
Right ØJHG
Lower Leg
Left ØJHP
Right ØJHN
Upper Arm
Left ØJHF
Right ØJHD
Upper Leg
Left ØJHM
Right ØJHL
Removal of device from
Lower Extremity ØJPW
Trunk ØJPT
Upper Extremity ØJPV
Revision of device in
Lower Extremity ØJWW
Trunk ØJWT
Upper Extremity ØJWV
Tunneled
Insertion of device in
Abdomen ØJH8
Chest ØJH6
Lower Arm
Left ØJHH
Right ØJHG
Lower Leg
Left ØJHP
Right ØJHN
Upper Arm
Left ØJHF
Right ØJHD
Upper Leg
Left ØJHM
Right ØJHL
Removal of device from
Lower Extremity ØJPW
Trunk ØJPT
Upper Extremity ØJPV
Revision of device in
Lower Extremity ØJWW
Trunk ØJWT
Upper Extremity ØJWV
Vasectomy see Excision, Male Reproductive System ØVB
Vasography
see Fluoroscopy, Male Reproductive System BV1
see Plain Radiography, Male Reproductive System BVØ
Vasoligation see Occlusion, Male Reproductive System ØVL
Vasorrhaphy see Repair, Male Reproductive System ØVQ
Vasostomy see Bypass, Male Reproductive System ØV1
Vasotomy
Drainage see Drainage, Male Reproductive System ØV9
With ligation see Occlusion, Male Reproductive System ØVL
Vasovasostomy see Repair, Male Reproductive System ØVQ
Vastus intermedius muscle
use Upper Leg Muscle, Left
use Upper Leg Muscle, Right
Vastus lateralis muscle
use Upper Leg Muscle, Left
use Upper Leg Muscle, Right
Vastus medialis muscle
use Upper Leg Muscle, Left
use Upper Leg Muscle, Right

VCG (vectorcardiogram) see Measurement, Cardiac 4A02
Vectra® Vascular Access Graft use Vascular Access Device, Tunneled in Subcutaneous Tissue and Fascia
Veklury use Remdesivir Anti-infective
Venclexta® use Venetoclax Antineoplastic
Venectomy
see Excision, Lower Veins 06B
see Excision, Upper Veins 05B
Venetoclax Antineoplastic XWØDXR5
Venography
see Fluoroscopy, Veins B51
see Plain Radiography, Veins B5Ø
Venorrhaphy
see Repair, Lower Veins 06Q
see Repair, Upper Veins 05Q
Venotripsy
see Occlusion, Lower Veins 06L
see Occlusion, Upper Veins 05L
Ventricular fold use Larynx
Ventriculoatriostomy see Bypass, Central Nervous System and Cranial Nerves 001
Ventriculocisternostomy see Bypass, Central Nervous System and Cranial Nerves 001
Ventriculogram, cardiac
Combined left and right heart see Fluoroscopy, Heart, Right and Left B216
Left ventricle see Fluoroscopy, Heart, Left B215
Right ventricle see Fluoroscopy, Heart, Right B214
Ventriculopuncture, through previously implanted catheter 8C01X6J
Ventriculoscopy 00J04ZZ
Ventriculostomy
External drainage see Drainage, Cerebral Ventricle 0096
Internal shunt see Bypass, Cerebral Ventricle 0016
Ventriculovenostomy see Bypass, Cerebral Ventricle 0016
Ventrio™ Hernia Patch use Synthetic Substitute
VEP (visual evoked potential) 4A07X0Z
Vermiform appendix use Appendix
Vermilion border
use Lower Lip
use Upper Lip
Versa use Pacemaker, Dual Chamber in ØJH
Version, obstetric
External 10S0XZZ
Internal 10S07ZZ
Vertebral arch
use Cervical Vertebra
use Lumbar Vertebra
use Thoracic Vertebra
Vertebral body
use Cervical Vertebra
use Lumbar Vertebra
use Thoracic Vertebra
Vertebral canal use Spinal Canal
Vertebral foramen
use Cervical Vertebra
use Lumbar Vertebra
use Thoracic Vertebra
Vertebral lamina
use Cervical Vertebra
use Lumbar Vertebra
use Thoracic Vertebra
Vertebral pedicle
use Cervical Vertebra
use Lumbar Vertebra
use Thoracic Vertebra
Vesical vein
use Hypogastric Vein, Left
use Hypogastric Vein, Right
Vesicotomy see Drainage, Urinary System ØT9
Vesiculectomy
see Excision, Male Reproductive System ØVB
see Resection, Male Reproductive System ØVT
Vesiculogram, seminal see Plain Radiography, Male Reproductive System BVØ
Vesiculotomy see Drainage, Male Reproductive System ØV9
Vestibular Assessment F15Z
Vestibular (Scarpa's) ganglion use Acoustic Nerve
Vestibular nerve use Acoustic Nerve
Vestibular Treatment F0C
Vestibulocochlear nerve use Acoustic Nerve

VH-IVUS (virtual histology intravascular ultrasound) *see* Ultrasonography, Heart B24
Virchow's (supraclavicular) lymph node
  use Lymphatic, Left Neck
  use Lymphatic, Right Neck
Virtuoso (II) (DR) (VR) *use* Defibrillator Generator in ØJH
Vistogard® *use* Uridine Triacetate
Visualase™ MRI-Guided Laser Ablation System *see* Destruction
Vitrectomy
  see Excision, Eye Ø8B
  see Resection, Eye Ø8T
Vitreous body
  use Vitreous, Left
  use Vitreous, Right
Viva (XT) (S) *use* Cardiac Resynchronization Defibrillator Pulse Generator in ØJH
Vivistim® Paired VNS System Lead *use* Neurostimulator Lead with Paired Stimulation System in New Technology
Vocal fold
  use Vocal Cord, Left
  use Vocal Cord, Right
Vocational
  Assessment *see* Activities of Daily Living Assessment, Rehabilitation FØ2
  Retraining *see* Activities of Daily Living Treatment, Rehabilitation FØ8
Volar (palmar) digital vein
  use Hand Vein, Left
  use Hand Vein, Right
Volar (palmar) metacarpal vein
  use Hand Vein, Left
  use Hand Vein, Right
Vomer bone *use* Nasal Septum
Vomer of nasal septum *use* Nasal Bone
Voraxaze *use* Glucarpidase
Vulvectomy
  see Excision, Female Reproductive System ØUB
  see Resection, Female Reproductive System ØUT
V-Wave Interatrial Shunt System *use* Synthetic Substitute
VYXEOS™ *use* Cytarabine and Daunorubicin Liposome Antineoplastic

W

WALLSTENT® Endoprosthesis *use* Intraluminal Device
Washing *see* Irrigation
WavelinQ EndoAVF system
  Radial Artery, Left Ø31C3ZF
  Radial Artery, Right Ø31B3ZF
  Ulnar Artery, Left Ø31A3ZF
  Ulnar Artery, Right Ø3193ZF
Wedge resection, pulmonary *see* Excision, Respiratory System ØBB
Whole Blood Nucleic Acid-base Microbial Detection XXE5XM5
Whole Blood Reverse Transcription and Quantitative Real-time Polymerase Chain Reaction XXE5X38
Window *see* Drainage
Wiring, dental 2W31X9Z

X

Xact Carotid Stent System *use* Intraluminal Device
XENLETA™ *use* Lefamulin Anti-infective
Xenograft *use* Zooplastic Tissue in Heart and Great Vessels
XENOVIEW™ BB34Z3Z
XIENCE Everolimus Eluting Coronary Stent System *use* Intraluminal Device, Drug-eluting in Heart and Great Vessels
Xiphoid process *use* Sternum
XLIF® System *use* Interbody Fusion Device in Lower Joints
XOSPATA® *use* Gilteritinib Antineoplastic
X-ray *see* Plain Radiography
X-Spine Axle Cage
  use Spinal Stabilization Device, Interspinous Process in ØRH
  use Spinal Stabilization Device, Interspinous Process in ØSH
X-STOP® Spacer
  use Spinal Stabilization Device, Interspinous Process in ØRH
  use Spinal Stabilization Device, Interspinous Process in ØSH

Y

Yescarta® *use* Axicabtagene Ciloleucel Immunotherapy
Yoga Therapy 8EØZXY4

Z

Zenith AAA Endovascular Graft *use* Intraluminal Device
Zenith Flex® AAA Endovascular Graft *use* Intraluminal Device
Zenith TX2® TAA Endovascular Graft *use* Intraluminal Device
Zenith® Fenestrated AAA Endovascular Graft
  use Intraluminal Device, Branched or Fenestrated, One or Two Arteries in Ø4V
  use Intraluminal Device, Branched or Fenestrated, Three or More Arteries in Ø4V
Zenith® Renu™ AAA Ancillary Graft *use* Intraluminal Device
ZEPZELCA™ *use* Lurbinectedin
ZERBAXA® *use* Ceftolozane/Tazobactam Anti-infective
Zilver® PTX® (paclitaxel) Drug-Eluting Peripheral Stent
  use Intraluminal Device, Drug-eluting in Lower Arteries
  use Intraluminal Device, Drug-eluting in Upper Arteries
Zimmer® NexGen® LPS Mobile Bearing Knee *use* Synthetic Substitute
Zimmer® NexGen® LPS-Flex Mobile Knee *use* Synthetic Substitute
ZINPLAVA™ infusion *see* Introduction with qualifier Other Therapeutic Monoclonal Antibody
Zonule of Zinn
  use Lens, Left
  use Lens, Right
Zotarolimus-eluting Coronary Stent *use* Intraluminal Device, Drug-eluting in Heart and Great Vessels
Z-plasty, skin for scar contracture *see* Release, Skin and Breast ØHN
ZULRESSO™ *use* Brexanolone
Zygomatic process of frontal bone *use* Frontal Bone
Zygomatic process of temporal bone
  use Temporal Bone, Left
  use Temporal Bone, Right
Zygomaticus muscle *use* Facial Muscle
Zyvox *use* Oxazolidinones

ICD-10-PCS Tables

Central Nervous System and Cranial Nerves 001–00X

Character Meanings

This Character Meaning table is provided as a guide to assist the user in the identification of character members that may be found in this section of code tables. It **SHOULD NOT** be used to build a PCS code.

Operation–Character 3		Body Part–Character 4		Approach–Character 5		Device–Character 6		Qualifier–Character 7	
1	Bypass	0	Brain	0	Open	0	Drainage Device	0	Nasopharynx
2	Change	1	Cerebral Meninges	3	Percutaneous	1	Radioactive Element	1	Mastoid Sinus
5	Destruction	2	Dura Mater	4	Percutaneous Endoscopic	2	Monitoring Device	2	Atrium
7	Dilation	3	Epidural Space, Intracranial	X	External	3	Infusion Device	3	Blood Vessel OR Laser Interstitial Thermal Therapy
8	Division	4	Subdural Space, Intracranial			4	Radioactive Element, Cesium-131 Collagen Implant	4	Pleural Cavity
9	Drainage	5	Subarachnoid Space, Intracranial			7	Autologous Tissue Substitute	5	Intestine
B	Excision	6	Cerebral Ventricle			J	Synthetic Substitute	6	Peritoneal Cavity
C	Extirpation	7	Cerebral Hemisphere			K	Nonautologous Tissue Substitute	7	Urinary Tract
D	Extraction	8	Basal Ganglia			M	Neurostimulator Lead	8	Bone Marrow
F	Fragmentation	9	Thalamus			Y	Other Device	9	Fallopian Tube
H	Insertion	A	Hypothalamus			Z	No Device	A	Subgaleal Space
J	Inspection	B	Pons					B	Cerebral Cisterns
K	Map	C	Cerebellum					F	Olfactory Nerve
N	Release	D	Medulla Oblongata					G	Optic Nerve
P	Removal	E	Cranial Nerve					H	Oculomotor Nerve
Q	Repair	F	Olfactory Nerve					J	Trochlear Nerve
R	Replacement	G	Optic Nerve					K	Trigeminal Nerve
S	Reposition	H	Oculomotor Nerve					L	Abducens Nerve
T	Resection	J	Trochlear Nerve					M	Facial Nerve
U	Supplement	K	Trigeminal Nerve					N	Acoustic Nerve
W	Revision	L	Abducens Nerve					P	Glossopharyngeal Nerve
X	Transfer	M	Facial Nerve					Q	Vagus Nerve
		N	Acoustic Nerve					R	Accessory Nerve
		P	Glossopharyngeal Nerve					S	Hypoglossal Nerve
		Q	Vagus Nerve					X	Diagnostic
		R	Accessory Nerve					Z	No Qualifier
		S	Hypoglossal Nerve						
		T	Spinal Meninges						
		U	Spinal Canal						
		V	Spinal Cord						
		W	Cervical Spinal Cord						
		X	Thoracic Spinal Cord						
		Y	Lumbar Spinal Cord						

AHA Coding Clinic for table 001

2021, 2Q, 19	Electromagnetic stealth guided ventriculoperitoneal shunt insertion with endoscopy
2019, 4Q, 21-22	Cerebral ventricle bypass Qualifier
2018, 4Q, 86	Placement of lumboatrial shunt
2017, 4Q, 39-41	Dilation and bypass of cerebral ventricle
2015, 2Q, 9	Revision of ventriculoperitoneal (VP) shunt
2013, 2Q, 36	Insertion of ventriculoperitoneal shunt with laparoscopic assistance

AHA Coding Clinic for table 005

2022, 1Q, 50	Percutaneous ganglion balloon compression
2021, 3Q, 16	Decompression of Chiari malformation by excision
2021, 2Q, 17	Dorsal root entry zone procedure

AHA Coding Clinic for table 007

2017, 4Q, 39-41	Dilation and bypass of cerebral ventricle

AHA Coding Clinic for table 009

2018, 4Q, 85	Externalization of lumboatrial shunt
2017, 1Q, 50	Failed lumbar puncture
2015, 3Q, 10	Open evacuation of subdural hematoma
2015, 3Q, 11	Percutaneous drainage of subdural hematoma
2015, 3Q, 12	Subdural evacuation portal system (SEPS) placement
2015, 3Q, 12	Placement of ventriculostomy catheter via burr hole
2015, 2Q, 30	Drainage of syrinx
2015, 1Q, 31	Intrathecal chemotherapy
2014, 1Q, 8	Diagnostic lumbar tap
2014, 1Q, 8	Lumbar drainage port aspiration

AHA Coding Clinic for table 00B

2021, 3Q, 16	Decompression of Chiari malformation by excision
2017, 3Q, 17	Resection of schwannoma and placement of DuraGen and Lorenz cranial plating system
2016, 2Q, 12	Resection of malignant neoplasm of infratemporal fossa
2016, 2Q, 18	Amygdalohippocampectomy
2014, 4Q, 34	Resection of brain malignancy with implantation of chemotherapeutic wafer
2014, 3Q, 24	Repair of lipomyelomeningocele and tethered cord

AHA Coding Clinic for table 00C

2019, 3Q, 4	Evacuation of subdural hematoma and control of bleeding artery
2019, 2Q, 36	Evacuation of hematoma using NICO Brainpath® technology
2017, 4Q, 48	New and revised body part values - Extirpation spinal canal
2016, 2Q, 29	Decompressive craniectomy with cryopreservation and storage of bone flap
2015, 3Q, 10	Open evacuation of subdural hematoma
2015, 3Q, 11	Percutaneous drainage of subdural hematoma
2015, 3Q, 13	Evacuation of intracerebral hematoma

AHA Coding Clinic for table 00D

2021, 4Q, 38-40	Ultrasonic surgical aspiration of brain
2015, 3Q, 13	Nonexcisional debridement of cranial wound with removal and replacement of hardware

AHA Coding Clinic for table 00H

2020, 4Q, 43-44	Insertion of radioactive element
2020, 2Q, 15	Ommaya reservoir with ventricular catheter placement
2020, 2Q, 16	Ommaya reservoir placement for cerebrospinal fluid infusion therapy
2017, 4Q, 30-31	Radiotherapeutic brain implant
2017, 3Q, 13	Implantation of bilateral neurostimulator electrodes
2014, 3Q, 19	End of life replacement of Baclofen pump

AHA Coding Clinic for table 00J

2021, 2Q, 19	Electromagnetic stealth guided ventriculoperitoneal shunt insertion with endoscopy
2019, 2Q, 36	Evacuation of hematoma using NICO Brainpath® technology
2017, 1Q, 50	Failed lumbar puncture

AHA Coding Clinic for table 00N

2019, 2Q, 19	Cervical spinal fusion, decompression and placement of interfacet stabilization device
2019, 1Q, 28	Decompressive laminectomy of both spinal cord and nerve roots
2018, 3Q, 30	Decompressive laminectomy (release of spinal cord versus release of spinal meninges)
2017, 3Q, 10	Repair of Chiari malformation
2017, 2Q, 23	Decompression of spinal cord and placement of instrumentation
2016, 2Q, 29	Decompressive craniectomy with cryopreservation and storage of bone flap
2015, 2Q, 20	Cervical laminoplasty
2015, 2Q, 21	Multiple decompressive cervical laminectomies
2015, 2Q, 34	Decompressive laminectomy
2014, 3Q, 24	Repair of lipomyelomeningocele and tethered cord

AHA Coding Clinic for table 00P

2014, 3Q, 19	End of life replacement of Baclofen pump

AHA Coding Clinic for table 00Q

2014, 3Q, 7	Hemi-cranioplasty for repair of cranial defect
2013, 3Q, 25	Fracture of frontal bone with repair and coagulation for hemostasis

AHA Coding Clinic for table 00S

2014, 4Q, 35	Reimplantation of buccal nerve

AHA Coding Clinic for table 00U

2021, 3Q, 16	Decompression of Chiari malformation by excision
2018, 1Q, 9	Craniectomy with DuraGaurd placement
2017, 4Q, 62	Added and revised device values - Nerve substitutes
2017, 3Q, 10	Repair of Chiari malformation
2017, 3Q, 17	Resection of schwannoma and placement of DuraGen and Lorenz cranial plating system
2015, 4Q, 39	Dural patch graft
2014, 3Q, 24	Repair of lipomyelomeningocele and tethered cord

AHA Coding Clinic for table 00W

2018, 4Q, 86	Placement of lumboatrial shunt

Brain

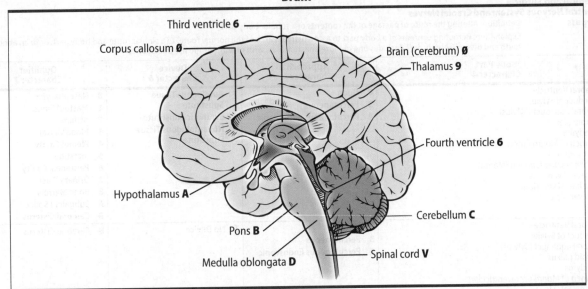

- Third ventricle **6**
- Corpus callosum **Ø**
- Brain (cerebrum) **Ø**
- Thalamus **9**
- Fourth ventricle **6**
- Hypothalamus **A**
- Cerebellum **C**
- Pons **B**
- Spinal cord **V**
- Medulla oblongata **D**

Cranial Nerves

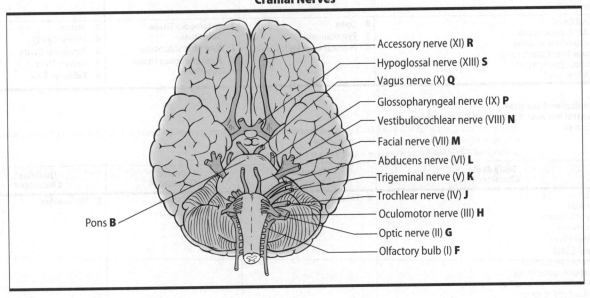

- Accessory nerve (XI) **R**
- Hypoglossal nerve (XIII) **S**
- Vagus nerve (X) **Q**
- Glossopharyngeal nerve (IX) **P**
- Vestibulocochlear nerve (VIII) **N**
- Facial nerve (VII) **M**
- Abducens nerve (VI) **L**
- Trigeminal nerve (V) **K**
- Trochlear nerve (IV) **J**
- Oculomotor nerve (III) **H**
- Optic nerve (II) **G**
- Olfactory bulb (I) **F**
- Pons **B**

Central Nervous System and Cranial Nerves

Ø   Medical and Surgical
Ø   Central Nervous System and Cranial Nerves
1   Bypass   Definition: Altering the route of passage of the contents of a tubular body part

                       Explanation: Rerouting contents of a body part to a downstream area of the normal route, to a similar route and body part, or to an abnormal route and dissimilar body part. Includes one or more anastomoses, with or without the use of a device.

Body Part Character 4	Approach Character 5	Device Character 6	Qualifier Character 7
6 Cerebral Ventricle Aqueduct of Sylvius Cerebral aqueduct (Sylvius) Choroid plexus Ependyma Foramen of Monro (intraventricular) Fourth ventricle Interventricular foramen (Monro) Left lateral ventricle Right lateral ventricle Third ventricle	**Ø** Open **3** Percutaneous **4** Percutaneous Endoscopic	**7** Autologous Tissue Substitute **J** Synthetic Substitute **K** Nonautologous Tissue Substitute	**Ø** Nasopharynx **1** Mastoid Sinus **2** Atrium **3** Blood Vessel **4** Pleural Cavity **5** Intestine **6** Peritoneal Cavity **7** Urinary Tract **8** Bone Marrow **A** Subgaleal Space **B** Cerebral Cisterns
6 Cerebral Ventricle Aqueduct of Sylvius Cerebral aqueduct (Sylvius) Choroid plexus Ependyma Foramen of Monro (intraventricular) Fourth ventricle Interventricular foramen (Monro) Left lateral ventricle Right lateral ventricle Third ventricle	**Ø** Open **3** Percutaneous **4** Percutaneous Endoscopic	**Z** No Device	**B** Cerebral Cisterns
U Spinal Canal Epidural space, spinal Extradural space, spinal Subarachnoid space, spinal Subdural space, spinal Vertebral canal	**Ø** Open **3** Percutaneous **4** Percutaneous Endoscopic	**7** Autologous Tissue Substitute **J** Synthetic Substitute **K** Nonautologous Tissue Substitute	**2** Atrium **4** Pleural Cavity **6** Peritoneal Cavity **7** Urinary Tract **9** Fallopian Tube

Ø   Medical and Surgical
Ø   Central Nervous System and Cranial Nerves
2   Change   Definition: Taking out or off a device from a body part and putting back an identical or similar device in or on the same body part without cutting or puncturing the skin or a mucous membrane

                       Explanation: All CHANGE procedures are coded using the approach EXTERNAL

Body Part Character 4	Approach Character 5	Device Character 6	Qualifier Character 7
Ø Brain Cerebrum Corpus callosum Encephalon **E Cranial Nerve** **U Spinal Canal** Epidural space, spinal Extradural space, spinal Subarachnoid space, spinal Subdural space, spinal Vertebral canal	**X** External	**Ø** Drainage Device **Y** Other Device	**Z** No Qualifier

Non-OR   All body part, approach, device, and qualifier values

Non-OR Procedure   DRG Non-OR Procedure   Valid OR Procedure   HAC Associated Procedure   Combination Only   New/Revised April   New/Revised October

134   ICD-10-PCS 2023

Ø   Medical and Surgical
Ø   Central Nervous System and Cranial Nerves
5   Destruction   Definition: Physical eradication of all or a portion of a body part by the direct use of energy, force, or a destructive agent
                       Explanation: None of the body part is physically taken out

Body Part Character 4		Approach Character 5	Device Character 6	Qualifier Character 7

Ø Brain
  Cerebrum
  Corpus callosum
  Encephalon
W Cervical Spinal Cord
  Dorsal root ganglion
	X Thoracic Spinal Cord
	  Dorsal root ganglion
	Y Lumbar Spinal Cord
	  Cauda equina
	  Conus medullaris
	  Dorsal root ganglion
		Ø Open
		3 Percutaneous
		4 Percutaneous Endoscopic
			Z No Device	**3 Laser Interstitial Thermal Therapy**
				Z No Qualifier

1 Cerebral Meninges
  Arachnoid mater,
    intracranial
  Leptomeninges,
    intracranial
  Pia mater, intracranial
2 Dura Mater
  Diaphragma sellae
  Dura mater, intracranial
  Falx cerebri
  Tentorium cerebelli
6 Cerebral Ventricle
  Aqueduct of Sylvius
  Cerebral aqueduct
    (Sylvius)
  Choroid plexus
  Ependyma
  Foramen of Monro
    (intraventricular)
  Fourth ventricle
  Interventricular foramen
    (Monro)
  Left lateral ventricle
  Right lateral ventricle
  Third ventricle
7 Cerebral Hemisphere
  Frontal lobe
  Occipital lobe
  Parietal lobe
  Temporal lobe
8 Basal Ganglia
  Basal nuclei
  Claustrum
  Corpus striatum
  Globus pallidus
  Substantia nigra
  Subthalamic nucleus
9 Thalamus
  Epithalamus
  Geniculate nucleus
  Metathalamus
  Pulvinar
A Hypothalamus
  Mammillary body
B Pons
  Apneustic center
  Basis pontis
  Locus ceruleus
  Pneumotaxic center
  Pontine tegmentum
  Superior olivary nucleus
C Cerebellum
  Culmen
D Medulla Oblongata
  Myelencephalon
F Olfactory Nerve
  First cranial nerve
  Olfactory bulb
G Optic Nerve
  Optic chiasma
  Second cranial nerve
	H Oculomotor Nerve
	  Third cranial nerve
	J Trochlear Nerve
	  Fourth cranial nerve
	K Trigeminal Nerve
	  Fifth cranial nerve
	  Gasserian ganglion
	  Mandibular nerve
	  Maxillary nerve
	  Ophthalmic nerve
	  Trifacial nerve
	L Abducens Nerve
	  Sixth cranial nerve
	M Facial Nerve
	  Chorda tympani
	  Geniculate ganglion
	  Greater superficial petrosal
	    nerve
	  Nerve to the stapedius
	  Parotid plexus
	  Posterior auricular nerve
	  Seventh cranial nerve
	  Submandibular ganglion
	N Acoustic Nerve
	  Cochlear nerve
	  Eighth cranial nerve
	  Scarpa's (vestibular)
	    ganglion
	  Spiral ganglion
	  Vestibular (Scarpa's)
	    ganglion
	  Vestibular nerve
	  Vestibulocochlear nerve
	P Glossopharyngeal Nerve
	  Carotid sinus nerve
	  Ninth cranial nerve
	  Tympanic nerve
	Q Vagus Nerve
	  Anterior vagal trunk
	  Pharyngeal plexus
	  Pneumogastric nerve
	  Posterior vagal trunk
	  Pulmonary plexus
	  Recurrent laryngeal nerve
	  Superior laryngeal nerve
	  Tenth cranial nerve
	R Accessory Nerve
	  Eleventh cranial nerve
	S Hypoglossal Nerve
	  Twelfth cranial nerve
	T Spinal Meninges
	  Arachnoid mater, spinal
	  Denticulate (dentate)
	    ligament
	  Dura mater, spinal
	  Filum terminale
	  Leptomeninges, spinal
	  Pia mater, spinal
		Ø Open
		3 Percutaneous
		4 Percutaneous Endoscopic
			Z No Device	**Z No Qualifier**

Non-OR   005[F,G,H,J,K,L,M,N,P,Q,R,S][Ø,3,4]ZZ

NC Noncovered Procedure   LC Limited Coverage   QA Questionable OB Admit   NT New Tech Add-on   ⊞ Combination Member   ♂ Male   ♀ Female

ICD-10-PCS 2023   135

Ø Medical and Surgical
Ø Central Nervous System and Cranial Nerves
7 Dilation   Definition: Expanding an orifice or the lumen of a tubular body part

Explanation: The orifice can be a natural orifice or an artificially created orifice. Accomplished by stretching a tubular body part using intraluminal pressure or by cutting part of the orifice or wall of the tubular body part.

Body Part Character 4	Approach Character 5	Device Character 6	Qualifier Character 7

6   Cerebral Ventricle
    Aqueduct of Sylvius
    Cerebral aqueduct (Sylvius)
    Choroid plexus
    Ependyma
    Foramen of Monro (intraventricular)
    Fourth ventricle
    Interventricular foramen (Monro)
    Left lateral ventricle
    Right lateral ventricle
    Third ventricle
	Ø Open
	3 Percutaneous
	4 Percutaneous Endoscopic
		Z No Device	Z No Qualifier

Ø Medical and Surgical
Ø Central Nervous System and Cranial Nerves
8 Division   Definition: Cutting into a body part, without draining fluids and/or gases from the body part, in order to separate or transect a body part

Explanation: All or a portion of the body part is separated into two or more portions

Body Part Character 4	Approach Character 5	Device Character 6	Qualifier Character 7

Ø   Brain
    Cerebrum
    Corpus callosum
    Encephalon
7   Cerebral Hemisphere
    Frontal lobe
    Occipital lobe
    Parietal lobe
    Temporal lobe
8   Basal Ganglia
    Basal nuclei
    Claustrum
    Corpus striatum
    Globus pallidus
    Substantia nigra
    Subthalamic nucleus
F   Olfactory Nerve
    First cranial nerve
    Olfactory bulb
G   Optic Nerve
    Optic chiasma
    Second cranial nerve
H   Oculomotor Nerve
    Third cranial nerve
J   Trochlear Nerve
    Fourth cranial nerve
K   Trigeminal Nerve
    Fifth cranial nerve
    Gasserian ganglion
    Mandibular nerve
    Maxillary nerve
    Ophthalmic nerve
    Trifacial nerve
L   Abducens Nerve
    Sixth cranial nerve
M   Facial Nerve
    Chorda tympani
    Geniculate ganglion
    Greater superficial petrosal
      nerve
    Nerve to the stapedius
    Parotid plexus
    Posterior auricular nerve
    Seventh cranial nerve
    Submandibular ganglion
	N Acoustic Nerve
	    Cochlear nerve
	    Eighth cranial nerve
	    Scarpa's (vestibular)
	      ganglion
	    Spiral ganglion
	    Vestibular (Scarpa's)
	      ganglion
	    Vestibular nerve
	    Vestibulocochlear nerve
	P Glossopharyngeal Nerve
	    Carotid sinus nerve
	    Ninth cranial nerve
	    Tympanic nerve
	Q Vagus Nerve
	    Anterior vagal trunk
	    Pharyngeal plexus
	    Pneumogastric nerve
	    Posterior vagal trunk
	    Pulmonary plexus
	    Recurrent laryngeal nerve
	    Superior laryngeal nerve
	    Tenth cranial nerve
	R Accessory Nerve
	    Eleventh cranial nerve
	S Hypoglossal Nerve
	    Twelfth cranial nerve
	W Cervical Spinal Cord
	    Dorsal root ganglion
	X Thoracic Spinal Cord
	    Dorsal root ganglion
	Y Lumbar Spinal Cord
	    Cauda equina
	    Conus medullaris
	    Dorsal root ganglion
		Ø Open
		3 Percutaneous
		4 Percutaneous Endoscopic
			Z No Device	Z No Qualifier

Non-OR Procedure   DRG Non-OR Procedure   Valid OR Procedure   HAC Associated Procedure   Combination Only   New/Revised April   New/Revised October

136

007–008

ICD-10-PCS 2023

Ø   **Medical and Surgical**
Ø   **Central Nervous System and Cranial Nerves**
9   **Drainage**   Definition: Taking or letting out fluids and/or gases from a body part
                 Explanation: The qualifier DIAGNOSTIC is used to identify drainage procedures that are biopsies

Body Part Character 4		Approach Character 5	Device Character 6	Qualifier Character 7

Ø Brain
  Cerebrum
  Corpus callosum
  Encephalon
1 Cerebral Meninges
  Arachnoid mater,
    intracranial
  Leptomeninges,
    intracranial
  Pia mater, intracranial
2 Dura Mater
  Diaphragma sellae
  Dura mater, intracranial
  Falx cerebri
  Tentorium cerebelli
3 Epidural Space,
** Intracranial**
  Extradural space,
    intracranial
4 Subdural Space,
** Intracranial**
5 Subarachnoid Space,
** Intracranial**
6 Cerebral Ventricle
  Aqueduct of Sylvius
  Cerebral aqueduct
    (Sylvius)
  Choroid plexus
  Ependyma
  Foramen of Monro
    (intraventricular)
  Fourth ventricle
  Interventricular foramen
    (Monro)
  Left lateral ventricle
  Right lateral ventricle
  Third ventricle
7 Cerebral Hemisphere
  Frontal lobe
  Occipital lobe
  Parietal lobe
  Temporal lobe
8 Basal Ganglia
  Basal nuclei
  Claustrum
  Corpus striatum
  Globus pallidus
  Substantia nigra
  Subthalamic nucleus
9 Thalamus
  Epithalamus
  Geniculate nucleus
  Metathalamus
  Pulvinar
A Hypothalamus
  Mammillary body
B Pons
  Apneustic center
  Basis pontis
  Locus ceruleus
  Pneumotaxic center
  Pontine tegmentum
  Superior olivary nucleus
C Cerebellum
  Culmen
D Medulla Oblongata
  Myelencephalon
F Olfactory Nerve
  First cranial nerve
  Olfactory bulb
	G Optic Nerve
	  Optic chiasma
	  Second cranial nerve
	H Oculomotor Nerve
	  Third cranial nerve
	J Trochlear Nerve
	  Fourth cranial nerve
	K Trigeminal Nerve
	  Fifth cranial nerve
	  Gasserian ganglion
	  Mandibular nerve
	  Maxillary nerve
	  Ophthalmic nerve
	  Trifacial nerve
	L Abducens Nerve
	  Sixth cranial nerve
	M Facial Nerve
	  Chorda tympani
	  Geniculate ganglion
	  Greater superficial petrosal
	    nerve
	  Nerve to the stapedius
	  Parotid plexus
	  Posterior auricular nerve
	  Seventh cranial nerve
	  Submandibular ganglion
	N Acoustic Nerve
	  Cochlear nerve
	  Eighth cranial nerve
	  Scarpa's (vestibular) ganglion
	  Spiral ganglion
	  Vestibular (Scarpa's) ganglion
	  Vestibular nerve
	  Vestibulocochlear nerve
	P Glossopharyngeal Nerve
	  Carotid sinus nerve
	  Ninth cranial nerve
	  Tympanic nerve
	Q Vagus Nerve
	  Anterior vagal trunk
	  Pharyngeal plexus
	  Pneumogastric nerve
	  Posterior vagal trunk
	  Pulmonary plexus
	  Recurrent laryngeal nerve
	  Superior laryngeal nerve
	  Tenth cranial nerve
	R Accessory Nerve
	  Eleventh cranial nerve
	S Hypoglossal Nerve
	  Twelfth cranial nerve
	T Spinal Meninges
	  Arachnoid mater, spinal
	  Denticulate (dentate)
	    ligament
	  Dura mater, spinal
	  Filum terminale
	  Leptomeninges, spinal
	  Pia mater, spinal
	U Spinal Canal
	  Epidural space, spinal
	  Extradural space, spinal
	  Subarachnoid space, spinal
	  Subdural space, spinal
	  Vertebral canal
	W Cervical Spinal Cord
	  Dorsal root ganglion
	X Thoracic Spinal Cord
	  Dorsal root ganglion
	Y Lumbar Spinal Cord
	  Cauda equina
	  Conus medullaris
	  Dorsal root ganglion
		Ø Open
		3 Percutaneous
		4 Percutaneous Endoscopic
			Ø Drainage Device	**Z No Qualifier**

Non-OR	ØØ9[T,W,X,Y]3ØZ
Non-OR	ØØ9U[3,4]ØZ

009 Continued on next page

NC Noncovered Procedure   **LC** Limited Coverage   **QA** Questionable OB Admit   **NT** New Tech Add-on   ⊞ Combination Member   ♂ Male   ♀ Female

ICD-10-PCS 2023   **137**

Central Nervous System and Cranial Nerves

Ø   **Medical and Surgical**
Ø   **Central Nervous System and Cranial Nerves**
9   **Drainage**   Definition: Taking or letting out fluids and/or gases from a body part

009 Continued

Explanation: The qualifier DIAGNOSTIC is used to identify drainage procedures that are biopsies

Body Part Character 4		Approach Character 5	Device Character 6	Qualifier Character 7
Ø Brain Cerebrum Corpus callosum Encephalon **1 Cerebral Meninges** Arachnoid mater, intracranial Leptomeninges, intracranial Pia mater, intracranial **2 Dura Mater** Diaphragma sellae Dura mater, intracranial Falx cerebri Tentorium cerebelli **3 Epidural Space, Intracranial** Extradural space, intracranial **4 Subdural Space, Intracranial** **5 Subarachnoid Space, Intracranial** **6 Cerebral Ventricle** Aqueduct of Sylvius Cerebral aqueduct (Sylvius) Choroid plexus Ependyma Foramen of Monro (intraventricular) Fourth ventricle Interventricular foramen (Monro) Left lateral ventricle Right lateral ventricle Third ventricle **7 Cerebral Hemisphere** Frontal lobe Occipital lobe Parietal lobe Temporal lobe **8 Basal Ganglia** Basal nuclei Claustrum Corpus striatum Globus pallidus Substantia nigra Subthalamic nucleus **9 Thalamus** Epithalamus Geniculate nucleus Metathalamus Pulvinar **A Hypothalamus** Mammillary body **B Pons** Apneustic center Basis pontis Locus ceruleus Pneumotaxic center Pontine tegmentum Superior olivary nucleus **C Cerebellum** Culmen **D Medulla Oblongata** Myelencephalon **F Olfactory Nerve** First cranial nerve Olfactory bulb	**G Optic Nerve** Optic chiasma Second cranial nerve **H Oculomotor Nerve** Third cranial nerve **J Trochlear Nerve** Fourth cranial nerve **K Trigeminal Nerve** Fifth cranial nerve Gasserian ganglion Mandibular nerve Maxillary nerve Ophthalmic nerve Trifacial nerve **L Abducens Nerve** Sixth cranial nerve **M Facial Nerve** Chorda tympani Geniculate ganglion Greater superficial petrosal nerve Nerve to the stapedius Parotid plexus Posterior auricular nerve Seventh cranial nerve Submandibular ganglion **N Acoustic Nerve** Cochlear nerve Eighth cranial nerve Scarpa's (vestibular) ganglion Spiral ganglion Vestibular (Scarpa's) ganglion Vestibular nerve Vestibulocochlear nerve **P Glossopharyngeal Nerve** Carotid sinus nerve Ninth cranial nerve Tympanic nerve **Q Vagus Nerve** Anterior vagal trunk Pharyngeal plexus Pneumogastric nerve Posterior vagal trunk Pulmonary plexus Recurrent laryngeal nerve Superior laryngeal nerve Tenth cranial nerve **R Accessory Nerve** Eleventh cranial nerve **S Hypoglossal Nerve** Twelfth cranial nerve **T Spinal Meninges** Arachnoid mater, spinal Denticulate (dentate) ligament Dura mater, spinal Filum terminale Leptomeninges, spinal Pia mater, spinal **U Spinal Canal** Epidural space, spinal Extradural space, spinal Subarachnoid space, spinal Subdural space, spinal Vertebral canal **W Cervical Spinal Cord** Dorsal root ganglion **X Thoracic Spinal Cord** Dorsal root ganglion **Y Lumbar Spinal Cord** Cauda equina Conus medullaris Dorsal root ganglion	**Ø Open** **3 Percutaneous** **4 Percutaneous Endoscopic**	**Z No Device**	**X Diagnostic** **Z No Qualifier**

Non-OR   009[Ø,1,2,3,4,5,6,7,8,9,A,B,C,D,F,G,H,J,K,L,M,N,P,Q,R,S][3,4]ZX
Non-OR   009[T,W,X,Y]3Z[X,Z]
Non-OR   009U[3,4]Z[X,Z]

Non-OR Procedure   DRG Non-OR Procedure   Valid OR Procedure   HAC Associated Procedure   Combination Only   New/Revised April   New/Revised October

0   **Medical and Surgical**
0   **Central Nervous System and Cranial Nerves**
B   **Excision**   Definition: Cutting out or off, without replacement, a portion of a body part
                      Explanation: The qualifier DIAGNOSTIC is used to identify excision procedures that are biopsies

Body Part Character 4		Approach Character 5	Device Character 6	Qualifier Character 7

0 Brain
  Cerebrum
  Corpus callosum
  Encephalon
1 Cerebral Meninges
  Arachnoid mater,
    intracranial
  Leptomeninges,
    intracranial
  Pia mater, intracranial
2 Dura Mater
  Diaphragma sellae
  Dura mater, intracranial
  Falx cerebri
  Tentorium cerebelli
6 Cerebral Ventricle
  Aqueduct of Sylvius
  Cerebral aqueduct
    (Sylvius)
  Choroid plexus
  Ependyma
  Foramen of Monro
    (intraventricular)
  Fourth ventricle
  Interventricular foramen
    (Monro)
  Left lateral ventricle
  Right lateral ventricle
  Third ventricle
7 Cerebral Hemisphere
  Frontal lobe
  Occipital lobe
  Parietal lobe
  Temporal lobe
8 Basal Ganglia
  Basal nuclei
  Claustrum
  Corpus striatum
  Globus pallidus
  Substantia nigra
  Subthalamic nucleus
9 Thalamus
  Epithalamus
  Geniculate nucleus
  Metathalamus
  Pulvinar
A Hypothalamus
  Mammillary body
B Pons
  Apneustic center
  Basis pontis
  Locus ceruleus
  Pneumotaxic center
  Pontine tegmentum
  Superior olivary nucleus
C Cerebellum
  Culmen
D Medulla Oblongata
  Myelencephalon
F Olfactory Nerve
  First cranial nerve
  Olfactory bulb
G Optic Nerve
  Optic chiasma
  Second cranial nerve
	H Oculomotor Nerve
	  Third cranial nerve
	J Trochlear Nerve
	  Fourth cranial nerve
	K Trigeminal Nerve
	  Fifth cranial nerve
	  Gasserian ganglion
	  Mandibular nerve
	  Maxillary nerve
	  Ophthalmic nerve
	  Trifacial nerve
	L Abducens Nerve
	  Sixth cranial nerve
	M Facial Nerve
	  Chorda tympani
	  Geniculate ganglion
	  Greater superficial petrosal
	    nerve
	  Nerve to the stapedius
	  Parotid plexus
	  Posterior auricular nerve
	  Seventh cranial nerve
	  Submandibular ganglion
	N Acoustic Nerve
	  Cochlear nerve
	  Eighth cranial nerve
	  Scarpa's (vestibular)
	    ganglion
	  Spiral ganglion
	  Vestibular (Scarpa's)
	    ganglion
	  Vestibular nerve
	  Vestibulocochlear nerve
	P Glossopharyngeal Nerve
	  Carotid sinus nerve
	  Ninth cranial nerve
	  Tympanic nerve
	Q Vagus Nerve
	  Anterior vagal trunk
	  Pharyngeal plexus
	  Pneumogastric nerve
	  Posterior vagal trunk
	  Pulmonary plexus
	  Recurrent laryngeal nerve
	  Superior laryngeal nerve
	  Tenth cranial nerve
	R Accessory Nerve
	  Eleventh cranial nerve
	S Hypoglossal Nerve
	  Twelfth cranial nerve
	T Spinal Meninges
	  Arachnoid mater, spinal
	  Denticulate (dentate)
	    ligament
	  Dura mater, spinal
	  Filum terminale
	  Leptomeninges, spinal
	  Pia mater, spinal
	W Cervical Spinal Cord
	  Dorsal root ganglion
	X Thoracic Spinal Cord
	  Dorsal root ganglion
	Y Lumbar Spinal Cord
	  Cauda equina
	  Conus medullaris
	  Dorsal root ganglion
		0 Open
		3 Percutaneous
		4 Percutaneous Endoscopic
			Z No Device	**X** Diagnostic
				Z No Qualifier

Non-OR   00B[F,G,H,J,K,L,M,N,P,Q,R,S][3,4]ZX

Central Nervous System and Cranial Nerves

Ø   **Medical and Surgical**
Ø   **Central Nervous System and Cranial Nerves**
C   **Extirpation**   Definition: Taking or cutting out solid matter from a body part

Explanation: The solid matter may be an abnormal byproduct of a biological function or a foreign body; it may be imbedded in a body part or in the lumen of a tubular body part. The solid matter may or may not have been previously broken into pieces.

Body Part Character 4		Approach Character 5	Device Character 6	Qualifier Character 7
Ø Brain Cerebrum Corpus callosum Encephalon **1 Cerebral Meninges** Arachnoid mater, intracranial Leptomeninges, intracranial Pia mater, intracranial **2 Dura Mater** Diaphragma sellae Dura mater, intracranial Falx cerebri Tentorium cerebelli **3 Epidural Space, Intracranial** Extradural space, intracranial **4 Subdural Space, Intracranial** **5 Subarachnoid Space, Intracranial** **6 Cerebral Ventricle** Aqueduct of Sylvius Cerebral aqueduct (Sylvius) Choroid plexus Ependyma Foramen of Monro (intraventricular) Fourth ventricle Interventricular foramen (Monro) Left lateral ventricle Right lateral ventricle Third ventricle **7 Cerebral Hemisphere** Frontal lobe Occipital lobe Parietal lobe Temporal lobe **8 Basal Ganglia** Basal nuclei Claustrum Corpus striatum Globus pallidus Substantia nigra Subthalamic nucleus **9 Thalamus** Epithalamus Geniculate nucleus Metathalamus Pulvinar **A Hypothalamus** Mammillary body **B Pons** Apneustic center Basis pontis Locus ceruleus Pneumotaxic center Pontine tegmentum Superior olivary nucleus **C Cerebellum** Culmen **D Medulla Oblongata** Myelencephalon **F Olfactory Nerve** First cranial nerve Olfactory bulb	**G Optic Nerve** Optic chiasma Second cranial nerve **H Oculomotor Nerve** Third cranial nerve **J Trochlear Nerve** Fourth cranial nerve **K Trigeminal Nerve** Fifth cranial nerve Gasserian ganglion Mandibular nerve Maxillary nerve Ophthalmic nerve Trifacial nerve **L Abducens Nerve** Sixth cranial nerve **M Facial Nerve** Chorda tympani Geniculate ganglion Greater superficial petrosal nerve Nerve to the stapedius Parotid plexus Posterior auricular nerve Seventh cranial nerve Submandibular ganglion **N Acoustic Nerve** Cochlear nerve Eighth cranial nerve Scarpa's (vestibular) ganglion Spiral ganglion Vestibular (Scarpa's) ganglion Vestibular nerve Vestibulocochlear nerve **P Glossopharyngeal Nerve** Carotid sinus nerve Ninth cranial nerve Tympanic nerve **Q Vagus Nerve** Anterior vagal trunk Pharyngeal plexus Pneumogastric nerve Posterior vagal trunk Pulmonary plexus Recurrent laryngeal nerve Superior laryngeal nerve Tenth cranial nerve **R Accessory Nerve** Eleventh cranial nerve **S Hypoglossal Nerve** Twelfth cranial nerve **T Spinal Meninges** Arachnoid mater, spinal Denticulate (dentate) ligament Dura mater, spinal Filum terminale Leptomeninges, spinal Pia mater, spinal **U Spinal Canal** **W Cervical Spinal Cord** Dorsal root ganglion **X Thoracic Spinal Cord** Dorsal root ganglion **Y Lumbar Spinal Cord** Cauda equina Conus medullaris Dorsal root ganglion	**Ø Open** **3 Percutaneous** **4 Percutaneous Endoscopic**	**Z No Device**	**Z No Qualifier**

Non-OR Procedure   DRG Non-OR Procedure   Valid OR Procedure   HAC Associated Procedure   Combination Only   New/Revised April   New/Revised October

140   ICD-10-PCS 2023

0   **Medical and Surgical**
0   **Central Nervous System and Cranial Nerves**
D   **Extraction**   Definition: Pulling or stripping out or off all or a portion of a body part by the use of force
                    Explanation: The qualifier DIAGNOSTIC is used to identify extraction procedures that are biopsies

Body Part Character 4		Approach Character 5	Device Character 6	Qualifier Character 7
0 Brain	**M Facial Nerve**	**0 Open**	**Z No Device**	**Z No Qualifier**
Cerebrum	Chorda tympani	**3 Percutaneous**		
Corpus callosum	Geniculate ganglion	**4 Percutaneous Endoscopic**		
Encephalon	Greater superficial petrosal nerve			
1 Cerebral Meninges	Nerve to the stapedius			
Arachnoid mater, intracranial	Parotid plexus			
Leptomeninges, intracranial	Posterior auricular nerve			
Pia mater, intracranial	Seventh cranial nerve			
2 Dura Mater	Submandibular ganglion			
Diaphragma sellae	**N Acoustic Nerve**			
Dura mater, intracranial	Cochlear nerve			
Falx cerebri	Eighth cranial nerve			
Tentorium cerebelli	Scarpa's (vestibular) ganglion			
7 Cerebral Hemisphere	Spiral ganglion			
Frontal lobe	Vestibular (Scarpa's) ganglion			
Occipital lobe	Vestibular nerve			
Parietal lobe	Vestibulocochlear nerve			
Temporal lobe	**P Glossopharyngeal Nerve**			
C Cerebellum	Carotid sinus nerve			
Culmen	Ninth cranial nerve			
F Olfactory Nerve	Tympanic nerve			
First cranial nerve	**Q Vagus Nerve**			
Olfactory bulb	Anterior vagal trunk			
G Optic Nerve	Pharyngeal plexus			
Optic chiasma	Pneumogastric nerve			
Second cranial nerve	Posterior vagal trunk			
H Oculomotor Nerve	Pulmonary plexus			
Third cranial nerve	Recurrent laryngeal nerve			
J Trochlear Nerve	Superior laryngeal nerve			
Fourth cranial nerve	Tenth cranial nerve			
K Trigeminal Nerve	**R Accessory Nerve**			
Fifth cranial nerve	Eleventh cranial nerve			
Gasserian ganglion	**S Hypoglossal Nerve**			
Mandibular nerve	Twelfth cranial nerve			
Maxillary nerve	**T Spinal Meninges**			
Ophthalmic nerve	Arachnoid mater, spinal			
Trifacial nerve	Denticulate (dentate) ligament			
L Abducens Nerve	Dura mater, spinal			
Sixth cranial nerve	Filum terminale			
	Leptomeninges, spinal			
	Pia mater, spinal			

0   **Medical and Surgical**
0   **Central Nervous System and Cranial Nerves**
F   **Fragmentation**   Definition: Breaking solid matter in a body part into pieces

Explanation: Physical force (e.g., manual, ultrasonic) applied directly or indirectly is used to break the solid matter into pieces. The solid matter may be an abnormal byproduct of a biological function or a foreign body. The pieces of solid matter are not taken out.

Body Part Character 4	Approach Character 5	Device Character 6	Qualifier Character 7

3   **Epidural Space, Intracranial**   NC
     Extradural space, intracranial
4   **Subdural Space, Intracranial**   NC
5   **Subarachnoid Space, Intracranial**   NC
6   **Cerebral Ventricle**   NC
     Aqueduct of Sylvius
     Cerebral aqueduct (Sylvius)
     Choroid plexus
     Ependyma
     Foramen of Monro (intraventricular)
     Fourth ventricle
     Interventricular foramen (Monro)
     Left lateral ventricle
     Right lateral ventricle
     Third ventricle
U   **Spinal Canal**
     Epidural space, spinal
     Extradural space, spinal
     Subarachnoid space, spinal
     Subdural space, spinal
     Vertebral canal
	0 Open
	3 Percutaneous
	4 Percutaneous Endoscopic
	X External
		Z No Device	**Z** No Qualifier

Non-OR	00F[3,4,5,6]XZZ
NC	00F[3,4,5,6]XZZ

0   **Medical and Surgical**
0   **Central Nervous System and Cranial Nerves**
H   **Insertion**   Definition: Putting in a nonbiological appliance that monitors, assists, performs, or prevents a physiological function but does not physically take the place of a body part

Explanation: None

Body Part Character 4	Approach Character 5	Device Character 6	Qualifier Character 7

0   **Brain**   ⊞
     Cerebrum
     Corpus callosum
     Encephalon
	0 Open	**1** Radioactive Element
		2 Monitoring Device
		3 Infusion Device
		4 Radioactive Element, Cesium-131 Collagen Implant
		M Neurostimulator Lead
		Y Other Device
			Z No Qualifier

0   **Brain**   ⊞
     Cerebrum
     Corpus callosum
     Encephalon
	3 Percutaneous
	4 Percutaneous Endoscopic
		1 Radioactive Element
		2 Monitoring Device
		3 Infusion Device
		M Neurostimulator Lead
		Y Other Device
			Z No Qualifier

6   **Cerebral Ventricle**   ⊞
     Aqueduct of Sylvius
     Cerebral aqueduct (Sylvius)
     Choroid plexus
     Ependyma
     Foramen of Monro (intraventricular)
     Fourth ventricle Interventricular foramen (Monro)
     Left lateral ventricle
     Right lateral ventricle
     Third ventricle
E   **Cranial Nerve**   ⊞
U   **Spinal Canal**   ⊞
     Epidural space, spinal
     Extradural space, spinal
     Subarachnoid space, spinal
     Subdural space, spinal
     Vertebral canal
V   **Spinal Cord**   ⊞
     Dorsal root ganglion
	0 Open
	3 Percutaneous
	4 Percutaneous Endoscopic
		1 Radioactive Element
		2 Monitoring Device
		3 Infusion Device
		M Neurostimulator Lead
		Y Other Device
			Z No Qualifier

DRG Non-OR	00H004Z
Non-OR	00H[E,U,V]32Z
Non-OR	00H[E,U][3,4]YZ
Non-OR	00H[U,V][0,3,4]3Z

See Appendix L for Procedure Combinations
⊞   00H00MZ
⊞   00H0[3,4]MZ
⊞   00H[6,E,U,V][0,3,4]MZ

Non-OR Procedure   DRG Non-OR Procedure   Valid OR Procedure   HAC Associated Procedure   Combination Only   New/Revised April   New/Revised October

142   ICD-10-PCS 2023

Central Nervous System and Cranial Nerves

00F–00H

Ø   **Medical and Surgical**
Ø   **Central Nervous System and Cranial Nerves**
J   **Inspection**   Definition: Visually and/or manually exploring a body part

                               Explanation: Visual exploration may be performed with or without optical instrumentation. Manual exploration may be performed directly or through intervening body layers.

Body Part Character 4	Approach Character 5	Device Character 6	Qualifier Character 7

Ø   **Brain**
    Cerebrum
    Corpus callosum
    Encephalon
E   **Cranial Nerve**
U   **Spinal Canal**
    Epidural space, spinal
    Extradural space, spinal
    Subarachnoid space, spinal
    Subdural space, spinal
    Vertebral canal
V   **Spinal Cord**
    Dorsal root ganglion
	Ø Open
	3 Percutaneous
	4 Percutaneous Endoscopic
		Z No Device	**Z** No Qualifier

Non-OR	ØØJ[Ø,E,U,V]3ZZ

Ø   **Medical and Surgical**
Ø   **Central Nervous System and Cranial Nerves**
K   **Map**   Definition: Locating the route of passage of electrical impulses and/or locating functional areas in a body part

                              Explanation: Applicable only to the cardiac conduction mechanism and the central nervous system

Body Part Character 4	Approach Character 5	Device Character 6	Qualifier Character 7

Ø   **Brain**
    Cerebrum
    Corpus callosum
    Encephalon
7   **Cerebral Hemisphere**
    Frontal lobe
    Occipital lobe
    Parietal lobe
    Temporal lobe
8   **Basal Ganglia**
    Basal nuclei
    Claustrum
    Corpus striatum
    Globus pallidus
    Substantia nigra
    Subthalamic nucleus
9   **Thalamus**
    Epithalamus
    Geniculate nucleus
    Metathalamus
    Pulvinar
A   **Hypothalamus**
    Mammillary body
B   **Pons**
    Apneustic center
    Basis pontis
    Locus ceruleus
    Pneumotaxic center
    Pontine tegmentum
    Superior olivary nucleus
C   **Cerebellum**
    Culmen
D   **Medulla Oblongata**
    Myelencephalon
	Ø Open
	3 Percutaneous
	4 Percutaneous Endoscopic
		Z No Device	**Z** No Qualifier

NC Noncovered Procedure   **LC** Limited Coverage   **QA** Questionable OB Admit   **NT** New Tech Add-on   ⊞ Combination Member   ♂ Male   ♀ Female

ICD-10-PCS 2023   **143**

Ø   Medical and Surgical
Ø   Central Nervous System and Cranial Nerves
N   Release   Definition: Freeing a body part from an abnormal physical constraint by cutting or by the use of force
Explanation: Some of the restraining tissue may be taken out but none of the body part is taken out

Body Part Character 4		Approach Character 5	Device Character 6	Qualifier Character 7

Ø Brain
   Cerebrum
   Corpus callosum
   Encephalon
1 Cerebral Meninges
   Arachnoid mater,
      intracranial
   Leptomeninges,
      intracranial
   Pia mater, intracranial
2 Dura Mater
   Diaphragma sellae
   Dura mater, intracranial
   Falx cerebri
   Tentorium cerebelli
6 Cerebral Ventricle
   Aqueduct of Sylvius
   Cerebral aqueduct
      (Sylvius)
   Choroid plexus
   Ependyma
   Foramen of Monro
      (intraventricular)
   Fourth ventricle
   Interventricular foramen
      (Monro)
   Left lateral ventricle
   Right lateral ventricle
   Third ventricle
7 Cerebral Hemisphere
   Frontal lobe
   Occipital lobe
   Parietal lobe
   Temporal lobe
8 Basal Ganglia
   Basal nuclei
   Claustrum
   Corpus striatum
   Globus pallidus
   Substantia nigra
   Subthalamic nucleus
9 Thalamus
   Epithalamus
   Geniculate nucleus
   Metathalamus
   Pulvinar
A Hypothalamus
   Mammillary body
B Pons
   Apneustic center
   Basis pontis
   Locus ceruleus
   Pneumotaxic center
   Pontine tegmentum
   Superior olivary nucleus
C Cerebellum
   Culmen
D Medulla Oblongata
   Myelencephalon
F Olfactory Nerve
   First cranial nerve
   Olfactory bulb
G Optic Nerve
   Optic chiasma
   Second cranial nerve
	H Oculomotor Nerve
	   Third cranial nerve
	J Trochlear Nerve
	   Fourth cranial nerve
	K Trigeminal Nerve
	   Fifth cranial nerve
	   Gasserian ganglion
	   Mandibular nerve
	   Maxillary nerve
	   Ophthalmic nerve
	   Trifacial nerve
	L Abducens Nerve
	   Sixth cranial nerve
	M Facial Nerve
	   Chorda tympani
	   Geniculate ganglion
	   Greater superficial petrosal
	      nerve
	   Nerve to the stapedius
	   Parotid plexus
	   Posterior auricular nerve
	   Seventh cranial nerve
	   Submandibular ganglion
	N Acoustic Nerve
	   Cochlear nerve
	   Eighth cranial nerve
	   Scarpa's (vestibular)
	      ganglion
	   Spiral ganglion
	   Vestibular (Scarpa's)
	      ganglion
	   Vestibular nerve
	   Vestibulocochlear nerve
	P Glossopharyngeal Nerve
	   Carotid sinus nerve
	   Ninth cranial nerve
	   Tympanic nerve
	Q Vagus Nerve
	   Anterior vagal trunk
	   Pharyngeal plexus
	   Pneumogastric nerve
	   Posterior vagal trunk
	   Pulmonary plexus
	   Recurrent laryngeal nerve
	   Superior laryngeal nerve
	   Tenth cranial nerve
	R Accessory Nerve
	   Eleventh cranial nerve
	S Hypoglossal Nerve
	   Twelfth cranial nerve
	T Spinal Meninges
	   Arachnoid mater, spinal
	   Denticulate (dentate)
	      ligament
	   Dura mater, spinal
	   Filum terminale
	   Leptomeninges, spinal
	   Pia mater, spinal
	W Cervical Spinal Cord
	   Dorsal root ganglion
	X Thoracic Spinal Cord
	   Dorsal root ganglion
	Y Lumbar Spinal Cord
	   Cauda equina
	   Conus medullaris
	   Dorsal root ganglion
		Ø Open
		3 Percutaneous
		4 Percutaneous Endoscopic
			Z No Device	**Z No Qualifier**

Non-OR Procedure   DRG Non-OR Procedure   Valid OR Procedure   HAC Associated Procedure   Combination Only   New/Revised April   New/Revised October

144
ICD-10-PCS 2023

0   **Medical and Surgical**
0   **Central Nervous System and Cranial Nerves**
P   **Removal**   Definition: Taking out or off a device from a body part

                     Explanation: If a device is taken out and a similar device put in without cutting or puncturing the skin or mucous membrane, the procedure is coded to the root operation CHANGE. Otherwise, the procedure for taking out a device is coded to the root operation REMOVAL.

Body Part Character 4	Approach Character 5	Device Character 6	Qualifier Character 7

0 Brain
  Cerebrum
  Corpus callosum
  Encephalon
V Spinal Cord
  Dorsal root ganglion
	0 Open
	3 Percutaneous
	4 Percutaneous Endoscopic
		0 Drainage Device
		2 Monitoring Device
		3 Infusion Device
		7 Autologous Tissue
		    Substitute
		J Synthetic Substitute
		K Nonautologous Tissue
		    Substitute
		M Neurostimulator Lead
		Y Other Device
			Z No Qualifier

0 Brain
  Cerebrum
  Corpus callosum
  Encephalon
V Spinal Cord
  Dorsal root ganglion
	X External	**0** Drainage Device
		2 Monitoring Device
		3 Infusion Device
		M Neurostimulator Lead
			Z No Qualifier

6 Cerebral Ventricle
  Aqueduct of Sylvius
  Cerebral aqueduct (Sylvius)
  Choroid plexus
  Ependyma
  Foramen of Monro (intraventricular)
  Fourth ventricle
  Interventricular foramen (Monro)
  Left lateral ventricle
  Right lateral ventricle
  Third ventricle
U Spinal Canal
  Epidural space, spinal
  Extradural space, spinal
  Subarachnoid space, spinal
  Subdural space, spinal
  Vertebral canal
	0 Open
	3 Percutaneous
	4 Percutaneous Endoscopic
		0 Drainage Device
		2 Monitoring Device
		3 Infusion Device
		J Synthetic Substitute
		M Neurostimulator Lead
		Y Other Device
			Z No Qualifier

6 Cerebral Ventricle
  Aqueduct of Sylvius
  Cerebral aqueduct (Sylvius)
  Choroid plexus
  Ependyma
  Foramen of Monro (intraventricular)
  Fourth ventricle
  Interventricular foramen (Monro)
  Left lateral ventricle
  Right lateral ventricle
  Third ventricle
U Spinal Canal
  Epidural space, spinal
  Extradural space, spinal
  Subarachnoid space, spinal
  Subdural space, spinal
  Vertebral canal
	X External	**0** Drainage Device
		2 Monitoring Device
		3 Infusion Device
		M Neurostimulator Lead
			Z No Qualifier

E Cranial Nerve	**0** Open **3** Percutaneous **4** Percutaneous Endoscopic	**0** Drainage Device **2** Monitoring Device **3** Infusion Device **7** Autologous Tissue Substitute **M** Neurostimulator Lead **Y** Other Device	**Z** No Qualifier
E Cranial Nerve	**X** External	**0** Drainage Device **2** Monitoring Device **3** Infusion Device **M** Neurostimulator Lead	**Z** No Qualifier

Non-OR	00P[0,V]3[0,2,3]Z
Non-OR	00P[0,V][3,4]YZ
Non-OR	00P[0,V]X[0,2,3,M]Z
Non-OR	00P[6,U]3[0,2,3]Z
Non-OR	00P[6,U][3,4]YZ
Non-OR	00P[6,U]X[0,2,3,M]Z
Non-OR	00PE3[0,2,3]Z
Non-OR	00PE[3,4]YZ
Non-OR	00PEX[0,2,3,M]Z

 Noncovered Procedure   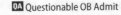 Limited Coverage   **QA** Questionable OB Admit   **NT** New Tech Add-on   ⊞ Combination Member   ♂ Male   ♀ Female

ICD-10-PCS 2023   **145**

Ø   Medical and Surgical
Ø   Central Nervous System and Cranial Nerves
Q   Repair   Definition: Restoring, to the extent possible, a body part to its normal anatomic structure and function

Explanation: Used only when the method to accomplish the repair is not one of the other root operations

Body Part Character 4		Approach Character 5	Device Character 6	Qualifier Character 7
Ø Brain	**H Oculomotor Nerve**	**Ø Open**	**Z No Device**	**Z No Qualifier**
Cerebrum	Third cranial nerve	**3 Percutaneous**		
Corpus callosum	**J Trochlear Nerve**	**4 Percutaneous Endoscopic**		
Encephalon	Fourth cranial nerve			
1 Cerebral Meninges	**K Trigeminal Nerve**			
Arachnoid mater,	Fifth cranial nerve			
intracranial	Gasserian ganglion			
Leptomeninges,	Mandibular nerve			
intracranial	Maxillary nerve			
Pia mater, intracranial	Ophthalmic nerve			
2 Dura Mater	Trifacial nerve			
Diaphragma sellae	**L Abducens Nerve**			
Dura mater, intracranial	Sixth cranial nerve			
Falx cerebri	**M Facial Nerve**			
Tentorium cerebelli	Chorda tympani			
6 Cerebral Ventricle	Geniculate ganglion			
Aqueduct of Sylvius	Greater superficial petrosal			
Cerebral aqueduct	nerve			
(Sylvius)	Nerve to the stapedius			
Choroid plexus	Parotid plexus			
Ependyma	Posterior auricular nerve			
Foramen of Monro	Seventh cranial nerve			
(intraventricular)	Submandibular ganglion			
Fourth ventricle	**N Acoustic Nerve**			
Interventricular foramen	Cochlear nerve			
(Monro)	Eighth cranial nerve			
Left lateral ventricle	Scarpa's (vestibular)			
Right lateral ventricle	ganglion			
Third ventricle	Spiral ganglion			
7 Cerebral Hemisphere	Vestibular (Scarpa's)			
Frontal lobe	ganglion			
Occipital lobe	Vestibular nerve			
Parietal lobe	Vestibulocochlear nerve			
Temporal lobe	**P Glossopharyngeal Nerve**			
8 Basal Ganglia	Carotid sinus nerve			
Basal nuclei	Ninth cranial nerve			
Claustrum	Tympanic nerve			
Corpus striatum	**Q Vagus Nerve**			
Globus pallidus	Anterior vagal trunk			
Substantia nigra	Pharyngeal plexus			
Subthalamic nucleus	Pneumogastric nerve			
9 Thalamus	Posterior vagal trunk			
Epithalamus	Pulmonary plexus			
Geniculate nucleus	Recurrent laryngeal nerve			
Metathalamus	Superior laryngeal nerve			
Pulvinar	Tenth cranial nerve			
A Hypothalamus	**R Accessory Nerve**			
Mammillary body	Eleventh cranial nerve			
B Pons	**S Hypoglossal Nerve**			
Apneustic center	Twelfth cranial nerve			
Basis pontis	**T Spinal Meninges**			
Locus ceruleus	Arachnoid mater, spinal			
Pneumotaxic center	Denticulate (dentate)			
Pontine tegmentum	ligament			
Superior olivary nucleus	Dura mater, spinal			
C Cerebellum	Filum terminale			
Culmen	Leptomeninges, spinal			
D Medulla Oblongata	Pia mater, spinal			
Myelencephalon	**W Cervical Spinal Cord**			
F Olfactory Nerve	Dorsal root ganglion			
First cranial nerve	**X Thoracic Spinal Cord**			
Olfactory bulb	Dorsal root ganglion			
G Optic Nerve	**Y Lumbar Spinal Cord**			
Optic chiasma	Cauda equina			
Second cranial nerve	Conus medullaris			
	Dorsal root ganglion			

Non-OR Procedure   DRG Non-OR Procedure   Valid OR Procedure   HAC Associated Procedure   Combination Only   New/Revised April   New/Revised October

146   ICD-10-PCS 2023

Ø   Medical and Surgical
Ø   Central Nervous System and Cranial Nerves
R   Replacement   Definition: Putting in or on biological or synthetic material that physically takes the place and/or function of all or a portion of a body part

       Explanation: The body part may have been taken out or replaced, or may be taken out, physically eradicated, or rendered nonfunctional during the REPLACEMENT procedure. A REMOVAL procedure is coded for taking out the device used in a previous replacement procedure.

Body Part Character 4		Approach Character 5	Device Character 6	Qualifier Character 7

1 Cerebral Meninges
  Arachnoid mater,
    intracranial
  Leptomeninges,
    intracranial
  Pia mater, intracranial
2 Dura Mater
  Diaphragma sellae
  Dura mater, intracranial
  Falx cerebri
  Tentorium cerebelli
6 Cerebral Ventricle
  Aqueduct of Sylvius
  Cerebral aqueduct
    (Sylvius)
  Choroid plexus
  Ependyma
  Foramen of Monro
    (intraventricular)
  Fourth ventricle
  Interventricular foramen
    (Monro)
  Left lateral ventricle
  Right lateral ventricle
  Third ventricle
F Olfactory Nerve
  First cranial nerve
  Olfactory bulb
G Optic Nerve
  Optic chiasma
  Second cranial nerve
H Oculomotor Nerve
  Third cranial nerve
J Trochlear Nerve
  Fourth cranial nerve
K Trigeminal Nerve
  Fifth cranial nerve
  Gasserian ganglion
  Mandibular nerve
  Maxillary nerve
  Ophthalmic nerve
  Trifacial nerve
L Abducens Nerve
  Sixth cranial nerve
	M Facial Nerve
	  Chorda tympani
	  Geniculate ganglion
	  Greater superficial petrosal
	    nerve
	  Nerve to the stapedius
	  Parotid plexus
	  Posterior auricular nerve
	  Seventh cranial nerve
	  Submandibular ganglion
	N Acoustic Nerve
	  Cochlear nerve
	  Eighth cranial nerve
	  Scarpa's (vestibular)
	    ganglion
	  Spiral ganglion
	  Vestibular (Scarpa's)
	    ganglion
	  Vestibular nerve
	  Vestibulocochlear nerve
	P Glossopharyngeal Nerve
	  Carotid sinus nerve
	  Ninth cranial nerve
	  Tympanic nerve
	Q Vagus Nerve
	  Anterior vagal trunk
	  Pharyngeal plexus
	  Pneumogastric nerve
	  Posterior vagal trunk
	  Pulmonary plexus
	  Recurrent laryngeal nerve
	  Superior laryngeal nerve
	  Tenth cranial nerve
	R Accessory Nerve
	  Eleventh cranial nerve
	S Hypoglossal Nerve
	  Twelfth cranial nerve
	T Spinal Meninges
	  Arachnoid mater, spinal
	  Denticulate (dentate)
	    ligament
	  Dura mater, spinal
	  Filum terminale
	  Leptomeninges, spinal
	  Pia mater, spinal
		Ø Open
		4 Percutaneous Endoscopic
			**7 Autologous Tissue
			  Substitute**
			J Synthetic Substitute
			**K Nonautologous Tissue
			  Substitute**
				Z No Qualifier

NC Noncovered Procedure   LC Limited Coverage   QA Questionable OB Admit   NT New Tech Add-on   ⊞ Combination Member   ♂ Male   ♀ Female

ICD-10-PCS 2023   147

ØØR–ØØR

0 Medical and Surgical
0 Central Nervous System and Cranial Nerves
S Reposition — Definition: Moving to its normal location, or other suitable location, all or a portion of a body part

Explanation: The body part is moved to a new location from an abnormal location, or from a normal location where it is not functioning correctly. The body part may or may not be cut out or off to be moved to the new location.

Body Part Character 4		Approach Character 5	Device Character 6	Qualifier Character 7

F **Olfactory Nerve**
First cranial nerve
Olfactory bulb
G **Optic Nerve**
Optic chiasma
Second cranial nerve
H **Oculomotor Nerve**
Third cranial nerve
J **Trochlear Nerve**
Fourth cranial nerve
K **Trigeminal Nerve**
Fifth cranial nerve
Gasserian ganglion
Mandibular nerve
Maxillary nerve
Ophthalmic nerve
Trifacial nerve
L **Abducens Nerve**
Sixth cranial nerve
M **Facial Nerve**
Chorda tympani
Geniculate ganglion
Greater superficial petrosal
  nerve
Nerve to the stapedius
Parotid plexus
Posterior auricular nerve
Seventh cranial nerve
Submandibular ganglion
	N **Acoustic Nerve**
	Cochlear nerve
	Eighth cranial nerve
	Scarpa's (vestibular)
	  ganglion
	Spiral ganglion
	Vestibular (Scarpa's)
	  ganglion
	Vestibular nerve
	Vestibulocochlear nerve
	P **Glossopharyngeal Nerve**
	Carotid sinus nerve
	Ninth cranial nerve
	Tympanic nerve
	Q **Vagus Nerve**
	Anterior vagal trunk
	Pharyngeal plexus
	Pneumogastric nerve
	Posterior vagal trunk
	Pulmonary plexus
	Recurrent laryngeal nerve
	Superior laryngeal nerve
	Tenth cranial nerve
	R **Accessory Nerve**
	Eleventh cranial nerve
	S **Hypoglossal Nerve**
	Twelfth cranial nerve
	W **Cervical Spinal Cord**
	Dorsal root ganglion
	X **Thoracic Spinal Cord**
	Dorsal root ganglion
	Y **Lumbar Spinal Cord**
	Cauda equina
	Conus medullaris
	Dorsal root ganglion
		0 Open
		3 Percutaneous
		4 Percutaneous Endoscopic
			Z No Device	**Z** No Qualifier

0 Medical and Surgical
0 Central Nervous System and Cranial Nerves
T Resection — Definition: Cutting out or off, without replacement, all of a body part

Explanation: None

Body Part Character 4	Approach Character 5	Device Character 6	Qualifier Character 7
7 **Cerebral Hemisphere** Frontal lobe Occipital lobe Parietal lobe Temporal lobe	**0** Open **3** Percutaneous **4** Percutaneous Endoscopic	**Z** No Device	**Z** No Qualifier

Central Nervous System and Cranial Nerves

Ø　Medical and Surgical
Ø　Central Nervous System and Cranial Nerves
U　Supplement　　Definition: Putting in or on biological or synthetic material that physically reinforces and/or augments the function of a portion of a body part

Explanation: The biological material is non-living, or is living and from the same individual. The body part may have been previously replaced, and the SUPPLEMENT procedure is performed to physically reinforce and/or augment the function of the replaced body part.

Body Part Character 4		Approach Character 5	Device Character 6	Qualifier Character 7
1 Cerebral Meninges Arachnoid mater, intracranial Leptomeninges, intracranial Pia mater, intracranial **2 Dura Mater** Diaphragma sellae Dura mater, intracranial Falx cerebri Tentorium cerebelli **6 Cerebral Ventricle** Aqueduct of Sylvius Cerebral aqueduct (Sylvius) Choroid plexus Ependyma Foramen of Monro (intraventricular) Fourth ventricle Interventricular foramen (Monro) Left lateral ventricle Right lateral ventricle Third ventricle **F Olfactory Nerve** First cranial nerve Olfactory bulb **G Optic Nerve** Optic chiasma Second cranial nerve **H Oculomotor Nerve** Third cranial nerve **J Trochlear Nerve** Fourth cranial nerve **K Trigeminal Nerve** Fifth cranial nerve Gasserian ganglion Mandibular nerve Maxillary nerve Ophthalmic nerve Trifacial nerve **L Abducens Nerve** Sixth cranial nerve	**M Facial Nerve** Chorda tympani Geniculate ganglion Greater superficial petrosal nerve Nerve to the stapedius Parotid plexus Posterior auricular nerve Seventh cranial nerve Submandibular ganglion **N Acoustic Nerve** Cochlear nerve Eighth cranial nerve Scarpa's (vestibular) ganglion Spiral ganglion Vestibular (Scarpa's) ganglion Vestibular nerve Vestibulocochlear nerve **P Glossopharyngeal Nerve** Carotid sinus nerve Ninth cranial nerve Tympanic nerve **Q Vagus Nerve** Anterior vagal trunk Pharyngeal plexus Pneumogastric nerve Posterior vagal trunk Pulmonary plexus Recurrent laryngeal nerve Superior laryngeal nerve Tenth cranial nerve **R Accessory Nerve** Eleventh cranial nerve **S Hypoglossal Nerve** Twelfth cranial nerve **T Spinal Meninges** Arachnoid mater, spinal Denticulate (dentate) ligament Dura mater, spinal Filum terminale Leptomeninges, spinal Pia mater, spinal	**Ø Open** **3 Percutaneous** **4 Percutaneous Endoscopic**	**7 Autologous Tissue Substitute** **J Synthetic Substitute** **K Nonautologous Tissue Substitute**	**Z No Qualifier**

NC Noncovered Procedure　　LC Limited Coverage　　OA Questionable OB Admit　　NT New Tech Add-on　　⊞ Combination Member　　♂ Male　　♀ Female

ICD-10-PCS 2023

149

0   **Medical and Surgical**
0   **Central Nervous System and Cranial Nerves**
W   **Revision**   Definition: Correcting, to the extent possible, a portion of a malfunctioning device or the position of a displaced device

Explanation: Revision can include correcting a malfunctioning or displaced device by taking out or putting in components of the device such as a screw or pin

Body Part Character 4	Approach Character 5	Device Character 6	Qualifier Character 7
0 **Brain** Cerebrum Corpus callosum Encephalon **V** **Spinal Cord** Dorsal root ganglion	**0** Open **3** Percutaneous **4** Percutaneous Endoscopic	**0** Drainage Device **2** Monitoring Device **3** Infusion Device **7** Autologous Tissue Substitute **J** Synthetic Substitute **K** Nonautologous Tissue Substitute **M** Neurostimulator Lead **Y** Other Device	**Z** No Qualifier
0 **Brain** Cerebrum Corpus callosum Encephalon **V** **Spinal Cord** Dorsal root ganglion	**X** External	**0** Drainage Device **2** Monitoring Device **3** Infusion Device **7** Autologous Tissue Substitute **J** Synthetic Substitute **K** Nonautologous Tissue Substitute **M** Neurostimulator Lead	**Z** No Qualifier
6 **Cerebral Ventricle** Aqueduct of Sylvius Cerebral aqueduct (Sylvius) Choroid plexus Ependyma Foramen of Monro (intraventricular) Fourth ventricle Interventricular foramen (Monro) Left lateral ventricle Right lateral ventricle Third ventricle **U** **Spinal Canal** Epidural space, spinal Extradural space, spinal Subarachnoid space, spinal Subdural space, spinal Vertebral canal	**0** Open **3** Percutaneous **4** Percutaneous Endoscopic	**0** Drainage Device **2** Monitoring Device **3** Infusion Device **J** Synthetic Substitute **M** Neurostimulator Lead **Y** Other Device	**Z** No Qualifier
6 **Cerebral Ventricle** Aqueduct of Sylvius Cerebral aqueduct (Sylvius) Choroid plexus Ependyma Foramen of Monro (intraventricular) Fourth ventricle Interventricular foramen (Monro) Left lateral ventricle Right lateral ventricle Third ventricle **U** **Spinal Canal** Epidural space, spinal Extradural space, spinal Subarachnoid space, spinal Subdural space, spinal Vertebral canal	**X** External	**0** Drainage Device **2** Monitoring Device **3** Infusion Device **J** Synthetic Substitute **M** Neurostimulator Lead	**Z** No Qualifier
E **Cranial Nerve**	**0** Open **3** Percutaneous **4** Percutaneous Endoscopic	**0** Drainage Device **2** Monitoring Device **3** Infusion Device **7** Autologous Tissue Substitute **M** Neurostimulator Lead **Y** Other Device	**Z** No Qualifier
E **Cranial Nerve**	**X** External	**0** Drainage Device **2** Monitoring Device **3** Infusion Device **7** Autologous Tissue Substitute **M** Neurostimulator Lead	**Z** No Qualifier

Non-OR   00W[0,V][3,4]YZ
Non-OR   00W[0,V]X[0,2,3,7,J,K,M]Z
Non-OR   00W[6,U][3,4]YZ
Non-OR   00W[6,U]X[0,2,3,J,M]Z
Non-OR   00WE[3,4]YZ
Non-OR   00WEX[0,2,3,7,M]Z

Ø   Medical and Surgical
Ø   Central Nervous System and Cranial Nerves
X   Transfer   Definition: Moving, without taking out, all or a portion of a body part to another location to take over the function of all or a portion of a body part
                  Explanation: The body part transferred remains connected to its vascular and nervous supply

Body Part Character 4	Approach Character 5	Device Character 6	Qualifier Character 7

F   **Olfactory Nerve**
    First cranial nerve
    Olfactory bulb
G   **Optic Nerve**
    Optic chiasma
    Second cranial nerve
H   **Oculomotor Nerve**
    Third cranial nerve
J   **Trochlear Nerve**
    Fourth cranial nerve
K   **Trigeminal Nerve**
    Fifth cranial nerve
    Gasserian ganglion
    Mandibular nerve
    Maxillary nerve
    Ophthalmic nerve
    Trifacial nerve
L   **Abducens Nerve**
    Sixth cranial nerve
M   **Facial Nerve**
    Chorda tympani
    Geniculate ganglion
    Greater superficial petrosal nerve
    Nerve to the stapedius
    Parotid plexus
    Posterior auricular nerve
    Seventh cranial nerve
    Submandibular ganglion
N   **Acoustic Nerve**
    Cochlear nerve
    Eighth cranial nerve
    Scarpa's (vestibular) ganglion
    Spiral ganglion
    Vestibular (Scarpa's) ganglion
    Vestibular nerve
    Vestibulocochlear nerve
P   **Glossopharyngeal Nerve**
    Carotid sinus nerve
    Ninth cranial nerve
    Tympanic nerve
Q   **Vagus Nerve**
    Anterior vagal trunk
    Pharyngeal plexus
    Pneumogastric nerve
    Posterior vagal trunk
    Pulmonary plexus
    Recurrent laryngeal nerve
    Superior laryngeal nerve
    Tenth cranial nerve
R   **Accessory Nerve**
    Eleventh cranial nerve
S   **Hypoglossal Nerve**
    Twelfth cranial nerve
	Ø Open
	4 Percutaneous Endoscopic
		Z No Device	**F** Olfactory Nerve
			G Optic Nerve
			H Oculomotor Nerve
			J Trochlear Nerve
			K Trigeminal Nerve
			L Abducens Nerve
			M Facial Nerve
			N Acoustic Nerve
			P Glossopharyngeal Nerve
			Q Vagus Nerve
			R Accessory Nerve
			S Hypoglossal Nerve

NC Noncovered Procedure   **LC** Limited Coverage   **QA** Questionable OB Admit   **NT** New Tech Add-on   ⊞ Combination Member   ♂ Male   ♀ Female

ICD-10-PCS 2023   151

0 Medical and Surgical
0 Central Nervous System and Cranial Nerves
X Transfer: Moving, without taking out, all or a portion of a body part to another location to take over the function of all or a portion of a body part

Body Part Character 4	Approach Character 5	Device Character 6	Qualifier Character 7
0 Olfactory Nerve 1 Optic Nerve 2 Oculomotor Nerve 3 Trochlear Nerve 4 Trigeminal Nerve 5 Abducens Nerve 6 Facial Nerve 7 Acoustic Nerve 8 Glossopharyngeal Nerve 9 Vagus Nerve A Accessory Nerve B Hypoglossal Nerve	0 Open	Z No Device	Z No Qualifier

Peripheral Nervous System Ø12–Ø1X

Character Meanings

This Character Meaning table is provided as a guide to assist the user in the identification of character members that may be found in this section of code tables. It **SHOULD NOT** be used to build a PCS code.

Operation–Character 3	Body Part–Character 4	Approach–Character 5	Device–Character 6	Qualifier–Character 7
2 Change	Ø Cervical Plexus	Ø Open	Ø Drainage Device	1 Cervical Nerve
5 Destruction	1 Cervical Nerve	3 Percutaneous	1 Radioactive Element	2 Phrenic Nerve
8 Division	2 Phrenic Nerve	4 Percutaneous Endoscopic	2 Monitoring Device	4 Ulnar Nerve
9 Drainage	3 Brachial Plexus	X External	7 Autologous Tissue Substitute	5 Median Nerve
B Excision	4 Ulnar Nerve		J Synthetic Substitute	6 Radial Nerve
C Extirpation	5 Median Nerve		K Nonautologous Tissue Substitute	8 Thoracic Nerve
D Extraction	6 Radial Nerve		M Neurostimulator Lead	B Lumbar Nerve
H Insertion	8 Thoracic Nerve		Y Other Device	C Perineal Nerve
J Inspection	9 Lumbar Plexus		Z No Device	D Femoral Nerve
N Release	A Lumbosacral Plexus			F Sciatic Nerve
P Removal	B Lumbar Nerve			G Tibial Nerve
Q Repair	C Pudendal Nerve			H Peroneal Nerve
R Replacement	D Femoral Nerve			X Diagnostic
S Reposition	F Sciatic Nerve			Z No Qualifier
U Supplement	G Tibial Nerve			
W Revision	H Peroneal Nerve			
X Transfer	K Head and Neck Sympathetic Nerve			
	L Thoracic Sympathetic Nerve			
	M Abdominal Sympathetic Nerve			
	N Lumbar Sympathetic Nerve			
	P Sacral Sympathetic Nerve			
	Q Sacral Plexus			
	R Sacral Nerve			
	Y Peripheral Nerve			

AHA Coding Clinic for table Ø1B
2018, 2Q, 22   Excision of synovial cyst
2017, 2Q, 19   Thoracic outlet decompression with sympathectomy

AHA Coding Clinic for table Ø1H
2020, 4Q, 43-44   Insertion of radioactive element

AHA Coding Clinic for table Ø1N
2019, 1Q, 28   Decompressive laminectomy of both spinal cord and nerve roots
2018, 2Q, 22   Excision of synovial cyst
2017, 2Q, 19   Thoracic outlet decompression with sympathectomy
2016, 2Q, 16   Decompressive laminectomy/foraminotomy and lumbar discectomy
2016, 2Q, 17   Removal of longitudinal ligament to decompress cervical nerve root
2016, 2Q, 23   Thoracic outlet syndrome and release of brachial plexus
2015, 2Q, 34   Decompressive laminectomy
2014, 3Q, 33   Radial fracture treatment with open reduction internal fixation, and release of carpal ligament

AHA Coding Clinic for table Ø1Q
2019, 3Q, 32   Breast reconstruction with neurotization

AHA Coding Clinic for table Ø1S
2021, 3Q, 19   Elbow amputation and targeted muscle reinnervation

AHA Coding Clinic for table Ø1U
2019, 3Q, 32   Breast reconstruction with neurotization
2017, 4Q, 62   Added and revised device values - Nerve substitutes

Median and Ulnar Nerves

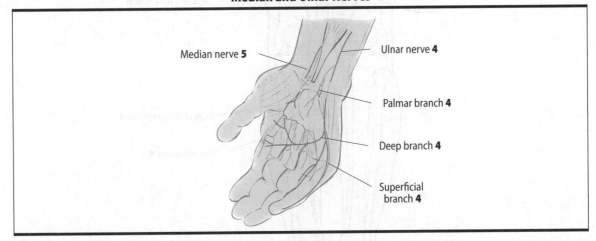

Median nerve **5**
Ulnar nerve **4**
Palmar branch **4**
Deep branch **4**
Superficial branch **4**

Peripheral Nervous System

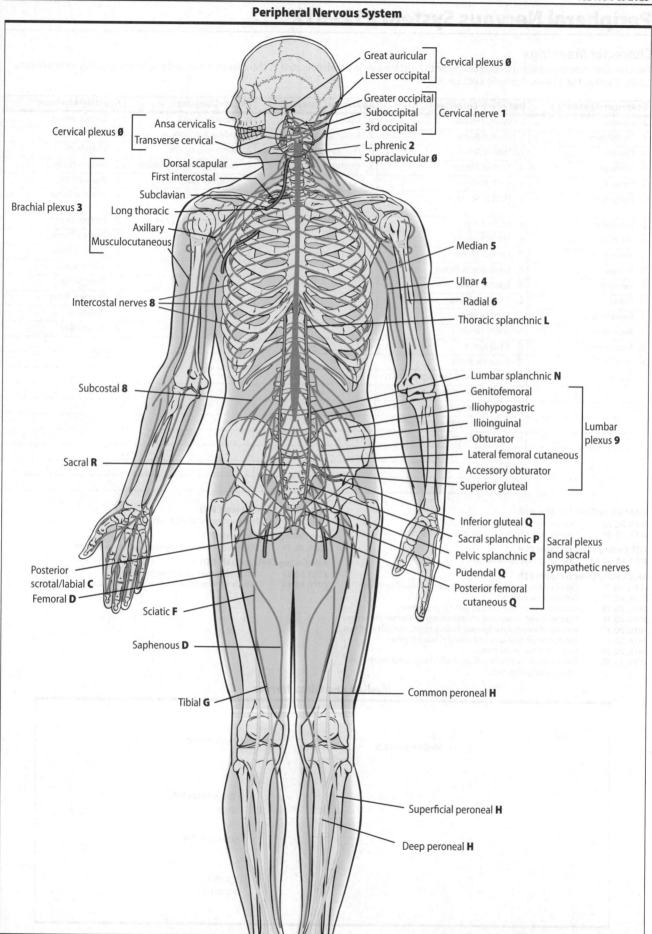

Great auricular
Lesser occipital
— Cervical plexus **Ø**

Greater occipital
Suboccipital
3rd occipital
— Cervical nerve **1**

Cervical plexus **Ø**

Ansa cervicalis
Transverse cervical

L. phrenic **2**
Supraclavicular **Ø**

Dorsal scapular
First intercostal
Subclavian
Long thoracic
Axillary
Musculocutaneous

Brachial plexus **3**

Median **5**

Ulnar **4**
Radial **6**
Thoracic splanchnic **L**

Intercostal nerves **8**

Subcostal **8**

Lumbar splanchnic **N**
Genitofemoral
Iliohypogastric
Ilioinguinal
Obturator
Lateral femoral cutaneous
Accessory obturator
Superior gluteal

Lumbar plexus **9**

Sacral **R**

Inferior gluteal **Q**
Sacral splanchnic **P**
Pelvic splanchnic **P**
Pudendal **Q**
Posterior femoral cutaneous **Q**

Sacral plexus and sacral sympathetic nerves

Posterior scrotal/labial **C**
Femoral **D**

Sciatic **F**

Saphenous **D**

Tibial **G**

Common peroneal **H**

Superficial peroneal **H**

Deep peroneal **H**

Ø   **Medical and Surgical**
1   **Peripheral Nervous System**
2   **Change**   Definition: Taking out or off a device from a body part and putting back an identical or similar device in or on the same body part without cutting or puncturing the skin or a mucous membrane
                                 Explanation: All CHANGE procedures are coded using the approach EXTERNAL

Body Part Character 4	Approach Character 5	Device Character 6	Qualifier Character 7
Y Peripheral Nerve	**X** External	**Ø** Drainage Device **Y** Other Device	**Z** No Qualifier

Non-OR   All body part, approach, device, and qualifier values

Ø   **Medical and Surgical**
1   **Peripheral Nervous System**   Definition: Physical eradication of all or a portion of a body part by the direct use of energy, force, or a destructive agent
5   **Destruction**   Explanation: None of the body part is physically taken out

Body Part Character 4		Approach Character 5	Device Character 6	Qualifier Character 7

Ø **Cervical Plexus**
    Ansa cervicalis
    Cutaneous (transverse) cervical nerve
    Great auricular nerve
    Lesser occipital nerve
    Supraclavicular nerve
    Transverse (cutaneous) cervical nerve
1 **Cervical Nerve**
    Greater occipital nerve
    Spinal nerve, cervical
    Suboccipital nerve
    Third occipital nerve
2 **Phrenic Nerve**
    Accessory phrenic nerve
3 **Brachial Plexus**
    Axillary nerve
    Dorsal scapular nerve
    First intercostal nerve
    Long thoracic nerve
    Musculocutaneous nerve
    Subclavius nerve
    Suprascapular nerve
4 **Ulnar Nerve**
    Cubital nerve
5 **Median Nerve**
    Anterior interosseous nerve
    Palmar cutaneous nerve
6 **Radial Nerve**
    Dorsal digital nerve
    Musculospiral nerve
    Palmar cutaneous nerve
    Posterior interosseous nerve
8 **Thoracic Nerve**
    Intercostal nerve
    Intercostobrachial nerve
    Spinal nerve, thoracic
    Subcostal nerve
9 **Lumbar Plexus**
    Accessory obturator nerve
    Genitofemoral nerve
    Iliohypogastric nerve
    Ilioinguinal nerve
    Lateral femoral cutaneous nerve
    Obturator nerve
    Superior gluteal nerve
A **Lumbosacral Plexus**
B **Lumbar Nerve**
    Lumbosacral trunk
    Spinal nerve, lumbar
    Superior clunic (cluneal) nerve
C **Pudendal Nerve**
    Posterior labial nerve
    Posterior scrotal nerve
D **Femoral Nerve**
    Anterior crural nerve
    Saphenous nerve
F **Sciatic Nerve**
    Ischiatic nerve
G **Tibial Nerve**
    Lateral plantar nerve
    Medial plantar nerve
    Medial popliteal nerve
    Medial sural cutaneous nerve
	H **Peroneal Nerve**
	    Common fibular nerve
	    Common peroneal nerve
	    External popliteal nerve
	    Lateral sural cutaneous nerve
	K **Head and Neck Sympathetic Nerve**
	    Cavernous plexus
	    Cervical ganglion
	    Ciliary ganglion
	    Internal carotid plexus
	    Otic ganglion
	    Pterygopalatine (sphenopalatine)
	      ganglion
	    Sphenopalatine (pterygopalatine)
	      ganglion
	    Stellate ganglion
	    Submandibular ganglion
	    Submaxillary ganglion
	L **Thoracic Sympathetic Nerve**
	    Cardiac plexus
	    Esophageal plexus
	    Greater splanchnic nerve
	    Inferior cardiac nerve
	    Least splanchnic nerve
	    Lesser splanchnic nerve
	    Middle cardiac nerve
	    Pulmonary plexus
	    Superior cardiac nerve
	    Thoracic aortic plexus
	    Thoracic ganglion
	M **Abdominal Sympathetic Nerve**
	    Abdominal aortic plexus
	    Auerbach's (myenteric) plexus
	    Celiac (solar) plexus
	    Celiac ganglion
	    Gastric plexus
	    Hepatic plexus
	    Inferior hypogastric plexus
	    Inferior mesenteric ganglion
	    Inferior mesenteric plexus
	    Meissner's (submucous) plexus
	    Myenteric (Auerbach's) plexus
	    Pancreatic plexus
	    Pelvic splanchnic nerve
	    Renal nerve
	    Renal plexus
	    Solar (celiac) plexus
	    Splenic plexus
	    Submucous (Meissner's) plexus
	    Superior hypogastric plexus
	    Superior mesenteric ganglion
	    Superior mesenteric plexus
	    Suprarenal plexus
	N **Lumbar Sympathetic Nerve**
	    Lumbar ganglion
	    Lumbar splanchnic nerve
	P **Sacral Sympathetic Nerve**
	    Ganglion impar (ganglion of
	      Walther)
	    Pelvic splanchnic nerve
	    Sacral ganglion
	    Sacral splanchnic nerve
	Q **Sacral Plexus**
	    Inferior gluteal nerve
	    Posterior femoral cutaneous nerve
	    Pudendal nerve
	R **Sacral Nerve**
	    Spinal nerve, sacral
		Ø Open
		3 Percutaneous
		4 Percutaneous
		    Endoscopic
			Z No Device	**Z** No Qualifier

Non-OR   Ø15[Ø,2,3,4,5,6,9,A,C,D,F,G,H,Q][Ø,3,4]ZZ   **Non-OR**   Ø15[1,8,B,R]3ZZ

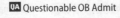

NC Noncovered Procedure   **LC** Limited Coverage   **UA** Questionable OB Admit   **NT** New Tech Add-on   ⊞ Combination Member   ♂ Male   ♀ Female

ICD-10-PCS 2023   **155**

Ø Medical and Surgical
1 Peripheral Nervous System
8 Division Definition: Cutting into a body part, without draining fluids and/or gases from the body part, in order to separate or transect a body part

Explanation: All or a portion of the body part is separated into two or more portions

Body Part Character 4	Approach Character 5	Device Character 6	Qualifier Character 7
Ø Cervical Plexus Ansa cervicalis Cutaneous (transverse) cervical nerve Great auricular nerve Lesser occipital nerve Supraclavicular nerve Transverse (cutaneous) cervical nerve **1 Cervical Nerve** Greater occipital nerve Spinal nerve, cervical Suboccipital nerve Third occipital nerve **2 Phrenic Nerve** Accessory phrenic nerve **3 Brachial Plexus** Axillary nerve Dorsal scapular nerve First intercostal nerve Long thoracic nerve Musculocutaneous nerve Subclavius nerve Suprascapular nerve **4 Ulnar Nerve** Cubital nerve **5 Median Nerve** Anterior interosseous nerve Palmar cutaneous nerve **6 Radial Nerve** Dorsal digital nerve Musculospiral nerve Palmar cutaneous nerve Posterior interosseous nerve **8 Thoracic Nerve** Intercostal nerve Intercostobrachial nerve Spinal nerve, thoracic Subcostal nerve **9 Lumbar Plexus** Accessory obturator nerve Genitofemoral nerve Iliohypogastric nerve Ilioinguinal nerve Lateral femoral cutaneous nerve Obturator nerve Superior gluteal nerve **A Lumbosacral Plexus** **B Lumbar Nerve** Lumbosacral trunk Spinal nerve, lumbar Superior clunic (cluneal) nerve **C Pudendal Nerve** Posterior labial nerve Posterior scrotal nerve **D Femoral Nerve** Anterior crural nerve Saphenous nerve **F Sciatic Nerve** Ischiatic nerve **G Tibial Nerve** Lateral plantar nerve Medial plantar nerve Medial popliteal nerve Medial sural cutaneous nerve **H Peroneal Nerve** Common fibular nerve Common peroneal nerve External popliteal nerve Lateral sural cutaneous nerve **K Head and Neck Sympathetic Nerve** Cavernous plexus Cervical ganglion Ciliary ganglion Internal carotid plexus Otic ganglion Pterygopalatine (sphenopalatine) ganglion Sphenopalatine (pterygopalatine) ganglion Stellate ganglion Submandibular ganglion Submaxillary ganglion **L Thoracic Sympathetic Nerve** Cardiac plexus Esophageal plexus Greater splanchnic nerve Inferior cardiac nerve Least splanchnic nerve Lesser splanchnic nerve Middle cardiac nerve Pulmonary plexus Superior cardiac nerve Thoracic aortic plexus Thoracic ganglion **M Abdominal Sympathetic Nerve** Abdominal aortic plexus Auerbach's (myenteric) plexus Celiac (solar) plexus Celiac ganglion Gastric plexus Hepatic plexus Inferior hypogastric plexus Inferior mesenteric ganglion Inferior mesenteric plexus Meissner's (submucous) plexus Myenteric (Auerbach's) plexus Pancreatic plexus Pelvic splanchnic nerve Renal nerve Renal plexus Solar (celiac) plexus Splenic plexus Submucous (Meissner's) plexus Superior hypogastric plexus Superior mesenteric ganglion Superior mesenteric plexus Suprarenal plexus **N Lumbar Sympathetic Nerve** Lumbar ganglion Lumbar splanchnic nerve **P Sacral Sympathetic Nerve** Ganglion impar (ganglion of Walther) Pelvic splanchnic nerve Sacral ganglion Sacral splanchnic nerve **Q Sacral Plexus** Inferior gluteal nerve Posterior femoral cutaneous nerve Pudendal nerve **R Sacral Nerve** Spinal nerve, sacral	**Ø Open** **3 Percutaneous** **4 Percutaneous Endoscopic**	**Z No Device**	**Z No Qualifier**

Ø	**Medical and Surgical**
1	**Peripheral Nervous System**
9	**Drainage**

Ø **Medical and Surgical**
1 **Peripheral Nervous System**
9 **Drainage**   Definition: Taking or letting out fluids and/or gases from a body part
Explanation: The qualifier DIAGNOSTIC is used to identify drainage procedures that are biopsies

Body Part		Approach	Device	Qualifier
Character 4		**Character 5**	**Character 6**	**Character 7**
Ø Cervical Plexus Ansa cervicalis Cutaneous (transverse) cervical nerve Great auricular nerve Lesser occipital nerve Supraclavicular nerve Transverse (cutaneous) cervical nerve **1** Cervical Nerve Greater occipital nerve Spinal nerve, cervical Suboccipital nerve Third occipital nerve **2** Phrenic Nerve Accessory phrenic nerve **3** Brachial Plexus Axillary nerve Dorsal scapular nerve First intercostal nerve Long thoracic nerve Musculocutaneous nerve Subclavius nerve Suprascapular nerve **4** Ulnar Nerve Cubital nerve **5** Median Nerve Anterior interosseous nerve Palmar cutaneous nerve **6** Radial Nerve Dorsal digital nerve Musculospiral nerve Palmar cutaneous nerve Posterior interosseous nerve **8** Thoracic Nerve Intercostal nerve Intercostobrachial nerve Spinal nerve, thoracic Subcostal nerve **9** Lumbar Plexus Accessory obturator nerve Genitofemoral nerve Iliohypogastric nerve Ilioinguinal nerve Lateral femoral cutaneous nerve Obturator nerve Superior gluteal nerve **A** Lumbosacral Plexus **B** Lumbar Nerve Lumbosacral trunk Spinal nerve, lumbar Superior clunic (cluneal) nerve **C** Pudendal Nerve Posterior labial nerve Posterior scrotal nerve **D** Femoral Nerve Anterior crural nerve Saphenous nerve **F** Sciatic Nerve Ischiatic nerve **G** Tibial Nerve Lateral plantar nerve Medial plantar nerve Medial popliteal nerve Medial sural cutaneous nerve	**H** Peroneal Nerve Common fibular nerve Common peroneal nerve External popliteal nerve Lateral sural cutaneous nerve **K** Head and Neck Sympathetic Nerve Cavernous plexus Cervical ganglion Ciliary ganglion Internal carotid plexus Otic ganglion Pterygopalatine (sphenopalatine) ganglion Sphenopalatine (pterygopalatine) ganglion Stellate ganglion Submandibular ganglion Submaxillary ganglion **L** Thoracic Sympathetic Nerve Cardiac plexus Esophageal plexus Greater splanchnic nerve Inferior cardiac nerve Least splanchnic nerve Lesser splanchnic nerve Middle cardiac nerve Pulmonary plexus Superior cardiac nerve Thoracic aortic plexus Thoracic ganglion **M** Abdominal Sympathetic Nerve Abdominal aortic plexus Auerbach's (myenteric) plexus Celiac (solar) plexus Celiac ganglion Gastric plexus Hepatic plexus Inferior hypogastric plexus Inferior mesenteric ganglion Inferior mesenteric plexus Meissner's (submucous) plexus Myenteric (Auerbach's) plexus Pancreatic plexus Pelvic splanchnic nerve Renal nerve Renal plexus Solar (celiac) plexus Splenic plexus Submucous (Meissner's) plexus Superior hypogastric plexus Superior mesenteric ganglion Superior mesenteric plexus Suprarenal plexus **N** Lumbar Sympathetic Nerve Lumbar ganglion Lumbar splanchnic nerve **P** Sacral Sympathetic Nerve Ganglion impar (ganglion of Walther) Pelvic splanchnic nerve Sacral ganglion Sacral splanchnic nerve **Q** Sacral Plexus Inferior gluteal nerve Posterior femoral cutaneous nerve Pudendal nerve **R** Sacral Nerve Spinal nerve, sacral	**Ø** Open **3** Percutaneous **4** Percutaneous Endoscopic	**Ø** Drainage Device	**Z** No Qualifier

Non-OR   Ø19[Ø,1,2,3,4,5,6,8,9,A,B,C,D,F,G,H,K,L,M,N,P,Q,R]3ØZ

Ø19 Continued on next page

Peripheral Nervous System

Ø   **Medical and Surgical**
1   **Peripheral Nervous System**
9   **Drainage**   Definition: Taking or letting out fluids and/or gases from a body part

Ø19 Continued

Explanation: The qualifier DIAGNOSTIC is used to identify drainage procedures that are biopsies

Body Part Character 4		Approach Character 5	Device Character 6	Qualifier Character 7
Ø Cervical Plexus Ansa cervicalis Cutaneous (transverse) cervical nerve Great auricular nerve Lesser occipital nerve Supraclavicular nerve Transverse (cutaneous) cervical nerve **1 Cervical Nerve** Greater occipital nerve Spinal nerve, cervical Suboccipital nerve Third occipital nerve **2 Phrenic Nerve** Accessory phrenic nerve **3 Brachial Plexus** Axillary nerve Dorsal scapular nerve First intercostal nerve Long thoracic nerve Musculocutaneous nerve Subclavius nerve Suprascapular nerve **4 Ulnar Nerve** Cubital nerve **5 Median Nerve** Anterior interosseous nerve Palmar cutaneous nerve **6 Radial Nerve** Dorsal digital nerve Musculospiral nerve Palmar cutaneous nerve Posterior interosseous nerve **8 Thoracic Nerve** Intercostal nerve Intercostobrachial nerve Spinal nerve, thoracic Subcostal nerve **9 Lumbar Plexus** Accessory obturator nerve Genitofemoral nerve Iliohypogastric nerve Ilioinguinal nerve Lateral femoral cutaneous nerve Obturator nerve Superior gluteal nerve **A Lumbosacral Plexus** **B Lumbar Nerve** Lumbosacral trunk Spinal nerve, lumbar Superior clunic (cluneal) nerve **C Pudendal Nerve** Posterior labial nerve Posterior scrotal nerve **D Femoral Nerve** Anterior crural nerve Saphenous nerve **F Sciatic Nerve** Ischiatic nerve **G Tibial Nerve** Lateral plantar nerve Medial plantar nerve Medial popliteal nerve Medial sural cutaneous nerve	**H Peroneal Nerve** Common fibular nerve Common peroneal nerve External popliteal nerve Lateral sural cutaneous nerve **K Head and Neck Sympathetic Nerve** Cavernous plexus Cervical ganglion Ciliary ganglion Internal carotid plexus Otic ganglion Pterygopalatine (sphenopalatine) ganglion Sphenopalatine (pterygopalatine) ganglion Stellate ganglion Submandibular ganglion Submaxillary ganglion **L Thoracic Sympathetic Nerve** Cardiac plexus Esophageal plexus Greater splanchnic nerve Inferior cardiac nerve Least splanchnic nerve Lesser splanchnic nerve Middle cardiac nerve Pulmonary plexus Superior cardiac nerve Thoracic aortic plexus Thoracic ganglion **M Abdominal Sympathetic Nerve** Abdominal aortic plexus Auerbach's (myenteric) plexus Celiac (solar) plexus Celiac ganglion Gastric plexus Hepatic plexus Inferior hypogastric plexus Inferior mesenteric ganglion Inferior mesenteric plexus Meissner's (submucous) plexus Myenteric (Auerbach's) plexus Pancreatic plexus Pelvic splanchnic nerve Renal nerve Renal plexus Solar (celiac) plexus Splenic plexus Submucous (Meissner's) plexus Superior hypogastric plexus Superior mesenteric ganglion Superior mesenteric plexus Suprarenal plexus **N Lumbar Sympathetic Nerve** Lumbar ganglion Lumbar splanchnic nerve **P Sacral Sympathetic Nerve** Ganglion impar (ganglion of Walther) Pelvic splanchnic nerve Sacral ganglion Sacral splanchnic nerve **Q Sacral Plexus** Inferior gluteal nerve Posterior femoral cutaneous nerve Pudendal nerve **R Sacral Nerve** Spinal nerve, sacral	**Ø Open** **3 Percutaneous** **4 Percutaneous Endoscopic**	**Z No Device**	**X Diagnostic** **Z No Qualifier**

Non-OR   Ø19[Ø,1,2,3,4,5,6,8,9,A,B,C,D,F,G,H,Q,R][3,4]ZX
Non-OR   Ø19[Ø,1,2,3,4,5,6,8,9,A,B,C,D,F,G,H,K,L,M,N,P,Q,R]3ZZ

Non-OR Procedure   DRG Non-OR Procedure   Valid OR Procedure   HAC Associated Procedure   Combination Only   New/Revised April   New/Revised October

158

ICD-10-PCS 2023

Ø19–Ø19

Peripheral Nervous System

Ø   **Medical and Surgical**
1   **Peripheral Nervous System**
B   **Excision**   Definition: Cutting out or off, without replacement, a portion of a body part
                            Explanation: The qualifier DIAGNOSTIC is used to identify excision procedures that are biopsies

Body Part Character 4		Approach Character 5	Device Character 6	Qualifier Character 7
Ø **Cervical Plexus** 　Ansa cervicalis 　Cutaneous (transverse) cervical 　　nerve 　Great auricular nerve 　Lesser occipital nerve 　Supraclavicular nerve 　Transverse (cutaneous) cervical 　　nerve **1** **Cervical Nerve** 　Greater occipital nerve 　Spinal nerve, cervical 　Suboccipital nerve 　Third occipital nerve **2** **Phrenic Nerve** 　Accessory phrenic nerve **3** **Brachial Plexus** 　Axillary nerve 　Dorsal scapular nerve 　First intercostal nerve 　Long thoracic nerve 　Musculocutaneous nerve 　Subclavius nerve 　Suprascapular nerve **4** **Ulnar Nerve** 　Cubital nerve **5** **Median Nerve** 　Anterior interosseous nerve 　Palmar cutaneous nerve **6** **Radial Nerve** 　Dorsal digital nerve 　Musculospiral nerve 　Palmar cutaneous nerve 　Posterior interosseous nerve **8** **Thoracic Nerve** 　Intercostal nerve 　Intercostobrachial nerve 　Spinal nerve, thoracic 　Subcostal nerve **9** **Lumbar Plexus** 　Accessory obturator nerve 　Genitofemoral nerve 　Iliohypogastric nerve 　Ilioinguinal nerve 　Lateral femoral cutaneous 　　nerve 　Obturator nerve 　Superior gluteal nerve **A** **Lumbosacral Plexus** **B** **Lumbar Nerve** 　Lumbosacral trunk 　Spinal nerve, lumbar 　Superior clunic (cluneal) nerve **C** **Pudendal Nerve** 　Posterior labial nerve 　Posterior scrotal nerve **D** **Femoral Nerve** 　Anterior crural nerve 　Saphenous nerve **F** **Sciatic Nerve** 　Ischiatic nerve **G** **Tibial Nerve** 　Lateral plantar nerve 　Medial plantar nerve 　Medial popliteal nerve 　Medial sural cutaneous nerve	**H** **Peroneal Nerve** 　Common fibular nerve 　Common peroneal nerve 　External popliteal nerve 　Lateral sural cutaneous nerve **K** **Head and Neck Sympathetic** **Nerve** 　Cavernous plexus 　Cervical ganglion 　Ciliary ganglion 　Internal carotid plexus 　Otic ganglion 　Pterygopalatine 　　(sphenopalatine) ganglion 　Sphenopalatine 　　(pterygopalatine) ganglion 　Stellate ganglion 　Submandibular ganglion 　Submaxillary ganglion **L** **Thoracic Sympathetic** **Nerve** 　Cardiac plexus 　Esophageal plexus 　Greater splanchnic nerve 　Inferior cardiac nerve 　Least splanchnic nerve 　Lesser splanchnic nerve 　Middle cardiac nerve 　Pulmonary plexus 　Superior cardiac nerve 　Thoracic aortic plexus 　Thoracic ganglion **M** **Abdominal Sympathetic** **Nerve** 　Abdominal aortic plexus 　Auerbach's (myenteric) plexus 　Celiac (solar) plexus 　Celiac ganglion 　Gastric plexus 　Hepatic plexus 　Inferior hypogastric plexus 　Inferior mesenteric ganglion 　Inferior mesenteric plexus 　Meissner's (submucous) plexus 　Myenteric (Auerbach's) plexus 　Pancreatic plexus 　Pelvic splanchnic nerve 　Renal nerve 　Renal plexus 　Solar (celiac) plexus 　Splenic plexus 　Submucous (Meissner's) plexus 　Superior hypogastric plexus 　Superior mesenteric ganglion 　Superior mesenteric plexus 　Suprarenal plexus **N** **Lumbar Sympathetic Nerve** 　Lumbar ganglion 　Lumbar splanchnic nerve **P** **Sacral Sympathetic Nerve** 　Ganglion impar (ganglion of 　　Walther) 　Pelvic splanchnic nerve 　Sacral ganglion 　Sacral splanchnic nerve **Q** **Sacral Plexus** 　Inferior gluteal nerve 　Posterior femoral cutaneous 　　nerve 　Pudendal nerve **R** **Sacral Nerve** 　Spinal nerve, sacral	**Ø** Open **3** Percutaneous **4** Percutaneous Endoscopic	**Z** No Device	**X** Diagnostic **Z** No Qualifier

Non-OR   Ø1B[Ø,1,2,3,4,5,6,8,9,A,B,C,D,F,G,H,Q,R][3,4]ZX

0   Medical and Surgical
1   Peripheral Nervous System
C   Extirpation   Definition: Taking or cutting out solid matter from a body part

Explanation: The solid matter may be an abnormal byproduct of a biological function or a foreign body; it may be imbedded in a body part or in the lumen of a tubular body part. The solid matter may or may not have been previously broken into pieces.

Body Part Character 4		Approach Character 5	Device Character 6	Qualifier Character 7

0 Cervical Plexus
Ansa cervicalis
Cutaneous (transverse) cervical
  nerve
Great auricular nerve
Lesser occipital nerve
Supraclavicular nerve
Transverse (cutaneous) cervical
  nerve
1 Cervical Nerve
Greater occipital nerve
Spinal nerve, cervical
Suboccipital nerve
Third occipital nerve
2 Phrenic Nerve
Accessory phrenic nerve
3 Brachial Plexus
Axillary nerve
Dorsal scapular nerve
First intercostal nerve
Long thoracic nerve
Musculocutaneous nerve
Subclavius nerve
Suprascapular nerve
4 Ulnar Nerve
Cubital nerve
5 Median Nerve
Anterior interosseous nerve
Palmar cutaneous nerve
6 Radial Nerve
Dorsal digital nerve
Musculospiral nerve
Palmar cutaneous nerve
Posterior interosseous nerve
8 Thoracic Nerve
Intercostal nerve
Intercostobrachial nerve
Spinal nerve, thoracic
Subcostal nerve
9 Lumbar Plexus
Accessory obturator nerve
Genitofemoral nerve
Iliohypogastric nerve
Ilioinguinal nerve
Lateral femoral cutaneous
  nerve
Obturator nerve
Superior gluteal nerve
A Lumbosacral Plexus
B Lumbar Nerve
Lumbosacral trunk
Spinal nerve, lumbar
Superior clunic (cluneal) nerve
C Pudendal Nerve
Posterior labial nerve
Posterior scrotal nerve
D Femoral Nerve
Anterior crural nerve
Saphenous nerve
F Sciatic Nerve
Ischiatic nerve
G Tibial Nerve
Lateral plantar nerve
Medial plantar nerve
Medial popliteal nerve
Medial sural cutaneous nerve
	H Peroneal Nerve
	Common fibular nerve
	Common peroneal nerve
	External popliteal nerve
	Lateral sural cutaneous nerve
	K Head and Neck Sympathetic
	Nerve
	Cavernous plexus
	Cervical ganglion
	Ciliary ganglion
	Internal carotid plexus
	Otic ganglion
	Pterygopalatine
	  (sphenopalatine) ganglion
	Sphenopalatine
	  (pterygopalatine) ganglion
	Stellate ganglion
	Submandibular ganglion
	Submaxillary ganglion
	L Thoracic Sympathetic Nerve
	Cardiac plexus
	Esophageal plexus
	Greater splanchnic nerve
	Inferior cardiac nerve
	Least splanchnic nerve
	Lesser splanchnic nerve
	Middle cardiac nerve
	Pulmonary plexus
	Superior cardiac nerve
	Thoracic aortic plexus
	Thoracic ganglion
	M Abdominal Sympathetic
	Nerve
	Abdominal aortic plexus
	Auerbach's (myenteric) plexus
	Celiac (solar) plexus
	Celiac ganglion
	Gastric plexus
	Hepatic plexus
	Inferior hypogastric plexus
	Inferior mesenteric ganglion
	Inferior mesenteric plexus
	Meissner's (submucous) plexus
	Myenteric (Auerbach's) plexus
	Pancreatic plexus
	Pelvic splanchnic nerve
	Renal nerve
	Renal plexus
	Solar (celiac) plexus
	Splenic plexus
	Submucous (Meissner's) plexus
	Superior hypogastric plexus
	Superior mesenteric ganglion
	Superior mesenteric plexus
	Suprarenal plexus
	N Lumbar Sympathetic Nerve
	Lumbar ganglion
	Lumbar splanchnic nerve
	P Sacral Sympathetic Nerve
	Ganglion impar (ganglion of
	  Walther)
	Pelvic splanchnic nerve
	Sacral ganglion
	Sacral splanchnic nerve
	Q Sacral Plexus
	Inferior gluteal nerve
	Posterior femoral cutaneous
	  nerve
	Pudendal nerve
	R Sacral Nerve
	Spinal nerve, sacral
		0 Open
		3 Percutaneous
		4 Percutaneous Endoscopic
			Z No Device	**Z No Qualifier**

Non-OR Procedure   **DRG Non-OR Procedure**   Valid OR Procedure   HAC Associated Procedure   **Combination Only**   New/Revised April   New/Revised October

160

ICD-10-PCS 2023

01C–01C

Ø   Medical and Surgical
1   Peripheral Nervous System
D   Extraction   Definition: Pulling or stripping out or off all or a portion of a body part by the use of force
                      Explanation: The qualifier DIAGNOSTIC is used to identify extraction procedures that are biopsies

Body Part Character 4		Approach Character 5	Device Character 6	Qualifier Character 7
Ø Cervical Plexus 　Ansa cervicalis 　Cutaneous (transverse) cervical 　　nerve 　Great auricular nerve 　Lesser occipital nerve 　Supraclavicular nerve 　Transverse (cutaneous) cervical 　　nerve **1 Cervical Nerve** 　Greater occipital nerve 　Spinal nerve, cervical 　Suboccipital nerve 　Third occipital nerve **2 Phrenic Nerve** 　Accessory phrenic nerve **3 Brachial Plexus** 　Axillary nerve 　Dorsal scapular nerve 　First intercostal nerve 　Long thoracic nerve 　Musculocutaneous nerve 　Subclavius nerve 　Suprascapular nerve **4 Ulnar Nerve** 　Cubital nerve **5 Median Nerve** 　Anterior interosseous nerve 　Palmar cutaneous nerve **6 Radial Nerve** 　Dorsal digital nerve 　Musculospiral nerve 　Palmar cutaneous nerve 　Posterior interosseous nerve **8 Thoracic Nerve** 　Intercostal nerve 　Intercostobrachial nerve 　Spinal nerve, thoracic 　Subcostal nerve **9 Lumbar Plexus** 　Accessory obturator nerve 　Genitofemoral nerve 　Iliohypogastric nerve 　Ilioinguinal nerve 　Lateral femoral cutaneous nerve 　Obturator nerve 　Superior gluteal nerve **A Lumbosacral Plexus** **B Lumbar Nerve** 　Lumbosacral trunk 　Spinal nerve, lumbar 　Superior clunic (cluneal) nerve **C Pudendal Nerve]** 　Posterior labial nerve 　Posterior scrotal nerve **D Femoral Nerve** 　Anterior crural nerve 　Saphenous nerve **F Sciatic Nerve** 　Ischiatic nerve **G Tibial Nerve** 　Lateral plantar nerve 　Medial plantar nerve 　Medial popliteal nerve 　Medial sural cutaneous nerve	**H Peroneal Nerve** 　Common fibular nerve 　Common peroneal nerve 　External popliteal nerve 　Lateral sural cutaneous nerve **K Head and Neck Sympathetic** 　**Nerve** 　Cavernous plexus 　Cervical ganglion 　Ciliary ganglion 　Internal carotid plexus 　Otic ganglion 　Pterygopalatine 　　(sphenopalatine) ganglion 　Sphenopalatine 　　(pterygopalatine) ganglion 　Stellate ganglion 　Submandibular ganglion 　Submaxillary ganglion **L Thoracic Sympathetic Nerve** 　Cardiac plexus 　Esophageal plexus 　Greater splanchnic nerve 　Inferior cardiac nerve 　Least splanchnic nerve 　Lesser splanchnic nerve 　Middle cardiac nerve 　Pulmonary plexus 　Superior cardiac nerve 　Thoracic aortic plexus 　Thoracic ganglion **M Abdominal Sympathetic Nerve** 　Abdominal aortic plexus 　Auerbach's (myenteric) plexus 　Celiac (solar) plexus 　Celiac ganglion 　Gastric plexus 　Hepatic plexus 　Inferior hypogastric plexus 　Inferior mesenteric ganglion 　Inferior mesenteric plexus 　Meissner's (submucous) plexus 　Myenteric (Auerbach's) plexus 　Pancreatic plexus 　Pelvic splanchnic nerve 　Renal nerve 　Renal plexus 　Solar (celiac) plexus 　Splenic plexus 　Submucous (Meissner's) plexus 　Superior hypogastric plexus 　Superior mesenteric ganglion 　Superior mesenteric plexus 　Suprarenal plexus **N Lumbar Sympathetic Nerve** 　Lumbar ganglion 　Lumbar splanchnic nerve **P Sacral Sympathetic Nerve** 　Ganglion impar (ganglion of 　　Walther) 　Pelvic splanchnic nerve 　Sacral ganglion 　Sacral splanchnic nerve **Q Sacral Plexus** 　Inferior gluteal nerve 　Posterior femoral cutaneous 　　nerve 　Pudendal nerve **R Sacral Nerve** 　Spinal nerve, sacral	**Ø Open** **3 Percutaneous** **4 Percutaneous Endoscopic**	**Z No Device**	**Z No Qualifier**

NC Noncovered Procedure   LC Limited Coverage   QA Questionable OB Admit   NT New Tech Add-on   ⊞ Combination Member   ♂ Male   ♀ Female

ICD-10-PCS 2023   **161**

Peripheral Nervous System

Ø **Medical and Surgical**
1 **Peripheral Nervous System**
H **Insertion**   Definition: Putting in a nonbiological appliance that monitors, assists, performs, or prevents a physiological function but does not physically take the place of a body part
Explanation: None

Body Part Character 4		Approach Character 5	Device Character 6	Qualifier Character 7
Y Peripheral Nerve	⊞	Ø Open 3 Percutaneous 4 Percutaneous Endoscopic	1 Radioactive Element 2 Monitoring Device M Neurostimulator Lead Y Other Device	Z No Qualifier

Non-OR	Ø1HY31Z	
Non-OR	Ø1HY[3,4]YZ	**See Appendix L for Procedure Combinations** ⊞ Ø1HY[Ø,3,4]MZ

Ø **Medical and Surgical**
1 **Peripheral Nervous System**
J **Inspection**   Definition: Visually and/or manually exploring a body part
Explanation: Visual exploration may be performed with or without optical instrumentation. Manual exploration may be performed directly or through intervening body layers.

Body Part Character 4	Approach Character 5	Device Character 6	Qualifier Character 7
Y Peripheral Nerve	Ø Open 3 Percutaneous 4 Percutaneous Endoscopic	Z No Device	Z No Qualifier

Non-OR	Ø1JY3ZZ

Non-OR Procedure   DRG Non-OR Procedure   Valid OR Procedure   HAC Associated Procedure   Combination Only   New/Revised April   New/Revised October

162   ICD-10-PCS 2023

Ø   **Medical and Surgical**
1   **Peripheral Nervous System**
N   **Release**   Definition: Freeing a body part from an abnormal physical constraint by cutting or by the use of force
                       Explanation: Some of the restraining tissue may be taken out but none of the body part is taken out

Body Part Character 4		Approach Character 5	Device Character 6	Qualifier Character 7
Ø Cervical Plexus Ansa cervicalis Cutaneous (transverse) cervical nerve Great auricular nerve Lesser occipital nerve Supraclavicular nerve Transverse (cutaneous) cervical nerve **1 Cervical Nerve** Greater occipital nerve Spinal nerve, cervical Suboccipital nerve Third occipital nerve **2 Phrenic Nerve** Accessory phrenic nerve **3 Brachial Plexus** Axillary nerve Dorsal scapular nerve First intercostal nerve Long thoracic nerve Musculocutaneous nerve Subclavius nerve Suprascapular nerve **4 Ulnar Nerve** Cubital nerve **5 Median Nerve** Anterior interosseous nerve Palmar cutaneous nerve **6 Radial Nerve** Dorsal digital nerve Musculospiral nerve Palmar cutaneous nerve Posterior interosseous nerve **8 Thoracic Nerve** Intercostal nerve Intercostobrachial nerve Spinal nerve, thoracic Subcostal nerve **9 Lumbar Plexus** Accessory obturator nerve Genitofemoral nerve Iliohypogastric nerve Ilioinguinal nerve Lateral femoral cutaneous nerve Obturator nerve Superior gluteal nerve **A Lumbosacral Plexus** **B Lumbar Nerve** Lumbosacral trunk Spinal nerve, lumbar Superior clunic (cluneal) nerve **C Pudendal Nerve** Posterior labial nerve Posterior scrotal nerve **D Femoral Nerve** Anterior crural nerve Saphenous nerve **F Sciatic Nerve** Ischiatic nerve **G Tibial Nerve** Lateral plantar nerve Medial plantar nerve Medial popliteal nerve Medial sural cutaneous nerve	**H Peroneal Nerve** Common fibular nerve Common peroneal nerve External popliteal nerve Lateral sural cutaneous nerve **K Head and Neck Sympathetic Nerve** Cavernous plexus Cervical ganglion Ciliary ganglion Internal carotid plexus Otic ganglion Pterygopalatine (sphenopalatine) ganglion Sphenopalatine (pterygopalatine) ganglion Stellate ganglion Submandibular ganglion Submaxillary ganglion **L Thoracic Sympathetic Nerve** Cardiac plexus Esophageal plexus Greater splanchnic nerve Inferior cardiac nerve Least splanchnic nerve Lesser splanchnic nerve Middle cardiac nerve Pulmonary plexus Superior cardiac nerve Thoracic aortic plexus Thoracic ganglion **M Abdominal Sympathetic Nerve** Abdominal aortic plexus Auerbach's (myenteric) plexus Celiac (solar) plexus Celiac ganglion Gastric plexus Hepatic plexus Inferior hypogastric plexus Inferior mesenteric ganglion Inferior mesenteric plexus Meissner's (submucous) plexus Myenteric (Auerbach's) plexus Pancreatic plexus Pelvic splanchnic nerve Renal nerve Renal plexus Solar (celiac) plexus Splenic plexus Submucous (Meissner's) plexus Superior hypogastric plexus Superior mesenteric ganglion Superior mesenteric plexus Suprarenal plexus **N Lumbar Sympathetic Nerve** Lumbar ganglion Lumbar splanchnic nerve **P Sacral Sympathetic Nerve** Ganglion impar (ganglion of Walther) Pelvic splanchnic nerve Sacral ganglion Sacral splanchnic nerve **Q Sacral Plexus** Inferior gluteal nerve Posterior femoral cutaneous nerve Pudendal nerve **R Sacral Nerve** Spinal nerve, sacral	**Ø Open** **3 Percutaneous** **4 Percutaneous Endoscopic**	**Z No Device**	**Z No Qualifier**

Ø   **Medical and Surgical**
1   **Peripheral Nervous System**
P   **Removal**   Definition: Taking out or off a device from a body part

Explanation: If a device is taken out and a similar device put in without cutting or puncturing the skin or mucous membrane, the procedure is coded to the root operation CHANGE. Otherwise, the procedure for taking out a device is coded to the root operation REMOVAL.

Body Part Character 4	Approach Character 5	Device Character 6	Qualifier Character 7
Y Peripheral Nerve	Ø Open 3 Percutaneous 4 Percutaneous Endoscopic	Ø Drainage Device 2 Monitoring Device 7 Autologous Tissue Substitute M Neurostimulator Lead Y Other Device	Z No Qualifier
Y Peripheral Nerve	X External	Ø Drainage Device 2 Monitoring Device M Neurostimulator Lead	Z No Qualifier

Non-OR   Ø1PY3[Ø,2]Z
Non-OR   Ø1PY[3,4]YZ
Non-OR   Ø1PYX[Ø,2,M]Z

0   Medical and Surgical
1   Peripheral Nervous System
Q   Repair   Definition: Restoring, to the extent possible, a body part to its normal anatomic structure and function

Explanation: Used only when the method to accomplish the repair is not one of the other root operations

Body Part Character 4		Approach Character 5	Device Character 6	Qualifier Character 7

0 Cervical Plexus
  Ansa cervicalis
  Cutaneous (transverse) cervical
    nerve
  Great auricular nerve
  Lesser occipital nerve
  Supraclavicular nerve
  Transverse (cutaneous) cervical
    nerve
1 Cervical Nerve
  Greater occipital nerve
  Spinal nerve, cervical
  Suboccipital nerve
  Third occipital nerve
2 Phrenic Nerve
  Accessory phrenic nerve
3 Brachial Plexus
  Axillary nerve
  Dorsal scapular nerve
  First intercostal nerve
  Long thoracic nerve
  Musculocutaneous nerve
  Subclavius nerve
  Suprascapular nerve
4 Ulnar Nerve
  Cubital nerve
5 Median Nerve
  Anterior interosseous nerve
  Palmar cutaneous nerve
6 Radial Nerve
  Dorsal digital nerve
  Musculospiral nerve
  Palmar cutaneous nerve
  Posterior interosseous nerve
8 Thoracic Nerve
  Intercostal nerve
  Intercostobrachial nerve
  Spinal nerve, thoracic
  Subcostal nerve
9 Lumbar Plexus
  Accessory obturator nerve
  Genitofemoral nerve
  Iliohypogastric nerve
  Ilioinguinal nerve
  Lateral femoral cutaneous
    nerve
  Obturator nerve
  Superior gluteal nerve
A Lumbosacral Plexus
B Lumbar Nerve
  Lumbosacral trunk
  Spinal nerve, lumbar
  Superior clunic (cluneal) nerve
C Pudendal Nerve
  Posterior labial nerve
  Posterior scrotal nerve
D Femoral Nerve
  Anterior crural nerve
  Saphenous nerve
F Sciatic Nerve
  Ischiatic nerve
G Tibial Nerve
  Lateral plantar nerve
  Medial plantar nerve
  Medial popliteal nerve
  Medial sural cutaneous nerve
	H Peroneal Nerve
	  Common fibular nerve
	  Common peroneal nerve
	  External popliteal nerve
	  Lateral sural cutaneous nerve
	K Head and Neck Sympathetic
	  Nerve
	  Cavernous plexus
	  Cervical ganglion
	  Ciliary ganglion
	  Internal carotid plexus
	  Otic ganglion
	  Pterygopalatine
	    (sphenopalatine) ganglion
	  Sphenopalatine
	    (pterygopalatine) ganglion
	  Stellate ganglion
	  Submandibular ganglion
	  Submaxillary ganglion
	L Thoracic Sympathetic Nerve
	  Cardiac plexus
	  Esophageal plexus
	  Greater splanchnic nerve
	  Inferior cardiac nerve
	  Least splanchnic nerve
	  Lesser splanchnic nerve
	  Middle cardiac nerve
	  Pulmonary plexus
	  Superior cardiac nerve
	  Thoracic aortic plexus
	  Thoracic ganglion
	M Abdominal Sympathetic
	  Nerve
	  Abdominal aortic plexus
	  Auerbach's (myenteric) plexus
	  Celiac (solar) plexus
	  Celiac ganglion
	  Gastric plexus
	  Hepatic plexus
	  Inferior hypogastric plexus
	  Inferior mesenteric ganglion
	  Inferior mesenteric plexus
	  Meissner's (submucous) plexus
	  Myenteric (Auerbach's) plexus
	  Pancreatic plexus
	  Pelvic splanchnic nerve
	  Renal nerve
	  Renal plexus
	  Solar (celiac) plexus
	  Splenic plexus
	  Submucous (Meissner's) plexus
	  Superior hypogastric plexus
	  Superior mesenteric ganglion
	  Superior mesenteric plexus
	  Suprarenal plexus
	N Lumbar Sympathetic Nerve
	  Lumbar ganglion
	  Lumbar splanchnic nerve
	P Sacral Sympathetic Nerve
	  Ganglion impar (ganglion of
	    Walther)
	  Pelvic splanchnic nerve
	  Sacral ganglion
	  Sacral splanchnic nerve
	Q Sacral Plexus
	  Inferior gluteal nerve
	  Posterior femoral cutaneous
	    nerve
	  Pudendal nerve
	R Sacral Nerve
	  Spinal nerve, sacral
		0 Open
		3 Percutaneous
		4 Percutaneous Endoscopic
			Z No Device	**Z** No Qualifier

NC Noncovered Procedure   **LC** Limited Coverage   **QA** Questionable OB Admit   **NT** New Tech Add-on   ⊞ Combination Member   ♂ Male   ♀ Female

ICD-10-PCS 2023   165

01Q–01Q

Peripheral Nervous System *(left margin)*

Ø   **Medical and Surgical**
1   **Peripheral Nervous System**
R   **Replacement**   Definition: Putting in or on biological or synthetic material that physically takes the place and/or function of all or a portion of a body part
                        Explanation: The body part may have been taken out or replaced, or may be taken out, physically eradicated, or rendered nonfunctional during
                        the REPLACEMENT procedure. A REMOVAL procedure is coded for taking out the device used in a previous replacement procedure.

Body Part Character 4	Approach Character 5	Device Character 6	Qualifier Character 7

1 Cervical Nerve
   Greater occipital nerve
   Spinal nerve, cervical
   Suboccipital nerve
   Third occipital nerve
2 Phrenic Nerve
   Accessory phrenic nerve
4 Ulnar Nerve
   Cubital nerve
5 Median Nerve
   Anterior interosseous nerve
   Palmar cutaneous nerve
6 Radial Nerve
   Dorsal digital nerve
   Musculospiral nerve
   Palmar cutaneous nerve
   Posterior interosseous nerve
8 Thoracic Nerve
   Intercostal nerve
   Intercostobrachial nerve
   Spinal nerve, thoracic
   Subcostal nerve
B Lumbar Nerve
   Lumbosacral trunk
   Spinal nerve, lumbar
   Superior clunic (cluneal) nerve
C Pudendal Nerve
   Posterior labial nerve
   Posterior scrotal nerve
D Femoral Nerve
   Anterior crural nerve
   Saphenous nerve
F Sciatic Nerve
   Ischiatic nerve
G Tibial Nerve
   Lateral plantar nerve
   Medial plantar nerve
   Medial popliteal nerve
   Medial sural cutaneous nerve
H Peroneal Nerve
   Common fibular nerve
   Common peroneal nerve
   External popliteal nerve
   Lateral sural cutaneous nerve
R Sacral Nerve
   Spinal nerve, sacral
	Ø Open
	4 Percutaneous Endoscopic
		7 Autologous Tissue Substitute
		J Synthetic Substitute
		K Nonautologous Tissue Substitute
			Z No Qualifier

Ø1R–Ø1R *(left margin bottom)*

0 Medical and Surgical
1 Peripheral Nervous System
S Reposition   Definition: Moving to its normal location, or other suitable location, all or a portion of a body part

Explanation: The body part is moved to a new location from an abnormal location, or from a normal location where it is not functioning correctly. The body part may or may not be cut out or off to be moved to the new location.

Body Part Character 4	Approach Character 5	Device Character 6	Qualifier Character 7
0 Cervical Plexus Ansa cervicalis Cutaneous (transverse) cervical nerve Great auricular nerve Lesser occipital nerve Supraclavicular nerve Transverse (cutaneous) cervical nerve **1 Cervical Nerve** Greater occipital nerve Spinal nerve, cervical Suboccipital nerve Third occipital nerve **2 Phrenic Nerve** Accessory phrenic nerve **3 Brachial Plexus** Axillary nerve Dorsal scapular nerve First intercostal nerve Long thoracic nerve Musculocutaneous nerve Subclavius nerve Suprascapular nerve **4 Ulnar Nerve** Cubital nerve **5 Median Nerve** Anterior interosseous nerve Palmar cutaneous nerve **6 Radial Nerve** Dorsal digital nerve Musculospiral nerve Palmar cutaneous nerve Posterior interosseous nerve **8 Thoracic Nerve** Intercostal nerve Intercostobrachial nerve Spinal nerve, thoracic Subcostal nerve **9 Lumbar Plexus** Accessory obturator nerve Genitofemoral nerve Iliohypogastric nerve Ilioinguinal nerve Lateral femoral cutaneous nerve Obturator nerve Superior gluteal nerve **A Lumbosacral Plexus** **B Lumbar Nerve** Lumbosacral trunk Spinal nerve, lumbar Superior clunic (cluneal) nerve **C Pudendal Nerve** Posterior labial nerve Posterior scrotal nerve **D Femoral Nerve** Anterior crural nerve Saphenous nerve **F Sciatic Nerve** Ischiatic nerve **G Tibial Nerve** Lateral plantar nerve Medial plantar nerve Medial popliteal nerve Medial sural cutaneous nerve **H Peroneal Nerve** Common fibular nerve Common peroneal nerve External popliteal nerve Lateral sural cutaneous nerve **Q Sacral Plexus** Inferior gluteal nerve Posterior femoral cutaneous nerve Pudendal nerve **R Sacral Nerve** Spinal nerve, sacral	**0 Open** **3 Percutaneous** **4 Percutaneous Endoscopic**	**Z No Device**	**Z No Qualifier**

NC Noncovered Procedure   **LC** Limited Coverage   **QA** Questionable OB Admit   **NT** New Tech Add-on   ⊞ Combination Member   ♂ Male   ♀ Female

ICD-10-PCS 2023   167

Ø   Medical and Surgical
1   Peripheral Nervous System
U   Supplement   Definition: Putting in or on biological or synthetic material that physically reinforces and/or augments the function of a portion of a body part

Explanation: The biological material is non-living, or is living and from the same individual. The body part may have been previously replaced, and the SUPPLEMENT procedure is performed to physically reinforce and/or augment the function of the replaced body part.

Body Part Character 4	Approach Character 5	Device Character 6	Qualifier Character 7

1 Cervical Nerve
   Greater occipital nerve
   Spinal nerve, cervical
   Suboccipital nerve
   Third occipital nerve
2 Phrenic Nerve
   Accessory phrenic nerve
4 Ulnar Nerve
   Cubital nerve
5 Median Nerve
   Anterior interosseous nerve
   Palmar cutaneous nerve
6 Radial Nerve
   Dorsal digital nerve
   Musculospiral nerve
   Palmar cutaneous nerve
   Posterior interosseous nerve
8 Thoracic Nerve
   Intercostal nerve
   Intercostobrachial nerve
   Spinal nerve, thoracic
   Subcostal nerve
B Lumbar Nerve
   Lumbosacral trunk
   Spinal nerve, lumbar
   Superior clunic (cluneal) nerve
C Pudendal Nerve
   Posterior labial nerve
   Posterior scrotal nerve
D Femoral Nerve
   Anterior crural nerve
   Saphenous nerve
F Sciatic Nerve
   Ischiatic nerve
G Tibial Nerve
   Lateral plantar nerve
   Medial plantar nerve
   Medial popliteal nerve
   Medial sural cutaneous nerve
H Peroneal Nerve
   Common fibular nerve
   Common peroneal nerve
   External popliteal nerve
   Lateral sural cutaneous nerve
R Sacral Nerve
   Spinal nerve, sacral
	Ø Open
	3 Percutaneous
	4 Percutaneous Endoscopic
		7 Autologous Tissue Substitute
		J Synthetic Substitute
		K Nonautologous Tissue Substitute
			Z No Qualifier

Ø   Medical and Surgical
1   Peripheral Nervous System
W   Revision   Definition: Correcting, to the extent possible, a portion of a malfunctioning device or the position of a displaced device

Explanation: Revision can include correcting a malfunctioning or displaced device by taking out or putting in components of the device such as a screw or pin

Body Part Character 4	Approach Character 5	Device Character 6	Qualifier Character 7
Y Peripheral Nerve	**Ø Open** **3 Percutaneous** **4 Percutaneous Endoscopic**	**Ø Drainage Device** **2 Monitoring Device** **7 Autologous Tissue Substitute** **M Neurostimulator Lead** **Y Other Device**	**Z No Qualifier**
Y Peripheral Nerve	**X External**	**Ø Drainage Device** **2 Monitoring Device** **7 Autologous Tissue Substitute** **M Neurostimulator Lead**	**Z No Qualifier**

Non-OR   Ø1WY[3,4]YZ
Non-OR   Ø1WYX[Ø,2,7,M]Z

Non-OR Procedure   DRG Non-OR Procedure   Valid OR Procedure   HAC Associated Procedure   Combination Only   New/Revised April   New/Revised October

Ø   **Medical and Surgical**
1   **Peripheral Nervous System**
X   **Transfer**   Definition: Moving, without taking out, all or a portion of a body part to another location to take over the function of all or a portion of a body part
                       Explanation: The body part transferred remains connected to its vascular and nervous supply

Body Part Character 4	Approach Character 5	Device Character 6	Qualifier Character 7
1 Cervical Nerve Greater occipital nerve Spinal nerve, cervical Suboccipital nerve Third occipital nerve **2 Phrenic Nerve** Accessory phrenic nerve	Ø Open 4 Percutaneous Endoscopic	Z No Device	1 Cervical Nerve 2 Phrenic Nerve
4 Ulnar Nerve Cubital nerve **5 Median Nerve** Anterior interosseous nerve Palmar cutaneous nerve **6 Radial Nerve** Dorsal digital nerve Musculospiral nerve Palmar cutaneous nerve Posterior interosseous nerve	Ø Open 4 Percutaneous Endoscopic	Z No Device	4 Ulnar Nerve 5 Median Nerve 6 Radial Nerve
8 Thoracic Nerve Intercostal nerve Intercostobrachial nerve Spinal nerve, thoracic Subcostal nerve	Ø Open 4 Percutaneous Endoscopic	Z No Device	8 Thoracic Nerve
B Lumbar Nerve Lumbosacral trunk Spinal nerve, lumbar Superior clunic (cluneal) nerve **C Pudendal Nerve** Posterior labial nerve Posterior scrotal nerve	Ø Open 4 Percutaneous Endoscopic	Z No Device	B Lumbar Nerve C Perineal Nerve
D Femoral Nerve Anterior crural nerve Saphenous nerve **F Sciatic Nerve** Ischiatic nerve **G Tibial Nerve** Lateral plantar nerve Medial plantar nerve Medial popliteal nerve Medial sural cutaneous nerve **H Peroneal Nerve** Common fibular nerve Common peroneal nerve External popliteal nerve Lateral sural cutaneous nerve	Ø Open 4 Percutaneous Endoscopic	Z No Device	D Femoral Nerve F Sciatic Nerve G Tibial Nerve H Peroneal Nerve

Heart and Great Vessels Ø21–Ø2Y

Character Meanings

This Character Meaning table is provided as a guide to assist the user in the identification of character members that may be found in this section of code tables. It **SHOULD NOT** be used to build a PCS code.

Operation–Character 3	Body Part–Character 4	Approach–Character 5	Device–Character 6	Qualifier–Character 7
1 Bypass	Ø Coronary Artery, One Artery	Ø Open	Ø Monitoring Device, Pressure Sensor	Ø Allogeneic OR Ultrasonic
4 Creation	1 Coronary Artery, Two Arteries	3 Percutaneous	2 Monitoring Device	1 Syngeneic
5 Destruction	2 Coronary Artery, Three Arteries	4 Percutaneous Endoscopic	3 Infusion Device	2 Zooplastic OR Common Atrioventricular Valve
7 Dilation	3 Coronary Artery, Four or More Arteries	X External	4 Intraluminal Device, Drug-eluting	3 Coronary Artery
8 Division	4 Coronary Vein		5 Intraluminal Device, Drug-eluting, Two	4 Coronary Vein
B Excision	5 Atrial Septum		6 Intraluminal Device, Drug-eluting, Three	5 Coronary Circulation
C Extirpation	6 Atrium, Right		7 Intraluminal Device, Drug-eluting, Four or More OR Autologous Tissue Substitute	6 Bifurcation OR Atrium, Right
F Fragmentation	7 Atrium, Left		8 Zooplastic Tissue	7 Atrium, Left OR Orbital Atherectomy Technique
H Insertion	8 Conduction Mechanism		9 Autologous Venous Tissue	8 Internal Mammary, Right
J Inspection	9 Chordae Tendineae		A Autologous Arterial Tissue	9 Internal Mammary, Left
K Map	A Heart		C Extraluminal Device	A Innominate Artery
L Occlusion	B Heart, Right		D Intraluminal Device	B Subclavian
N Release	C Heart, Left		E Intraluminal Device, Two OR Intraluminal Device, Branched or Fenestrated, One or Two Arteries	C Thoracic Artery
P Removal	D Papillary Muscle		F Intraluminal Device, Three OR Intraluminal Device, Branched or Fenestrated, Three or More Arteries	D Carotid
Q Repair	F Aortic Valve		G Intraluminal Device, Four or More	E Atrioventricular Valve, Left
R Replacement	G Mitral Valve		J Synthetic Substitute OR Cardiac Lead, Pacemaker	F Abdominal Artery
S Reposition	H Pulmonary Valve		K Nonautologous Tissue Substitute OR Cardiac Lead, Defibrillator	G Atrioventricular Valve, Right OR Axillary Artery
T Resection	J Tricuspid Valve		L Biologic with Synthetic Substitute, Autoregulated Electrohydraulic	H Transapical OR Brachial Artery
U Supplement	K Ventricle, Right		M Cardiac Lead OR Synthetic Substitute, Pneumatic	J Truncal Valve OR Temporary OR Intraoperative
V Restriction	L Ventricle, Left		N Intracardiac Pacemaker	K Left Atrial Appendage
			Q Implantable Heart Assist System	L In Existing Conduit
			R Short-term External Heart Assist System	M Native Site
W Revision	M Ventricular Septum		T Intraluminal Device, Radioactive	N Rapid Deployment Technique
Y Transplantation	N Pericardium		Y Other Device	P Pulmonary Trunk
	P Pulmonary Trunk		Z No Device	Q Pulmonary Artery, Right
	Q Pulmonary Artery, Right			R Pulmonary Artery, Left
	R Pulmonary Artery, Left			S Pulmonary Vein, Right OR Biventricular
	S Pulmonary Vein, Right			T Pulmonary Vein, Left OR Ductus Arteriosus
	T Pulmonary Vein, Left			U Pulmonary Vein, Confluence
	V Superior Vena Cava			V Lower Extremity Artery
	W Thoracic Aorta, Descending			W Aorta
	X Thoracic Aorta, Ascending/Arch			X Diagnostic
	Y Great Vessel			Z No Qualifier

AHA Coding Clinic for Heart and Great Vessels

2022, 1Q, 10-13	Procedures performed on a continuous vessel, ICD-10-PCS Guideline B4.1c

AHA Coding Clinic for table Ø21

2022, 1Q, 54	Coronary artery bypass graft surgery
2021, 3Q, 22	Left internal mammary artery free graft between obtuse marginal saphenous vein graft and left anterior descending artery
2020, 4Q, 44-45	Atrium bypass qualifier
2020, 1Q, 24	Pulmonary artery unifocalization
2020, 1Q, 37	Bypass of ascending aorta to brachiocephalic artery
2019, 4Q, 23	Bypass thoracic aorta to innominate artery
2019, 3Q, 30	Aortic aneurysm repair with debranching of common carotid and brachiocephalic arteries
2018, 4Q, 45-46	Descending thoracic aorta bypass
2018, 3Q, 8	Coronary artery bypass graft surgery (revision versus total redo)
2018, 3Q, 26	Coronary artery bypass graft with endarterectomy
2017, 4Q, 56	Added approach values - Percutaneous heart valve procedures
2017, 1Q, 19	Norwood Sano procedure
2016, 4Q, 80-81	Thoracic aorta, ascending/arch and descending
2016, 4Q, 82-83	Coronary artery, number of arteries
2016, 4Q, 102-109	Correction of congenital heart defects
2016, 4Q, 144	Repair of atrial septal defect and anomalous pulmonary venous return
2016, 4Q, 145	Modified Warden procedure for repair of septal defect and right partial anomalous pulmonary venous return
2016, 1Q, 27	Aortocoronary bypass graft utilizing Y-graft
2015, 4Q, 22, 24	Congenital heart corrective procedures
2015, 3Q, 16	Revision of previous truncus arteriosus surgery with ventricle to pulmonary artery conduit
2014, 3Q, 3	Blalock-Taussig shunt procedure
2014, 3Q, 8	Coronary artery bypass graft utilizing internal mammary as pedicle graft
2014, 3Q, 20	MAZE procedure performed with coronary artery bypass graft
2014, 3Q, 29	Fontan completion procedure stage II
2014, 3Q, 30	Creation of conduit from right ventricle to pulmonary artery
2014, 1Q, 10	Repair of thoracic aortic aneurysm & coronary artery bypass graft
2013, 2Q, 37	Coronary artery release performed during coronary artery bypass graft

AHA Coding Clinic for table Ø24

2016, 4Q, 101	Root operation Creation
2016, 4Q, 102-109	Correction of congenital heart defects

AHA Coding Clinic for table Ø25

2020, 1Q, 32	Ablation convergent procedure (catheter-based and thoracoscopic ablations)
2018, 3Q, 27	Alcohol septal ablation
2016, 4Q, 80-81	Thoracic aorta, ascending/arch and descending
2016, 3Q, 43-44	Peri-pulmonary catheter ablation
2016, 3Q, 44-45	Maze procedure
2016, 2Q, 17	Photodynamic therapy for treatment of malignant mesothelioma
2014, 4Q, 47	Catheter ablation of peripulmonary veins
2014, 3Q, 19	Ablation of ventricular tachycardia with Impella® support
2014, 3Q, 20	MAZE procedure performed with coronary artery bypass graft
2013, 2Q, 38	Catheter ablation to treat atrial fibrillation

AHA Coding Clinic for table Ø27

2018, 3Q, 7	Coronary brachytherapy with angioplasty
2018, 3Q, 10	Disruption of perma-catheter fibrin sheath via angioplasty of superior vena cava
2018, 2Q, 24	Coronary artery bifurcation
2017, 4Q, 32-33	Corrective surgery of left ventricular outflow tract obstruction
2016, 4Q, 80-81	Thoracic aorta, ascending/arch and descending
2016, 4Q, 82-83	Coronary artery, number of arteries
2016, 4Q, 84-85	Coronary artery, number of stents
2016, 4Q, 86-88	Coronary and peripheral artery bifurcation
2016, 1Q, 16	Pulmonary valvotomy and dilation of annulus
2015, 4Q, 13	New Section X codes—New Technology procedures
2015, 3Q, 9	Failed attempt to treat coronary artery occlusion
2015, 3Q, 10	Coronary angioplasty with unsuccessful stent insertion
2015, 3Q, 16	Revision of previous truncus arteriosus surgery with ventricle to pulmonary artery conduit
2015, 2Q, 3-5	Coronary artery intervention site
2014, 2Q, 4	Coronary angioplasty of bypassed vessel

AHA Coding Clinic for table Ø2B

2019, 3Q, 32	Endomyocardial biopsy and right heart catheterization
2019, 2Q, 20	Pericardiectomy for constrictive pericarditis
2017, 1Q, 38	Mitral valve repair and chordae tendineae transfer
2016, 4Q, 80-81	Thoracic aorta, ascending/arch and descending
2015, 2Q, 23	Annuloplasty ring

AHA Coding Clinic for table Ø2C

2021, 4Q, 41	Coronary orbital atherectomy
2019, 4Q, 25	Coronary artery to root operation Supplement
2018, 3Q, 26	Coronary artery bypass graft surgery with endarterectomy
2018, 2Q, 24	Coronary artery bifurcation
2017, 2Q, 23	Thrombectomy via Fogarty catheter
2016, 4Q, 80-81	Thoracic aorta, ascending/arch and descending
2016, 4Q, 82-83	Coronary artery, number of arteries
2016, 4Q, 86-87	Coronary and peripheral artery bifurcation
2016, 2Q, 24	Repair/decalcification of mitral valve
2016, 2Q, 25	Aortic valve surgery with excision of calcium deposits

AHA Coding Clinic for table Ø2F

2021, 4Q, 41-42	Coronary intravascular lithotripsy
2020, 4Q, 45-49	New fragmentation tables
2020, 4Q, 49-50	Intravascular ultrasound assisted thrombolysis
2020, 4Q, 50	Intravascular lithotripsy

AHA Coding Clinic for table Ø2H

2022, 2Q, 25	Temporary-permanent pacemaker placement
2021, 2Q, 23	Clarification of lead placement in bundle of HIS
2019, 4Q, 23-24	Coronary artery Body Part to root operation Insertion
2019, 3Q, 19	Insertion of left ventricular catheter
2019, 3Q, 23	Placement of pacemaker lead in Bundle of HIS
2019, 1Q, 24	Replacement of left ventricular assist device with retention of outflow graft
2018, 4Q, 94	Insertion and removal of failed Watchman™ device
2018, 2Q, 3-5	Intra-aortic balloon pump
2018, 2Q, 19	Pacing lead attached to automatic implantable cardioverter defibrillator
2017, 4Q, 42-45	Insertion of external heart assist devices
2017, 4Q, 63-64	Added and revised device values - Vascular access reservoir
2017, 4Q, 104	Placement of Watchman™ left atrial appendage device
2017, 3Q, 11	Placement of peripherally inserted central catheter using 3CG ECG technology
2017, 2Q, 24	Tunneled catheter versus totally implantable catheter
2017, 2Q, 26	Exchange of tunneled catheter
2017, 1Q, 10-11	External heart assist device
2016, 4Q, 80-81	Thoracic aorta, ascending/arch and descending
2016, 4Q, 95	Intracardiac pacemaker
2016, 4Q, 137-138	Heart assist device systems
2016, 2Q, 15	Removal and replacement of tunneled internal jugular catheter
2015, 4Q, 14	New Section X codes—New Technology procedures
2015, 4Q, 26-31	Vascular access devices
2015, 3Q, 35	Swan Ganz catheterization
2015, 2Q, 31	Leadless pacemaker insertion
2015, 2Q, 33	Totally implantable central venous access device (Port-a-Cath)
2013, 3Q, 18	Placement of peripherally inserted central catheter (PICC)

AHA Coding Clinic for table Ø2J

2015, 3Q, 9	Failed attempt to treat coronary artery occlusion

AHA Coding Clinic for table Ø2K

2020, 1Q, 32	Ablation convergent procedure (catheter-based and thoracoscopic ablations)

AHA Coding Clinic for table Ø2L

2018, 4Q, 94	Insertion and removal of failed Watchman™ device
2017, 4Q, 31	Resuscitative endovascular balloon occlusion of the aorta
2017, 4Q, 33-34	Occlusion/ligation of pulmonary trunk & right pulmonary artery
2016, 4Q, 102-109	Correction of congenital heart defects
2016, 2Q, 26	Embolization of pulmonary arteriovenous fistula
2015, 4Q, 23	Congenital heart corrective procedures
2014, 3Q, 20	MAZE procedure performed with coronary artery bypass graft

AHA Coding Clinic for table Ø2N

2021, 3Q, 26	Cavoatrial junction tear with repair and relief of cardiac tamponade
2019, 2Q, 13	Unroofing of anomalous coronary artery
2019, 2Q, 20	Pericardiectomy for constrictive pericarditis
2017, 4Q, 35	Release of myocardial bridge
2016, 4Q, 80-81	Thoracic aorta, ascending/arch and descending
2014, 3Q, 16	Repair of Tetralogy of Fallot

AHA Coding Clinic for table Ø2P

2022, 2Q, 25	Temporary-permanent pacemaker placement
2019, 1Q, 24	Replacement of left ventricular assist device with retention of outflow graft
2018, 4Q, 52-54	Percutaneous extracorporeal membrane oxygenation
2018, 4Q, 85	Externalization of lumboatrial shunt
2018, 4Q, 94	Insertion and removal of failed Watchman™ device
2018, 2Q, 3-5	Intra-aortic balloon pump
2017, 4Q, 42-45	Insertion of external heart assist devices
2017, 4Q, 104	Placement of Watchman™ left atrial appendage device
2017, 3Q, 18	Intra-aortic balloon pump removal
2017, 2Q, 24	Tunneled catheter versus totally implantable catheter
2017, 2Q, 26	Exchange of tunneled catheter
2017, 1Q, 11	External heart assist device
2017, 1Q, 13	SynCardia total artificial heart
2016, 4Q, 95-96	Intracardiac pacemaker
2016, 4Q, 137-139	Heart assist device systems
2016, 3Q, 19	Nonoperative removal of peripherally inserted central catheter
2016, 2Q, 15	Removal and replacement of tunneled internal jugular catheter
2015, 4Q, 31	Vascular access devices
2015, 3Q, 33	Approach values for repositioning and removal of cardiac lead

AHA Coding Clinic for table 02Q

2022, 1Q, 40	Repair of common atrioventricular valve using Alfieri stitch
2022, 1Q, 41	Common atrioventricular valve repair with commissuroplasty sutures
2021, 3Q, 26	Cavoatrial junction tear with repair and relief of cardiac tamponade
2018, 1Q, 12	Percutaneous balloon valvuloplasty & cardiac catheterization with ventriculogram
2017, 1Q, 18	Sutureless repair of pulmonary vein stenosis
2016, 4Q, 80-81	Thoracic aorta, ascending/arch and descending
2016, 4Q, 82-83	Coronary artery, number of arteries
2016, 4Q, 101	Root operation Creation
2016, 4Q, 102-109	Correction of congenital heart defects
2015, 4Q, 23	Congenital heart corrective procedures
2015, 3Q, 16	Vascular ring surgery and double aortic arch
2015, 2Q, 23	Annuloplasty ring
2013, 3Q, 26	Transcatheter replacement of heart valve (TAVR) with measurements

AHA Coding Clinic for table 02R

2021, 4Q, 42-43	Total artificial heart systems
2021, 4Q, 43	Transcatheter replacement of pulmonary valve
2020, 1Q, 25	Elephant trunk repair of aortic dissection
2019, 4Q, 24	Coronary artery Body Part to root operation Insertion
2019, 4Q, 46	Cerebral embolic filtration
2019, 3Q, 23	Replacement of atrioventricular valve
2019, 3Q, 24	Valve sparing aortic root replacement with modified Gleason Vascutek® graft to ascending aorta
2019, 1Q, 31	Transcatheter aortic valve in valve replacement
2018, 3Q, 11	Transcatheter aortic valve replacement via transaortic approach
2018, 1Q, 12	Percutaneous balloon valvuloplasty & cardiac catheterization with ventriculogram
2017, 4Q, 55-56	Added approach values - Percutaneous heart valve procedures
2017, 1Q, 13	SynCardia total artificial heart
2016, 4Q, 80-81	Thoracic aorta, ascending/arch and descending
2016, 3Q, 32	Transcatheter tricuspid valve replacement
2014, 1Q, 10	Repair of thoracic aortic aneurysm & coronary artery bypass graft

AHA Coding Clinic for table 02S

2016, 4Q, 80-81	Thoracic aorta, ascending/arch and descending
2016, 4Q, 82-83	Coronary artery, number of arteries
2016, 4Q, 102-109	Correction of congenital heart defects
2015, 4Q, 23	Congenital heart corrective procedures

AHA Coding Clinic for table 02U

2022, 1Q, 37	Insertion of amplatzer occluder device into atrium
2022, 1Q, 38	Reconstruction of aorto-mitral curtain using bovine pericardium
2021, 3Q, 28	Repair mitral valve with Pascal® system
2020, 4Q, 52	Transapical mitral valve repair with device
2020, 1Q, 24	Pulmonary artery unifocalization
2019, 4Q, 25	Coronary artery to root operation Supplement
2018, 1Q, 12	Percutaneous balloon valvuloplasty & cardiac catheterization with ventriculogram
2017, 4Q, 36	Alfieri stitch procedure
2017, 3Q, 7	Senning procedure (arterial switch)
2017, 1Q, 19	Norwood Sano procedure
2016, 4Q, 80-81	Thoracic aorta, ascending/arch and descending
2016, 4Q, 101	Root operation Creation
2016, 4Q, 102-109	Correction of congenital heart defects
2016, 2Q, 23	Repair of tetralogy of Fallot with autologous pericardial patch graft
2016, 2Q, 26	Aortic valve replacement with aortic root enlargement
2015, 4Q, 22-24	Congenital heart corrective procedures
2015, 3Q, 16	Revision of previous truncus arteriosus surgery with ventricle to pulmonary artery conduit
2015, 2Q, 23	Annuloplasty ring
2014, 3Q, 16	Repair of tetralogy of Fallot

AHA Coding Clinic for table 02V

2022, 1Q, 40	Repair of common atrioventricular valve using Alfieri stitch
2021, 4Q, 44	Restriction of left ventricle
2020, 1Q, 25	Elephant trunk repair of aortic dissection
2017, 4Q, 35-36	Alfieri stitch procedure
2016, 4Q, 80-81	Thoracic aorta, ascending/arch and descending
2016, 4Q, 89-92	Branched and fenestrated endograft repair of aneurysms

AHA Coding Clinic for table 02W

2019, 1Q, 24	Replacement of left ventricular assist device with retention of outflow graft
2018, 3Q, 8	Coronary artery bypass graft surgery (revision versus total redo)
2018, 3Q, 9	Fibrin sheath stripping of malfunctioning port-a-cath
2018, 1Q, 17	Repositioning of Impella short-term external heart assist device
2017, 4Q, 42-45	Insertion of external heart assist devices
2017, 4Q, 55-56	Added approach values - Percutaneous heart valve procedures
2016, 4Q, 85	Coronary artery, number of stents
2016, 4Q, 95-96	Intracardiac pacemaker
2015, 3Q, 32	Approach values for repositioning and removal of cardiac lead
2014, 3Q, 31	Closure of paravalvular leak using Amplatzer® vascular plug

AHA Coding Clinic for table 02Y

2013, 3Q, 18	Heart transplant surgery

Coronary Arteries

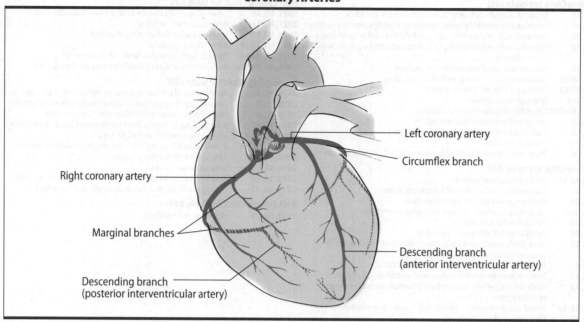

Left coronary artery

Circumflex branch

Right coronary artery

Marginal branches

Descending branch
(anterior interventricular artery)

Descending branch
(posterior interventricular artery)

Heart Anatomy

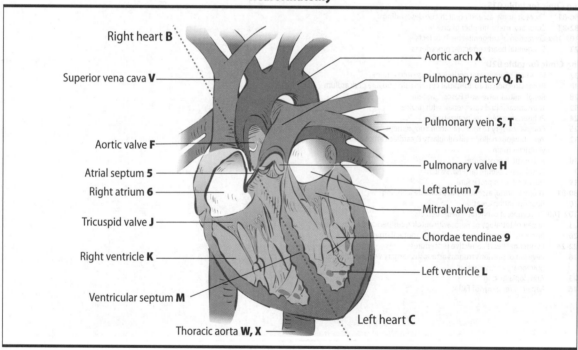

Right heart **B**

Superior vena cava **V**

Aortic valve **F**

Atrial septum **5**

Right atrium **6**

Tricuspid valve **J**

Right ventricle **K**

Ventricular septum **M**

Thoracic aorta **W, X**

Aortic arch **X**

Pulmonary artery **Q, R**

Pulmonary vein **S, T**

Pulmonary valve **H**

Left atrium **7**

Mitral valve **G**

Chordae tendinae **9**

Left ventricle **L**

Left heart **C**

Ø Medical and Surgical
2 Heart and Great Vessels
1 Bypass   Definition: Altering the route of passage of the contents of a tubular body part

Explanation: Rerouting contents of a body part to a downstream area of the normal route, to a similar route and body part, or to an abnormal route and dissimilar body part. Includes one or more anastomoses, with or without the use of a device.

Body Part Character 4	Approach Character 5	Device Character 6	Qualifier Character 7
Ø Coronary Artery, One Artery 1 Coronary Artery, Two Arteries 2 Coronary Artery, Three Arteries 3 Coronary Artery, Four or More Arteries	Ø Open	8 Zooplastic Tissue 9 Autologous Venous Tissue A Autologous Arterial Tissue J Synthetic Substitute K Nonautologous Tissue Substitute	3 Coronary Artery 8 Internal Mammary, Right 9 Internal Mammary, Left C Thoracic Artery F Abdominal Artery W Aorta
Ø Coronary Artery, One Artery 1 Coronary Artery, Two Arteries 2 Coronary Artery, Three Arteries 3 Coronary Artery, Four or More Arteries	Ø Open	Z No Device	3 Coronary Artery 8 Internal Mammary, Right 9 Internal Mammary, Left C Thoracic Artery F Abdominal Artery
Ø Coronary Artery, One Artery 1 Coronary Artery, Two Arteries 2 Coronary Artery, Three Arteries 3 Coronary Artery, Four or More Arteries	3 Percutaneous	4 Intraluminal Device, Drug-eluting D Intraluminal Device	4 Coronary Vein
Ø Coronary Artery, One Artery 1 Coronary Artery, Two Arteries 2 Coronary Artery, Three Arteries 3 Coronary Artery, Four or More Arteries	4 Percutaneous Endoscopic	4 Intraluminal Device, Drug-eluting D Intraluminal Device	4 Coronary Vein
Ø Coronary Artery, One Artery 1 Coronary Artery, Two Arteries 2 Coronary Artery, Three Arteries 3 Coronary Artery, Four or More Arteries	4 Percutaneous Endoscopic	8 Zooplastic Tissue 9 Autologous Venous Tissue A Autologous Arterial Tissue J Synthetic Substitute K Nonautologous Tissue Substitute	3 Coronary Artery 8 Internal Mammary, Right 9 Internal Mammary, Left C Thoracic Artery F Abdominal Artery W Aorta
Ø Coronary Artery, One Artery 1 Coronary Artery, Two Arteries 2 Coronary Artery, Three Arteries 3 Coronary Artery, Four or More Arteries	4 Percutaneous Endoscopic	Z No Device	3 Coronary Artery 8 Internal Mammary, Right 9 Internal Mammary, Left C Thoracic Artery F Abdominal Artery
6 Atrium, Right Atrium dextrum cordis Right auricular appendix Sinus venosus	Ø Open 4 Percutaneous Endoscopic	8 Zooplastic Tissue 9 Autologous Venous Tissue A Autologous Arterial Tissue J Synthetic Substitute K Nonautologous Tissue Substitute	P Pulmonary Trunk Q Pulmonary Artery, Right R Pulmonary Artery, Left
6 Atrium, Right Atrium dextrum cordis Right auricular appendix Sinus venosus	Ø Open 4 Percutaneous Endoscopic	Z No Device	7 Atrium, Left P Pulmonary Trunk Q Pulmonary Artery, Right R Pulmonary Artery, Left
6 Atrium, Right Atrium dextrum cordis Right auricular appendix Sinus venosus	3 Percutaneous	Z No Device	7 Atrium, Left
7 Atrium, Left Atrium pulmonale Left auricular appendix	Ø Open 4 Percutaneous Endoscopic	8 Zooplastic Tissue 9 Autologous Venous Tissue A Autologous Arterial Tissue J Synthetic Substitute K Nonautologous Tissue Substitute Z No Device	P Pulmonary Trunk Q Pulmonary Artery, Right R Pulmonary Artery, Left S Pulmonary Vein, Right T Pulmonary Vein, Left U Pulmonary Vein, Confluence
7 Atrium, Left Atrium pulmonale Left auricular appendix	3 Percutaneous	J Synthetic Substitute	6 Atrium, Right
K Ventricle, Right Conus arteriosus L Ventricle, Left	Ø Open 4 Percutaneous Endoscopic	8 Zooplastic Tissue 9 Autologous Venous Tissue A Autologous Arterial Tissue J Synthetic Substitute K Nonautologous Tissue Substitute	P Pulmonary Trunk Q Pulmonary Artery, Right R Pulmonary Artery, Left

HAC Ø21[Ø,1,2,3]Ø[8,9,A,J,K][3,8,9,C,F,W] when reported with SDx J98.51 or J98.59
HAC Ø21[Ø,1,2,3]ØZ[3,8,9,C,F] when reported with SDx J98.51 or J98.59
HAC Ø21[Ø,1,2,3]4[8,9,A,J,K][3,8,9,C,F,W] when reported with SDx J98.51 or J98.59
HAC Ø21[Ø,1,2,3]4Z[3,8,9,C,F] when reported with SDx J98.51 or J98.59

Ø21 Continued on next page

NC Noncovered Procedure LC Limited Coverage QA Questionable OB Admit NT New Tech Add-on ⊞ Combination Member ♂Male ♀Female

ICD-10-PCS 2023 175

Heart and Great Vessels

Ø21 Continued

Ø	Medical and Surgical
2	Heart and Great Vessels
1	Bypass

Definition: Altering the route of passage of the contents of a tubular body part

Explanation: Rerouting contents of a body part to a downstream area of the normal route, to a similar route and body part, or to an abnormal route and dissimilar body part. Includes one or more anastomoses, with or without the use of a device.

Body Part Character 4	Approach Character 5	Device Character 6	Qualifier Character 7
K Ventricle, Right Conus arteriosus L Ventricle, Left	Ø Open 4 Percutaneous Endoscopic	Z No Device	5 Coronary Circulation 8 Internal Mammary, Right 9 Internal Mammary, Left C Thoracic Artery F Abdominal Artery P Pulmonary Trunk Q Pulmonary Artery, Right R Pulmonary Artery, Left W Aorta

P Pulmonary Trunk
Q Pulmonary Artery, Right
R Pulmonary Artery, Left
  Arterial canal (duct)
  Botallo's duct
  Pulmoaortic canal
	Ø Open
	4 Percutaneous Endoscopic
		8 Zooplastic Tissue
		9 Autologous Venous Tissue
		A Autologous Arterial Tissue
		J Synthetic Substitute
		K Nonautologous Tissue Substitute
		Z No Device
			A Innominate Artery
			B Subclavian
			D Carotid

V Superior Vena Cava
  Cavoatrial junction
  Precava
	Ø Open
	4 Percutaneous Endoscopic
		8 Zooplastic Tissue
		9 Autologous Venous Tissue
		A Autologous Arterial Tissue
		J Synthetic Substitute
		K Nonautologous Tissue Substitute
		Z No Device
			P Pulmonary Trunk
			Q Pulmonary Artery, Right
			R Pulmonary Artery, Left
			S Pulmonary Vein, Right
			T Pulmonary Vein, Left
			U Pulmonary Vein, Confluence

W Thoracic Aorta, Descending	Ø Open	8 Zooplastic Tissue 9 Autologous Venous Tissue A Autologous Arterial Tissue J Synthetic Substitute K Nonautologous Tissue Substitute	A Innominate Artery B Subclavian D Carotid F Abdominal Artery G Axillary Artery H Brachial Artery P Pulmonary Trunk Q Pulmonary Artery, Right R Pulmonary Artery, Left V Lower Extremity Artery
W Thoracic Aorta, Descending	Ø Open	Z No Device	A Innominate Artery B Subclavian D Carotid P Pulmonary Trunk Q Pulmonary Artery, Right R Pulmonary Artery, Left
W Thoracic Aorta, Descending	4 Percutaneous Endoscopic	8 Zooplastic Tissue 9 Autologous Venous Tissue A Autologous Arterial Tissue J Synthetic Substitute K Nonautologous Tissue Substitute Z No Device	A Innominate Artery B Subclavian D Carotid P Pulmonary Trunk Q Pulmonary Artery, Right R Pulmonary Artery, Left

X Thoracic Aorta, Ascending/Arch
  Aortic arch
  Ascending aorta
	Ø Open
	4 Percutaneous Endoscopic
		8 Zooplastic Tissue
		9 Autologous Venous Tissue
		A Autologous Arterial Tissue
		J Synthetic Substitute
		K Nonautologous Tissue Substitute
		Z No Device
			A Innominate Artery
			B Subclavian
			D Carotid
			P Pulmonary Trunk
			Q Pulmonary Artery, Right
			R Pulmonary Artery, Left

Ø	Medical and Surgical
2	Heart and Great Vessels
4	Creation

Definition: Putting in or on biological or synthetic material to form a new body part that to the extent possible replicates the anatomic structure or function of an absent body part

Explanation: Used for gender reassignment surgery and corrective procedures in individuals with congenital anomalies

Body Part Character 4	Approach Character 5	Device Character 6	Qualifier Character 7
F Aortic Valve Aortic annulus	Ø Open	7 Autologous Tissue 8 Zooplastic Tissue J Synthetic Substitute K Nonautologous Tissue Substitute	J Truncal Valve

G Mitral Valve
  Bicuspid valve
  Left atrioventricular valve
  Mitral annulus
J Tricuspid Valve
  Right atrioventricular valve
  Tricuspid annulus
	Ø Open	7 Autologous Tissue
		8 Zooplastic Tissue
		J Synthetic Substitute
		K Nonautologous Tissue Substitute
			2 Common Atrioventricular Valve

Non-OR Procedure   DRG Non-OR Procedure   Valid OR Procedure   HAC Associated Procedure   Combination Only   New/Revised April   New/Revised October

176   ICD-10-PCS 2023

Ø   **Medical and Surgical**
2   **Heart and Great Vessels**
5   **Destruction**   Definition: Physical eradication of all or a portion of a body part by the direct use of energy, force, or a destructive agent
                        Explanation: None of the body part is physically taken out

Body Part Character 4	Approach Character 5	Device Character 6	Qualifier Character 7
4 Coronary Vein	Ø Open	Z No Device	Z No Qualifier
5 Atrial Septum Interatrial septum	3 Percutaneous 4 Percutaneous Endoscopic		

6 Atrium, Right
    Atrium dextrum cordis
    Right auricular appendix
    Sinus venosus			

8 Conduction Mechanism
    Atrioventricular node
    Bundle of His
    Bundle of Kent
    Sinoatrial node			

9 Chordae Tendineae			
D Papillary Muscle			
F Aortic Valve Aortic annulus			

G Mitral Valve
    Bicuspid valve
    Left atrioventricular valve
    Mitral annulus			

H Pulmonary Valve
    Pulmonary annulus
    Pulmonic valve			

J Tricuspid Valve
    Right atrioventricular valve
    Tricuspid annulus			

K Ventricle, Right Conus arteriosus			
L Ventricle, Left			
M Ventricular Septum Interventricular septum			
N Pericardium			
P Pulmonary Trunk			
Q Pulmonary Artery, Right			

R Pulmonary Artery, Left
    Arterial canal (duct)
    Botallo's duct
    Pulmoaortic canal			

S Pulmonary Vein, Right
    Right inferior pulmonary vein
    Right superior pulmonary vein			

T Pulmonary Vein, Left
    Left inferior pulmonary vein
    Left superior pulmonary vein			

V Superior Vena Cava
    Cavoatrial junction
    Precava			

W Thoracic Aorta, Descending			

X Thoracic Aorta, Ascending/Arch
    Aortic arch
    Ascending aorta			

7 Atrium, Left
    Atrium pulmonale
    Left auricular appendix
	Ø Open
	3 Percutaneous
	4 Percutaneous Endoscopic
		Z No Device	K Left Atrial Appendage
			Z No Qualifier

DRG Non-OR   Ø257[Ø,3,4]ZK

Ø   **Medical and Surgical**
2   **Heart and Great Vessels**
7   **Dilation**   Definition: Expanding an orifice or the lumen of a tubular body part

Explanation: The orifice can be a natural orifice or an artificially created orifice. Accomplished by stretching a tubular body part using intraluminal pressure or by cutting part of the orifice or wall of the tubular body part.

Body Part Character 4	Approach Character 5	Device Character 6	Qualifier Character 7
Ø Coronary Artery, One Artery **1** Coronary Artery, Two Arteries **2** Coronary Artery, Three Arteries **3** Coronary Artery, Four or More Arteries	**Ø** Open **3** Percutaneous **4** Percutaneous Endoscopic	**4** Intraluminal Device, Drug-eluting **5** Intraluminal Device, Drug-eluting, Two **6** Intraluminal Device, Drug-eluting, Three **7** Intraluminal Device, Drug-eluting, Four or More **D** Intraluminal Device **E** Intraluminal Device, Two **F** Intraluminal Device, Three **G** Intraluminal Device, Four or More **T** Intraluminal Device, Radioactive **Z** No Device	**6** Bifurcation **Z** No Qualifier

F Aortic Valve
  Aortic annulus
G Mitral Valve
  Bicuspid valve
  Left atrioventricular valve
  Mitral annulus
H Pulmonary Valve
  Pulmonary annulus
  Pulmonic valve
J Tricuspid Valve
  Right atrioventricular valve
  Tricuspid annulus
K Ventricle, Right
  Conus arteriosus
L Ventricle, Left
P Pulmonary Trunk
Q Pulmonary Artery, Right
S Pulmonary Vein, Right
  Right inferior pulmonary vein
  Right superior pulmonary vein
T Pulmonary Vein, Left
  Left inferior pulmonary vein
  Left superior pulmonary vein
V Superior Vena Cava
  Cavoatrial junction
  Precava
W Thoracic Aorta, Descending
X Thoracic Aorta, Ascending/Arch
  Aortic arch
  Ascending aorta
	Ø Open
	3 Percutaneous
	4 Percutaneous Endoscopic
		4 Intraluminal Device, Drug-eluting
		D Intraluminal Device
		Z No Device
			Z No Qualifier

R Pulmonary Artery, Left
  Arterial canal (duct)
  Botallo's duct
  Pulmoaortic canal
	Ø Open
	3 Percutaneous
	4 Percutaneous Endoscopic
		4 Intraluminal Device, Drug-eluting
		D Intraluminal Device
		Z No Device
			T Ductus Arteriosus
			Z No Qualifier

Ø   **Medical and Surgical**
2   **Heart and Great Vessels**
8   **Division**   Definition: Cutting into a body part, without draining fluids and/or gases from the body part, in order to separate or transect a body part

Explanation: All or a portion of the body part is separated into two or more portions

Body Part Character 4	Approach Character 5	Device Character 6	Qualifier Character 7

8 Conduction Mechanism
  Atrioventricular node
  Bundle of His
  Bundle of Kent
  Sinoatrial node
9 Chordae Tendineae
D Papillary Muscle
	Ø Open
	3 Percutaneous
	4 Percutaneous Endoscopic
		Z No Device	**Z** No Qualifier

Non-OR Procedure   DRG Non-OR Procedure   Valid OR Procedure   HAC Associated Procedure   Combination Only   New/Revised April   New/Revised October

178   ICD-10-PCS 2023

0   Medical and Surgical
2   Heart and Great Vessels
B   Excision   Definition: Cutting out or off, without replacement, a portion of a body part
                Explanation: The qualifier DIAGNOSTIC is used to identify excision procedures that are biopsies

Body Part Character 4	Approach Character 5	Device Character 6	Qualifier Character 7
4 **Coronary Vein**	Ø Open	Z No Device	X Diagnostic
5 **Atrial Septum**	3 Percutaneous		Z No Qualifier
Interatrial septum	4 Percutaneous Endoscopic		
6 **Atrium, Right**			
Atrium dextrum cordis			
Right auricular appendix			
Sinus venosus			
8 **Conduction Mechanism**			
Atrioventricular node			
Bundle of His			
Bundle of Kent			
Sinoatrial node			
9 **Chordae Tendineae**			
D **Papillary Muscle**			
F **Aortic Valve**			
Aortic annulus			
G **Mitral Valve**			
Bicuspid valve			
Left atrioventricular valve			
Mitral annulus			
H **Pulmonary Valve**			
Pulmonary annulus			
Pulmonic valve			
J **Tricuspid Valve**			
Right atrioventricular valve			
Tricuspid annulus			
K **Ventricle, Right** NC			
Conus arteriosus			
L **Ventricle, Left** NC			
M **Ventricular Septum**			
Interventricular septum			
N **Pericardium**			
P **Pulmonary Trunk**			
Q **Pulmonary Artery, Right**			
R **Pulmonary Artery, Left**			
Arterial canal (duct)			
Botallo's duct			
Pulmoaortic canal			
S **Pulmonary Vein, Right**			
Right inferior pulmonary vein			
Right superior pulmonary vein			
T **Pulmonary Vein, Left**			
Left inferior pulmonary vein			
Left superior pulmonary vein			
V **Superior Vena Cava**			
Cavoatrial junction			
Precava			
W **Thoracic Aorta, Descending**			
X **Thoracic Aorta, Ascending/Arch**			
Aortic arch			
Ascending aorta			
7 **Atrium, Left**	Ø Open	Z No Device	K Left Atrial Appendage
Atrium pulmonale	3 Percutaneous		X Diagnostic
Left auricular appendage	4 Percutaneous Endoscopic		Z No Qualifier

DRG Non-OR   02B7[Ø,3,4]ZK
Non-OR   02B[4,5,6,8,9,D,F,G,H,J,K,L,M][Ø,3,4]ZX
NC   02B[K,L][Ø,3,4]ZZ

Heart and Great Vessels

Ø   Medical and Surgical
2   Heart and Great Vessels
C   Extirpation   Definition: Taking or cutting out solid matter from a body part

Explanation: The solid matter may be an abnormal byproduct of a biological function or a foreign body; it may be imbedded in a body part or in the lumen of a tubular body part. The solid matter may or may not have been previously broken into pieces.

Body Part Character 4	Approach Character 5	Device Character 6	Qualifier Character 7
Ø **Coronary Artery, One Artery** **1** **Coronary Artery, Two Arteries** **2** **Coronary Artery, Three Arteries** **3** **Coronary Artery, Four or More Arteries**	**Ø** Open **4** Percutaneous Endoscopic	**Z** No Device	**6** Bifurcation **Z** No Qualifier
Ø **Coronary Artery, One Artery** **1** **Coronary Artery, Two Arteries** **2** **Coronary Artery, Three Arteries** **3** **Coronary Artery, Four or More Arteries**	**3** Percutaneous	**Z** No Device	**6** Bifurcation **7** Orbital Atherectomy Technique **Z** No Qualifier

4   **Coronary Vein**
5   **Atrial Septum**
     Interatrial septum
6   **Atrium, Right**
     Atrium dextrum cordis
     Right auricular appendix
     Sinus venosus
7   **Atrium, Left**
     Atrium pulmonale
     Left auricular appendix
8   **Conduction Mechanism**
     Atrioventricular node
     Bundle of His
     Bundle of Kent
     Sinoatrial node
9   **Chordae Tendineae**
D   **Papillary Muscle**
F   **Aortic Valve**
     Aortic annulus
G   **Mitral Valve**
     Bicuspid valve
     Left atrioventricular valve
     Mitral annulus
H   **Pulmonary Valve**
     Pulmonary annulus
     Pulmonic valve
J   **Tricuspid Valve**
     Right atrioventricular valve
     Tricuspid annulus
K   **Ventricle, Right**
     Conus arteriosus
L   **Ventricle, Left**
M   **Ventricular Septum**
     Interventricular septum
N   **Pericardium**
P   **Pulmonary Trunk**
Q   **Pulmonary Artery, Right**
R   **Pulmonary Artery, Left**
     Arterial canal (duct)
     Botallo's duct
     Pulmoaortic canal
S   **Pulmonary Vein, Right**
     Right inferior pulmonary vein
     Right superior pulmonary vein
T   **Pulmonary Vein, Left**
     Left inferior pulmonary vein
     Left superior pulmonary vein
V   **Superior Vena Cava**
     Cavoatrial junction
     Precava
W   **Thoracic Aorta, Descending**
X   **Thoracic Aorta, Ascending/Arch**
     Aortic arch
     Ascending aorta
	Ø Open
	3 Percutaneous
	4 Percutaneous Endoscopic
		Z No Device	**Z** No Qualifier

Non-OR Procedure   DRG Non-OR Procedure   Valid OR Procedure   HAC Associated Procedure   Combination Only   New/Revised April   New/Revised October

180   ICD-10-PCS 2023

Ø   **Medical and Surgical**
2   **Heart and Great Vessels**
F   **Fragmentation**   Definition: Breaking solid matter in a body part into pieces

                Explanation: Physical force (e.g., manual, ultrasonic) applied directly or indirectly is used to break the solid matter into pieces. The solid matter may be an abnormal byproduct of a biological function or a foreign body. The pieces of solid matter are not taken out.

Body Part Character 4	Approach Character 5	Device Character 6	Qualifier Character 7
Ø Coronary Artery, One Artery **1** Coronary Artery, Two Arteries **2** Coronary Artery, Three Arteries **3** Coronary Artery, Four or More Arteries	**3** Percutaneous	**Z** No Device **NT**	**Z** No Qualifier
N Pericardium **NC**	**Ø** Open **3** Percutaneous **4** Percutaneous Endoscopic **X** External	**Z** No Device	**Z** No Qualifier

P   Pulmonary Trunk
Q   Pulmonary Artery, Right
R   Pulmonary Artery, Left
     Arterial canal (duct)
     Botallo's duct
     Pulmoaortic canal
S   Pulmonary Vein, Right
     Right inferior pulmonary vein
     Right superior pulmonary vein
T   Pulmonary Vein, Left
     Left inferior pulmonary vein
     Left superior pulmonary vein
	3 Percutaneous	**Z** No Device	**Ø** Ultrasonic
			Z No Qualifier

Non-OR	Ø2FNXZZ
NC	Ø2FNXZZ
NT	Ø2F[Ø,1,2,3]3ZZ for Shockwave C2 Intravascular Lithotripsy (IVL) System

NC Noncovered Procedure   **LC** Limited Coverage   **QA** Questionable OB Admit   **NT** New Tech Add-on   ⊞ Combination Member   ♂ Male   ♀ Female

ICD-10-PCS 2023   **181**

Heart and Great Vessels *(left margin)*

Ø   Medical and Surgical
2   Heart and Great Vessels
H   Insertion   Definition: Putting in a nonbiological appliance that monitors, assists, performs, or prevents a physiological function but does not physically take the place of a body part
                             Explanation: None

Body Part Character 4	Approach Character 5	Device Character 6	Qualifier Character 7
Ø Coronary Artery, One Artery 1 Coronary Artery, Two Arteries 2 Coronary Artery, Three Arteries 3 Coronary Artery, Four or More Arteries	Ø Open 3 Percutaneous 4 Percutaneous Endoscopic	D Intraluminal Device Y Other Device	Z No Qualifier

4 Coronary Vein ⊞
6 Atrium, Right ⊞
  Atrium dextrum cordis
  Right auricular appendix
  Sinus venosus
7 Atrium, Left ⊞
  Atrium pulmonale
  Left auricular appendix
K Ventricle, Right ⊞
  Conus arteriosus
L Ventricle, Left ⊞
	Ø Open
	3 Percutaneous
	4 Percutaneous Endoscopic
		Ø Monitoring Device, Pressure Sensor
		2 Monitoring Device
		3 Infusion Device
		D Intraluminal Device
		J Cardiac Lead, Pacemaker
		K Cardiac Lead, Defibrillator
		M Cardiac Lead
		N Intracardiac Pacemaker
		Y Other Device
			Z No Qualifier

A Heart NC	Ø Open 3 Percutaneous 4 Percutaneous Endoscopic	Q Implantable Heart Assist System Y Other Device	Z No Qualifier
A Heart ⊞	Ø Open 3 Percutaneous 4 Percutaneous Endoscopic	R Short-term External Heart Assist System	J Intraoperative S Biventricular Z No Qualifier
N Pericardium ⊞	Ø Open 3 Percutaneous 4 Percutaneous Endoscopic	Ø Monitoring Device, Pressure Sensor 2 Monitoring Device J Cardiac Lead, Pacemaker K Cardiac Lead, Defibrillator M Cardiac Lead Y Other Device	Z No Qualifier

P Pulmonary Trunk
Q Pulmonary Artery, Right
R Pulmonary Artery, Left
  Arterial canal (duct)
  Botallo's duct
  Pulmoaortic canal
S Pulmonary Vein, Right
  Right inferior pulmonary vein
  Right superior pulmonary vein
T Pulmonary Vein, Left
  Left inferior pulmonary vein
  Left superior pulmonary vein
V Superior Vena Cava
  Cavoatrial junction
  Precava
W Thoracic Aorta, Descending
	Ø Open
	3 Percutaneous
	4 Percutaneous Endoscopic
		Ø Monitoring Device, Pressure Sensor
		2 Monitoring Device
		3 Infusion Device
		D Intraluminal Device
		Y Other Device
			Z No Qualifier

X Thoracic Aorta, Ascending/Arch
  Aortic arch
  Ascending aorta
	Ø Open
	3 Percutaneous
	4 Percutaneous Endoscopic
		Ø Monitoring Device, Pressure Sensor
		2 Monitoring Device
		3 Infusion Device
		D Intraluminal Device
			Z No Qualifier

DRG Non-OR Ø2H[4,6,7,K,L][Ø,3,4][J,M]Z	HAC Ø2H43[J,K,M]Z when reported with SDx K68.11 or T81.4Ø-T81.49, T82.7 with 7th character A
DRG Non-OR Ø2HK32Z	HAC Ø2H[6,K]33Z when reported with SDx J95.811
DRG Non-OR Ø2HN[Ø,3,4][J,M]Z	HAC Ø2H[6,7]3[J,M]Z when reported with SDx K68.11 or T81.4Ø-T81.49, T82.7 with 7th character A
Non-OR Ø2H[4,6,7,L]3[2,3]Z	
Non-OR Ø2H[6,7]3MZ	HAC Ø2H[K,L]3JZ when reported with SDx K68.11 or T81.4Ø-T81.49, T82.7 with 7th character A
Non-OR Ø2HK3[Ø,3]Z	
Non-OR Ø2HN32Z	HAC Ø2HN[Ø,3,4][J,M]Z when reported with SDx K68.11 or T81.4Ø-T81.49, T82.7 with 7th character A
Non-OR Ø2HP[Ø,3,4][Ø,2,3]Z	
Non-OR Ø2H[Q,R][Ø,3,4][2,3]Z	HAC Ø2H[S,T,V][3,4]3Z when reported with SDx J95.811
Non-OR Ø2H[S,T,V,W][Ø,3,4]3Z	NC Ø2HA[3,4]QZ
Non-OR Ø2H[S,T,V,W]32Z	
Non-OR Ø2HW[Ø,3]ØZ	**See Appendix L for Procedure Combinations**
Non-OR Ø2HX[Ø,3,4][Ø,3]Z	⊞ Ø2H[4,6,7,K,L][Ø,3,4][J,K,M]Z
	⊞ Ø2HA[Ø,4]R[S,Z]
	⊞ Ø2HA3RS
	⊞ Ø2HN[Ø,3,4][J,K,M]Z

Ø　**Medical and Surgical**
2　**Heart and Great Vessels**
J　**Inspection**　　Definition: Visually and/or manually exploring a body part

Explanation: Visual exploration may be performed with or without optical instrumentation. Manual exploration may be performed directly or through intervening body layers.

Body Part Character 4	Approach Character 5	Device Character 6	Qualifier Character 7
A　Heart Y　Great Vessel	Ø　Open 3　Percutaneous 4　Percutaneous Endoscopic	Z　No Device	Z　No Qualifier

Non-OR　Ø2J[A,Y]3ZZ

Ø　**Medical and Surgical**
2　**Heart and Great Vessels**
K　**Map**　　Definition: Locating the route of passage of electrical impulses and/or locating functional areas in a body part

Explanation: Applicable only to the cardiac conduction mechanism and the central nervous system

Body Part Character 4	Approach Character 5	Device Character 6	Qualifier Character 7
8　Conduction Mechanism 　　Atrioventricular node 　　Bundle of His 　　Bundle of Kent 　　Sinoatrial node	Ø　Open 3　Percutaneous 4　Percutaneous Endoscopic	Z　No Device	Z　No Qualifier

DRG Non-OR　Ø2K8[Ø,3,4]ZZ

Ø　**Medical and Surgical**
2　**Heart and Great Vessels**
L　**Occlusion**　　Definition: Completely closing an orifice or the lumen of a tubular body part

Explanation: The orifice can be a natural orifice or an artificially created orifice

Body Part Character 4	Approach Character 5	Device Character 6	Qualifier Character 7
7　Atrium, Left 　　Atrium pulmonale 　　Left auricular appendix	Ø　Open 3　Percutaneous 4　Percutaneous Endoscopic	C　Extraluminal Device D　Intraluminal Device Z　No Device	K　Left Atrial Appendage
H　Pulmonary Valve 　　Pulmonary annulus 　　Pulmonic valve P　Pulmonary Trunk Q　Pulmonary Artery, Right S　Pulmonary Vein, Right 　　Right inferior pulmonary vein 　　Right superior pulmonary vein T　Pulmonary Vein, Left 　　Left inferior pulmonary vein 　　Left superior pulmonary vein V　Superior Vena Cava 　　Cavoatrial junction 　　Precava	Ø　Open 3　Percutaneous 4　Percutaneous Endoscopic	C　Extraluminal Device D　Intraluminal Device Z　No Device	Z　No Qualifier
R　Pulmonary Artery, Left 　　Arterial canal (duct) 　　Botallo's duct 　　Pulmoaortic canal	Ø　Open 3　Percutaneous 4　Percutaneous Endoscopic	C　Extraluminal Device D　Intraluminal Device Z　No Device	T　Ductus Arteriosus Z　No Qualifier
W　Thoracic Aorta, Descending	3　Percutaneous	D　Intraluminal Device	J　Temporary

DRG Non-OR　Ø2L7[Ø,3,4][C,D,Z]K

NC Noncovered Procedure　　LC Limited Coverage　　QA Questionable OB Admit　　NT New Tech Add-on　　⊞ Combination Member　　♂Male　　♀Female

ICD-10-PCS 2023　　　183

02J–02L

Heart and Great Vessels

Ø **Medical and Surgical**
2 **Heart and Great Vessels**
N **Release**   Definition: Freeing a body part from an abnormal physical constraint by cutting or by the use of force
                Explanation: Some of the restraining tissue may be taken out but none of the body part is taken out

Body Part Character 4	Approach Character 5	Device Character 6	Qualifier Character 7

Ø Coronary Artery, One Artery
1 Coronary Artery, Two Arteries
2 Coronary Artery, Three Arteries
3 Coronary Artery, Four or More Arteries
4 Coronary Vein
5 Atrial Septum
   Interatrial septum
6 Atrium, Right
   Atrium dextrum cordis
   Right auricular appendix
   Sinus venosus
7 Atrium, Left
   Atrium pulmonale
   Left auricular appendix
8 Conduction Mechanism
   Atrioventricular node
   Bundle of His
   Bundle of Kent
   Sinoatrial node
9 Chordae Tendineae
D Papillary Muscle
F Aortic Valve
   Aortic annulus
G Mitral Valve
   Bicuspid valve
   Left atrioventricular valve
   Mitral annulus
H Pulmonary Valve
   Pulmonary annulus
   Pulmonic valve
J Tricuspid Valve
   Right atrioventricular valve
   Tricuspid annulus
K Ventricle, Right
   Conus arteriosus
L Ventricle, Left
M Ventricular Septum
   Interventricular septum
N Pericardium
P Pulmonary Trunk
Q Pulmonary Artery, Right
R Pulmonary Artery, Left
   Arterial canal (duct)
   Botallo's duct
   Pulmoaortic canal
S Pulmonary Vein, Right
   Right inferior pulmonary vein
   Right superior pulmonary vein
T Pulmonary Vein, Left
   Left inferior pulmonary vein
   Left superior pulmonary vein
V Superior Vena Cava
   Cavoatrial junction
   Precava
W Thoracic Aorta, Descending
X Thoracic Aorta, Ascending/Arch
   Aortic arch
   Ascending aorta
	Ø Open
	3 Percutaneous
	4 Percutaneous Endoscopic
		Z No Device	**Z** No Qualifier

Non-OR Procedure   DRG Non-OR Procedure   Valid OR Procedure   HAC Associated Procedure   Combination Only   New/Revised April   New/Revised October

184   ICD-10-PCS 2023

Ø Medical and Surgical
2 Heart and Great Vessels
P Removal   Definition: Taking out or off a device from a body part

Explanation: If a device is taken out and a similar device put in without cutting or puncturing the skin or mucous membrane, the procedure is coded to the root operation CHANGE. Otherwise, the procedure for taking out a device is coded to the root operation REMOVAL.

Body Part Character 4	Approach Character 5	Device Character 6	Qualifier Character 7
A Heart	Ø Open 3 Percutaneous 4 Percutaneous Endoscopic	2 Monitoring Device 3 Infusion Device 7 Autologous Tissue Substitute 8 Zooplastic Tissue C Extraluminal Device D Intraluminal Device J Synthetic Substitute K Nonautologous Tissue Substitute M Cardiac Lead N Intracardiac Pacemaker Q Implantable Heart Assist System Y Other Device	Z No Qualifier
A Heart ⊞	Ø Open 3 Percutaneous 4 Percutaneous Endoscopic	R Short-term External Heart Assist System	S Biventricular Z No Qualifier
A Heart	X External	2 Monitoring Device 3 Infusion Device D Intraluminal Device M Cardiac Lead	Z No Qualifier
Y Great Vessel	Ø Open 3 Percutaneous 4 Percutaneous Endoscopic	2 Monitoring Device 3 Infusion Device 7 Autologous Tissue Substitute 8 Zooplastic Tissue C Extraluminal Device D Intraluminal Device J Synthetic Substitute K Nonautologous Tissue Substitute Y Other Device	Z No Qualifier
Y Great Vessel	X External	2 Monitoring Device 3 Infusion Device D Intraluminal Device	Z No Qualifier

Non-OR 02PA3[2,3,D]Z	**See Appendix L for Procedure Combinations**
Non-OR 02PA[3,4]YZ	⊞ 02PA[Ø,3,4]RZ
Non-OR 02PAX[2,3,D,M]Z	
Non-OR 02PY3[2,3,D]Z	
Non-OR 02PY[3,4]YZ	
Non-OR 02PYX[2,3,D]Z	
HAC 02PA[Ø,3,4]MZ when reported with SDx K68.11 or T81.40-T81.49, T82.7 with 7th character A	
HAC 02PAXMZ when reported with SDx K68.11 or T81.40-T81.49, T82.7 with 7th character A	

Heart and Great Vessels

Ø **Medical and Surgical**
2 **Heart and Great Vessels**
Q **Repair**   Definition: Restoring, to the extent possible, a body part to its normal anatomic structure and function
                    Explanation: Used only when the method to accomplish the repair is not one of the other root operations

Body Part Character 4	Approach Character 5	Device Character 6	Qualifier Character 7

Ø Coronary Artery, One Artery
1 Coronary Artery, Two Arteries
2 Coronary Artery, Three Arteries
3 Coronary Artery, Four or More
    Arteries
4 Coronary Vein
5 Atrial Septum
    Interatrial septum
6 Atrium, Right
    Atrium dextrum cordis
    Right auricular appendix
    Sinus venosus
7 Atrium, Left
    Atrium pulmonale
    Left auricular appendix
8 Conduction Mechanism
    Atrioventricular node
    Bundle of His
    Bundle of Kent
    Sinoatrial node
9 Chordae Tendineae
A Heart
B Heart, Right
    Right coronary sulcus
C Heart, Left
    Left coronary sulcus
    Obtuse margin
D Papillary Muscle
H Pulmonary Valve
    Pulmonary annulus
    Pulmonic valve
K Ventricle, Right
    Conus arteriosus
L Ventricle, Left
M Ventricular Septum
    Interventricular septum
N Pericardium
P Pulmonary Trunk
Q Pulmonary Artery, Right
R Pulmonary Artery, Left
    Arterial canal (duct)
    Botallo's duct
    Pulmoaortic canal
S Pulmonary Vein, Right
    Right inferior pulmonary vein
    Right superior pulmonary vein
T Pulmonary Vein, Left
    Left inferior pulmonary vein
    Left superior pulmonary vein
V Superior Vena Cava
    Cavoatrial junction
    Precava
W Thoracic Aorta, Descending
X Thoracic Aorta, Ascending/Arch
    Aortic arch
    Ascending aorta
	Ø Open
	3 Percutaneous
	4 Percutaneous Endoscopic
		Z No Device	Z No Qualifier

F Aortic Valve Aortic annulus	Ø Open 3 Percutaneous 4 Percutaneous Endoscopic	Z No Device	J Truncal Valve Z No Qualifier

G Mitral Valve
    Bicuspid valve
    Left atrioventricular valve
    Mitral annulus
	Ø Open
	3 Percutaneous
	4 Percutaneous Endoscopic
		Z No Device	E Atrioventricular Valve, Left
			Z No Qualifier

J Tricuspid Valve
    Right atrioventricular valve
    Tricuspid annulus
	Ø Open
	3 Percutaneous
	4 Percutaneous Endoscopic
		Z No Device	G Atrioventricular Valve, Right
			Z No Qualifier

Non-OR Procedure   DRG Non-OR Procedure   Valid OR Procedure   HAC Associated Procedure   Combination Only   New/Revised April   New/Revised October

186   ICD-10-PCS 2023

02Q–02Q

0 Medical and Surgical
2 Heart and Great Vessels
R Replacement   Definition: Putting in or on biological or synthetic material that physically takes the place and/or function of all or a portion of a body part
         Explanation: The body part may have been taken out or replaced, or may be taken out, physically eradicated, or rendered nonfunctional during the REPLACEMENT procedure. A REMOVAL procedure is coded for taking out the device used in a previous replacement procedure.

Body Part Character 4	Approach Character 5	Device Character 6	Qualifier Character 7

5 Atrial Septum
   Interatrial septum
6 Atrium, Right
   Atrium dextrum cordis
   Right auricular appendix
   Sinus venosus
7 Atrium, Left
   Atrium pulmonale
   Left auricular appendix
9 Chordae Tendineae
D Papillary Muscle
K Ventricle, Right ⊞
   Conus arteriosus
L Ventricle, Left ⊞
M Ventricular Septum
   Interventricular septum
N Pericardium
P Pulmonary Trunk
Q Pulmonary Artery, Right
R Pulmonary Artery, Left
   Arterial canal (duct)
   Botallo's duct
   Pulmoaortic canal
S Pulmonary Vein, Right
   Right inferior pulmonary vein
   Right superior pulmonary vein
T Pulmonary Vein, Left
   Left inferior pulmonary vein
   Left superior pulmonary vein
V Superior Vena Cava
   Cavoatrial junction
   Precava
W Thoracic Aorta, Descending
X Thoracic Aorta, Ascending/Arch
   Aortic arch
   Ascending aorta
	0 Open
	4 Percutaneous Endoscopic
		7 Autologous Tissue Substitute
		8 Zooplastic Tissue
		J Synthetic Substitute
		K Nonautologous Tissue Substitute
			Z No Qualifier

A Heart	**0 Open**	**L Biologic with Synthetic Substitute, Autoregulated Electrohydraulic** **M Synthetic Substitute, Pneumatic**	**Z No Qualifier**
F Aortic Valve Aortic annulus	**0 Open** **4 Percutaneous Endoscopic**	**7 Autologous Tissue Substitute** **J Synthetic Substitute** **K Nonautologous Tissue Substitute**	**Z No Qualifier**
F Aortic Valve Aortic annulus	**0 Open** **4 Percutaneous Endoscopic**	**8 Zooplastic Tissue**	**N Rapid Deployment Technique** **Z No Qualifier**
F Aortic Valve Aortic annulus	**3 Percutaneous**	**7 Autologous Tissue Substitute** **J Synthetic Substitute** **K Nonautologous Tissue Substitute**	**H Transapical** **Z No Qualifier**
F Aortic Valve Aortic annulus	**3 Percutaneous**	**8 Zooplastic Tissue**	**H Transapical** **N Rapid Deployment Technique** **Z No Qualifier**

G Mitral Valve
   Bicuspid valve
   Left atrioventricular valve
   Mitral annulus
J Tricuspid Valve
   Right atrioventricular valve
   Tricuspid annulus
	0 Open
	4 Percutaneous Endoscopic
		7 Autologous Tissue Substitute
		8 Zooplastic Tissue
		J Synthetic Substitute
		K Nonautologous Tissue Substitute
			Z No Qualifier

G Mitral Valve
   Bicuspid valve
   Left atrioventricular valve
   Mitral annulus
J Tricuspid Valve
   Right atrioventricular valve
   Tricuspid annulus
	3 Percutaneous	**7 Autologous Tissue Substitute**
		8 Zooplastic Tissue
		J Synthetic Substitute
		K Nonautologous Tissue Substitute
			H Transapical
			Z No Qualifier

H Pulmonary Valve
   Pulmonary annulus
   Pulmonic valve
	0 Open
	4 Percutaneous Endoscopic
		7 Autologous Tissue Substitute
		8 Zooplastic Tissue
		J Synthetic Substitute
		K Nonautologous Tissue Substitute
			Z No Qualifier

H Pulmonary Valve
   Pulmonary annulus
   Pulmonic valve
	3 Percutaneous	**7 Autologous Tissue Substitute**
		J Synthetic Substitute
		K Nonautologous Tissue Substitute
			H Transapical
			Z No Qualifier

H Pulmonary Valve
   Pulmonary annulus
   Pulmonic valve
	3 Percutaneous	**8 Zooplastic Tissue** ⓃⓉ	**H Transapical**
			L In Existing Conduit
			M Native Site
			Z No Qualifier

ⓃⓉ   02RH38M for Harmony™ Transcatheter Pulmonary Valve (TPV) System   **See Appendix L for Procedure Combinations**
                                                 ⊞   02R[K,L]0JZ

ⓃⒸ Noncovered Procedure   ⓁⒸ Limited Coverage   ⓊⒶ Questionable OB Admit   ⓃⓉ New Tech Add-on   ⊞ Combination Member   ♂ Male   ♀ Female

ICD-10-PCS 2023   **187**

Heart and Great Vessels (side tab, left margin)

Ø **Medical and Surgical**
2 **Heart and Great Vessels**
S **Reposition**   Definition: Moving to its normal location, or other suitable location, all or a portion of a body part

Explanation: The body part is moved to a new location from an abnormal location, or from a normal location where it is not functioning correctly. The body part may or may not be cut out or off to be moved to the new location.

Body Part Character 4	Approach Character 5	Device Character 6	Qualifier Character 7
Ø **Coronary Artery, One Artery**	Ø **Open**	Z **No Device**	Z **No Qualifier**
1 **Coronary Artery, Two Arteries**			
P **Pulmonary Trunk**			
Q **Pulmonary Artery, Right**			
R **Pulmonary Artery, Left**			
Arterial canal (duct)			
Botallo's duct			
Pulmoaortic canal			
S **Pulmonary Vein, Right**			
Right inferior pulmonary vein			
Right superior pulmonary vein			
T **Pulmonary Vein, Left**			
Left inferior pulmonary vein			
Left superior pulmonary vein			
V **Superior Vena Cava**			
Cavoatrial junction			
Precava			
W **Thoracic Aorta, Descending**			
X **Thoracic Aorta, Ascending/Arch**			
Aortic arch			
Ascending aorta			

Ø **Medical and Surgical**
2 **Heart and Great Vessels**
T **Resection**   Definition: Cutting out or off, without replacement, all of a body part

Explanation: None

Body Part Character 4	Approach Character 5	Device Character 6	Qualifier Character 7
5 **Atrial Septum**	Ø **Open**	Z **No Device**	Z **No Qualifier**
Interatrial septum	3 **Percutaneous**		
8 **Conduction Mechanism**	4 **Percutaneous Endoscopic**		
Atrioventricular node			
Bundle of His			
Bundle of Kent			
Sinoatrial node			
9 **Chordae Tendineae**			
D **Papillary Muscle**			
H **Pulmonary Valve**			
Pulmonary annulus			
Pulmonic valve			
M **Ventricular Septum**			
Interventricular septum			
N **Pericardium**			

Non-OR Procedure   DRG Non-OR Procedure   Valid OR Procedure   HAC Associated Procedure   Combination Only   New/Revised April   New/Revised October

188

ICD-10-PCS 2023

02S–02T

Ø **Medical and Surgical**
2 **Heart and Great Vessels**
U **Supplement**   Definition: Putting in or on biological or synthetic material that physically reinforces and/or augments the function of a portion of a body part

       Explanation: The biological material is non-living, or is living and from the same individual. The body part may have been previously replaced, and the SUPPLEMENT procedure is performed to physically reinforce and/or augment the function of the replaced body part.

Body Part Character 4	Approach Character 5	Device Character 6	Qualifier Character 7

Ø Coronary Artery, One Artery
1 Coronary Artery, Two Arteries
2 Coronary Artery, Three Arteries
3 Coronary Artery, Four or More
   Arteries
5 Atrial Septum
   Interatrial septum
6 Atrium, Right
   Atrium dextrum cordis
   Right auricular appendix
   Sinus venosus
7 Atrium, Left
   Atrium pulmonale
   Left auricular appendix
9 Chordae Tendineae
A Heart
D Papillary Muscle
H Pulmonary Valve
   Pulmonary annulus
   Pulmonic valve
K Ventricle, Right
   Conus arteriosus
L Ventricle, Left
M Ventricular Septum
   Interventricular septum
N Pericardium
P Pulmonary Trunk
Q Pulmonary Artery, Right
R Pulmonary Artery, Left
   Arterial canal (duct)
   Botallo's duct
   Pulmoaortic canal
S Pulmonary Vein, Right
   Right inferior pulmonary vein
   Right superior pulmonary vein
T Pulmonary Vein, Left
   Left inferior pulmonary vein
   Left superior pulmonary vein
V Superior Vena Cava
   Cavoatrial junction
   Precava
W Thoracic Aorta, Descending
X Thoracic Aorta, Ascending/Arch
   Aortic arch
   Ascending aorta
	Ø Open
	3 Percutaneous
	4 Percutaneous Endoscopic
		7 Autologous Tissue Substitute
		8 Zooplastic Tissue
		J Synthetic Substitute
		K Nonautologous Tissue Substitute
			Z No Qualifier

F Aortic Valve Aortic annulus	Ø Open 3 Percutaneous 4 Percutaneous Endoscopic	7 Autologous Tissue Substitute 8 Zooplastic Tissue J Synthetic Substitute K Nonautologous Tissue Substitute	J Truncal Valve Z No Qualifier

G Mitral Valve
   Bicuspid valve
   Left atrioventricular valve
   Mitral annulus
	Ø Open
	4 Percutaneous Endoscopic
		7 Autologous Tissue Substitute
		8 Zooplastic Tissue
		J Synthetic Substitute
		K Nonautologous Tissue Substitute
			E Atrioventricular Valve, Left
			Z No Qualifier

G Mitral Valve
   Bicuspid valve
   Left atrioventricular valve
   Mitral annulus
	3 Percutaneous	7 Autologous Tissue Substitute
		8 Zooplastic Tissue
		K Nonautologous Tissue Substitute
			E Atrioventricular Valve, Left
			Z No Qualifier

G Mitral Valve
   Bicuspid valve
   Left atrioventricular valve
   Mitral annulus
	3 Percutaneous	J Synthetic Substitute	E Atrioventricular Valve, Left
			H Transapical
			Z No Qualifier

J Tricuspid Valve
   Right atrioventricular valve
   Tricuspid annulus
	Ø Open
	3 Percutaneous
	4 Percutaneous Endoscopic
		7 Autologous Tissue Substitute
		8 Zooplastic Tissue
		J Synthetic Substitute
		K Nonautologous Tissue Substitute
			G Atrioventricular Valve, Right
			Z No Qualifier

DRG Non-OR   Ø2U7[3,4]JZ

NC Noncovered Procedure   **LC** Limited Coverage   **QA** Questionable OB Admit   **NT** New Tech Add-on   ⊞ Combination Member   ♂ Male   ♀ Female

ICD-10-PCS 2023   189

Ø2U–Ø2U

Heart and Great Vessels

Ø   **Medical and Surgical**
2   **Heart and Great Vessels**
V   **Restriction**   Definition: Partially closing an orifice or the lumen of a tubular body part
                        Explanation: The orifice can be a natural orifice or an artificially created orifice

Body Part Character 4	Approach Character 5	Device Character 6	Qualifier Character 7
A Heart	**Ø** Open **3** Percutaneous **4** Percutaneous Endoscopic	**C** Extraluminal Device **Z** No Device	**Z** No Qualifier
G Mitral Valve Bicuspid valve Left atrioventricular valve Mitral annulus	**Ø** Open **3** Percutaneous **4** Percutaneous Endoscopic	**Z** No Device	**Z** No Qualifier
L Ventricle, Left **P Pulmonary Trunk** **Q Pulmonary Artery, Right** **S Pulmonary Vein, Right** Right inferior pulmonary vein Right superior pulmonary vein **T Pulmonary Vein, Left** Left inferior pulmonary vein Left superior pulmonary vein **V Superior Vena Cava** Cavoatrial junction Precava	**Ø** Open **3** Percutaneous **4** Percutaneous Endoscopic	**C** Extraluminal Device **D** Intraluminal Device **Z** No Device	**Z** No Qualifier
R Pulmonary Artery, Left Arterial canal (duct) Botallo's duct Pulmoaortic canal	**Ø** Open **3** Percutaneous **4** Percutaneous Endoscopic	**C** Extraluminal Device **D** Intraluminal Device **Z** No Device	**T** Ductus Arteriosus **Z** No Qualifier

W Thoracic Aorta, Descending
X Thoracic Aorta, Ascending/Arch
Aortic arch
Ascending aorta
	Ø Open
	3 Percutaneous
	4 Percutaneous Endoscopic
		C Extraluminal Device
		D Intraluminal Device
		E Intraluminal Device, Branched or
		    Fenestrated, One or Two Arteries
		F Intraluminal Device, Branched or
		    Fenestrated, Three or More Arteries
		Z No Device
			Z No Qualifier

Non-OR Procedure   DRG Non-OR Procedure   Valid OR Procedure   HAC Associated Procedure   Combination Only   New/Revised April   New/Revised October

190   ICD-10-PCS 2023

0 Medical and Surgical
2 Heart and Great Vessels
W Revision   Definition: Correcting, to the extent possible, a portion of a malfunctioning device or the position of a displaced device

Explanation: Revision can include correcting a malfunctioning or displaced device by taking out or putting in components of the device such as a screw or pin

Body Part Character 4	Approach Character 5	Device Character 6	Qualifier Character 7
5 Atrial Septum Interatrial septum **M Ventricular Septum** Interventricular septum	**0 Open** **4 Percutaneous Endoscopic**	**J Synthetic Substitute**	**Z No Qualifier**
A Heart LC ⊞	**0 Open** **3 Percutaneous** **4 Percutaneous Endoscopic**	**2 Monitoring Device** **3 Infusion Device** **7 Autologous Tissue Substitute** **8 Zooplastic Tissue** **C Extraluminal Device** **D Intraluminal Device** **J Synthetic Substitute** **K Nonautologous Tissue Substitute** **M Cardiac Lead** **N Intracardiac Pacemaker** **Q Implantable Heart Assist System** **Y Other Device**	**Z No Qualifier**
A Heart ⊞	**0 Open** **3 Percutaneous** **4 Percutaneous Endoscopic**	**R Short-term External Heart Assist System**	**S Biventricular** **Z No Qualifier**
A Heart	**X External**	**2 Monitoring Device** **3 Infusion Device** **7 Autologous Tissue Substitute** **8 Zooplastic Tissue** **C Extraluminal Device** **D Intraluminal Device** **J Synthetic Substitute** **K Nonautologous Tissue Substitute** **M Cardiac Lead** **N Intracardiac Pacemaker** **Q Implantable Heart Assist System**	**Z No Qualifier**
A Heart	**X External**	**R Short-term External Heart Assist System**	**S Biventricular** **Z No Qualifier**
F Aortic Valve Aortic annulus **G Mitral Valve** Bicuspid valve Left atrioventricular valve Mitral annulus **H Pulmonary Valve** Pulmonary annulus Pulmonic valve **J Tricuspid Valve** Right atrioventricular valve Tricuspid annulus	**0 Open** **3 Percutaneous** **4 Percutaneous Endoscopic**	**7 Autologous Tissue Substitute** **8 Zooplastic Tissue** **J Synthetic Substitute** **K Nonautologous Tissue Substitute**	**Z No Qualifier**
Y Great Vessel	**0 Open** **3 Percutaneous** **4 Percutaneous Endoscopic**	**2 Monitoring Device** **3 Infusion Device** **7 Autologous Tissue Substitute** **8 Zooplastic Tissue** **C Extraluminal Device** **D Intraluminal Device** **J Synthetic Substitute** **K Nonautologous Tissue Substitute** **Y Other Device**	**Z No Qualifier**
Y Great Vessel	**X External**	**2 Monitoring Device** **3 Infusion Device** **7 Autologous Tissue Substitute** **8 Zooplastic Tissue** **C Extraluminal Device** **D Intraluminal Device** **J Synthetic Substitute** **K Nonautologous Tissue Substitute**	**Z No Qualifier**

Non-OR 02WA3[2,3,D]Z	**HAC**	02WA[0,3,4]MZ when reported with T81.40–T81.49, T82.7 with 7th character A
Non-OR 02WA[3,4]YZ	**LC**	02WA[3,4]QZ
Non-OR 02WAX[2,3,7,8,C,D,J,K,M,N,Q]Z		
Non-OR 02WAXRZ	**See Appendix L for Procedure Combinations**	
Non-OR 02WY3[2,3]Z	⊞	02WA[0,3,4]QZ
Non-OR 02WY[3,4]YZ	⊞	02WA[0,3,4]RZ
Non-OR 02WYX[2,3,7,8,C,D,J,K]Z		

NC Noncovered Procedure   LC Limited Coverage   QA Questionable OB Admit   NT New Tech Add-on   ⊞ Combination Member   ♂ Male   ♀ Female

ICD-10-PCS 2023   191

02W–02W

Ø Medical and Surgical
2 Heart and Great Vessels
Y Transplantation Definition: Putting in or on all or a portion of a living body part taken from another individual or animal to physically take the place and/or function of all or a portion of a similar body part

Explanation: The native body part may or may not be taken out, and the transplanted body part may take over all or a portion of its function

Body Part Character 4	Approach Character 5	Device Character 6	Qualifier Character 7
A Heart LC	Ø Open	Z No Device	Ø Allogeneic 1 Syngeneic 2 Zooplastic

LC   Ø2YAØZ[Ø,1,2]

Non-OR Procedure   DRG Non-OR Procedure   Valid OR Procedure   HAC Associated Procedure   Combination Only   New/Revised April   New/Revised October

192   ICD-10-PCS 2023

Upper Arteries Ø31–Ø3W

Character Meanings

This Character Meaning table is provided as a guide to assist the user in the identification of character members that may be found in this section of code tables. It **SHOULD NOT** be used to build a PCS code.

Operation–Character 3	Body Part–Character 4	Approach–Character 5	Device–Character 6	Qualifier–Character 7
1 Bypass	Ø Internal Mammary Artery, Right	Ø Open	Ø Drainage Device	Ø Upper Arm Artery, Right OR Ultrasonic
5 Destruction	1 Internal Mammary Artery, Left	3 Percutaneous	2 Monitoring Device	1 Upper Arm Artery, Left OR Drug-Coated Balloon
7 Dilation	2 Innominate Artery	4 Percutaneous Endoscopic	3 Infusion Device	2 Upper Arm Artery, Bilateral
9 Drainage	3 Subclavian Artery, Right	X External	4 Intraluminal Device, Drug-eluting	3 Lower Arm Artery, Right
B Excision	4 Subclavian Artery, Left		5 Intraluminal Device, Drug-eluting, Two	4 Lower Arm Artery, Left
C Extirpation	5 Axillary Artery, Right		6 Intraluminal Device, Drug-eluting, Three	5 Lower Arm Artery, Bilateral
F Fragmentation	6 Axillary Artery, Left		7 Intraluminal Device, Drug-eluting, Four or More OR Autologous Tissue Substitute	6 Upper Leg Artery, Right
H Insertion	7 Brachial Artery, Right		9 Autologous Venous Tissue	7 Upper Leg Artery, Left OR Stent Retriever
J Inspection	8 Brachial Artery, Left		A Autologous Arterial Tissue	8 Upper Leg Artery, Bilateral
L Occlusion	9 Ulnar Artery, Right		B Intraluminal Device, Bioactive	9 Lower Leg Artery, Right
N Release	A Ulnar Artery, Left		C Extraluminal Device	B Lower Leg Artery, Left
P Removal	B Radial Artery, Right		D Intraluminal Device	C Lower Leg Artery, Bilateral
Q Repair	C Radial Artery, Left		E Intraluminal Device, Two	D Upper Arm Vein
R Replacement	D Hand Artery, Right		F Intraluminal Device, Three	F Lower Arm Vein
S Reposition	F Hand Artery, Left		G Intraluminal Device, Four or More	G Intracranial Artery
U Supplement	G Intracranial Artery		H Intraluminal Device, Flow Diverter	J Extracranial Artery, Right
V Restriction	H Common Carotid Artery, Right		J Synthetic Substitute	K Extracranial Artery, Left
W Revision	J Common Carotid Artery, Left		K Nonautologous Tissue Substitute	M Pulmonary Artery, Right
	K Internal Carotid Artery, Right		M Stimulator Lead	N Pulmonary Artery, Left
	L Internal Carotid Artery, Left		Y Other Device	T Abdominal Artery
	M External Carotid Artery, Right		Z No Device	V Superior Vena Cava
	N External Carotid Artery, Left			W Lower Extremity Vein
	P Vertebral Artery, Right			X Diagnostic
	Q Vertebral Artery, Left			Y Upper Artery
	R Face Artery			Z No Qualifier
	S Temporal Artery, Right			
	T Temporal Artery, Left			
	U Thyroid Artery, Right			
	V Thyroid Artery, Left			
	Y Upper Artery			

AHA Coding Clinic for Upper Arteries

2022, 1Q, 10-13	Procedures performed on a continuous vessel, ICD-10-PCS Guideline B4.1c

AHA Coding Clinic for table Ø31

2021, 4Q, 45-46	Percutaneous bypass of brachial artery for arteriovenous fistula creation
2021, 3Q, 14	Arteriovenous fistula revision with graft to cephalic vein stump
2019, 4Q, 26	Upper artery bypass Qualifier
2019, 4Q, 26	Percutaneous approach upper artery bypass
2017, 4Q, 64-65	New qualifier values - Left to right carotid bypass
2017, 2Q, 22	Carotid artery to subclavian artery transposition
2017, 1Q, 31	Left to right common carotid artery bypass
2016, 3Q, 37	Insertion of arteriovenous graft using HeRO device
2016, 3Q, 39	Revision of arteriovenous graft
2013, 4Q, 125	Stage II cephalic vein transposition (superficialization) of arteriovenous fistula
2013, 1Q, 27	Creation of radial artery fistula

AHA Coding Clinic for table Ø37

2020, 4Q, 70-71	Cerebral embolic filtration extracorporeal flow reversal circuit
2019, 4Q, 27	Bifurcation Qualifier
2019, 3Q, 29	Transcarotid arterial catheterization
2018, 2Q, 24	Coronary artery bifurcation
2016, 4Q, 86	Peripheral artery, number of stents
2016, 4Q, 86-87	Coronary and peripheral artery bifurcation
2015, 1Q, 32	Deployment of stent for herniated/migrated coil in basilar artery

AHA Coding Clinic for table Ø3B

2016, 2Q, 12	Resection of malignant neoplasm of infratemporal fossa

AHA Coding Clinic for table Ø3C

2022, 1Q, 43	Cerebral thrombectomy with failed stent retriever deployment and aspiration of thrombus
2021, 2Q, 13	Thromboendarterectomy with deconstruction of internal carotid artery
2020, 3Q, 38	Thrombectomy of arteriovenous fistula with angioplasty and stent placement
2019, 4Q, 27	Bifurcation Qualifier
2018, 4Q, 47-48	Endovascular thrombectomy with stent retriever
2018, 2Q, 24	Coronary artery bifurcation
2017, 4Q, 64-65	New qualifier values - Left to right carotid bypass
2017, 2Q, 23	Thrombectomy via Fogarty catheter
2016, 4Q, 86-87	Coronary and peripheral artery bifurcation
2016, 2Q, 11	Carotid endarterectomy with patch angioplasty
2015, 1Q, 29	Discontinued carotid endarterectomy

AHA Coding Clinic for table Ø3F

2021, 4Q, 46	Fragmentation of intracranial artery
2020, 4Q, 45-49	New fragmentation tables
2020, 4Q, 49-50	Intravascular ultrasound assisted thrombolysis
2020, 4Q, 50	Intravascular lithotripsy

AHA Coding Clinic for table Ø3H

2020, 1Q, 25	Elephant trunk repair of aortic dissection
2016, 2Q, 32	Arterial catheter placement

AHA Coding Clinic for table Ø3J

2021, 1Q, 16	Placement of Sentinel™ embolic protection device with deployment of single filter
2015, 1Q, 29	Discontinued carotid endarterectomy

AHA Coding Clinic for table Ø3L

2021, 2Q, 13	Thromboendarterectomy with deconstruction of internal carotid artery
2016, 2Q, 30	Clipping (occlusion) of cerebral artery, decompressive craniectomy and storage of bone flap in abdominal wall
2014, 4Q, 20	Control of epistaxis
2014, 4Q, 37	Endovascular embolization of arteriovenous malformation using Onyx-18 liquid

AHA Coding Clinic for table Ø3Q

2017, 1Q, 31	Left to right common carotid artery bypass

AHA Coding Clinic for table Ø3S

2017, 2Q, 22	Carotid artery to subclavian artery transposition
2015, 3Q, 27	Moyamoya disease and hemispheric pial synangiosis with craniotomy

AHA Coding Clinic for table Ø3U

2019, 1Q, 22	Cerebral artery fusiform aneurysm repair via wrapping
2016, 2Q, 11	Carotid endarterectomy with patch angioplasty

AHA Coding Clinic for table Ø3V

2019, 4Q, 27-28	Aneurysm treatment using flow diverter stent
2019, 1Q, 22	Cerebral artery fusiform aneurysm repair via wrapping
2016, 1Q, 19	Embolization of superior hypophyseal aneurysm using stent-assisted coil

AHA Coding Clinic for table Ø3W

2016, 3Q, 39	Revision of arteriovenous graft
2015, 1Q, 32	Deployment of stent for herniated/migrated coil in basilar artery

Upper Arteries

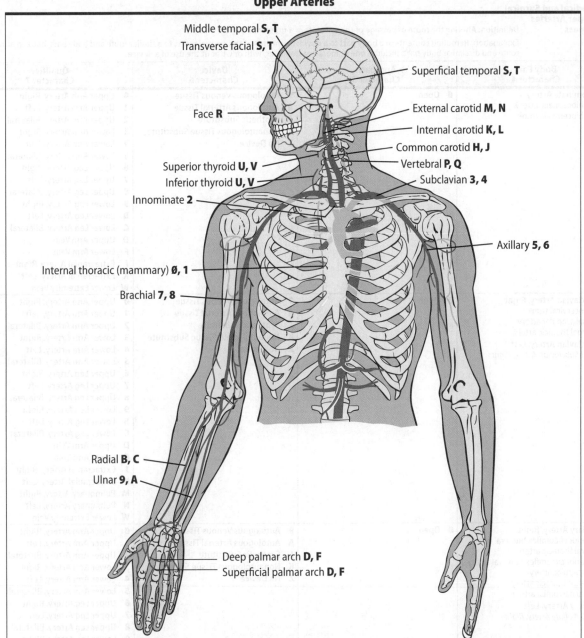

Middle temporal **S, T**
Transverse facial **S, T**
Superficial temporal **S, T**
Face **R**
External carotid **M, N**
Internal carotid **K, L**
Common carotid **H, J**
Superior thyroid **U, V**
Inferior thyroid **U, V**
Vertebral **P, Q**
Subclavian **3, 4**
Innominate **2**
Axillary **5, 6**
Internal thoracic (mammary) **Ø, 1**
Brachial **7, 8**
Radial **B, C**
Ulnar **9, A**
Deep palmar arch **D, F**
Superficial palmar arch **D, F**

Head and Neck Arteries

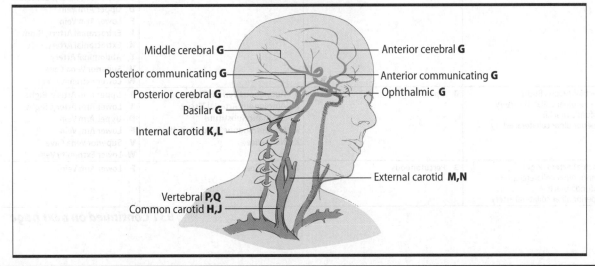

Middle cerebral **G**
Anterior cerebral **G**
Posterior communicating **G**
Anterior communicating **G**
Posterior cerebral **G**
Ophthalmic **G**
Basilar **G**
Internal carotid **K,L**
External carotid **M, N**
Vertebral **P,Q**
Common carotid **H,J**

Ø   Medical and Surgical
3   Upper Arteries
1   Bypass   Definition: Altering the route of passage of the contents of a tubular body part

                Explanation: Rerouting contents of a body part to a downstream area of the normal route, to a similar route and body part, or to an abnormal route and dissimilar body part. Includes one or more anastomoses, with or without the use of a device.

Body Part Character 4	Approach Character 5	Device Character 6	Qualifier Character 7

2 Innominate Artery
   Brachiocephalic artery
   Brachiocephalic trunk
	Ø Open	9 Autologous Venous Tissue
		A Autologous Arterial Tissue
		J Synthetic Substitute
		K Nonautologous Tissue Substitute
		Z No Device
			Ø Upper Arm Artery, Right
			1 Upper Arm Artery, Left
			2 Upper Arm Artery, Bilateral
			3 Lower Arm Artery, Right
			4 Lower Arm Artery, Left
			5 Lower Arm Artery, Bilateral
			6 Upper Leg Artery, Right
			7 Upper Leg Artery, Left
			8 Upper Leg Artery, Bilateral
			9 Lower Leg Artery, Right
			B Lower Leg Artery, Left
			C Lower Leg Artery, Bilateral
			D Upper Arm Vein
			F Lower Arm Vein
			J Extracranial Artery, Right
			K Extracranial Artery, Left
			W Lower Extremity Vein

3 Subclavian Artery, Right
   Costocervical trunk
   Dorsal scapular artery
   Internal thoracic artery
4 Subclavian Artery, Left
   See 3 Subclavian Artery, Right
	Ø Open	9 Autologous Venous Tissue
		A Autologous Arterial Tissue
		J Synthetic Substitute
		K Nonautologous Tissue Substitute
		Z No Device
			Ø Upper Arm Artery, Right
			1 Upper Arm Artery, Left
			2 Upper Arm Artery, Bilateral
			3 Lower Arm Artery, Right
			4 Lower Arm Artery, Left
			5 Lower Arm Artery, Bilateral
			6 Upper Leg Artery, Right
			7 Upper Leg Artery, Left
			8 Upper Leg Artery, Bilateral
			9 Lower Leg Artery, Right
			B Lower Leg Artery, Left
			C Lower Leg Artery, Bilateral
			D Upper Arm Vein
			F Lower Arm Vein
			J Extracranial Artery, Right
			K Extracranial Artery, Left
			M Pulmonary Artery, Right
			N Pulmonary Artery, Left
			W Lower Extremity Vein

5 Axillary Artery, Right
   Anterior circumflex humeral artery
   Lateral thoracic artery
   Posterior circumflex humeral artery
   Subscapular artery
   Superior thoracic artery
   Thoracoacromial artery
6 Axillary Artery, Left
   See 5 Axillary Artery, Right
	Ø Open	9 Autologous Venous Tissue
		A Autologous Arterial Tissue
		J Synthetic Substitute
		K Nonautologous Tissue Substitute
		Z No Device
			Ø Upper Arm Artery, Right
			1 Upper Arm Artery, Left
			2 Upper Arm Artery, Bilateral
			3 Lower Arm Artery, Right
			4 Lower Arm Artery, Left
			5 Lower Arm Artery, Bilateral
			6 Upper Leg Artery, Right
			7 Upper Leg Artery, Left
			8 Upper Leg Artery, Bilateral
			9 Lower Leg Artery, Right
			B Lower Leg Artery, Left
			C Lower Leg Artery, Bilateral
			D Upper Arm Vein
			F Lower Arm Vein
			J Extracranial Artery, Right
			K Extracranial Artery, Left
			T Abdominal Artery
			V Superior Vena Cava
			W Lower Extremity Vein

7 Brachial Artery, Right
   Inferior ulnar collateral artery
   Profunda brachii
   Superior ulnar collateral artery
	Ø Open	9 Autologous Venous Tissue
		A Autologous Arterial Tissue
		J Synthetic Substitute
		K Nonautologous Tissue Substitute
		Z No Device
			Ø Upper Arm Artery, Right
			3 Lower Arm Artery, Right
			D Upper Arm Vein
			F Lower Arm Vein
			V Superior Vena Cava
			W Lower Extremity Vein

7 Brachial Artery, Right
   Inferior ulnar collateral artery
   Profunda brachii
   Superior ulnar collateral artery
	3 Percutaneous	Z No Device	F Lower Arm Vein

Ø31 Continued on next page

Non-OR Procedure   DRG Non-OR Procedure   Valid OR Procedure   HAC Associated Procedure   Combination Only   New/Revised April   New/Revised October

196   ICD-10-PCS 2023

Ø   **Medical and Surgical**   *Ø31 Continued*
3   **Upper Arteries**
1   **Bypass**   Definition: Altering the route of passage of the contents of a tubular body part
                 Explanation: Rerouting contents of a body part to a downstream area of the normal route, to a similar route and body part, or to an abnormal
                 route and dissimilar body part. Includes one or more anastomoses, with or without the use of a device.

Body Part Character 4	Approach Character 5	Device Character 6	Qualifier Character 7
8 Brachial Artery, Left Inferior ulnar collateral artery Profunda brachii Superior ulnar collateral artery	**Ø** Open	**9** Autologous Venous Tissue **A** Autologous Arterial Tissue **J** Synthetic Substitute **K** Nonautologous Tissue Substitute **Z** No Device	**1** Upper Arm Artery, Left **4** Lower Arm Artery, Left **D** Upper Arm Vein **F** Lower Arm Vein **V** Superior Vena Cava **W** Lower Extremity Vein
8 Brachial Artery, Left Inferior ulnar collateral artery Profunda brachii Superior ulnar collateral artery	**3** Percutaneous	**Z** No Device	**F** Lower Arm Vein
9 Ulnar Artery, Right Anterior ulnar recurrent artery Common interosseous artery Posterior ulnar recurrent artery **B** Radial Artery, Right Radial recurrent artery	**Ø** Open	**9** Autologous Venous Tissue **A** Autologous Arterial Tissue **J** Synthetic Substitute **K** Nonautologous Tissue Substitute **Z** No Device	**3** Lower Arm Artery, Right **F** Lower Arm Vein
9 Ulnar Artery, Right Anterior ulnar recurrent artery Common interosseous artery Posterior ulnar recurrent artery **B** Radial Artery, Right Radial recurrent artery	**3** Percutaneous	**Z** No Device	**F** Lower Arm Vein
A Ulnar Artery, Left Anterior ulnar recurrent artery Common interosseous artery Posterior ulnar recurrent artery **C** Radial Artery, Left Radial recurrent artery	**Ø** Open	**9** Autologous Venous Tissue **A** Autologous Arterial Tissue **J** Synthetic Substitute **K** Nonautologous Tissue Substitute **Z** No Device	**4** Lower Arm Artery, Left **F** Lower Arm Vein
A Ulnar Artery, Left Anterior ulnar recurrent artery Common interosseous artery Posterior ulnar recurrent artery **C** Radial Artery, Left Radial recurrent artery	**3** Percutaneous	**Z** No Device	**F** Lower Arm Vein

G Intracranial Artery
Anterior cerebral artery
Anterior choroidal artery
Anterior communicating artery
Basilar artery
Circle of Willis
Internal carotid artery, intracranial
   portion
Middle cerebral artery
Ophthalmic artery
Posterior cerebral artery
Posterior communicating artery
Posterior inferior cerebellar artery
   (PICA)
S Temporal Artery, Right
Middle temporal artery
Superficial temporal artery
Transverse facial artery
T Temporal Artery, Left
See S Temporal Artery, Right
	Ø Open	**9** Autologous Venous Tissue
		A Autologous Arterial Tissue
		J Synthetic Substitute
		K Nonautologous Tissue Substitute
		Z No Device
			G Intracranial Artery

H Common Carotid Artery, Right **J** Common Carotid Artery, Left	**Ø** Open	**9** Autologous Venous Tissue **A** Autologous Arterial Tissue **J** Synthetic Substitute **K** Nonautologous Tissue Substitute **Z** No Device	**G** Intracranial Artery **J** Extracranial Artery, Right **K** Extracranial Artery, Left **Y** Upper Artery

Ø31 Continued on next page

NC Noncovered Procedure   **LC** Limited Coverage   **QA** Questionable OB Admit   **NT** New Tech Add-on   ⊞ Combination Member   ♂ Male   ♀ Female

ICD-10-PCS 2023   197

Ø31–Ø31

Upper Arteries

Ø31 Continued

Ø   **Medical and Surgical**
3   **Upper Arteries**
1   **Bypass**   Definition: Altering the route of passage of the contents of a tubular body part

Explanation: Rerouting contents of a body part to a downstream area of the normal route, to a similar route and body part, or to an abnormal route and dissimilar body part. Includes one or more anastomoses, with or without the use of a device.

Body Part Character 4	Approach Character 5	Device Character 6	Qualifier Character 7

K **Internal Carotid Artery, Right**
    Caroticotympanic artery
    Carotid sinus
 L **Internal Carotid Artery, Left**
    Caroticotympanic artery
    Carotid sinus
 M **External Carotid Artery, Right**
    Ascending pharyngeal artery
    Internal maxillary artery
    Lingual artery
    Maxillary artery
    Occipital artery
    Posterior auricular artery
    Superior thyroid artery
 N **External Carotid Artery, Left**
    Ascending pharyngeal artery
    Internal maxillary artery
    Lingual artery
    Maxillary artery
    Occipital artery
    Posterior auricular artery
    Superior thyroid artery
	Ø Open	**9** Autologous Venous Tissue
		 A Autologous Arterial Tissue
		 J Synthetic Substitute
		 K Nonautologous Tissue Substitute
		 Z No Device
			J Extracranial Artery, Right
			 K Extracranial Artery, Left

Ø31–Ø31

Non-OR Procedure   DRG Non-OR Procedure   Valid OR Procedure   HAC Associated Procedure   Combination Only   New/Revised April   New/Revised October

198   ICD-10-PCS 2023

Ø   Medical and Surgical
3   Upper Arteries
5   Destruction   Definition: Physical eradication of all or a portion of a body part by the direct use of energy, force, or a destructive agent
                          Explanation: None of the body part is physically taken out

Body Part Character 4		Approach Character 5	Device Character 6	Qualifier Character 7
Ø Internal Mammary Artery, Right Anterior intercostal artery Internal thoracic artery Musculophrenic artery Pericardiophrenic artery Superior epigastric artery **1 Internal Mammary Artery, Left** *See Ø Internal Mammary Artery, Right* **2 Innominate Artery** Brachiocephalic artery Brachiocephalic trunk **3 Subclavian Artery, Right** Costocervical trunk Dorsal scapular artery Internal thoracic artery **4 Subclavian Artery, Left** *See 3 Subclavian Artery, Right* **5 Axillary Artery, Right** Anterior circumflex humeral artery Lateral thoracic artery Posterior circumflex humeral artery Subscapular artery Superior thoracic artery Thoracoacromial artery **6 Axillary Artery, Left** *See 5 Axillary Artery, Right* **7 Brachial Artery, Right** Inferior ulnar collateral artery Profunda brachii Superior ulnar collateral artery **8 Brachial Artery, Left** *See 7 Brachial Artery, Right* **9 Ulnar Artery, Right** Anterior ulnar recurrent artery Common interosseous artery Posterior ulnar recurrent artery **A Ulnar Artery, Left** *See 9 Ulnar Artery, Right* **B Radial Artery, Right** Radial recurrent artery **C Radial Artery, Left** *See B Radial Artery, Right* **D Hand Artery, Right** Deep palmar arch Princeps pollicis artery Radialis indicis Superficial palmar arch **F Hand Artery, Left** *See D Hand Artery, Right* **G Intracranial Artery** Anterior cerebral artery Anterior choroidal artery Anterior communicating artery Basilar artery Circle of Willis Internal carotid artery, intracranial portion Middle cerebral artery Ophthalmic artery Posterior cerebral artery Posterior communicating artery Posterior inferior cerebellar artery (PICA)	**H Common Carotid Artery, Right** **J Common Carotid Artery, Left** **K Internal Carotid Artery, Right** Caroticotympanic artery Carotid sinus **L Internal Carotid Artery, Left** *See K Internal Carotid Artery, Right* **M External Carotid Artery, Right** Ascending pharyngeal artery Internal maxillary artery Lingual artery Maxillary artery Occipital artery Posterior auricular artery Superior thyroid artery **N External Carotid Artery, Left** *See M External Carotid Artery, Right* **P Vertebral Artery, Right** Anterior spinal artery Posterior spinal artery **Q Vertebral Artery, Left** *See P Vertebral Artery, Right* **R Face Artery** Angular artery Ascending palatine artery External maxillary artery Facial artery Inferior labial artery Submental artery Superior labial artery **S Temporal Artery, Right** Middle temporal artery Superficial temporal artery Transverse facial artery **T Temporal Artery, Left** *See S Temporal Artery, Right* **U Thyroid Artery, Right** Cricothyroid artery Hyoid artery Sternocleidomastoid artery Superior laryngeal artery Superior thyroid artery Thyrocervical trunk **V Thyroid Artery, Left** *See U Thyroid Artery, Right* **Y Upper Artery** Aortic intercostal artery Bronchial artery Esophageal artery Subcostal artery	**Ø Open** **3 Percutaneous** **4 Percutaneous Endoscopic**	**Z No Device**	**Z No Qualifier**

NC Noncovered Procedure   **LC** Limited Coverage   **QA** Questionable OB Admit   **NT** New Tech Add-on   ⊞ Combination Member   ♂ Male   ♀ Female

ICD-10-PCS 2023   **199**

Ø35–Ø35

Ø   Medical and Surgical
3   Upper Arteries
7   Dilation   Definition: Expanding an orifice or the lumen of a tubular body part

Explanation: The orifice can be a natural orifice or an artificially created orifice. Accomplished by stretching a tubular body part using intraluminal pressure or by cutting part of the orifice or wall of the tubular body part.

Body Part Character 4		Approach Character 5	Device Character 6	Qualifier Character 7
Ø Internal Mammary Artery, Right Anterior intercostal artery Internal thoracic artery Musculophrenic artery Pericardiophrenic artery Superior epigastric artery **1 Internal Mammary Artery, Left** *See Ø Internal Mammary Artery, Right* **2 Innominate Artery** Brachiocephalic artery Brachiocephalic trunk **3 Subclavian Artery, Right** Costocervical trunk Dorsal scapular artery Internal thoracic artery **4 Subclavian Artery, Left** *See 3 Subclavian Artery, Right* **5 Axillary Artery, Right** Anterior circumflex humeral artery Lateral thoracic artery Posterior circumflex humeral artery Subscapular artery Superior thoracic artery Thoracoacromial artery	**6 Axillary Artery, Left** *See 5 Axillary Artery, Right* **7 Brachial Artery, Right** Inferior ulnar collateral artery Profunda brachii Superior ulnar collateral artery **8 Brachial Artery, Left** *See 7 Brachial Artery, Right* **9 Ulnar Artery, Right** Anterior ulnar recurrent artery Common interosseous artery Posterior ulnar recurrent artery **A Ulnar Artery, Left** *See 9 Ulnar Artery, Right* **B Radial Artery, Right** Radial recurrent artery **C Radial Artery, Left** *See B Radial Artery, Right*	**Ø Open** **3 Percutaneous** **4 Percutaneous Endoscopic**	**4 Intraluminal Device, Drug-eluting** **5 Intraluminal Device, Drug-eluting, Two** **6 Intraluminal Device, Drug-eluting, Three** **7 Intraluminal Device, Drug-eluting, Four or More** **E Intraluminal Device, Two** **F Intraluminal Device, Three** **G Intraluminal Device, Four or More**	**Z No Qualifier**
Ø Internal Mammary Artery, Right Anterior intercostal artery Internal thoracic artery Musculophrenic artery Pericardiophrenic artery Superior epigastric artery **1 Internal Mammary Artery, Left** *See Ø Internal Mammary Artery, Right* **2 Innominate Artery** Brachiocephalic artery Brachiocephalic trunk **3 Subclavian Artery, Right** Costocervical trunk Dorsal scapular artery Internal thoracic artery **4 Subclavian Artery, Left** *See 3 Subclavian Artery, Right* **5 Axillary Artery, Right** Anterior circumflex humeral artery Lateral thoracic artery Posterior circumflex humeral artery Subscapular artery Superior thoracic artery Thoracoacromial artery	**6 Axillary Artery, Left** *See 5 Axillary Artery, Right* **7 Brachial Artery, Right** Inferior ulnar collateral artery Profunda brachii Superior ulnar collateral artery **8 Brachial Artery, Left** *See 7 Brachial Artery, Right* **9 Ulnar Artery, Right** Anterior ulnar recurrent artery Common interosseous artery Posterior ulnar recurrent artery **A Ulnar Artery, Left** *See 9 Ulnar Artery, Right* **B Radial Artery, Right** Radial recurrent artery **C Radial Artery, Left** *See B Radial Artery, Right*	**Ø Open** **3 Percutaneous** **4 Percutaneous Endoscopic**	**D Intraluminal Device** **Z No Device**	**1 Drug-Coated Balloon** **Z No Qualifier**

Ø37 Continued on next page

Non-OR Procedure   DRG Non-OR Procedure   Valid OR Procedure   HAC Associated Procedure   Combination Only   New/Revised April   New/Revised October

Ø　**Medical and Surgical**
3　**Upper Arteries**　　　　　　　　　　　　　　　　　　　　　　*Ø37 Continued*
7　**Dilation**　　　Definition: Expanding an orifice or the lumen of a tubular body part

Explanation: The orifice can be a natural orifice or an artificially created orifice. Accomplished by stretching a tubular body part using intraluminal pressure or by cutting part of the orifice or wall of the tubular body part.

Body Part Character 4		Approach Character 5	Device Character 6	Qualifier Character 7
D Hand Artery, Right Deep palmar arch Princeps pollicis artery Radialis indicis Superficial palmar arch **F Hand Artery, Left** *See D Hand Artery, Right* **G Intracranial Artery** NC Anterior cerebral artery Anterior choroidal artery Anterior communicating artery Basilar artery Circle of Willis Internal carotid artery, 　intracranial portion Middle cerebral artery Ophthalmic artery Posterior cerebral artery Posterior communicating 　artery Posterior inferior cerebellar 　artery (PICA) **H Common Carotid Artery, Right** **J Common Carotid Artery, Left** **K Internal Carotid Artery, Right** Caroticotympanic artery Carotid sinus **L Internal Carotid Artery, Left** *See K Internal Carotid Artery, Right* **M External Carotid Artery, Right** Ascending pharyngeal artery Internal maxillary artery Lingual artery Maxillary artery Occipital artery Posterior auricular artery Superior thyroid artery	**N External Carotid Artery, Left** *See M External Carotid Artery, Right* **P Vertebral Artery, Right** Anterior spinal artery Posterior spinal artery **Q Vertebral Artery, Left** *See P Vertebral Artery, Right* **R Face Artery** Angular artery Ascending palatine artery External maxillary artery Facial artery Inferior labial artery Submental artery Superior labial artery **S Temporal Artery, Right** Middle temporal artery Superficial temporal artery Transverse facial artery **T Temporal Artery, Left** *See S Temporal Artery, Right* **U Thyroid Artery, Right** Cricothyroid artery Hyoid artery Sternocleidomastoid artery Superior laryngeal artery Superior thyroid artery Thyrocervical trunk **V Thyroid Artery, Left** *See U Thyroid Artery, Right* **Y Upper Artery** Aortic intercostal artery Bronchial artery Esophageal artery Subcostal artery	**Ø Open** **3 Percutaneous** **4 Percutaneous Endoscopic**	**4 Intraluminal Device, Drug-eluting** **5 Intraluminal Device, Drug- eluting, Two** **6 Intraluminal Device, Drug- eluting, Three** **7 Intraluminal Device, Drug- eluting, Four or More** **D Intraluminal Device** **E Intraluminal Device, Two** **F Intraluminal Device, Three** **G Intraluminal Device, Four or More** **Z No Device**	**Z No Qualifier**

NC　Ø37G[3,4]ZZ

NC Noncovered Procedure　　LC Limited Coverage　　QA Questionable OB Admit　　NT New Tech Add-on　　✚ Combination Member　　♂ Male　　♀ Female

ICD-10-PCS 2023　　　　　　　　　　　　　　　　　　　　　　　　　　　　　　　　　　　　　**201**

Upper Arteries

Ø Medical and Surgical
3 Upper Arteries
9 Drainage   Definition: Taking or letting out fluids and/or gases from a body part
               Explanation: The qualifier DIAGNOSTIC is used to identify drainage procedures that are biopsies

Body Part Character 4		Approach Character 5	Device Character 6	Qualifier Character 7
Ø Internal Mammary Artery, Right Anterior intercostal artery Internal thoracic artery Musculophrenic artery Pericardiophrenic artery Superior epigastric artery **1 Internal Mammary Artery, Left** *See Ø Internal Mammary Artery, Right above* **2 Innominate Artery** Brachiocephalic artery Brachiocephalic trunk **3 Subclavian Artery, Right** Costocervical trunk Dorsal scapular artery Internal thoracic artery **4 Subclavian Artery, Left** *See 3 Subclavian Artery, Right* **5 Axillary Artery, Right** Anterior circumflex humeral artery Lateral thoracic artery Posterior circumflex humeral artery Subscapular artery Superior thoracic artery Thoracoacromial artery **6 Axillary Artery, Left** *See 5 Axillary Artery, Right* **7 Brachial Artery, Right** Inferior ulnar collateral artery Profunda brachii Superior ulnar collateral artery **8 Brachial Artery, Left** *See 7 Brachial Artery, Right* **9 Ulnar Artery, Right** Anterior ulnar recurrent artery Common interosseous artery Posterior ulnar recurrent artery **A Ulnar Artery, Left** *See 9 Ulnar Artery, Right* **B Radial Artery, Right** Radial recurrent artery **C Radial Artery, Left** *See B Radial Artery, Right* **D Hand Artery, Right** Deep palmar arch Princeps pollicis artery Radialis indicis Superficial palmar arch **F Hand Artery, Left** *See D Hand Artery, Right* **G Intracranial Artery** Anterior cerebral artery Anterior choroidal artery Anterior communicating artery Basilar artery Circle of Willis Internal carotid artery, intracranial portion Middle cerebral artery Ophthalmic artery Posterior cerebral artery Posterior communicating artery Posterior inferior cerebellar artery (PICA)	**H Common Carotid Artery, Right** **J Common Carotid Artery, Left** **K Internal Carotid Artery, Right** Caroticotympanic artery Carotid sinus **L Internal Carotid Artery, Left** *See K Internal Carotid Artery, Right* **M External Carotid Artery, Right** Ascending pharyngeal artery Internal maxillary artery Lingual artery Maxillary artery Occipital artery Posterior auricular artery Superior thyroid artery **N External Carotid Artery, Left** *See M External Carotid Artery, Right* **P Vertebral Artery, Right** Anterior spinal artery Posterior spinal artery **Q Vertebral Artery, Left** *See P Vertebral Artery, Right* **R Face Artery** Angular artery Ascending palatine artery External maxillary artery Facial artery Inferior labial artery Submental artery Superior labial artery **S Temporal Artery, Right** Middle temporal artery Superficial temporal artery Transverse facial artery **T Temporal Artery, Left** *See S Temporal Artery, Right* **U Thyroid Artery, Right** Cricothyroid artery Hyoid artery Sternocleidomastoid artery Superior laryngeal artery Superior thyroid artery Thyrocervical trunk **V Thyroid Artery, Left** *See U Thyroid Artery, Right* **Y Upper Artery** Aortic intercostal artery Bronchial artery Esophageal artery Subcostal artery	**Ø Open** **3 Percutaneous** **4 Percutaneous Endoscopic**	**Ø Drainage Device**	**Z No Qualifier**

Non-OR   Ø39[Ø,1,2,3,4,5,6,7,8,9,A,B,C,D,F,G,H,J,K,L,M,N,P,Q,R,S,T,U,V,Y][Ø,3,4]ØZ

Ø39 Continued on next page

Non-OR Procedure   DRG Non-OR Procedure   Valid OR Procedure   HAC Associated Procedure   Combination Only   New/Revised April   New/Revised October

202   ICD-10-PCS 2023

Ø **Medical and Surgical**　　　　　　　　　　　　　　　　　　　　　　*Ø39 Continued*
3 **Upper Arteries**
9 **Drainage**　　　　Definition: Taking or letting out fluids and/or gases from a body part

Explanation: The qualifier DIAGNOSTIC is used to identify drainage procedures that are biopsies

Body Part Character 4		Approach Character 5	Device Character 6	Qualifier Character 7
Ø Internal Mammary Artery, Right Anterior intercostal artery Internal thoracic artery Musculophrenic artery Pericardiophrenic artery Superior epigastric artery	**H Common Carotid Artery, Right** **J Common Carotid Artery, Left** **K Internal Carotid Artery, Right** Caroticotympanic artery Carotid sinus	**Ø Open** **3 Percutaneous** **4 Percutaneous Endoscopic**	**Z No Device**	**X Diagnostic** **Z No Qualifier**
1 Internal Mammary Artery, Left *See Ø Internal Mammary Artery, Right*	**L Internal Carotid Artery, Left** *See K Internal Carotid Artery, Right*			
2 Innominate Artery Brachiocephalic artery Brachiocephalic trunk	**M External Carotid Artery, Right** Ascending pharyngeal artery Internal maxillary artery Lingual artery			
3 Subclavian Artery, Right Costocervical trunk Dorsal scapular artery Internal thoracic artery	Maxillary artery Occipital artery Posterior auricular artery Superior thyroid artery			
4 Subclavian Artery, Left *See 3 Subclavian Artery, Right*	**N External Carotid Artery, Left** *See M External Carotid Artery, Right*			
5 Axillary Artery, Right Anterior circumflex humeral artery Lateral thoracic artery Posterior circumflex humeral artery Subscapular artery Superior thoracic artery Thoracoacromial artery	**P Vertebral Artery, Right** Anterior spinal artery Posterior spinal artery **Q Vertebral Artery, Left** *See P Vertebral Artery, Right* **R Face Artery** Angular artery Ascending palatine artery External maxillary artery			
6 Axillary Artery, Left *See 5 Axillary Artery, Right*	Facial artery Inferior labial artery Submental artery Superior labial artery			
7 Brachial Artery, Right Inferior ulnar collateral artery Profunda brachii Superior ulnar collateral artery	**S Temporal Artery, Right** Middle temporal artery Superficial temporal artery Transverse facial artery			
8 Brachial Artery, Left *See 7 Brachial Artery, Right*	**T Temporal Artery, Left** *See S Temporal Artery, Right*			
9 Ulnar Artery, Right Anterior ulnar recurrent artery Common interosseous artery Posterior ulnar recurrent artery	**U Thyroid Artery, Right** Cricothyroid artery Hyoid artery Sternocleidomastoid artery Superior laryngeal artery			
A Ulnar Artery, Left *See 9 Ulnar Artery, Right*	Superior thyroid artery Thyrocervical trunk			
B Radial Artery, Right Radial recurrent artery	**V Thyroid Artery, Left** *See U Thyroid Artery, Right*			
C Radial Artery, Left *See B Radial Artery, Right*	**Y Upper Artery** Aortic intercostal artery Bronchial artery			
D Hand Artery, Right Deep palmar arch Princeps pollicis artery Radialis indicis Superficial palmar arch	Esophageal artery Subcostal artery			
F Hand Artery, Left *See D Hand Artery, Right*				
G Intracranial Artery Anterior cerebral artery Anterior choroidal artery Anterior communicating artery Basilar artery Circle of Willis Internal carotid artery, intracranial portion Middle cerebral artery Ophthalmic artery Posterior cerebral artery Posterior communicating artery Posterior inferior cerebellar artery (PICA)				

Non-OR　Ø39[Ø,1,2,3,4,5,6,7,8,9,A,B,C,D,F,G,H,J,K,L,M,N,P,Q,R,S,T,U,V,Y]3ZX
Non-OR　Ø39[Ø,1,2,3,4,5,6,7,8,9,A,B,C,D,F,G,H,J,K,L,M,N,P,Q,R,S,T,U,V,Y][Ø,3,4]ZZ

NC Noncovered Procedure　**LC** Limited Coverage　**QA** Questionable OB Admit　**NT** New Tech Add-on　⊞ Combination Member　♂ Male　♀ Female

ICD-10-PCS 2023　　　　　　　　　　　　　　　　　　　　　　　　　　　　　　　　　　　**203**

Ø39–Ø39

Upper Arteries

Ø   **Medical and Surgical**
3   **Upper Arteries**
B   **Excision**   Definition: Cutting out or off, without replacement, a portion of a body part
                  Explanation: The qualifier DIAGNOSTIC is used to identify excision procedures that are biopsies

Body Part Character 4		Approach Character 5	Device Character 6	Qualifier Character 7
Ø Internal Mammary Artery, Right	**H Common Carotid Artery, Right**	**Ø Open**	**Z No Device**	**X Diagnostic**
Anterior intercostal artery	**J Common Carotid Artery, Left**	**3 Percutaneous**		**Z No Qualifier**
Internal thoracic artery	**K Internal Carotid Artery, Right**	**4 Percutaneous Endoscopic**		
Musculophrenic artery	Caroticotympanic artery			
Pericardiophrenic artery	Carotid sinus			
Superior epigastric artery	**L Internal Carotid Artery, Left**			
1 Internal Mammary Artery, Left	*See K Internal Carotid Artery, Right*			
See Ø Internal Mammary Artery, Right	**M External Carotid Artery, Right**			
2 Innominate Artery	Ascending pharyngeal artery			
Brachiocephalic artery	Internal maxillary artery			
Brachiocephalic trunk	Lingual artery			
3 Subclavian Artery, Right	Maxillary artery			
Costocervical trunk	Occipital artery			
Dorsal scapular artery	Posterior auricular artery			
Internal thoracic artery	Superior thyroid artery			
4 Subclavian Artery, Left	**N External Carotid Artery, Left**			
See 3 Subclavian Artery, Right	*See M External Carotid Artery, Right*			
5 Axillary Artery, Right	**P Vertebral Artery, Right**			
Anterior circumflex humeral artery	Anterior spinal artery			
Lateral thoracic artery	Posterior spinal artery			
Posterior circumflex humeral artery	**Q Vertebral Artery, Left**			
Subscapular artery	*See P Vertebral Artery, Right*			
Superior thoracic artery	**R Face Artery**			
Thoracoacromial artery	Angular artery			
6 Axillary Artery, Left	Ascending palatine artery			
See 5 Axillary Artery, Right	External maxillary artery			
7 Brachial Artery, Right	Facial artery			
Inferior ulnar collateral artery	Inferior labial artery			
Profunda brachii	Submental artery			
Superior ulnar collateral artery	Superior labial artery			
8 Brachial Artery, Left	**S Temporal Artery, Right**			
See 7 Brachial Artery, Right	Middle temporal artery			
9 Ulnar Artery, Right	Superficial temporal artery			
Anterior ulnar recurrent artery	Transverse facial artery			
Common interosseous artery	**T Temporal Artery, Left**			
Posterior ulnar recurrent artery	*See S Temporal Artery, Right*			
A Ulnar Artery, Left	**U Thyroid Artery, Right**			
See 9 Ulnar Artery, Right	Cricothyroid artery			
B Radial Artery, Right	Hyoid artery			
Radial recurrent artery	Sternocleidomastoid artery			
C Radial Artery, Left	Superior laryngeal artery			
See B Radial Artery, Right	Superior thyroid artery			
D Hand Artery, Right	Thyrocervical trunk			
Deep palmar arch	**V Thyroid Artery, Left**			
Princeps pollicis artery	*See U Thyroid Artery, Right*			
Radialis indicis	**Y Upper Artery**			
Superficial palmar arch	Aortic intercostal artery			
F Hand Artery, Left	Bronchial artery			
See D Hand Artery, Right	Esophageal artery			
G Intracranial Artery	Subcostal artery			
Anterior cerebral artery				
Anterior choroidal artery				
Anterior communicating artery				
Basilar artery				
Circle of Willis				
Internal carotid artery, intracranial portion				
Middle cerebral artery				
Ophthalmic artery				
Posterior cerebral artery				
Posterior communicating artery				
Posterior inferior cerebellar artery (PICA)				

Non-OR Procedure   DRG Non-OR Procedure   Valid OR Procedure   HAC Associated Procedure   Combination Only   New/Revised April   New/Revised October

204   ICD-10-PCS 2023

Ø   **Medical and Surgical**
3   **Upper Arteries**
C   **Extirpation**   Definition: Taking or cutting out solid matter from a body part

Explanation: The solid matter may be an abnormal byproduct of a biological function or a foreign body; it may be imbedded in a body part or in the lumen of a tubular body part. The solid matter may or may not have been previously broken into pieces.

Body Part Character 4		Approach Character 5	Device Character 6	Qualifier Character 7
Ø Internal Mammary Artery, Right Anterior intercostal artery Internal thoracic artery Musculophrenic artery Pericardiophrenic artery Superior epigastric artery **1 Internal Mammary Artery, Left** *See Ø Internal Mammary Artery, Right* **2 Innominate Artery** Brachiocephalic artery Brachiocephalic trunk **3 Subclavian Artery, Right** Costocervical trunk Dorsal scapular artery Internal thoracic artery **4 Subclavian Artery, Left** *See 3 Subclavian Artery, Right* **5 Axillary Artery, Right** Anterior circumflex humeral artery Lateral thoracic artery Posterior circumflex humeral artery Subscapular artery Superior thoracic artery Thoracoacromial artery **6 Axillary Artery, Left** *See 5 Axillary Artery, Right* **7 Brachial Artery, Right** Inferior ulnar collateral artery Profunda brachii Superior ulnar collateral artery **8 Brachial Artery, Left** *See 7 Brachial Artery, Right* **9 Ulnar Artery, Right** Anterior ulnar recurrent artery Common interosseous artery Posterior ulnar recurrent artery	**A Ulnar Artery, Left** *See 9 Ulnar Artery, Right* **B Radial Artery, Right** Radial recurrent artery **C Radial Artery, Left** *See B Radial Artery, Right* **D Hand Artery, Right** Deep palmar arch Princeps pollicis artery Radialis indicis Superficial palmar arch **F Hand Artery, Left** *See D Hand Artery, Right* **R Face Artery** Angular artery Ascending palatine artery External maxillary artery Facial artery Inferior labial artery Submental artery Superior labial artery **S Temporal Artery, Right** Middle temporal artery Superficial temporal artery Transverse facial artery **T Temporal Artery, Left** *See S Temporal Artery, Right* **U Thyroid Artery, Right** Cricothyroid artery Hyoid artery Sternocleidomastoid artery Superior laryngeal artery Superior thyroid artery Thyrocervical trunk **V Thyroid Artery, Left** *See U Thyroid Artery, Right* **Y Upper Artery** Aortic intercostal artery Bronchial artery Esophageal artery Subcostal artery	**Ø Open** **3 Percutaneous** **4 Percutaneous Endoscopic**	**Z No Device**	**Z No Qualifier**
G Intracranial Artery Anterior cerebral artery Anterior choroidal artery Anterior communicating artery Basilar artery Circle of Willis Internal carotid artery, intracranial portion Middle cerebral artery Ophthalmic artery Posterior cerebral artery Posterior communicating artery Posterior inferior cerebellar artery (PICA) **H Common Carotid Artery, Right** **J Common Carotid Artery, Left** **K Internal Carotid Artery, Right** Caroticotympanic artery Carotid sinus	**L Internal Carotid Artery, Left** *See K Internal Carotid Artery, Right* **M External Carotid Artery, Right** Ascending pharyngeal artery Internal maxillary artery Lingual artery Maxillary artery Occipital artery Posterior auricular artery Superior thyroid artery **N External Carotid Artery, Left** *See M External Carotid Artery, Right* **P Vertebral Artery, Right** Anterior spinal artery Posterior spinal artery **Q Vertebral Artery, Left** *See P Vertebral Artery, Right*	**Ø Open** **4 Percutaneous Endoscopic**	**Z No Device**	**Z No Qualifier**

Ø3C Continued on next page

NC Noncovered Procedure   **LC** Limited Coverage   **QA** Questionable OB Admit   **NT** New Tech Add-on   ⊞ Combination Member   ♂ Male   ♀ Female

ICD-10-PCS 2023   **205**

03C–03C

Upper Arteries

03C Continued

0 Medical and Surgical
3 Upper Arteries
C Extirpation   Definition: Taking or cutting out solid matter from a body part

Explanation: The solid matter may be an abnormal byproduct of a biological function or a foreign body; it may be imbedded in a body part or in the lumen of a tubular body part. The solid matter may or may not have been previously broken into pieces.

Body Part Character 4		Approach Character 5	Device Character 6	Qualifier Character 7

G Intracranial Artery
  Anterior cerebral artery
  Anterior choroidal artery
  Anterior communicating
    artery
  Basilar artery
  Circle of Willis
  Internal carotid artery,
    intracranial portion
  Middle cerebral artery
  Ophthalmic artery
  Posterior cerebral artery
  Posterior communicating
    artery
  Posterior inferior cerebellar
    artery (PICA)
**H Common Carotid Artery,
  Right**
J Common Carotid Artery, Left
K Internal Carotid Artery, Right
  Caroticotympanic artery
  Carotid sinus
	L Internal Carotid Artery, Left
	  *See K Internal Carotid Artery,
	  Right*
	M External Carotid Artery, Right
	  Ascending pharyngeal artery
	  Internal maxillary artery
	  Lingual artery
	  Maxillary artery
	  Occipital artery
	  Posterior auricular artery
	  Superior thyroid artery
	N External Carotid Artery, Left
	  *See M External Carotid Artery,
	  Right*
	P Vertebral Artery, Right
	  Anterior spinal artery
	  Posterior spinal artery
	Q Vertebral Artery, Left
	  See P Vertebral Artery, Right
		3 Percutaneous	**Z No Device**	**7 Stent Retriever**
				Z No Qualifier

0 Medical and Surgical
3 Upper Arteries
F Fragmentation   Definition: Breaking solid matter in a body part into pieces

Explanation: Physical force (e.g., manual, ultrasonic) applied directly or indirectly is used to break the solid matter into pieces. The solid matter may be an abnormal byproduct of a biological function or a foreign body. The pieces of solid matter are not taken out.

Body Part Character 4		Approach Character 5	Device Character 6	Qualifier Character 7

2 Innominate Artery
  Brachiocephalic artery
  Brachiocephalic trunk
3 Subclavian Artery, Right
  Costocervical trunk
  Dorsal scapular artery
  Internal thoracic artery
4 Subclavian Artery, Left
  See 3 Subclavian Artery, Right
5 Axillary Artery, Right
  Anterior circumflex humeral
    artery
  Lateral thoracic artery
  Posterior circumflex humeral
    artery
  Subscapular artery
  Superior thoracic artery
  Thoracoacromial artery
6 Axillary Artery, Left
  See 5 Axillary Artery, Right
7 Brachial Artery, Right
  Inferior ulnar collateral artery
  Profunda brachii
  Superior ulnar collateral artery
8 Brachial Artery, Left
  See 7 Brachial Artery, Right
	9 Ulnar Artery, Right
	  Anterior ulnar recurrent artery
	  Common interosseous artery
	  Posterior ulnar recurrent artery
	A Ulnar Artery, Left
	  See 9 Ulnar Artery, Right
	B Radial Artery, Right
	  Radial recurrent artery
	C Radial Artery, Left
	  See B Radial Artery, Right
	G Intracranial Artery
	  Anterior cerebral artery
	  Anterior choroidal artery
	  Anterior communicating artery
	  Basilar artery
	  Circle of Willis
	  Internal carotid artery,
	    intracranial portion
	  Middle cerebral artery
	  Ophthalmic artery
	  Posterior cerebral artery
	  Posterior communicating
	    artery
	  Posterior inferior cerebellar
	    artery (PICA)
	Y Upper Artery
	  Aortic intercostal artery
	  Bronchial artery
	  Esophageal artery
	  Subcostal artery
		3 Percutaneous	**Z No Device**	**0 Ultrasonic**
				Z No Qualifier

0   **Medical and Surgical**
3   **Upper Arteries**
H   **Insertion**   Definition: Putting in a nonbiological appliance that monitors, assists, performs, or prevents a physiological function but does not physically take the place of a body part
         Explanation: None

Body Part Character 4		Approach Character 5	Device Character 6	Qualifier Character 7
0 Internal Mammary Artery, Right Anterior intercostal artery Internal thoracic artery Musculophrenic artery Pericardiophrenic artery Superior epigastric artery **1 Internal Mammary Artery, Left** *See 0 Internal Mammary Artery, Right* **2 Innominate Artery** Brachiocephalic artery Brachiocephalic trunk **3 Subclavian Artery, Right** Costocervical trunk Dorsal scapular artery Internal thoracic artery **4 Subclavian Artery, Left** *See 3 Subclavian Artery, Right* **5 Axillary Artery, Right** Anterior circumflex humeral artery Lateral thoracic artery Posterior circumflex humeral artery Subscapular artery Superior thoracic artery Thoracoacromial artery **6 Axillary Artery, Left** *See 5 Axillary Artery, Right* **7 Brachial Artery, Right** Inferior ulnar collateral artery Profunda brachii Superior ulnar collateral artery **8 Brachial Artery, Left** *See 7 Brachial Artery, Right* **9 Ulnar Artery, Right** Anterior ulnar recurrent artery Common interosseous artery Posterior ulnar recurrent artery **A Ulnar Artery, Left** *See 9 Ulnar Artery, Right* **B Radial Artery, Right** Radial recurrent artery **C Radial Artery, Left** *See B Radial Artery, Right* **D Hand Artery, Right** Deep palmar arch Princeps pollicis artery Radialis indicis Superficial palmar arch **F Hand Artery, Left** *See D Hand Artery, Right*	**G Intracranial Artery** Anterior cerebral artery Anterior choroidal artery Anterior communicating artery Basilar artery Circle of Willis Internal carotid artery, intracranial portion Middle cerebral artery Ophthalmic artery Posterior cerebral artery Posterior communicating artery Posterior inferior cerebellar artery (PICA) **H Common Carotid Artery, Right** **J Common Carotid Artery, Left** **M External Carotid Artery, Right** Ascending pharyngeal artery Internal maxillary artery Lingual artery Maxillary artery Occipital artery Posterior auricular artery Superior thyroid artery **N External Carotid Artery, Left** *See M External Carotid Artery, Right* **P Vertebral Artery, Right** Anterior spinal artery Posterior spinal artery **Q Vertebral Artery, Left** *See P Vertebral Artery, Right* **R Face Artery** Angular artery Ascending palatine artery External maxillary artery Facial artery Inferior labial artery Submental artery Superior labial artery **S Temporal Artery, Right** Middle temporal artery Superficial temporal artery Transverse facial artery **T Temporal Artery, Left** *See S Temporal Artery, Right* **U Thyroid Artery, Right** Cricothyroid artery Hyoid artery Sternocleidomastoid artery Superior laryngeal artery Superior thyroid artery Thyrocervical trunk **V Thyroid Artery, Left** *See U Thyroid Artery, Right*	**0** Open **3** Percutaneous **4** Percutaneous Endoscopic	**3** Infusion Device **D** Intraluminal Device	**Z** No Qualifier
K Internal Carotid Artery, Right Caroticotympanic artery Carotid sinus **L Internal Carotid Artery, Left** *See K Internal Carotid Artery, Right*		**0** Open **3** Percutaneous **4** Percutaneous Endoscope	**3** Infusion Device **D** Intraluminal Device **M** Stimulator Lead	**Z** No Qualifier
Y Upper Artery Aortic intercostal artery Bronchial artery Esophageal artery Subcostal artery		**0** Open **3** Percutaneous **4** Percutaneous Endoscopic	**2** Monitoring Device **3** Infusion Device **D** Intraluminal Device **Y** Other Device	**Z** No Qualifier

Non-OR	03H[0,1,2,3,4,5,6,7,8,9,A,B,C,D,F,G,H,J,M,N,P,Q,R,S,T,U,V][0,3,4]3Z
Non-OR	03H[K,L][0,3,4]3Z
Non-OR	03HY[0,3,4]3Z
Non-OR	03HY32Z
Non-OR	03HY[3,4]YZ

NC Noncovered Procedure   LC Limited Coverage   QA Questionable OB Admit   NT New Tech Add-on   ⊞ Combination Member   ♂ Male   ♀ Female

ICD-10-PCS 2023   207   03H–03H

Ø   Medical and Surgical
3   Upper Arteries
J   Inspection   Definition: Visually and/or manually exploring a body part

Explanation: Visual exploration may be performed with or without optical instrumentation. Manual exploration may be performed directly or through intervening body layers.

Body Part Character 4	Approach Character 5	Device Character 6	Qualifier Character 7

Y   Upper Artery
    Aortic intercostal artery
    Bronchial artery
    Esophageal artery
    Subcostal artery
	Ø Open
	3 Percutaneous
	4 Percutaneous Endoscopic
	X External
		Z No Device	Z No Qualifier

Non-OR   Ø3JY[3,4,X]ZZ

Ø Medical and Surgical
3 Upper Arteries
L Occlusion   Definition: Completely closing an orifice or the lumen of a tubular body part
                 Explanation: The orifice can be a natural orifice or an artificially created orifice

Body Part Character 4		Approach Character 5	Device Character 6	Qualifier Character 7
Ø Internal Mammary Artery, Right Anterior intercostal artery Internal thoracic artery Musculophrenic artery Pericardiophrenic artery Superior epigastric artery **1 Internal Mammary Artery, Left** *See Ø Internal Mammary Artery, Left* **2 Innominate Artery** Brachiocephalic artery Brachiocephalic trunk **3 Subclavian Artery, Right** Costocervical trunk Dorsal scapular artery Internal thoracic artery **4 Subclavian Artery, Left** *See 3 Subclavian Artery, Right* **5 Axillary Artery, Right** Anterior circumflex humeral artery Lateral thoracic artery Posterior circumflex humeral artery Subscapular artery Superior thoracic artery Thoracoacromial artery **6 Axillary Artery, Left** *See 5 Axillary Artery, Right* **7 Brachial Artery, Right** Inferior ulnar collateral artery Profunda brachii Superior ulnar collateral artery **8 Brachial Artery, Left** *See 7 Brachial Artery, Right* **9 Ulnar Artery, Right** Anterior ulnar recurrent artery Common interosseous artery Posterior ulnar recurrent artery	**A Ulnar Artery, Left** *See 9 Ulnar Artery, Right* **B Radial Artery, Right** Radial recurrent artery **C Radial Artery, Left** *See B Radial Artery, Right* **D Hand Artery, Right** Deep palmar arch Princeps pollicis artery Radialis indicis Superficial palmar arch **F Hand Artery, Left** *See D Hand Artery, Right* **R Face Artery** Angular artery Ascending palatine artery External maxillary artery Facial artery Inferior labial artery Submental artery Superior labial artery **S Temporal Artery, Right** Middle temporal artery Superficial temporal artery Transverse facial artery **T Temporal Artery, Left** *See S Temporal Artery, Right* **U Thyroid Artery, Right** Cricothyroid artery Hyoid artery Sternocleidomastoid artery Superior laryngeal artery Superior thyroid artery Thyrocervical trunk **V Thyroid Artery, Left** *See U Thyroid Artery, Right* **Y Upper Artery** Aortic intercostal artery Bronchial artery Esophageal artery Subcostal artery	**Ø Open** **3 Percutaneous** **4 Percutaneous Endoscopic**	**C Extraluminal Device** **D Intraluminal Device** **Z No Device**	**Z No Qualifier**
G Intracranial Artery Anterior cerebral artery Anterior choroidal artery Anterior communicating artery Basilar artery Circle of Willis Internal carotid artery, intracranial portion Middle cerebral artery Ophthalmic artery Posterior cerebral artery Posterior communicating artery Posterior inferior cerebellar artery (PICA) **H Common Carotid Artery, Right** **J Common Carotid Artery, Left** **K Internal Carotid Artery, Right** Caroticotympanic artery Carotid sinus	**L Internal Carotid Artery, Left** *See K Internal Carotid Artery, Right* **M External Carotid Artery, Right** Ascending pharyngeal artery Internal maxillary artery Lingual artery Maxillary artery Occipital artery Posterior auricular artery Superior thyroid artery **N External Carotid Artery, Left** *See M External Carotid Artery, Right* **P Vertebral Artery, Right** Anterior spinal artery Posterior spinal artery **Q Vertebral Artery, Left** *See P Vertebral Artery, Right*	**Ø Open** **3 Percutaneous** **4 Percutaneous Endoscopic**	**B Intraluminal Device, Bioactive** **C Extraluminal Device** **D Intraluminal Device** **Z No Device**	**Z No Qualifier**

NC Noncovered Procedure   **LC** Limited Coverage   **QA** Questionable OB Admit   **NT** New Tech Add-on   ⊞ Combination Member   ♂ Male   ♀ Female

ICD-10-PCS 2023   **209**

03L–03L

Upper Arteries

Ø	Medical and Surgical
3	Upper Arteries
N	Release

Definition: Freeing a body part from an abnormal physical constraint by cutting or by the use of force

Explanation: Some of the restraining tissue may be taken out but none of the body part is taken out

Body Part Character 4		Approach Character 5	Device Character 6	Qualifier Character 7
Ø **Internal Mammary Artery, Right** Anterior intercostal artery Internal thoracic artery Musculophrenic artery Pericardiophrenic artery Superior epigastric artery 1 **Internal Mammary Artery, Left** *See Ø Internal Mammary Artery, Right* 2 **Innominate Artery** Brachiocephalic artery Brachiocephalic trunk 3 **Subclavian Artery, Right** Costocervical trunk Dorsal scapular artery Internal thoracic artery 4 **Subclavian Artery, Left** *See 3 Subclavian Artery, Right* 5 **Axillary Artery, Right** Anterior circumflex humeral artery Lateral thoracic artery Posterior circumflex humeral artery Subscapular artery Superior thoracic artery Thoracoacromial artery 6 **Axillary Artery, Left** *See 5 Axillary Artery, Right* 7 **Brachial Artery, Right** Inferior ulnar collateral artery Profunda brachii Superior ulnar collateral artery 8 **Brachial Artery, Left** *See 7 Brachial Artery, Right* 9 **Ulnar Artery, Right** Anterior ulnar recurrent artery Common interosseous artery Posterior ulnar recurrent artery A **Ulnar Artery, Left** *See 9 Ulnar Artery, Right* B **Radial Artery, Right** Radial recurrent artery C **Radial Artery, Left** *See B Radial Artery, Right* D **Hand Artery, Right** Deep palmar arch Princeps pollicis artery Radialis indicis Superficial palmar arch F **Hand Artery, Left** *See D Hand Artery, Right* G **Intracranial Artery** Anterior cerebral artery Anterior choroidal artery Anterior communicating artery Basilar artery Circle of Willis Internal carotid artery, intracranial portion Middle cerebral artery Ophthalmic artery Posterior cerebral artery Posterior communicating artery Posterior inferior cerebellar artery (PICA)	H **Common Carotid Artery, Right** J **Common Carotid Artery, Left** K **Internal Carotid Artery, Right** Caroticotympanic artery Carotid sinus L **Internal Carotid Artery, Left** *See K Internal Carotid Artery, Right* M **External Carotid Artery, Right** Ascending pharyngeal artery Internal maxillary artery Lingual artery Maxillary artery Occipital artery Posterior auricular artery Superior thyroid artery N **External Carotid Artery, Left** *See M External Carotid Artery, Right* P **Vertebral Artery, Right** Anterior spinal artery Posterior spinal artery Q **Vertebral Artery, Left** *See P Vertebral Artery, Right* R **Face Artery** Angular artery Ascending palatine artery External maxillary artery Facial artery Inferior labial artery Submental artery Superior labial artery S **Temporal Artery, Right** Middle temporal artery Superficial temporal artery Transverse facial artery T **Temporal Artery, Left** *See S Temporal Artery, Right* U **Thyroid Artery, Right** Cricothyroid artery Hyoid artery Sternocleidomastoid artery Superior laryngeal artery Superior thyroid artery Thyrocervical trunk V **Thyroid Artery, Left** *See U Thyroid Artery, Right* Y **Upper Artery** Aortic intercostal artery Bronchial artery Esophageal artery Subcostal artery	Ø Open 3 Percutaneous 4 Percutaneous Endoscopic	Z No Device	Z No Qualifier

Non-OR Procedure　　DRG Non-OR Procedure　　Valid OR Procedure　　HAC Associated Procedure　　Combination Only　　New/Revised April　　New/Revised October

210　　ICD-10-PCS 2023

Ø	**Medical and Surgical**
3	**Upper Arteries**
P	**Removal** Definition: Taking out or off a device from a body part

Explanation: If a device is taken out and a similar device put in without cutting or puncturing the skin or mucous membrane, the procedure is coded to the root operation CHANGE. Otherwise, the procedure for taking out a device is coded to the root operation REMOVAL.

Body Part Character 4	Approach Character 5	Device Character 6	Qualifier Character 7

Y   Upper Artery
    Aortic intercostal artery
    Bronchial artery
    Esophageal artery
    Subcostal artery
	Ø Open
	3 Percutaneous
	4 Percutaneous Endoscopic
		Ø Drainage Device
		2 Monitoring Device
		3 Infusion Device
		7 Autologous Tissue Substitute
		C Extraluminal Device
		D Intraluminal Device
		J Synthetic Substitute
		K Nonautologous Tissue Substitute
		M Stimulator Lead
		Y Other Device
			Z No Qualifier

Y   Upper Artery
    Aortic intercostal artery
    Bronchial artery
    Esophageal artery
    Subcostal artery
	X External	Ø Drainage Device
		2 Monitoring Device
		3 Infusion Device
		D Intraluminal Device
		M Stimulator Lead
			Z No Qualifier

Non-OR	Ø3PY3[Ø,2,3,D]Z
Non-OR	Ø3PY[3,4]YZ
Non-OR	Ø3PYX[Ø,2,3,D,M]Z

Upper Arteries

Ø Medical and Surgical
3 Upper Arteries
Q Repair   Definition: Restoring, to the extent possible, a body part to its normal anatomic structure and function
           Explanation: Used only when the method to accomplish the repair is not one of the other root operations

Body Part Character 4		Approach Character 5	Device Character 6	Qualifier Character 7
Ø Internal Mammary Artery, Right Anterior intercostal artery Internal thoracic artery Musculophrenic artery Pericardiophrenic artery Superior epigastric artery **1 Internal Mammary Artery, Left** *See Ø Internal Mammary Artery, Right* **2 Innominate Artery** Brachiocephalic artery Brachiocephalic trunk **3 Subclavian Artery, Right** Costocervical trunk Dorsal scapular artery Internal thoracic artery **4 Subclavian Artery, Left** *See 3 Subclavian Artery, Right* **5 Axillary Artery, Right** Anterior circumflex humeral artery Lateral thoracic artery Posterior circumflex humeral artery Subscapular artery Superior thoracic artery Thoracoacromial artery **6 Axillary Artery, Left** *See 5 Axillary Artery, Right* **7 Brachial Artery, Right** Inferior ulnar collateral artery Profunda brachii Superior ulnar collateral artery **8 Brachial Artery, Left** *See 7 Brachial Artery, Right* **9 Ulnar Artery, Right** Anterior ulnar recurrent artery Common interosseous artery Posterior ulnar recurrent artery **A Ulnar Artery, Left** *See 9 Ulnar Artery, Right* **B Radial Artery, Right** Radial recurrent artery **C Radial Artery, Left** *See B Radial Artery, Right* **D Hand Artery, Right** Deep palmar arch Princeps pollicis artery Radialis indicis Superficial palmar arch **F Hand Artery, Left** *See D Hand Artery, Right* **G Intracranial Artery** Anterior cerebral artery Anterior choroidal artery Anterior communicating artery Basilar artery Circle of Willis Internal carotid artery, intracranial portion Middle cerebral artery Ophthalmic artery Posterior cerebral artery Posterior communicating artery Posterior inferior cerebellar artery (PICA)	**H Common Carotid Artery, Right** **J Common Carotid Artery, Left** **K Internal Carotid Artery, Right** Caroticotympanic artery Carotid sinus **L Internal Carotid Artery, Left** *See K Internal Carotid Artery, Right* **M External Carotid Artery, Right** Ascending pharyngeal artery Internal maxillary artery Lingual artery Maxillary artery Occipital artery Posterior auricular artery Superior thyroid artery **N External Carotid Artery, Left** *See M External Carotid Artery, Right* **P Vertebral Artery, Right** Anterior spinal artery Posterior spinal artery **Q Vertebral Artery, Left** *See P Vertebral Artery, Right* **R Face Artery** Angular artery Ascending palatine artery External maxillary artery Facial artery Inferior labial artery Submental artery Superior labial artery **S Temporal Artery, Right** Middle temporal artery Superficial temporal artery Transverse facial artery **T Temporal Artery, Left** *See S Temporal Artery, Right* **U Thyroid Artery, Right** Cricothyroid artery Hyoid artery Sternocleidomastoid artery Superior laryngeal artery Superior thyroid artery Thyrocervical trunk **V Thyroid Artery, Left** *See U Thyroid Artery, Right* **Y Upper Artery** Aortic intercostal artery Bronchial artery Esophageal artery Subcostal artery	**Ø Open** **3 Percutaneous** **4 Percutaneous Endoscopic**	**Z No Device**	**Z No Qualifier**

Non-OR Procedure   DRG Non-OR Procedure   Valid OR Procedure   HAC Associated Procedure   Combination Only   New/Revised April   New/Revised October

212   ICD-10-PCS 2023

Ø　**Medical and Surgical**
3　**Upper Arteries**
R　**Replacement**　　Definition: Putting in or on biological or synthetic material that physically takes the place and/or function of all or a portion of a body part
　　　　　　　　　　Explanation: The body part may have been taken out or replaced, or may be taken out, physically eradicated, or rendered nonfunctional during
　　　　　　　　　　the REPLACEMENT procedure. A REMOVAL procedure is coded for taking out the device used in a previous replacement procedure.

Body Part Character 4		Approach Character 5	Device Character 6	Qualifier Character 7
Ø **Internal Mammary Artery, Right** 　Anterior intercostal artery 　Internal thoracic artery 　Musculophrenic artery 　Pericardiophrenic artery 　Superior epigastric artery **1** **Internal Mammary Artery, Left** 　*See Ø Internal Mammary Artery, Right* **2** **Innominate Artery** 　Brachiocephalic artery 　Brachiocephalic trunk **3** **Subclavian Artery, Right** 　Costocervical trunk 　Dorsal scapular artery 　Internal thoracic artery **4** **Subclavian Artery, Left** 　*See 3 Subclavian Artery, Right* **5** **Axillary Artery, Right** 　Anterior circumflex humeral artery 　Lateral thoracic artery 　Posterior circumflex humeral artery 　Subscapular artery 　Superior thoracic artery 　Thoracoacromial artery **6** **Axillary Artery, Left** 　*See 5 Axillary Artery, Right* **7** **Brachial Artery, Right** 　Inferior ulnar collateral artery 　Profunda brachii 　Superior ulnar collateral artery **8** **Brachial Artery, Left** 　*See 7 Brachial Artery, Right* **9** **Ulnar Artery, Right** 　Anterior ulnar recurrent artery 　Common interosseous artery 　Posterior ulnar recurrent artery **A** **Ulnar Artery, Left** 　*See 9 Ulnar Artery, Right* **B** **Radial Artery, Right** 　Radial recurrent artery **C** **Radial Artery, Left** 　*See B Radial Artery, Right* **D** **Hand Artery, Right** 　Deep palmar arch 　Princeps pollicis artery 　Radialis indicis 　Superficial palmar arch **F** **Hand Artery, Left** 　*See D Hand Artery, Right* **G** **Intracranial Artery** 　Anterior cerebral artery 　Anterior choroidal artery 　Anterior communicating artery 　Basilar artery 　Circle of Willis 　Internal carotid artery, intracranial portion 　Middle cerebral artery 　Ophthalmic artery 　Posterior cerebral artery 　Posterior communicating artery 　Posterior inferior cerebellar artery (PICA)	**H** **Common Carotid Artery, Right** **J** **Common Carotid Artery, Left** **K** **Internal Carotid Artery, Right** 　Caroticotympanic artery 　Carotid sinus **L** **Internal Carotid Artery, Left** 　*See K Internal Carotid Artery, Right* **M** **External Carotid Artery, Right** 　Ascending pharyngeal artery 　Internal maxillary artery 　Lingual artery 　Maxillary artery 　Occipital artery 　Posterior auricular artery 　Superior thyroid artery **N** **External Carotid Artery, Left** 　*See M External Carotid Artery, Right* **P** **Vertebral Artery, Right** 　Anterior spinal artery 　Posterior spinal artery **Q** **Vertebral Artery, Left** 　*See P Vertebral Artery, Right* **R** **Face Artery** 　Angular artery 　Ascending palatine artery 　External maxillary artery 　Facial artery 　Inferior labial artery 　Submental artery 　Superior labial artery **S** **Temporal Artery, Right** 　Middle temporal artery 　Superficial temporal artery 　Transverse facial artery **T** **Temporal Artery, Left** 　*See S Temporal Artery, Right* **U** **Thyroid Artery, Right** 　Cricothyroid artery 　Hyoid artery 　Sternocleidomastoid artery 　Superior laryngeal artery 　Superior thyroid artery 　Thyrocervical trunk **V** **Thyroid Artery, Left** 　*See U Thyroid Artery, Right* **Y** **Upper Artery** 　Aortic intercostal artery 　Bronchial artery 　Esophageal artery 　Subcostal artery	**Ø** Open **4** Percutaneous Endoscopic	**7** Autologous Tissue Substitute **J** Synthetic Substitute **K** Nonautologous Tissue Substitute	**Z** No Qualifier

NC Noncovered Procedure　　LC Limited Coverage　　QA Questionable OB Admit　　NT New Tech Add-on　　⊞ Combination Member　　♂ Male　　♀ Female

ICD-10-PCS 2023　　**213**

Ø3R–Ø3R

Upper Arteries

Ø Medical and Surgical
3 Upper Arteries
S Reposition   Definition: Moving to its normal location, or other suitable location, all or a portion of a body part

Explanation: The body part is moved to a new location from an abnormal location, or from a normal location where it is not functioning correctly. The body part may or may not be cut out or off to be moved to the new location.

Body Part Character 4		Approach Character 5	Device Character 6	Qualifier Character 7

Ø **Internal Mammary Artery, Right**
  Anterior intercostal artery
  Internal thoracic artery
  Musculophrenic artery
  Pericardiophrenic artery
  Superior epigastric artery
1 **Internal Mammary Artery, Left**
  See Ø Internal Mammary Artery, Right
2 **Innominate Artery**
  Brachiocephalic artery
  Brachiocephalic trunk
3 **Subclavian Artery, Right**
  Costocervical trunk
  Dorsal scapular artery
  Internal thoracic artery
4 **Subclavian Artery, Left**
  See 3 Subclavian Artery, Right
5 **Axillary Artery, Right**
  Anterior circumflex humeral artery
  Lateral thoracic artery
  Posterior circumflex humeral artery
  Subscapular artery
  Superior thoracic artery
  Thoracoacromial artery
6 **Axillary Artery, Left**
  See 5 Axillary Artery, Right
7 **Brachial Artery, Right**
  Inferior ulnar collateral artery
  Profunda brachii
  Superior ulnar collateral artery
8 **Brachial Artery, Left**
  See 7 Brachial Artery, Right
9 **Ulnar Artery, Right**
  Anterior ulnar recurrent artery
  Common interosseous artery
  Posterior ulnar recurrent artery
A **Ulnar Artery, Left**
  See 9 Ulnar Artery, Right
B **Radial Artery, Right**
  Radial recurrent artery
C **Radial Artery, Left**
  See B Radial Artery, Right
D **Hand Artery, Right**
  Deep palmar arch
  Princeps pollicis artery
  Radialis indicis
  Superficial palmar arch
F **Hand Artery, Left**
  See D Hand Artery, Right
G **Intracranial Artery**
  Anterior cerebral artery
  Anterior choroidal artery
  Anterior communicating artery
  Basilar artery
  Circle of Willis
  Internal carotid artery, intracranial portion
  Middle cerebral artery
  Ophthalmic artery
  Posterior cerebral artery
  Posterior communicating artery
  Posterior inferior cerebellar artery (PICA)
	H **Common Carotid Artery, Right**
	J **Common Carotid Artery, Left**
	K **Internal Carotid Artery, Right**
	  Caroticotympanic artery
	  Carotid sinus
	L **Internal Carotid Artery, Left**
	  See K Internal Carotid Artery, Right
	M **External Carotid Artery, Right**
	  Ascending pharyngeal artery
	  Internal maxillary artery
	  Lingual artery
	  Maxillary artery
	  Occipital artery
	  Posterior auricular artery
	  Superior thyroid artery
	N **External Carotid Artery, Left**
	  See M External Carotid Artery, Right
	P **Vertebral Artery, Right**
	  Anterior spinal artery
	  Posterior spinal artery
	Q **Vertebral Artery, Left**
	  See P Vertebral Artery, Right
	R **Face Artery**
	  Angular artery
	  Ascending palatine artery
	  External maxillary artery
	  Facial artery
	  Inferior labial artery
	  Submental artery
	  Superior labial artery
	S **Temporal Artery, Right**
	  Middle temporal artery
	  Superficial temporal artery
	  Transverse facial artery
	T **Temporal Artery, Left**
	  See S Temporal Artery, Right
	U **Thyroid Artery, Right**
	  Cricothyroid artery
	  Hyoid artery
	  Sternocleidomastoid artery
	  Superior laryngeal artery
	  Superior thyroid artery
	  Thyrocervical trunk
	V **Thyroid Artery, Left**
	  See U Thyroid Artery, Right
	Y **Upper Artery**
	  Aortic intercostal artery
	  Bronchial artery
	  Esophageal artery
	  Subcostal artery
		Ø Open
		3 Percutaneous
		4 Percutaneous Endoscopic
			Z No Device	**Z** No Qualifier

Non-OR Procedure   DRG Non-OR Procedure   Valid OR Procedure   HAC Associated Procedure   Combination Only   New/Revised April   New/Revised October

214   ICD-10-PCS 2023

0   **Medical and Surgical**
3   **Upper Arteries**
U   **Supplement**   Definition: Putting in or on biological or synthetic material that physically reinforces and/or augments the function of a portion of a body part

Explanation: The biological material is non-living, or is living and from the same individual. The body part may have been previously replaced, and the SUPPLEMENT procedure is performed to physically reinforce and/or augment the function of the replaced body part.

Body Part Character 4		Approach Character 5	Device Character 6	Qualifier Character 7
0 **Internal Mammary Artery, Right** Anterior intercostal artery Internal thoracic artery Musculophrenic artery Pericardiophrenic artery Superior epigastric artery **1** **Internal Mammary Artery, Left** *See 0 Internal Mammary Artery, Right* **2** **Innominate Artery** Brachiocephalic artery Brachiocephalic trunk **3** **Subclavian Artery, Right** Costocervical trunk Dorsal scapular artery Internal thoracic artery **4** **Subclavian Artery, Left** *See 3 Subclavian Artery, Right* **5** **Axillary Artery, Right** Anterior circumflex humeral artery Lateral thoracic artery Posterior circumflex humeral artery Subscapular artery Superior thoracic artery Thoracoacromial artery **6** **Axillary Artery, Left** *See 5 Axillary Artery, Right* **7** **Brachial Artery, Right** Inferior ulnar collateral artery Profunda brachii Superior ulnar collateral artery **8** **Brachial Artery, Left** *See 7 Brachial Artery, Right* **9** **Ulnar Artery, Right** Anterior ulnar recurrent artery Common interosseous artery Posterior ulnar recurrent artery **A** **Ulnar Artery, Left** *See 9 Ulnar Artery, Right* **B** **Radial Artery, Right** Radial recurrent artery **C** **Radial Artery, Left** *See B Radial Artery, Right* **D** **Hand Artery, Right** Deep palmar arch Princeps pollicis artery Radialis indicis Superficial palmar arch **F** **Hand Artery, Left** *See D Hand Artery, Right* **G** **Intracranial Artery** Anterior cerebral artery Anterior choroidal artery Anterior communicating artery Basilar artery Circle of Willis Internal carotid artery, intracranial portion Middle cerebral artery Ophthalmic artery Posterior cerebral artery Posterior communicating artery Posterior inferior cerebellar artery (PICA)	**H** **Common Carotid Artery, Right** **J** **Common Carotid Artery, Left** **K** **Internal Carotid Artery, Right** Caroticotympanic artery Carotid sinus **L** **Internal Carotid Artery, Left** *See K Internal Carotid Artery, Right* **M** **External Carotid Artery, Right** Ascending pharyngeal artery Internal maxillary artery Lingual artery Maxillary artery Occipital artery Posterior auricular artery Superior thyroid artery **N** **External Carotid Artery, Left** *See M External Carotid Artery, Right* **P** **Vertebral Artery, Right** Anterior spinal artery Posterior spinal artery **Q** **Vertebral Artery, Left** *See P Vertebral Artery, Right* **R** **Face Artery** Angular artery Ascending palatine artery External maxillary artery Facial artery Inferior labial artery Submental artery Superior labial artery **S** **Temporal Artery, Right** Middle temporal artery Superficial temporal artery Transverse facial artery **T** **Temporal Artery, Left** *See S Temporal Artery, Right* **U** **Thyroid Artery, Right** Cricothyroid artery Hyoid artery Sternocleidomastoid artery Superior laryngeal artery Superior thyroid artery Thyrocervical trunk **V** **Thyroid Artery, Left** *See U Thyroid Artery, Right* **Y** **Upper Artery** Aortic intercostal artery Bronchial artery Esophageal artery Subcostal artery	**0** Open **3** Percutaneous **4** Percutaneous Endoscopic	**7** Autologous Tissue Substitute **J** Synthetic Substitute **K** Nonautologous Tissue Substitute	**Z** No Qualifier

NC Noncovered Procedure   **LC** Limited Coverage   **QA** Questionable OB Admit   **NT** New Tech Add-on   ⊞ Combination Member   ♂ Male   ♀ Female

ICD-10-PCS 2023   **215**

03U–03U

Upper Arteries

0   **Medical and Surgical**
3   **Upper Arteries**
V   **Restriction**   Definition: Partially closing an orifice or the lumen of a tubular body part
           Explanation: The orifice can be a natural orifice or an artificially created orifice

Body Part Character 4		Approach Character 5	Device Character 6	Qualifier Character 7

0 Internal Mammary Artery, Right
  Anterior intercostal artery
  Internal thoracic artery
  Musculophrenic artery
  Pericardiophrenic artery
  Superior epigastric artery
1 Internal Mammary Artery, Left
  See 0 Internal Mammary Artery,
    Right
2 Innominate Artery
  Brachiocephalic artery
  Brachiocephalic trunk
3 Subclavian Artery, Right
  Costocervical trunk
  Dorsal scapular artery
  Internal thoracic artery
4 Subclavian Artery, Left
  See 3 Subclavian Artery, Right
5 Axillary Artery, Right
  Anterior circumflex humeral artery
  Lateral thoracic artery
  Posterior circumflex humeral artery
  Subscapular artery
  Superior thoracic artery
  Thoracoacromial artery
6 Axillary Artery, Left
  See 5 Axillary Artery, Right
7 Brachial Artery, Right
  Inferior ulnar collateral artery
  Profunda brachii
  Superior ulnar collateral artery
8 Brachial Artery, Left
  See 7 Brachial Artery, Right
9 Ulnar Artery, Right
  Anterior ulnar recurrent artery
  Common interosseous artery
  Posterior ulnar recurrent artery
A Ulnar Artery, Left
  See 9 Ulnar Artery, Right
	B Radial Artery, Right
	  Radial recurrent artery
	C Radial Artery, Left
	  See B Radial Artery, Right
	D Hand Artery, Right
	  Deep palmar arch
	  Princeps pollicis artery
	  Radialis indicis
	  Superficial palmar arch
	F Hand Artery, Left
	  See D Hand Artery, Right
	R Face Artery
	  Angular artery
	  Ascending palatine artery
	  External maxillary artery
	  Facial artery
	  Inferior labial artery
	  Submental artery
	  Superior labial artery
	S Temporal Artery, Right
	  Middle temporal artery
	  Superficial temporal artery
	  Transverse facial artery
	T Temporal Artery, Left
	  See S Temporal Artery, Right
	U Thyroid Artery, Right
	  Cricothyroid artery
	  Hyoid artery
	  Sternocleidomastoid artery
	  Superior laryngeal artery
	  Superior thyroid artery
	  Thyrocervical trunk
	V Thyroid Artery, Left
	  See U Thyroid Artery, Right
	Y Upper Artery
	  Aortic intercostal artery
	  Bronchial artery
	  Esophageal artery
	  Subcostal artery
		0 Open
		3 Percutaneous
		4 Percutaneous
		  Endoscopic
			C Extraluminal Device
			D Intraluminal Device
			Z No Device
				Z No Qualifier

G Intracranial Artery
  Anterior cerebral artery
  Anterior choroidal artery
  Anterior communicating artery
  Basilar artery
  Circle of Willis
  Internal carotid artery,
    intracranial portion
  Middle cerebral artery
  Ophthalmic artery
  Posterior cerebral artery
  Posterior communicating artery
  Posterior inferior cerebellar artery
    (PICA)
H Common Carotid Artery, Right
J Common Carotid Artery, Left
K Internal Carotid Artery, Right
  Caroticotympanic artery
  Carotid sinus
	L Internal Carotid Artery, Left
	  See K Internal Carotid Artery, Right
	M External Carotid Artery, Right
	  Ascending pharyngeal artery
	  Internal maxillary artery
	  Lingual artery
	  Maxillary artery
	  Occipital artery
	  Posterior auricular artery
	  Superior thyroid artery
	N External Carotid Artery, Left
	  See M External Carotid Artery, Right
	P Vertebral Artery, Right
	  Anterior spinal artery
	  Posterior spinal artery
	Q Vertebral Artery, Left
	  See P Vertebral Artery, Right
		0 Open
		3 Percutaneous
		4 Percutaneous
		  Endoscopic
			B Intraluminal Device,
			  Bioactive
			C Extraluminal Device
			D Intraluminal Device
			H Intraluminal Device,
			  Flow Diverter
			Z No Device
				Z No Qualifier

Non-OR Procedure   DRG Non-OR Procedure   Valid OR Procedure   HAC Associated Procedure   Combination Only   New/Revised April   New/Revised October

216   ICD-10-PCS 2023

0   **Medical and Surgical**
3   **Upper Arteries**
W   **Revision**   Definition: Correcting, to the extent possible, a portion of a malfunctioning device or the position of a displaced device

Explanation: Revision can include correcting a malfunctioning or displaced device by taking out or putting in components of the device such as a screw or pin

Body Part Character 4	Approach Character 5	Device Character 6	Qualifier Character 7

Y   Upper Artery
     Aortic intercostal artery
     Bronchial artery
     Esophageal artery
     Subcostal artery
	0 Open
	3 Percutaneous
	4 Percutaneous Endoscopic
		0 Drainage Device
		2 Monitoring Device
		3 Infusion Device
		7 Autologous Tissue Substitute
		C Extraluminal Device
		D Intraluminal Device
		J Synthetic Substitute
		K Nonautologous Tissue Substitute
		M Stimulator Lead
		Y Other Device
			Z No Qualifier

Y   Upper Artery
     Aortic intercostal artery
     Bronchial artery
     Esophageal artery
     Subcostal artery
	X External	**0** Drainage Device
		2 Monitoring Device
		3 Infusion Device
		7 Autologous Tissue Substitute
		C Extraluminal Device
		D Intraluminal Device
		J Synthetic Substitute
		K Nonautologous Tissue Substitute
		M Stimulator Lead
			Z No Qualifier

Non-OR   03WY3[0,2,3]Z
Non-OR   03WY[3,4]YZ
Non-OR   03WYX[0,2,3,7,C,D,J,K,M]Z

Lower Arteries Ø41–Ø4W

Character Meanings

This Character Meaning table is provided as a guide to assist the user in the identification of character members that may be found in this section of code tables. It **SHOULD NOT** be used to build a PCS code.

Operation–Character 3	Body Part–Character 4	Approach–Character 5	Device–Character 6	Qualifier–Character 7
1 Bypass	Ø Abdominal Aorta	Ø Open	Ø Drainage Device	Ø Abdominal Aorta OR Ultrasonic
5 Destruction	1 Celiac Artery	3 Percutaneous	1 Radioactive Element	1 Celiac Artery OR Drug-Coated Balloon
7 Dilation	2 Gastric Artery	4 Percutaneous Endoscopic	2 Monitoring Device	2 Mesenteric Artery
9 Drainage	3 Hepatic Artery	X External	3 Infusion Device	3 Renal Artery, Right
B Excision	4 Splenic Artery		4 Intraluminal Device, Drug-eluting	4 Renal Artery, Left
C Extirpation	5 Superior Mesenteric Artery		5 Intraluminal Device, Drug-eluting, Two	5 Renal Artery, Bilateral
F Fragmentation	6 Colic Artery, Right		6 Intraluminal Device, Drug-eluting, Three	6 Common Iliac Artery, Right
H Insertion	7 Colic Artery, Left		7 Intraluminal Device, Drug-eluting, Four or More OR Autologous Tissue Substitute	7 Common Iliac Artery, Left
J Inspection	8 Colic Artery, Middle		9 Autologous Venous Tissue	8 Common Iliac Arteries, Bilateral
L Occlusion	9 Renal Artery, Right		A Autologous Arterial Tissue	9 Internal Iliac Artery, Right
N Release	A Renal Artery, Left		C Extraluminal Device	B Internal Iliac Artery, Left
P Removal	B Inferior Mesenteric Artery		D Intraluminal Device	C Internal Iliac Arteries, Bilateral
Q Repair	C Common Iliac Artery, Right		E Intraluminal Device, Two OR Intraluminal Device, Branched or Fenestrated, One or Two Arteries	D External Iliac Artery, Right
R Replacement	D Common Iliac Artery, Left		F Intraluminal Device, Three OR Intraluminal Device, Branched or Fenestrated, Three or More Arteries	F External Iliac Artery, Left
S Reposition	E Internal Iliac Artery, Right		G Intraluminal Device, Four or More	G External Iliac Arteries, Bilateral
U Supplement	F Internal Iliac Artery, Left		J Synthetic Substitute	H Femoral Artery, Right
V Restriction	H External Iliac Artery, Right		K Nonautologous Tissue Substitute	J Femoral Artery, Left OR Temporary
W Revision	J External Iliac Artery, Left		Y Other Device	K Femoral Arteries, Bilateral
	K Femoral Artery, Right		Z No Device	L Popliteal Artery
	L Femoral Artery, Left			M Peroneal Artery
	M Popliteal Artery, Right			N Posterior Tibial Artery
	N Popliteal Artery, Left			P Foot Artery
	P Anterior Tibial Artery, Right			Q Lower Extremity Artery
	Q Anterior Tibial Artery, Left			R Lower Artery
	R Posterior Tibial Artery, Right			S Lower Extremity Vein
	S Posterior Tibial Artery, Left			T Uterine Artery, Right
	T Peroneal Artery, Right			U Uterine Artery, Left
	U Peroneal Artery, Left			V Prostatic Artery, Right
	V Foot Artery, Right			W Prostatic Artery, Left
	W Foot Artery, Left			X Diagnostic
	Y Lower Artery			Z No Qualifier

Lower Arteries

AHA Coding Clinic for Lower Arteries

2022, 1Q, 10-13	Procedures performed on a continuous vessel, ICD-10-PCS Guideline B4.1c

AHA Coding Clinic for table Ø41

2019, 1Q, 23	Endovascular repair of shaggy aorta and deployment of chimney stent grafts
2018, 3Q, 25	Femoral artery to tibioperoneal trunk bypass
2017, 4Q, 46-47	New and revised body part values - Bypass hepatic artery to renal artery
2017, 3Q, 5	Femoral artery to posterior tibial artery bypass using autologous and synthetic grafts
2017, 3Q, 16	Abdominal aortic debranching with bypass of external iliac artery to bilateral renal arteries and superior mesenteric artery
2017, 1Q, 32	Peroneal artery to dorsalis pedis artery bypass using saphenous vein graft
2016, 2Q, 18	Femoral-tibial artery bypass and saphenous vein graft
2015, 3Q, 28	Bilateral renal artery bypass

AHA Coding Clinic for table Ø47

2020, 4Q, 50	Intravascular lithotripsy
2019, 4Q, 27	Bifurcation Qualifier
2019, 2Q, 14	Revision of occluded femoral-popliteal bypass graft
2018, 2Q, 24	Coronary artery bifurcation
2016, 4Q, 86	Peripheral artery, number of stents
2016, 4Q, 86-88	Coronary and peripheral artery bifurcation
2016, 3Q, 39	Infrarenal abdominal aortic aneurysm repair with iliac graft extension
2015, 4Q, 4-7, 15	Drug-coated balloon angioplasty in peripheral vessels
2015, 3Q, 9	Aborted endovascular stenting of superficial femoral artery

AHA Coding Clinic for table Ø4C

2021, 1Q, 15	Iliofemoral endarterectomy and furthest point of entry
2019, 4Q, 27	Bifurcation Qualifier
2019, 1Q, 23	Endovascular repair of shaggy aorta and deployment of chimney stent grafts
2018, 2Q, 24	Coronary artery bifurcation
2017, 2Q, 23	Thrombectomy via Fogarty catheter
2016, 4Q, 86-88	Coronary and peripheral artery bifurcation
2016, 1Q, 31	Iliofemoral endarterectomy with patch repair
2015, 1Q, 29	Discontinued carotid endarterectomy
2015, 1Q, 36	Percutaneous mechanical thrombectomy of femoropopliteal bypass graft

AHA Coding Clinic for table Ø4F

2020, 4Q, 45-49	New fragmentation tables
2020, 4Q, 49-50	Intravascular ultrasound assisted thrombolysis
2020, 4Q, 50-51	Intravascular lithotripsy

AHA Coding Clinic for table Ø4H

2019, 3Q, 20	Removal and revision of ECMO component
2019, 1Q, 23	Endovascular repair of shaggy aorta and deployment of chimney stent grafts
2017, 1Q, 30	Insertion of umbilical artery catheter

AHA Coding Clinic for table Ø4L

2020, 3Q, 43	Staged laparoscopic gastric conduit and placement of feeding tube
2018, 2Q, 18	Transverse rectus abdominis myocutaneous (TRAM) delay
2017, 4Q, 31	Resuscitative endovascular balloon occlusion of the aorta
2015, 2Q, 27	Uterine artery embolization using Gelfoam
2014, 3Q, 26	Coil embolization of gastroduodenal artery with chemoembolization of hepatic artery
2014, 1Q, 24	Endovascular embolization for gastrointestinal bleeding

AHA Coding Clinic for table Ø4N

2015, 2Q, 28	Release and replacement of celiac artery

AHA Coding Clinic for table Ø4P

2019, 3Q, 20	Removal and revision of ECMO component

AHA Coding Clinic for table Ø4Q

2014, 1Q, 21	Repair of femoral artery pseudoaneurysm

AHA Coding Clinic for table Ø4R

2019, 1Q, 22	Abdominal aortic aneurysm repair using tube graft
2015, 2Q, 28	Release and replacement of celiac artery

AHA Coding Clinic for table Ø4U

2019, 1Q, 22	Abdominal aortic aneurysm repair using tube graft
2016, 2Q, 18	Femoral-tibial artery bypass and saphenous vein graft
2016, 1Q, 31	Iliofemoral endarterectomy with patch repair
2014, 4Q, 37	Bovine patch arterioplasty
2014, 1Q, 22	Repair of pseudoaneurysm of femoral-popliteal bypass graft

AHA Coding Clinic for table Ø4V

2021, 3Q, 23	Transcatheter embolization of splenic artery
2019, 4Q, 27	Bifurcation Qualifier
2019, 1Q, 22	Abdominal aortic aneurysm repair using tube graft
2018, 2Q, 24	Coronary artery bifurcation
2016, 4Q, 86-87	Coronary and peripheral artery bifurcation
2016, 4Q, 89-93	Branched and fenestrated endograft repair of aneurysms
2016, 3Q, 39	Infrarenal abdominal aortic aneurysm repair with iliac graft extension
2014, 1Q, 9	Endovascular repair of abdominal aortic aneurysm

AHA Coding Clinic for table Ø4W

2020, 3Q, 5	Types of endoleaks following endovascular aneurysm repair
2019, 2Q, 14	Revision of occluded femoral-popliteal bypass graft
2015, 1Q, 36	Revision of femoropopliteal bypass graft
2014, 1Q, 9	Endovascular repair of endoleak
2014, 1Q, 22	Repair of pseudoaneurysm of femoral-popliteal bypass graft

Lower Arteries

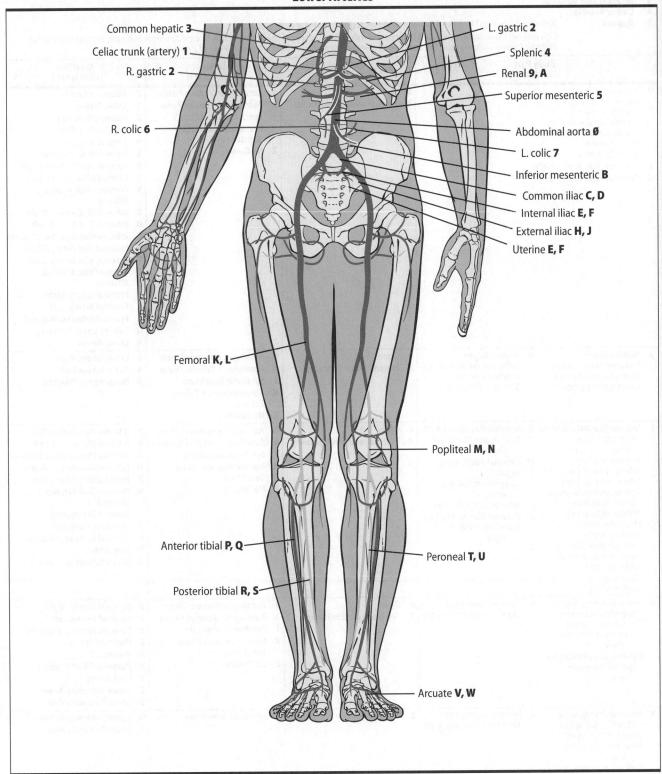

Common hepatic **3**

Celiac trunk (artery) **1**

R. gastric **2**

R. colic **6**

L. gastric **2**

Splenic **4**

Renal **9, A**

Superior mesenteric **5**

Abdominal aorta **Ø**

L. colic **7**

Inferior mesenteric **B**

Common iliac **C, D**

Internal iliac **E, F**

External iliac **H, J**

Uterine **E, F**

Femoral **K, L**

Popliteal **M, N**

Anterior tibial **P, Q**

Peroneal **T, U**

Posterior tibial **R, S**

Arcuate **V, W**

Lower Arteries

Ø	Medical and Surgical
4	Lower Arteries
1	Bypass

Definition: Altering the route of passage of the contents of a tubular body part

Explanation: Rerouting contents of a body part to a downstream area of the normal route, to a similar route and body part, or to an abnormal route and dissimilar body part. Includes one or more anastomoses, with or without the use of a device.

Body Part Character 4		Approach Character 5	Device Character 6	Qualifier Character 7

Ø Abdominal Aorta
   Inferior phrenic artery
   Lumbar artery
   Median sacral artery
   Middle suprarenal artery
   Ovarian artery
   Testicular artery
C Common Iliac Artery, Right
D Common Iliac Artery, Left
		Ø Open
		4 Percutaneous Endoscopic
			9 Autologous Venous Tissue
			A Autologous Arterial Tissue
			J Synthetic Substitute
			K Nonautologous Tissue Substitute
			Z No Device
				Ø Abdominal Aorta
				1 Celiac Artery
				2 Mesenteric Artery
				3 Renal Artery, Right
				4 Renal Artery, Left
				5 Renal Artery, Bilateral
				6 Common Iliac Artery, Right
				7 Common Iliac Artery, Left
				8 Common Iliac Arteries, Bilateral
				9 Internal Iliac Artery, Right
				B Internal Iliac Artery, Left
				C Internal Iliac Arteries, Bilateral
				D External Iliac Artery, Right
				F External Iliac Artery, Left
				G External Iliac Arteries, Bilateral
				H Femoral Artery, Right
				J Femoral Artery, Left
				K Femoral Arteries, Bilateral
				Q Lower Extremity Artery
				R Lower Artery

3 Hepatic Artery
   Common hepatic artery
   Gastroduodenal artery
   Hepatic artery proper
	4 Splenic Artery
	   Left gastroepiploic artery
	   Pancreatic artery
	   Short gastric artery
		Ø Open
		4 Percutaneous Endoscopic
			9 Autologous Venous Tissue
			A Autologous Arterial Tissue
			J Synthetic Substitute
			K Nonautologous Tissue Substitute
			Z No Device
				3 Renal Artery, Right
				4 Renal Artery, Left
				5 Renal Artery, Bilateral

E Internal Iliac Artery, Right
   Deferential artery
   Hypogastric artery
   Iliolumbar artery
   Inferior gluteal artery
   Inferior vesical artery
   Internal pudendal artery
   Lateral sacral artery
   Middle rectal artery
   Obturator artery
   Prostatic artery
   Superior gluteal artery
   Superior vesical artery
   Umbilical artery
   Uterine artery
   Vaginal artery
	F Internal Iliac Artery, Left
	   See E Internal Iliac Artery, Right
	H External Iliac Artery, Right
	   Deep circumflex iliac artery
	   Inferior epigastric artery
	J External Iliac Artery, Left
	   See H External Iliac Artery, Right
		Ø Open
		4 Percutaneous Endoscopic
			9 Autologous Venous Tissue
			A Autologous Arterial Tissue
			J Synthetic Substitute
			K Nonautologous Tissue Substitute
			Z No Device
				9 Internal Iliac Artery, Right
				B Internal Iliac Artery, Left
				C Internal Iliac Arteries, Bilateral
				D External Iliac Artery, Right
				F External Iliac Artery, Left
				G External Iliac Arteries, Bilateral
				H Femoral Artery, Right
				J Femoral Artery, Left
				K Femoral Arteries, Bilateral
				P Foot Artery
				Q Lower Extremity Artery

K Femoral Artery, Right
   Circumflex iliac artery
   Deep femoral artery
   Descending genicular artery
   External pudendal artery
   Superficial epigastric artery
	L Femoral Artery, Left
	   See K Femoral Artery, Right
		Ø Open
		4 Percutaneous Endoscopic
			9 Autologous Venous Tissue
			A Autologous Arterial Tissue
			J Synthetic Substitute
			K Nonautologous Tissue Substitute
			Z No Device
				H Femoral Artery, Right
				J Femoral Artery, Left
				K Femoral Arteries, Bilateral
				L Popliteal Artery
				M Peroneal Artery
				N Posterior Tibial Artery
				P Foot Artery
				Q Lower Extremity Artery
				S Lower Extremity Vein

K Femoral Artery, Right
   Circumflex iliac artery
   Deep femoral artery
   Descending genicular artery
   External pudendal artery
   Superficial epigastric artery
	L Femoral Artery, Left
	   See K Femoral Artery, Right
		3 Percutaneous	J Synthetic Substitute	Q Lower Extremity Artery
				S Lower Extremity Vein

M Popliteal Artery, Right
   Inferior genicular artery
   Middle genicular artery
   Superior genicular artery
   Sural artery
   Tibioperoneal trunk
	N Popliteal Artery, Left
	   See M Popliteal Artery, Right
		Ø Open
		4 Percutaneous Endoscopic
			9 Autologous Venous Tissue
			A Autologous Arterial Tissue
			J Synthetic Substitute
			K Nonautologous Tissue Substitute
			Z No Device
				L Popliteal Artery
				M Peroneal Artery
				P Foot Artery
				Q Lower Extremity Artery
				S Lower Extremity Vein

Ø41 Continued on next page

Non-OR Procedure   DRG Non-OR Procedure   Valid OR Procedure   HAC Associated Procedure   Combination Only   New/Revised April   New/Revised October

222   ICD-10-PCS 2023

Ø   Medical and Surgical
4   Lower Arteries
1   Bypass   Definition: Altering the route of passage of the contents of a tubular body part

041 Continued

Explanation: Rerouting contents of a body part to a downstream area of the normal route, to a similar route and body part, or to an abnormal route and dissimilar body part. Includes one or more anastomoses, with or without the use of a device.

Body Part Character 4		Approach Character 5	Device Character 6	Qualifier Character 7
M Popliteal Artery, Right Inferior genicular artery Middle genicular artery Superior genicular artery Sural artery Tibioperoneal trunk	**N Popliteal Artery, Left** *See M Popliteal Artery, Right*	**3 Percutaneous**	**J Synthetic Substitute**	**Q Lower Extremity Artery** **S Lower Extremity Vein**
P Anterior Tibial Artery, Right Anterior lateral malleolar artery Anterior medial malleolar artery Anterior tibial recurrent artery Dorsalis pedis artery Posterior tibial recurrent artery	**Q Anterior Tibial Artery, Left** *See P Anterior Tibial Artery, Right* **R Posterior Tibial Artery, Right** **S Posterior Tibial Artery, Left**	**Ø Open** **3 Percutaneous** **4 Percutaneous Endoscopic**	**J Synthetic Substitute**	**Q Lower Extremity Artery** **S Lower Extremity Vein**
T Peroneal Artery, Right Fibular artery **U Peroneal Artery, Left** *See T Peroneal Artery, Right*	**V Foot Artery, Right** Arcuate artery Dorsal metatarsal artery Lateral plantar artery Lateral tarsal artery Medial plantar artery **W Foot Artery, Left** *See V Foot Artery, Right*	**Ø Open** **4 Percutaneous Endoscopic**	**9 Autologous Venous Tissue** **A Autologous Arterial Tissue** **J Synthetic Substitute** **K Nonautologous Tissue Substitute** **Z No Device**	**P Foot Artery** **Q Lower Extremity Artery** **S Lower Extremity Vein**
T Peroneal Artery, Right Fibular artery **U Peroneal Artery, Left** *See T Peroneal Artery, Right*	**V Foot Artery, Right** Arcuate artery Dorsal metatarsal artery Lateral plantar artery Lateral tarsal artery Medial plantar artery **W Foot Artery, Left** *See V Foot Artery, Right*	**3 Percutaneous**	**J Synthetic Substitute**	**Q Lower Extremity Artery** **S Lower Extremity Vein**

NC Noncovered Procedure   **LC** Limited Coverage   **QA** Questionable OB Admit   **NT** New Tech Add-on   ⊞ Combination Member   ♂ Male   ♀ Female

ICD-10-PCS 2023   223

041–041

Lower Arteries

Ø   Medical and Surgical
4   Lower Arteries
5   Destruction   Definition: Physical eradication of all or a portion of a body part by the direct use of energy, force, or a destructive agent
                  Explanation: None of the body part is physically taken out

Body Part Character 4		Approach Character 5	Device Character 6	Qualifier Character 7
Ø Abdominal Aorta	**F Internal Iliac Artery, Left**	**Ø Open**	**Z No Device**	**Z No Qualifier**
Inferior phrenic artery	*See E Internal Iliac Artery, Right*	**3 Percutaneous**		
Lumbar artery	**H External Iliac Artery, Right**	**4 Percutaneous Endoscopic**		
Median sacral artery	Deep circumflex iliac artery			
Middle suprarenal artery	Inferior epigastric artery			
Ovarian artery	**J External Iliac Artery, Left**			
Testicular artery	*See H External Iliac Artery, Right*			
1 Celiac Artery	**K Femoral Artery, Right**			
Celiac trunk	Circumflex iliac artery			
2 Gastric Artery	Deep femoral artery			
Left gastric artery	Descending genicular artery			
Right gastric artery	External pudendal artery			
3 Hepatic Artery	Superficial epigastric artery			
Common hepatic artery	**L Femoral Artery, Left**			
Gastroduodenal artery	*See K Femoral Artery, Right*			
Hepatic artery proper	**M Popliteal Artery, Right**			
4 Splenic Artery	Inferior genicular artery			
Left gastroepiploic artery	Middle genicular artery			
Pancreatic artery	Superior genicular artery			
Short gastric artery	Sural artery			
5 Superior Mesenteric Artery	Tibioperoneal trunk			
Ileal artery	**N Popliteal Artery, Left**			
Ileocolic artery	*See M Popliteal Artery, Right*			
Inferior pancreaticoduodenal artery	**P Anterior Tibial Artery, Right**			
Jejunal artery	Anterior lateral malleolar artery			
6 Colic Artery, Right	Anterior medial malleolar artery			
7 Colic Artery, Left	Anterior tibial recurrent artery			
8 Colic Artery, Middle	Dorsalis pedis artery			
9 Renal Artery, Right	Posterior tibial recurrent artery			
Inferior suprarenal artery	**Q Anterior Tibial Artery, Left**			
Renal segmental artery	*See P Anterior Tibial Artery, Right*			
A Renal Artery, Left	**R Posterior Tibial Artery, Right**			
See 9 Renal Artery, Right	**S Posterior Tibial Artery, Left**			
B Inferior Mesenteric Artery	**T Peroneal Artery, Right**			
Sigmoid artery	Fibular artery			
Superior rectal artery	**U Peroneal Artery, Left**			
C Common Iliac Artery, Right	*See T Peroneal Artery, Right*			
D Common Iliac Artery, Left	**V Foot Artery, Right**			
E Internal Iliac Artery, Right	Arcuate artery			
Deferential artery	Dorsal metatarsal artery			
Hypogastric artery	Lateral plantar artery			
Iliolumbar artery	Lateral tarsal artery			
Inferior gluteal artery	Medial plantar artery			
Inferior vesical artery	**W Foot Artery, Left**			
Internal pudendal artery	*See V Foot Artery, Right*			
Lateral sacral artery	**Y Lower Artery**			
Middle rectal artery	Umbilical artery			
Obturator artery				
Prostatic artery				
Superior gluteal artery				
Superior vesical artery				
Umbilical artery				
Uterine artery				
Vaginal artery				

Ø Medical and Surgical
4 Lower Arteries
7 Dilation   Definition: Expanding an orifice or the lumen of a tubular body part

Explanation: The orifice can be a natural orifice or an artificially created orifice. Accomplished by stretching a tubular body part using intraluminal pressure or by cutting part of the orifice or wall of the tubular body part.

Body Part — Character 4		Approach — Character 5	Device — Character 6	Qualifier — Character 7
Ø Abdominal Aorta Inferior phrenic artery Lumbar artery Median sacral artery Middle suprarenal artery Ovarian artery Testicular artery **1 Celiac Artery** Celiac trunk **2 Gastric Artery** Left gastric artery Right gastric artery **3 Hepatic Artery** Common hepatic artery Gastroduodenal artery Hepatic artery proper **4 Splenic Artery** Left gastroepiploic artery Pancreatic artery Short gastric artery **5 Superior Mesenteric Artery** Ileal artery Ileocolic artery Inferior pancreaticoduodenal artery Jejunal artery **6 Colic Artery, Right** **7 Colic Artery, Left** **8 Colic Artery, Middle** **9 Renal Artery, Right** Inferior suprarenal artery Renal segmental artery **A Renal Artery, Left** See 9 Renal Artery, Right **B Inferior Mesenteric Artery** Sigmoid artery Superior rectal artery **C Common Iliac Artery, Right** **D Common Iliac Artery, Left** **E Internal Iliac Artery, Right** Deferential artery Hypogastric artery Iliolumbar artery Inferior gluteal artery Inferior vesical artery Internal pudendal artery Lateral sacral artery Middle rectal artery Obturator artery Prostatic artery Superior gluteal artery Superior vesical artery Umbilical artery Uterine artery Vaginal artery	**F Internal Iliac Artery, Left** See E Internal Iliac Artery, Right **H External Iliac Artery, Right** Deep circumflex iliac artery Inferior epigastric artery **J External Iliac Artery, Left** See H External Iliac Artery, Right **K Femoral Artery, Right** Circumflex iliac artery Deep femoral artery Descending genicular artery External pudendal artery Superficial epigastric artery **L Femoral Artery, Left** See K Femoral Artery, Right **M Popliteal Artery, Right** Inferior genicular artery Middle genicular artery Superior genicular artery Sural artery Tibioperoneal trunk **N Popliteal Artery, Left** See M Popliteal Artery, Right **P Anterior Tibial Artery, Right** Anterior lateral malleolar artery Anterior medial malleolar artery Anterior tibial recurrent artery Dorsalis pedis artery Posterior tibial recurrent artery **Q Anterior Tibial Artery, Left** See P Anterior Tibial Artery, Right **R Posterior Tibial Artery, Right** **S Posterior Tibial Artery, Left** **T Peroneal Artery, Right** Fibular artery **U Peroneal Artery, Left** See T Peroneal Artery, Right **V Foot Artery, Right** Arcuate artery Dorsal metatarsal artery Lateral plantar artery Lateral tarsal artery Medial plantar artery **W Foot Artery, Left** See V Foot Artery, Right **Y Lower Artery** Umbilical artery	**Ø Open** **3 Percutaneous** **4 Percutaneous Endoscopic**	**4 Intraluminal Device, Drug-eluting** **D Intraluminal Device** **Z No Device**	**1 Drug-Coated Balloon** **Z No Qualifier**

Ø47 Continued on next page

NC Noncovered Procedure   **LC** Limited Coverage   **QA** Questionable OB Admit   **NT** New Tech Add-on   ⊞ Combination Member   ♂ Male   ♀ Female

ICD-10-PCS 2023   225

Ø47–Ø47

Lower Arteries

0	Medical and Surgical		*047 Continued*
4	Lower Arteries		
7	Dilation		

Definition: Expanding an orifice or the lumen of a tubular body part

Explanation: The orifice can be a natural orifice or an artificially created orifice. Accomplished by stretching a tubular body part using intraluminal pressure or by cutting part of the orifice or wall of the tubular body part.

Body Part — Character 4		Approach — Character 5	Device — Character 6	Qualifier — Character 7
0 Abdominal Aorta Inferior phrenic artery Lumbar artery Median sacral artery Middle suprarenal artery Ovarian artery Testicular artery **1 Celiac Artery** Celiac trunk **2 Gastric Artery** Left gastric artery Right gastric artery **3 Hepatic Artery** Common hepatic artery Gastroduodenal artery Hepatic artery proper **4 Splenic Artery** Left gastroepiploic artery Pancreatic artery Short gastric artery **5 Superior Mesenteric Artery** Ileal artery Ileocolic artery Inferior pancreaticoduodenal artery Jejunal artery **6 Colic Artery, Right** **7 Colic Artery, Left** **8 Colic Artery, Middle** **9 Renal Artery, Right** Inferior suprarenal artery Renal segmental artery **A Renal Artery, Left** *See 9 Renal Artery, Right* **B Inferior Mesenteric Artery** Sigmoid artery Superior rectal artery **C Common Iliac Artery, Right** **D Common Iliac Artery, Left** **E Internal Iliac Artery, Right** Deferential artery Hypogastric artery Iliolumbar artery Inferior gluteal artery Inferior vesical artery Internal pudendal artery Lateral sacral artery Middle rectal artery Obturator artery Prostatic artery Superior gluteal artery Superior vesical artery Umbilical artery Uterine artery Vaginal artery	**F Internal Iliac Artery, Left** *See E Internal Iliac Artery, Right* **H External Iliac Artery, Right** Deep circumflex iliac artery Inferior epigastric artery **J External Iliac Artery, Left** *See H External Iliac Artery, Right* **K Femoral Artery, Right** Circumflex iliac artery Deep femoral artery Descending genicular artery External pudendal artery Superficial epigastric artery **L Femoral Artery, Left** *See K Femoral Artery, Right* **M Popliteal Artery, Right** Inferior genicular artery Middle genicular artery Superior genicular artery Sural artery Tibioperoneal trunk **N Popliteal Artery, Left** *See M Popliteal Artery, Right* **P Anterior Tibial Artery, Right** Anterior lateral malleolar artery Anterior medial malleolar artery Anterior tibial recurrent artery Dorsalis pedis artery Posterior tibial recurrent artery **Q Anterior Tibial Artery, Left** *See P Anterior Tibial Artery, Right* **R Posterior Tibial Artery, Right** **S Posterior Tibial Artery, Left** **T Peroneal Artery, Right** Fibular artery **U Peroneal Artery, Left** *See T Peroneal Artery, Right* **V Foot Artery, Right** Arcuate artery Dorsal metatarsal artery Lateral plantar artery Lateral tarsal artery Medial plantar artery **W Foot Artery, Left** *See V Foot Artery, Right* **Y Lower Artery** Umbilical artery	**0** Open **3** Percutaneous **4** Percutaneous Endoscopic	**5** Intraluminal Device, Drug-eluting, Two **6** Intraluminal Device, Drug-eluting, Three **7** Intraluminal Device, Drug-eluting, Four or More **E** Intraluminal Device, Two **F** Intraluminal Device, Three **G** Intraluminal Device, Four or More	**Z** No Qualifier

Non-OR Procedure   DRG Non-OR Procedure   Valid OR Procedure   HAC Associated Procedure   Combination Only   New/Revised April   New/Revised October

Ø   Medical and Surgical
4   Lower Arteries
9   Drainage   Definition: Taking or letting out fluids and/or gases from a body part
                 Explanation: The qualifier DIAGNOSTIC is used to identify drainage procedures that are biopsies

Body Part Character 4		Approach Character 5	Device Character 6	Qualifier Character 7

Ø Abdominal Aorta
Inferior phrenic artery
Lumbar artery
Median sacral artery
Middle suprarenal artery
Ovarian artery
Testicular artery
1 Celiac Artery
Celiac trunk
2 Gastric Artery
Left gastric artery
Right gastric artery
3 Hepatic Artery
Common hepatic artery
Gastroduodenal artery
Hepatic artery proper
4 Splenic Artery
Left gastroepiploic artery
Pancreatic artery
Short gastric artery
5 Superior Mesenteric Artery
Ileal artery
Ileocolic artery
Inferior pancreaticoduodenal
   artery
Jejunal artery
6 Colic Artery, Right
7 Colic Artery, Left
8 Colic Artery, Middle
9 Renal Artery, Right
Inferior suprarenal artery
Renal segmental artery
A Renal Artery, Left
See 9 Renal Artery, Right
B Inferior Mesenteric Artery
Sigmoid artery
Superior rectal artery
C Common Iliac Artery, Right
D Common Iliac Artery, Left
E Internal Iliac Artery, Right
Deferential artery
Hypogastric artery
Iliolumbar artery
Inferior gluteal artery
Inferior vesical artery
Internal pudendal artery
Lateral sacral artery
Middle rectal artery
Obturator artery
Prostatic artery
Superior gluteal artery
Superior vesical artery
Umbilical artery
Uterine artery
Vaginal artery
	F Internal Iliac Artery, Left
	See E Internal Iliac Artery, Right
	H External Iliac Artery, Right
	Deep circumflex iliac artery
	Inferior epigastric artery
	J External Iliac Artery, Left
	See H External Iliac Artery, Right
	K Femoral Artery, Right
	Circumflex iliac artery
	Deep femoral artery
	Descending genicular artery
	External pudendal artery
	Superficial epigastric artery
	L Femoral Artery, Left
	See K Femoral Artery, Right
	M Popliteal Artery, Right
	Inferior genicular artery
	Middle genicular artery
	Superior genicular artery
	Sural artery
	Tibioperoneal trunk
	N Popliteal Artery, Left
	See M Popliteal Artery, Right
	P Anterior Tibial Artery, Right
	Anterior lateral malleolar
	   artery
	Anterior medial malleolar
	   artery
	Anterior tibial recurrent artery
	Dorsalis pedis artery
	Posterior tibial recurrent artery
	Q Anterior Tibial Artery, Left
	See P Anterior Tibial Artery,
	Right
	R Posterior Tibial Artery, Right
	S Posterior Tibial Artery, Left
	T Peroneal Artery, Right
	Fibular artery
	U Peroneal Artery, Left
	See T Peroneal Artery, Right
	V Foot Artery, Right
	Arcuate artery
	Dorsal metatarsal artery
	Lateral plantar artery
	Lateral tarsal artery
	Medial plantar artery
	W Foot Artery, Left
	See V Foot Artery, Right
	Y Lower Artery
	Umbilical artery
		Ø Open
		3 Percutaneous
		4 Percutaneous Endoscopic
			Ø Drainage Device	**Z No Qualifier**

Non-OR   Ø49[Ø,1,2,3,4,5,6,7,8,9,A,B,C,D,E,F,H,J,K,L,M,N,P,Q,R,S,T,U,V,W,Y][Ø,3,4]ØZ

Ø49 Continued on next page

NC Noncovered Procedure   LC Limited Coverage   QA Questionable OB Admit   NT New Tech Add-on   ⊞ Combination Member   ♂ Male   ♀ Female

ICD-10-PCS 2023   227

Lower Arteries

Ø **Medical and Surgical**
4 **Lower Arteries**
9 **Drainage**

049 Continued

Definition: Taking or letting out fluids and/or gases from a body part

Explanation: The qualifier DIAGNOSTIC is used to identify drainage procedures that are biopsies

Body Part Character 4		Approach Character 5	Device Character 6	Qualifier Character 7
Ø **Abdominal Aorta** Inferior phrenic artery Lumbar artery Median sacral artery Middle suprarenal artery Ovarian artery Testicular artery 1 **Celiac Artery** Celiac trunk 2 **Gastric Artery** Left gastric artery Right gastric artery 3 **Hepatic Artery** Common hepatic artery Gastroduodenal artery Hepatic artery proper 4 **Splenic Artery** Left gastroepiploic artery Pancreatic artery Short gastric artery 5 **Superior Mesenteric Artery** Ileal artery Ileocolic artery Inferior pancreaticoduodenal artery Jejunal artery 6 **Colic Artery, Right** 7 **Colic Artery, Left** 8 **Colic Artery, Middle** 9 **Renal Artery, Right** Inferior suprarenal artery Renal segmental artery A **Renal Artery, Left** *See 9 Renal Artery, Right* B **Inferior Mesenteric Artery** Sigmoid artery Superior rectal artery C **Common Iliac Artery, Right** D **Common Iliac Artery, Left** E **Internal Iliac Artery, Right** Deferential artery Hypogastric artery Iliolumbar artery Inferior gluteal artery Inferior vesical artery Internal pudendal artery Lateral sacral artery Middle rectal artery Obturator artery Prostatic artery Superior gluteal artery Superior vesical artery Umbilical artery Uterine artery Vaginal artery	F **Internal Iliac Artery, Left** *See E Internal Iliac Artery, Right* H **External Iliac Artery, Right** Deep circumflex iliac artery Inferior epigastric artery J **External Iliac Artery, Left** *See H External Iliac Artery, Right* K **Femoral Artery, Right** Circumflex iliac artery Deep femoral artery Descending genicular artery External pudendal artery Superficial epigastric artery L **Femoral Artery, Left** *See K Femoral Artery, Right* M **Popliteal Artery, Right** Inferior genicular artery Middle genicular artery Superior genicular artery Sural artery Tibioperoneal trunk N **Popliteal Artery, Left** *See M Popliteal Artery, Right* P **Anterior Tibial Artery, Right** Anterior lateral malleolar artery Anterior medial malleolar artery Anterior tibial recurrent artery Dorsalis pedis artery Posterior tibial recurrent artery Q **Anterior Tibial Artery, Left** *See P Anterior Tibial Artery, Right* R **Posterior Tibial Artery, Right** S **Posterior Tibial Artery, Left** T **Peroneal Artery, Right** Fibular artery U **Peroneal Artery, Left** *See T Peroneal Artery, Right* V **Foot Artery, Right** Arcuate artery Dorsal metatarsal artery Lateral plantar artery Lateral tarsal artery Medial plantar artery W **Foot Artery, Left** *See V Foot Artery, Right* Y **Lower Artery** Umbilical artery	Ø **Open** 3 **Percutaneous** 4 **Percutaneous Endoscopic**	Z **No Device**	X **Diagnostic** Z **No Qualifier**

Non-OR 049[Ø,1,2,3,4,5,6,7,8,9,A,B,C,D,E,F,H,J,K,L,M,N,P,Q,R,S,T,U,V,W,Y]3ZX
Non-OR 049[Ø,1,2,3,4,5,6,7,8,9,A,B,C,D,E,F,H,J,K,L,M,N,P,Q,R,S,T,U,V,W,Y][Ø,3,4]ZZ

Non-OR Procedure   DRG Non-OR Procedure   Valid OR Procedure   HAC Associated Procedure   Combination Only   New/Revised April   New/Revised October

228   ICD-10-PCS 2023

049–049

Ø   **Medical and Surgical**
4   **Lower Arteries**
B   **Excision**   Definition: Cutting out or off, without replacement, a portion of a body part
                Explanation: The qualifier DIAGNOSTIC is used to identify excision procedures that are biopsies

Body Part Character 4		Approach Character 5	Device Character 6	Qualifier Character 7

Ø Abdominal Aorta
  Inferior phrenic artery
  Lumbar artery
  Median sacral artery
  Middle suprarenal artery
  Ovarian artery
  Testicular artery
1 Celiac Artery
  Celiac trunk
2 Gastric Artery
  Left gastric artery
  Right gastric artery
3 Hepatic Artery
  Common hepatic artery
  Gastroduodenal artery
  Hepatic artery proper
4 Splenic Artery
  Left gastroepiploic artery
  Pancreatic artery
  Short gastric artery
5 Superior Mesenteric Artery
  Ileal artery
  Ileocolic artery
  Inferior pancreaticoduodenal
    artery
  Jejunal artery
6 Colic Artery, Right
7 Colic Artery, Left
8 Colic Artery, Middle
9 Renal Artery, Right
  Inferior suprarenal artery
  Renal segmental artery
A Renal Artery, Left
  See 9 Renal Artery, Right
B Inferior Mesenteric Artery
  Sigmoid artery
  Superior rectal artery
C Common Iliac Artery, Right
D Common Iliac Artery, Left
E Internal Iliac Artery, Right
  Deferential artery
  Hypogastric artery
  Iliolumbar artery
  Inferior gluteal artery
  Inferior vesical artery
  Internal pudendal artery
  Lateral sacral artery
  Middle rectal artery
  Obturator artery
  Prostatic artery
  Superior gluteal artery
  Superior vesical artery
  Umbilical artery
  Uterine artery
  Vaginal artery
	F Internal Iliac Artery, Left
	  See E Internal Iliac Artery, Right
	H External Iliac Artery, Right
	  Deep circumflex iliac artery
	  Inferior epigastric artery
	J External Iliac Artery, Left
	  See H External Iliac Artery, Right
	K Femoral Artery, Right
	  Circumflex iliac artery
	  Deep femoral artery
	  Descending genicular artery
	  External pudendal artery
	  Superficial epigastric artery
	L Femoral Artery, Left
	  See K Femoral Artery, Right
	M Popliteal Artery, Right
	  Inferior genicular artery
	  Middle genicular artery
	  Superior genicular artery
	  Sural artery
	  Tibioperoneal trunk
	N Popliteal Artery, Left
	  See M Popliteal Artery, Right
	P Anterior Tibial Artery, Right
	  Anterior lateral malleolar
	    artery
	  Anterior medial malleolar
	    artery
	  Anterior tibial recurrent artery
	  Dorsalis pedis artery
	  Posterior tibial recurrent artery
	Q Anterior Tibial Artery, Left
	  *See P Anterior Tibial Artery,
	    Right*
	R Posterior Tibial Artery, Right
	S Posterior Tibial Artery, Left
	T Peroneal Artery, Right
	  Fibular artery
	U Peroneal Artery, Left
	  See T Peroneal Artery, Right
	V Foot Artery, Right
	  Arcuate artery
	  Dorsal metatarsal artery
	  Lateral plantar artery
	  Lateral tarsal artery
	  Medial plantar artery
	W Foot Artery, Left
	  See V Foot Artery, Right
	Y Lower Artery
	  Umbilical artery
		Ø Open
		3 Percutaneous
		4 Percutaneous Endoscopic
			Z No Device	**X** Diagnostic
				Z No Qualifier

NC Noncovered Procedure   **LC** Limited Coverage   **QA** Questionable OB Admit   **NT** New Tech Add-on   ⊞ Combination Member   ♂ Male   ♀ Female
ICD-10-PCS 2023   229

04B–04B

Lower Arteries

0   **Medical and Surgical**
4   **Lower Arteries**
C   **Extirpation**   Definition: Taking or cutting out solid matter from a body part

Explanation: The solid matter may be an abnormal byproduct of a biological function or a foreign body; it may be imbedded in a body part or in the lumen of a tubular body part. The solid matter may or may not have been previously broken into pieces.

Body Part Character 4		Approach Character 5	Device Character 6	Qualifier Character 7

0   **Abdominal Aorta**
    Inferior phrenic artery
    Lumbar artery
    Median sacral artery
    Middle suprarenal artery
    Ovarian artery
    Testicular artery
 1   **Celiac Artery**
    Celiac trunk
 2   **Gastric Artery**
    Left gastric artery
    Right gastric artery
 3   **Hepatic Artery**
    Common hepatic artery
    Gastroduodenal artery
    Hepatic artery proper
 4   **Splenic Artery**
    Left gastroepiploic artery
    Pancreatic artery
    Short gastric artery
 5   **Superior Mesenteric Artery**
    Ileal artery
    Ileocolic artery
    Inferior pancreaticoduodenal artery
    Jejunal artery
 6   **Colic Artery, Right**
 7   **Colic Artery, Left**
 8   **Colic Artery, Middle**
 9   **Renal Artery, Right**
    Inferior suprarenal artery
    Renal segmental artery
 A   **Renal Artery, Left**
    See 9 Renal Artery, Right
 B   **Inferior Mesenteric Artery**
    Sigmoid artery
    Superior rectal artery
 C   **Common Iliac Artery, Right**
 D   **Common Iliac Artery, Left**
 E   **Internal Iliac Artery, Right**
    Deferential artery
    Hypogastric artery
    Iliolumbar artery
    Inferior gluteal artery
    Inferior vesical artery
    Internal pudendal artery
    Lateral sacral artery
    Middle rectal artery
    Obturator artery
    Prostatic artery
    Superior gluteal artery
    Superior vesical artery
    Umbilical artery
    Uterine artery
    Vaginal artery
	F **Internal Iliac Artery, Left**
	    See E Internal Iliac Artery, Right
	 H **External Iliac Artery, Right**
	    Deep circumflex iliac artery
	    Inferior epigastric artery
	 J **External Iliac Artery, Left**
	    See H External Iliac Artery, Right
	 K **Femoral Artery, Right**
	    Circumflex iliac artery
	    Deep femoral artery
	    Descending genicular artery
	    External pudendal artery
	    Superficial epigastric artery
	 L **Femoral Artery, Left**
	    See K Femoral Artery, Right
	 M **Popliteal Artery, Right**
	    Inferior genicular artery
	    Middle genicular artery
	    Superior genicular artery
	    Sural artery
	    Tibioperoneal trunk
	 N **Popliteal Artery, Left**
	    See M Popliteal Artery, Right
	 P **Anterior Tibial Artery, Right**
	    Anterior lateral malleolar artery
	    Anterior medial malleolar artery
	    Anterior tibial recurrent artery
	    Dorsalis pedis artery
	    Posterior tibial recurrent artery
	 Q **Anterior Tibial Artery, Left**
	    See P Anterior Tibial Artery, Right
	 R **Posterior Tibial Artery, Right**
	 S **Posterior Tibial Artery, Left**
	 T **Peroneal Artery, Right**
	    Fibular artery
	 U **Peroneal Artery, Left**
	    See T Peroneal Artery, Right
	 V **Foot Artery, Right**
	    Arcuate artery
	    Dorsal metatarsal artery
	    Lateral plantar artery
	    Lateral tarsal artery
	    Medial plantar artery
	 W **Foot Artery, Left**
	    See V Foot Artery, Right
	 Y **Lower Artery**
	    Umbilical artery
		0 Open
		 3 Percutaneous
		 4 Percutaneous Endoscopic
			Z No Device	**Z** No Qualifier

Non-OR Procedure   DRG Non-OR Procedure   Valid OR Procedure   HAC Associated Procedure   Combination Only   New/Revised April   New/Revised October

230   ICD-10-PCS 2023

Ø   **Medical and Surgical**
4   **Lower Arteries**
F   **Fragmentation**   Definition: Breaking solid matter in a body part into pieces

Explanation: Physical force (e.g., manual, ultrasonic) applied directly or indirectly is used to break the solid matter into pieces. The solid matter may be an abnormal byproduct of a biological function or a foreign body. The pieces of solid matter are not taken out.

Body Part Character 4	Approach Character 5	Device Character 6	Qualifier Character 7
C **Common Iliac Artery, Right**	**3** Percutaneous	**Z** No Device	**Ø** Ultrasonic
D **Common Iliac Artery, Left**			**Z** No Qualifier
E **Internal Iliac Artery, Right**			
Deferential artery			
Hypogastric artery			
Iliolumbar artery			
Inferior gluteal artery			
Inferior vesical artery			
Internal pudendal artery			
Lateral sacral artery			
Middle rectal artery			
Obturator artery			
Prostatic artery			
Superior gluteal artery			
Superior vesical artery			
Umbilical artery			
Uterine artery			
Vaginal artery			
F **Internal Iliac Artery, Left**			
See E Internal Iliac Artery, Right			
H **External Iliac Artery, Right**			
Deep circumflex iliac artery			
Inferior epigastric artery			
J **External Iliac Artery, Left**			
See H External Iliac Artery, Right			
K **Femoral Artery, Right**			
Circumflex iliac artery			
Deep femoral artery			
Descending genicular artery			
External pudendal artery			
Superficial epigastric artery			
L **Femoral Artery, Left**			
See K Femoral Artery, Right			
M **Popliteal Artery, Right**			
Inferior genicular artery			
Middle genicular artery			
Superior genicular artery			
Sural artery			
Tibioperoneal trunk			
N **Popliteal Artery, Left**			
See M Popliteal Artery, Right			
P **Anterior Tibial Artery, Right**			
Anterior lateral malleolar artery			
Anterior medial malleolar artery			
Anterior tibial recurrent artery			
Dorsalis pedis artery			
Posterior tibial recurrent artery			
Q **Anterior Tibial Artery, Left**			
See P Anterior Tibial Artery, Right			
R **Posterior Tibial Artery, Right**			
S **Posterior Tibial Artery, Left**			
T **Peroneal Artery, Right**			
Fibular artery			
U **Peroneal Artery, Left**			
See T Peroneal Artery, Right			
Y **Lower Artery**			
Umbilical artery			

NC Noncovered Procedure   **LC** Limited Coverage   **QA** Questionable OB Admit   **NT** New Tech Add-on   ⊞ Combination Member   ♂ Male   ♀ Female

ICD-10-PCS 2023   231

04F–04F

Lower Arteries

Ø **Medical and Surgical**
4 **Lower Arteries**
H **Insertion**

Definition: Putting in a nonbiological appliance that monitors, assists, performs, or prevents a physiological function but does not physically take the place of a body part

Explanation: None

Body Part Character 4		Approach Character 5	Device Character 6	Qualifier Character 7
Ø Abdominal Aorta		**Ø Open**	**2 Monitoring Device**	**Z No Qualifier**
Inferior phrenic artery		**3 Percutaneous**	**3 Infusion Device**	
Lumbar artery		**4 Percutaneous Endoscopic**	**D Intraluminal Device**	
Median sacral artery				
Middle suprarenal artery				
Ovarian artery				
Testicular artery				
1 Celiac Artery	**F Internal Iliac Artery, Left**	**Ø Open**	**3 Infusion Device**	**Z No Qualifier**
Celiac trunk	*See E Internal Iliac Artery, Right*	**3 Percutaneous**	**D Intraluminal Device**	
2 Gastric Artery	**H External Iliac Artery, Right**	**4 Percutaneous Endoscopic**		
Left gastric artery	Deep circumflex iliac artery			
Right gastric artery	Inferior epigastric artery			
3 Hepatic Artery	**J External Iliac Artery, Left**			
Common hepatic artery	*See H External Iliac Artery, Right*			
Gastroduodenal artery	**K Femoral Artery, Right**			
Hepatic artery proper	Circumflex iliac artery			
4 Splenic Artery	Deep femoral artery			
Left gastroepiploic artery	Descending genicular artery			
Pancreatic artery	External pudendal artery			
Short gastric artery	Superficial epigastric artery			
5 Superior Mesenteric Artery	**L Femoral Artery, Left**			
Ileal artery	*See K Femoral Artery, Right*			
Ileocolic artery	**M Popliteal Artery, Right**			
Inferior pancreaticoduodenal artery	Inferior genicular artery			
Jejunal artery	Middle genicular artery			
6 Colic Artery, Right	Superior genicular artery			
7 Colic Artery, Left	Sural artery			
8 Colic Artery, Middle	Tibioperoneal trunk			
9 Renal Artery, Right	**N Popliteal Artery, Left**			
Inferior suprarenal artery	*See M Popliteal Artery, Right*			
Renal segmental artery	**P Anterior Tibial Artery, Right**			
A Renal Artery, Left	Anterior lateral malleolar artery			
See 9 Renal Artery, Right	Anterior medial malleolar artery			
B Inferior Mesenteric Artery	Anterior tibial recurrent artery			
Sigmoid artery	Dorsalis pedis artery			
Superior rectal artery	Posterior tibial recurrent artery			
C Common Iliac Artery, Right	**Q Anterior Tibial Artery, Left**			
D Common Iliac Artery, Left	*See P Anterior Tibial Artery, Right*			
E Internal Iliac Artery, Right	**R Posterior Tibial Artery, Right**			
Deferential artery	**S Posterior Tibial Artery, Left**			
Hypogastric artery	**T Peroneal Artery, Right**			
Iliolumbar artery	Fibular artery			
Inferior gluteal artery	**U Peroneal Artery, Left**			
Inferior vesical artery	*See T Peroneal Artery, Right*			
Internal pudendal artery	**V Foot Artery, Right**			
Lateral sacral artery	Arcuate artery			
Middle rectal artery	Dorsal metatarsal artery			
Obturator artery	Lateral plantar artery			
Prostatic artery	Lateral tarsal artery			
Superior gluteal artery	Medial plantar artery			
Superior vesical artery	**W Foot Artery, Left**			
Umbilical artery	*See V Foot Artery, Right*			
Uterine artery				
Vaginal artery				
Y Lower Artery		**Ø Open**	**2 Monitoring Device**	**Z No Qualifier**
Umbilical artery		**3 Percutaneous**	**3 Infusion Device**	
		4 Percutaneous Endoscopic	**D Intraluminal Device**	
			Y Other Device	

Non-OR   Ø4HØ[Ø,3,4][2,3]Z
Non-OR   Ø4H[1,2,3,4,5,6,7,8,9,A,B,C,D,E,F,H,J,K,L,M,N,P,Q,R,S,T,U,V,W][Ø,3,4]3Z
Non-OR   Ø4HY32Z
Non-OR   Ø4HY[Ø,3,4]3Z
Non-OR   Ø4HY[3,4]YZ

Non-OR Procedure   DRG Non-OR Procedure   Valid OR Procedure   HAC Associated Procedure   Combination Only   New/Revised April   New/Revised October

Ø   Medical and Surgical
4   Lower Arteries
J   Inspection   Definition: Visually and/or manually exploring a body part

Explanation: Visual exploration may be performed with or without optical instrumentation. Manual exploration may be performed directly or through intervening body layers.

Body Part Character 4	Approach Character 5	Device Character 6	Qualifier Character 7
Y Lower Artery Umbilical artery	Ø Open 3 Percutaneous 4 Percutaneous Endoscopic X External	Z No Device	Z No Qualifier

Non-OR	Ø4JY[3,4,X]ZZ

Ø   Medical and Surgical
4   Lower Arteries
L   Occlusion   Definition: Completely closing an orifice or the lumen of a tubular body part

Explanation: The orifice can be a natural orifice or an artificially created orifice

Body Part Character 4	Approach Character 5	Device Character 6	Qualifier Character 7

Ø **Abdominal Aorta**
   Inferior phrenic artery
   Lumbar artery
   Median sacral artery
   Middle suprarenal artery
   Ovarian artery
   Testicular artery
	Ø Open
	4 Percutaneous Endoscopic
		C Extraluminal Device
		D Intraluminal Device
		Z No Device
			Z No Qualifier

Ø **Abdominal Aorta**
   Inferior phrenic artery
   Lumbar artery
   Median sacral artery
   Middle suprarenal artery
   Ovarian artery
   Testicular artery
	3 Percutaneous	C Extraluminal Device
		Z No Device
			Z No Qualifier

Ø **Abdominal Aorta**
   Inferior phrenic artery
   Lumbar artery
   Median sacral artery
   Middle suprarenal artery
   Ovarian artery
   Testicular artery
	3 Percutaneous	D Intraluminal Device	J Temporary
			Z No Qualifier

04L Continued on next page

NC Noncovered Procedure   **LC** Limited Coverage   **QA** Questionable OB Admit   **NT** New Tech Add-on   ⊞ Combination Member   ♂ Male   ♀ Female

04L Continued

Ø **Medical and Surgical**
4 **Lower Arteries**
L **Occlusion**

Definition: Completely closing an orifice or the lumen of a tubular body part

Explanation: The orifice can be a natural orifice or an artificially created orifice

Body Part Character 4		Approach Character 5	Device Character 6	Qualifier Character 7
1 **Celiac Artery** Celiac trunk	K **Femoral Artery, Right** Circumflex iliac artery Deep femoral artery Descending genicular artery External pudendal artery Superficial epigastric artery	Ø Open 3 Percutaneous 4 Percutaneous Endoscopic	C Extraluminal Device D Intraluminal Device Z No Device	Z No Qualifier
2 **Gastric Artery** Left gastric artery Right gastric artery				
3 **Hepatic Artery** Common hepatic artery Gastroduodenal artery Hepatic artery proper	L **Femoral Artery, Left** *See K Femoral Artery, Right*			
4 **Splenic Artery** Left gastroepiploic artery Pancreatic artery Short gastric artery	M **Popliteal Artery, Right** Inferior genicular artery Middle genicular artery Superior genicular artery Sural artery Tibioperoneal trunk			
5 **Superior Mesenteric Artery** Ileal artery Ileocolic artery Inferior pancreaticoduodenal artery Jejunal artery	N **Popliteal Artery, Left** *See M Popliteal Artery, Right* P **Anterior Tibial Artery, Right** Anterior lateral malleolar artery Anterior medial malleolar artery Anterior tibial recurrent artery Dorsalis pedis artery Posterior tibial recurrent artery			
6 **Colic Artery, Right**				
7 **Colic Artery, Left**				
8 **Colic Artery, Middle**				
9 **Renal Artery, Right** Inferior suprarenal artery Renal segmental artery	Q **Anterior Tibial Artery, Left** *See P Anterior Tibial Artery, Right* R **Posterior Tibial Artery, Right**			
A **Renal Artery, Left** *See 9 Renal Artery, Right*	S **Posterior Tibial Artery, Left** T **Peroneal Artery, Right** Fibular artery			
B **Inferior Mesenteric Artery** Sigmoid artery Superior rectal artery	U **Peroneal Artery, Left** *See T Peroneal Artery, Right*			
C **Common Iliac Artery, Right**	V **Foot Artery, Right** Arcuate artery Dorsal metatarsal artery Lateral plantar artery Lateral tarsal artery Medial plantar artery			
D **Common Iliac Artery, Left**				
H **External Iliac Artery, Right** Deep circumflex iliac artery Inferior epigastric artery				
J **External Iliac Artery, Left** *See H External Iliac Artery, Right*	W **Foot Artery, Left** *See V Foot Artery, Right* Y **Lower Artery** Umbilical artery			
E **Internal Iliac Artery, Right** Deferential artery Hypogastric artery Iliolumbar artery Inferior gluteal artery Inferior vesical artery Internal pudendal artery Lateral sacral artery Middle rectal artery Obturator artery Prostatic artery Superior gluteal artery Superior vesical artery Umbilical artery Uterine artery Vaginal artery		Ø Open 3 Percutaneous 4 Percutaneous Endoscopic	C Extraluminal Device D Intraluminal Device Z No Device	T Uterine Artery, Right ♀ V Prostatic Artery, Right ♂ Z No Qualifier
F **Internal Iliac Artery, Left** Deferential artery Hypogastric artery Iliolumbar artery Inferior gluteal artery Inferior vesical artery Internal pudendal artery Lateral sacral artery Middle rectal artery Obturator artery Prostatic artery Superior gluteal artery Superior vesical artery Umbilical artery Uterine artery Vaginal artery		Ø Open 3 Percutaneous 4 Percutaneous Endoscopic	C Extraluminal Device D Intraluminal Device Z No Device	U Uterine Artery, Left ♀ W Prostatic Artery, Left ♂ Z No Qualifier

♀ 04LE[Ø,3,4][C,D,Z]T
♀ 04LF[Ø,3,4][C,D,Z]U
♂ 04LE[Ø,3,4][C,D,Z]V
♂ 04LF[Ø,3,4][C,D,Z]W

Non-OR Procedure   DRG Non-OR Procedure   Valid OR Procedure   HAC Associated Procedure   Combination Only   New/Revised April   New/Revised October

Ø   **Medical and Surgical**
4   **Lower Arteries**
N   **Release**   Definition: Freeing a body part from an abnormal physical constraint by cutting or by the use of force
                 Explanation: Some of the restraining tissue may be taken out but none of the body part is taken out

Body Part Character 4		Approach Character 5	Device Character 6	Qualifier Character 7
Ø **Abdominal Aorta** Inferior phrenic artery Lumbar artery Median sacral artery Middle suprarenal artery Ovarian artery Testicular artery **1** **Celiac Artery** Celiac trunk **2** **Gastric Artery** Left gastric artery Right gastric artery **3** **Hepatic Artery** Common hepatic artery Gastroduodenal artery Hepatic artery proper **4** **Splenic Artery** Left gastroepiploic artery Pancreatic artery Short gastric artery **5** **Superior Mesenteric Artery** Ileal artery Ileocolic artery Inferior pancreaticoduodenal artery Jejunal artery **6** **Colic Artery, Right** **7** **Colic Artery, Left** **8** **Colic Artery, Middle** **9** **Renal Artery, Right** Inferior suprarenal artery Renal segmental artery **A** **Renal Artery, Left** *See 9 Renal Artery, Right* **B** **Inferior Mesenteric Artery** Sigmoid artery Superior rectal artery **C** **Common Iliac Artery, Right** **D** **Common Iliac Artery, Left** **E** **Internal Iliac Artery, Right** Deferential artery Hypogastric artery Iliolumbar artery Inferior gluteal artery Inferior vesical artery Internal pudendal artery Lateral sacral artery Middle rectal artery Obturator artery Prostatic artery Superior gluteal artery Superior vesical artery Umbilical artery Uterine artery Vaginal artery	**F** **Internal Iliac Artery, Left** *See E Internal Iliac Artery, Right* **H** **External Iliac Artery, Right** Deep circumflex iliac artery Inferior epigastric artery **J** **External Iliac Artery, Left** *See H External Iliac Artery, Right* **K** **Femoral Artery, Right** Circumflex iliac artery Deep femoral artery Descending genicular artery External pudendal artery Superficial epigastric artery **L** **Femoral Artery, Left** *See K Femoral Artery, Right* **M** **Popliteal Artery, Right** Inferior genicular artery Middle genicular artery Superior genicular artery Sural artery Tibioperoneal trunk **N** **Popliteal Artery, Left** *See M Popliteal Artery, Right* **P** **Anterior Tibial Artery, Right** Anterior lateral malleolar artery Anterior medial malleolar artery Anterior tibial recurrent artery Dorsalis pedis artery Posterior tibial recurrent artery **Q** **Anterior Tibial Artery, Left** *See P Anterior Tibial Artery, Right* **R** **Posterior Tibial Artery, Right** **S** **Posterior Tibial Artery, Left** **T** **Peroneal Artery, Right** Fibular artery **U** **Peroneal Artery, Left** *See T Peroneal Artery, Right* **V** **Foot Artery, Right** Arcuate artery Dorsal metatarsal artery Lateral plantar artery Lateral tarsal artery Medial plantar artery **W** **Foot Artery, Left** *See V Foot Artery, Right* **Y** **Lower Artery** Umbilical artery	**Ø** Open **3** Percutaneous **4** Percutaneous Endoscopic	**Z** No Device	**Z** No Qualifier

NC Noncovered Procedure   LC Limited Coverage   QA Questionable OB Admit   NT New Tech Add-on   ⊞ Combination Member   ♂ Male   ♀ Female

ICD-10-PCS 2023   235

Ø4N–Ø4N

Lower Arteries

Ø   **Medical and Surgical**
4   **Lower Arteries**
P   **Removal**   Definition: Taking out or off a device from a body part

Explanation: If a device is taken out and a similar device put in without cutting or puncturing the skin or mucous membrane, the procedure is coded to the root operation CHANGE. Otherwise, the procedure for taking out a device is coded to the root operation REMOVAL.

Body Part Character 4	Approach Character 5	Device Character 6	Qualifier Character 7
Y Lower Artery Umbilical artery	Ø Open 3 Percutaneous 4 Percutaneous Endoscopic	Ø Drainage Device 2 Monitoring Device 3 Infusion Device 7 Autologous Tissue Substitute C Extraluminal Device D Intraluminal Device J Synthetic Substitute K Nonautologous Tissue Substitute Y Other Device	Z No Qualifier
Y Lower Artery Umbilical artery	X External	Ø Drainage Device 1 Radioactive Element 2 Monitoring Device 3 Infusion Device D Intraluminal Device	Z No Qualifier

Non-OR   04PY3[Ø,2,3,D]Z
Non-OR   04PY[3,4]YZ
Non-OR   04PYX[Ø,1,2,3,D]Z

Ø   Medical and Surgical
4   Lower Arteries
Q   Repair   Definition: Restoring, to the extent possible, a body part to its normal anatomic structure and function
                    Explanation: Used only when the method to accomplish the repair is not one of the other root operations

Body Part Character 4		Approach Character 5	Device Character 6	Qualifier Character 7

Ø Abdominal Aorta
 Inferior phrenic artery
 Lumbar artery
 Median sacral artery
 Middle suprarenal artery
 Ovarian artery
 Testicular artery
 1 Celiac Artery
 Celiac trunk
 2 Gastric Artery
 Left gastric artery
 Right gastric artery
 3 Hepatic Artery
 Common hepatic artery
 Gastroduodenal artery
 Hepatic artery proper
 4 Splenic Artery
 Left gastroepiploic artery
 Pancreatic artery
 Short gastric artery
 5 Superior Mesenteric Artery
 Ileal artery
 Ileocolic artery
 Inferior pancreaticoduodenal
     artery
 Jejunal artery
 6 Colic Artery, Right
 7 Colic Artery, Left
 8 Colic Artery, Middle
 9 Renal Artery, Right
 Inferior suprarenal artery
 Renal segmental artery
 A Renal Artery, Left
 See 9 Renal Artery, Right
 B Inferior Mesenteric Artery
 Sigmoid artery
 Superior rectal artery
 C Common Iliac Artery, Right
 D Common Iliac Artery, Left
 E Internal Iliac Artery, Right
 Deferential artery
 Hypogastric artery
 Iliolumbar artery
 Inferior gluteal artery
 Inferior vesical artery
 Internal pudendal artery
 Lateral sacral artery
 Middle rectal artery
 Obturator artery
 Prostatic artery
 Superior gluteal artery
 Superior vesical artery
 Umbilical artery
 Uterine artery
 Vaginal artery
	F Internal Iliac Artery, Left
	 See E Internal Iliac Artery, Right
	 H External Iliac Artery, Right
	 Deep circumflex iliac artery
	 Inferior epigastric artery
	 J External Iliac Artery, Left
	 See H External Iliac Artery, Right
	 K Femoral Artery, Right
	 Circumflex iliac artery
	 Deep femoral artery
	 Descending genicular artery
	 External pudendal artery
	 Superficial epigastric artery
	 L Femoral Artery, Left
	 See K Femoral Artery, Right
	 M Popliteal Artery, Right
	 Inferior genicular artery
	 Middle genicular artery
	 Superior genicular artery
	 Sural artery
	 Tibioperoneal trunk
	 N Popliteal Artery, Left
	 See M Popliteal Artery, Right
	 P Anterior Tibial Artery, Right
	 Anterior lateral malleolar
	     artery
	 Anterior medial malleolar
	     artery
	 Anterior tibial recurrent
	     artery
	 Dorsalis pedis artery
	 Posterior tibial recurrent
	     artery
	 Q Anterior Tibial Artery, Left
	 See P Anterior Tibial Artery, Right
	 R Posterior Tibial Artery, Right
	 S Posterior Tibial Artery, Left
	 T Peroneal Artery, Right
	 Fibular artery
	 U Peroneal Artery, Left
	 See T Peroneal Artery, Right
	 V Foot Artery, Right
	 Arcuate artery
	 Dorsal metatarsal artery
	 Lateral plantar artery
	 Lateral tarsal artery
	 Medial plantar artery
	 W Foot Artery, Left
	 See V Foot Artery, Right
	 Y Lower Artery
	 Umbilical artery
		Ø Open
		 3 Percutaneous
		 4 Percutaneous Endoscopic
			Z No Device	**Z No Qualifier**

NC Noncovered Procedure   LC Limited Coverage   QA Questionable OB Admit   NT New Tech Add-on   ⊞ Combination Member   ♂ Male   ♀ Female

ICD-10-PCS 2023   237

Ø4Q–Ø4Q

Ø   Medical and Surgical
4   Lower Arteries
R   Replacement   Definition: Putting in or on biological or synthetic material that physically takes the place and/or function of all or a portion of a body part
                  Explanation: The body part may have been taken out or replaced, or may be taken out, physically eradicated, or rendered nonfunctional during the REPLACEMENT procedure. A REMOVAL procedure is coded for taking out the device used in a previous replacement procedure.

Body Part Character 4		Approach Character 5	Device Character 6	Qualifier Character 7

Ø Abdominal Aorta
  Inferior phrenic artery
  Lumbar artery
  Median sacral artery
  Middle suprarenal artery
  Ovarian artery
  Testicular artery
1 Celiac Artery
  Celiac trunk
2 Gastric Artery
  Left gastric artery
  Right gastric artery
3 Hepatic Artery
  Common hepatic artery
  Gastroduodenal artery
  Hepatic artery proper
4 Splenic Artery
  Left gastroepiploic artery
  Pancreatic artery
  Short gastric artery
5 Superior Mesenteric Artery
  Ileal artery
  Ileocolic artery
  Inferior pancreaticoduodenal
    artery
  Jejunal artery
6 Colic Artery, Right
7 Colic Artery, Left
8 Colic Artery, Middle
9 Renal Artery, Right
  Inferior suprarenal artery
  Renal segmental artery
A Renal Artery, Left
  See 9 Renal Artery, Right
B Inferior Mesenteric Artery
  Sigmoid artery
  Superior rectal artery
C Common Iliac Artery, Right
D Common Iliac Artery, Left
E Internal Iliac Artery, Right
  Deferential artery
  Hypogastric artery
  Iliolumbar artery
  Inferior gluteal artery
  Inferior vesical artery
  Internal pudendal artery
  Lateral sacral artery
  Middle rectal artery
  Obturator artery
  Prostatic artery
  Superior gluteal artery
  Superior vesical artery
  Umbilical artery
  Uterine artery
  Vaginal artery
	F Internal Iliac Artery, Left
	  See E Internal Iliac Artery, Right
	H External Iliac Artery, Right
	  Deep circumflex iliac artery
	  Inferior epigastric artery
	J External Iliac Artery, Left
	  See H External Iliac Artery, Right
	K Femoral Artery, Right
	  Circumflex iliac artery
	  Deep femoral artery
	  Descending genicular artery
	  External pudendal artery
	  Superficial epigastric artery
	L Femoral Artery, Left
	  See K Femoral Artery, Right
	M Popliteal Artery, Right
	  Inferior genicular artery
	  Middle genicular artery
	  Superior genicular artery
	  Sural artery
	  Tibioperoneal trunk
	N Popliteal Artery, Left
	  See M Popliteal Artery, Right
	P Anterior Tibial Artery, Right
	  Anterior lateral malleolar
	    artery
	  Anterior medial malleolar
	    artery
	  Anterior tibial recurrent artery
	  Dorsalis pedis artery
	  Posterior tibial recurrent artery
	Q Anterior Tibial Artery, Left
	  See P Anterior Tibial Artery,
	    Right
	R Posterior Tibial Artery, Right
	S Posterior Tibial Artery, Left
	T Peroneal Artery, Right
	  Fibular artery
	U Peroneal Artery, Left
	  See T Peroneal Artery, Right
	V Foot Artery, Right
	  Arcuate artery
	  Dorsal metatarsal artery
	  Lateral plantar artery
	  Lateral tarsal artery
	  Medial plantar artery
	W Foot Artery, Left
	  See V Foot Artery, Right
	Y Lower Artery
	  Umbilical artery
		Ø Open
		4 Percutaneous Endoscopic
			7 Autologous Tissue
			  Substitute
			J Synthetic Substitute
			K Nonautologous Tissue
			  Substitute
				Z No Qualifier

Non-OR Procedure   DRG Non-OR Procedure   Valid OR Procedure   HAC Associated Procedure   Combination Only   New/Revised April   New/Revised October

238

Ø4R–Ø4R

ICD-10-PCS 2023

Ø   Medical and Surgical
4   Lower Arteries
S   Reposition   Definition: Moving to its normal location, or other suitable location, all or a portion of a body part

Explanation: The body part is moved to a new location from an abnormal location, or from a normal location where it is not functioning correctly. The body part may or may not be cut out or off to be moved to the new location.

Body Part Character 4		Approach Character 5	Device Character 6	Qualifier Character 7

Ø Abdominal Aorta
  Inferior phrenic artery
  Lumbar artery
  Median sacral artery
  Middle suprarenal artery
  Ovarian artery
  Testicular artery
1 Celiac Artery
  Celiac trunk
2 Gastric Artery
  Left gastric artery
  Right gastric artery
3 Hepatic Artery
  Common hepatic artery
  Gastroduodenal artery
  Hepatic artery proper
4 Splenic Artery
  Left gastroepiploic artery
  Pancreatic artery
  Short gastric artery
5 Superior Mesenteric Artery
  Ileal artery
  Ileocolic artery
  Inferior pancreaticoduodenal
    artery
  Jejunal artery
6 Colic Artery, Right
7 Colic Artery, Left
8 Colic Artery, Middle
9 Renal Artery, Right
  Inferior suprarenal artery
  Renal segmental artery
A Renal Artery, Left
  See 9 Renal Artery, Right
B Inferior Mesenteric Artery
  Sigmoid artery
  Superior rectal artery
C Common Iliac Artery, Right
D Common Iliac Artery, Left
E Internal Iliac Artery, Right
  Deferential artery
  Hypogastric artery
  Iliolumbar artery
  Inferior gluteal artery
  Inferior vesical artery
  Internal pudendal artery
  Lateral sacral artery
  Middle rectal artery
  Obturator artery
  Prostatic artery
  Superior gluteal artery
  Superior vesical artery
  Umbilical artery
  Uterine artery
  Vaginal artery
	F Internal Iliac Artery, Left
	  See E Internal Iliac Artery, Right
	H External Iliac Artery, Right
	  Deep circumflex iliac artery
	  Inferior epigastric artery
	J External Iliac Artery, Left
	  See H External Iliac Artery, Right
	K Femoral Artery, Right
	  Circumflex iliac artery
	  Deep femoral artery
	  Descending genicular artery
	  External pudendal artery
	  Superficial epigastric artery
	L Femoral Artery, Left
	  See K Femoral Artery, Right
	M Popliteal Artery, Right
	  Inferior genicular artery
	  Middle genicular artery
	  Superior genicular artery
	  Sural artery
	  Tibioperoneal trunk
	N Popliteal Artery, Left
	  See M Popliteal Artery, Right
	P Anterior Tibial Artery, Right
	  Anterior lateral malleolar
	    artery
	  Anterior medial malleolar
	    artery
	  Anterior tibial recurrent artery
	  Dorsalis pedis artery
	  Posterior tibial recurrent artery
	Q Anterior Tibial Artery, Left
	  See P Anterior Tibial Artery,
	  Right
	R Posterior Tibial Artery, Right
	S Posterior Tibial Artery, Left
	T Peroneal Artery, Right
	  Fibular artery
	U Peroneal Artery, Left
	  See T Peroneal Artery, Right
	V Foot Artery, Right
	  Arcuate artery
	  Dorsal metatarsal artery
	  Lateral plantar artery
	  Lateral tarsal artery
	  Medial plantar artery
	W Foot Artery, Left
	  See V Foot Artery, Right
	Y Lower Artery
	  Umbilical artery
		Ø Open
		3 Percutaneous
		4 Percutaneous Endoscopic
			Z No Device	**Z No Qualifier**

NC Noncovered Procedure   LC Limited Coverage   QA Questionable OB Admit   NT New Tech Add-on   ⊞ Combination Member   ♂ Male   ♀ Female

ICD-10-PCS 2023   **239**

Lower Arteries

0 Medical and Surgical
4 Lower Arteries
U Supplement

Definition: Putting in or on biological or synthetic material that physically reinforces and/or augments the function of a portion of a body part

Explanation: The biological material is non-living, or is living and from the same individual. The body part may have been previously replaced, and the SUPPLEMENT procedure is performed to physically reinforce and/or augment the function of the replaced body part.

Body Part Character 4		Approach Character 5	Device Character 6	Qualifier Character 7
0 Abdominal Aorta Inferior phrenic artery Lumbar artery Median sacral artery Middle suprarenal artery Ovarian artery Testicular artery	**F Internal Iliac Artery, Left** *See E Internal Iliac Artery, Right* **H External Iliac Artery, Right** Deep circumflex iliac artery Inferior epigastric artery	**0 Open** **3 Percutaneous** **4 Percutaneous Endoscopic**	**7 Autologous Tissue Substitute** **J Synthetic Substitute** **K Nonautologous Tissue Substitute**	**Z No Qualifier**
1 Celiac Artery Celiac trunk	**J External Iliac Artery, Left** *See H External Iliac Artery, Right*			
2 Gastric Artery Left gastric artery Right gastric artery	**K Femoral Artery, Right** Circumflex iliac artery Deep femoral artery Descending genicular artery External pudendal artery Superficial epigastric artery			
3 Hepatic Artery Common hepatic artery Gastroduodenal artery Hepatic artery proper	**L Femoral Artery, Left** *See K Femoral Artery, Right*			
4 Splenic Artery Left gastroepiploic artery Pancreatic artery Short gastric artery	**M Popliteal Artery, Right** Inferior genicular artery Middle genicular artery Superior genicular artery Sural artery Tibioperoneal trunk			
5 Superior Mesenteric Artery Ileal artery Ileocolic artery Inferior pancreaticoduodenal artery Jejunal artery	**N Popliteal Artery, Left** *See M Popliteal Artery, Right* **P Anterior Tibial Artery, Right** Anterior lateral malleolar artery Anterior medial malleolar artery Anterior tibial recurrent artery Dorsalis pedis artery Posterior tibial recurrent artery			
6 Colic Artery, Right				
7 Colic Artery, Left				
8 Colic Artery, Middle				
9 Renal Artery, Right Inferior suprarenal artery Renal segmental artery	**Q Anterior Tibial Artery, Left** *See P Anterior Tibial Artery, Right*			
A Renal Artery, Left *See 9 Renal Artery, Right*	**R Posterior Tibial Artery, Right** **S Posterior Tibial Artery, Left**			
B Inferior Mesenteric Artery Sigmoid artery Superior rectal artery	**T Peroneal Artery, Right** Fibular artery			
C Common Iliac Artery, Right	**U Peroneal Artery, Left** *See T Peroneal Artery, Right*			
D Common Iliac Artery, Left	**V Foot Artery, Right** Arcuate artery Dorsal metatarsal artery Lateral plantar artery Lateral tarsal artery Medial plantar artery			
E Internal Iliac Artery, Right Deferential artery Hypogastric artery Iliolumbar artery Inferior gluteal artery Inferior vesical artery Internal pudendal artery Lateral sacral artery Middle rectal artery Obturator artery Prostatic artery Superior gluteal artery Superior vesical artery Umbilical artery Uterine artery Vaginal artery	**W Foot Artery, Left** *See V Foot Artery, Right* **Y Lower Artery** Umbilical artery			

Non-OR Procedure   DRG Non-OR Procedure   Valid OR Procedure   HAC Associated Procedure   Combination Only   New/Revised April   New/Revised October

240

ICD-10-PCS 2023

04U–04U

0   Medical and Surgical
4   Lower Arteries
V   Restriction   Definition: Partially closing an orifice or the lumen of a tubular body part
                     Explanation: The orifice can be a natural orifice or an artificially created orifice

Body Part Character 4		Approach Character 5	Device Character 6	Qualifier Character 7
0 **Abdominal Aorta** Inferior phrenic artery Lumbar artery Median sacral artery Middle suprarenal artery Ovarian artery Testicular artery		**0** Open **3** Percutaneous **4** Percutaneous Endoscopic	**C** Extraluminal Device **E** Intraluminal Device, Branched or Fenestrated, One or Two Arteries **F** Intraluminal Device, Branched or Fenestrated, Three or More Arteries **Z** No Device	**Z** No Qualifier
0 **Abdominal Aorta** Inferior phrenic artery Lumbar artery Median sacral artery Middle suprarenal artery Ovarian artery Testicular artery		**0** Open **3** Percutaneous **4** Percutaneous Endoscopic	**D** Intraluminal Device	**J** Temporary **Z** No Qualifier

1 **Celiac Artery**
Celiac trunk
2 **Gastric Artery**
Left gastric artery
Right gastric artery
3 **Hepatic Artery**
Common hepatic artery
Gastroduodenal artery
Hepatic artery proper
4 **Splenic Artery**
Left gastroepiploic artery
Pancreatic artery
Short gastric artery
5 **Superior Mesenteric Artery**
Ileal artery
Ileocolic artery
Inferior pancreaticoduodenal
   artery
Jejunal artery
6 **Colic Artery, Right**
7 **Colic Artery, Left**
8 **Colic Artery, Middle**
9 **Renal Artery, Right**
Inferior suprarenal artery
Renal segmental artery
A **Renal Artery, Left**
See 9 Renal Artery, Right
B **Inferior Mesenteric Artery**
Sigmoid artery
Superior rectal artery
E **Internal Iliac Artery, Right**
Deferential artery
Hypogastric artery
Iliolumbar artery
Inferior gluteal artery
Inferior vesical artery
Internal pudendal artery
Lateral sacral artery
Middle rectal artery
Obturator artery
Prostatic artery
Superior gluteal artery
Superior vesical artery
Umbilical artery
Uterine artery
Vaginal artery
F **Internal Iliac Artery, Left**
See E Internal Iliac Artery, Right
	H **External Iliac Artery, Right**
	Deep circumflex iliac artery
	Inferior epigastric artery
	J **External Iliac Artery, Left**
	See H External Iliac Artery, Right
	K **Femoral Artery, Right**
	Circumflex iliac artery
	Deep femoral artery
	Descending genicular artery
	External pudendal artery
	Superficial epigastric artery
	L **Femoral Artery, Left**
	See K Femoral Artery, Right
	M **Popliteal Artery, Right**
	Inferior genicular artery
	Middle genicular artery
	Superior genicular artery
	Sural artery
	Tibioperoneal trunk
	N **Popliteal Artery, Left**
	See M Popliteal Artery, Right
	P **Anterior Tibial Artery, Right**
	Anterior lateral malleolar
	   artery
	Anterior medial malleolar
	   artery
	Anterior tibial recurrent artery
	Dorsalis pedis artery
	Posterior tibial recurrent artery
	Q **Anterior Tibial Artery, Left**
	See P Anterior Tibial Artery,
	Right
	R **Posterior Tibial Artery, Right**
	S **Posterior Tibial Artery, Left**
	T **Peroneal Artery, Right**
	Fibular artery
	U **Peroneal Artery, Left**
	See T Peroneal Artery, Right
	V **Foot Artery, Right**
	Arcuate artery
	Dorsal metatarsal artery
	Lateral plantar artery
	Lateral tarsal artery
	Medial plantar artery
	W **Foot Artery, Left**
	See V Foot Artery, Right
	Y **Lower Artery**
	Umbilical artery
		0 Open
		3 Percutaneous
		4 Percutaneous Endoscopic
			C Extraluminal Device
			D Intraluminal Device
			Z No Device
				Z No Qualifier

C **Common Iliac Artery, Right** **D** **Common Iliac Artery, Left**		**0** Open **3** Percutaneous **4** Percutaneous Endoscopic	**C** Extraluminal Device **D** Intraluminal Device **E** Intraluminal Device, Branched or Fenestrated, One or Two Arteries **Z** No Device	**Z** No Qualifier

NC Noncovered Procedure   **LC** Limited Coverage   **QA** Questionable OB Admit   **NT** New Tech Add-on   ⊞ Combination Member   ♂Male   ♀Female

ICD-10-PCS 2023   241

Lower Arteries

Ø   **Medical and Surgical**
4   **Lower Arteries**
W   **Revision**

Definition: Correcting, to the extent possible, a portion of a malfunctioning device or the position of a displaced device

Explanation: Revision can include correcting a malfunctioning or displaced device by taking out or putting in components of the device such as a screw or pin

Body Part Character 4	Approach Character 5	Device Character 6	Qualifier Character 7
Y Lower Artery Umbilical artery	Ø Open 3 Percutaneous 4 Percutaneous Endoscopic	Ø Drainage Device 2 Monitoring Device 3 Infusion Device 7 Autologous Tissue Substitute C Extraluminal Device D Intraluminal Device J Synthetic Substitute K Nonautologous Tissue Substitute Y Other Device	Z No Qualifier
Y Lower Artery Umbilical artery	X External	Ø Drainage Device 2 Monitoring Device 3 Infusion Device 7 Autologous Tissue Substitute C Extraluminal Device D Intraluminal Device J Synthetic Substitute K Nonautologous Tissue Substitute	Z No Qualifier

Non-OR   Ø4WY3[Ø,2,3]Z
Non-OR   Ø4WY[3,4]YZ
Non-OR   Ø4WYX[Ø,2,3,7,C,D,J,K]Z

Upper Veins Ø51–Ø5W

Character Meanings

This Character Meaning table is provided as a guide to assist the user in the identification of character members that may be found in this section of code tables. It **SHOULD NOT** be used to build a PCS code.

Operation–Character 3		Body Part–Character 4		Approach–Character 5		Device–Character 6		Qualifier–Character 7	
1	Bypass	Ø	Azygos Vein	Ø	Open	Ø	Drainage Device	Ø	Ultrasonic
5	Destruction	1	Hemiazygos Vein	3	Percutaneous	2	Monitoring Device	1	Drug-Coated Balloon
7	Dilation	3	Innominate Vein, Right	4	Percutaneous Endoscopic	3	Infusion Device	X	Diagnostic
9	Drainage	4	Innominate Vein, Left	X	External	7	Autologous Tissue Substitute	Y	Upper Vein
B	Excision	5	Subclavian Vein, Right			9	Autologous Venous Tissue	Z	No Qualifier
C	Extirpation	6	Subclavian Vein, Left			A	Autologous Arterial Tissue		
D	Extraction	7	Axillary Vein, Right			C	Extraluminal Device		
F	Fragmentation	8	Axillary Vein, Left			D	Intraluminal Device		
H	Insertion	9	Brachial Vein, Right			J	Synthetic Substitute		
J	Inspection	A	Brachial Vein, Left			K	Nonautologous Tissue Substitute		
L	Occlusion	B	Basilic Vein, Right			M	Neurostimulator Lead		
N	Release	C	Basilic Vein, Left			Y	Other Device		
P	Removal	D	Cephalic Vein, Right			Z	No Device		
Q	Repair	F	Cephalic Vein, Left						
R	Replacement	G	Hand Vein, Right						
S	Reposition	H	Hand Vein, Left						
U	Supplement	L	Intracranial Vein						
V	Restriction	M	Internal Jugular Vein, Right						
W	Revision	N	Internal Jugular Vein, Left						
		P	External Jugular Vein, Right						
		Q	External Jugular Vein, Left						
		R	Vertebral Vein, Right						
		S	Vertebral Vein, Left						
		T	Face Vein, Right						
		V	Face Vein, Left						
		Y	Upper Vein						

AHA Coding Clinic for Upper Veins
2022, 1Q, 10-13   Procedures performed on a continuous vessel, ICD-10-PCS Guideline B4.1c

AHA Coding Clinic for table Ø51
2020, 1Q, 28   Free flap microvascular breast reconstruction
2017, 3Q, 15   Bypass of innominate vein to atrial appendage

AHA Coding Clinic for table Ø57
2020, 3Q, 38   Thrombectomy of arteriovenous fistula with angioplasty and stent placement

AHA Coding Clinic for table Ø59
2018, 3Q, 7   Catheter placement for treatment of congestive heart failure

AHA Coding Clinic for table Ø5B
2021, 2Q, 15   Excision of pituitary macroadenoma within cavernous sinus
2020, 3Q, 40   Excision of ulceration of arteriovenous fistula
2020, 1Q, 24   Resection of vascular malformation, likely cavernoma
2016, 2Q, 12   Resection of malignant neoplasm of infratemporal fossa

AHA Coding Clinic for table Ø5C
2020, 3Q, 37   Repair of aneurysm of arteriovenous fistula with endovenectomy
2020, 3Q, 38   Thrombectomy of arteriovenous fistula with angioplasty and stent placement

AHA Coding Clinic for table Ø5F
2020, 4Q, 45-49   New fragmentation tables
2020, 4Q, 49-50   Intravascular ultrasound assisted thrombolysis
2020, 4Q, 50   Intravascular lithotripsy

AHA Coding Clinic for table Ø5H
2016, 4Q, 97-98   Phrenic neurostimulator

AHA Coding Clinic for table Ø5P
2016, 4Q, 97-98   Phrenic neurostimulator

AHA Coding Clinic for table Ø5Q
2017, 3Q, 15   Bypass of innominate vein to atrial appendage

AHA Coding Clinic for table Ø5S
2013, 4Q, 125   Stage II cephalic vein transposition (superficialization) of arteriovenous fistula

AHA Coding Clinic for table Ø5V
2020, 3Q, 37   Repair of aneurysm of arteriovenous fistula with endovenectomy

AHA Coding Clinic for table Ø5W
2016, 4Q, 97-98   Phrenic neurostimulator

Head and Neck Veins

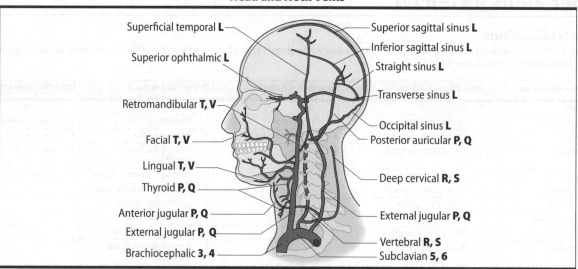

Superficial temporal **L**
Superior ophthalmic **L**
Retromandibular **T, V**
Facial **T, V**
Lingual **T, V**
Thyroid **P, Q**
Anterior jugular **P, Q**
External jugular **P, Q**
Brachiocephalic **3, 4**

Superior sagittal sinus **L**
Inferior sagittal sinus **L**
Straight sinus **L**
Transverse sinus **L**
Occipital sinus **L**
Posterior auricular **P, Q**
Deep cervical **R, S**
External jugular **P, Q**
Vertebral **R, S**
Subclavian **5, 6**

Upper Veins

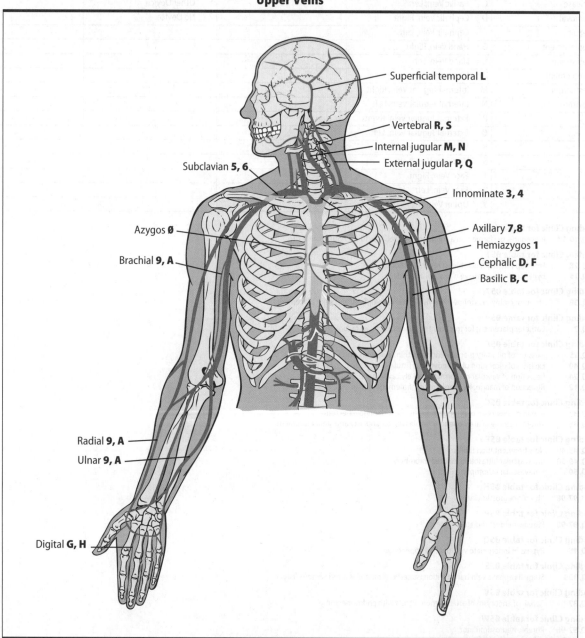

Superficial temporal **L**
Vertebral **R, S**
Internal jugular **M, N**
External jugular **P, Q**
Subclavian **5, 6**
Innominate **3, 4**
Azygos **Ø**
Axillary **7,8**
Hemiazygos **1**
Brachial **9, A**
Cephalic **D, F**
Basilic **B, C**
Radial **9, A**
Ulnar **9, A**
Digital **G, H**

0   **Medical and Surgical**
5   **Upper Veins**
1   **Bypass**   Definition: Altering the route of passage of the contents of a tubular body part

                   Explanation: Rerouting contents of a body part to a downstream area of the normal route, to a similar route and body part, or to an abnormal route and dissimilar body part. Includes one or more anastomoses, with or without the use of a device.

Body Part Character 4	Approach Character 5	Device Character 6	Qualifier Character 7

0   **Azygos Vein**
     Right ascending lumbar vein
     Right subcostal vein
	0 Open
	4 Percutaneous Endoscopic
		7 Autologous Tissue Substitute
		9 Autologous Venous Tissue
		A Autologous Arterial Tissue
		J Synthetic Substitute
		K Nonautologous Tissue Substitute
		Z No Device
			Y Upper Vein

1   **Hemiazygos Vein**
     Left ascending lumbar vein
     Left subcostal vein			

3   **Innominate Vein, Right**
     Brachiocephalic vein
     Inferior thyroid vein			

4 **Innominate Vein, Left** *See 3 Innominate Vein, Right*			
5 **Subclavian Vein, Right**			
6 **Subclavian Vein, Left**			
7 **Axillary Vein, Right**			
8 **Axillary Vein, Left**			

9   **Brachial Vein, Right**
     Radial vein
     Ulnar vein			

A **Brachial Vein, Left** *See 9 Brachial Vein, Right*			

B   **Basilic Vein, Right**
     Median antebrachial vein
     Median cubital vein			

C **Basilic Vein, Left** *See B Basilic Vein, Right*			
D **Cephalic Vein, Right** Accessory cephalic vein			
F **Cephalic Vein, Left** *See D Cephalic Vein, Right*			

G   **Hand Vein, Right**
     Dorsal metacarpal vein
     Palmar (volar) digital vein
     Palmar (volar) metacarpal vein
     Superficial palmar venous arch
     Volar (palmar) digital vein
     Volar (palmar) metacarpal vein			

H **Hand Vein, Left** *See G Hand Vein, Right*			

L   **Intracranial Vein**
     Anterior cerebral vein
     Basal (internal) cerebral vein
     Dural venous sinus
     Great cerebral vein
     Inferior cerebellar vein
     Inferior cerebral vein
     Internal (basal) cerebral vein
     Middle cerebral vein
     Ophthalmic vein
     Superior cerebellar vein
     Superior cerebral vein			

M **Internal Jugular Vein, Right**			
N **Internal Jugular Vein, Left**			
P **External Jugular Vein, Right** Posterior auricular vein			
Q **External Jugular Vein, Left** *See P External Jugular Vein, Right*			

R   **Vertebral Vein, Right**
     Deep cervical vein
     Suboccipital venous plexus			

S **Vertebral Vein, Left** *See R Vertebral Vein, Right*			

T   **Face Vein, Right**
     Angular vein
     Anterior facial vein
     Common facial vein
     Deep facial vein
     Frontal vein
     Posterior facial (retromandibular) vein
     Supraorbital vein			

V **Face Vein, Left** *See T Face Vein, Right*			

Ø **Medical and Surgical**
5 **Upper Veins**
5 **Destruction**   Definition: Physical eradication of all or a portion of a body part by the direct use of energy, force, or a destructive agent
                      Explanation: None of the body part is physically taken out

Body Part Character 4	Approach Character 5	Device Character 6	Qualifier Character 7
Ø **Azygos Vein** Right ascending lumbar vein Right subcostal vein	**Ø** Open **3** Percutaneous **4** Percutaneous Endoscopic	**Z** No Device	**Z** No Qualifier
1 **Hemiazygos Vein** Left ascending lumbar vein Left subcostal vein			
3 **Innominate Vein, Right** Brachiocephalic vein Inferior thyroid vein			
4 **Innominate Vein, Left** *See 3 Innominate Vein, Right*			
5 **Subclavian Vein, Right**			
6 **Subclavian Vein, Left**			
7 **Axillary Vein, Right**			
8 **Axillary Vein, Left**			
9 **Brachial Vein, Right** Radial vein Ulnar vein			
A **Brachial Vein, Left** *See 9 Brachial Vein, Right*			
B **Basilic Vein, Right** Median antebrachial vein Median cubital vein			
C **Basilic Vein, Left** *See B Basilic Vein, Right*			
D **Cephalic Vein, Right** Accessory cephalic vein			
F **Cephalic Vein, Left** *See D Cephalic Vein, Right*			
G **Hand Vein, Right** Dorsal metacarpal vein Palmar (volar) digital vein Palmar (volar) metacarpal vein Superficial palmar venous arch Volar (palmar) digital vein Volar (palmar) metacarpal vein			
H **Hand Vein, Left** *See G Hand Vein, Right*			
L **Intracranial Vein** Anterior cerebral vein Basal (internal) cerebral vein Dural venous sinus Great cerebral vein Inferior cerebellar vein Inferior cerebral vein Internal (basal) cerebral vein Middle cerebral vein Ophthalmic vein Superior cerebellar vein Superior cerebral vein			
M **Internal Jugular Vein, Right**			
N **Internal Jugular Vein, Left**			
P **External Jugular Vein, Right** Posterior auricular vein			
Q **External Jugular Vein, Left** *See P External Jugular Vein, Right*			
R **Vertebral Vein, Right** Deep cervical vein Suboccipital venous plexus			
S **Vertebral Vein, Left** *See R Vertebral Vein, Right*			
T **Face Vein, Right** Angular vein Anterior facial vein Common facial vein Deep facial vein Frontal vein Posterior facial (retromandibular) vein Supraorbital vein			
V **Face Vein, Left** *See T Face Vein, Right*			
Y **Upper Vein**			

Non-OR Procedure   DRG Non-OR Procedure   Valid OR Procedure   HAC Associated Procedure   Combination Only   New/Revised April   New/Revised October

246   ICD-10-PCS 2023

Upper Veins
Ø55–Ø55

Ø Medical and Surgical
5 Upper Veins
7 Dilation   Definition: Expanding an orifice or the lumen of a tubular body part

Explanation: The orifice can be a natural orifice or an artificially created orifice. Accomplished by stretching a tubular body part using intraluminal pressure or by cutting part of the orifice or wall of the tubular body part.

Body Part Character 4	Approach Character 5	Device Character 6	Qualifier Character 7
Ø Azygos Vein Right ascending lumbar vein Right subcostal vein **1 Hemiazygos Vein** Left ascending lumbar vein Left subcostal vein **G Hand Vein, Right** Dorsal metacarpal vein Palmar (volar) digital vein Palmar (volar) metacarpal vein Superficial palmar venous arch Volar (palmar) digital vein Volar (palmar) metacarpal vein **H Hand Vein, Left** See G Hand Vein, Right **L Intracranial Vein** `NC` Anterior cerebral vein Basal (internal) cerebral vein Dural venous sinus Great cerebral vein Inferior cerebellar vein Inferior cerebral vein Internal (basal) cerebral vein Middle cerebral vein Ophthalmic vein Superior cerebellar vein Superior cerebral vein **M Internal Jugular Vein, Right** **N Internal Jugular Vein, Left** **P External Jugular Vein, Right** Posterior auricular vein **Q External Jugular Vein, Left** See P External Jugular Vein, Right **R Vertebral Vein, Right** Deep cervical vein Suboccipital venous plexus **S Vertebral Vein, Left** See R Vertebral Vein, Right **T Face Vein, Right** Angular vein Anterior facial vein Common facial vein Deep facial vein Frontal vein Posterior facial (retromandibular) vein Supraorbital vein **V Face Vein, Left** See T Face Vein, Right **Y Upper Vein**	**Ø Open** **3 Percutaneous** **4 Percutaneous Endoscopic**	**D Intraluminal Device** **Z No Device**	**Z No Qualifier**
3 Innominate Vein, Right Brachiocephalic vein Inferior thyroid vein **4 Innominate Vein, Left** See 3 Innominate Vein, Right **5 Subclavian Vein, Right** **6 Subclavian Vein, Left** **7 Axillary Vein, Right** **8 Axillary Vein, Left** **9 Brachial Vein, Right** Radial vein Ulnar vein **A Brachial Vein, Left** See 9 Brachial Vein, Right **B Basilic Vein, Right** Median antebrachial vein Median cubital vein **C Basilic Vein, Left** See B Basilic Vein, Right **D Cephalic Vein, Right** Accessory cephalic vein **F Cephalic Vein, Left** See D Cephalic Vein, Right	**Ø Open** **3 Percutaneous** **4 Percutaneous Endoscopic**	**D Intraluminal Device** **Z No Device**	**1 Drug-Coated Balloon** **Z No Qualifier**

`NC`   Ø57L[3,4]ZZ

`NC` Noncovered Procedure   `LC` Limited Coverage   `QA` Questionable OB Admit   `NT` New Tech Add-on   ➕ Combination Member   ♂ Male   ♀ Female

Upper Veins

Ø Medical and Surgical
5 Upper Veins
9 Drainage   Definition: Taking or letting out fluids and/or gases from a body part

                       Explanation: The qualifier DIAGNOSTIC is used to identify drainage procedures that are biopsies

Body Part Character 4		Approach Character 5	Device Character 6	Qualifier Character 7
Ø Azygos Vein Right ascending lumbar vein Right subcostal vein **1 Hemiazygos Vein** Left ascending lumbar vein Left subcostal vein **3 Innominate Vein, Right** Brachiocephalic vein Inferior thyroid vein **4 Innominate Vein, Left** See 3 Innominate Vein, Right **5 Subclavian Vein, Right** **6 Subclavian Vein, Left** **7 Axillary Vein, Right** **8 Axillary Vein, Left** **9 Brachial Vein, Right** Radial vein Ulnar vein **A Brachial Vein, Left** See 9 Brachial Vein, Right **B Basilic Vein, Right** Median antebrachial vein Median cubital vein **C Basilic Vein, Left** See B Basilic Vein, Right **D Cephalic Vein, Right** Accessory cephalic vein **F Cephalic Vein, Left** See D Cephalic Vein, Right **G Hand Vein, Right** Dorsal metacarpal vein Palmar (volar) digital vein Palmar (volar) metacarpal vein Superficial palmar venous arch Volar (palmar) digital vein Volar (palmar) metacarpal vein	**H Hand Vein, Left** See G Hand Vein, Right **L Intracranial Vein** Anterior cerebral vein Basal (internal) cerebral vein Dural venous sinus Great cerebral vein Inferior cerebellar vein Inferior cerebral vein Internal (basal) cerebral vein Middle cerebral vein Ophthalmic vein Superior cerebellar vein Superior cerebral vein **M Internal Jugular Vein, Right** **N Internal Jugular Vein, Left** **P External Jugular Vein, Right** Posterior auricular vein **Q External Jugular Vein, Left** See P External Jugular Vein, Right **R Vertebral Vein, Right** Deep cervical vein Suboccipital venous plexus **S Vertebral Vein, Left** See R Vertebral Vein, Right **T Face Vein, Right** Angular vein Anterior facial vein Common facial vein Deep facial vein Frontal vein Posterior facial (retromandibular) vein Supraorbital vein **V Face Vein, Left** See T Face Vein, Right **Y Upper Vein**	**Ø Open** **3 Percutaneous** **4 Percutaneous Endoscopic**	**Ø Drainage Device**	**Z No Qualifier**
Ø Azygos Vein Right ascending lumbar vein Right subcostal vein **1 Hemiazygos Vein** Left ascending lumbar vein Left subcostal vein **3 Innominate Vein, Right** Brachiocephalic vein Inferior thyroid vein **4 Innominate Vein, Left** See 3 Innominate Vein, Right **5 Subclavian Vein, Right** **6 Subclavian Vein, Left** **7 Axillary Vein, Right** **8 Axillary Vein, Left** **9 Brachial Vein, Right** Radial vein Ulnar vein **A Brachial Vein, Left** See 9 Brachial Vein, Right **B Basilic Vein, Right** Median antebrachial vein Median cubital vein **C Basilic Vein, Left** See B Basilic Vein, Right **D Cephalic Vein, Right** Accessory cephalic vein **F Cephalic Vein, Left** See D Cephalic Vein, Right **G Hand Vein, Right** Dorsal metacarpal vein Palmar (volar) digital vein Palmar (volar) metacarpal vein Superficial palmar venous arch Volar (palmar) digital vein Volar (palmar) metacarpal vein	**H Hand Vein, Left** See G Hand Vein, Right **L Intracranial Vein** Anterior cerebral vein Basal (internal) cerebral vein Dural venous sinus Great cerebral vein Inferior cerebellar vein Inferior cerebral vein Internal (basal) cerebral vein Middle cerebral vein Ophthalmic vein Superior cerebellar vein Superior cerebral vein **M Internal Jugular Vein, Right** **N Internal Jugular Vein, Left** **P External Jugular Vein, Right** Posterior auricular vein **Q External Jugular Vein, Left** See P External Jugular Vein, Right **R Vertebral Vein, Right** Deep cervical vein Suboccipital venous plexus **S Vertebral Vein, Left** See R Vertebral Vein, Right **T Face Vein, Right** Angular vein Anterior facial vein Common facial vein Deep facial vein Frontal vein Posterior facial (retromandibular) vein Supraorbital vein **V Face Vein, Left** See T Face Vein, Right **Y Upper Vein**	**Ø Open** **3 Percutaneous** **4 Percutaneous Endoscopic**	**Z No Device**	**X Diagnostic** **Z No Qualifier**

Non-OR   Ø59[Ø,1,3,4,5,6,7,8,9,A,B,C,D,F,G,H,L,M,N,P,Q,R,S,T,V,Y][Ø,3,4]ØZ
Non-OR   Ø59[Ø,1,3,4,5,6,7,8,9,A,B,C,D,F,G,H,L,M,N,P,Q,R,S,T,V,Y]3ZX
Non-OR   Ø59[Ø,1,3,4,5,6,7,8,9,A,B,C,D,F,G,H,L,M,N,P,Q,R,S,T,V,Y][Ø,3,4]ZZ

Non-OR Procedure   DRG Non-OR Procedure   Valid OR Procedure   HAC Associated Procedure   Combination Only   New/Revised April   New/Revised October

0　Medical and Surgical
5　Upper Veins
B　Excision　　　Definition: Cutting out or off, without replacement, a portion of a body part

Explanation: The qualifier DIAGNOSTIC is used to identify excision procedures that are biopsies

Body Part Character 4	Approach Character 5	Device Character 6	Qualifier Character 7
0　Azygos Vein 　　Right ascending lumbar vein 　　Right subcostal vein **1　Hemiazygos Vein** 　　Left ascending lumbar vein 　　Left subcostal vein **3　Innominate Vein, Right** 　　Brachiocephalic vein 　　Inferior thyroid vein **4　Innominate Vein, Left** 　　*See 3 Innominate Vein, Right* **5　Subclavian Vein, Right** **6　Subclavian Vein, Left** **7　Axillary Vein, Right** **8　Axillary Vein, Left** **9　Brachial Vein, Right** 　　Radial vein 　　Ulnar vein **A　Brachial Vein, Left** 　　*See 9 Brachial Vein, Right* **B　Basilic Vein, Right** 　　Median antebrachial vein 　　Median cubital vein **C　Basilic Vein, Left** 　　*See B Basilic Vein, Right* **D　Cephalic Vein, Right** 　　Accessory cephalic vein **F　Cephalic Vein, Left** 　　*See D Cephalic Vein, Right* **G　Hand Vein, Right** 　　Dorsal metacarpal vein 　　Palmar (volar) digital vein 　　Palmar (volar) metacarpal vein 　　Superficial palmar venous arch 　　Volar (palmar) digital vein 　　Volar (palmar) metacarpal vein **H　Hand Vein, Left** 　　*See G Hand Vein, Right* **L　Intracranial Vein** 　　Anterior cerebral vein 　　Basal (internal) cerebral vein 　　Dural venous sinus 　　Great cerebral vein 　　Inferior cerebellar vein 　　Inferior cerebral vein 　　Internal (basal) cerebral vein 　　Middle cerebral vein 　　Ophthalmic vein 　　Superior cerebellar vein 　　Superior cerebral vein **M　Internal Jugular Vein, Right** **N　Internal Jugular Vein, Left** **P　External Jugular Vein, Right** 　　Posterior auricular vein **Q　External Jugular Vein, Left** 　　*See P External Jugular Vein, Right* **R　Vertebral Vein, Right** 　　Deep cervical vein 　　Suboccipital venous plexus **S　Vertebral Vein, Left** 　　*See R Vertebral Vein, Right* **T　Face Vein, Right** 　　Angular vein 　　Anterior facial vein 　　Common facial vein 　　Deep facial vein 　　Frontal vein 　　Posterior facial (retromandibular) vein 　　Supraorbital vein **V　Face Vein, Left** 　　*See T Face Vein, Right* **Y　Upper Vein**	**0　Open** **3　Percutaneous** **4　Percutaneous Endoscopic**	**Z　No Device**	**X　Diagnostic** **Z　No Qualifier**

NC Noncovered Procedure　　**LC** Limited Coverage　　**QA** Questionable OB Admit　　**NT** New Tech Add-on　　⊞ Combination Member　　♂ Male　　♀ Female

ICD-10-PCS 2023　　　　　　　　　　　　　　　　　　　　　　　　　　　　　　　　　　　　　　249

Upper Veins (side tab)

0   **Medical and Surgical**
5   **Upper Veins**
C   **Extirpation**   Definition: Taking or cutting out solid matter from a body part

Explanation: The solid matter may be an abnormal byproduct of a biological function or a foreign body; it may be imbedded in a body part or in the lumen of a tubular body part. The solid matter may or may not have been previously broken into pieces.

Body Part Character 4	Approach Character 5	Device Character 6	Qualifier Character 7

0 **Azygos Vein**
   Right ascending lumbar vein
   Right subcostal vein
1 **Hemiazygos Vein**
   Left ascending lumbar vein
   Left subcostal vein
3 **Innominate Vein, Right**
   Brachiocephalic vein
   Inferior thyroid vein
4 **Innominate Vein, Left**
   See 3 Innominate Vein, Right
5 **Subclavian Vein, Right**
6 **Subclavian Vein, Left**
7 **Axillary Vein, Right**
8 **Axillary Vein, Left**
9 **Brachial Vein, Right**
   Radial vein
   Ulnar vein
A **Brachial Vein, Left**
   See 9 Brachial Vein, Right
B **Basilic Vein, Right**
   Median antebrachial vein
   Median cubital vein
C **Basilic Vein, Left**
   See B Basilic Vein, Right
D **Cephalic Vein, Right**
   Accessory cephalic vein
F **Cephalic Vein, Left**
   See D Cephalic Vein, Right
G **Hand Vein, Right**
   Dorsal metacarpal vein
   Palmar (volar) digital vein
   Palmar (volar) metacarpal vein
   Superficial palmar venous arch
   Volar (palmar) digital vein
   Volar (palmar) metacarpal vein
H **Hand Vein, Left**
   See G Hand Vein, Right
L **Intracranial Vein**
   Anterior cerebral vein
   Basal (internal) cerebral vein
   Dural venous sinus
   Great cerebral vein
   Inferior cerebellar vein
   Inferior cerebral vein
   Internal (basal) cerebral vein
   Middle cerebral vein
   Ophthalmic vein
   Superior cerebellar vein
   Superior cerebral vein
M **Internal Jugular Vein, Right**
N **Internal Jugular Vein, Left**
P **External Jugular Vein, Right**
   Posterior auricular vein
Q **External Jugular Vein, Left**
   See P External Jugular Vein, Right
R **Vertebral Vein, Right**
   Deep cervical vein
   Suboccipital venous plexus
S **Vertebral Vein, Left**
   See R Vertebral Vein, Right
T **Face Vein, Right**
   Angular vein
   Anterior facial vein
   Common facial vein
   Deep facial vein
   Frontal vein
   Posterior facial (retromandibular) vein
   Supraorbital vein
V **Face Vein, Left**
   See T Face Vein, Right
Y **Upper Vein**
	0 Open
	3 Percutaneous
	4 Percutaneous Endoscopic
		Z No Device	**Z** No Qualifier

Non-OR Procedure   DRG Non-OR Procedure   Valid OR Procedure   HAC Associated Procedure   Combination Only   New/Revised April   New/Revised October

250

05C–05C

ICD-10-PCS 2023

0   **Medical and Surgical**
5   **Upper Veins**
D   **Extraction**   Definition: Pulling or stripping out or off all or a portion of a body part by the use of force
                      Explanation: The qualifier DIAGNOSTIC is used to identify extraction procedures that are biopsies

Body Part Character 4	Approach Character 5	Device Character 6	Qualifier Character 7

9   **Brachial Vein, Right**
    Radial vein
    Ulnar vein
A   **Brachial Vein, Left**
    See 9 Brachial Vein, Right
B   **Basilic Vein, Right**
    Median antebrachial vein
    Median cubital vein
C   **Basilic Vein, Left**
    See B Basilic Vein, Right
D   **Cephalic Vein, Right**
    Accessory cephalic vein
F   **Cephalic Vein, Left**
    See D Cephalic Vein, Right
G   **Hand Vein, Right**
    Dorsal metacarpal vein
    Palmar (volar) digital vein
    Palmar (volar) metacarpal vein
    Superficial palmar venous arch
    Volar (palmar) digital vein
    Volar (palmar) metacarpal vein
H   **Hand Vein, Left**
    See G Hand Vein, Right
Y   **Upper Vein**
	0 Open
	3 Percutaneous
		Z No Device	**Z** No Qualifier

0   **Medical and Surgical**
5   **Upper Veins**
F   **Fragmentation**   Definition: Breaking solid matter in a body part into pieces
                      Explanation: Physical force (e.g., manual, ultrasonic) applied directly or indirectly is used to break the solid matter into pieces. The solid matter may be an abnormal byproduct of a biological function or a foreign body. The pieces of solid matter are not taken out.

Body Part Character 4	Approach Character 5	Device Character 6	Qualifier Character 7

3   **Innominate Vein, Right**
    Brachiocephalic vein
    Inferior thyroid vein
4   **Innominate Vein, Left**
    See 3 Innominate Vein, Right
5   **Subclavian Vein, Right**
6   **Subclavian Vein, Left**
7   **Axillary Vein, Right**
8   **Axillary Vein, Left**
9   **Brachial Vein, Right**
    Radial vein
    Ulnar vein
A   **Brachial Vein, Left**
    See 9 Brachial Vein, Right
B   **Basilic Vein, Right**
    Median antebrachial vein
    Median cubital vein
C   **Basilic Vein, Left**
    See B Basilic Vein, Right
D   **Cephalic Vein, Right**
    Accessory cephalic vein
F   **Cephalic Vein, Left**
    See D Cephalic Vein, Right
Y   **Upper Vein**
	3 Percutaneous	**Z** No Device	**0** Ultrasonic
			Z No Qualifier

NC Noncovered Procedure   **LC** Limited Coverage   **QA** Questionable OB Admit   **NT** New Tech Add-on   ⊞ Combination Member   ♂ Male   ♀ Female

ICD-10-PCS 2023   251

05D–05F

Ø   Medical and Surgical
5   Upper Veins
H   Insertion   Definition: Putting in a nonbiological appliance that monitors, assists, performs, or prevents a physiological function but does not physically take the place of a body part
                    Explanation: None

Body Part Character 4		Approach Character 5	Device Character 6	Qualifier Character 7
Ø **Azygos Vein** ⊞ Right ascending lumbar vein Right subcostal vein		**Ø** Open **3** Percutaneous **4** Percutaneous Endoscopic	**2** Monitoring Device **3** Infusion Device **D** Intraluminal Device **M** Neurostimulator Lead	**Z** No Qualifier
1 **Hemiazygos Vein** Left ascending lumbar vein Left subcostal vein **5** **Subclavian Vein, Right** **6** **Subclavian Vein, Left** **7** **Axillary Vein, Right** **8** **Axillary Vein, Left** **9** **Brachial Vein, Right** Radial vein Ulnar vein **A** **Brachial Vein, Left** *See 9 Brachial Vein, Right* **B** **Basilic Vein, Right** Median antebrachial vein Median cubital vein **C** **Basilic Vein, Left** *See B Basilic Vein, Right* **D** **Cephalic Vein, Right** Accessory cephalic vein **F** **Cephalic Vein, Left** *See D Cephalic Vein, Right* **G** **Hand Vein, Right** Dorsal metacarpal vein Palmar (volar) digital vein Palmar (volar) metacarpal vein Superficial palmar venous arch Volar (palmar) digital vein Volar (palmar) metacarpal vein **H** **Hand Vein, Left** *See G Hand Vein, Right*	**L** **Intracranial Vein** Anterior cerebral vein Basal (internal) cerebral vein Dural venous sinus Great cerebral vein Inferior cerebellar vein Inferior cerebral vein Internal (basal) cerebral vein Middle cerebral vein Ophthalmic vein Superior cerebellar vein Superior cerebral vein **M** **Internal Jugular Vein, Right** **N** **Internal Jugular Vein, Left** **P** **External Jugular Vein, Right** Posterior auricular vein **Q** **External Jugular Vein, Left** *See P External Jugular Vein, Right* **R** **Vertebral Vein, Right** Deep cervical vein Suboccipital venous plexus **S** **Vertebral Vein, Left** *See R Vertebral Vein, Right* **T** **Face Vein, Right** Angular vein Anterior facial vein Common facial vein Deep facial vein Frontal vein Posterior facial (retromandibular) vein Supraorbital vein **V** **Face Vein, Left** *See T Face Vein, Right*	**Ø** Open **3** Percutaneous **4** Percutaneous Endoscopic	**3** Infusion Device **D** Intraluminal Device	**Z** No Qualifier
3 **Innominate Vein, Right** ⊞ Brachiocephalic vein Inferior thyroid vein **4** **Innominate Vein, Left** ⊞ *See 3 Innominate Vein, Right*		**Ø** Open **3** Percutaneous **4** Percutaneous Endoscopic	**3** Infusion Device **D** Intraluminal Device **M** Neurostimulator Lead	**Z** No Qualifier
Y **Upper Vein**		**Ø** Open **3** Percutaneous **4** Percutaneous Endoscopic	**2** Monitoring Device **3** Infusion Device **D** Intraluminal Device **Y** Other Device	**Z** No Qualifier

Non-OR	Ø5HØ[Ø,3,4]3Z	
Non-OR	Ø5H[1,5,6,7,8,9,A,B,C,D,F,G,H,L,M,N,P,Q,R,S,T,V][Ø,3,4]3Z	
Non-OR	Ø5H[3,4][Ø,3,4]3Z	
Non-OR	Ø5HY[Ø,3,4]3Z	
Non-OR	Ø5HY32Z	
Non-OR	Ø5HY[3,4]YZ	
HAC	Ø5HØ[3,4]3Z when reported with SDx J95.811	
HAC	Ø5H[1,5,6][3,4]3Z when reported with SDx J95.811	
HAC	Ø5H[M,N,P,Q]33Z when reported with SDx J95.811	
HAC	Ø5H[3,4][3,4]3Z when reported with SDx J95.811	

See Appendix L for Procedure Combinations
⊞   Ø5HØ[Ø,3,4]MZ
⊞   Ø5H[3,4][Ø,3,4]MZ

Ø   Medical and Surgical
5   Upper Veins
J   Inspection   Definition: Visually and/or manually exploring a body part
                     Explanation: Visual exploration may be performed with or without optical instrumentation. Manual exploration may be performed directly or through intervening body layers.

Body Part Character 4	Approach Character 5	Device Character 6	Qualifier Character 7
Y **Upper Vein**	**Ø** Open **3** Percutaneous **4** Percutaneous Endoscopic **X** External	**Z** No Device	**Z** No Qualifier

Non-OR	Ø5JY[3,X]ZZ

Non-OR Procedure   DRG Non-OR Procedure   Valid OR Procedure   HAC Associated Procedure   Combination Only   New/Revised April   New/Revised October

252   ICD-10-PCS 2023

Ø   Medical and Surgical
5   Upper Veins
L   Occlusion   Definition: Completely closing an orifice or the lumen of a tubular body part
                           Explanation: The orifice can be a natural orifice or an artificially created orifice

Body Part Character 4	Approach Character 5	Device Character 6	Qualifier Character 7

Ø Azygos Vein
   Right ascending lumbar vein
   Right subcostal vein
	Ø Open
	3 Percutaneous
	4 Percutaneous Endoscopic
		C Extraluminal Device
		D Intraluminal Device
		Z No Device
			Z No Qualifier

1 Hemiazygos Vein
   Left ascending lumbar vein
   Left subcostal vein			

3 Innominate Vein, Right
   Brachiocephalic vein
   Inferior thyroid vein			

4 Innominate Vein, Left *See 3 Innominate Vein, Right*			
5 Subclavian Vein, Right			
6 Subclavian Vein, Left			
7 Axillary Vein, Right			
8 Axillary Vein, Left			

9 Brachial Vein, Right
   Radial vein
   Ulnar vein			

A Brachial Vein, Left *See 9 Brachial Vein, Right*			

B Basilic Vein, Right
   Median antebrachial vein
   Median cubital vein			

C Basilic Vein, Left *See B Basilic Vein, Right*			
D Cephalic Vein, Right Accessory cephalic vein			
F Cephalic Vein, Left *See D Cephalic Vein, Right*			

G Hand Vein, Right
   Dorsal metacarpal vein
   Palmar (volar) digital vein
   Palmar (volar) metacarpal vein
   Superficial palmar venous arch
   Volar (palmar) digital vein
   Volar (palmar) metacarpal vein			

H Hand Vein, Left *See G Hand Vein, Right*			

L Intracranial Vein
   Anterior cerebral vein
   Basal (internal) cerebral vein
   Dural venous sinus
   Great cerebral vein
   Inferior cerebellar vein
   Inferior cerebral vein
   Internal (basal) cerebral vein
   Middle cerebral vein
   Ophthalmic vein
   Superior cerebellar vein
   Superior cerebral vein			

M Internal Jugular Vein, Right			
N Internal Jugular Vein, Left			
P External Jugular Vein, Right Posterior auricular vein			
Q External Jugular Vein, Left *See P External Jugular Vein, Right*			

R Vertebral Vein, Right
   Deep cervical vein
   Suboccipital venous plexus			

S Vertebral Vein, Left *See R Vertebral Vein, Right*			

T Face Vein, Right
   Angular vein
   Anterior facial vein
   Common facial vein
   Deep facial vein
   Frontal vein
   Posterior facial (retromandibular) vein
   Supraorbital vein			

V Face Vein, Left *See T Face Vein, Right*			
Y Upper Vein			

NC Noncovered Procedure   **LC** Limited Coverage   **QA** Questionable OB Admit   **NT** New Tech Add-on   ⊞ Combination Member   ♂ Male   ♀ Female

ICD-10-PCS 2023   253

Ø5L–Ø5L

Ø Medical and Surgical
5 Upper Veins
N Release   Definition: Freeing a body part from an abnormal physical constraint by cutting or by the use of force
                      Explanation: Some of the restraining tissue may be taken out but none of the body part is taken out

Body Part Character 4	Approach Character 5	Device Character 6	Qualifier Character 7

Ø Azygos Vein
   Right ascending lumbar vein
   Right subcostal vein
1 Hemiazygos Vein
   Left ascending lumbar vein
   Left subcostal vein
3 Innominate Vein, Right
   Brachiocephalic vein
   Inferior thyroid vein
4 Innominate Vein, Left
   See 3 Innominate Vein, Right
5 Subclavian Vein, Right
6 Subclavian Vein, Left
7 Axillary Vein, Right
8 Axillary Vein, Left
9 Brachial Vein, Right
   Radial vein
   Ulnar vein
A Brachial Vein, Left
   See 9 Brachial Vein, Right
B Basilic Vein, Right
   Median antebrachial vein
   Median cubital vein
C Basilic Vein, Left
   See B Basilic Vein, Right
D Cephalic Vein, Right
   Accessory cephalic vein
F Cephalic Vein, Left
   See D Cephalic Vein, Right
G Hand Vein, Right
   Dorsal metacarpal vein
   Palmar (volar) digital vein
   Palmar (volar) metacarpal vein
   Superficial palmar venous arch
   Volar (palmar) digital vein
   Volar (palmar) metacarpal vein
H Hand Vein, Left
   See G Hand Vein, Right
L Intracranial Vein
   Anterior cerebral vein
   Basal (internal) cerebral vein
   Dural venous sinus
   Great cerebral vein
   Inferior cerebellar vein
   Inferior cerebral vein
   Internal (basal) cerebral vein
   Middle cerebral vein
   Ophthalmic vein
   Superior cerebellar vein
   Superior cerebral vein
M Internal Jugular Vein, Right
N Internal Jugular Vein, Left
P External Jugular Vein, Right
   Posterior auricular vein
Q External Jugular Vein, Left
   See P External Jugular Vein, Right
R Vertebral Vein, Right
   Deep cervical vein
   Suboccipital venous plexus
S Vertebral Vein, Left
   See R Vertebral Vein, Right
T Face Vein, Right
   Angular vein
   Anterior facial vein
   Common facial vein
   Deep facial vein
   Frontal vein
   Posterior facial (retromandibular) vein
   Supraorbital vein
V Face Vein, Left
   See T Face Vein, Right
Y Upper Vein
	Ø Open
	3 Percutaneous
	4 Percutaneous Endoscopic
		Z No Device	**Z No Qualifier**

Non-OR Procedure   DRG Non-OR Procedure   Valid OR Procedure   HAC Associated Procedure   Combination Only   New/Revised April   New/Revised October

Ø   **Medical and Surgical**
5   **Upper Veins**
P   **Removal**   Definition: Taking out or off a device from a body part

Explanation: If a device is taken out and a similar device put in without cutting or puncturing the skin or mucous membrane, the procedure is coded to the root operation CHANGE. Otherwise, the procedure for taking out a device is coded to the root operation REMOVAL.

Body Part Character 4	Approach Character 5	Device Character 6	Qualifier Character 7
Ø Azygos Vein Right ascending lumbar vein Right subcostal vein	**Ø** Open **3** Percutaneous **4** Percutaneous Endoscopic **X** External	**2** Monitoring Device **M** Neurostimulator Lead	**Z** No Qualifier
3 Innominate Vein, Right Brachiocephalic vein Inferior thyroid vein **4 Innominate Vein, Left** *See 3 Innominate Vein, Right*	**Ø** Open **3** Percutaneous **4** Percutaneous Endoscopic **X** External	**M** Neurostimulator Lead	**Z** No Qualifier
Y Upper Vein	**Ø** Open **3** Percutaneous **4** Percutaneous Endoscopic	**Ø** Drainage Device **2** Monitoring Device **3** Infusion Device **7** Autologous Tissue Substitute **C** Extraluminal Device **D** Intraluminal Device **J** Synthetic Substitute **K** Nonautologous Tissue Substitute **Y** Other Device	**Z** No Qualifier
Y Upper Vein	**X** External	**Ø** Drainage Device **2** Monitoring Device **3** Infusion Device **D** Intraluminal Device	**Z** No Qualifier

Non-OR	Ø5PØ[Ø,3,4,X]2Z
Non-OR	Ø5PY3[Ø,2,3]Z
Non-OR	Ø5PY[3,4]YZ
Non-OR	Ø5PYX[Ø,2,3,D]Z

NC Noncovered Procedure   **LC** Limited Coverage   **QA** Questionable OB Admit   **NT** New Tech Add-on   ⊞ Combination Member   ♂ Male   ♀ Female

ICD-10-PCS 2023   255

Upper Veins (side tab)

Ø Medical and Surgical
5 Upper Veins
Q Repair   Definition: Restoring, to the extent possible, a body part to its normal anatomic structure and function
                       Explanation: Used only when the method to accomplish the repair is not one of the other root operations

Body Part Character 4	Approach Character 5	Device Character 6	Qualifier Character 7

Ø Azygos Vein
   Right ascending lumbar vein
   Right subcostal vein
1 Hemiazygos Vein
   Left ascending lumbar vein
   Left subcostal vein
3 Innominate Vein, Right
   Brachiocephalic vein
   Inferior thyroid vein
4 Innominate Vein, Left
   See 3 Innominate Vein, Right
5 Subclavian Vein, Right
6 Subclavian Vein, Left
7 Axillary Vein, Right
8 Axillary Vein, Left
9 Brachial Vein, Right
   Radial vein
   Ulnar vein
A Brachial Vein, Left
   See 9 Brachial Vein, Right
B Basilic Vein, Right
   Median antebrachial vein
   Median cubital vein
C Basilic Vein, Left
   See B Basilic Vein, Right
D Cephalic Vein, Right
   Accessory cephalic vein
F Cephalic Vein, Left
   See D Cephalic Vein, Right
G Hand Vein, Right
   Dorsal metacarpal vein
   Palmar (volar) digital vein
   Palmar (volar) metacarpal vein
   Superficial palmar venous arch
   Volar (palmar) digital vein
   Volar (palmar) metacarpal vein
H Hand Vein, Left
   See G Hand Vein, Right
L Intracranial Vein
   Anterior cerebral vein
   Basal (internal) cerebral vein
   Dural venous sinus
   Great cerebral vein
   Inferior cerebellar vein
   Inferior cerebral vein
   Internal (basal) cerebral vein
   Middle cerebral vein
   Ophthalmic vein
   Superior cerebellar vein
   Superior cerebral vein
M Internal Jugular Vein, Right
N Internal Jugular Vein, Left
P External Jugular Vein, Right
   Posterior auricular vein
Q External Jugular Vein, Left
   See P External Jugular Vein, Right
R Vertebral Vein, Right
   Deep cervical vein
   Suboccipital venous plexus
S Vertebral Vein, Left
   See R Vertebral Vein, Right
T Face Vein, Right
   Angular vein
   Anterior facial vein
   Common facial vein
   Deep facial vein
   Frontal vein
   Posterior facial (retromandibular) vein
   Supraorbital vein
V Face Vein, Left
   See T Face Vein, Right
Y Upper Vein
	Ø Open
	3 Percutaneous
	4 Percutaneous Endoscopic
		Z No Device	**Z No Qualifier**

Non-OR Procedure   DRG Non-OR Procedure   Valid OR Procedure   HAC Associated Procedure   Combination Only   New/Revised April   New/Revised October

256   ICD-10-PCS 2023

Ø5Q–Ø5Q (side tab)

0   **Medical and Surgical**
5   **Upper Veins**
R   **Replacement**   Definition: Putting in or on biological or synthetic material that physically takes the place and/or function of all or a portion of a body part
          Explanation: The body part may have been taken out or replaced, or may be taken out, physically eradicated, or rendered nonfunctional during the REPLACEMENT procedure. A REMOVAL procedure is coded for taking out the device used in a previous replacement procedure.

Body Part Character 4	Approach Character 5	Device Character 6	Qualifier Character 7

0   **Azygos Vein**
     Right ascending lumbar vein
     Right subcostal vein
	0 Open
	4 Percutaneous Endoscopic
		7 Autologous Tissue Substitute
		J Synthetic Substitute
		K Nonautologous Tissue Substitute
			Z No Qualifier

1   **Hemiazygos Vein**
     Left ascending lumbar vein
     Left subcostal vein			

3   **Innominate Vein, Right**
     Brachiocephalic vein
     Inferior thyroid vein			

4 **Innominate Vein, Left** *See 3 Innominate Vein, Right*			
5 **Subclavian Vein, Right**			
6 **Subclavian Vein, Left**			
7 **Axillary Vein, Right**			
8 **Axillary Vein, Left**			

9   **Brachial Vein, Right**
     Radial vein
     Ulnar vein			

A **Brachial Vein, Left** *See 9 Brachial Vein, Right*			

B   **Basilic Vein, Right**
     Median antebrachial vein
     Median cubital vein			

C **Basilic Vein, Left** *See B Basilic Vein, Right*			
D **Cephalic Vein, Right** Accessory cephalic vein			
F **Cephalic Vein, Left** *See D Cephalic Vein, Right*			

G   **Hand Vein, Right**
     Dorsal metacarpal vein
     Palmar (volar) digital vein
     Palmar (volar) metacarpal vein
     Superficial palmar venous arch
     Volar (palmar) digital vein
     Volar (palmar) metacarpal vein			

H **Hand Vein, Left** *See G Hand Vein, Right*			

L   **Intracranial Vein**
     Anterior cerebral vein
     Basal (internal) cerebral vein
     Dural venous sinus
     Great cerebral vein
     Inferior cerebellar vein
     Inferior cerebral vein
     Internal (basal) cerebral vein
     Middle cerebral vein
     Ophthalmic vein
     Superior cerebellar vein
     Superior cerebral vein			

M **Internal Jugular Vein, Right**			
N **Internal Jugular Vein, Left**			
P **External Jugular Vein, Right** Posterior auricular vein			
Q **External Jugular Vein, Left** *See P External Jugular Vein, Right*			

R   **Vertebral Vein, Right**
     Deep cervical vein
     Suboccipital venous plexus			

S **Vertebral Vein, Left** *See R Vertebral Vein, Right*			

T   **Face Vein, Right**
     Angular vein
     Anterior facial vein
     Common facial vein
     Deep facial vein
     Frontal vein
     Posterior facial (retromandibular) vein
     Supraorbital vein			

V **Face Vein, Left** *See T Face Vein, Right*			
Y **Upper Vein**			

NC Noncovered Procedure   **LC** Limited Coverage   **QA** Questionable OB Admit   **NT** New Tech Add-on   ⊞ Combination Member   ♂ Male   ♀ Female

ICD-10-PCS 2023   257

0 Medical and Surgical
5 Upper Veins
S Reposition   Definition: Moving to its normal location, or other suitable location, all or a portion of a body part

Explanation: The body part is moved to a new location from an abnormal location, or from a normal location where it is not functioning correctly. The body part may or may not be cut out or off to be moved to the new location.

Body Part Character 4	Approach Character 5	Device Character 6	Qualifier Character 7

0 Azygos Vein
   Right ascending lumbar vein
   Right subcostal vein
	0 Open
	3 Percutaneous
	4 Percutaneous Endoscopic
		Z No Device	**Z No Qualifier**

1 Hemiazygos Vein
   Left ascending lumbar vein
   Left subcostal vein			

3 Innominate Vein, Right
   Brachiocephalic vein
   Inferior thyroid vein			

4 Innominate Vein, Left *See 3 Innominate Vein, Right*			
5 Subclavian Vein, Right			
6 Subclavian Vein, Left			
7 Axillary Vein, Right			
8 Axillary Vein, Left			

9 Brachial Vein, Right
   Radial vein
   Ulnar vein			

A Brachial Vein, Left *See 9 Brachial Vein, Right*			

B Basilic Vein, Right
   Median antebrachial vein
   Median cubital vein			

C Basilic Vein, Left *See B Basilic Vein, Right*			
D Cephalic Vein, Right Accessory cephalic vein			
F Cephalic Vein, Left *See D Cephalic Vein, Right*			

G Hand Vein, Right
   Dorsal metacarpal vein
   Palmar (volar) digital vein
   Palmar (volar) metacarpal vein
   Superficial palmar venous arch
   Volar (palmar) digital vein
   Volar (palmar) metacarpal vein			

H Hand Vein, Left *See G Hand Vein, Right*			

L Intracranial Vein
   Anterior cerebral vein
   Basal (internal) cerebral vein
   Dural venous sinus
   Great cerebral vein
   Inferior cerebellar vein
   Inferior cerebral vein
   Internal (basal) cerebral vein
   Middle cerebral vein
   Ophthalmic vein
   Superior cerebellar vein
   Superior cerebral vein			

M Internal Jugular Vein, Right			
N Internal Jugular Vein, Left			
P External Jugular Vein, Right Posterior auricular vein			
Q External Jugular Vein, Left *See P External Jugular Vein, Right*			

R Vertebral Vein, Right
   Deep cervical vein
   Suboccipital venous plexus			

S Vertebral Vein, Left *See R Vertebral Vein, Right*			

T Face Vein, Right
   Angular vein
   Anterior facial vein
   Common facial vein
   Deep facial vein
   Frontal vein
   Posterior facial (retromandibular) vein
   Supraorbital vein			

V Face Vein, Left *See T Face Vein, Right*			
Y Upper Vein			

Non-OR Procedure   DRG Non-OR Procedure   Valid OR Procedure   HAC Associated Procedure   Combination Only   New/Revised April   New/Revised October

258   ICD-10-PCS 2023

Ø **Medical and Surgical**
5 **Upper Veins**
U **Supplement** Definition: Putting in or on biological or synthetic material that physically reinforces and/or augments the function of a portion of a body part
Explanation: The biological material is non-living, or is living and from the same individual. The body part may have been previously replaced, and the SUPPLEMENT procedure is performed to physically reinforce and/or augment the function of the replaced body part.

Body Part Character 4	Approach Character 5	Device Character 6	Qualifier Character 7
Ø **Azygos Vein** Right ascending lumbar vein Right subcostal vein	**Ø** Open **3** Percutaneous **4** Percutaneous Endoscopic	**7** Autologous Tissue Substitute **J** Synthetic Substitute **K** Nonautologous Tissue Substitute	**Z** No Qualifier
1 **Hemiazygos Vein** Left ascending lumbar vein Left subcostal vein			
3 **Innominate Vein, Right** Brachiocephalic vein Inferior thyroid vein			
4 **Innominate Vein, Left** *See 3 Innominate Vein, Right*			
5 **Subclavian Vein, Right**			
6 **Subclavian Vein, Left**			
7 **Axillary Vein, Right**			
8 **Axillary Vein, Left**			
9 **Brachial Vein, Right** Radial vein Ulnar vein			
A **Brachial Vein, Left** *See 9 Brachial Vein, Right*			
B **Basilic Vein, Right** Median antebrachial vein Median cubital vein			
C **Basilic Vein, Left** *See B Basilic Vein, Right*			
D **Cephalic Vein, Right** Accessory cephalic vein			
F **Cephalic Vein, Left** *See D Cephalic Vein, Right*			
G **Hand Vein, Right** Dorsal metacarpal vein Palmar (volar) digital vein Palmar (volar) metacarpal vein Superficial palmar venous arch Volar (palmar) digital vein Volar (palmar) metacarpal vein			
H **Hand Vein, Left** *See G Hand Vein, Right*			
L **Intracranial Vein** Anterior cerebral vein Basal (internal) cerebral vein Dural venous sinus Great cerebral vein Inferior cerebellar vein Inferior cerebral vein Internal (basal) cerebral vein Middle cerebral vein Ophthalmic vein Superior cerebellar vein Superior cerebral vein			
M **Internal Jugular Vein, Right**			
N **Internal Jugular Vein, Left**			
P **External Jugular Vein, Right** Posterior auricular vein			
Q **External Jugular Vein, Left** *See P External Jugular Vein, Right*			
R **Vertebral Vein, Right** Deep cervical vein Suboccipital venous plexus			
S **Vertebral Vein, Left** *See R Vertebral Vein, Right*			
T **Face Vein, Right** Angular vein Anterior facial vein Common facial vein Deep facial vein Frontal vein Posterior facial (retromandibular) vein Supraorbital vein			
V **Face Vein, Left** *See T Face Vein, Right*			
Y **Upper Vein**			

Ø Medical and Surgical
5 Upper Veins
V Restriction   Definition: Partially closing an orifice or the lumen of a tubular body part
                    Explanation: The orifice can be a natural orifice or an artificially created orifice

Body Part Character 4	Approach Character 5	Device Character 6	Qualifier Character 7
Ø Azygos Vein Right ascending lumbar vein Right subcostal vein	**Ø Open** **3 Percutaneous** **4 Percutaneous Endoscopic**	**C Extraluminal Device** **D Intraluminal Device** **Z No Device**	**Z No Qualifier**
1 Hemiazygos Vein Left ascending lumbar vein Left subcostal vein			
3 Innominate Vein, Right Brachiocephalic vein Inferior thyroid vein			
4 Innominate Vein, Left *See 3 Innominate Vein, Right*			
5 Subclavian Vein, Right			
6 Subclavian Vein, Left			
7 Axillary Vein, Right			
8 Axillary Vein, Left			
9 Brachial Vein, Right Radial vein Ulnar vein			
A Brachial Vein, Left *See 9 Brachial Vein, Right*			
B Basilic Vein, Right Median antebrachial vein Median cubital vein			
C Basilic Vein, Left *See B Basilic Vein, Right*			
D Cephalic Vein, Right Accessory cephalic vein			
F Cephalic Vein, Left *See D Cephalic Vein, Right*			
G Hand Vein, Right Dorsal metacarpal vein Palmar (volar) digital vein Palmar (volar) metacarpal vein Superficial palmar venous arch Volar (palmar) digital vein Volar (palmar) metacarpal vein			
H Hand Vein, Left *See G Hand Vein, Right*			
L Intracranial Vein Anterior cerebral vein Basal (internal) cerebral vein Dural venous sinus Great cerebral vein Inferior cerebellar vein Inferior cerebral vein Internal (basal) cerebral vein Middle cerebral vein Ophthalmic vein Superior cerebellar vein Superior cerebral vein			
M Internal Jugular Vein, Right			
N Internal Jugular Vein, Left			
P External Jugular Vein, Right Posterior auricular vein			
Q External Jugular Vein, Left *See P External Jugular Vein, Right*			
R Vertebral Vein, Right Deep cervical vein Suboccipital venous plexus			
S Vertebral Vein, Left *See R Vertebral Vein, Right*			
T Face Vein, Right Angular vein Anterior facial vein Common facial vein Deep facial vein Frontal vein Posterior facial (retromandibular) vein Supraorbital vein			
V Face Vein, Left *See T Face Vein, Right*			
Y Upper Vein			

Non-OR Procedure   DRG Non-OR Procedure   Valid OR Procedure   HAC Associated Procedure   Combination Only   New/Revised April   New/Revised October

260   ICD-10-PCS 2023

Ø   Medical and Surgical
5   Upper Veins
W   Revision   Definition: Correcting, to the extent possible, a portion of a malfunctioning device or the position of a displaced device

                         Explanation: Revision can include correcting a malfunctioning or displaced device by taking out or putting in components of the device such as a screw or pin

Body Part Character 4	Approach Character 5	Device Character 6	Qualifier Character 7
Ø **Azygos Vein** Right ascending lumbar vein Right subcostal vein	**Ø** Open **3** Percutaneous **4** Percutaneous Endoscopic **X** External	**2** Monitoring Device **M** Neurostimulator Lead	**Z** No Qualifier
3 **Innominate Vein, Right** Brachiocephalic vein Inferior thyroid vein **4** **Innominate Vein, Left** *See 3 Innominate Vein, Right*	**Ø** Open **3** Percutaneous **4** Percutaneous Endoscopic **X** External	**M** Neurostimulator Lead	**Z** No Qualifier
Y **Upper Vein**	**Ø** Open **3** Percutaneous **4** Percutaneous Endoscopic	**Ø** Drainage Device **2** Monitoring Device **3** Infusion Device **7** Autologous Tissue Substitute **C** Extraluminal Device **D** Intraluminal Device **J** Synthetic Substitute **K** Nonautologous Tissue Substitute **Y** Other Device	**Z** No Qualifier
Y **Upper Vein**	**X** External	**Ø** Drainage Device **2** Monitoring Device **3** Infusion Device **7** Autologous Tissue Substitute **C** Extraluminal Device **D** Intraluminal Device **J** Synthetic Substitute **K** Nonautologous Tissue Substitute	**Z** No Qualifier

Non-OR	Ø5WØXMZ
Non-OR	Ø5W[3,4]XMZ
Non-OR	Ø5WY3[Ø,2,3]Z
Non-OR	Ø5WY[3,4]YZ
Non-OR	Ø5WYX[Ø,2,3,7,C,D,J,K]Z

NC Noncovered Procedure   LC Limited Coverage   UA Questionable OB Admit   NT New Tech Add-on   ⊞ Combination Member   ♂ Male   ♀ Female

ICD-10-PCS 2023   **261**

Lower Veins Ø61–Ø6W

Character Meanings

This Character Meaning table is provided as a guide to assist the user in the identification of character members that may be found in this section of code tables. It **SHOULD NOT** be used to build a PCS code.

Operation–Character 3		Body Part–Character 4		Approach–Character 5		Device–Character 6		Qualifier–Character 7	
1	Bypass	Ø	Inferior Vena Cava	Ø	Open	Ø	Drainage Device	Ø	Ultrasonic
5	Destruction	1	Splenic Vein	3	Percutaneous	2	Monitoring Device	4	Hepatic Vein
7	Dilation	2	Gastric Vein	4	Percutaneous Endoscopic	3	Infusion Device	5	Superior Mesenteric Vein
9	Drainage	3	Esophageal Vein	7	Via Natural or Artificial Opening	7	Autologous Tissue Substitute	6	Inferior Mesenteric Vein
B	Excision	4	Hepatic Vein	8	Via Natural or Artificial Opening Endoscopic	9	Autologous Venous Tissue	9	Renal Vein, Right
C	Extirpation	5	Superior Mesenteric Vein	X	External	A	Autologous Arterial Tissue	B	Renal Vein, Left
D	Extraction	6	Inferior Mesenteric Vein			C	Extraluminal Device	C	Hemorrhoidal Plexus
F	Fragmentation	7	Colic Vein			D	Intraluminal Device	P	Pulmonary Trunk
H	Insertion	8	Portal Vein			J	Synthetic Substitute	Q	Pulmonary Artery, Right
J	Inspection	9	Renal Vein, Right			K	Nonautologous Tissue Substitute	R	Pulmonary Artery, Left
L	Occlusion	B	Renal Vein, Left			Y	Other Device	T	Via Umbilical Vein
N	Release	C	Common Iliac Vein, Right			Z	No Device	X	Diagnostic
P	Removal	D	Common Iliac Vein, Left					Y	Lower Vein
Q	Repair	F	External Iliac Vein, Right					Z	No Qualifier
R	Replacement	G	External Iliac Vein, Left						
S	Reposition	H	Hypogastric Vein, Right						
U	Supplement	J	Hypogastric Vein, Left						
V	Restriction	M	Femoral Vein, Right						
W	Revision	N	Femoral Vein, Left						
		P	Saphenous Vein, Right						
		Q	Saphenous Vein, Left						
		T	Foot Vein, Right						
		V	Foot Vein, Left						
		Y	Lower Vein						

AHA Coding Clinic for Lower Veins
2022, 1Q, 10-13   Procedures performed on a continuous vessel, ICD-10-PCS Guideline B4.1c

AHA Coding Clinic for table Ø61
2017, 4Q, 36-38   Fontan completion procedure
2017, 4Q, 66-67   New qualifier values - Portal to hepatic shunt

AHA Coding Clinic for table Ø6B
2020, 1Q, 28   Free flap microvascular breast reconstruction
2017, 3Q, 5   Femoral artery to posterior tibial artery bypass using autologous and synthetic grafts
2017, 1Q, 31   Left to right common carotid artery bypass
2017, 1Q, 32   Peroneal artery to dorsalis pedis artery bypass using saphenous vein graft
2016, 3Q, 31   Femoral to peroneal artery bypass with in-situ saphenous vein graft and lysis of valves
2016, 2Q, 18   Femoral-tibial artery bypass and saphenous vein graft
2016, 1Q, 27   Aortocoronary bypass graft utilizing Y-graft
2014, 3Q, 8   Excision of saphenous vein for coronary artery bypass graft
2014, 3Q, 20   MAZE procedure performed with coronary artery bypass graft
2014, 1Q, 10   Repair of thoracic aortic aneurysm & coronary artery bypass graft

AHA Coding Clinic for table Ø6F
2020, 4Q, 45-49   New fragmentation tables
2020, 4Q, 49-50   Intravascular ultrasound assisted thrombolysis
2020, 4Q, 50   Intravascular lithotripsy

AHA Coding Clinic for table Ø6H
2021, 3Q, 18   Placement and removal of cannulas for extracorporeal membrane oxygenation
2017, 3Q, 11   Placement of peripherally inserted central catheter using 3CG ECG technology
2017, 1Q, 31   Umbilical vein catheterization
2017, 1Q, 31   Central catheter placement in femoral vein
2013, 3Q, 18   Heart transplant surgery

AHA Coding Clinic for table Ø6L
2021, 4Q, 47   Endoscopic banding of hemorrhoidal plexus
2021, 4Q, 49   Division of liver for staged hepatectomy
2020, 3Q, 44   Cardiophrenic vein embolization
2019, 4Q, 28   Transorifice occlusion of gastric varices
2018, 2Q, 18   Transverse rectus abdominis myocutaneous (TRAM) delay
2017, 4Q, 57-58   Added approach values - Transorifice esophageal vein banding
2013, 4Q, 112   Endoscopic banding of esophageal varices

AHA Coding Clinic for table Ø6P
2021, 3Q, 18   Placement and removal of cannulas for extracorporeal membrane oxygenation

AHA Coding Clinic for table Ø6V
2018, 3Q, 11   Transvenous transcatheter placement of valve in inferior vena cava
2018, 1Q, 10   Revision of transjugular intrahepatic portosystemic shunt

AHA Coding Clinic for table Ø6W
2019, 2Q, 39   Transjugular intrahepatic portosystemic shunt revision
2018, 1Q, 10   Revision of transjugular intrahepatic portosystemic shunt
2014, 3Q, 25   Revision of transjugular intrahepatic portosystemic shunt (TIPS)

Lower Veins

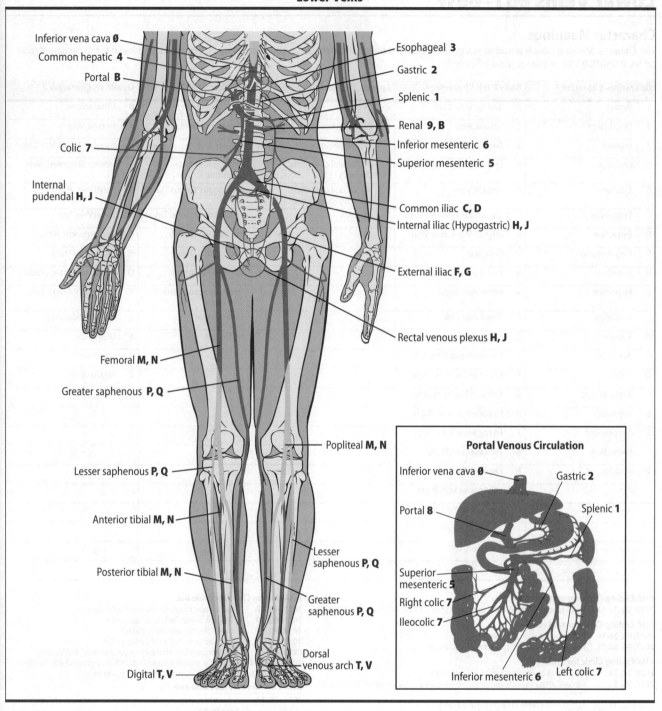

Inferior vena cava **Ø**
Common hepatic **4**
Portal **B**

Esophageal **3**
Gastric **2**
Splenic **1**
Renal **9, B**
Inferior mesenteric **6**
Superior mesenteric **5**

Colic **7**

Internal
pudendal **H, J**

Common iliac **C, D**
Internal iliac (Hypogastric) **H, J**

External iliac **F, G**

Rectal venous plexus **H, J**

Femoral **M, N**

Greater saphenous **P, Q**

Popliteal **M, N**

Lesser saphenous **P, Q**

Anterior tibial **M, N**

Lesser
saphenous **P, Q**

Posterior tibial **M, N**

Greater
saphenous **P, Q**

Dorsal
venous arch **T, V**

Digital **T, V**

Portal Venous Circulation

Inferior vena cava **Ø**

Gastric **2**

Portal **8**

Splenic **1**

Superior
mesenteric **5**

Right colic **7**

Ileocolic **7**

Inferior mesenteric **6**

Left colic **7**

Ø   Medical and Surgical
6   Lower Veins
1   Bypass   **Definition:** Altering the route of passage of the contents of a tubular body part

Explanation: Rerouting contents of a body part to a downstream area of the normal route, to a similar route and body part, or to an abnormal route and dissimilar body part. Includes one or more anastomoses, with or without the use of a device.

Body Part Character 4		Approach Character 5	Device Character 6	Qualifier Character 7
Ø Inferior Vena Cava Postcava Right inferior phrenic vein Right ovarian vein Right second lumbar vein Right suprarenal vein Right testicular vein		**Ø Open** **4 Percutaneous Endoscopic**	**7 Autologous Tissue Substitute** **9 Autologous Venous Tissue** **A Autologous Arterial Tissue** **J Synthetic Substitute** **K Nonautologous Tissue Substitute** **Z No Device**	**5 Superior Mesenteric Vein** **6 Inferior Mesenteric Vein** **P Pulmonary Trunk** **Q Pulmonary Artery, Right** **R Pulmonary Artery, Left** **Y Lower Vein**
1 Splenic Vein Left gastroepiploic vein Pancreatic vein		**Ø Open** **4 Percutaneous Endoscopic**	**7 Autologous Tissue Substitute** **9 Autologous Venous Tissue** **A Autologous Arterial Tissue** **J Synthetic Substitute** **K Nonautologous Tissue Substitute** **Z No Device**	**9 Renal Vein, Right** **B Renal Vein, Left** **Y Lower Vein**

2 Gastric Vein
3 Esophageal Vein
4 Hepatic Vein
5 Superior Mesenteric Vein
Right gastroepiploic vein
6 Inferior Mesenteric Vein
Sigmoid vein
Superior rectal vein
7 Colic Vein
Ileocolic vein
Left colic vein
Middle colic vein
Right colic vein
9 Renal Vein, Right
B Renal Vein, Left
Left inferior phrenic vein
Left ovarian vein
Left second lumbar vein
Left suprarenal vein
Left testicular vein
C Common Iliac Vein, Right
D Common Iliac Vein, Left
F External Iliac Vein, Right
G External Iliac Vein, Left
H Hypogastric Vein, Right
Gluteal vein
Internal iliac vein
Internal pudendal vein
Lateral sacral vein
Middle hemorrhoidal vein
Obturator vein
Uterine vein
Vaginal vein
Vesical vein
	J Hypogastric Vein, Left
	   See H Hypogastric Vein, Right
	M Femoral Vein, Right
	   Deep femoral (profunda femoris) vein
	   Popliteal vein
	   Profunda femoris (deep femoral) vein
	N Femoral Vein, Left
	   See M Femoral Vein, Right
	P Saphenous Vein, Right
	   External pudendal vein
	   Great(er) saphenous vein
	   Lesser saphenous vein
	   Small saphenous vein
	   Superficial circumflex iliac vein
	   Superficial epigastric vein
	Q Saphenous Vein, Left
	   See P Saphenous Vein, Right
	T Foot Vein, Right
	   Common digital vein
	   Dorsal metatarsal vein
	   Dorsal venous arch
	   Plantar digital vein
	   Plantar metatarsal vein
	   Plantar venous arch
	V Foot Vein, Left
	   See T Foot Vein, Right
		Ø Open
		4 Percutaneous Endoscopic
			7 Autologous Tissue Substitute
			9 Autologous Venous Tissue
			A Autologous Arterial Tissue
			J Synthetic Substitute
			K Nonautologous Tissue Substitute
			Z No Device
				Y Lower Vein

8 Portal Vein Hepatic portal vein		**Ø Open**	**7 Autologous Tissue Substitute** **9 Autologous Venous Tissue** **A Autologous Arterial Tissue** **J Synthetic Substitute** **K Nonautologous Tissue Substitute** **Z No Device**	**9 Renal Vein, Right** **B Renal Vein, Left** **Y Lower Vein**
8 Portal Vein Hepatic portal vein		**3 Percutaneous**	**J Synthetic Substitute**	**4 Hepatic Vein** **Y Lower Vein**
8 Portal Vein Hepatic portal vein		**4 Percutaneous Endoscopic**	**7 Autologous Tissue Substitute** **9 Autologous Venous Tissue** **A Autologous Arterial Tissue** **K Nonautologous Tissue Substitute** **Z No Device**	**9 Renal Vein, Right** **B Renal Vein, Left** **Y Lower Vein**
8 Portal Vein Hepatic portal vein		**4 Percutaneous Endoscopic**	**J Synthetic Substitute**	**4 Hepatic Vein** **9 Renal Vein, Right** **B Renal Vein, Left** **Y Lower Vein**

Lower Veins

Ø   **Medical and Surgical**
6   **Lower Veins**
5   **Destruction**   Definition: Physical eradication of all or a portion of a body part by the direct use of energy, force, or a destructive agent
                              Explanation: None of the body part is physically taken out

Body Part Character 4	Approach Character 5	Device Character 6	Qualifier Character 7

Ø **Inferior Vena Cava**
    Postcava
    Right inferior phrenic vein
    Right ovarian vein
    Right second lumbar vein
    Right suprarenal vein
    Right testicular vein
1 **Splenic Vein**
    Left gastroepiploic vein
    Pancreatic vein
2 **Gastric Vein**
3 **Esophageal Vein**
4 **Hepatic Vein**
5 **Superior Mesenteric Vein**
    Right gastroepiploic vein
6 **Inferior Mesenteric Vein**
    Sigmoid vein
    Superior rectal vein
7 **Colic Vein**
    Ileocolic vein
    Left colic vein
    Middle colic vein
    Right colic vein
8 **Portal Vein**
    Hepatic portal vein
9 **Renal Vein, Right**
B **Renal Vein, Left**
    Left inferior phrenic vein
    Left ovarian vein
    Left second lumbar vein
    Left suprarenal vein
    Left testicular vein
C **Common Iliac Vein, Right**
D **Common Iliac Vein, Left**
F **External Iliac Vein, Right**
G **External Iliac Vein, Left**
H **Hypogastric Vein, Right**
    Gluteal vein
    Internal iliac vein
    Internal pudendal vein
    Lateral sacral vein
    Middle hemorrhoidal vein
    Obturator vein
    Uterine vein
    Vaginal vein
    Vesical vein
J **Hypogastric Vein, Left**
    See H Hypogastric Vein, Right
M **Femoral Vein, Right**
    Deep femoral (profunda femoris) vein
    Popliteal vein
    Profunda femoris (deep femoral) vein
N **Femoral Vein, Left**
    See M Femoral Vein, Right
P **Saphenous Vein, Right**
    External pudendal vein
    Great(er) saphenous vein
    Lesser saphenous vein
    Small saphenous vein
    Superficial circumflex iliac vein
    Superficial epigastric vein
Q **Saphenous Vein, Left**
    See P Saphenous Vein, Right
T **Foot Vein, Right**
    Common digital vein
    Dorsal metatarsal vein
    Dorsal venous arch
    Plantar digital vein
    Plantar metatarsal vein
    Plantar venous arch
V **Foot Vein, Left**
    See T Foot Vein, Right
	Ø **Open**
	3 **Percutaneous**
	4 **Percutaneous Endoscopic**
		Z **No Device**	**Z** **No Qualifier**

Y **Lower Vein**	**Ø** **Open** **3** **Percutaneous** **4** **Percutaneous Endoscopic**	**Z** **No Device**	**C** **Hemorrhoidal Plexus** **Z** **No Qualifier**

Non-OR Procedure   DRG Non-OR Procedure   Valid OR Procedure   HAC Associated Procedure   Combination Only   New/Revised April   New/Revised October

266   ICD-10-PCS 2023

Ø   **Medical and Surgical**
6   **Lower Veins**
7   **Dilation**   Definition: Expanding an orifice or the lumen of a tubular body part

Explanation: The orifice can be a natural orifice or an artificially created orifice. Accomplished by stretching a tubular body part using intraluminal pressure or by cutting part of the orifice or wall of the tubular body part.

Body Part Character 4	Approach Character 5	Device Character 6	Qualifier Character 7

Ø   **Inferior Vena Cava**
    Postcava
    Right inferior phrenic vein
    Right ovarian vein
    Right second lumbar vein
    Right suprarenal vein
    Right testicular vein
1   **Splenic Vein**
    Left gastroepiploic vein
    Pancreatic vein
2   **Gastric Vein**
3   **Esophageal Vein**
4   **Hepatic Vein**
5   **Superior Mesenteric Vein**
    Right gastroepiploic vein
6   **Inferior Mesenteric Vein**
    Sigmoid vein
    Superior rectal vein
7   **Colic Vein**
    Ileocolic vein
    Left colic vein
    Middle colic vein
    Right colic vein
8   **Portal Vein**
    Hepatic portal vein
9   **Renal Vein, Right**
B   **Renal Vein, Left**
    Left inferior phrenic vein
    Left ovarian vein
    Left second lumbar vein
    Left suprarenal vein
    Left testicular vein
C   **Common Iliac Vein, Right**
D   **Common Iliac Vein, Left**
F   **External Iliac Vein, Right**
G   **External Iliac Vein, Left**
H   **Hypogastric Vein, Right**
    Gluteal vein
    Internal iliac vein
    Internal pudendal vein
    Lateral sacral vein
    Middle hemorrhoidal vein
    Obturator vein
    Uterine vein
    Vaginal vein
    Vesical vein
J   **Hypogastric Vein, Left**
    See H Hypogastric Vein, Right
M   **Femoral Vein, Right**
    Deep femoral (profunda femoris) vein
    Popliteal vein
    Profunda femoris (deep femoral) vein
N   **Femoral Vein, Left**
    See M Femoral Vein, Right
P   **Saphenous Vein, Right**
    External pudendal vein
    Great(er) saphenous vein
    Lesser saphenous vein
    Small saphenous vein
    Superficial circumflex iliac vein
    Superficial epigastric vein
Q   **Saphenous Vein, Left**
    See P Saphenous Vein, Right
T   **Foot Vein, Right**
    Common digital vein
    Dorsal metatarsal vein
    Dorsal venous arch
    Plantar digital vein
    Plantar metatarsal vein
    Plantar venous arch
V   **Foot Vein, Left**
    See T Foot Vein, Right
Y   **Lower Vein**
	Ø Open
	3 Percutaneous
	4 Percutaneous Endoscopic
		D Intraluminal Device
		Z No Device
			Z No Qualifier

Ø67 Continued on next page

NC Noncovered Procedure   **LC** Limited Coverage   **QA** Questionable OB Admit   **NT** New Tech Add-on   ⊞ Combination Member   ♂ Male   ♀ Female

ICD-10-PCS 2023   267

Lower Veins

069–069

0   **Medical and Surgical**
6   **Lower Veins**
9   **Drainage**   Definition: Taking or letting out fluids and/or gases from a body part
                        Explanation: The qualifier DIAGNOSTIC is used to identify drainage procedures that are biopsies

Body Part Character 4	Approach Character 5	Device Character 6	Qualifier Character 7
0 **Inferior Vena Cava** Postcava Right inferior phrenic vein Right ovarian vein Right second lumbar vein Right suprarenal vein Right testicular vein **1** **Splenic Vein** Left gastroepiploic vein Pancreatic vein **2** **Gastric Vein** **3** **Esophageal Vein** **4** **Hepatic Vein** **5** **Superior Mesenteric Vein** Right gastroepiploic vein **6** **Inferior Mesenteric Vein** Sigmoid vein Superior rectal vein **7** **Colic Vein** Ileocolic vein Left colic vein Middle colic vein Right colic vein **8** **Portal Vein** Hepatic portal vein **9** **Renal Vein, Right** **B** **Renal Vein, Left** Left inferior phrenic vein Left ovarian vein Left second lumbar vein Left suprarenal vein Left testicular vein **C** **Common Iliac Vein, Right** **D** **Common Iliac Vein, Left** **F** **External Iliac Vein, Right** **G** **External Iliac Vein, Left** **H** **Hypogastric Vein, Right** Gluteal vein Internal iliac vein Internal pudendal vein Lateral sacral vein Middle hemorrhoidal vein Obturator vein Uterine vein Vaginal vein Vesical vein **J** **Hypogastric Vein, Left** *See H Hypogastric Vein, Right* **M** **Femoral Vein, Right** Deep femoral (profunda femoris) vein Popliteal vein Profunda femoris (deep femoral) vein **N** **Femoral Vein, Left** *See M Femoral Vein, Right* **P** **Saphenous Vein, Right** External pudendal vein Great(er) saphenous vein Lesser saphenous vein Small saphenous vein Superficial circumflex iliac vein Superficial epigastric vein **Q** **Saphenous Vein, Left** *See P Saphenous Vein, Right* **T** **Foot Vein, Right** Common digital vein Dorsal metatarsal vein Dorsal venous arch Plantar digital vein Plantar metatarsal vein Plantar venous arch **V** **Foot Vein, Left** *See T Foot Vein, Right* **Y** **Lower Vein**	**0** Open **3** Percutaneous **4** Percutaneous Endoscopic	**0** Drainage Device	**Z** No Qualifier

Non-OR   069[0,1,2,4,5,6,7,8,9,B,C,D,F,G,H,J,M,N,P,Q,T,V,Y][0,3,4]0Z
Non-OR   069330Z

069 Continued on next page

Non-OR Procedure   DRG Non-OR Procedure   Valid OR Procedure   HAC Associated Procedure   Combination Only   New/Revised April   New/Revised October

268   ICD-10-PCS 2023

			Ø69 Continued

Ø **Medical and Surgical**
6 **Lower Veins**
9 **Drainage**　　Definition: Taking or letting out fluids and/or gases from a body part

Explanation: The qualifier DIAGNOSTIC is used to identify drainage procedures that are biopsies

Body Part Character 4	Approach Character 5	Device Character 6	Qualifier Character 7
Ø **Inferior Vena Cava**	**Ø** Open	**Z** No Device	**X** Diagnostic
Postcava	**3** Percutaneous		**Z** No Qualifier
Right inferior phrenic vein	**4** Percutaneous Endoscopic		
Right ovarian vein			
Right second lumbar vein			
Right suprarenal vein			
Right testicular vein			
1 **Splenic Vein**			
Left gastroepiploic vein			
Pancreatic vein			
2 **Gastric Vein**			
3 **Esophageal Vein**			
4 **Hepatic Vein**			
5 **Superior Mesenteric Vein**			
Right gastroepiploic vein			
6 **Inferior Mesenteric Vein**			
Sigmoid vein			
Superior rectal vein			
7 **Colic Vein**			
Ileocolic vein			
Left colic vein			
Middle colic vein			
Right colic vein			
8 **Portal Vein**			
Hepatic portal vein			
9 **Renal Vein, Right**			
B **Renal Vein, Left**			
Left inferior phrenic vein			
Left ovarian vein			
Left second lumbar vein			
Left suprarenal vein			
Left testicular vein			
C **Common Iliac Vein, Right**			
D **Common Iliac Vein, Left**			
F **External Iliac Vein, Right**			
G **External Iliac Vein, Left**			
H **Hypogastric Vein, Right**			
Gluteal vein			
Internal iliac vein			
Internal pudendal vein			
Lateral sacral vein			
Middle hemorrhoidal vein			
Obturator vein			
Uterine vein			
Vaginal vein			
Vesical vein			
J **Hypogastric Vein, Left**			
See H Hypogastric Vein, Right			
M **Femoral Vein, Right**			
Deep femoral (profunda femoris) vein			
Popliteal vein			
Profunda femoris (deep femoral) vein			
N **Femoral Vein, Left**			
See M Femoral Vein, Right			
P **Saphenous Vein, Right**			
External pudendal vein			
Great(er) saphenous vein			
Lesser saphenous vein			
Small saphenous vein			
Superficial circumflex iliac vein			
Superficial epigastric vein			
Q **Saphenous Vein, Left**			
See P Saphenous Vein, Right			
T **Foot Vein, Right**			
Common digital vein			
Dorsal metatarsal vein			
Dorsal venous arch			
Plantar digital vein			
Plantar metatarsal vein			
Plantar venous arch			
V **Foot Vein, Left**			
See T Foot Vein, Right			
Y **Lower Vein**			

Non-OR　Ø69[Ø,1,2,3,4,5,6,7,8,9,B,C,D,F,G,H,J,M,N,P,Q,T,V,Y]3ZX
Non-OR　Ø69[Ø,1,2,4,5,6,7,8,9,B,C,D,F,G,H,J,M,N,P,Q,T,V,Y][Ø,3,4]ZZ
Non-OR　Ø6933ZZ

NC Noncovered Procedure　　**LC** Limited Coverage　　**QA** Questionable OB Admit　　**NT** New Tech Add-on　　⊞ Combination Member　　♂ Male　　♀ Female

ICD-10-PCS 2023

269

Lower Veins

0   Medical and Surgical
6   Lower Veins
B   Excision   Definition: Cutting out or off, without replacement, a portion of a body part

Explanation: The qualifier DIAGNOSTIC is used to identify excision procedures that are biopsies

Body Part Character 4	Approach Character 5	Device Character 6	Qualifier Character 7

0   **Inferior Vena Cava**
    Postcava
    Right inferior phrenic vein
    Right ovarian vein
    Right second lumbar vein
    Right suprarenal vein
    Right testicular vein
	0 Open
	3 Percutaneous
	4 Percutaneous Endoscopic
		Z No Device	**X** Diagnostic
			Z No Qualifier

1   **Splenic Vein**
    Left gastroepiploic vein
    Pancreatic vein			

2 **Gastric Vein**			
3 **Esophageal Vein**			
4 **Hepatic Vein**			
5 **Superior Mesenteric Vein** Right gastroepiploic vein			

6   **Inferior Mesenteric Vein**
    Sigmoid vein
    Superior rectal vein			

7   **Colic Vein**
    Ileocolic vein
    Left colic vein
    Middle colic vein
    Right colic vein			

8 **Portal Vein** Hepatic portal vein			
9 **Renal Vein, Right**			

B   **Renal Vein, Left**
    Left inferior phrenic vein
    Left ovarian vein
    Left second lumbar vein
    Left suprarenal vein
    Left testicular vein			

C **Common Iliac Vein, Right**			
D **Common Iliac Vein, Left**			
F **External Iliac Vein, Right**			
G **External Iliac Vein, Left**			

H   **Hypogastric Vein, Right**
    Gluteal vein
    Internal iliac vein
    Internal pudendal vein
    Lateral sacral vein
    Middle hemorrhoidal vein
    Obturator vein
    Uterine vein
    Vaginal vein
    Vesical vein			

J **Hypogastric Vein, Left** *See H Hypogastric Vein, Right*			

M   **Femoral Vein, Right**
    Deep femoral (profunda femoris) vein
    Popliteal vein
    Profunda femoris (deep femoral) vein			

N **Femoral Vein, Left** *See M Femoral Vein, Right*			

P   **Saphenous Vein, Right**
    External pudendal vein
    Great(er) saphenous vein
    Lesser saphenous vein
    Small saphenous vein
    Superficial circumflex iliac vein
    Superficial epigastric vein			

Q **Saphenous Vein, Left** *See P Saphenous Vein, Right*			

T   **Foot Vein, Right**
    Common digital vein
    Dorsal metatarsal vein
    Dorsal venous arch
    Plantar digital vein
    Plantar metatarsal vein
    Plantar venous arch			

V **Foot Vein, Left** *See T Foot Vein, Right*			
Y **Lower Vein**	**0** Open **3** Percutaneous **4** Percutaneous Endoscopic	**Z** No Device	**C** Hemorrhoidal Plexus **X** Diagnostic **Z** No Qualifier

Non-OR Procedure   DRG Non-OR Procedure   Valid OR Procedure   HAC Associated Procedure   Combination Only   New/Revised April   New/Revised October

270   ICD-10-PCS 2023

Ø	**Medical and Surgical**
6	**Lower Veins**
C	**Extirpation**

Definition: Taking or cutting out solid matter from a body part

Explanation: The solid matter may be an abnormal byproduct of a biological function or a foreign body; it may be imbedded in a body part or in the lumen of a tubular body part. The solid matter may or may not have been previously broken into pieces.

Body Part Character 4	Approach Character 5	Device Character 6	Qualifier Character 7
Ø Inferior Vena Cava Postcava Right inferior phrenic vein Right ovarian vein Right second lumbar vein Right suprarenal vein Right testicular vein **1 Splenic Vein** Left gastroepiploic vein Pancreatic vein **2 Gastric Vein** **3 Esophageal Vein** **4 Hepatic Vein** **5 Superior Mesenteric Vein** Right gastroepiploic vein **6 Inferior Mesenteric Vein** Sigmoid vein Superior rectal vein **7 Colic Vein** Ileocolic vein Left colic vein Middle colic vein Right colic vein **8 Portal Vein** Hepatic portal vein **9 Renal Vein, Right** **B Renal Vein, Left** Left inferior phrenic vein Left ovarian vein Left second lumbar vein Left suprarenal vein Left testicular vein **C Common Iliac Vein, Right** **D Common Iliac Vein, Left** **F External Iliac Vein, Right** **G External Iliac Vein, Left** **H Hypogastric Vein, Right** Gluteal vein Internal iliac vein Internal pudendal vein Lateral sacral vein Middle hemorrhoidal vein Obturator vein Uterine vein Vaginal vein Vesical vein **J Hypogastric Vein, Left** *See H Hypogastric Vein, Right* **M Femoral Vein, Right** Deep femoral (profunda femoris) vein Popliteal vein Profunda femoris (deep femoral) vein **N Femoral Vein, Left** *See M Femoral Vein, Right* **P Saphenous Vein, Right** External pudendal vein Great(er) saphenous vein Lesser saphenous vein Small saphenous vein Superficial circumflex iliac vein Superficial epigastric vein **Q Saphenous Vein, Left** *See P Saphenous Vein, Right* **T Foot Vein, Right** Common digital vein Dorsal metatarsal vein Dorsal venous arch Plantar digital vein Plantar metatarsal vein Plantar venous arch **V Foot Vein, Left** *See T Foot Vein, Right* **Y Lower Vein**	**Ø Open** **3 Percutaneous** **4 Percutaneous Endoscopic**	**Z No Device**	**Z No Qualifier**

NC Noncovered Procedure   **LC** Limited Coverage   **QA** Questionable OB Admit   **NT** New Tech Add-on   ⊞ Combination Member   ♂ Male   ♀ Female

ICD-10-PCS 2023   271

Ø   Medical and Surgical
6   Lower Veins
D   Extraction   Definition: Pulling or stripping out or off all or a portion of a body part by the use of force

Explanation: The qualifier DIAGNOSTIC is used to identify extraction procedures that are biopsies

Body Part Character 4	Approach Character 5	Device Character 6	Qualifier Character 7

M **Femoral Vein, Right**
   Deep femoral (profunda femoris) vein
   Popliteal vein
   Profunda femoris (deep femoral) vein
N **Femoral Vein, Left**
   See M Femoral Vein, Right
P **Saphenous Vein, Right**
   External pudendal vein
   Great(er) saphenous vein
   Lesser saphenous vein
   Small saphenous vein
   Superficial circumflex iliac vein
   Superficial epigastric vein
Q **Saphenous Vein, Left**
   See P Saphenous Vein, Right
T **Foot Vein, Right**
   Common digital vein
   Dorsal metatarsal vein
   Dorsal venous arch
   Plantar digital vein
   Plantar metatarsal vein
   Plantar venous arch
V **Foot Vein, Left**
   See T Foot Vein, Right
Y **Lower Vein**
	Ø Open
	3 Percutaneous
	4 Percutaneous Endoscopic
		Z No Device	**Z** No Qualifier

Ø   Medical and Surgical
6   Lower Veins
F   Fragmentation   Definition: Breaking solid matter in a body part into pieces

Explanation: Physical force (e.g., manual, ultrasonic) applied directly or indirectly is used to break the solid matter into pieces. The solid matter may be an abnormal byproduct of a biological function or a foreign body. The pieces of solid matter are not taken out.

Body Part Character 4	Approach Character 5	Device Character 6	Qualifier Character 7

C **Common Iliac Vein, Right**
D **Common Iliac Vein, Left**
F **External Iliac Vein, Right**
G **External Iliac Vein, Left**
H **Hypogastric Vein, Right**
   Gluteal vein
   Internal iliac vein
   Internal pudendal vein
   Lateral sacral vein
   Middle hemorrhoidal vein
   Obturator vein
   Uterine vein
   Vaginal vein
   Vesical vein
J **Hypogastric Vein, Left**
   See H Hypogastric Vein, Right
M **Femoral Vein, Right**
   Deep femoral (profunda femoris) vein
   Popliteal vein
   Profunda femoris (deep femoral) vein
N **Femoral Vein, Left**
   See M Femoral Vein, Right
P **Saphenous Vein, Right**
   External pudendal vein
   Great(er) saphenous vein
   Lesser saphenous vein
   Small saphenous vein
   Superficial circumflex iliac vein
   Superficial epigastric vein
Q **Saphenous Vein, Left**
   See P Saphenous Vein, Right
Y **Lower Vein**
	3 Percutaneous	**Z** No Device	**Ø** Ultrasonic
			Z No Qualifier

Non-OR Procedure   DRG Non-OR Procedure   Valid OR Procedure   HAC Associated Procedure   Combination Only   New/Revised April   New/Revised October

272

Ø6D–Ø6F

ICD-10-PCS 2023

Ø   **Medical and Surgical**
6   **Lower Veins**
H   **Insertion**   Definition: Putting in a nonbiological appliance that monitors, assists, performs, or prevents a physiological function but does not physically take the place of a body part
                 Explanation: None

Body Part — Character 4		Approach — Character 5	Device — Character 6	Qualifier — Character 7
Ø Inferior Vena Cava Postcava Right inferior phrenic vein Right ovarian vein Right second lumbar vein Right suprarenal vein Right testicular vein		**Ø** Open **3** Percutaneous	**3** Infusion Device	**T** Via Umbilical Vein **Z** No Qualifier
Ø Inferior Vena Cava Postcava Right inferior phrenic vein Right ovarian vein Right second lumbar vein Right suprarenal vein Right testicular vein		**Ø** Open **3** Percutaneous	**D** Intraluminal Device	**Z** No Qualifier
Ø Inferior Vena Cava Postcava Right inferior phrenic vein Right ovarian vein Right second lumbar vein Right suprarenal vein Right testicular vein		**4** Percutaneous Endoscopic	**3** Infusion Device **D** Intraluminal Device	**Z** No Qualifier
1 Splenic Vein Left gastroepiploic vein Pancreatic vein **2 Gastric Vein** **3 Esophageal Vein** **4 Hepatic Vein** **5 Superior Mesenteric Vein** Right gastroepiploic vein **6 Inferior Mesenteric Vein** Sigmoid vein Superior rectal vein **7 Colic Vein** Ileocolic vein Left colic vein Middle colic vein Right colic vein **8 Portal Vein** Hepatic portal vein **9 Renal Vein, Right** **B Renal Vein, Left** Left inferior phrenic vein Left ovarian vein Left second lumbar vein Left suprarenal vein Left testicular vein **C Common Iliac Vein, Right** **D Common Iliac Vein, Left** **F External Iliac Vein, Right** **G External Iliac Vein, Left**	**H Hypogastric Vein, Right** Gluteal vein Internal iliac vein Internal pudendal vein Lateral sacral vein Middle hemorrhoidal vein Obturator vein Uterine vein Vaginal vein Vesical vein **J Hypogastric Vein, Left** *See H Hypogastric Vein, Right* **M Femoral Vein, Right** Deep femoral (profunda femoris) vein Popliteal vein Profunda femoris (deep femoral) vein **N Femoral Vein, Left** *See M Femoral Vein, Right* **P Saphenous Vein, Right** External pudendal vein Great(er) saphenous vein Lesser saphenous vein Small saphenous vein Superficial circumflex iliac vein Superficial epigastric vein **Q Saphenous Vein, Left** *See P Saphenous Vein, Right* **T Foot Vein, Right** Common digital vein Dorsal metatarsal vein Dorsal venous arch Plantar digital vein Plantar metatarsal vein Plantar venous arch **V Foot Vein, Left** *See T Foot Vein, Right*	**Ø** Open **3** Percutaneous **4** Percutaneous Endoscopic	**3** Infusion Device **D** Intraluminal Device	**Z** No Qualifier
Y Lower Vein		**Ø** Open **3** Percutaneous **4** Percutaneous Endoscopic	**2** Monitoring Device **3** Infusion Device **D** Intraluminal Device **Y** Other Device	**Z** No Qualifier

Non-OR	06HØ[Ø,3]3[T,Z]
Non-OR	06HØ3DZ
Non-OR	06HØ43Z
Non-OR	06H[1,2,3,4,5,6,7,8,9,B,C,D,F,G,H,J,M,N,P,Q,T,V][Ø,3,4]3Z
Non-OR	06HY[Ø,3,4]3Z
Non-OR	06HY32Z
Non-OR	06HY[3,4]YZ

NC Noncovered Procedure   **LC** Limited Coverage   **QA** Questionable OB Admit   **NT** New Tech Add-on   ⊞ Combination Member   ♂ Male   ♀ Female

ICD-10-PCS 2023   **273**

06H–06H

0   **Medical and Surgical**
6   **Lower Veins**
J   **Inspection**   Definition: Visually and/or manually exploring a body part

Explanation: Visual exploration may be performed with or without optical instrumentation. Manual exploration may be performed directly or through intervening body layers.

Body Part Character 4	Approach Character 5	Device Character 6	Qualifier Character 7
Y Lower Vein	Ø Open 3 Percutaneous 4 Percutaneous Endoscopic X External	Z No Device	Z No Qualifier

Non-OR   06JY[3,X]ZZ

---

0   **Medical and Surgical**
6   **Lower Veins**
L   **Occlusion**   Definition: Completely closing an orifice or the lumen of a tubular body part

Explanation: The orifice can be a natural orifice or an artificially created orifice

Body Part Character 4	Approach Character 5	Device Character 6	Qualifier Character 7

Ø   **Inferior Vena Cava**
    Postcava
    Right inferior phrenic vein
    Right ovarian vein
    Right second lumbar vein
    Right suprarenal vein
    Right testicular vein
1   **Splenic Vein**
    Left gastroepiploic vein
    Pancreatic vein
4   **Hepatic Vein**
5   **Superior Mesenteric Vein**
    Right gastroepiploic vein
6   **Inferior Mesenteric Vein**
    Sigmoid vein
    Superior rectal vein
7   **Colic Vein**
    Ileocolic vein
    Left colic vein
    Middle colic vein
    Right colic vein
8   **Portal Vein**
    Hepatic portal vein
9   **Renal Vein, Right**
B   **Renal Vein, Left**
    Left inferior phrenic vein
    Left ovarian vein
    Left second lumbar vein
    Left suprarenal vein
    Left testicular vein
C   **Common Iliac Vein, Right**
D   **Common Iliac Vein, Left**
F   **External Iliac Vein, Right**
G   **External Iliac Vein, Left**
 	
H   **Hypogastric Vein, Right**
    Gluteal vein
    Internal iliac vein
    Internal pudendal vein
    Lateral sacral vein
    Middle hemorrhoidal vein
    Obturator vein
    Uterine vein
    Vaginal vein
    Vesical vein
J   **Hypogastric Vein, Left**
    See H Hypogastric Vein, Right
M   **Femoral Vein, Right**
    Deep femoral (profunda
    femoris) vein
    Popliteal vein
    Profunda femoris (deep
    femoral) vein
N   **Femoral Vein, Left**
    See M Femoral Vein, Right
P   **Saphenous Vein, Right**
    External pudendal vein
    Great(er) saphenous vein
    Lesser saphenous vein
    Small saphenous vein
    Superficial circumflex iliac vein
    Superficial epigastric vein
Q   **Saphenous Vein, Left**
    See P Saphenous Vein, Right
T   **Foot Vein, Right**
    Common digital vein
    Dorsal metatarsal vein
    Dorsal venous arch
    Plantar digital vein
    Plantar metatarsal vein
    Plantar venous arch
V   **Foot Vein, Left**
    See T Foot Vein, Right
	Ø Open
	3 Percutaneous
	4 Percutaneous Endoscopic
		C Extraluminal Device
		D Intraluminal Device
		Z No Device
			Z No Qualifier

2   **Gastric Vein**
3   **Esophageal Vein**
	Ø Open
	3 Percutaneous
	4 Percutaneous Endoscopic
	7 Via Natural or Artificial
	    Opening
	8 Via Natural or Artificial
	    Opening Endoscopic
		C Extraluminal Device
		D Intraluminal Device
		Z No Device
			Z No Qualifier

Y **Lower Vein**	Ø Open
	3 Percutaneous
	4 Percutaneous Endoscopic
	7 Via Natural or Artificial
	    Opening
	8 Via Natural or Artificial
	    Opening Endoscopic
		C Extraluminal Device
		D Intraluminal Device
		Z No Device
			C Hemorrhoidal Plexus
			Z No Qualifier

Non-OR   06L2[7,8][C,D,Z]Z
Non-OR   06L3[3,4,7,8][C,D,Z]Z

Non-OR Procedure   DRG Non-OR Procedure   Valid OR Procedure   HAC Associated Procedure   Combination Only   New/Revised April   New/Revised October

0   Medical and Surgical
6   Lower Veins
N   Release   Definition: Freeing a body part from an abnormal physical constraint by cutting or by the use of force

                        Explanation: Some of the restraining tissue may be taken out but none of the body part is taken out

Body Part Character 4		Approach Character 5	Device Character 6	Qualifier Character 7
0 **Inferior Vena Cava** Postcava Right inferior phrenic vein Right ovarian vein Right second lumbar vein Right suprarenal vein Right testicular vein	**H** **Hypogastric Vein, Right** Gluteal vein Internal iliac vein Internal pudendal vein Lateral sacral vein Middle hemorrhoidal vein Obturator vein Uterine vein Vaginal vein Vesical vein	**0** **Open** **3** **Percutaneous** **4** **Percutaneous Endoscopic**	**Z** **No Device**	**Z** **No Qualifier**
1 **Splenic Vein** Left gastroepiploic vein Pancreatic vein	**J** **Hypogastric Vein, Left** *See H Hypogastric Vein, Right*			
2 **Gastric Vein**	**M** **Femoral Vein, Right** Deep femoral (profunda femoris) vein Popliteal vein Profunda femoris (deep femoral) vein			
3 **Esophageal Vein**				
4 **Hepatic Vein**				
5 **Superior Mesenteric Vein** Right gastroepiploic vein				
6 **Inferior Mesenteric Vein** Sigmoid vein Superior rectal vein	**N** **Femoral Vein, Left** *See M Femoral Vein, Right*			
7 **Colic Vein** Ileocolic vein Left colic vein Middle colic vein Right colic vein	**P** **Saphenous Vein, Right** External pudendal vein Great(er) saphenous vein Lesser saphenous vein Small saphenous vein Superficial circumflex iliac vein Superficial epigastric vein			
8 **Portal Vein** Hepatic portal vein	**Q** **Saphenous Vein, Left** *See P Saphenous Vein, Right*			
9 **Renal Vein, Right**				
B **Renal Vein, Left** Left inferior phrenic vein Left ovarian vein Left second lumbar vein Left suprarenal vein Left testicular vein	**T** **Foot Vein, Right** Common digital vein Dorsal metatarsal vein Dorsal venous arch Plantar digital vein Plantar metatarsal vein Plantar venous arch			
C **Common Iliac Vein, Right**				
D **Common Iliac Vein, Left**	**V** **Foot Vein, Left** *See T Foot Vein, Right*			
F **External Iliac Vein, Right**				
G **External Iliac Vein, Left**	**Y** **Lower Vein**			

0   Medical and Surgical
6   Lower Veins
P   Removal   Definition: Taking out or off a device from a body part

                        Explanation: If a device is taken out and a similar device put in without cutting or puncturing the skin or mucous membrane, the procedure is coded to the root operation CHANGE. Otherwise, the procedure for taking out a device is coded to the root operation REMOVAL.

Body Part Character 4	Approach Character 5	Device Character 6	Qualifier Character 7
Y Lower Vein	**0** **Open** **3** **Percutaneous** **4** **Percutaneous Endoscopic**	**0** **Drainage Device** **2** **Monitoring Device** **3** **Infusion Device** **7** **Autologous Tissue Substitute** **C** **Extraluminal Device** **D** **Intraluminal Device** **J** **Synthetic Substitute** **K** **Nonautologous Tissue Substitute** **Y** **Other Device**	**Z** **No Qualifier**
Y Lower Vein	**X** **External**	**0** **Drainage Device** **2** **Monitoring Device** **3** **Infusion Device** **D** **Intraluminal Device**	**Z** **No Qualifier**

Non-OR	06PY3[0,2,3]Z
Non-OR	06PY[3,4]YZ
Non-OR	06PYX[0,2,3,D]Z

NC Noncovered Procedure   **LC** Limited Coverage   **QA** Questionable OB Admit   **NT** New Tech Add-on   ⊞ Combination Member   ♂ Male   ♀ Female

ICD-10-PCS 2023   **275**

Lower Veins

0 Medical and Surgical
6 Lower Veins
Q Repair

Definition: Restoring, to the extent possible, a body part to its normal anatomic structure and function
Explanation: Used only when the method to accomplish the repair is not one of the other root operations

Body Part Character 4	Approach Character 5	Device Character 6	Qualifier Character 7
0 Inferior Vena Cava Postcava Right inferior phrenic vein Right ovarian vein Right second lumbar vein Right suprarenal vein Right testicular vein	0 Open 3 Percutaneous 4 Percutaneous Endoscopic	Z No Device	Z No Qualifier
1 Splenic Vein Left gastroepiploic vein Pancreatic vein			
2 Gastric Vein			
3 Esophageal Vein			
4 Hepatic Vein			
5 Superior Mesenteric Vein Right gastroepiploic vein			
6 Inferior Mesenteric Vein Sigmoid vein Superior rectal vein			
7 Colic Vein Ileocolic vein Left colic vein Middle colic vein Right colic vein			
8 Portal Vein Hepatic portal vein			
9 Renal Vein, Right			
B Renal Vein, Left Left inferior phrenic vein Left ovarian vein Left second lumbar vein Left suprarenal vein Left testicular vein			
C Common Iliac Vein, Right			
D Common Iliac Vein, Left			
F External Iliac Vein, Right			
G External Iliac Vein, Left			
H Hypogastric Vein, Right Gluteal vein Internal iliac vein Internal pudendal vein Lateral sacral vein Middle hemorrhoidal vein Obturator vein Uterine vein Vaginal vein Vesical vein			
J Hypogastric Vein, Left See H Hypogastric Vein, Right			
M Femoral Vein, Right Deep femoral (profunda femoris) vein Popliteal vein Profunda femoris (deep femoral) vein			
N Femoral Vein, Left See M Femoral Vein, Right			
P Saphenous Vein, Right External pudendal vein Great(er) saphenous vein Lesser saphenous vein Small saphenous vein Superficial circumflex iliac vein Superficial epigastric vein			
Q Saphenous Vein, Left See P Saphenous Vein, Right			
T Foot Vein, Right Common digital vein Dorsal metatarsal vein Dorsal venous arch Plantar digital vein Plantar metatarsal vein Plantar venous arch			
V Foot Vein, Left See T Foot Vein, Right			
Y Lower Vein			

Ø   **Medical and Surgical**
6   **Lower Veins**
R   **Replacement**   Definition: Putting in or on biological or synthetic material that physically takes the place and/or function of all or a portion of a body part
          Explanation: The body part may have been taken out or replaced, or may be taken out, physically eradicated, or rendered nonfunctional during the REPLACEMENT procedure. A REMOVAL procedure is coded for taking out the device used in a previous replacement procedure.

Body Part Character 4	Approach Character 5	Device Character 6	Qualifier Character 7

Ø **Inferior Vena Cava**
   Postcava
   Right inferior phrenic vein
   Right ovarian vein
   Right second lumbar vein
   Right suprarenal vein
   Right testicular vein
1 **Splenic Vein**
   Left gastroepiploic vein
   Pancreatic vein
2 **Gastric Vein**
3 **Esophageal Vein**
4 **Hepatic Vein**
5 **Superior Mesenteric Vein**
   Right gastroepiploic vein
6 **Inferior Mesenteric Vein**
   Sigmoid vein
   Superior rectal vein
7 **Colic Vein**
   Ileocolic vein
   Left colic vein
   Middle colic vein
   Right colic vein
8 **Portal Vein**
   Hepatic portal vein
9 **Renal Vein, Right**
B **Renal Vein, Left**
   Left inferior phrenic vein
   Left ovarian vein
   Left second lumbar vein
   Left suprarenal vein
   Left testicular vein
C **Common Iliac Vein, Right**
D **Common Iliac Vein, Left**
F **External Iliac Vein, Right**
G **External Iliac Vein, Left**
H **Hypogastric Vein, Right**
   Gluteal vein
   Internal iliac vein
   Internal pudendal vein
   Lateral sacral vein
   Middle hemorrhoidal vein
   Obturator vein
   Uterine vein
   Vaginal vein
   Vesical vein
J **Hypogastric Vein, Left**
   See H Hypogastric Vein, Right
M **Femoral Vein, Right**
   Deep femoral (profunda femoris) vein
   Popliteal vein
   Profunda femoris (deep femoral) vein
N **Femoral Vein, Left**
   See M Femoral Vein, Right
P **Saphenous Vein, Right**
   External pudendal vein
   Great(er) saphenous vein
   Lesser saphenous vein
   Small saphenous vein
   Superficial circumflex iliac vein
   Superficial epigastric vein
Q **Saphenous Vein, Left**
   See P Saphenous Vein, Right
T **Foot Vein, Right**
   Common digital vein
   Dorsal metatarsal vein
   Dorsal venous arch
   Plantar digital vein
   Plantar metatarsal vein
   Plantar venous arch
V **Foot Vein, Left**
   See T Foot Vein, Right
Y **Lower Vein**
	Ø Open
	4 Percutaneous Endoscopic
		7 Autologous Tissue Substitute
		J Synthetic Substitute
		K Nonautologous Tissue Substitute
			Z No Qualifier

NC Noncovered Procedure   LC Limited Coverage   QA Questionable OB Admit   NT New Tech Add-on   ⊞ Combination Member   ♂ Male   ♀ Female

ICD-10-PCS 2023   277

Ø6R–Ø6R

Lower Veins

0   **Medical and Surgical**
6   **Lower Veins**
S   **Reposition**   Definition: Moving to its normal location, or other suitable location, all or a portion of a body part

Explanation: The body part is moved to a new location from an abnormal location, or from a normal location where it is not functioning correctly. The body part may or may not be cut out or off to be moved to the new location.

Body Part Character 4	Approach Character 5	Device Character 6	Qualifier Character 7

0   **Inferior Vena Cava**
    Postcava
    Right inferior phrenic vein
    Right ovarian vein
    Right second lumbar vein
    Right suprarenal vein
    Right testicular vein
	0 Open
	3 Percutaneous
	4 Percutaneous Endoscopic
		Z No Device	**Z** No Qualifier

1   **Splenic Vein**
    Left gastroepiploic vein
    Pancreatic vein			

2 **Gastric Vein**			
3 **Esophageal Vein**			
4 **Hepatic Vein**			
5 **Superior Mesenteric Vein** Right gastroepiploic vein			

6   **Inferior Mesenteric Vein**
    Sigmoid vein
    Superior rectal vein			

7   **Colic Vein**
    Ileocolic vein
    Left colic vein
    Middle colic vein
    Right colic vein			

8 **Portal Vein** Hepatic portal vein			
9 **Renal Vein, Right**			

B   **Renal Vein, Left**
    Left inferior phrenic vein
    Left ovarian vein
    Left second lumbar vein
    Left suprarenal vein
    Left testicular vein			

C **Common Iliac Vein, Right**			
D **Common Iliac Vein, Left**			
F **External Iliac Vein, Right**			
G **External Iliac Vein, Left**			

H   **Hypogastric Vein, Right**
    Gluteal vein
    Internal iliac vein
    Internal pudendal vein
    Lateral sacral vein
    Middle hemorrhoidal vein
    Obturator vein
    Uterine vein
    Vaginal vein
    Vesical vein			

J **Hypogastric Vein, Left** *See H Hypogastric Vein, Right*			

M   **Femoral Vein, Right**
    Deep femoral (profunda femoris) vein
    Popliteal vein
    Profunda femoris (deep femoral) vein			

N **Femoral Vein, Left** *See M Femoral Vein, Right*			

P   **Saphenous Vein, Right**
    External pudendal vein
    Great(er) saphenous vein
    Lesser saphenous vein
    Small saphenous vein
    Superficial circumflex iliac vein
    Superficial epigastric vein			

Q **Saphenous Vein, Left** *See P Saphenous Vein, Right*			

T   **Foot Vein, Right**
    Common digital vein
    Dorsal metatarsal vein
    Dorsal venous arch
    Plantar digital vein
    Plantar metatarsal vein
    Plantar venous arch			

V **Foot Vein, Left** *See T Foot Vein, Right*			
Y **Lower Vein**			

Non-OR Procedure   DRG Non-OR Procedure   Valid OR Procedure   HAC Associated Procedure   Combination Only   New/Revised April   New/Revised October

278   ICD-10-PCS 2023

Ø   Medical and Surgical
6   Lower Veins
U   Supplement   Definition: Putting in or on biological or synthetic material that physically reinforces and/or augments the function of a portion of a body part
           Explanation: The biological material is non-living, or is living and from the same individual. The body part may have been previously replaced, and the SUPPLEMENT procedure is performed to physically reinforce and/or augment the function of the replaced body part.

Body Part Character 4	Approach Character 5	Device Character 6	Qualifier Character 7

Ø   Inferior Vena Cava
    Postcava
    Right inferior phrenic vein
    Right ovarian vein
    Right second lumbar vein
    Right suprarenal vein
    Right testicular vein
1   Splenic Vein
    Left gastroepiploic vein
    Pancreatic vein
2   Gastric Vein
3   Esophageal Vein
4   Hepatic Vein
5   Superior Mesenteric Vein
    Right gastroepiploic vein
6   Inferior Mesenteric Vein
    Sigmoid vein
    Superior rectal vein
7   Colic Vein
    Ileocolic vein
    Left colic vein
    Middle colic vein
    Right colic vein
8   Portal Vein
    Hepatic portal vein
9   Renal Vein, Right
B   Renal Vein, Left
    Left inferior phrenic vein
    Left ovarian vein
    Left second lumbar vein
    Left suprarenal vein
    Left testicular vein
C   Common Iliac Vein, Right
D   Common Iliac Vein, Left
F   External Iliac Vein, Right
G   External Iliac Vein, Left
H   Hypogastric Vein, Right
    Gluteal vein
    Internal iliac vein
    Internal pudendal vein
    Lateral sacral vein
    Middle hemorrhoidal vein
    Obturator vein
    Uterine vein
    Vaginal vein
    Vesical vein
J   Hypogastric Vein, Left
    See H Hypogastric Vein, Right
M   Femoral Vein, Right
    Deep femoral (profunda femoris) vein
    Popliteal vein
    Profunda femoris (deep femoral) vein
N   Femoral Vein, Left
    See M Femoral Vein, Right
P   Saphenous Vein, Right
    External pudendal vein
    Great(er) saphenous vein
    Lesser saphenous vein
    Small saphenous vein
    Superficial circumflex iliac vein
    Superficial epigastric vein
Q   Saphenous Vein, Left
    See P Saphenous Vein, Right
T   Foot Vein, Right
    Common digital vein
    Dorsal metatarsal vein
    Dorsal venous arch
    Plantar digital vein
    Plantar metatarsal vein
    Plantar venous arch
V   Foot Vein, Left
    See T Foot Vein, Right
Y   Lower Vein
	Ø Open
	3 Percutaneous
	4 Percutaneous Endoscopic
		7 Autologous Tissue Substitute
		J Synthetic Substitute
		K Nonautologous Tissue Substitute
			Z No Qualifier

NC Noncovered Procedure   LC Limited Coverage   UA Questionable OB Admit   NT New Tech Add-on   ⊞ Combination Member   ♂ Male   ♀ Female

Lower Veins

Ø6V–Ø6V

Ø	**Medical and Surgical**
6	**Lower Veins**
V	**Restriction** Definition: Partially closing an orifice or the lumen of a tubular body part
	Explanation: The orifice can be a natural orifice or an artificially created orifice

Body Part Character 4	Approach Character 5	Device Character 6	Qualifier Character 7

Ø Inferior Vena Cava
  Postcava
  Right inferior phrenic vein
  Right ovarian vein
  Right second lumbar vein
  Right suprarenal vein
  Right testicular vein
	Ø Open
	3 Percutaneous
	4 Percutaneous Endoscopic
		C Extraluminal Device
		D Intraluminal Device
		Z No Device
			Z No Qualifier

1 Splenic Vein
  Left gastroepiploic vein
  Pancreatic vein			

2 Gastric Vein			
3 Esophageal Vein			
4 Hepatic Vein			
5 Superior Mesenteric Vein Right gastroepiploic vein			

6 Inferior Mesenteric Vein
  Sigmoid vein
  Superior rectal vein			

7 Colic Vein
  Ileocolic vein
  Left colic vein
  Middle colic vein
  Right colic vein			

8 Portal Vein Hepatic portal vein			
9 Renal Vein, Right			

B Renal Vein, Left
  Left inferior phrenic vein
  Left ovarian vein
  Left second lumbar vein
  Left suprarenal vein
  Left testicular vein			

C Common Iliac Vein, Right			
D Common Iliac Vein, Left			
F External Iliac Vein, Right			
G External Iliac Vein, Left			

H Hypogastric Vein, Right
  Gluteal vein
  Internal iliac vein
  Internal pudendal vein
  Lateral sacral vein
  Middle hemorrhoidal vein
  Obturator vein
  Uterine vein
  Vaginal vein
  Vesical vein			

J Hypogastric Vein, Left *See* H Hypogastric Vein, Right			

M Femoral Vein, Right
  Deep femoral (profunda femoris) vein
  Popliteal vein
  Profunda femoris (deep femoral) vein			

N Femoral Vein, Left *See* M Femoral Vein, Right			

P Saphenous Vein, Right
  External pudendal vein
  Great(er) saphenous vein
  Lesser saphenous vein
  Small saphenous vein
  Superficial circumflex iliac vein
  Superficial epigastric vein			

Q Saphenous Vein, Left *See* P Saphenous Vein, Right			

T Foot Vein, Right
  Common digital vein
  Dorsal metatarsal vein
  Dorsal venous arch
  Plantar digital vein
  Plantar metatarsal vein
  Plantar venous arch			

V Foot Vein, Left *See* T Foot Vein, Right			
Y Lower Vein			

Non-OR Procedure   DRG Non-OR Procedure   Valid OR Procedure   HAC Associated Procedure   Combination Only   New/Revised April   New/Revised October

280   ICD-10-PCS 2023

Ø   **Medical and Surgical**
6   **Lower Veins**
W   **Revision**   Definition: Correcting, to the extent possible, a portion of a malfunctioning device or the position of a displaced device

Explanation: Revision can include correcting a malfunctioning or displaced device by taking out or putting in components of the device such as a screw or pin

Body Part Character 4	Approach Character 5	Device Character 6	Qualifier Character 7
Y Lower Vein	Ø Open 3 Percutaneous 4 Percutaneous Endoscopic	Ø Drainage Device 2 Monitoring Device 3 Infusion Device 7 Autologous Tissue Substitute C Extraluminal Device D Intraluminal Device J Synthetic Substitute K Nonautologous Tissue Substitute Y Other Device	Z No Qualifier
Y Lower Vein	X External	Ø Drainage Device 2 Monitoring Device 3 Infusion Device 7 Autologous Tissue Substitute C Extraluminal Device D Intraluminal Device J Synthetic Substitute K Nonautologous Tissue Substitute	Z No Qualifier

Non-OR   Ø6WY3[Ø,2,3]Z
Non-OR   Ø6WY[3,4]YZ
Non-OR   Ø6WYX[Ø,2,3,7,C,D,J,K]Z

NC Noncovered Procedure   LC Limited Coverage   QA Questionable OB Admit   NT New Tech Add-on   ⊞ Combination Member   ♂ Male   ♀ Female

ICD-10-PCS 2023   281

Lymphatic and Hemic Systems Ø72–Ø7Y

Character Meanings*

This Character Meaning table is provided as a guide to assist the user in the identification of character members that may be found in this section of code tables. It **SHOULD NOT** be used to build a PCS code.

Operation–Character 3	Body Part–Character 4	Approach–Character 5	Device–Character 6	Qualifier–Character 7
2 Change	Ø Lymphatic, Head	Ø Open	Ø Drainage Device	Ø Allogeneic
5 Destruction	1 Lymphatic, Right Neck	3 Percutaneous	1 Radioactive Element	1 Syngeneic
9 Drainage	2 Lymphatic, Left Neck	4 Percutaneous Endoscopic	3 Infusion Device	2 Zooplastic
B Excision	3 Lymphatic, Right Upper Extremity	8 Via Natural or Artificial Opening Endoscopic	7 Autologous Tissue Substitute	X Diagnostic
C Extirpation	4 Lymphatic, Left Upper Extremity	X External	C Extraluminal Device	Z No Qualifier
D Extraction	5 Lymphatic, Right Axillary		D Intraluminal Device	
H Insertion	6 Lymphatic, Left Axillary		J Synthetic Substitute	
J Inspection	7 Lymphatic, Thorax		K Nonautologous Tissue Substitute	
L Occlusion	8 Lymphatic, Internal Mammary, Right		Y Other Device	
N Release	9 Lymphatic, Internal Mammary, Left		Z No Device	
P Removal	B Lymphatic, Mesenteric			
Q Repair	C Lymphatic, Pelvis			
S Reposition	D Lymphatic, Aortic			
T Resection	F Lymphatic, Right Lower Extremity			
U Supplement	G Lymphatic, Left Lower Extremity			
V Restriction	H Lymphatic, Right Inguinal			
W Revision	J Lymphatic, Left Inguinal			
Y Transplantation	K Thoracic Duct			
	L Cisterna Chyli			
	M Thymus			
	N Lymphatic			
	P Spleen			
	Q Bone Marrow, Sternum			
	R Bone Marrow, Iliac			
	S Bone Marrow, Vertebral			
	T Bone Marrow			

* Includes lymph vessels and lymph nodes.

AHA Coding Clinic for table Ø79

2021, 4Q, 47	Extraction of bone marrow from other sites
2018, 4Q, 84	Fine needle aspiration biopsy of lymphatic tissue
2017, 1Q, 34	Lymphovenous bypass following mastectomy
2014, 1Q, 26	Transbronchial needle aspiration lymph node biopsy
2013, 4Q, 111	Transbronchial needle aspiration lymph node biopsy

AHA Coding Clinic for table Ø7B

2022, 1Q, 14	Reduction mammoplasty for breast symmetry
2019, 1Q, 3-8	Whipple procedure
2018, 4Q, 84	Fine needle aspiration biopsy of lymphatic tissue
2018, 1Q, 22	Resection of lymph node chains
2016, 1Q, 30	Axillary lymph node resection with modified radical mastectomy
2014, 3Q, 10	Selective excision of paratracheal lymph nodes
2014, 1Q, 20	Fiducial marker placement
2014, 1Q, 26	Transbronchial endoscopic lymph node aspiration biopsy

AHA Coding Clinic for table Ø7D

2022, 1Q, 54	Extraction of bone marrow from other sites
2021, 4Q, 47	Extraction of bone marrow from other sites
2018, 4Q, 84	Fine needle aspiration biopsy of lymphatic tissue
2013, 4Q, 111	Root operation for bone marrow biopsy

AHA Coding Clinic for table Ø7H

| 2020, 4Q, 43-44 | Insertion of radioactive element |
| 2020, 4Q, 53 | Bone marrow body part |

AHA Coding Clinic for table Ø7Q

| 2017, 1Q, 34 | Lymphovenous bypass following mastectomy |

AHA Coding Clinic for table Ø7S

| 2019, 3Q, 29 | Thymus transplant for T-Cell production |

AHA Coding Clinic for table Ø7T

2018, 1Q, 22	Resection of lymph node chains
2016, 2Q, 12	Resection of malignant neoplasm of infratemporal fossa
2016, 1Q, 30	Axillary lymph node resection with modified radical mastectomy
2015, 4Q, 13	New Section X codes—New Technology procedures
2014, 3Q, 9	Radical resection of level I lymph nodes
2014, 3Q, 16	Repair of Tetralogy of Fallot

AHA Coding Clinic for table Ø7Y

| 2019, 3Q, 29 | Thymus transplant for T-Cell production |

Lymphatic System

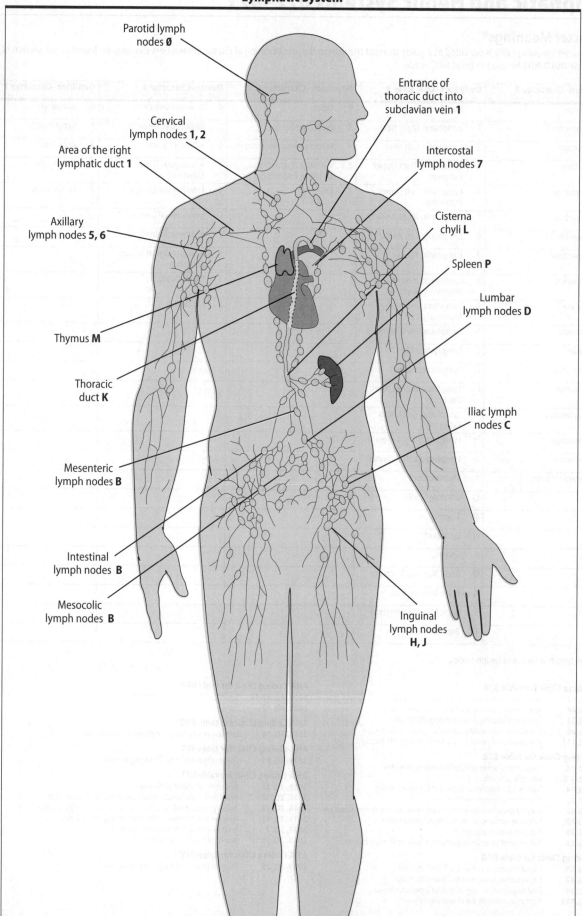

Parotid lymph nodes **Ø**

Entrance of thoracic duct into subclavian vein **1**

Cervical lymph nodes **1, 2**

Area of the right lymphatic duct **1**

Intercostal lymph nodes **7**

Cisterna chyli **L**

Axillary lymph nodes **5, 6**

Spleen **P**

Lumbar lymph nodes **D**

Thymus **M**

Thoracic duct **K**

Iliac lymph nodes **C**

Mesenteric lymph nodes **B**

Intestinal lymph nodes **B**

Mesocolic lymph nodes **B**

Inguinal lymph nodes **H, J**

Ø Medical and Surgical
7 Lymphatic and Hemic Systems
2 Change   Definition: Taking out or off a device from a body part and putting back an identical or similar device in or on the same body part without cutting or puncturing the skin or a mucous membrane

          Explanation: All CHANGE procedures are coded using the approach EXTERNAL

Body Part Character 4		Approach Character 5	Device Character 6	Qualifier Character 7
K Thoracic Duct Left jugular trunk Left subclavian trunk **L Cisterna Chyli** Intestinal lymphatic trunk Lumbar lymphatic trunk	**M Thymus** Thymus gland **N Lymphatic** **P Spleen** Accessory spleen **T Bone Marrow**	X External	Ø Drainage Device Y Other Device	Z No Qualifier

Non-OR   All body part, approach, device, and qualifier values

Ø Medical and Surgical
7 Lymphatic and Hemic Systems
5 Destruction   Definition: Physical eradication of all or a portion of a body part by the direct use of energy, force, or a destructive agent

          Explanation: None of the body part is physically taken out

Body Part Character 4		Approach Character 5	Device Character 6	Qualifier Character 7
Ø Lymphatic, Head Buccinator lymph node Infraauricular lymph node Infraparotid lymph node Parotid lymph node Preauricular lymph node Submandibular lymph node Submaxillary lymph node Submental lymph node Subparotid lymph node Suprahyoid lymph node **1 Lymphatic, Right Neck** Cervical lymph node Jugular lymph node Mastoid (postauricular) lymph node Occipital lymph node Postauricular (mastoid) lymph node Retropharyngeal lymph node Right jugular trunk Right lymphatic duct Right subclavian trunk Supraclavicular (Virchow's) lymph node Virchow's (supraclavicular) lymph node **2 Lymphatic, Left Neck** Cervical lymph node Jugular lymph node Mastoid (postauricular) lymph node Occipital lymph node Postauricular (mastoid) lymph node Retropharyngeal lymph node Supraclavicular (Virchow's) lymph node Virchow's (supraclavicular) lymph node **3 Lymphatic, Right Upper Extremity** Cubital lymph node Deltopectoral (infraclavicular) lymph node Epitrochlear lymph node Infraclavicular (deltopectoral) lymph node Supratrochlear lymph node **4 Lymphatic, Left Upper Extremity** *See 3 Lymphatic, Right Upper Extremity* **5 Lymphatic, Right Axillary** Anterior (pectoral) lymph node Apical (subclavicular) lymph node Brachial (lateral) lymph node Central axillary lymph node Lateral (brachial) lymph node Pectoral (anterior) lymph node Posterior (subscapular) lymph node Subclavicular (apical) lymph node Subscapular (posterior) lymph node	**6 Lymphatic, Left Axillary** *See 5 Lymphatic, Right Axillary* **7 Lymphatic, Thorax** Intercostal lymph node Mediastinal lymph node Parasternal lymph node Paratracheal lymph node Tracheobronchial lymph node **8 Lymphatic, Internal Mammary, Right** **9 Lymphatic, Internal Mammary, Left** **B Lymphatic, Mesenteric** Inferior mesenteric lymph node Pararectal lymph node Superior mesenteric lymph node **C Lymphatic, Pelvis** Common iliac (subaortic) lymph node Gluteal lymph node Iliac lymph node Inferior epigastric lymph node Obturator lymph node Sacral lymph node Subaortic (common iliac) lymph node Suprainguinal lymph node **D Lymphatic, Aortic** Celiac lymph node Gastric lymph node Hepatic lymph node Lumbar lymph node Pancreaticosplenic lymph node Paraaortic lymph node Retroperitoneal lymph node **F Lymphatic, Right Lower Extremity** Femoral lymph node Popliteal lymph node **G Lymphatic, Left Lower Extremity** *See F Lymphatic, Right Lower Extremity* **H Lymphatic, Right Inguinal** **J Lymphatic, Left Inguinal** **K Thoracic Duct** Left jugular trunk Left subclavian trunk **L Cisterna Chyli** Intestinal lymphatic trunk Lumbar lymphatic trunk **M Thymus** Thymus gland **P Spleen** Accessory spleen	Ø Open 3 Percutaneous 4 Percutaneous Endoscopic	Z No Device	Z No Qualifier

NC Noncovered Procedure   **LC** Limited Coverage   **QA** Questionable OB Admit   **NT** New Tech Add-on   ⊞ Combination Member   ♂ Male   ♀ Female

ICD-10-PCS 2023   **285**

Ø   Medical and Surgical
7   Lymphatic and Hemic Systems
9   Drainage   Definition: Taking or letting out fluids and/or gases from a body part
                   Explanation: The qualifier DIAGNOSTIC is used to identify drainage procedures that are biopsies

Body Part Character 4		Approach Character 5	Device Character 6	Qualifier Character 7

Ø Lymphatic, Head
Buccinator lymph node
Infraauricular lymph node
Infraparotid lymph node
Parotid lymph node
Preauricular lymph node
Submandibular lymph node
Submaxillary lymph node
Submental lymph node
Subparotid lymph node
Suprahyoid lymph node
1 Lymphatic, Right Neck
Cervical lymph node
Jugular lymph node
Mastoid (postauricular) lymph node
Occipital lymph node
Postauricular (mastoid) lymph node
Retropharyngeal lymph node
Right jugular trunk
Right lymphatic duct
Right subclavian trunk
Supraclavicular (Virchow's) lymph
    node
Virchow's (supraclavicular) lymph
    node
2 Lymphatic, Left Neck
Cervical lymph node
Jugular lymph node
Mastoid (postauricular) lymph node
Occipital lymph node
Postauricular (mastoid) lymph node
Retropharyngeal lymph node
Supraclavicular (Virchow's) lymph
    node
Virchow's (supraclavicular) lymph
    node
3 Lymphatic, Right Upper Extremity
Cubital lymph node
Deltopectoral (infraclavicular) lymph
    node
Epitrochlear lymph node
Infraclavicular (deltopectoral) lymph
    node
Supratrochlear lymph node
4 Lymphatic, Left Upper Extremity
See 3 Lymphatic, Right Upper Extremity
5 Lymphatic, Right Axillary
Anterior (pectoral) lymph node
Apical (subclavicular) lymph node
Brachial (lateral) lymph node
Central axillary lymph node
Lateral (brachial) lymph node
Pectoral (anterior) lymph node
Posterior (subscapular) lymph node
Subclavicular (apical) lymph node
Subscapular (posterior) lymph node
	6 Lymphatic, Left Axillary
	See 5 Lymphatic, Right Axillary
	7 Lymphatic, Thorax
	Intercostal lymph node
	Mediastinal lymph node
	Parasternal lymph node
	Paratracheal lymph node
	Tracheobronchial lymph node
	8 Lymphatic, Internal Mammary, Right
	9 Lymphatic, Internal Mammary, Left
	B Lymphatic, Mesenteric
	Inferior mesenteric lymph node
	Pararectal lymph node
	Superior mesenteric lymph node
	C Lymphatic, Pelvis
	Common iliac (subaortic) lymph node
	Gluteal lymph node
	Iliac lymph node
	Inferior epigastric lymph node
	Obturator lymph node
	Sacral lymph node
	Subaortic (common iliac) lymph node
	Suprainguinal lymph node
	D Lymphatic, Aortic
	Celiac lymph node
	Gastric lymph node
	Hepatic lymph node
	Lumbar lymph node
	Pancreaticosplenic lymph node
	Paraaortic lymph node
	Retroperitoneal lymph node
	F Lymphatic, Right Lower Extremity
	Femoral lymph node
	Popliteal lymph node
	G Lymphatic, Left Lower Extremity
	See F Lymphatic, Right Lower Extremity
	H Lymphatic, Right Inguinal
	J Lymphatic, Left Inguinal
	K Thoracic Duct
	Left jugular trunk
	Left subclavian trunk
	L Cisterna Chyli
	Intestinal lymphatic trunk
	Lumbar lymphatic trunk
		Ø Open
		3 Percutaneous
		**4 Percutaneous
		    Endoscopic**
		**8 Via Natural or
		    Artificial Opening
		    Endoscopic**
			Ø Drainage Device	**Z No Qualifier**

Non-OR   Ø79[Ø,1,2,3,4,5,6,7,8,9,B,C,D,F,G,H,J,K,L][3,8]ØZ

Ø79 Continued on next page

Non-OR Procedure   DRG Non-OR Procedure   Valid OR Procedure   HAC Associated Procedure   Combination Only   New/Revised April   New/Revised October
286   ICD-10-PCS 2023

Ø79–Ø79

Ø79 Continued

Ø **Medical and Surgical**
7 **Lymphatic and Hemic Systems**
9 **Drainage** Definition: Taking or letting out fluids and/or gases from a body part
Explanation: The qualifier DIAGNOSTIC is used to identify drainage procedures that are biopsies

Body Part Character 4		Approach Character 5	Device Character 6	Qualifier Character 7
Ø **Lymphatic, Head** Buccinator lymph node Infraauricular lymph node Infraparotid lymph node Parotid lymph node Preauricular lymph node Submandibular lymph node Submaxillary lymph node Submental lymph node Subparotid lymph node Suprahyoid lymph node 1 **Lymphatic, Right Neck** Cervical lymph node Jugular lymph node Mastoid (postauricular) lymph node Occipital lymph node Postauricular (mastoid) lymph node Retropharyngeal lymph node Right jugular trunk Right lymphatic duct Right subclavian trunk Supraclavicular (Virchow's) lymph node Virchow's (supraclavicular) lymph node 2 **Lymphatic, Left Neck** Cervical lymph node Jugular lymph node Mastoid (postauricular) lymph node Occipital lymph node Postauricular (mastoid) lymph node Retropharyngeal lymph node Supraclavicular (Virchow's) lymph node Virchow's (supraclavicular) lymph node 3 **Lymphatic, Right Upper Extremity** Cubital lymph node Deltopectoral (infraclavicular) lymph node Epitrochlear lymph node Infraclavicular (deltopectoral) lymph node Supratrochlear lymph node 4 **Lymphatic, Left Upper Extremity** *See 3 Lymphatic, Right Upper Extremity* 5 **Lymphatic, Right Axillary** Anterior (pectoral) lymph node Apical (subclavicular) lymph node Brachial (lateral) lymph node Central axillary lymph node Lateral (brachial) lymph node Pectoral (anterior) lymph node Posterior (subscapular) lymph node Subclavicular (apical) lymph node Subscapular (posterior) lymph node	6 **Lymphatic, Left Axillary** *See 5 Lymphatic, Right Axillary* 7 **Lymphatic, Thorax** Intercostal lymph node Mediastinal lymph node Parasternal lymph node Paratracheal lymph node Tracheobronchial lymph node 8 **Lymphatic, Internal Mammary, Right** 9 **Lymphatic, Internal Mammary, Left** B **Lymphatic, Mesenteric** Inferior mesenteric lymph node Pararectal lymph node Superior mesenteric lymph node C **Lymphatic, Pelvis** Common iliac (subaortic) lymph node Gluteal lymph node Iliac lymph node Inferior epigastric lymph node Obturator lymph node Sacral lymph node Subaortic (common iliac) lymph node Suprainguinal lymph node D **Lymphatic, Aortic** Celiac lymph node Gastric lymph node Hepatic lymph node Lumbar lymph node Pancreaticosplenic lymph node Paraaortic lymph node Retroperitoneal lymph node F **Lymphatic, Right Lower Extremity** Femoral lymph node Popliteal lymph node G **Lymphatic, Left Lower Extremity** *See F Lymphatic, Right Lower Extremity* H **Lymphatic, Right Inguinal** J **Lymphatic, Left Inguinal** K **Thoracic Duct** Left jugular trunk Left subclavian trunk L **Cisterna Chyli** Intestinal lymphatic trunk Lumbar lymphatic trunk	Ø **Open** 3 **Percutaneous** 4 **Percutaneous Endoscopic** 8 **Via Natural or Artificial Opening Endoscopic**	Z **No Device**	X **Diagnostic** Z **No Qualifier**
M **Thymus** Thymus gland P **Spleen** Accessory spleen T **Bone Marrow**		Ø **Open** 3 **Percutaneous** 4 **Percutaneous Endoscopic**	Ø **Drainage Device**	Z **No Qualifier**
M **Thymus** Thymus gland P **Spleen** Accessory spleen T **Bone Marrow**		Ø **Open** 3 **Percutaneous** 4 **Percutaneous Endoscopic**	Z **No Device**	X **Diagnostic** Z **No Qualifier**

Non-OR	Ø79[Ø,1,2,3,4,5,6,7,8,9,B,C,D,F,G,H,J,K,L]8ZX
Non-OR	Ø79[Ø,1,2,3,4,5,6,7,8,9,B,C,D,F,G,H,J,K,L][3,8]ZZ
Non-OR	Ø79M3ØZ
Non-OR	Ø79P[3,4]ØZ
Non-OR	Ø79T[Ø,3,4]ØZ
Non-OR	Ø79M3ZZ
Non-OR	Ø79P[3,4]Z[X,Z]
Non-OR	Ø79T[Ø,3,4]Z[X,Z]

NC Noncovered Procedure LC Limited Coverage QA Questionable OB Admit NT New Tech Add-on ⊞ Combination Member ♂ Male ♀ Female

Lymphatic and Hemic Systems

0 Medical and Surgical
7 Lymphatic and Hemic Systems
B Excision   Definition: Cutting out or off, without replacement, a portion of a body part
       Explanation: The qualifier DIAGNOSTIC is used to identify excision procedures that are biopsies

Body Part Character 4		Approach Character 5	Device Character 6	Qualifier Character 7
0 Lymphatic, Head Buccinator lymph node Infraauricular lymph node Infraparotid lymph node Parotid lymph node Preauricular lymph node Submandibular lymph node Submaxillary lymph node Submental lymph node Subparotid lymph node Suprahyoid lymph node **1 Lymphatic, Right Neck** Cervical lymph node Jugular lymph node Mastoid (postauricular) lymph node Occipital lymph node Postauricular (mastoid) lymph node Retropharyngeal lymph node Right jugular trunk Right lymphatic duct Right subclavian trunk Supraclavicular (Virchow's) lymph node Virchow's (supraclavicular) lymph node **2 Lymphatic, Left Neck** Cervical lymph node Jugular lymph node Mastoid (postauricular) lymph node Occipital lymph node Postauricular (mastoid) lymph node Retropharyngeal lymph node Supraclavicular (Virchow's) lymph node Virchow's (supraclavicular) lymph node **3 Lymphatic, Right Upper Extremity** Cubital lymph node Deltopectoral (infraclavicular) lymph node Epitrochlear lymph node Infraclavicular (deltopectoral) lymph node Supratrochlear lymph node **4 Lymphatic, Left Upper Extremity** See 3 Lymphatic, Right Upper Extremity **5 Lymphatic, Right Axillary** Anterior (pectoral) lymph node Apical (subclavicular) lymph node Brachial (lateral) lymph node Central axillary lymph node Lateral (brachial) lymph node Pectoral (anterior) lymph node Posterior (subscapular) lymph node Subclavicular (apical) lymph node Subscapular (posterior) lymph node	**6 Lymphatic, Left Axillary** See 5 Lymphatic, Right Axillary **7 Lymphatic, Thorax** Intercostal lymph node Mediastinal lymph node Parasternal lymph node Paratracheal lymph node Tracheobronchial lymph node **8 Lymphatic, Internal Mammary, Right** **9 Lymphatic, Internal Mammary, Left** **B Lymphatic, Mesenteric** Inferior mesenteric lymph node Pararectal lymph node Superior mesenteric lymph node **C Lymphatic, Pelvis** Common iliac (subaortic) lymph node Gluteal lymph node Iliac lymph node Inferior epigastric lymph node Obturator lymph node Sacral lymph node Subaortic (common iliac) lymph node Suprainguinal lymph node **D Lymphatic, Aortic** Celiac lymph node Gastric lymph node Hepatic lymph node Lumbar lymph node Pancreaticosplenic lymph node Paraaortic lymph node Retroperitoneal lymph node **F Lymphatic, Right Lower Extremity** Femoral lymph node Popliteal lymph node **G Lymphatic, Left Lower Extremity** See F Lymphatic, Right Lower Extremity **H Lymphatic, Right Inguinal** ⊞ **J Lymphatic, Left Inguinal** ⊞ **K Thoracic Duct** Left jugular trunk Left subclavian trunk **L Cisterna Chyli** Intestinal lymphatic trunk Lumbar lymphatic trunk **M Thymus** Thymus gland **P Spleen** Accessory spleen	**0** Open **3** Percutaneous **4** Percutaneous Endoscopic	**Z** No Device	**X** Diagnostic **Z** No Qualifier

Non-OR 07BP[3,4]ZX

See Appendix L for Procedure Combinations
⊞ 07B[H,J][0,4]ZZ

0   **Medical and Surgical**
7   **Lymphatic and Hemic Systems**
C   **Extirpation**   Definition: Taking or cutting out solid matter from a body part

Explanation: The solid matter may be an abnormal byproduct of a biological function or a foreign body; it may be imbedded in a body part or in the lumen of a tubular body part. The solid matter may or may not have been previously broken into pieces.

Body Part Character 4		Approach Character 5	Device Character 6	Qualifier Character 7
0 Lymphatic, Head Buccinator lymph node Infraauricular lymph node Infraparotid lymph node Parotid lymph node Preauricular lymph node Submandibular lymph node Submaxillary lymph node Submental lymph node Subparotid lymph node Suprahyoid lymph node **1 Lymphatic, Right Neck** Cervical lymph node Jugular lymph node Mastoid (postauricular) lymph node Occipital lymph node Postauricular (mastoid) lymph node Retropharyngeal lymph node Right jugular trunk Right lymphatic duct Right subclavian trunk Supraclavicular (Virchow's) lymph node Virchow's (supraclavicular) lymph node **2 Lymphatic, Left Neck** Cervical lymph node Jugular lymph node Mastoid (postauricular) lymph node Occipital lymph node Postauricular (mastoid) lymph node Retropharyngeal lymph node Supraclavicular (Virchow's) lymph node Virchow's (supraclavicular) lymph node **3 Lymphatic, Right Upper Extremity** Cubital lymph node Deltopectoral (infraclavicular) lymph node Epitrochlear lymph node Infraclavicular (deltopectoral) lymph node Supratrochlear lymph node **4 Lymphatic, Left Upper Extremity** *See 3 Lymphatic, Right Upper Extremity* **5 Lymphatic, Right Axillary** Anterior (pectoral) lymph node Apical (subclavicular) lymph node Brachial (lateral) lymph node Central axillary lymph node Lateral (brachial) lymph node Pectoral (anterior) lymph node Posterior (subscapular) lymph node Subclavicular (apical) lymph node Subscapular (posterior) lymph node	**6 Lymphatic, Left Axillary** *See 5 Lymphatic, Right Axillary* **7 Lymphatic, Thorax** Intercostal lymph node Mediastinal lymph node Parasternal lymph node Paratracheal lymph node Tracheobronchial lymph node **8 Lymphatic, Internal Mammary, Right** **9 Lymphatic, Internal Mammary, Left** **B Lymphatic, Mesenteric** Inferior mesenteric lymph node Pararectal lymph node Superior mesenteric lymph node **C Lymphatic, Pelvis** Common iliac (subaortic) lymph node Gluteal lymph node Iliac lymph node Inferior epigastric lymph node Obturator lymph node Sacral lymph node Subaortic (common iliac) lymph node Suprainguinal lymph node **D Lymphatic, Aortic** Celiac lymph node Gastric lymph node Hepatic lymph node Lumbar lymph node Pancreaticosplenic lymph node Paraaortic lymph node Retroperitoneal lymph node **F Lymphatic, Right Lower Extremity** Femoral lymph node Popliteal lymph node **G Lymphatic, Left Lower Extremity** *See F Lymphatic, Right Lower Extremity* **H Lymphatic, Right Inguinal** **J Lymphatic, Left Inguinal** **K Thoracic Duct** Left jugular trunk Left subclavian trunk **L Cisterna Chyli** Intestinal lymphatic trunk Lumbar lymphatic trunk **M Thymus** Thymus gland **P Spleen** Accessory spleen	**0 Open** **3 Percutaneous** **4 Percutaneous Endoscopic**	**Z No Device**	**Z No Qualifier**

Non-OR   07CP[3,4]ZZ

NC Noncovered Procedure   **LC** Limited Coverage   **QA** Questionable OB Admit   **NT** New Tech Add-on   ⊞ Combination Member   ♂ Male   ♀ Female

ICD-10-PCS 2023   289

Lymphatic and Hemic Systems

Ø   **Medical and Surgical**
7   **Lymphatic and Hemic Systems**
D   **Extraction**   Definition: Pulling or stripping out or off all or a portion of a body part by the use of force

Explanation: The qualifier DIAGNOSTIC is used to identify extraction procedures that are biopsies

Body Part Character 4		Approach Character 5	Device Character 6	Qualifier Character 7
Ø Lymphatic, Head Buccinator lymph node Infraauricular lymph node Infraparotid lymph node Parotid lymph node Preauricular lymph node Submandibular lymph node Submaxillary lymph node Submental lymph node Subparotid lymph node Suprahyoid lymph node **1 Lymphatic, Right Neck** Cervical lymph node Jugular lymph node Mastoid (postauricular) lymph node Occipital lymph node Postauricular (mastoid) lymph node Retropharyngeal lymph node Right jugular trunk Right lymphatic duct Right subclavian trunk Supraclavicular (Virchow's) lymph node Virchow's (supraclavicular) lymph node **2 Lymphatic, Left Neck** Cervical lymph node Jugular lymph node Mastoid (postauricular) lymph node Occipital lymph node Postauricular (mastoid) lymph node Retropharyngeal lymph node Supraclavicular (Virchow's) lymph node Virchow's (supraclavicular) lymph node **3 Lymphatic, Right Upper Extremity** Cubital lymph node Deltopectoral (infraclavicular) lymph node Epitrochlear lymph node Infraclavicular (deltopectoral) lymph node Supratrochlear lymph node **4 Lymphatic, Left Upper Extremity** *See 3 Lymphatic, Right Upper Extremity* **5 Lymphatic, Right Axillary** Anterior (pectoral) lymph node Apical (subclavicular) lymph node Brachial (lateral) lymph node Central axillary lymph node Lateral (brachial) lymph node Pectoral (anterior) lymph node Posterior (subscapular) lymph node Subclavicular (apical) lymph node Subscapular (posterior) lymph node	**6 Lymphatic, Left Axillary** *See 5 Lymphatic, Right Axillary* **7 Lymphatic, Thorax** Intercostal lymph node Mediastinal lymph node Parasternal lymph node Paratracheal lymph node Tracheobronchial lymph node **8 Lymphatic, Internal Mammary, Right** **9 Lymphatic, Internal Mammary, Left** **B Lymphatic, Mesenteric** Inferior mesenteric lymph node Pararectal lymph node Superior mesenteric lymph node **C Lymphatic, Pelvis** Common iliac (subaortic) lymph node Gluteal lymph node Iliac lymph node Inferior epigastric lymph node Obturator lymph node Sacral lymph node Subaortic (common iliac) lymph node Suprainguinal lymph node **D Lymphatic, Aortic** Celiac lymph node Gastric lymph node Hepatic lymph node Lumbar lymph node Pancreaticosplenic lymph node Paraaortic lymph node Retroperitoneal lymph node **F Lymphatic, Right Lower Extremity** Femoral lymph node Popliteal lymph node **G Lymphatic, Left Lower Extremity** *See F Lymphatic, Right Lower Extremity* **H Lymphatic, Right Inguinal** **J Lymphatic, Left Inguinal** **K Thoracic Duct** Left jugular trunk Left subclavian trunk **L Cisterna Chyli** Intestinal lymphatic trunk Lumbar lymphatic trunk	**3 Percutaneous** **4 Percutaneous Endoscopic** **8 Via Natural or Artificial Opening Endoscopic**	**Z No Device**	**X Diagnostic**
M Thymus Thymus gland **P Spleen** Accessory spleen		**3 Percutaneous** **4 Percutaneous Endoscopic**	**Z No Device**	**X Diagnostic**
Q Bone Marrow, Sternum **R Bone Marrow, Iliac** **S Bone Marrow, Vertebral** **T Bone Marrow**		**Ø Open** **3 Percutaneous**	**Z No Device**	**X Diagnostic** **Z No Qualifier**

Non-OR   All body part, approach, device, and qualifier values

Non-OR Procedure   DRG Non-OR Procedure   Valid OR Procedure   HAC Associated Procedure   Combination Only   New/Revised April   New/Revised October

Ø   **Medical and Surgical**
7   **Lymphatic and Hemic Systems**
H   **Insertion**   Definition: Putting in a nonbiological appliance that monitors, assists, performs, or prevents a physiological function but does not physically take the place of a body part
                            Explanation: None

Body Part Character 4	Approach Character 5	Device Character 6	Qualifier Character 7

K Thoracic Duct
    Left jugular trunk
    Left subclavian trunk
L Cisterna Chyli
    Intestinal lymphatic trunk
    Lumbar lymphatic trunk
M Thymus
    Thymus gland
N Lymphatic
P Spleen
    Accessory spleen
T Bone Marrow
	Ø Open
	3 Percutaneous
	4 Percutaneous Endoscopic
		1 Radioactive Element
		3 Infusion Device
		Y Other Device
			Z No Qualifier

Non-OR	Ø7H[K,L,M,N,P][Ø,4]3Z
Non-OR	Ø7H[K,L,M,N,P,T]3[1,3,Y]Z
Non-OR	Ø7H[N,P]4YZ
Non-OR	Ø7HT[Ø,4][1,3,Y]Z

Ø   **Medical and Surgical**
7   **Lymphatic and Hemic Systems**
J   **Inspection**   Definition: Visually and/or manually exploring a body part
                            Explanation: Visual exploration may be performed with or without optical instrumentation. Manual exploration may be performed directly or through intervening body layers.

Body Part Character 4	Approach Character 5	Device Character 6	Qualifier Character 7

K Thoracic Duct
    Left jugular trunk
    Left subclavian trunk
L Cisterna Chyli
    Intestinal lymphatic trunk
    Lumbar lymphatic trunk
M Thymus
    Thymus gland
T Bone Marrow
	Ø Open
	3 Percutaneous
	4 Percutaneous Endoscopic
		Z No Device	**Z** No Qualifier

N Lymphatic	**Ø** Open **3** Percutaneous **4** Percutaneous Endoscopic **8** Via Natural or Artificial Opening Endoscopic **X** External	**Z** No Device	**Z** No Qualifier
P Spleen Accessory spleen	**Ø** Open **3** Percutaneous **4** Percutaneous Endoscopic **X** External	**Z** No Device	**Z** No Qualifier

Non-OR	Ø7J[K,L,M]3ZZ
Non-OR	Ø7JT[Ø,3,4]ZZ
Non-OR	Ø7JN[3,8,X]ZZ
Non-OR	Ø7JP[3,4,X]ZZ

Lymphatic and Hemic Systems

0   **Medical and Surgical**
7   **Lymphatic and Hemic Systems**
L   **Occlusion**   Definition: Completely closing an orifice or the lumen of a tubular body part
                       Explanation: The orifice can be a natural orifice or an artificially created orifice

Body Part Character 4		Approach Character 5	Device Character 6	Qualifier Character 7

0 Lymphatic, Head
Buccinator lymph node
Infraauricular lymph node
Infraparotid lymph node
Parotid lymph node
Preauricular lymph node
Submandibular lymph node
Submaxillary lymph node
Submental lymph node
Subparotid lymph node
Suprahyoid lymph node
1 Lymphatic, Right Neck
Cervical lymph node
Jugular lymph node
Mastoid (postauricular) lymph node
Occipital lymph node
Postauricular (mastoid) lymph node
Retropharyngeal lymph node
Right jugular trunk
Right lymphatic duct
Right subclavian trunk
Supraclavicular (Virchow's) lymph
   node
Virchow's (supraclavicular) lymph
   node
2 Lymphatic, Left Neck
Cervical lymph node
Jugular lymph node
Mastoid (postauricular) lymph node
Occipital lymph node
Postauricular (mastoid) lymph node
Retropharyngeal lymph node
Supraclavicular (Virchow's) lymph
   node
Virchow's (supraclavicular) lymph
   node
3 Lymphatic, Right Upper Extremity
Cubital lymph node
Deltopectoral (infraclavicular) lymph
   node
Epitrochlear lymph node
Infraclavicular (deltopectoral) lymph
   node
Supratrochlear lymph node
4 Lymphatic, Left Upper Extremity
See 3 Lymphatic, Right Upper Extremity
5 Lymphatic, Right Axillary
Anterior (pectoral) lymph node
Apical (subclavicular) lymph node
Brachial (lateral) lymph node
Central axillary lymph node
Lateral (brachial) lymph node
Pectoral (anterior) lymph node
Posterior (subscapular) lymph node
Subclavicular (apical) lymph node
Subscapular (posterior) lymph node
	6 Lymphatic, Left Axillary
	See 5 Lymphatic, Right Axillary
	7 Lymphatic, Thorax
	Intercostal lymph node
	Mediastinal lymph node
	Parasternal lymph node
	Paratracheal lymph node
	Tracheobronchial lymph node
	8 Lymphatic, Internal Mammary, Right
	9 Lymphatic, Internal Mammary, Left
	B Lymphatic, Mesenteric
	Inferior mesenteric lymph node
	Pararectal lymph node
	Superior mesenteric lymph node
	C Lymphatic, Pelvis
	Common iliac (subaortic) lymph node
	Gluteal lymph node
	Iliac lymph node
	Inferior epigastric lymph node
	Obturator lymph node
	Sacral lymph node
	Subaortic (common iliac) lymph node
	Suprainguinal lymph node
	D Lymphatic, Aortic
	Celiac lymph node
	Gastric lymph node
	Hepatic lymph node
	Lumbar lymph node
	Pancreaticosplenic lymph node
	Paraaortic lymph node
	Retroperitoneal lymph node
	F Lymphatic, Right Lower Extremity
	Femoral lymph node
	Popliteal lymph node
	G Lymphatic, Left Lower Extremity
	See F Lymphatic, Right Lower Extremity
	H Lymphatic, Right Inguinal
	J Lymphatic, Left Inguinal
	K Thoracic Duct
	Left jugular trunk
	Left subclavian trunk
	L Cisterna Chyli
	Intestinal lymphatic trunk
	Lumbar lymphatic trunk
		0 Open
		3 Percutaneous
		**4 Percutaneous
		   Endoscopic**
			C Extraluminal Device
			D Intraluminal Device
			Z No Device
				Z No Qualifier

Non-OR Procedure   DRG Non-OR Procedure   Valid OR Procedure   HAC Associated Procedure   Combination Only   New/Revised April   New/Revised October

292   ICD-10-PCS 2023

Ø   **Medical and Surgical**
7   **Lymphatic and Hemic Systems**
N   **Release**   Definition: Freeing a body part from an abnormal physical constraint by cutting or by the use of force
                     Explanation: Some of the restraining tissue may be taken out but none of the body part is taken out

Body Part Character 4		Approach Character 5	Device Character 6	Qualifier Character 7

Ø **Lymphatic, Head**
    Buccinator lymph node
    Infraauricular lymph node
    Infraparotid lymph node
    Parotid lymph node
    Preauricular lymph node
    Submandibular lymph node
    Submaxillary lymph node
    Submental lymph node
    Subparotid lymph node
    Suprahyoid lymph node
1 **Lymphatic, Right Neck**
    Cervical lymph node
    Jugular lymph node
    Mastoid (postauricular) lymph node
    Occipital lymph node
    Postauricular (mastoid) lymph node
    Retropharyngeal lymph node
    Right jugular trunk
    Right lymphatic duct
    Right subclavian trunk
    Supraclavicular (Virchow's) lymph
      node
    Virchow's (supraclavicular) lymph
      node
2 **Lymphatic, Left Neck**
    Cervical lymph node
    Jugular lymph node
    Mastoid (postauricular) lymph node
    Occipital lymph node
    Postauricular (mastoid) lymph node
    Retropharyngeal lymph node
    Supraclavicular (Virchow's) lymph
      node
    Virchow's (supraclavicular) lymph
      node
3 **Lymphatic, Right Upper Extremity**
    Cubital lymph node
    Deltopectoral (infraclavicular) lymph
      node
    Epitrochlear lymph node
    Infraclavicular (deltopectoral) lymph
      node
    Supratrochlear lymph node
4 **Lymphatic, Left Upper Extremity**
    See 3 Lymphatic, Right Upper Extremity
5 **Lymphatic, Right Axillary**
    Anterior (pectoral) lymph node
    Apical (subclavicular) lymph node
    Brachial (lateral) lymph node
    Central axillary lymph node
    Lateral (brachial) lymph node
    Pectoral (anterior) lymph node
    Posterior (subscapular) lymph node
    Subclavicular (apical) lymph node
    Subscapular (posterior) lymph node
	6 **Lymphatic, Left Axillary**
	    See 5 Lymphatic, Right Axillary
	7 **Lymphatic, Thorax**
	    Intercostal lymph node
	    Mediastinal lymph node
	    Parasternal lymph node
	    Paratracheal lymph node
	    Tracheobronchial lymph node
	8 **Lymphatic, Internal Mammary, Right**
	9 **Lymphatic, Internal Mammary, Left**
	B **Lymphatic, Mesenteric**
	    Inferior mesenteric lymph node
	    Pararectal lymph node
	    Superior mesenteric lymph node
	C **Lymphatic, Pelvis**
	    Common iliac (subaortic) lymph node
	    Gluteal lymph node
	    Iliac lymph node
	    Inferior epigastric lymph node
	    Obturator lymph node
	    Sacral lymph node
	    Subaortic (common iliac) lymph node
	    Suprainguinal lymph node
	D **Lymphatic, Aortic**
	    Celiac lymph node
	    Gastric lymph node
	    Hepatic lymph node
	    Lumbar lymph node
	    Pancreaticosplenic lymph node
	    Paraaortic lymph node
	    Retroperitoneal lymph node
	F **Lymphatic, Right Lower Extremity**
	    Femoral lymph node
	    Popliteal lymph node
	G **Lymphatic, Left Lower Extremity**
	    See F Lymphatic, Right Lower Extremity
	H **Lymphatic, Right Inguinal**
	J **Lymphatic, Left Inguinal**
	K **Thoracic Duct**
	    Left jugular trunk
	    Left subclavian trunk
	L **Cisterna Chyli**
	    Intestinal lymphatic trunk
	    Lumbar lymphatic trunk
	M **Thymus**
	    Thymus gland
	P **Spleen**
	    Accessory spleen
		Ø Open
		3 Percutaneous
		4 Percutaneous
		    Endoscopic
			Z No Device	**Z** No Qualifier

NC Noncovered Procedure   **LC** Limited Coverage   **QA** Questionable OB Admit   **NT** New Tech Add-on   ⊞ Combination Member   ♂ Male   ♀ Female

ICD-10-PCS 2023   **293**

0 **Medical and Surgical**
7 **Lymphatic and Hemic Systems**
P **Removal**

Definition: Taking out or off a device from a body part

Explanation: If a device is taken out and a similar device put in without cutting or puncturing the skin or mucous membrane, the procedure is coded to the root operation CHANGE. Otherwise, the procedure for taking out a device is coded to the root operation REMOVAL.

Body Part Character 4		Approach Character 5	Device Character 6	Qualifier Character 7
K Thoracic Duct Left jugular trunk Left subclavian trunk **L** Cisterna Chyli Intestinal lymphatic trunk Lumbar lymphatic trunk **N** Lymphatic		**0** Open **3** Percutaneous **4** Percutaneous Endoscopic	**0** Drainage Device **3** Infusion Device **7** Autologous Tissue Substitute **C** Extraluminal Device **D** Intraluminal Device **J** Synthetic Substitute **K** Nonautologous Tissue Substitute **Y** Other Device	**Z** No Qualifier
K Thoracic Duct Left jugular trunk Left subclavian trunk **L** Cisterna Chyli Intestinal lymphatic trunk Lumbar lymphatic trunk **N** Lymphatic		**X** External	**0** Drainage Device **3** Infusion Device **D** Intraluminal Device	**Z** No Qualifier
M Thymus Thymus gland **P** Spleen Accessory spleen		**0** Open **3** Percutaneous **4** Percutaneous Endoscopic	**0** Drainage Device **3** Infusion Device **Y** Other Device	**Z** No Qualifier
M Thymus Thymus gland **P** Spleen Accessory spleen		**X** External	**0** Drainage Device **3** Infusion Device	**Z** No Qualifier
T Bone Marrow		**0** Open **3** Percutaneous **4** Percutaneous Endoscopic **X** External	**0** Drainage Device	**Z** No Qualifier

Non-OR	07P[K,L,N][3,4]YZ
Non-OR	07P[K,L,N]X[0,3,D]Z
Non-OR	07P[M,P][3,4]YZ
Non-OR	07P[M,P]X[0,3]Z
Non-OR	07PT[0,3,4,X]0Z

Non-OR Procedure   DRG Non-OR Procedure   Valid OR Procedure   HAC Associated Procedure   Combination Only   New/Revised April   New/Revised October

294   ICD-10-PCS 2023

Ø **Medical and Surgical**
7 **Lymphatic and Hemic Systems**
Q **Repair**   Definition: Restoring, to the extent possible, a body part to its normal anatomic structure and function
Explanation: Used only when the method to accomplish the repair is not one of the other root operations

Body Part Character 4		Approach Character 5	Device Character 6	Qualifier Character 7

Ø **Lymphatic, Head**
   Buccinator lymph node
   Infraauricular lymph node
   Infraparotid lymph node
   Parotid lymph node
   Preauricular lymph node
   Submandibular lymph node
   Submaxillary lymph node
   Submental lymph node
   Subparotid lymph node
   Suprahyoid lymph node
1 **Lymphatic, Right Neck**
   Cervical lymph node
   Jugular lymph node
   Mastoid (postauricular) lymph node
   Occipital lymph node
   Postauricular (mastoid) lymph node
   Retropharyngeal lymph node
   Right jugular trunk
   Right lymphatic duct
   Right subclavian trunk
   Supraclavicular (Virchow's) lymph
     node
   Virchow's (supraclavicular) lymph
     node
2 **Lymphatic, Left Neck**
   Cervical lymph node
   Jugular lymph node
   Mastoid (postauricular) lymph node
   Occipital lymph node
   Postauricular (mastoid) lymph node
   Retropharyngeal lymph node
   Supraclavicular (Virchow's) lymph
     node
   Virchow's (supraclavicular) lymph
     node
3 **Lymphatic, Right Upper Extremity**
   Cubital lymph node
   Deltopectoral (infraclavicular) lymph
     node
   Epitrochlear lymph node
   Infraclavicular (deltopectoral) lymph
     node
   Supratrochlear lymph node
4 **Lymphatic, Left Upper Extremity**
   See 3 Lymphatic, Right Upper Extremity
5 **Lymphatic, Right Axillary**
   Anterior (pectoral) lymph node
   Apical (subclavicular) lymph node
   Brachial (lateral) lymph node
   Central axillary lymph node
   Lateral (brachial) lymph node
   Pectoral (anterior) lymph node
   Posterior (subscapular) lymph node
   Subclavicular (apical) lymph node
   Subscapular (posterior) lymph node
	6 **Lymphatic, Left Axillary**
	   See 5 Lymphatic, Right Axillary
	7 **Lymphatic, Thorax**
	   Intercostal lymph node
	   Mediastinal lymph node
	   Parasternal lymph node
	   Paratracheal lymph node
	   Tracheobronchial lymph node
	8 **Lymphatic, Internal Mammary, Right**
	9 **Lymphatic, Internal Mammary, Left**
	B **Lymphatic, Mesenteric**
	   Inferior mesenteric lymph node
	   Pararectal lymph node
	   Superior mesenteric lymph node
	C **Lymphatic, Pelvis**
	   Common iliac (subaortic) lymph node
	   Gluteal lymph node
	   Iliac lymph node
	   Inferior epigastric lymph node
	   Obturator lymph node
	   Sacral lymph node
	   Subaortic (common iliac) lymph node
	   Suprainguinal lymph node
	D **Lymphatic, Aortic**
	   Celiac lymph node
	   Gastric lymph node
	   Hepatic lymph node
	   Lumbar lymph node
	   Pancreaticosplenic lymph node
	   Paraaortic lymph node
	   Retroperitoneal lymph node
	F **Lymphatic, Right Lower Extremity**
	   Femoral lymph node
	   Popliteal lymph node
	G **Lymphatic, Left Lower Extremity**
	   See F Lymphatic, Right Lower Extremity
	H **Lymphatic, Right Inguinal**
	J **Lymphatic, Left Inguinal**
	K **Thoracic Duct**
	   Left jugular trunk
	   Left subclavian trunk
	L **Cisterna Chyli**
	   Intestinal lymphatic trunk
	   Lumbar lymphatic trunk
		Ø **Open**
		3 **Percutaneous**
		4 **Percutaneous**
		   Endoscopic
		8 **Via Natural or**
		   Artificial Opening
		   Endoscopic
			Z No Device	Z No Qualifier

M **Thymus**
   Thymus gland
P **Spleen**
   Accessory spleen
		Ø **Open**
		3 **Percutaneous**
		4 **Percutaneous**
		   Endoscopic
			Z No Device	Z No Qualifier

Ø   Medical and Surgical
7   Lymphatic and Hemic Systems
S   Reposition   Definition: Moving to its normal location, or other suitable location, all or a portion of a body part

Explanation: The body part is moved to a new location from an abnormal location, or from a normal location where it is not functioning correctly. The body part may or may not be cut out or off to be moved to the new location.

Body Part Character 4	Approach Character 5	Device Character 6	Qualifier Character 7
M Thymus Thymus gland **P** Spleen Accessory spleen	**Ø** Open	**Z** No Device	**Z** No Qualifier

Ø   Medical and Surgical
7   Lymphatic and Hemic Systems
T   Resection   Definition: Cutting out or off, without replacement, all of a body part

Explanation: None

Body Part Character 4	Approach Character 5	Device Character 6	Qualifier Character 7
Ø Lymphatic, Head Buccinator lymph node Infraauricular lymph node Infraparotid lymph node Parotid lymph node Preauricular lymph node Submandibular lymph node Submaxillary lymph node Submental lymph node Subparotid lymph node Suprahyoid lymph node **1** Lymphatic, Right Neck Cervical lymph node Jugular lymph node Mastoid (postauricular) lymph node Occipital lymph node Postauricular (mastoid) lymph node Retropharyngeal lymph node Right jugular trunk Right lymphatic duct Right subclavian trunk Supraclavicular (Virchow's) lymph node Virchow's (supraclavicular) lymph node **2** Lymphatic, Left Neck Cervical lymph node Jugular lymph node Mastoid (postauricular) lymph node Occipital lymph node Postauricular (mastoid) lymph node Retropharyngeal lymph node Supraclavicular (Virchow's) lymph node Virchow's (supraclavicular) lymph node **3** Lymphatic, Right Upper Extremity Cubital lymph node Deltopectoral (infraclavicular) lymph node Epitrochlear lymph node Infraclavicular (deltopectoral) lymph node Supratrochlear lymph node **4** Lymphatic, Left Upper Extremity *See 3 Lymphatic, Right Upper Extremity* **5** Lymphatic, Right Axillary ⊞ Anterior (pectoral) lymph node Apical (subclavicular) lymph node Brachial (lateral) lymph node Central axillary lymph node Lateral (brachial) lymph node Pectoral (anterior) lymph node Posterior (subscapular) lymph node Subclavicular (apical) lymph node Subscapular (posterior) lymph node **6** Lymphatic, Left Axillary ⊞ *See 5 Lymphatic, Right Axillary* **7** Lymphatic, Thorax ⊞ Intercostal lymph node Mediastinal lymph node Parasternal lymph node Paratracheal lymph node Tracheobronchial lymph node **8** Lymphatic, Internal ⊞ Mammary, Right **9** Lymphatic, Internal ⊞ Mammary, Left **B** Lymphatic, Mesenteric Inferior mesenteric lymph node Pararectal lymph node Superior mesenteric lymph node **C** Lymphatic, Pelvis Common iliac (subaortic) lymph node Gluteal lymph node Iliac lymph node Inferior epigastric lymph node Obturator lymph node Sacral lymph node Subaortic (common iliac) lymph node Suprainguinal lymph node **D** Lymphatic, Aortic Celiac lymph node Gastric lymph node Hepatic lymph node Lumbar lymph node Pancreaticosplenic lymph node Paraaortic lymph node Retroperitoneal lymph node **F** Lymphatic, Right Lower Extremity Femoral lymph node Popliteal lymph node **G** Lymphatic, Left Lower Extremity *See F Lymphatic, Right Lower Extremity* **H** Lymphatic, Right Inguinal **J** Lymphatic, Left Inguinal **K** Thoracic Duct Left jugular trunk Left subclavian trunk **L** Cisterna Chyli Intestinal lymphatic trunk Lumbar lymphatic trunk **M** Thymus Thymus gland **P** Spleen Accessory spleen	**Ø** Open **4** Percutaneous Endoscopic	**Z** No Device	**Z** No Qualifier

See Appendix L for Procedure Combinations
⊞   Ø7T[5,6,7,8,9]ØZZ

Ø   **Medical and Surgical**
7   **Lymphatic and Hemic Systems**
U   **Supplement**   Definition: Putting in or on biological or synthetic material that physically reinforces and/or augments the function of a portion of a body part

                              Explanation: The biological material is non-living, or is living and from the same individual. The body part may have been previously replaced, and the SUPPLEMENT procedure is performed to physically reinforce and/or augment the function of the replaced body part.

Body Part Character 4		Approach Character 5	Device Character 6	Qualifier Character 7

Ø   **Lymphatic, Head**
    Buccinator lymph node
    Infraauricular lymph node
    Infraparotid lymph node
    Parotid lymph node
    Preauricular lymph node
    Submandibular lymph node
    Submaxillary lymph node
    Submental lymph node
    Subparotid lymph node
    Suprahyoid lymph node
1   **Lymphatic, Right Neck**
    Cervical lymph node
    Jugular lymph node
    Mastoid (postauricular) lymph node
    Occipital lymph node
    Postauricular (mastoid) lymph node
    Retropharyngeal lymph node
    Right jugular trunk
    Right lymphatic duct
    Right subclavian trunk
    Supraclavicular (Virchow's) lymph
       node
    Virchow's (supraclavicular) lymph
       node
2   **Lymphatic, Left Neck**
    Cervical lymph node
    Jugular lymph node
    Mastoid (postauricular) lymph node
    Occipital lymph node
    Postauricular (mastoid) lymph node
    Retropharyngeal lymph node
    Supraclavicular (Virchow's) lymph
       node
    Virchow's (supraclavicular) lymph
       node
3   **Lymphatic, Right Upper Extremity**
    Cubital lymph node
    Deltopectoral (infraclavicular) lymph
       node
    Epitrochlear lymph node
    Infraclavicular (deltopectoral) lymph
       node
    Supratrochlear lymph node
4   **Lymphatic, Left Upper Extremity**
    See 3 Lymphatic, Right Upper Extremity
5   **Lymphatic, Right Axillary**
    Anterior (pectoral) lymph node
    Apical (subclavicular) lymph node
    Brachial (lateral) lymph node
    Central axillary lymph node
    Lateral (brachial) lymph node
    Pectoral (anterior) lymph node
    Posterior (subscapular) lymph node
    Subclavicular (apical) lymph node
    Subscapular (posterior) lymph node
	6 **Lymphatic, Left Axillary**
	    See 5 Lymphatic, Right Axillary
	7 **Lymphatic, Thorax**
	    Intercostal lymph node
	    Mediastinal lymph node
	    Parasternal lymph node
	    Paratracheal lymph node
	    Tracheobronchial lymph node
	8 **Lymphatic, Internal Mammary, Right**
	9 **Lymphatic, Internal Mammary, Left**
	B **Lymphatic, Mesenteric**
	    Inferior mesenteric lymph node
	    Pararectal lymph node
	    Superior mesenteric lymph node
	C **Lymphatic, Pelvis**
	    Common iliac (subaortic) lymph node
	    Gluteal lymph node
	    Iliac lymph node
	    Inferior epigastric lymph node
	    Obturator lymph node
	    Sacral lymph node
	    Subaortic (common iliac) lymph node
	    Suprainguinal lymph node
	D **Lymphatic, Aortic**
	    Celiac lymph node
	    Gastric lymph node
	    Hepatic lymph node
	    Lumbar lymph node
	    Pancreaticosplenic lymph node
	    Paraaortic lymph node
	    Retroperitoneal lymph node
	F **Lymphatic, Right Lower Extremity**
	    Femoral lymph node
	    Popliteal lymph node
	G **Lymphatic, Left Lower Extremity**
	    See F Lymphatic, Right Lower Extremity
	H **Lymphatic, Right Inguinal**
	J **Lymphatic, Left Inguinal**
	K **Thoracic Duct**
	    Left jugular trunk
	    Left subclavian trunk
	L **Cisterna Chyli**
	    Intestinal lymphatic trunk
	    Lumbar lymphatic trunk
		Ø Open
		4 Percutaneous
		    Endoscopic
			7 Autologous Tissue
			    Substitute
			J Synthetic Substitute
			K Nonautologous
			    Tissue Substitute
				Z No Qualifier

Ø **Medical and Surgical**
7 **Lymphatic and Hemic Systems**
V **Restriction**   Definition: Partially closing an orifice or the lumen of a tubular body part
                      Explanation: The orifice can be a natural orifice or an artificially created orifice

Body Part Character 4		Approach Character 5	Device Character 6	Qualifier Character 7

Ø **Lymphatic, Head**
Buccinator lymph node
Infraauricular lymph node
Infraparotid lymph node
Parotid lymph node
Preauricular lymph node
Submandibular lymph node
Submaxillary lymph node
Submental lymph node
Subparotid lymph node
Suprahyoid lymph node
1 **Lymphatic, Right Neck**
Cervical lymph node
Jugular lymph node
Mastoid (postauricular) lymph node
Occipital lymph node
Postauricular (mastoid) lymph node
Retropharyngeal lymph node
Right jugular trunk
Right lymphatic duct
Right subclavian trunk
Supraclavicular (Virchow's) lymph
   node
Virchow's (supraclavicular) lymph
   node
2 **Lymphatic, Left Neck**
Cervical lymph node
Jugular lymph node
Mastoid (postauricular) lymph node
Occipital lymph node
Postauricular (mastoid) lymph node
Retropharyngeal lymph node
Supraclavicular (Virchow's) lymph
   node
Virchow's (supraclavicular) lymph
   node
3 **Lymphatic, Right Upper Extremity**
Cubital lymph node
Deltopectoral (infraclavicular) lymph
   node
Epitrochlear lymph node
Infraclavicular (deltopectoral) lymph
   node
Supratrochlear lymph node
4 **Lymphatic, Left Upper Extremity**
See 3 Lymphatic, Right Upper Extremity
5 **Lymphatic, Right Axillary**
Anterior (pectoral) lymph node
Apical (subclavicular) lymph node
Brachial (lateral) lymph node
Central axillary lymph node
Lateral (brachial) lymph node
Pectoral (anterior) lymph node
Posterior (subscapular) lymph node
Subclavicular (apical) lymph node
Subscapular (posterior) lymph node
	6 **Lymphatic, Left Axillary**
	See 5 Lymphatic, Right Axillary
	7 **Lymphatic, Thorax**
	Intercostal lymph node
	Mediastinal lymph node
	Parasternal lymph node
	Paratracheal lymph node
	Tracheobronchial lymph node
	8 **Lymphatic, Internal Mammary, Right**
	9 **Lymphatic, Internal Mammary, Left**
	B **Lymphatic, Mesenteric**
	Inferior mesenteric lymph node
	Pararectal lymph node
	Superior mesenteric lymph node
	C **Lymphatic, Pelvis**
	Common iliac (subaortic) lymph node
	Gluteal lymph node
	Iliac lymph node
	Inferior epigastric lymph node
	Obturator lymph node
	Sacral lymph node
	Subaortic (common iliac) lymph node
	Suprainguinal lymph node
	D **Lymphatic, Aortic**
	Celiac lymph node
	Gastric lymph node
	Hepatic lymph node
	Lumbar lymph node
	Pancreaticosplenic lymph node
	Paraaortic lymph node
	Retroperitoneal lymph node
	F **Lymphatic, Right Lower Extremity**
	Femoral lymph node
	Popliteal lymph node
	G **Lymphatic, Left Lower Extremity**
	See F Lymphatic, Right Lower Extremity
	H **Lymphatic, Right Inguinal**
	J **Lymphatic, Left Inguinal**
	K **Thoracic Duct**
	Left jugular trunk
	Left subclavian trunk
	L **Cisterna Chyli**
	Intestinal lymphatic trunk
	Lumbar lymphatic trunk
		Ø **Open**
		3 **Percutaneous**
		4 **Percutaneous Endoscopic**
			C **Extraluminal Device**
			D **Intraluminal Device**
			Z **No Device**
				Z **No Qualifier**

0   Medical and Surgical
7   Lymphatic and Hemic Systems
W   Revision   Definition: Correcting, to the extent possible, a portion of a malfunctioning device or the position of a displaced device

Explanation: Revision can include correcting a malfunctioning or displaced device by taking out or putting in components of the device such as a screw or pin

Body Part Character 4	Approach Character 5	Device Character 6	Qualifier Character 7

K Thoracic Duct
   Left jugular trunk
   Left subclavian trunk
L Cisterna Chyli
   Intestinal lymphatic trunk
   Lumbar lymphatic trunk
N Lymphatic
	0 Open
	3 Percutaneous
	4 Percutaneous Endoscopic
		0 Drainage Device
		3 Infusion Device
		7 Autologous Tissue
		   Substitute
		C Extraluminal Device
		D Intraluminal Device
		J Synthetic Substitute
		K Nonautologous Tissue
		   Substitute
		Y Other Device
			Z No Qualifier

K Thoracic Duct
   Left jugular trunk
   Left subclavian trunk
L Cisterna Chyli
   Intestinal lymphatic trunk
   Lumbar lymphatic trunk
N Lymphatic
	X External	0 Drainage Device
		3 Infusion Device
		7 Autologous Tissue
		   Substitute
		C Extraluminal Device
		D Intraluminal Device
		J Synthetic Substitute
		K Nonautologous Tissue
		   Substitute
			Z No Qualifier

M Thymus
   Thymus gland
P Spleen
   Accessory spleen
	0 Open
	3 Percutaneous
	4 Percutaneous Endoscopic
		0 Drainage Device
		3 Infusion Device
		Y Other Device
			Z No Qualifier

M Thymus
   Thymus gland
P Spleen
   Accessory spleen
	X External	0 Drainage Device
		3 Infusion Device
			Z No Qualifier

T Bone Marrow	0 Open 3 Percutaneous 4 Percutaneous Endoscopic X External	0 Drainage Device	Z No Qualifier

Non-OR	07W[K,L,N][3,4]YZ
Non-OR	07W[K,L,N]X[0,3,7,C,D,J,K]Z
Non-OR	07W[M,P][3,4]YZ
Non-OR	07W[M,P]X[0,3]Z
Non-OR	07WT[0,3,4,X]0Z

0   Medical and Surgical
7   Lymphatic and Hemic Systems
Y   Transplantation   Definition: Putting in or on all or a portion of a living body part taken from another individual or animal to physically take the place and/or function of all or a portion of a similar body part

Explanation: The native body part may or may not be taken out, and the transplanted body part may take over all or a portion of its function

Body Part Character 4	Approach Character 5	Device Character 6	Qualifier Character 7

M Thymus
   Thymus gland
P Spleen
   Accessory spleen
	0 Open	Z No Device	0 Allogeneic
			1 Syngeneic
			2 Zooplastic

NC Noncovered Procedure   LC Limited Coverage   QA Questionable OB Admit   NT New Tech Add-on   ⊞ Combination Member   ♂ Male   ♀ Female

ICD-10-PCS 2023   299

07W–07Y

Eye Ø8Ø–Ø8X

Character Meanings

This Character Meaning table is provided as a guide to assist the user in the identification of character members that may be found in this section of code tables. It **SHOULD NOT** be used to build a PCS code.

Operation–Character 3	Body Part–Character 4	Approach–Character 5	Device–Character 6	Qualifier–Character 7
Ø Alteration	Ø Eye, Right	Ø Open	Ø Drainage Device OR Synthetic Substitute, Intraocular Telescope	3 Nasal Cavity
1 Bypass	1 Eye, Left	3 Percutaneous	1 Radioactive Element	4 Sclera
2 Change	2 Anterior Chamber, Right	7 Via Natural or Artificial Opening	3 Infusion Device	X Diagnostic
5 Destruction	3 Anterior Chamber, Left	8 Via Natural or Artificial Opening Endoscopic	5 Epiretinal Visual Prosthesis	Z No Qualifier
7 Dilation	4 Vitreous, Right	X External	7 Autologous Tissue Substitute	
9 Drainage	5 Vitreous, Left		C Extraluminal Device	
B Excision	6 Sclera, Right		D Intraluminal Device	
C Extirpation	7 Sclera, Left		J Synthetic Substitute	
D Extraction	8 Cornea, Right		K Nonautologous Tissue Substitute	
F Fragmentation	9 Cornea, Left		Y Other Device	
H Insertion	A Choroid, Right		Z No Device	
J Inspection	B Choroid, Left			
L Occlusion	C Iris, Right			
M Reattachment	D Iris, Left			
N Release	E Retina, Right			
P Removal	F Retina, Left			
Q Repair	G Retinal Vessel, Right			
R Replacement	H Retinal Vessel, Left			
S Reposition	J Lens, Right			
T Resection	K Lens, Left			
U Supplement	L Extraocular Muscle, Right			
V Restriction	M Extraocular Muscle, Left			
W Revision	N Upper Eyelid, Right			
X Transfer	P Upper Eyelid, Left			
	Q Lower Eyelid, Right			
	R Lower Eyelid, Left			
	S Conjunctiva, Right			
	T Conjunctiva, Left			
	V Lacrimal Gland, Right			
	W Lacrimal Gland, Left			
	X Lacrimal Duct, Right			
	Y Lacrimal Duct, Left			

AHA Coding Clinic for table Ø81
2019, 1Q, 27   Glaucoma tube shunt

AHA Coding Clinic for table Ø89
2016, 2Q, 21   Laser trabeculoplasty

AHA Coding Clinic for table Ø8B
2014, 4Q, 35   Vitrectomy with air/fluid exchange
2014, 4Q, 36   Pars plans vitrectomy without mention of instillation of oil, air or fluid

AHA Coding Clinic for table Ø8J
2015, 1Q, 35   Attempted removal of foreign body from cornea

AHA Coding Clinic for table Ø8N
2015, 2Q, 24   Penetrating keratoplasty and anterior segment reconstruction

AHA Coding Clinic for table Ø8Q
2018, 3Q, 13   Repair of ruptured globe

AHA Coding Clinic for table Ø8R
2015, 2Q, 24   Penetrating keratoplasty and anterior segment reconstruction
2015, 2Q, 25   Penetrating keratoplasty and placement of viscoelastic eye with paracentesis

AHA Coding Clinic for table Ø8T
2015, 2Q, 12   Orbital exenteration

AHA Coding Clinic for table Ø8U
2014, 3Q, 31   Corneal amniotic membrane transplantation

Eye

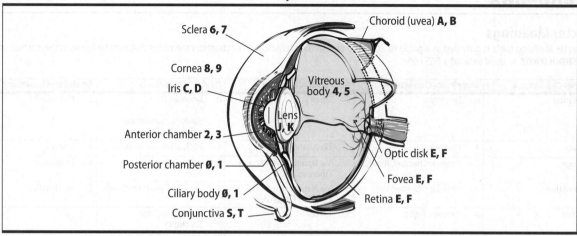

Sclera **6, 7**
Cornea **8, 9**
Iris **C, D**
Lens **J, K**
Anterior chamber **2, 3**
Posterior chamber **Ø, 1**
Ciliary body **Ø, 1**
Conjunctiva **S, T**
Choroid (uvea) **A, B**
Vitreous body **4, 5**
Optic disk **E, F**
Fovea **E, F**
Retina **E, F**

Eye Musculature

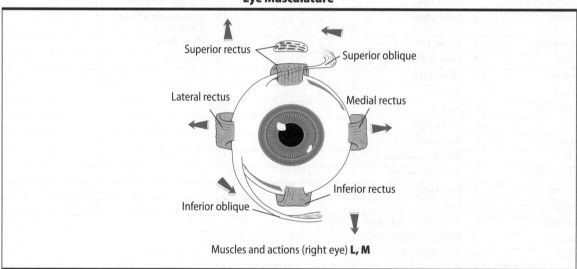

Superior rectus
Superior oblique
Lateral rectus
Medial rectus
Inferior oblique
Inferior rectus
Muscles and actions (right eye) **L, M**

Lacrimal System

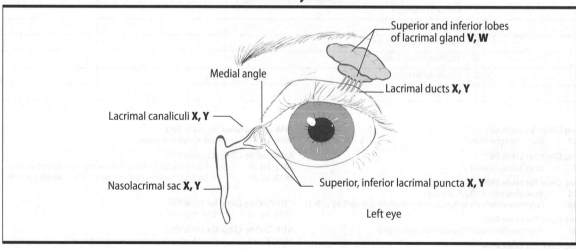

Superior and inferior lobes of lacrimal gland **V, W**
Medial angle
Lacrimal ducts **X, Y**
Lacrimal canaliculi **X, Y**
Nasolacrimal sac **X, Y**
Superior, inferior lacrimal puncta **X, Y**
Left eye

Ø   Medical and Surgical
8   Eye
Ø   Alteration   Definition: Modifying the anatomic structure of a body part without affecting the function of the body part
Explanation: Principal purpose is to improve appearance

Body Part Character 4	Approach Character 5	Device Character 6	Qualifier Character 7
N **Upper Eyelid, Right** Lateral canthus Levator palpebrae superioris muscle Orbicularis oculi muscle Superior tarsal plate **P** **Upper Eyelid, Left** *See N Upper Eyelid, Right* **Q** **Lower Eyelid, Right** Inferior tarsal plate Medial canthus **R** **Lower Eyelid, Left** *See Q Lower Eyelid, Right*	**Ø** Open **3** Percutaneous **X** External	**7** Autologous Tissue Substitute **J** Synthetic Substitute **K** Nonautologous Tissue Substitute **Z** No Device	**Z** No Qualifier

Non-OR	All body part, approach, device, and qualifier values

Ø   Medical and Surgical
8   Eye
1   Bypass   Definition: Altering the route of passage of the contents of a tubular body part
Explanation: Rerouting contents of a body part to a downstream area of the normal route, to a similar route and body part, or to an abnormal route and dissimilar body part. Includes one or more anastomoses, with or without the use of a device.

Body Part Character 4	Approach Character 5	Device Character 6	Qualifier Character 7
2 **Anterior Chamber, Right** Aqueous humour **3** **Anterior Chamber, Left** *See 2 Anterior Chamber, Right*	**3** Percutaneous	**J** Synthetic Substitute **K** Nonautologous Tissue Substitute **Z** No Device	**4** Sclera
X **Lacrimal Duct, Right** Lacrimal canaliculus Lacrimal punctum Lacrimal sac Nasolacrimal duct **Y** **Lacrimal Duct, Left** *See X Lacrimal Duct, Right*	**Ø** Open **3** Percutaneous	**J** Synthetic Substitute **K** Nonautologous Tissue Substitute **Z** No Device	**3** Nasal Cavity

Ø   Medical and Surgical
8   Eye
2   Change   Definition: Taking out or off a device from a body part and putting back an identical or similar device in or on the same body part without cutting or puncturing the skin or a mucous membrane
Explanation: All CHANGE procedures are coded using the approach EXTERNAL

Body Part Character 4	Approach Character 5	Device Character 6	Qualifier Character 7
Ø **Eye, Right** Ciliary body Posterior chamber **1** **Eye, Left** *See Ø Eye, Right*	**X** External	**Ø** Drainage Device **Y** Other Device	**Z** No Qualifier

Non-OR	All body part, approach, device, and qualifier values

NC Noncovered Procedure   **LC** Limited Coverage   **QA** Questionable OB Admit   **NT** New Tech Add-on   ⊞ Combination Member   ♂ Male   ♀ Female
ICD-10-PCS 2023   303

Ø8Ø–Ø82

0   Medical and Surgical
8   Eye
5   Destruction   Definition: Physical eradication of all or a portion of a body part by the direct use of energy, force, or a destructive agent
                        Explanation: None of the body part is physically taken out

Body Part Character 4		Approach Character 5	Device Character 6	Qualifier Character 7
0 Eye, Right Ciliary body Posterior chamber **1** Eye, Left *See 0 Eye, Right* **6** Sclera, Right **7** Sclera, Left	**8** Cornea, Right **9** Cornea, Left **S** Conjunctiva, Right Plica semilunaris **T** Conjunctiva, Left *See S Conjunctiva, Right*	**X** External	**Z** No Device	**Z** No Qualifier
2 Anterior Chamber, Right Aqueous humour **3** Anterior Chamber, Left *See 2 Anterior Chamber, Right* **4** Vitreous, Right Vitreous body **5** Vitreous, Left *See 4 Vitreous, Right* **C** Iris, Right **D** Iris, Left	**E** Retina, Right Fovea Macula Optic disc **F** Retina, Left *See E Retina, Right* **G** Retinal Vessel, Right **H** Retinal Vessel, Left **J** Lens, Right Zonule of Zinn **K** Lens, Left *See J Lens, Right*	**3** Percutaneous	**Z** No Device	**Z** No Qualifier
A Choroid, Right **B** Choroid, Left **L** Extraocular Muscle, Right Inferior oblique muscle Inferior rectus muscle Lateral rectus muscle Medial rectus muscle Superior oblique muscle Superior rectus muscle	**M** Extraocular Muscle, Left *See L Extraocular Muscle, Right* **V** Lacrimal Gland, Right **W** Lacrimal Gland, Left	**0** Open **3** Percutaneous	**Z** No Device	**Z** No Qualifier
N Upper Eyelid, Right Lateral canthus Levator palpebrae superioris muscle Orbicularis oculi muscle Superior tarsal plate **P** Upper Eyelid, Left *See N Upper Eyelid, Right*	**Q** Lower Eyelid, Right Inferior tarsal plate Medial canthus **R** Lower Eyelid, Left *See Q Lower Eyelid, Right*	**0** Open **3** Percutaneous **X** External	**Z** No Device	**Z** No Qualifier
X Lacrimal Duct, Right Lacrimal canaliculus Lacrimal punctum Lacrimal sac Nasolacrimal duct	**Y** Lacrimal Duct, Left *See X Lacrimal Duct, Right*	**0** Open **3** Percutaneous **7** Via Natural or Artificial Opening **8** Via Natural or Artificial Opening Endoscopic	**Z** No Device	**Z** No Qualifier

Non-OR	085[E,F]3ZZ

0   Medical and Surgical
8   Eye
7   Dilation   Definition: Expanding an orifice or the lumen of a tubular body part
                     Explanation: The orifice can be a natural orifice or an artificially created orifice. Accomplished by stretching a tubular body part using
                     intraluminal pressure or by cutting part of the orifice or wall of the tubular body part.

Body Part Character 4	Approach Character 5	Device Character 6	Qualifier Character 7
X Lacrimal Duct, Right Lacrimal canaliculus Lacrimal punctum Lacrimal sac Nasolacrimal duct **Y** Lacrimal Duct, Left *See X Lacrimal Duct, Right*	**0** Open **3** Percutaneous **7** Via Natural or Artificial Opening **8** Via Natural or Artificial Opening Endoscopic	**D** Intraluminal Device **Z** No Device	**Z** No Qualifier

Non-OR Procedure   DRG Non-OR Procedure   Valid OR Procedure   HAC Associated Procedure   Combination Only   New/Revised April   New/Revised October

304   ICD-10-PCS 2023

085–087

Ø   Medical and Surgical
8   Eye
9   Drainage   Definition: Taking or letting out fluids and/or gases from a body part
                       Explanation: The qualifier DIAGNOSTIC is used to identify drainage procedures that are biopsies

Body Part Character 4		Approach Character 5	Device Character 6	Qualifier Character 7

Ø Eye, Right
  Ciliary body
  Posterior chamber
1 Eye, Left
  See Ø Eye, Right
6 Sclera, Right
7 Sclera, Left
	8 Cornea, Right
	9 Cornea, Left
	S Conjunctiva, Right
	  Plica semilunaris
	T Conjunctiva, Left
	  See S Conjunctiva, Right
		X External	Ø Drainage Device	Z No Qualifier

Ø Eye, Right
  Ciliary body
  Posterior chamber
1 Eye, Left
  See Ø Eye, Right
6 Sclera, Right
7 Sclera, Left
	8 Cornea, Right
	9 Cornea, Left
	S Conjunctiva, Right
	  Plica semilunaris
	T Conjunctiva, Left
	  See S Conjunctiva, Right
		X External	Z No Device	X Diagnostic
				Z No Qualifier

2 Anterior Chamber, Right
  Aqueous humour
3 Anterior Chamber, Left
  See 2 Anterior Chamber, Right
4 Vitreous, Right
  Vitreous body
5 Vitreous, Left
  See 4 Vitreous, Right
C Iris, Right
D Iris, Left
	E Retina, Right
	  Fovea
	  Macula
	  Optic disc
	F Retina, Left
	  See E Retina, Right
	G Retinal Vessel, Right
	H Retinal Vessel, Left
	J Lens, Right
	  Zonule of Zinn
	K Lens, Left
	  See J Lens, Right
		3 Percutaneous	Ø Drainage Device	Z No Qualifier

2 Anterior Chamber, Right
  Aqueous humour
3 Anterior Chamber, Left
  See 2 Anterior Chamber, Right
4 Vitreous, Right
  Vitreous body
5 Vitreous, Left
  See 4 Vitreous, Right
C Iris, Right
D Iris, Left
	E Retina, Right
	  Fovea
	  Macula
	  Optic disc
	F Retina, Left
	  See E Retina, Right
	G Retinal Vessel, Right
	H Retinal Vessel, Left
	J Lens, Right
	  Zonule of Zinn
	K Lens, Left
	  See J Lens, Right
		3 Percutaneous	Z No Device	X Diagnostic
				Z No Qualifier

A Choroid, Right
B Choroid, Left
L Extraocular Muscle, Right
  Inferior oblique muscle
  Inferior rectus muscle
  Lateral rectus muscle
  Medial rectus muscle
  Superior oblique muscle
  Superior rectus muscle
	M Extraocular Muscle, Left
	  See L Extraocular Muscle, Right
	V Lacrimal Gland, Right
	W Lacrimal Gland, Left
		Ø Open
		3 Percutaneous
			Ø Drainage Device	Z No Qualifier

A Choroid, Right
B Choroid, Left
L Extraocular Muscle, Right
  Inferior oblique muscle
  Inferior rectus muscle
  Lateral rectus muscle
  Medial rectus muscle
  Superior oblique muscle
  Superior rectus muscle
	M Extraocular Muscle, Left
	  See L Extraocular Muscle, Right
	V Lacrimal Gland, Right
	W Lacrimal Gland, Left
		Ø Open
		3 Percutaneous
			Z No Device	X Diagnostic
				Z No Qualifier

N Upper Eyelid, Right
  Lateral canthus
  Levator palpebrae superioris
    muscle
  Orbicularis oculi muscle
  Superior tarsal plate
P Upper Eyelid, Left
  See N Upper Eyelid, Right
	Q Lower Eyelid, Right
	  Inferior tarsal plate
	  Medial canthus
	R Lower Eyelid, Left
	  See Q Lower Eyelid, Right
		Ø Open
		3 Percutaneous
		X External
			Ø Drainage Device	Z No Qualifier

Non-OR	Ø89[Ø,1,6,7,8,9,S,T]XZ[X,Z]
Non-OR	Ø89[N,P,Q,R][Ø,3,X]ØZ

Ø89 Continued on next page

NC Noncovered Procedure   **LC** Limited Coverage   **QA** Questionable OB Admit   **NT** New Tech Add-on   ⊞ Combination Member   ♂ Male   ♀ Female

ICD-10-PCS 2023   305

Ø89–Ø89

Ø Medical and Surgical
8 Eye
9 Drainage

Definition: Taking or letting out fluids and/or gases from a body part

Explanation: The qualifier DIAGNOSTIC is used to identify drainage procedures that are biopsies

Body Part Character 4		Approach Character 5	Device Character 6	Qualifier Character 7
N Upper Eyelid, Right Lateral canthus Levator palpebrae superioris muscle Orbicularis oculi muscle Superior tarsal plate **P Upper Eyelid, Left** *See N Upper Eyelid, Right*	**Q Lower Eyelid, Right** Inferior tarsal plate Medial canthus **R Lower Eyelid, Left** *See Q Lower Eyelid, Right*	**Ø** Open **3** Percutaneous **X** External	**Z** No Device	**X** Diagnostic **Z** No Qualifier
X Lacrimal Duct, Right Lacrimal canaliculus Lacrimal punctum Lacrimal sac Nasolacrimal duct	**Y Lacrimal Duct, Left** *See X Lacrimal Duct, Right*	**Ø** Open **3** Percutaneous **7** Via Natural or Artificial Opening **8** Via Natural or Artificial Opening Endoscopic	**Ø** Drainage Device	**Z** No Qualifier
X Lacrimal Duct, Right Lacrimal canaliculus Lacrimal punctum Lacrimal sac Nasolacrimal duct	**Y Lacrimal Duct, Left** *See X Lacrimal Duct, Right*	**Ø** Open **3** Percutaneous **7** Via Natural or Artificial Opening **8** Via Natural or Artificial Opening Endoscopic	**Z** No Device	**X** Diagnostic **Z** No Qualifier

Non-OR	Ø89[N,P,Q,R]ØZZ
Non-OR	Ø89[N,P,Q,R][3,X]Z[X,Z]

Ø Medical and Surgical
8 Eye
B Excision

Definition: Cutting out or off, without replacement, a portion of a body part

Explanation: The qualifier DIAGNOSTIC is used to identify excision procedures that are biopsies

Body Part Character 4		Approach Character 5	Device Character 6	Qualifier Character 7
Ø Eye, Right Ciliary body Posterior chamber **1 Eye, Left** *See Ø Eye, Right* **N Upper Eyelid, Right** Lateral canthus Levator palpebrae superioris muscle Orbicularis oculi muscle Superior tarsal plate	**P Upper Eyelid, Left** *See N Upper Eyelid, Right* **Q Lower Eyelid, Right** Inferior tarsal plate Medial canthus **R Lower Eyelid, Left** *See Q Lower Eyelid, Right*	**Ø** Open **3** Percutaneous **X** External	**Z** No Device	**X** Diagnostic **Z** No Qualifier
4 Vitreous, Right Vitreous body **5 Vitreous, Left** *See 4 Vitreous, Right* **C Iris, Right** **D Iris, Left** **E Retina, Right** Fovea Macula Optic disc	**F Retina, Left** *See E Retina, Right* **J Lens, Right** Zonule of Zinn **K Lens, Left** *See J Lens, Right*	**3** Percutaneous	**Z** No Device	**X** Diagnostic **Z** No Qualifier
6 Sclera, Right **7 Sclera, Left** **8 Cornea, Right** **9 Cornea, Left**	**S Conjunctiva, Right** Plica semilunaris **T Conjunctiva, Left** *See S Conjunctiva, Right*	**X** External	**Z** No Device	**X** Diagnostic **Z** No Qualifier
A Choroid, Right **B Choroid, Left** **L Extraocular Muscle, Right** Inferior oblique muscle Inferior rectus muscle Lateral rectus muscle Medial rectus muscle Superior oblique muscle Superior rectus muscle	**M Extraocular Muscle, Left** *See L Extraocular Muscle, Right* **V Lacrimal Gland, Right** **W Lacrimal Gland, Left**	**Ø** Open **3** Percutaneous	**Z** No Device	**X** Diagnostic **Z** No Qualifier
X Lacrimal Duct, Right Lacrimal canaliculus Lacrimal punctum Lacrimal sac Nasolacrimal duct	**Y Lacrimal Duct, Left** *See X Lacrimal Duct, Right*	**Ø** Open **3** Percutaneous **7** Via Natural or Artificial Opening **8** Via Natural or Artificial Opening Endoscopic	**Z** No Device	**X** Diagnostic **Z** No Qualifier

Non-OR Procedure   DRG Non-OR Procedure   Valid OR Procedure   HAC Associated Procedure   Combination Only   New/Revised April   New/Revised October

306

ICD-10-PCS 2023

Ø89–Ø8B

0   **Medical and Surgical**
8   **Eye**
C   **Extirpation**   Definition: Taking or cutting out solid matter from a body part

Explanation: The solid matter may be an abnormal byproduct of a biological function or a foreign body; it may be imbedded in a body part or in the lumen of a tubular body part. The solid matter may or may not have been previously broken into pieces.

Body Part Character 4	Approach Character 5	Device Character 6	Qualifier Character 7

0   **Eye, Right**
    Ciliary body
    Posterior chamber
1   **Eye, Left**
    See 0 Eye, Right
6   **Sclera, Right**
7   **Sclera, Left**
8   **Cornea, Right**
9   **Cornea, Left**
S   **Conjunctiva, Right**
    Plica semilunaris
T   **Conjunctiva, Left**
    See S Conjunctiva, Right
	X External	**Z** No Device	**Z** No Qualifier

2   **Anterior Chamber, Right**
    Aqueous humour
3   **Anterior Chamber, Left**
    See 2 Anterior Chamber, Right
4   **Vitreous, Right**
    Vitreous body
5   **Vitreous, Left**
    See 4 Vitreous, Right
C   **Iris, Right**
D   **Iris, Left**
E   **Retina, Right**
    Fovea
    Macula
    Optic disc
F   **Retina, Left**
    See E Retina, Right
G   **Retinal Vessel, Right**
H   **Retinal Vessel, Left**
J   **Lens, Right**
    Zonule of Zinn
K   **Lens, Left**
    See J Lens, Right
	3 Percutaneous
	X External
		Z No Device	**Z** No Qualifier

A   **Choroid, Right**
B   **Choroid, Left**
L   **Extraocular Muscle, Right**
    Inferior oblique muscle
    Inferior rectus muscle
    Lateral rectus muscle
    Medial rectus muscle
    Superior oblique muscle
    Superior rectus muscle
M   **Extraocular Muscle, Left**
    See L Extraocular Muscle, Right
N   **Upper Eyelid, Right**
    Lateral canthus
    Levator palpebrae superioris muscle
    Orbicularis oculi muscle
    Superior tarsal plate
P   **Upper Eyelid, Left**
    See N Upper Eyelid, Right
Q   **Lower Eyelid, Right**
    Inferior tarsal plate
    Medial canthus
R   **Lower Eyelid, Left**
    See Q Lower Eyelid, Right
V   **Lacrimal Gland, Right**
W   **Lacrimal Gland, Left**
	0 Open
	3 Percutaneous
	X External
		Z No Device	**Z** No Qualifier

X   **Lacrimal Duct, Right**
    Lacrimal canaliculus
    Lacrimal punctum
    Lacrimal sac
    Nasolacrimal duct
Y   **Lacrimal Duct, Left**
    See X Lacrimal Duct, Right
	0 Open
	3 Percutaneous
	7 Via Natural or Artificial Opening
	8 Via Natural or Artificial Opening Endoscopic
		Z No Device	**Z** No Qualifier

Non-OR	08C[0,1,6,7,S,T]XZZ
Non-OR	08C[2,3]XZZ
Non-OR	08C[N,P,Q,R][0,3,X]ZZ

NC Noncovered Procedure   **LC** Limited Coverage   **QA** Questionable OB Admit   **NT** New Tech Add-on   ⊞ Combination Member   ♂ Male   ♀ Female

Ø   Medical and Surgical
8   Eye
D   Extraction   Definition: Pulling or stripping out or off all or a portion of a body part by the use of force
             Explanation: The qualifier DIAGNOSTIC is used to identify extraction procedures that are biopsies

Body Part Character 4	Approach Character 5	Device Character 6	Qualifier Character 7
8 Cornea, Right 9 Cornea, Left	X External	Z No Device	X Diagnostic Z No Qualifier

J Lens, Right
   Zonule of Zinn
K Lens, Left
   See J Lens, Right
	3 Percutaneous	Z No Device	Z No Qualifier

Ø   Medical and Surgical
8   Eye
F   Fragmentation   Definition: Breaking solid matter in a body part into pieces
                 Explanation: Physical force (e.g., manual, ultrasonic) applied directly or indirectly is used to break the solid matter into pieces. The solid matter may be an abnormal byproduct of a biological function or a foreign body. The pieces of solid matter are not taken out.

Body Part Character 4	Approach Character 5	Device Character 6	Qualifier Character 7

4 Vitreous, Right   **NC**
   Vitreous body
5 Vitreous, Left   **NC**
   See 4 Vitreous, Right
	3 Percutaneous
	X External
		Z No Device	Z No Qualifier

Non-OR	Ø8F[4,5]XZZ
NC	Ø8F[4,5]XZZ

Ø   Medical and Surgical
8   Eye
H   Insertion   Definition: Putting in a nonbiological appliance that monitors, assists, performs, or prevents a physiological function but does not physically take the place of a body part
             Explanation: None

Body Part Character 4	Approach Character 5	Device Character 6	Qualifier Character 7

Ø Eye, Right
   Ciliary body
   Posterior chamber
1 Eye, Left
   See Ø Eye, Right
	Ø Open	5 Epiretinal Visual Prosthesis
		Y Other Device
			Z No Qualifier

Ø Eye, Right
   Ciliary body
   Posterior chamber
1 Eye, Left
   See Ø Eye, Right
	3 Percutaneous	1 Radioactive Element
		3 Infusion Device
		Y Other Device
			Z No Qualifier

Ø Eye, Right
   Ciliary body
   Posterior chamber
1 Eye, Left
   See Ø Eye, Right
	7 Via Natural or Artificial Opening
	8 Via Natural or Artificial Opening Endoscopic
		Y Other Device	Z No Qualifier

Ø Eye, Right
   Ciliary body
   Posterior chamber
1 Eye, Left
   See Ø Eye, Right
	X External	1 Radioactive Element
		3 Infusion Device
			Z No Qualifier

Non-OR	Ø8H[Ø,1]3YZ
Non-OR	Ø8H[Ø,1][7,8]YZ

Non-OR Procedure   DRG Non-OR Procedure   Valid OR Procedure   HAC Associated Procedure   Combination Only   New/Revised April   New/Revised October

Ø8D–Ø8H

308   ICD-10-PCS 2023

Ø   Medical and Surgical
8   Eye
J   Inspection   Definition: Visually and/or manually exploring a body part

Explanation: Visual exploration may be performed with or without optical instrumentation. Manual exploration may be performed directly or through intervening body layers.

Body Part Character 4	Approach Character 5	Device Character 6	Qualifier Character 7
Ø Eye, Right Ciliary body Posterior chamber **1 Eye, Left** *See Ø Eye, Right* **J Lens, Right** Zonule of Zinn **K Lens, Left** *See J Lens, Right*	**X** External	**Z** No Device	**Z** No Qualifier
L Extraocular Muscle, Right Inferior oblique muscle Inferior rectus muscle Lateral rectus muscle Medial rectus muscle Superior oblique muscle Superior rectus muscle **M Extraocular Muscle, Left** *See L Extraocular Muscle, Right*	**Ø** Open **X** External	**Z** No Device	**Z** No Qualifier

Non-OR   Ø8J[Ø,1,J,K]XZZ
Non-OR   Ø8J[L,M]XZZ

Ø   Medical and Surgical
8   Eye
L   Occlusion   Definition: Completely closing an orifice or the lumen of a tubular body part

Explanation: The orifice can be a natural orifice or an artificially created orifice

Body Part Character 4	Approach Character 5	Device Character 6	Qualifier Character 7
X Lacrimal Duct, Right Lacrimal canaliculus Lacrimal punctum Lacrimal sac Nasolacrimal duct **Y Lacrimal Duct, Left** *See X Lacrimal Duct, Right*	**Ø** Open **3** Percutaneous	**C** Extraluminal Device **D** Intraluminal Device **Z** No Device	**Z** No Qualifier
X Lacrimal Duct, Right Lacrimal canaliculus Lacrimal punctum Lacrimal sac Nasolacrimal duct **Y Lacrimal Duct, Left** *See X Lacrimal Duct, Right*	**7** Via Natural or Artificial Opening **8** Via Natural or Artificial Opening Endoscopic	**D** Intraluminal Device **Z** No Device	**Z** No Qualifier

Ø   Medical and Surgical
8   Eye
M   Reattachment   Definition: Putting back in or on all or a portion of a separated body part to its normal location or other suitable location

Explanation: Vascular circulation and nervous pathways may or may not be reestablished

Body Part Character 4	Approach Character 5	Device Character 6	Qualifier Character 7
N Upper Eyelid, Right Lateral canthus Levator palpebrae superioris muscle Orbicularis oculi muscle Superior tarsal plate **P Upper Eyelid, Left** *See N Upper Eyelid, Right* **Q Lower Eyelid, Right** Inferior tarsal plate Medial canthus **R Lower Eyelid, Left** *See Q Lower Eyelid, Right*	**X** External	**Z** No Device	**Z** No Qualifier

NC Noncovered Procedure   **LC** Limited Coverage   **QA** Questionable OB Admit   **NT** New Tech Add-on   ⊞ Combination Member   ♂ Male   ♀ Female

ICD-10-PCS 2023

309

08J–08M

Ø Medical and Surgical
8 Eye
N Release Definition: Freeing a body part from an abnormal physical constraint by cutting or by the use of force

Explanation: Some of the restraining tissue may be taken out but none of the body part is taken out

Body Part Character 4	Approach Character 5	Device Character 6	Qualifier Character 7
Ø Eye, Right Ciliary body Posterior chamber **1 Eye, Left** *See Ø Eye, Right* **6 Sclera, Right** **7 Sclera, Left** **8 Cornea, Right** **9 Cornea, Left** **S Conjunctiva, Right** Plica semilunaris **T Conjunctiva, Left** *See S Conjunctiva, Right*	**X External**	**Z No Device**	**Z No Qualifier**
2 Anterior Chamber, Right Aqueous humour **3 Anterior Chamber, Left** *See 2 Anterior Chamber, Right* **4 Vitreous, Right** Vitreous body **5 Vitreous, Left** *See 4 Vitreous, Right* **C Iris, Right** **D Iris, Left** **E Retina, Right** Fovea Macula Optic disc **F Retina, Left** *See E Retina, Right* **G Retinal Vessel, Right** **H Retinal Vessel, Left** **J Lens, Right** Zonule of Zinn **K Lens, Left** *See J Lens, Right*	**3 Percutaneous**	**Z No Device**	**Z No Qualifier**
A Choroid, Right **B Choroid, Left** **L Extraocular Muscle, Right** Inferior oblique muscle Inferior rectus muscle Lateral rectus muscle Medial rectus muscle Superior oblique muscle Superior rectus muscle **M Extraocular Muscle, Left** *See L Extraocular Muscle, Right* **V Lacrimal Gland, Right** **W Lacrimal Gland, Left**	**Ø Open** **3 Percutaneous**	**Z No Device**	**Z No Qualifier**
N Upper Eyelid, Right Lateral canthus Levator palpebrae superioris muscle Orbicularis oculi muscle Superior tarsal plate **P Upper Eyelid, Left** *See N Upper Eyelid, Right* **Q Lower Eyelid, Right** Inferior tarsal plate Medial canthus **R Lower Eyelid, Left** *See Q Lower Eyelid, Right*	**Ø Open** **3 Percutaneous** **X External**	**Z No Device**	**Z No Qualifier**
X Lacrimal Duct, Right Lacrimal canaliculus Lacrimal punctum Lacrimal sac Nasolacrimal duct **Y Lacrimal Duct, Left** *See X Lacrimal Duct, Right*	**Ø Open** **3 Percutaneous** **7 Via Natural or Artificial Opening** **8 Via Natural or Artificial Opening Endoscopic**	**Z No Device**	**Z No Qualifier**

Non-OR Procedure   DRG Non-OR Procedure   Valid OR Procedure   HAC Associated Procedure   Combination Only   New/Revised April   New/Revised October

310

ICD-10-PCS 2023

Ø Medical and Surgical
8 Eye
P Removal   Definition: Taking out or off a device from a body part

Explanation: If a device is taken out and a similar device put in without cutting or puncturing the skin or mucous membrane, the procedure is coded to the root operation CHANGE. Otherwise, the procedure for taking out a device is coded to the root operation REMOVAL.

Body Part Character 4	Approach Character 5	Device Character 6	Qualifier Character 7

Ø Eye, Right
   Ciliary body
   Posterior chamber
1 Eye, Left
   See Ø Eye, Right
	Ø Open
	3 Percutaneous
	7 Via Natural or Artificial Opening
	8 Via Natural or Artificial Opening
	   Endoscopic
		Ø Drainage Device
		1 Radioactive Element
		3 Infusion Device
		7 Autologous Tissue Substitute
		C Extraluminal Device
		D Intraluminal Device
		J Synthetic Substitute
		K Nonautologous Tissue Substitute
		Y Other Device
			Z No Qualifier

Ø Eye, Right
   Ciliary body
   Posterior chamber
1 Eye, Left
   See Ø Eye, Right
	X External	Ø Drainage Device
		1 Radioactive Element
		3 Infusion Device
		7 Autologous Tissue Substitute
		C Extraluminal Device
		D Intraluminal Device
		J Synthetic Substitute
		K Nonautologous Tissue Substitute
			Z No Qualifier

J Lens, Right
   Zonule of Zinn
K Lens, Left
   See J Lens, Right
	3 Percutaneous	J Synthetic Substitute
		Y Other Device
			Z No Qualifier

L Extraocular Muscle, Right
   Inferior oblique muscle
   Inferior rectus muscle
   Lateral rectus muscle
   Medial rectus muscle
   Superior oblique muscle
   Superior rectus muscle
M Extraocular Muscle, Left
   See L Extraocular Muscle, Right
	Ø Open
	3 Percutaneous
		Ø Drainage Device
		7 Autologous Tissue Substitute
		J Synthetic Substitute
		K Nonautologous Tissue Substitute
		Y Other Device
			Z No Qualifier

Non-OR   Ø8P[Ø,1]3YZ
Non-OR   Ø8P[Ø,1][7,8][Ø,3,D,Y]Z
Non-OR   Ø8P[Ø,1]X[Ø,1,3,C,D,J]Z
Non-OR   Ø8P[J,K]3YZ
Non-OR   Ø8P[L,M]3YZ

NC Noncovered Procedure   LC Limited Coverage   QA Questionable OB Admit   NT New Tech Add-on   ⊞ Combination Member   ♂ Male   ♀ Female

ICD-10-PCS 2023   311

Ø8P–Ø8P

Ø   Medical and Surgical
8   Eye
Q   Repair   Definition: Restoring, to the extent possible, a body part to its normal anatomic structure and function
   Explanation: Used only when the method to accomplish the repair is not one of the other root operations

Body Part Character 4	Approach Character 5	Device Character 6	Qualifier Character 7

Ø Eye, Right
   Ciliary body
   Posterior chamber
1 Eye, Left
   See Ø Eye, Right
6 Sclera, Right
7 Sclera, Left
8 Cornea, Right   **NC**
9 Cornea, Left   **NC**
S Conjunctiva, Right
   Plica semilunaris
T Conjunctiva, Left
   See S Conjunctiva, Right
	X External	Z No Device	Z No Qualifier

2 Anterior Chamber, Right
   Aqueous humour
3 Anterior Chamber, Left
   See 2 Anterior Chamber, Right
4 Vitreous, Right
   Vitreous body
5 Vitreous, Left
   See 4 Vitreous, Right
C Iris, Right
D Iris, Left
E Retina, Right
   Fovea
   Macula
   Optic disc
F Retina, Left
   See E Retina, Right
G Retinal Vessel, Right
H Retinal Vessel, Left
J Lens, Right
   Zonule of Zinn
K Lens, Left
   See J Lens, Right
	3 Percutaneous	Z No Device	Z No Qualifier

A Choroid, Right
B Choroid, Left
L Extraocular Muscle, Right
   Inferior oblique muscle
   Inferior rectus muscle
   Lateral rectus muscle
   Medial rectus muscle
   Superior oblique muscle
   Superior rectus muscle
M Extraocular Muscle, Left
   See L Extraocular Muscle, Right
V Lacrimal Gland, Right
W Lacrimal Gland, Left
	Ø Open
	3 Percutaneous
		Z No Device	Z No Qualifier

N Upper Eyelid, Right
   Lateral canthus
   Levator palpebrae superioris muscle
   Orbicularis oculi muscle
   Superior tarsal plate
P Upper Eyelid, Left
   See N Upper Eyelid, Right
Q Lower Eyelid, Right
   Inferior tarsal plate
   Medial canthus
R Lower Eyelid, Left
   See Q Lower Eyelid, Right
	Ø Open
	3 Percutaneous
	X External
		Z No Device	Z No Qualifier

X Lacrimal Duct, Right
   Lacrimal canaliculus
   Lacrimal punctum
   Lacrimal sac
   Nasolacrimal duct
Y Lacrimal Duct, Left
   See X Lacrimal Duct, Right
	Ø Open
	3 Percutaneous
	7 Via Natural or Artificial Opening
	8 Via Natural or Artificial Opening
	   Endoscopic
		Z No Device	Z No Qualifier

Non-OR Ø8Q[N,P,Q,R][Ø,3,X]ZZ
NC Ø8Q[8,9]XZZ

Non-OR Procedure   DRG Non-OR Procedure   Valid OR Procedure   HAC Associated Procedure   Combination Only   New/Revised April   New/Revised October

312 ICD-10-PCS 2023

Ø   Medical and Surgical
8   Eye
R   Replacement   Definition: Putting in or on biological or synthetic material that physically takes the place and/or function of all or a portion of a body part

Explanation: The body part may have been taken out or replaced, or may be taken out, physically eradicated, or rendered nonfunctional during the REPLACEMENT procedure. A REMOVAL procedure is coded for taking out the device used in a previous replacement procedure.

Body Part Character 4	Approach Character 5	Device Character 6	Qualifier Character 7

Ø Eye, Right
    Ciliary body
    Posterior chamber
1 Eye, Left
    See Ø Eye, Right
A Choroid, Right
B Choroid, Left
	Ø Open
	3 Percutaneous
		7 Autologous Tissue Substitute
		J Synthetic Substitute
		K Nonautologous Tissue Substitute
			Z No Qualifier

4 Vitreous, Right
    Vitreous body
5 Vitreous, Left
    See 4 Vitreous, Right
C Iris, Right
D Iris, Left
G Retinal Vessel, Right
H Retinal Vessel, Left
	3 Percutaneous	7 Autologous Tissue Substitute
		J Synthetic Substitute
		K Nonautologous Tissue Substitute
			Z No Qualifier

6 Sclera, Right
7 Sclera, Left
S Conjunctiva, Right
    Plica semilunaris
T Conjunctiva, Left
    See S Conjunctiva, Right
	X External	7 Autologous Tissue Substitute
		J Synthetic Substitute
		K Nonautologous Tissue Substitute
			Z No Qualifier

8 Cornea, Right 9 Cornea, Left	3 Percutaneous X External	7 Autologous Tissue Substitute J Synthetic Substitute K Nonautologous Tissue Substitute	Z No Qualifier

J Lens, Right
    Zonule of Zinn
K Lens, Left
    See J Lens, Right
	3 Percutaneous	Ø Synthetic Substitute, Intraocular
		    Telescope
		7 Autologous Tissue Substitute
		J Synthetic Substitute
		K Nonautologous Tissue Substitute
			Z No Qualifier

N Upper Eyelid, Right
    Lateral canthus
    Levator palpebrae superioris muscle
    Orbicularis oculi muscle
    Superior tarsal plate
P Upper Eyelid, Left
    See N Upper Eyelid, Right
Q Lower Eyelid, Right
    Inferior tarsal plate
    Medial canthus
R Lower Eyelid, Left
    See Q Lower Eyelid, Right
	Ø Open
	3 Percutaneous
	X External
		7 Autologous Tissue Substitute
		J Synthetic Substitute
		K Nonautologous Tissue Substitute
			Z No Qualifier

X Lacrimal Duct, Right
    Lacrimal canaliculus
    Lacrimal punctum
    Lacrimal sac
    Nasolacrimal duct
Y Lacrimal Duct, Left
    See X Lacrimal Duct, Right
	Ø Open
	3 Percutaneous
	7 Via Natural or Artificial Opening
	8 Via Natural or Artificial Opening
	    Endoscopic
		7 Autologous Tissue Substitute
		J Synthetic Substitute
		K Nonautologous Tissue Substitute
			Z No Qualifier

NC Noncovered Procedure   LC Limited Coverage   OA Questionable OB Admit   NT New Tech Add-on   ⊞ Combination Member   ♂ Male   ♀ Female

ICD-10-PCS 2023   313

Ø8R–Ø8R

0   Medical and Surgical
8   Eye
S   Reposition   Definition: Moving to its normal location, or other suitable location, all or a portion of a body part

Explanation: The body part is moved to a new location from an abnormal location, or from a normal location where it is not functioning correctly. The body part may or may not be cut out or off to be moved to the new location.

Body Part Character 4	Approach Character 5	Device Character 6	Qualifier Character 7

C Iris, Right
D Iris, Left
G Retinal Vessel, Right
H Retinal Vessel, Left
J Lens, Right
   Zonule of Zinn
K Lens, Left
   See J Lens, Right
	3 Percutaneous	**Z** No Device	**Z** No Qualifier

L Extraocular Muscle, Right
   Inferior oblique muscle
   Inferior rectus muscle
   Lateral rectus muscle
   Medial rectus muscle
   Superior oblique muscle
   Superior rectus muscle
M Extraocular Muscle, Left
   See L Extraocular Muscle, Right
V Lacrimal Gland, Right
W Lacrimal Gland, Left
	0 Open
	3 Percutaneous
		Z No Device	**Z** No Qualifier

N Upper Eyelid, Right
   Lateral canthus
   Levator palpebrae superioris muscle
   Orbicularis oculi muscle
   Superior tarsal plate
P Upper Eyelid, Left
   See N Upper Eyelid, Right
Q Lower Eyelid, Right
   Inferior tarsal plate
   Medial canthus
R Lower Eyelid, Left
   See Q Lower Eyelid, Right
	0 Open
	3 Percutaneous
	X External
		Z No Device	**Z** No Qualifier

X Lacrimal Duct, Right
   Lacrimal canaliculus
   Lacrimal punctum
   Lacrimal sac
   Nasolacrimal duct
Y Lacrimal Duct, Left
   See X Lacrimal Duct, Right
	0 Open
	3 Percutaneous
	7 Via Natural or Artificial Opening
	8 Via Natural or Artificial Opening Endoscopic
		Z No Device	**Z** No Qualifier

Non-OR Procedure   DRG Non-OR Procedure   Valid OR Procedure   HAC Associated Procedure   Combination Only   New/Revised April   New/Revised October

314   ICD-10-PCS 2023

Ø   Medical and Surgical
8   Eye
T   Resection   Definition: Cutting out or off, without replacement, all of a body part
                      Explanation: None

Body Part Character 4	Approach Character 5	Device Character 6	Qualifier Character 7

Ø **Eye, Right**
    Ciliary body
    Posterior chamber
1 **Eye, Left**
    See Ø Eye, Right
8 **Cornea, Right**
9 **Cornea, Left**
	X External	**Z** No Device	**Z** No Qualifier

4 **Vitreous, Right**
    Vitreous body
5 **Vitreous, Left**
    See 4 Vitreous, Right
C **Iris, Right**
D **Iris, Left**
J **Lens, Right**
    Zonule of Zinn
K **Lens, Left**
    See J Lens, Right
	3 Percutaneous	**Z** No Device	**Z** No Qualifier

L **Extraocular Muscle, Right**
    Inferior oblique muscle
    Inferior rectus muscle
    Lateral rectus muscle
    Medial rectus muscle
    Superior oblique muscle
    Superior rectus muscle
M **Extraocular Muscle, Left**
    See L Extraocular Muscle, Right
V **Lacrimal Gland, Right**
W **Lacrimal Gland, Left**
	Ø Open
	3 Percutaneous
		Z No Device	**Z** No Qualifier

N **Upper Eyelid, Right**
    Lateral canthus
    Levator palpebrae superioris muscle
    Orbicularis oculi muscle
    Superior tarsal plate
P **Upper Eyelid, Left**
    See N Upper Eyelid, Right
Q **Lower Eyelid, Right**
    Inferior tarsal plate
    Medial canthus
R **Lower Eyelid, Left**
    See Q Lower Eyelid, Right
	Ø Open
	X External
		Z No Device	**Z** No Qualifier

X **Lacrimal Duct, Right**
    Lacrimal canaliculus
    Lacrimal punctum
    Lacrimal sac
    Nasolacrimal duct
Y **Lacrimal Duct, Left**
    See X Lacrimal Duct, Right
	Ø Open
	3 Percutaneous
	7 Via Natural or Artificial Opening
	8 Via Natural or Artificial Opening
	    Endoscopic
		Z No Device	**Z** No Qualifier

NC Noncovered Procedure   **LC** Limited Coverage   **QA** Questionable OB Admit   **NT** New Tech Add-on   ⊞ Combination Member   ♂ Male   ♀ Female

ICD-10-PCS 2023   **315**

Ø **Medical and Surgical**
8 **Eye**
U **Supplement**   Definition: Putting in or on biological or synthetic material that physically reinforces and/or augments the function of a portion of a body part
     Explanation: The biological material is non-living, or is living and from the same individual. The body part may have been previously replaced, and the SUPPLEMENT procedure is performed to physically reinforce and/or augment the function of the replaced body part.

Body Part Character 4	Approach Character 5	Device Character 6	Qualifier Character 7
Ø Eye, Right Ciliary body Posterior chamber **1** Eye, Left *See Ø Eye, Right* **C** Iris, Right **D** Iris, Left **E** Retina, Right Fovea Macula Optic disc **F** Retina, Left *See E Retina, Right* **G** Retinal Vessel, Right **H** Retinal Vessel, Left **L** Extraocular Muscle, Right Inferior oblique muscle Inferior rectus muscle Lateral rectus muscle Medial rectus muscle Superior oblique muscle Superior rectus muscle **M** Extraocular Muscle, Left *See L Extraocular Muscle, Right*	**Ø** Open **3** Percutaneous	**7** Autologous Tissue Substitute **J** Synthetic Substitute **K** Nonautologous Tissue Substitute	**Z** No Qualifier
8 Cornea, Right ⁿᶜ **9** Cornea, Left ⁿᶜ **N** Upper Eyelid, Right Lateral canthus Levator palpebrae superioris muscle Orbicularis oculi muscle Superior tarsal plate **P** Upper Eyelid, Left *See N Upper Eyelid, Right* **Q** Lower Eyelid, Right Inferior tarsal plate Medial canthus **R** Lower Eyelid, Left *See Q Lower Eyelid, Right*	**Ø** Open **3** Percutaneous **X** External	**7** Autologous Tissue Substitute **J** Synthetic Substitute **K** Nonautologous Tissue Substitute	**Z** No Qualifier
X Lacrimal Duct, Right Lacrimal canaliculus Lacrimal punctum Lacrimal sac Nasolacrimal duct **Y** Lacrimal Duct, Left *See X Lacrimal Duct, Right*	**Ø** Open **3** Percutaneous **7** Via Natural or Artificial Opening **8** Via Natural or Artificial Opening Endoscopic	**7** Autologous Tissue Substitute **J** Synthetic Substitute **K** Nonautologous Tissue Substitute	**Z** No Qualifier

ⁿᶜ Ø8U[8,9][Ø,3,X]KZ

Ø **Medical and Surgical**
8 **Eye**
V **Restriction**   Definition: Partially closing an orifice or the lumen of a tubular body part
     Explanation: The orifice can be a natural orifice or an artificially created orifice

Body Part Character 4	Approach Character 5	Device Character 6	Qualifier Character 7
X Lacrimal Duct, Right Lacrimal canaliculus Lacrimal punctum Lacrimal sac Nasolacrimal duct **Y** Lacrimal Duct, Left *See X Lacrimal Duct, Right*	**Ø** Open **3** Percutaneous	**C** Extraluminal Device **D** Intraluminal Device **Z** No Device	**Z** No Qualifier
X Lacrimal Duct, Right Lacrimal canaliculus Lacrimal punctum Lacrimal sac Nasolacrimal duct **Y** Lacrimal Duct, Left *See X Lacrimal Duct, Right*	**7** Via Natural or Artificial Opening **8** Via Natural or Artificial Opening Endoscopic	**D** Intraluminal Device **Z** No Device	**Z** No Qualifier

Non-OR Procedure   DRG Non-OR Procedure   Valid OR Procedure   HAC Associated Procedure   Combination Only   New/Revised April   New/Revised October

Ø   Medical and Surgical
8   Eye
W   Revision   Definition: Correcting, to the extent possible, a portion of a malfunctioning device or the position of a displaced device

Explanation: Revision can include correcting a malfunctioning or displaced device by taking out or putting in components of the device such as a screw or pin

Body Part Character 4	Approach Character 5	Device Character 6	Qualifier Character 7

Ø Eye, Right
   Ciliary body
   Posterior chamber
1 Eye, Left
   See Ø Eye, Right
	Ø Open
	3 Percutaneous
	7 Via Natural or Artificial Opening
	8 Via Natural or Artificial Opening
	   Endoscopic
		Ø Drainage Device
		3 Infusion Device
		7 Autologous Tissue Substitute
		C Extraluminal Device
		D Intraluminal Device
		J Synthetic Substitute
		K Nonautologous Tissue Substitute
		Y Other Device
			Z No Qualifier

Ø Eye, Right
   Ciliary body
   Posterior chamber
1 Eye, Left
   See Ø Eye, Right
	X External	**Ø** Drainage Device
		3 Infusion Device
		7 Autologous Tissue Substitute
		C Extraluminal Device
		D Intraluminal Device
		J Synthetic Substitute
		K Nonautologous Tissue Substitute
			Z No Qualifier

J Lens, Right
   Zonule of Zinn
K Lens, Left
   See J Lens, Right
	3 Percutaneous	**J** Synthetic Substitute
		Y Other Device
			Z No Qualifier

J Lens, Right
   Zonule of Zinn
K Lens, Left
   See J Lens, Right
	X External	**J** Synthetic Substitute	**Z** No Qualifier

L Extraocular Muscle, Right
   Inferior oblique muscle
   Inferior rectus muscle
   Lateral rectus muscle
   Medial rectus muscle
   Superior oblique muscle
   Superior rectus muscle
M Extraocular Muscle, Left
   See L Extraocular Muscle, Right
	Ø Open
	3 Percutaneous
		Ø Drainage Device
		7 Autologous Tissue Substitute
		J Synthetic Substitute
		K Nonautologous Tissue Substitute
		Y Other Device
			Z No Qualifier

Non-OR	08W[Ø,1][3,7,8]YZ
Non-OR	08W[Ø,1]X[Ø,3,7,C,D,J,K]Z
Non-OR	08W[J,K]3YZ
Non-OR	08W[J,K]XJZ
Non-OR	08W[L,M]3YZ

Ø   Medical and Surgical
8   Eye
X   Transfer   Definition: Moving, without taking out, all or a portion of a body part to another location to take over the function of all or a portion of a body part

Explanation: The body part transferred remains connected to its vascular and nervous supply

Body Part Character 4	Approach Character 5	Device Character 6	Qualifier Character 7

L Extraocular Muscle, Right
   Inferior oblique muscle
   Inferior rectus muscle
   Lateral rectus muscle
   Medial rectus muscle
   Superior oblique muscle
   Superior rectus muscle
M Extraocular Muscle, Left
   See L Extraocular Muscle, Right
	Ø Open
	3 Percutaneous
		Z No Device	**Z** No Qualifier

NC Noncovered Procedure   **LC** Limited Coverage   **QA** Questionable OB Admit   **NT** New Tech Add-on   ⊞ Combination Member   ♂ Male   ♀ Female

ICD-10-PCS 2023   317

Ear, Nose, Sinus Ø9Ø–Ø9W

Character Meanings*

This Character Meaning table is provided as a guide to assist the user in the identification of character members that may be found in this section of code tables. It **SHOULD NOT** be used to build a PCS code.

Operation–Character 3		Body Part–Character 4		Approach–Character 5		Device–Character 6		Qualifier–Character 7	
Ø	Alteration	Ø	External Ear, Right	Ø	Open	Ø	Drainage Device	Ø	Endolymphatic
1	Bypass	1	External Ear, Left	3	Percutaneous	1	Radioactive Element	X	Diagnostic
2	Change	2	External Ear, Bilateral	4	Percutaneous Endoscopic	4	Hearing Device, Bone Conduction	Z	No Qualifier
3	Control	3	External Auditory Canal, Right	7	Via Natural or Artificial Opening	5	Hearing Device, Single Channel Cochlear Prosthesis		
5	Destruction	4	External Auditory Canal, Left	8	Via Natural or Artificial Opening Endoscopic	6	Hearing Device, Multiple Channel Cochlear Prosthesis		
7	Dilation	5	Middle Ear, Right	X	External	7	Autologous Tissue Substitute		
8	Division	6	Middle Ear, Left			B	Intraluminal Device, Airway		
9	Drainage	7	Tympanic Membrane, Right			D	Intraluminal Device		
B	Excision	8	Tympanic Membrane, Left			J	Synthetic Substitute		
C	Extirpation	9	Auditory Ossicle, Right			K	Nonautologous Tissue Substitute		
D	Extraction	A	Auditory Ossicle, Left			S	Hearing Device		
H	Insertion	B	Mastoid Sinus, Right			Y	Other Device		
J	Inspection	C	Mastoid Sinus, Left			Z	No Device		
M	Reattachment	D	Inner Ear, Right						
N	Release	E	Inner Ear, Left						
P	Removal	F	Eustachian Tube, Right						
Q	Repair	G	Eustachian Tube, Left						
R	Replacement	H	Ear, Right						
S	Reposition	J	Ear, Left						
T	Resection	K	Nasal Mucosa and Soft Tissue						
U	Supplement	L	Nasal Turbinate						
W	Revision	M	Nasal Septum						
		N	Nasopharynx						
		P	Accessory Sinus						
		Q	Maxillary Sinus, Right						
		R	Maxillary Sinus, Left						
		S	Frontal Sinus, Right						
		T	Frontal Sinus, Left						
		U	Ethmoid Sinus, Right						
		V	Ethmoid Sinus, Left						
		W	Sphenoid Sinus, Right						
		X	Sphenoid Sinus, Left						
		Y	Sinus						

* Includes sinus ducts.

AHA Coding Clinic for table Ø93
2018, 4Q, 38   Control of epistaxis

AHA Coding Clinic for table Ø95
2018, 1Q, 19   Control of epistaxis via silver nitrate cauterization

AHA Coding Clinic for table Ø9H
2022, 2Q, 17   Congenital nasal pyriform aperture stenosis and repair
2020, 4Q, 43-44   Insertion of radioactive element

AHA Coding Clinic for table Ø9Q
2018, 1Q, 19   Control of epistaxis via silver nitrate cauterization
2017, 4Q, 106   Control of bleeding of external naris using suture
2014, 4Q, 20   Control of epistaxis
2014, 3Q, 22   Transsphenoidal removal of pituitary tumor and fat graft placement
2013, 4Q, 114   Balloon sinuplasty

AHA Coding Clinic for table Ø9U
2022, 1Q, 48   Repair of facial fractures of frontal sinus and orbital roof
2019, 4Q, 28-29   Sinus supplement

Ear Anatomy

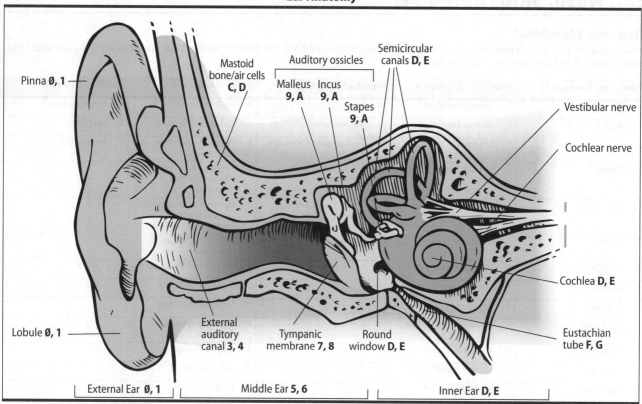

Pinna Ø, 1

Mastoid bone/air cells C, D

Auditory ossicles

Malleus 9, A   Incus 9, A

Stapes 9, A

Semicircular canals D, E

Vestibular nerve

Cochlear nerve

Cochlea D, E

Lobule Ø, 1

External auditory canal 3, 4

Tympanic membrane 7, 8

Round window D, E

Eustachian tube F, G

External Ear Ø, 1   Middle Ear 5, 6   Inner Ear D, E

Nasal Turbinates

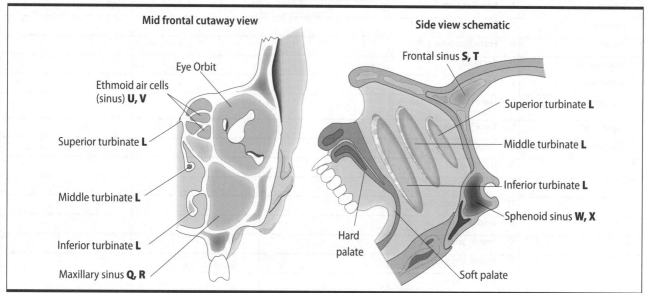

Mid frontal cutaway view

Eye Orbit

Ethmoid air cells (sinus) U, V

Superior turbinate L

Middle turbinate L

Inferior turbinate L

Maxillary sinus Q, R

Side view schematic

Frontal sinus S, T

Superior turbinate L

Middle turbinate L

Inferior turbinate L

Sphenoid sinus W, X

Hard palate

Soft palate

Paranasal Sinuses

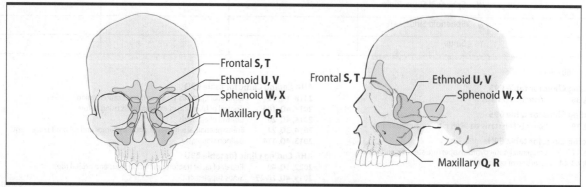

Frontal S, T
Ethmoid U, V
Sphenoid W, X
Maxillary Q, R

Frontal S, T

Ethmoid U, V

Sphenoid W, X

Maxillary Q, R

Ø   **Medical and Surgical**
9   **Ear, Nose, Sinus**
Ø   **Alteration**   Definition: Modifying the anatomic structure of a body part without affecting the function of the body part

                      Explanation: Principal purpose is to improve appearance

Body Part Character 4		Approach Character 5	Device Character 6	Qualifier Character 7

Ø External Ear, Right
  Antihelix
  Antitragus
  Auricle
  Earlobe
  Helix
  Pinna
  Tragus
1 External Ear, Left
  See Ø External Ear, Right
	2 External Ear, Bilateral
	  See Ø External Ear, Right
	K Nasal Mucosa and Soft Tissue
	  Columella
	  External naris
	  Greater alar cartilage
	  Internal naris
	  Lateral nasal cartilage
	  Lesser alar cartilage
	  Nasal cavity
	  Nostril
		Ø Open
		3 Percutaneous
		4 Percutaneous Endoscopic
		X External
			7 Autologous Tissue
			  Substitute
			J Synthetic Substitute
			K Nonautologous Tissue
			  Substitute
			Z No Device
				Z No Qualifier

Ø   **Medical and Surgical**
9   **Ear, Nose, Sinus**
1   **Bypass**   Definition: Altering the route of passage of the contents of a tubular body part

                      Explanation: Rerouting contents of a body part to a downstream area of the normal route, to a similar route and body part, or to an abnormal route and dissimilar body part. Includes one or more anastomoses, with or without the use of a device.

Body Part Character 4	Approach Character 5	Device Character 6	Qualifier Character 7

D Inner Ear, Right
  Bony labyrinth
  Bony vestibule
  Cochlea
  Round window
  Semicircular canal
E Inner Ear, Left
  See D Inner Ear, Right
	Ø Open	**7** Autologous Tissue
		  Substitute
		J Synthetic Substitute
		K Nonautologous Tissue
		  Substitute
		Z No Device
			Ø Endolymphatic

Ø   **Medical and Surgical**
9   **Ear, Nose, Sinus**
2   **Change**   Definition: Taking out or off a device from a body part and putting back an identical or similar device in or on the same body part without cutting or puncturing the skin or a mucous membrane

                      Explanation: All CHANGE procedures are coded using the approach EXTERNAL

Body Part Character 4	Approach Character 5	Device Character 6	Qualifier Character 7

H Ear, Right
J Ear, Left
K Nasal Mucosa and Soft Tissue
  Columella
  External naris
  Greater alar cartilage
  Internal naris
  Lateral nasal cartilage
  Lesser alar cartilage
  Nasal cavity
  Nostril
Y Sinus
	X External	**Ø** Drainage Device
		Y Other Device
			Z No Qualifier

Non-OR   All body part, approach, device, and qualifier values

Ø   **Medical and Surgical**
9   **Ear, Nose, Sinus**
3   **Control**   Definition: Stopping, or attempting to stop, postprocedural or other acute bleeding

                      Explanation: None

Body Part Character 4	Approach Character 5	Device Character 6	Qualifier Character 7

K Nasal Mucosa and Soft Tissue
  Columella
  External naris
  Greater alar cartilage
  Internal naris
  Lateral nasal cartilage
  Lesser alar cartilage
  Nasal cavity
  Nostril
	7 Via Natural or Artificial
	  Opening
	8 Via Natural or Artificial
	  Opening Endoscopic
		Z No Device	**Z** No Qualifier

Non-OR   Ø93K[7,8]ZZ

NC Noncovered Procedure   **LC** Limited Coverage   **QA** Questionable OB Admit   **NT** New Tech Add-on   ⊞ Combination Member   ♂ Male   ♀ Female

ICD-10-PCS 2023   321

Ø   Medical and Surgical
9   Ear, Nose, Sinus
5   Destruction   Definition: Physical eradication of all or a portion of a body part by the direct use of energy, force, or a destructive agent
                        Explanation: None of the body part is physically taken out

Body Part Character 4		Approach Character 5	Device Character 6	Qualifier Character 7
Ø External Ear, Right Antihelix Antitragus Auricle Earlobe Helix Pinna Tragus	**1 External Ear, Left** *See Ø External Ear, Right*	**Ø Open** **3 Percutaneous** **4 Percutaneous Endoscopic** **X External**	**Z No Device**	**Z No Qualifier**
3 External Auditory Canal, Right External auditory meatus	**4 External Auditory Canal, Left** *See 3 External Auditory Canal, Right*	**Ø Open** **3 Percutaneous** **4 Percutaneous Endoscopic** **7 Via Natural or Artificial Opening** **8 Via Natural or Artificial Opening Endoscopic** **X External**	**Z No Device**	**Z No Qualifier**
5 Middle Ear, Right Oval window Tympanic cavity **6 Middle Ear, Left** *See 5 Middle Ear, Right* **9 Auditory Ossicle, Right** Incus Malleus Stapes **A Auditory Ossicle, Left** *See 9 Auditory Ossicle, Right*	**D Inner Ear, Right** Bony labyrinth Bony vestibule Cochlea Round window Semicircular canal **E Inner Ear, Left** *See D Inner Ear, Right*	**Ø Open** **8 Via Natural or Artificial Opening Endoscopic**	**Z No Device**	**Z No Qualifier**
7 Tympanic Membrane, Right Pars flaccida **8 Tympanic Membrane, Left** *See 7 Tympanic Membrane, Right* **F Eustachian Tube, Right** Auditory tube Pharyngotympanic tube **G Eustachian Tube, Left** *See F Eustachian Tube, Right*	**L Nasal Turbinate** Inferior turbinate Middle turbinate Nasal concha Superior turbinate **N Nasopharynx** Choana Fossa of Rosenmuller Pharyngeal recess Rhinopharynx	**Ø Open** **3 Percutaneous** **4 Percutaneous Endoscopic** **7 Via Natural or Artificial Opening** **8 Via Natural or Artificial Opening Endoscopic**	**Z No Device**	**Z No Qualifier**
B Mastoid Sinus, Right Mastoid air cells **C Mastoid Sinus, Left** *See B Mastoid Sinus, Right* **M Nasal Septum** Quadrangular cartilage Septal cartilage Vomer bone **P Accessory Sinus** **Q Maxillary Sinus, Right** Antrum of Highmore	**R Maxillary Sinus, Left** *See Q Maxillary Sinus, Right* **S Frontal Sinus, Right** **T Frontal Sinus, Left** **U Ethmoid Sinus, Right** Ethmoidal air cell **V Ethmoid Sinus, Left** *See U Ethmoid Sinus, Right* **W Sphenoid Sinus, Right** **X Sphenoid Sinus, Left**	**Ø Open** **3 Percutaneous** **4 Percutaneous Endoscopic** **8 Via Natural or Artificial Opening Endoscopic**	**Z No Device**	**Z No Qualifier**
K Nasal Mucosa and Soft Tissue Columella External naris Greater alar cartilage Internal naris Lateral nasal cartilage Lesser alar cartilage Nasal cavity Nostril		**Ø Open** **3 Percutaneous** **4 Percutaneous Endoscopic** **8 Via Natural or Artificial Opening Endoscopic** **X External**	**Z No Device**	**Z No Qualifier**

Non-OR	Ø95[Ø,1][Ø,3,4,X]ZZ
Non-OR	Ø95[3,4][Ø,3,4,7,8,X]ZZ
Non-OR	Ø95[F,G][Ø,3,4,7,8]ZZ
Non-OR	Ø95M[Ø,3,4,8]ZZ
Non-OR	Ø95K[Ø,3,4,8,X]ZZ

Non-OR Procedure   DRG Non-OR Procedure   Valid OR Procedure   HAC Associated Procedure   Combination Only   New/Revised April   New/Revised October

Ø   **Medical and Surgical**
9   **Ear, Nose, Sinus**
7   **Dilation**   Definition: Expanding an orifice or the lumen of a tubular body part

Explanation: The orifice can be a natural orifice or an artificially created orifice. Accomplished by stretching a tubular body part using intraluminal pressure or by cutting part of the orifice or wall of the tubular body part.

Body Part Character 4	Approach Character 5	Device Character 6	Qualifier Character 7

F Eustachian Tube, Right
   Auditory tube
   Pharyngotympanic tube
G Eustachian Tube, Left
   See F Eustachian Tube, Right
	Ø Open
	7 Via Natural or Artificial Opening
	8 Via Natural or Artificial Opening
	   Endoscopic
		D Intraluminal Device
		Z No Device
			Z No Qualifier

F Eustachian Tube, Right
   Auditory tube
   Pharyngotympanic tube
G Eustachian Tube, Left
   See F Eustachian Tube, Right
	3 Percutaneous
	4 Percutaneous Endoscopic
		Z No Device	**Z** No Qualifier

Non-OR   All body part, approach, device, and qualifier values

Ø   **Medical and Surgical**
9   **Ear, Nose, Sinus**
8   **Division**   Definition: Cutting into a body part, without draining fluids and/or gases from the body part, in order to separate or transect a body part

Explanation: All or a portion of the body part is separated into two or more portions

Body Part Character 4	Approach Character 5	Device Character 6	Qualifier Character 7

L Nasal Turbinate
   Inferior turbinate
   Middle turbinate
   Nasal concha
   Superior turbinate
	Ø Open
	3 Percutaneous
	4 Percutaneous Endoscopic
	7 Via Natural or Artificial Opening
	8 Via Natural or Artificial Opening
	   Endoscopic
		Z No Device	**Z** No Qualifier

Ø   **Medical and Surgical**
9   **Ear, Nose, Sinus**
9   **Drainage**   Definition: Taking or letting out fluids and/or gases from a body part

                           Explanation: The qualifier DIAGNOSTIC is used to identify drainage procedures that are biopsies

Body Part Character 4		Approach Character 5	Device Character 6	Qualifier Character 7
Ø External Ear, Right Antihelix Antitragus Auricle Earlobe Helix Pinna Tragus	**1 External Ear, Left** *See Ø External Ear, Right*	**Ø** Open **3** Percutaneous **4** Percutaneous Endoscopic **X** External	**Ø** Drainage Device	**Z** No Qualifier
Ø External Ear, Right Antihelix Antitragus Auricle Earlobe Helix Pinna Tragus	**1 External Ear, Left** *See Ø External Ear, Right*	**Ø** Open **3** Percutaneous **4** Percutaneous Endoscopic **X** External	**Z** No Device	**X** Diagnostic **Z** No Qualifier
3 External Auditory Canal, Right External auditory meatus **4 External Auditory Canal, Left** *See 3 External Auditory Canal, Right*	**K Nasal Mucosa and Soft Tissue** Columella External naris Greater alar cartilage Internal naris Lateral nasal cartilage Lesser alar cartilage Nasal cavity Nostril	**Ø** Open **3** Percutaneous **4** Percutaneous Endoscopic **7** Via Natural or Artificial Opening **8** Via Natural or Artificial Opening Endoscopic **X** External	**Ø** Drainage Device	**Z** No Qualifier
3 External Auditory Canal, Right External auditory meatus **4 External Auditory Canal, Left** *See 3 External Auditory Canal, Right*	**K Nasal Mucosa and Soft Tissue** Columella External naris Greater alar cartilage Internal naris Lateral nasal cartilage Lesser alar cartilage Nasal cavity Nostril	**Ø** Open **3** Percutaneous **4** Percutaneous Endoscopic **7** Via Natural or Artificial Opening **8** Via Natural or Artificial Opening Endoscopic **X** External	**Z** No Device	**X** Diagnostic **Z** No Qualifier
5 Middle Ear, Right Oval window Tympanic cavity **6 Middle Ear, Left** *See 5 Middle Ear, Right* **9 Auditory Ossicle, Right** Incus Malleus Stapes	**A Auditory Ossicle, Left** *See 9 Auditory Ossicle, Right* **D Inner Ear, Right** Bony labyrinth Bony vestibule Cochlea Round window Semicircular canal **E Inner Ear, Left** *See D Inner Ear, Right*	**Ø** Open **7** Via Natural or Artificial Opening **8** Via Natural or Artificial Opening Endoscopic	**Ø** Drainage Device	**Z** No Qualifier
5 Middle Ear, Right Oval window Tympanic cavity **6 Middle Ear, Left** *See 5 Middle Ear, Right* **9 Auditory Ossicle, Right** Incus Malleus Stapes	**A Auditory Ossicle, Left** *See 9 Auditory Ossicle, Right* **D Inner Ear, Right** Bony labyrinth Bony vestibule Cochlea Round window Semicircular canal **E Inner Ear, Left** *See D Inner Ear, Right*	**Ø** Open **7** Via Natural or Artificial Opening **8** Via Natural or Artificial Opening Endoscopic	**Z** No Device	**X** Diagnostic **Z** No Qualifier

Non-OR   Ø99[Ø,1][Ø,3,4,X]ØZ
Non-OR   Ø99[Ø,1][Ø,3,4,X]Z[X,Z]
Non-OR   Ø99[3,4,K][Ø,3,4,7,8,X]ØZ
Non-OR   Ø99[3,4,K][Ø,3,4,7,8,X]Z[X,Z]
Non-OR   Ø99[5,6]8ØZ
Non-OR   Ø99[9,A,D,E][7,8]ØZ
Non-OR   Ø99[5,6]ØZZ
Non-OR   Ø99[5,6,9,A,D,E][7,8]Z[X,Z]

Ø99 Continued on next page

Non-OR Procedure   DRG Non-OR Procedure   Valid OR Procedure   HAC Associated Procedure   Combination Only   New/Revised April   New/Revised October

324   ICD-10-PCS 2023

Ø   **Medical and Surgical**
9   **Ear, Nose, Sinus**
9   **Drainage**   Definition: Taking or letting out fluids and/or gases from a body part

Ø99 Continued

Explanation: The qualifier DIAGNOSTIC is used to identify drainage procedures that are biopsies

Body Part Character 4		Approach Character 5	Device Character 6	Qualifier Character 7
7 Tympanic Membrane, Right Pars flaccida **8 Tympanic Membrane, Left** *See 7 Tympanic Membrane, Right* **B Mastoid Sinus, Right** Mastoid air cells **C Mastoid Sinus, Left** *See B Mastoid Sinus, Right* **F Eustachian Tube, Right** Auditory tube Pharyngotympanic tube **G Eustachian Tube, Left** *See F Eustachian Tube, Right* **L Nasal Turbinate** Inferior turbinate Middle turbinate Nasal concha Superior turbinate **M Nasal Septum** Quadrangular cartilage Septal cartilage Vomer bone	**N Nasopharynx** Choana Fossa of Rosenmuller Pharyngeal recess Rhinopharynx **P Accessory Sinus** **Q Maxillary Sinus, Right** Antrum of Highmore **R Maxillary Sinus, Left** *See Q Maxillary Sinus, Right* **S Frontal Sinus, Right** **T Frontal Sinus, Left** **U Ethmoid Sinus, Right** Ethmoidal air cell **V Ethmoid Sinus, Left** *See U Ethmoid Sinus, Right* **W Sphenoid Sinus, Right** **X Sphenoid Sinus, Left**	**Ø Open** **3 Percutaneous** **4 Percutaneous Endoscopic** **7 Via Natural or Artificial Opening** **8 Via Natural or Artificial Opening Endoscopic**	**Ø Drainage Device**	**Z No Qualifier**
7 Tympanic Membrane, Right Pars flaccida **8 Tympanic Membrane, Left** *See 7 Tympanic Membrane, Right* **B Mastoid Sinus, Right** Mastoid air cells **C Mastoid Sinus, Left** *See B Mastoid Sinus, Right* **F Eustachian Tube, Right** Auditory tube Pharyngotympanic tube **G Eustachian Tube, Left** *See F Eustachian Tube, Right* **L Nasal Turbinate** Inferior turbinate Middle turbinate Nasal concha Superior turbinate **M Nasal Septum** Quadrangular cartilage Septal cartilage Vomer bone	**N Nasopharynx** Choana Fossa of Rosenmuller Pharyngeal recess Rhinopharynx **P Accessory Sinus** **Q Maxillary Sinus, Right** Antrum of Highmore **R Maxillary Sinus, Left** *See Q Maxillary Sinus, Right* **S Frontal Sinus, Right** **T Frontal Sinus, Left** **U Ethmoid Sinus, Right** Ethmoidal air cell **V Ethmoid Sinus, Left** *See U Ethmoid Sinus, Right* **W Sphenoid Sinus, Right** **X Sphenoid Sinus, Left**	**Ø Open** **3 Percutaneous** **4 Percutaneous Endoscopic** **7 Via Natural or Artificial Opening** **8 Via Natural or Artificial Opening Endoscopic**	**Z No Device**	**X Diagnostic** **Z No Qualifier**

Non-OR	Ø99[B,C][3,7,8]ØZ
Non-OR	Ø99[F,G,L,M][Ø,3,4,7,8]ØZ
Non-OR	Ø99N3ØZ
Non-OR	Ø99[P,Q,R,S,T,U,V,W,X][3,4,7,8]ØZ
Non-OR	Ø99[7,8][Ø,3,4,7,8]ZZ
Non-OR	Ø99[7,8][7,8]ZX
Non-OR	Ø99[B,C]3ZZ
Non-OR	Ø99[B,C][7,8]Z[X,Z]
Non-OR	Ø99[F,G][Ø,3,4,7,8]ZZ
Non-OR	Ø99[F,G][7,8]ZX
Non-OR	Ø99[L,M][Ø,3,4,7,8]Z[X,Z]
Non-OR	Ø99N[Ø,3,4,7,8]ZX
Non-OR	Ø99N3ZZ
Non-OR	Ø99[P,Q,R,S,T,U,V,W,X][3,4,7,8]Z[X,Z]

NC Noncovered Procedure   LC Limited Coverage   QA Questionable OB Admit   NT New Tech Add-on   ⊞ Combination Member   ♂ Male   ♀ Female

ICD-10-PCS 2023   **325**

Ø99–Ø99

Ear, Nose, Sinus

0   **Medical and Surgical**
9   **Ear, Nose, Sinus**
B   **Excision**

             Definition: Cutting out or off, without replacement, a portion of a body part
             Explanation: The qualifier DIAGNOSTIC is used to identify excision procedures that are biopsies

Body Part — Character 4		Approach — Character 5	Device — Character 6	Qualifier — Character 7
0 External Ear, Right Antihelix Antitragus Auricle Earlobe Helix Pinna Tragus	**1** External Ear, Left *See 0 External Ear, Right*	**0** Open **3** Percutaneous **4** Percutaneous Endoscopic **X** External	**Z** No Device	**X** Diagnostic **Z** No Qualifier
3 External Auditory Canal, Right External auditory meatus	**4** External Auditory Canal, Left *See 3 External Auditory Canal, Right*	**0** Open **3** Percutaneous **4** Percutaneous Endoscopic **7** Via Natural or Artificial Opening **8** Via Natural or Artificial Opening Endoscopic **X** External	**Z** No Device	**X** Diagnostic **Z** No Qualifier
5 Middle Ear, Right Oval window Tympanic cavity **6** Middle Ear, Left *See 5 Middle Ear, Right* **9** Auditory Ossicle, Right Incus Malleus Stapes	**A** Auditory Ossicle, Left *See 9 Auditory Ossicle, Right* **D** Inner Ear, Right Bony labyrinth Bony vestibule Cochlea Round window Semicircular canal **E** Inner Ear, Left *See D Inner Ear, Right*	**0** Open **8** Via Natural or Artificial Opening Endoscopic	**Z** No Device	**X** Diagnostic **Z** No Qualifier
7 Tympanic Membrane, Right Pars flaccida **8** Tympanic Membrane, Left *See 7 Tympanic Membrane, Right* **F** Eustachian Tube, Right Auditory tube Pharyngotympanic tube **G** Eustachian Tube, Left *See F Eustachian Tube, Right*	**L** Nasal Turbinate Inferior turbinate Middle turbinate Nasal concha Superior turbinate **N** Nasopharynx Choana Fossa of Rosenmuller Pharyngeal recess Rhinopharynx	**0** Open **3** Percutaneous **4** Percutaneous Endoscopic **7** Via Natural or Artificial Opening **8** Via Natural or Artificial Opening Endoscopic	**Z** No Device	**X** Diagnostic **Z** No Qualifier
B Mastoid Sinus, Right Mastoid air cells **C** Mastoid Sinus, Left *See B Mastoid Sinus, Right* **M** Nasal Septum Quadrangular cartilage Septal cartilage Vomer bone **P** Accessory Sinus **Q** Maxillary Sinus, Right Antrum of Highmore	**R** Maxillary Sinus, Left *See Q Maxillary Sinus, Right* **S** Frontal Sinus, Right **T** Frontal Sinus, Left **U** Ethmoid Sinus, Right Ethmoidal air cell **V** Ethmoid Sinus, Left *See U Ethmoid Sinus, Right* **W** Sphenoid Sinus, Right **X** Sphenoid Sinus, Left	**0** Open **3** Percutaneous **4** Percutaneous Endoscopic **8** Via Natural or Artificial Opening Endoscopic	**Z** No Device	**X** Diagnostic **Z** No Qualifier
K Nasal Mucosa and Soft Tissue Columella External naris Greater alar cartilage Internal naris Lateral nasal cartilage Lesser alar cartilage Nasal cavity Nostril		**0** Open **3** Percutaneous **4** Percutaneous Endoscopic **8** Via Natural or Artificial Opening Endoscopic **X** External	**Z** No Device	**X** Diagnostic **Z** No Qualifier

Non-OR   09B[0,1][0,3,4,X]Z[X,Z]
Non-OR   09B[3,4][0,3,4,7,8,X]Z[X,Z]
Non-OR   09B[F,G,L,N][0,3,4,7,8]Z[X,Z]
Non-OR   09BM[0,3,4,8]ZX
Non-OR   09B[P,Q,R,S,T,U,V,W,X][3,4,8]ZX
Non-OR   09BK8Z[X,Z]

Non-OR Procedure   DRG Non-OR Procedure   Valid OR Procedure   HAC Associated Procedure   Combination Only   New/Revised April   New/Revised October

326   ICD-10-PCS 2023

Ø   **Medical and Surgical**
9   **Ear, Nose, Sinus**
C   **Extirpation**   Definition: Taking or cutting out solid matter from a body part

Explanation: The solid matter may be an abnormal byproduct of a biological function or a foreign body; it may be imbedded in a body part or in the lumen of a tubular body part. The solid matter may or may not have been previously broken into pieces.

Body Part Character 4		Approach Character 5	Device Character 6	Qualifier Character 7
Ø External Ear, Right Antihelix Antitragus Auricle Earlobe Helix Pinna Tragus	**1 External Ear, Left** *See Ø External Ear, Right*	**Ø Open** **3 Percutaneous** **4 Percutaneous Endoscopic** **X External**	**Z No Device**	**Z No Qualifier**
3 External Auditory Canal, Right External auditory meatus	**4 External Auditory Canal, Left** *See 3 External Auditory Canal, Right*	**Ø Open** **3 Percutaneous** **4 Percutaneous Endoscopic** **7 Via Natural or Artificial Opening** **8 Via Natural or Artificial Opening Endoscopic** **X External**	**Z No Device**	**Z No Qualifier**
5 Middle Ear, Right Oval window Tympanic cavity **6 Middle Ear, Left** *See 5 Middle Ear, Right* **9 Auditory Ossicle, Right** Incus Malleus Stapes	**A Auditory Ossicle, Left** *See 9 Auditory Ossicle, Right* **D Inner Ear, Right** Bony labyrinth Bony vestibule Cochlea Round window Semicircular canal **E Inner Ear, Left** *See D Inner Ear, Right*	**Ø Open** **8 Via Natural or Artificial Opening Endoscopic**	**Z No Device**	**Z No Qualifier**
7 Tympanic Membrane, Right Pars flaccida **8 Tympanic Membrane, Left** *See 7 Tympanic Membrane, Right* **F Eustachian Tube, Right** Auditory tube Pharyngotympanic tube **G Eustachian Tube, Left** *See F Eustachian Tube, Right*	**L Nasal Turbinate** Inferior turbinate Middle turbinate Nasal concha Superior turbinate **N Nasopharynx** Choana Fossa of Rosenmuller Pharyngeal recess Rhinopharynx	**Ø Open** **3 Percutaneous** **4 Percutaneous Endoscopic** **7 Via Natural or Artificial Opening** **8 Via Natural or Artificial Opening Endoscopic**	**Z No Device**	**Z No Qualifier**
B Mastoid Sinus, Right Mastoid air cells **C Mastoid Sinus, Left** *See B Mastoid Sinus, Right* **M Nasal Septum** Quadrangular cartilage Septal cartilage Vomer bone **P Accessory Sinus** **Q Maxillary Sinus, Right** Antrum of Highmore	**R Maxillary Sinus, Left** *See Q Maxillary Sinus, Right* **S Frontal Sinus, Right** **T Frontal Sinus, Left** **U Ethmoid Sinus, Right** Ethmoidal air cell **V Ethmoid Sinus, Left** *See U Ethmoid Sinus, Right* **W Sphenoid Sinus, Right** **X Sphenoid Sinus, Left**	**Ø Open** **3 Percutaneous** **4 Percutaneous Endoscopic** **8 Via Natural or Artificial Opening Endoscopic**	**Z No Device**	**Z No Qualifier**
K Nasal Mucosa and Soft Tissue Columella External naris Greater alar cartilage Internal naris Lateral nasal cartilage Lesser alar cartilage Nasal cavity Nostril		**Ø Open** **3 Percutaneous** **4 Percutaneous Endoscopic** **8 Via Natural or Artificial Opening Endoscopic** **X External**	**Z No Device**	**Z No Qualifier**

Non-OR	Ø9C[Ø,1][Ø,3,4,X]ZZ
Non-OR	Ø9C[3,4][Ø,3,4,7,8,X]ZZ
Non-OR	Ø9C[7,8,F,G,L][Ø,3,4,7,8]ZZ
Non-OR	Ø9CM[Ø,3,4,8]ZZ
Non-OR	Ø9CK8ZZ

NC Noncovered Procedure   **LC** Limited Coverage   **QA** Questionable OB Admit   **NT** New Tech Add-on   ⊞ Combination Member   ♂ Male   ♀ Female

ICD-10-PCS 2023   **327**

Ø9C–Ø9C

Ear, Nose, Sinus

Ø   **Medical and Surgical**
9   **Ear, Nose, Sinus**
D   **Extraction**   Definition: Pulling or stripping out or off all or a portion of a body part by the use of force
                 Explanation: The qualifier DIAGNOSTIC is used to identify extraction procedures that are biopsies

Body Part Character 4	Approach Character 5	Device Character 6	Qualifier Character 7
7 Tympanic Membrane, Right Pars flaccida **8 Tympanic Membrane, Left** *See 7 Tympanic Membrane, Right* **L Nasal Turbinate** Inferior turbinate Middle turbinate Nasal concha Superior turbinate	**Ø** Open **3** Percutaneous **4** Percutaneous Endoscopic **7** Via Natural or Artificial Opening **8** Via Natural or Artificial Opening Endoscopic	**Z** No Device	**Z** No Qualifier
9 Auditory Ossicle, Right Incus Malleus Stapes **A Auditory Ossicle, Left** *See 9 Auditory Ossicle, Right*	**Ø** Open	**Z** No Device	**Z** No Qualifier
B Mastoid Sinus, Right Mastoid air cells **C Mastoid Sinus, Left** *See B Mastoid Sinus, Right* **M Nasal Septum** Quadrangular cartilage Septal cartilage Vomer bone **P Accessory Sinus** **Q Maxillary Sinus, Right** Antrum of Highmore **R Maxillary Sinus, Left** *See Q Maxillary Sinus, Right* **S Frontal Sinus, Right** **T Frontal Sinus, Left** **U Ethmoid Sinus, Right** Ethmoidal air cell **V Ethmoid Sinus, Left** *See U Ethmoid Sinus, Right* **W Sphenoid Sinus, Right** **X Sphenoid Sinus, Left**	**Ø** Open **3** Percutaneous **4** Percutaneous Endoscopic	**Z** No Device	**Z** No Qualifier

Ø   **Medical and Surgical**
9   **Ear, Nose, Sinus**
H   **Insertion**   Definition: Putting in a nonbiological appliance that monitors, assists, performs, or prevents a physiological function but does not physically
                 take the place of a body part
                 Explanation: None

Body Part Character 4	Approach Character 5	Device Character 6	Qualifier Character 7

D Inner Ear, Right
Bony labyrinth
Bony vestibule
Cochlea
Round window
Semicircular canal
E Inner Ear, Left
See D Inner Ear, Right
	Ø Open
	3 Percutaneous
	4 Percutaneous Endoscopic
		1 Radioactive Element
		4 Hearing Device, Bone Conduction
		5 Hearing Device, Single Channel
		    Cochlear Prosthesis
		6 Hearing Device, Multiple Channel
		    Cochlear Prosthesis
		S Hearing Device
			Z No Qualifier

H Ear, Right **J Ear, Left** **K Nasal Mucosa and Soft Tissue** Columella External naris Greater alar cartilage Internal naris Lateral nasal cartilage Lesser alar cartilage Nasal cavity Nostril **Y Sinus**	**Ø** Open **3** Percutaneous **4** Percutaneous Endoscopic **7** Via Natural or Artificial Opening **8** Via Natural or Artificial Opening Endoscopic	**1** Radioactive Element **Y** Other Device	**Z** No Qualifier
N Nasopharynx Choana Fossa of Rosenmuller Pharyngeal recess Rhinopharynx	**7** Via Natural or Artificial Opening **8** Via Natural or Artificial Opening Endoscopic	**1** Radioactive Element **B** Intraluminal Device, Airway	**Z** No Qualifier

Non-OR Ø9H[H,J,K]Ø1Z		**Non-OR** Ø9H[H,J,K,Y][3,4,7,8][1,Y]Z	
Non-OR Ø9HKØYZ		**Non-OR** Ø9HN[7,8][1,B]Z	

Non-OR Procedure   DRG Non-OR Procedure   Valid OR Procedure   HAC Associated Procedure   Combination Only   New/Revised April   New/Revised October

328

ICD-10-PCS 2023

Ø   **Medical and Surgical**
9   **Ear, Nose, Sinus**
J   **Inspection**   Definition: Visually and/or manually exploring a body part

Explanation: Visual exploration may be performed with or without optical instrumentation. Manual exploration may be performed directly or through intervening body layers.

Body Part Character 4	Approach Character 5	Device Character 6	Qualifier Character 7
7 **Tympanic Membrane, Right** Pars flaccida 8 **Tympanic Membrane, Left** *See 7 Tympanic Membrane, Right* H **Ear, Right** J **Ear, Left**	Ø Open 3 Percutaneous 4 Percutaneous Endoscopic 7 Via Natural or Artificial Opening 8 Via Natural or Artificial Opening Endoscopic X External	Z No Device	Z No Qualifier
D **Inner Ear, Right** Bony labyrinth Bony vestibule Cochlea Round window Semicircular canal E **Inner Ear, Left** *See D Inner Ear, Right* K **Nasal Mucosa and Soft Tissue** Columella External naris Greater alar cartilage Internal naris Lateral nasal cartilage Lesser alar cartilage Nasal cavity Nostril Y **Sinus**	Ø Open 3 Percutaneous 4 Percutaneous Endoscopic 8 Via Natural or Artificial Opening Endoscopic X External	Z No Device	Z No Qualifier

Non-OR   09J[7,8][3,7,8,X]ZZ
Non-OR   09J[H,J][Ø,3,4,7,8,X]ZZ
Non-OR   09J[D,E][3,8,X]ZZ
Non-OR   09J[K,Y][Ø,3,4,8,X]ZZ

Ø   **Medical and Surgical**
9   **Ear, Nose, Sinus**
M   **Reattachment**   Definition: Putting back in or on all or a portion of a separated body part to its normal location or other suitable location

Explanation: Vascular circulation and nervous pathways may or may not be reestablished

Body Part Character 4	Approach Character 5	Device Character 6	Qualifier Character 7
Ø **External Ear, Right** Antihelix Antitragus Auricle Earlobe Helix Pinna Tragus 1 **External Ear, Left** *See Ø External Ear, Right* K **Nasal Mucosa and Soft Tissue** Columella External naris Greater alar cartilage Internal naris Lateral nasal cartilage Lesser alar cartilage Nasal cavity Nostril	X External	Z No Device	Z No Qualifier

NC Noncovered Procedure   **LC** Limited Coverage   **QA** Questionable OB Admit   **NT** New Tech Add-on   ⊞ Combination Member   ♂ Male   ♀ Female

ICD-10-PCS 2023   329

09J–09M

Ø   **Medical and Surgical**
9   **Ear, Nose, Sinus**
N   **Release**   Definition: Freeing a body part from an abnormal physical constraint by cutting or by the use of force

                         Explanation: Some of the restraining tissue may be taken out but none of the body part is taken out

Body Part Character 4		Approach Character 5	Device Character 6	Qualifier Character 7
Ø External Ear, Right Antihelix Antitragus Auricle Earlobe Helix Pinna Tragus	**1 External Ear, Left** *See Ø External Ear, Right*	**Ø** Open **3** Percutaneous **4** Percutaneous Endoscopic **X** External	**Z** No Device	**Z** No Qualifier
3 External Auditory Canal, Right External auditory meatus	**4 External Auditory Canal, Left** *See 3 External Auditory Canal, Right*	**Ø** Open **3** Percutaneous **4** Percutaneous Endoscopic **7** Via Natural or Artificial Opening **8** Via Natural or Artificial Opening Endoscopic **X** External	**Z** No Device	**Z** No Qualifier
5 Middle Ear, Right Oval window Tympanic cavity **6 Middle Ear, Left** *See 5 Middle Ear, Right* **9 Auditory Ossicle, Right** Incus Malleus Stapes	**A Auditory Ossicle, Left** *See 9 Auditory Ossicle, Right* **D Inner Ear, Right** Bony labyrinth Bony vestibule Cochlea Round window Semicircular canal **E Inner Ear, Left** *See D Inner Ear, Right*	**Ø** Open **8** Via Natural or Artificial Opening Endoscopic	**Z** No Device	**Z** No Qualifier
7 Tympanic Membrane, Right Pars flaccida **8 Tympanic Membrane, Left** *See 7 Tympanic Membrane, Right* **F Eustachian Tube, Right** Auditory tube Pharyngotympanic tube **G Eustachian Tube, Left** *See F Eustachian Tube, Right*	**L Nasal Turbinate** Inferior turbinate Middle turbinate Nasal concha Superior turbinate **N Nasopharynx** Choana Fossa of Rosenmuller Pharyngeal recess Rhinopharynx	**Ø** Open **3** Percutaneous **4** Percutaneous Endoscopic **7** Via Natural or Artificial Opening **8** Via Natural or Artificial Opening Endoscopic	**Z** No Device	**Z** No Qualifier
B Mastoid Sinus, Right Mastoid air cells **C Mastoid Sinus, Left** *See B Mastoid Sinus, Right* **M Nasal Septum** Quadrangular cartilage Septal cartilage Vomer bone **P Accessory Sinus** **Q Maxillary Sinus, Right** Antrum of Highmore	**R Maxillary Sinus, Left** *See Q Maxillary Sinus, Right* **S Frontal Sinus, Right** **T Frontal Sinus, Left** **U Ethmoid Sinus, Right** Ethmoidal air cell **V Ethmoid Sinus, Left** *See U Ethmoid Sinus, Right* **W Sphenoid Sinus, Right** **X Sphenoid Sinus, Left**	**Ø** Open **3** Percutaneous **4** Percutaneous Endoscopic **8** Via Natural or Artificial Opening Endoscopic	**Z** No Device	**Z** No Qualifier
K Nasal Mucosa and Soft Tissue Columella External naris Greater alar cartilage Internal naris Lateral nasal cartilage Lesser alar cartilage Nasal cavity Nostril		**Ø** Open **3** Percutaneous **4** Percutaneous Endoscopic **8** Via Natural or Artificial Opening Endoscopic **X** External	**Z** No Device	**Z** No Qualifier

Non-OR	Ø9N[Ø,1]XZZ
Non-OR	Ø9N[3,4]XZZ
Non-OR	Ø9N[F,G,L][Ø,3,4,7,8]ZZ
Non-OR	Ø9NM[Ø,3,4,8]ZZ
Non-OR	Ø9NK[Ø,3,4,8,X]ZZ

Non-OR Procedure   DRG Non-OR Procedure   Valid OR Procedure   HAC Associated Procedure   Combination Only   New/Revised April   New/Revised October

330   ICD-10-PCS 2023

Ø	Medical and Surgical
9	Ear, Nose, Sinus
P	Removal

Definition: Taking out or off a device from a body part

Explanation: If a device is taken out and a similar device put in without cutting or puncturing the skin or mucous membrane, the procedure is coded to the root operation CHANGE. Otherwise, the procedure for taking out a device is coded to the root operation REMOVAL.

Body Part Character 4		Approach Character 5	Device Character 6	Qualifier Character 7
7 8	**Tympanic Membrane, Right** 　Pars flaccida **Tympanic Membrane, Left** 　*See 7 Tympanic Membrane, Right*	Ø　Open 7　Via Natural or Artificial Opening 8　Via Natural or Artificial Opening 　　Endoscopic X　External	Ø　Drainage Device	Z　No Qualifier
D E	**Inner Ear, Right** 　Bony labyrinth 　Bony vestibule 　Cochlea 　Round window 　Semicircular canal **Inner Ear, Left** 　*See D Inner Ear, Right*	Ø　Open 7　Via Natural or Artificial Opening 8　Via Natural or Artificial Opening 　　Endoscopic	S　Hearing Device	Z　No Qualifier
H J K	**Ear, Right** **Ear, Left** **Nasal Mucosa and Soft Tissue** 　Columella 　External naris 　Greater alar cartilage 　Internal naris 　Lateral nasal cartilage 　Lesser alar cartilage 　Nasal cavity 　Nostril	Ø　Open 3　Percutaneous 4　Percutaneous Endoscopic 7　Via Natural or Artificial Opening 8　Via Natural or Artificial Opening 　　Endoscopic	Ø　Drainage Device 7　Autologous Tissue Substitute D　Intraluminal Device J　Synthetic Substitute K　Nonautologous Tissue Substitute Y　Other Device	Z　No Qualifier
H J K	**Ear, Right** **Ear, Left** **Nasal Mucosa and Soft Tissue** 　Columella 　External naris 　Greater alar cartilage 　Internal naris 　Lateral nasal cartilage 　Lesser alar cartilage 　Nasal cavity 　Nostril	X　External	Ø　Drainage Device 7　Autologous Tissue Substitute D　Intraluminal Device J　Synthetic Substitute K　Nonautologous Tissue Substitute	Z　No Qualifier
Y	**Sinus**	Ø　Open 3　Percutaneous 4　Percutaneous Endoscopic	Ø　Drainage Device Y　Other Device	Z　No Qualifier
Y	**Sinus**	7　Via Natural or Artificial Opening 8　Via Natural or Artificial Opening 　　Endoscopic	Y　Other Device	Z　No Qualifier
Y	**Sinus**	X　External	Ø　Drainage Device	Z　No Qualifier

Non-OR	Ø9P[7,8][Ø,7,8,X]ØZ
Non-OR	Ø9P[H,J][3,4][Ø,J,K,Y]Z
Non-OR	Ø9P[H,J][7,8][Ø,D,Y]Z
Non-OR	Ø9PK[Ø,3,4,7,8][Ø,7,D,J,K,Y]Z
Non-OR	Ø9P[H,J]X[Ø,7,D,J,K]Z
Non-OR	Ø9PKX[Ø,7,D,J,K]Z
Non-OR	Ø9PY[3,4]YZ
Non-OR	Ø9PY[7,8]YZ
Non-OR	Ø9PYXØZ

NC Noncovered Procedure　　**LC** Limited Coverage　　**QA** Questionable OB Admit　　**NT** New Tech Add-on　　⊞ Combination Member　　♂ Male　　♀ Female

ICD-10-PCS 2023　　　331

Ø9P–Ø9P

Ø   **Medical and Surgical**
9   **Ear, Nose, Sinus**
Q   **Repair**   Definition: Restoring, to the extent possible, a body part to its normal anatomic structure and function
                        Explanation: Used only when the method to accomplish the repair is not one of the other root operations

Body Part Character 4		Approach Character 5	Device Character 6	Qualifier Character 7
Ø External Ear, Right Antihelix Antitragus Auricle Earlobe Helix Pinna Tragus	**1 External Ear, Left** *See Ø External Ear, Right* **2 External Ear, Bilateral** *See Ø External Ear, Right*	**Ø** Open **3** Percutaneous **4** Percutaneous Endoscopic **X** External	**Z** No Device	**Z** No Qualifier
3 External Auditory Canal, Right External auditory meatus **4 External Auditory Canal, Left** *See 3 External Auditory Canal, Right*	**F Eustachian Tube, Right** Auditory tube Pharyngotympanic tube **G Eustachian Tube, Left** *See F Eustachian Tube, Right*	**Ø** Open **3** Percutaneous **4** Percutaneous Endoscopic **7** Via Natural or Artificial Opening **8** Via Natural or Artificial Opening Endoscopic **X** External	**Z** No Device	**Z** No Qualifier
5 Middle Ear, Right Oval window Tympanic cavity **6 Middle Ear, Left** *See 5 Middle Ear, Right* **9 Auditory Ossicle, Right** Incus Malleus Stapes	**A Auditory Ossicle, Left** *See 9 Auditory Ossicle, Right* **D Inner Ear, Right** Bony labyrinth Bony vestibule Cochlea Round window Semicircular canal **E Inner Ear, Left** *See D Inner Ear, Right*	**Ø** Open **8** Via Natural or Artificial Opening Endoscopic	**Z** No Device	**Z** No Qualifier
7 Tympanic Membrane, Right Pars flaccida **8 Tympanic Membrane, Left** *See 7 Tympanic Membrane, Right* **L Nasal Turbinate** Inferior turbinate Middle turbinate Nasal concha Superior turbinate	**N Nasopharynx** Choana Fossa of Rosenmuller Pharyngeal recess Rhinopharynx	**Ø** Open **3** Percutaneous **4** Percutaneous Endoscopic **7** Via Natural or Artificial Opening **8** Via Natural or Artificial Opening Endoscopic	**Z** No Device	**Z** No Qualifier
B Mastoid Sinus, Right Mastoid air cells **C Mastoid Sinus, Left** *See B Mastoid Sinus, Right* **M Nasal Septum** Quadrangular cartilage Septal cartilage Vomer bone **P Accessory Sinus** **Q Maxillary Sinus, Right** Antrum of Highmore	**R Maxillary Sinus, Left** *See Q Maxillary Sinus, Right* **S Frontal Sinus, Right** **T Frontal Sinus, Left** **U Ethmoid Sinus, Right** Ethmoidal air cell **V Ethmoid Sinus, Left** *See U Ethmoid Sinus, Right* **W Sphenoid Sinus, Right** **X Sphenoid Sinus, Left**	**Ø** Open **3** Percutaneous **4** Percutaneous Endoscopic **8** Via Natural or Artificial Opening Endoscopic	**Z** No Device	**Z** No Qualifier
K Nasal Mucosa and Soft Tissue Columella External naris Greater alar cartilage Internal naris Lateral nasal cartilage Lesser alar cartilage Nasal cavity Nostril		**Ø** Open **3** Percutaneous **4** Percutaneous Endoscopic **8** Via Natural or Artificial Opening Endoscopic **X** External	**Z** No Device	**Z** No Qualifier

Non-OR	Ø9Q[Ø,1,2]XZZ
Non-OR	Ø9Q[3,4]XZZ
Non-OR	Ø9Q[F,G][Ø,3,4,7,8,X]ZZ
Non-OR	Ø9QKXZZ

Non-OR Procedure   DRG Non-OR Procedure   Valid OR Procedure   HAC Associated Procedure   Combination Only   New/Revised April   New/Revised October

332   ICD-10-PCS 2023

0   **Medical and Surgical**
9   **Ear, Nose, Sinus**
R   **Replacement**   Definition: Putting in or on biological or synthetic material that physically takes the place and/or function of all or a portion of a body part

Explanation: The body part may have been taken out or replaced, or may be taken out, physically eradicated, or rendered nonfunctional during the REPLACEMENT procedure. A REMOVAL procedure is coded for taking out the device used in a previous replacement procedure.

Body Part Character 4	Approach Character 5	Device Character 6	Qualifier Character 7

0 **External Ear, Right**
   Antihelix
   Antitragus
   Auricle
   Earlobe
   Helix
   Pinna
   Tragus
1 **External Ear, Left**
   See 0 External Ear, Right
2 **External Ear, Bilateral**
   See 0 External Ear, Right
K **Nasal Mucosa and Soft Tissue**
   Columella
   External naris
   Greater alar cartilage
   Internal naris
   Lateral nasal cartilage
   Lesser alar cartilage
   Nasal cavity
   Nostril
	0 Open
	X External
		7 Autologous Tissue Substitute
		J Synthetic Substitute
		K Nonautologous Tissue Substitute
			Z No Qualifier

5 **Middle Ear, Right**
   Oval window
   Tympanic cavity
6 **Middle Ear, Left**
   See 5 Middle Ear, Right
9 **Auditory Ossicle, Right**
   Incus
   Malleus
   Stapes
A **Auditory Ossicle, Left**
   See 9 Auditory Ossicle, Right
D **Inner Ear, Right**
   Bony labyrinth
   Bony vestibule
   Cochlea
   Round window
   Semicircular canal
E **Inner Ear, Left**
   See D Inner Ear, Right
	0 Open	**7** Autologous Tissue Substitute
		J Synthetic Substitute
		K Nonautologous Tissue Substitute
			Z No Qualifier

7 **Tympanic Membrane, Right**
   Pars flaccida
8 **Tympanic Membrane, Left**
   See 7 Tympanic Membrane, Right
N **Nasopharynx**
   Choana
   Fossa of Rosenmuller
   Pharyngeal recess
   Rhinopharynx
	0 Open
	7 Via Natural or Artificial Opening
	8 Via Natural or Artificial Opening Endoscopic
		7 Autologous Tissue Substitute
		J Synthetic Substitute
		K Nonautologous Tissue Substitute
			Z No Qualifier

L **Nasal Turbinate**
   Inferior turbinate
   Middle turbinate
   Nasal concha
   Superior turbinate
	0 Open
	3 Percutaneous
	4 Percutaneous Endoscopic
	7 Via Natural or Artificial Opening
	8 Via Natural or Artificial Opening Endoscopic
		7 Autologous Tissue Substitute
		J Synthetic Substitute
		K Nonautologous Tissue Substitute
			Z No Qualifier

M **Nasal Septum**
   Quadrangular cartilage
   Septal cartilage
   Vomer bone
	0 Open
	3 Percutaneous
	4 Percutaneous Endoscopic
		7 Autologous Tissue Substitute
		J Synthetic Substitute
		K Nonautologous Tissue Substitute
			Z No Qualifier

NC Noncovered Procedure   LC Limited Coverage   QA Questionable OB Admit   NT New Tech Add-on   ⊞ Combination Member   ♂ Male   ♀ Female

ICD-10-PCS 2023   333

09R–09R

Ø   Medical and Surgical
9   Ear, Nose, Sinus
S   Reposition   Definition: Moving to its normal location, or other suitable location, all or a portion of a body part

Explanation: The body part is moved to a new location from an abnormal location, or from a normal location where it is not functioning correctly. The body part may or may not be cut out or off to be moved to the new location.

Body Part Character 4	Approach Character 5	Device Character 6	Qualifier Character 7
Ø External Ear, Right Antihelix Antitragus Auricle Earlobe Helix Pinna Tragus **1 External Ear, Left** *See Ø External Ear, Right* **2 External Ear, Bilateral** *See Ø External Ear, Right* **K Nasal Mucosa and Soft Tissue** Columella External naris Greater alar cartilage Internal naris Lateral nasal cartilage Lesser alar cartilage Nasal cavity Nostril	**Ø Open** **4 Percutaneous Endoscopic** **X External**	**Z No Device**	**Z No Qualifier**
7 Tympanic Membrane, Right Pars flaccida **8 Tympanic Membrane, Left** *See 7 Tympanic Membrane, Right* **F Eustachian Tube, Right** Auditory tube Pharyngotympanic tube **G Eustachian Tube, Left** *See F Eustachian Tube, Right* **L Nasal Turbinate** Inferior turbinate Middle turbinate Nasal concha Superior turbinate	**Ø Open** **4 Percutaneous Endoscopic** **7 Via Natural or Artificial Opening** **8 Via Natural or Artificial Opening Endoscopic**	**Z No Device**	**Z No Qualifier**
9 Auditory Ossicle, Right Incus Malleus Stapes **A Auditory Ossicle, Left** *See 9 Auditory Ossicle, Right* **M Nasal Septum** Quadrangular cartilage Septal cartilage Vomer bone	**Ø Open** **4 Percutaneous Endoscopic**	**Z No Device**	**Z No Qualifier**

Non-OR   09S[F,G][Ø,4,7,8]ZZ

Non-OR Procedure   DRG Non-OR Procedure   Valid OR Procedure   HAC Associated Procedure   Combination Only   New/Revised April   New/Revised October

334

ICD-10-PCS 2023

0   **Medical and Surgical**
9   **Ear, Nose, Sinus**
T   **Resection**   Definition: Cutting out or off, without replacement, all of a body part
                  Explanation: None

Body Part Character 4		Approach Character 5	Device Character 6	Qualifier Character 7

0 External Ear, Right
   Antihelix
   Antitragus
   Auricle
   Earlobe
   Helix
   Pinna
   Tragus
	1 External Ear, Left
	   See 0 External Ear, Right
		0 Open
		4 Percutaneous Endoscopic
		X External
			Z No Device	**Z** No Qualifier

5 Middle Ear, Right
   Oval window
   Tympanic cavity
6 Middle Ear, Left
   See 5 Middle Ear, Right
9 Auditory Ossicle, Right
   Incus
   Malleus
   Stapes
	A Auditory Ossicle, Left
	   See 9 Auditory Ossicle, Right
	D Inner Ear, Right
	   Bony labyrinth
	   Bony vestibule
	   Cochlea
	   Round window
	   Semicircular canal
	E Inner Ear, Left
	   See D Inner Ear, Right
		0 Open
		8 Via Natural or Artificial Opening Endoscopic
			Z No Device	**Z** No Qualifier

7 Tympanic Membrane, Right
   Pars flaccida
8 Tympanic Membrane, Left
   See 7 Tympanic Membrane, Right
F Eustachian Tube, Right
   Auditory tube
   Pharyngotympanic tube
G Eustachian Tube, Left
   See F Eustachian Tube, Right
	L Nasal Turbinate
	   Inferior turbinate
	   Middle turbinate
	   Nasal concha
	   Superior turbinate
	N Nasopharynx
	   Choana
	   Fossa of Rosenmuller
	   Pharyngeal recess
	   Rhinopharynx
		0 Open
		4 Percutaneous Endoscopic
		7 Via Natural or Artificial Opening
		8 Via Natural or Artificial Opening Endoscopic
			Z No Device	**Z** No Qualifier

B Mastoid Sinus, Right
   Mastoid air cells
C Mastoid Sinus, Left
   See B Mastoid Sinus, Right
M Nasal Septum
   Quadrangular cartilage
   Septal cartilage
   Vomer bone
P Accessory Sinus
Q Maxillary Sinus, Right
   Antrum of Highmore
	R Maxillary Sinus, Left
	   See Q Maxillary Sinus, Right
	S Frontal Sinus, Right
	T Frontal Sinus, Left
	U Ethmoid Sinus, Right
	   Ethmoidal air cell
	V Ethmoid Sinus, Left
	   See U Ethmoid Sinus, Right
	W Sphenoid Sinus, Right
	X Sphenoid Sinus, Left
		0 Open
		4 Percutaneous Endoscopic
		8 Via Natural or Artificial Opening Endoscopic
			Z No Device	**Z** No Qualifier

K Nasal Mucosa and Soft Tissue
   Columella
   External naris
   Greater alar cartilage
   Internal naris
   Lateral nasal cartilage
   Lesser alar cartilage
   Nasal cavity
   Nostril
		0 Open
		4 Percutaneous Endoscopic
		8 Via Natural or Artificial Opening Endoscopic
		X External
			Z No Device	**Z** No Qualifier

Non-OR   09T[F,G][0,4,7,8]ZZ

NC Noncovered Procedure   **LC** Limited Coverage   **QA** Questionable OB Admit   **NT** New Tech Add-on   ⊞ Combination Member   ♂ Male   ♀ Female

ICD-10-PCS 2023   **335**

Ø   Medical and Surgical
9   Ear, Nose, Sinus
U   Supplement

Definition: Putting in or on biological or synthetic material that physically reinforces and/or augments the function of a portion of a body part

Explanation: The biological material is non-living, or is living and from the same individual. The body part may have been previously replaced, and the SUPPLEMENT procedure is performed to physically reinforce and/or augment the function of the replaced body part.

Body Part — Character 4		Approach — Character 5	Device — Character 6	Qualifier — Character 7

Ø **External Ear, Right**
  Antihelix
  Antitragus
  Auricle
  Earlobe
  Helix
  Pinna
  Tragus
	1 **External Ear, Left**
	  See Ø External Ear, Right
	2 **External Ear, Bilateral**
	  See Ø External Ear, Right
		Ø Open
		X External
			7 Autologous Tissue Substitute
			J Synthetic Substitute
			K Nonautologous Tissue Substitute
				Z No Qualifier

5 **Middle Ear, Right**
  Oval window
  Tympanic cavity
6 **Middle Ear, Left**
  See 5 Middle Ear, Right
9 **Auditory Ossicle, Right**
  Incus
  Malleus
  Stapes
A **Auditory Ossicle, Left**
  See 9 Auditory Ossicle, Right
	D **Inner Ear, Right**
	  Bony labyrinth
	  Bony vestibule
	  Cochlea
	  Round window
	  Semicircular canal
	E **Inner Ear, Left**
	  See D Inner Ear, Right
		Ø Open
		8 Via Natural or Artificial Opening Endoscopic
			7 Autologous Tissue Substitute
			J Synthetic Substitute
			K Nonautologous Tissue Substitute
				Z No Qualifier

7 **Tympanic Membrane, Right**
  Pars flaccida
8 **Tympanic Membrane, Left**
  See 7 Tympanic Membrane, Right
	N **Nasopharynx**
	  Choana
	  Fossa of Rosenmuller
	  Pharyngeal recess
	  Rhinopharynx
		Ø Open
		7 Via Natural or Artificial Opening
		8 Via Natural or Artificial Opening Endoscopic
			7 Autologous Tissue Substitute
			J Synthetic Substitute
			K Nonautologous Tissue Substitute
				Z No Qualifier

B **Mastoid Sinus, Right**
  Mastoid air cells
C **Mastoid Sinus, Left**
  See B Mastoid Sinus, Right
L **Nasal Turbinate**
  Inferior turbinate
  Middle turbinate
  Nasal concha
  Superior turbinate
P **Accessory Sinus**
Q **Maxillary Sinus, Right**
  Antrum of Highmore
	R **Maxillary Sinus, Left**
	  See Q Maxillary Sinus, Right
	S **Frontal Sinus, Right**
	T **Frontal Sinus, Left**
	U **Ethmoid Sinus, Right**
	  Ethmoidal air cell
	V **Ethmoid Sinus, Left**
	  See U Ethmoid Sinus, Right
	W **Sphenoid Sinus, Right**
	X **Sphenoid Sinus, Left**
		Ø Open
		3 Percutaneous
		4 Percutaneous Endoscopic
		7 Via Natural or Artificial Opening
		8 Via Natural or Artificial Opening Endoscopic
			7 Autologous Tissue Substitute
			J Synthetic Substitute
			K Nonautologous Tissue Substitute
				Z No Qualifier

K **Nasal Mucosa and Soft Tissue**
  Columella
  External naris
  Greater alar cartilage
  Internal naris
  Lateral nasal cartilage
  Lesser alar cartilage
  Nasal cavity
  Nostril
		Ø Open
		8 Via Natural or Artificial Opening Endoscopic
		X External
			7 Autologous Tissue Substitute
			J Synthetic Substitute
			K Nonautologous Tissue Substitute
				Z No Qualifier

M **Nasal Septum**
  Quadrangular cartilage
  Septal cartilage
  Vomer bone
		Ø Open
		3 Percutaneous
		4 Percutaneous Endoscopic
		8 Via Natural or Artificial Opening Endoscopic
			7 Autologous Tissue Substitute
			J Synthetic Substitute
			K Nonautologous Tissue Substitute
				Z No Qualifier

Non-OR Procedure   DRG Non-OR Procedure   Valid OR Procedure   HAC Associated Procedure   Combination Only   New/Revised April   New/Revised October

336   ICD-10-PCS 2023

Ø9U–Ø9U

Ø   Medical and Surgical
9   Ear, Nose, Sinus
W   Revision   Definition: Correcting, to the extent possible, a portion of a malfunctioning device or the position of a displaced device

Explanation: Revision can include correcting a malfunctioning or displaced device by taking out or putting in components of the device such as a screw or pin

Body Part Character 4	Approach Character 5	Device Character 6	Qualifier Character 7

7   Tympanic Membrane, Right
    Pars flaccida
8   Tympanic Membrane, Left
    See 7 Tympanic Membrane, Right
9   Auditory Ossicle, Right
    Incus
    Malleus
    Stapes
A   Auditory Ossicle, Left
    See 9 Auditory Ossicle, Right
	Ø Open
	7 Via Natural or Artificial Opening
	**8 Via Natural or Artificial Opening
	    Endoscopic**
		7 Autologous Tissue Substitute
		J Synthetic Substitute
		K Nonautologous Tissue Substitute
			Z No Qualifier

D   Inner Ear, Right
    Bony labyrinth
    Bony vestibule
    Cochlea
    Round window
    Semicircular canal
E   Inner Ear, Left
    See D Inner Ear, Right
	Ø Open
	7 Via Natural or Artificial Opening
	**8 Via Natural or Artificial Opening
	    Endoscopic**
		S Hearing Device	**Z No Qualifier**

H   Ear, Right
J   Ear, Left
K   Nasal Mucosa and Soft Tissue
    Columella
    External naris
    Greater alar cartilage
    Internal naris
    Lateral nasal cartilage
    Lesser alar cartilage
    Nasal cavity
    Nostril
	Ø Open
	3 Percutaneous
	4 Percutaneous Endoscopic
	7 Via Natural or Artificial Opening
	**8 Via Natural or Artificial Opening
	    Endoscopic**
		Ø Drainage Device
		7 Autologous Tissue Substitute
		D Intraluminal Device
		J Synthetic Substitute
		K Nonautologous Tissue Substitute
		Y Other Device
			Z No Qualifier

H   Ear, Right
J   Ear, Left
K   Nasal Mucosa and Soft Tissue
    Columella
    External naris
    Greater alar cartilage
    Internal naris
    Lateral nasal cartilage
    Lesser alar cartilage
    Nasal cavity
    Nostril
	X External	**Ø Drainage Device**
		7 Autologous Tissue Substitute
		D Intraluminal Device
		J Synthetic Substitute
		K Nonautologous Tissue Substitute
			Z No Qualifier

Y Sinus	**Ø Open** **3 Percutaneous** **4 Percutaneous Endoscopic**	**Ø Drainage Device** **Y Other Device**	**Z No Qualifier**
Y Sinus	**7 Via Natural or Artificial Opening** **8 Via Natural or Artificial Opening Endoscopic**	**Y Other Device**	**Z No Qualifier**
Y Sinus	**X External**	**Ø Drainage Device**	**Z No Qualifier**

Non-OR	Ø9W[H,J][3,4][J,K,Y]Z
Non-OR	Ø9W[H,J][7,8][D,Y]Z
Non-OR	Ø9WK[Ø,3,4,7,8][Ø,7,D,J,K,Y]Z
Non-OR	Ø9W[H,J,K]X[Ø,7,D,J,K]Z
Non-OR	Ø9WY[3,4]YZ
Non-OR	Ø9WY[7,8]YZ
Non-OR	Ø9WYXØZ

NC Noncovered Procedure   **LC** Limited Coverage   **QA** Questionable OB Admit   **NT** New Tech Add-on   ⊞ Combination Member   ♂ Male   ♀ Female

ICD-10-PCS 2023   337

Respiratory System ØB1–ØBY

Character Meanings

This Character Meaning table is provided as a guide to assist the user in the identification of character members that may be found in this section of code tables. It **SHOULD NOT** be used to build a PCS code.

Operation–Character 3	Body Part–Character 4	Approach–Character 5	Device–Character 6	Qualifier–Character 7
1 Bypass	Ø Tracheobronchial Tree	Ø Open	Ø Drainage Device	Ø Allogeneic
2 Change	1 Trachea	3 Percutaneous	1 Radioactive Element	1 Syngeneic
5 Destruction	2 Carina	4 Percutaneous Endoscopic	2 Monitoring Device	2 Zooplastic
7 Dilation	3 Main Bronchus, Right	7 Via Natural or Artificial Opening	3 Infusion Device	3 Laser Interstitial Thermal Therapy
9 Drainage	4 Upper Lobe Bronchus, Right	8 Via Natural or Artificial Opening Endoscopic	7 Autologous Tissue Substitute	4 Cutaneous
B Excision	5 Middle Lobe Bronchus, Right	X External	C Extraluminal Device	6 Esophagus
C Extirpation	6 Lower Lobe Bronchus, Right		D Intraluminal Device	X Diagnostic
D Extraction	7 Main Bronchus, Left		E Intraluminal Device, Endotracheal Airway	Z No Qualifier
F Fragmentation	8 Upper Lobe Bronchus, Left		F Tracheostomy Device	
H Insertion	9 Lingula Bronchus		G Intraluminal Device, Endobronchial Valve	
J Inspection	B Lower Lobe Bronchus, Left		J Synthetic Substitute	
L Occlusion	C Upper Lung Lobe, Right		K Nonautologous Tissue Substitute	
M Reattachment	D Middle Lung Lobe, Right		M Diaphragmatic Pacemaker Lead	
N Release	F Lower Lung Lobe, Right		Y Other Device	
P Removal	G Upper Lung Lobe, Left		Z No Device	
Q Repair	H Lung Lingula			
R Replacement	J Lower Lung Lobe, Left			
S Reposition	K Lung, Right			
T Resection	L Lung, Left			
U Supplement	M Lungs, Bilateral			
V Restriction	N Pleura, Right			
W Revision	P Pleura, Left			
Y Transplantation	Q Pleura			
	T Diaphragm			

AHA Coding Clinic for table ØB5
2016, 2Q, 17   Photodynamic therapy for treatment of malignant mesothelioma
2015, 2Q, 31   Thoracoscopic talc pleurodesis

AHA Coding Clinic for table ØB7
2020, 3Q, 43   Tracheobronchomalacia with placement of tracheobronchial stent

AHA Coding Clinic for table ØB9
2017, 3Q, 15   Bronchoscopy with suctioning for removal of retained secretions
2017, 1Q, 51   Bronchoalveolar lavage
2016, 1Q, 26   Bronchoalveolar lavage, endobronchial biopsy and transbronchial biopsy
2016, 1Q, 27   Fiberoptic bronchoscopy with brushings and bronchoalveolar lavage

AHA Coding Clinic for table ØBB
2022, 2Q, 19   Transbronchial lung biopsy using alligator forceps
2016, 1Q, 26   Bronchoalveolar lavage, endobronchial biopsy and transbronchial biopsy
2016, 1Q, 27   Fiberoptic bronchoscopy with brushings and bronchoalveolar lavage
2014, 1Q, 20   Fiducial marker placement

AHA Coding Clinic for table ØBC
2017, 3Q, 14   Bronchoscopy with suctioning and washings for removal of mucus plug

AHA Coding Clinic for table ØBD
2020, 3Q, 40   Transbronchial cryobiopsy of upper, middle and lower lobes of lung
2018, 3Q, 28   Lung decortication for empyema

AHA Coding Clinic for table ØBH
2019, 3Q, 33   Insertion of endobronchial valve
2014, 4Q, 3-10   Mechanical ventilation

AHA Coding Clinic for table ØBJ
2015, 2Q, 31   Thoracoscopic talc pleurodesis
2014, 1Q, 20   Fiducial marker placement

AHA Coding Clinic for table ØBL
2019, 3Q, 33   Insertion of endobronchial valve

AHA Coding Clinic for table ØBN
2019, 2Q, 20   Pericardiectomy for constrictive pericarditis
2018, 3Q, 28   Lung decortication
2018, 3Q, 28   Lung decortication for empyema
2015, 3Q, 15   Vascular ring surgery with release of esophagus and trachea

AHA Coding Clinic for table ØBQ
2020, 3Q, 41   Plication of diaphragm
2016, 2Q, 22   Esophageal lengthening Collis gastroplasty with Nissen fundoplication and hiatal hernia
2014, 3Q, 28   Laparoscopic Nissen fundoplication and diaphragmatic hernia repair

AHA Coding Clinic for table ØBU
2020, 3Q, 43   Tracheobronchomalacia with placement of tracheobronchial stent
2015, 1Q, 28   Repair of bronchopleural fistula using omental pedicle graft

AHA Coding Clinic for table ØBV
2020, 3Q, 41   Plication of diaphragm

Respiratory System

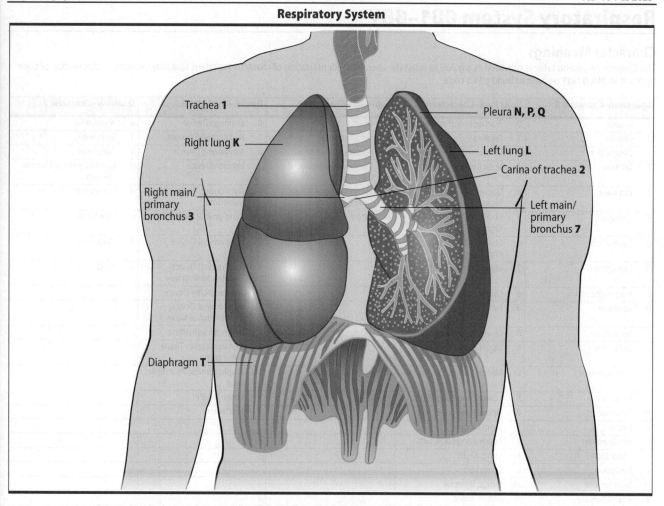

Trachea **1**

Right lung **K**

Right main/primary bronchus **3**

Diaphragm **T**

Pleura **N, P, Q**

Left lung **L**

Carina of trachea **2**

Left main/primary bronchus **7**

Right Lung Bronchi

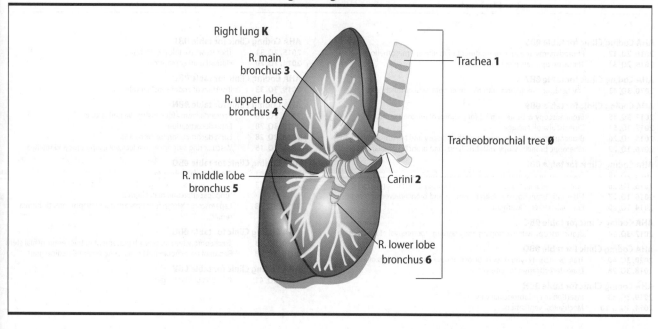

Right lung **K**

R. main bronchus **3**

R. upper lobe bronchus **4**

R. middle lobe bronchus **5**

R. lower lobe bronchus **6**

Trachea **1**

Tracheobronchial tree **Ø**

Carini **2**

Ø   Medical and Surgical
B   Respiratory System
1   Bypass   Definition: Altering the route of passage of the contents of a tubular body part

           Explanation: Rerouting contents of a body part to a downstream area of the normal route, to a similar route and body part, or to an abnormal route and dissimilar body part. Includes one or more anastomoses, with or without the use of a device.

Body Part Character 4	Approach Character 5	Device Character 6	Qualifier Character 7
1 Trachea Cricoid cartilage	**Ø** Open	**D** Intraluminal Device	**6** Esophagus
1 Trachea Cricoid cartilage	**Ø** Open	**F** Tracheostomy Device **Z** No Device	**4** Cutaneous
1 Trachea Cricoid cartilage	**3** Percutaneous **4** Percutaneous Endoscopic	**F** Tracheostomy Device **Z** No Device	**4** Cutaneous

DRG Non-OR   ØB113[F,Z]4
Non-OR   ØB11ØD6

Ø   Medical and Surgical
B   Respiratory System
2   Change   Definition: Taking out or off a device from a body part and putting back an identical or similar device in or on the same body part without cutting or puncturing the skin or a mucous membrane

           Explanation: All CHANGE procedures are coded using the approach EXTERNAL

Body Part Character 4	Approach Character 5	Device Character 6	Qualifier Character 7
Ø Tracheobronchial Tree **K** Lung, Right **L** Lung, Left **Q** Pleura **T** Diaphragm	**X** External	**Ø** Drainage Device **Y** Other Device	**Z** No Qualifier
1 Trachea Cricoid cartilage	**X** External	**Ø** Drainage Device **E** Intraluminal Device, Endotracheal Airway **F** Tracheostomy Device **Y** Other Device	**Z** No Qualifier

Non-OR   All body part, approach, device, and qualifier values

NC Noncovered Procedure   **LC** Limited Coverage   **QA** Questionable OB Admit   **NT** New Tech Add-on   ⊞ Combination Member   ♂ Male   ♀ Female

ICD-10-PCS 2023   341

Ø Medical and Surgical
B Respiratory System
5 Destruction　Definition: Physical eradication of all or a portion of a body part by the direct use of energy, force, or a destructive agent

Explanation: None of the body part is physically taken out

Body Part Character 4	Approach Character 5	Device Character 6	Qualifier Character 7
1 Trachea Cricoid cartilage 2 Carina 3 Main Bronchus, Right Bronchus intermedius Intermediate bronchus 4 Upper Lobe Bronchus, Right 5 Middle Lobe Bronchus, Right 6 Lower Lobe Bronchus, Right 7 Main Bronchus, Left 8 Upper Lobe Bronchus, Left 9 Lingula Bronchus B Lower Lobe Bronchus, Left	Ø Open 3 Percutaneous 4 Percutaneous Endoscopic 7 Via Natural or Artificial Opening 8 Via Natural or Artificial Opening Endoscopic	Z No Device	Z No Qualifier
C Upper Lung Lobe, Right D Middle Lung Lobe, Right F Lower Lung Lobe, Right G Upper Lung Lobe, Left H Lung Lingula J Lower Lung Lobe, Left K Lung, Right L Lung, Left M Lungs, Bilateral	Ø Open 3 Percutaneous 4 Percutaneous Endoscopic	Z No Device	3 Laser Interstitial Thermal Therapy Z No Qualifier
C Upper Lung Lobe, Right D Middle Lung Lobe, Right F Lower Lung Lobe, Right G Upper Lung Lobe, Left H Lung Lingula J Lower Lung Lobe, Left K Lung, Right L Lung, Left M Lungs, Bilateral	7 Via Natural or Artificial Opening 8 Via Natural or Artificial Opening Endoscopic	Z No Device	Z No Qualifier
N Pleura, Right P Pleura, Left T Diaphragm	Ø Open 3 Percutaneous 4 Percutaneous Endoscopic	Z No Device	Z No Qualifier

Non-OR　ØB5[3,4,5,6,7,8,9,B]4ZZ
Non-OR　ØB5[C,D,F,G,H,J,K,L,M]8ZZ

Ø Medical and Surgical
B Respiratory System
7 Dilation　Definition: Expanding an orifice or the lumen of a tubular body part

Explanation: The orifice can be a natural orifice or an artificially created orifice. Accomplished by stretching a tubular body part using intraluminal pressure or by cutting part of the orifice or wall of the tubular body part.

Body Part Character 4	Approach Character 5	Device Character 6	Qualifier Character 7
1 Trachea Cricoid cartilage 2 Carina 3 Main Bronchus, Right Bronchus intermedius Intermediate bronchus 4 Upper Lobe Bronchus, Right 5 Middle Lobe Bronchus, Right 6 Lower Lobe Bronchus, Right 7 Main Bronchus, Left 8 Upper Lobe Bronchus, Left 9 Lingula Bronchus B Lower Lobe Bronchus, Left	Ø Open 3 Percutaneous 4 Percutaneous Endoscopic 7 Via Natural or Artificial Opening 8 Via Natural or Artificial Opening Endoscopic	D Intraluminal Device Z No Device	Z No Qualifier

Non-OR　ØB7[3,4,5,6,7,8,9,B][Ø,3,4,7,8][D,Z]Z

Ø   Medical and Surgical
B   Respiratory System
9   Drainage   Definition: Taking or letting out fluids and/or gases from a body part
                Explanation: The qualifier DIAGNOSTIC is used to identify drainage procedures that are biopsies

Body Part Character 4		Approach Character 5	Device Character 6	Qualifier Character 7

1 Trachea
  Cricoid cartilage
2 Carina
3 Main Bronchus, Right
  Bronchus intermedius
  Intermediate bronchus
4 Upper Lobe Bronchus, Right
5 Middle Lobe Bronchus, Right
6 Lower Lobe Bronchus, Right
7 Main Bronchus, Left
	8 Upper Lobe Bronchus, Left
	9 Lingula Bronchus
	B Lower Lobe Bronchus, Left
	C Upper Lung Lobe, Right
	D Middle Lung Lobe, Right
	F Lower Lung Lobe, Right
	G Upper Lung Lobe, Left
	H Lung Lingula
	J Lower Lung Lobe, Left
	K Lung, Right
	L Lung, Left
	M Lungs, Bilateral
		Ø Open
		3 Percutaneous
		4 Percutaneous Endoscopic
		7 Via Natural or Artificial Opening
		8 Via Natural or Artificial Opening Endoscopic
			Ø Drainage Device	Z No Qualifier

1 Trachea
  Cricoid cartilage
2 Carina
3 Main Bronchus, Right
  Bronchus intermedius
  Intermediate bronchus
4 Upper Lobe Bronchus, Right
5 Middle Lobe Bronchus, Right
6 Lower Lobe Bronchus, Right
7 Main Bronchus, Left
	8 Upper Lobe Bronchus, Left
	9 Lingula Bronchus
	B Lower Lobe Bronchus, Left
	C Upper Lung Lobe, Right
	D Middle Lung Lobe, Right
	F Lower Lung Lobe, Right
	G Upper Lung Lobe, Left
	H Lung Lingula
	J Lower Lung Lobe, Left
	K Lung, Right
	L Lung, Left
	M Lungs, Bilateral
		Ø Open
		3 Percutaneous
		4 Percutaneous Endoscopic
		7 Via Natural or Artificial Opening
		8 Via Natural or Artificial Opening Endoscopic
			Z No Device	X Diagnostic
				Z No Qualifier

N Pleura, Right P Pleura, Left		Ø Open 3 Percutaneous 4 Percutaneous Endoscopic 8 Via Natural or Artificial Opening Endoscopic	Ø Drainage Device	Z No Qualifier
N Pleura, Right P Pleura, Left		Ø Open 3 Percutaneous 4 Percutaneous Endoscopic 8 Via Natural or Artificial Opening Endoscopic	Z No Device	X Diagnostic Z No Qualifier
T Diaphragm		Ø Open 3 Percutaneous 4 Percutaneous Endoscopic	Ø Drainage Device	Z No Qualifier
T Diaphragm		Ø Open 3 Percutaneous 4 Percutaneous Endoscopic	Z No Device	X Diagnostic Z No Qualifier

Non-OR   ØB9[1,2,3,4,5,6,7,8,9,B][7,8]ØZ
Non-OR   ØB9[1,2,3,4,5,6,7,8,9,B][3,4]ZX
Non-OR   ØB9[1,2,3,4,5,6,7,8,9,B][7,8]Z[X,Z]
Non-OR   ØB9[C,D,F,G,H,J,K,L,M][3,4,7]ZX
Non-OR   ØB9[C,D,F,G,H,J,K,L,M]8Z[X,Z]

Non-OR   ØB9[N,P][Ø,3,8]ØZ
Non-OR   ØB9[N,P][Ø,3,8]Z[X,Z]
Non-OR   ØB9[N,P]4ZX
Non-OR   ØB9T[3,4]ØZ
Non-OR   ØB9T[3,4]Z[X,Z]

NC Noncovered Procedure   LC Limited Coverage   QA Questionable OB Admit   NT New Tech Add-on   ✚ Combination Member   ♂ Male   ♀ Female

ICD-10-PCS 2023   343

ØB9–ØB9

Ø   **Medical and Surgical**
B   **Respiratory System**
B   **Excision**   Definition: Cutting out or off, without replacement, a portion of a body part

       Explanation: The qualifier DIAGNOSTIC is used to identify excision procedures that are biopsies

Body Part Character 4	Approach Character 5	Device Character 6	Qualifier Character 7

1   Trachea
     Cricoid cartilage
2   Carina
3   Main Bronchus, Right
     Bronchus intermedius
     Intermediate bronchus
4   Upper Lobe Bronchus, Right
5   Middle Lobe Bronchus, Right
6   Lower Lobe Bronchus, Right
7   Main Bronchus, Left
8   Upper Lobe Bronchus, Left
9   Lingula Bronchus
B   Lower Lobe Bronchus, Left
C   Upper Lung Lobe, Right
D   Middle Lung Lobe, Right
F   Lower Lung Lobe, Right
G   Upper Lung Lobe, Left
H   Lung Lingula
J   Lower Lung Lobe, Left
K   Lung, Right
L   Lung, Left
M   Lungs, Bilateral
	Ø Open
	3 Percutaneous
	4 Percutaneous Endoscopic
	7 Via Natural or Artificial Opening
	8 Via Natural or Artificial Opening
	     Endoscopic
		Z No Device	X Diagnostic
			Z No Qualifier

N Pleura, Right P Pleura, Left	Ø Open 3 Percutaneous 4 Percutaneous Endoscopic 8 Via Natural or Artificial Opening Endoscopic	Z No Device	X Diagnostic Z No Qualifier
T Diaphragm	Ø Open 3 Percutaneous 4 Percutaneous Endoscopic	Z No Device	X Diagnostic Z No Qualifier

Non-OR   ØBB[1,2,3,4,5,6,7,8,9,B][3,4,7,8]ZX   Non-OR   ØBB[C,D,F,G,H,J,K,L]8ZZ
Non-OR   ØBB[3,4,5,6,7,8,9,B,M][4,8]ZZ   Non-OR   ØBB[N,P]3ZX
Non-OR   ØBB[C,D,F,G,H,J,K,L,M]3ZX

Ø   **Medical and Surgical**
B   **Respiratory System**
C   **Extirpation**   Definition: Taking or cutting out solid matter from a body part

       Explanation: The solid matter may be an abnormal byproduct of a biological function or a foreign body; it may be imbedded in a body part or in the lumen of a tubular body part. The solid matter may or may not have been previously broken into pieces.

Body Part Character 4	Approach Character 5	Device Character 6	Qualifier Character 7

1   Trachea
     Cricoid cartilage
2   Carina
3   Main Bronchus, Right
     Bronchus intermedius
     Intermediate bronchus
4   Upper Lobe Bronchus, Right
5   Middle Lobe Bronchus, Right
6   Lower Lobe Bronchus, Right
7   Main Bronchus, Left
8   Upper Lobe Bronchus, Left
9   Lingula Bronchus
B   Lower Lobe Bronchus, Left
C   Upper Lung Lobe, Right
D   Middle Lung Lobe, Right
F   Lower Lung Lobe, Right
G   Upper Lung Lobe, Left
H   Lung Lingula
J   Lower Lung Lobe, Left
K   Lung, Right
L   Lung, Left
M   Lungs, Bilateral
	Ø Open
	3 Percutaneous
	4 Percutaneous Endoscopic
	7 Via Natural or Artificial Opening
	8 Via Natural or Artificial Opening
	     Endoscopic
		Z No Device	Z No Qualifier

N Pleura, Right P Pleura, Left T Diaphragm	Ø Open 3 Percutaneous 4 Percutaneous Endoscopic	Z No Device	Z No Qualifier

Non-OR   ØBC[1,2,3,4,5,6,7,8,9,B][7,8]ZZ
Non-OR   ØBC[N,P]3ZZ

Non-OR Procedure   DRG Non-OR Procedure   Valid OR Procedure   HAC Associated Procedure   Combination Only   New/Revised April   New/Revised October

344   ICD-10-PCS 2023

Ø   Medical and Surgical
B   Respiratory System
D   Extraction   Definition: Pulling or stripping out or off all or a portion of a body part by the use of force

Explanation: The qualifier DIAGNOSTIC is used to identify extraction procedures that are biopsies

Body Part Character 4	Approach Character 5	Device Character 6	Qualifier Character 7

1   Trachea
     Cricoid cartilage
2   Carina
3   Main Bronchus, Right
     Bronchus intermedius
     Intermediate bronchus
4   Upper Lobe Bronchus, Right
5   Middle Lobe Bronchus, Right
6   Lower Lobe Bronchus, Right
7   Main Bronchus, Left
8   Upper Lobe Bronchus, Left
9   Lingula Bronchus
B   Lower Lobe Bronchus, Left
C   Upper Lung Lobe, Right
D   Middle Lung Lobe, Right
F   Lower Lung Lobe, Right
G   Upper Lung Lobe, Left
H   Lung Lingula
J   Lower Lung Lobe, Left
K   Lung, Right
L   Lung, Left
M   Lungs, Bilateral
	4 Percutaneous Endoscopic
	8 Via Natural or Artificial Opening
	     Endoscopic
		Z No Device	X Diagnostic

N Pleura, Right P Pleura, Left	Ø Open 3 Percutaneous 4 Percutaneous Endoscopic	Z No Device	X Diagnostic Z No Qualifier

Non-OR   ØBD[1,2,3,4,5,6,7,8,9,B,C,D,F,G,H,J,K,L,M][4,8]ZX

Ø   Medical and Surgical
B   Respiratory System
F   Fragmentation   Definition: Breaking solid matter in a body part into pieces

Explanation: Physical force (e.g., manual, ultrasonic) applied directly or indirectly is used to break the solid matter into pieces. The solid matter may be an abnormal byproduct of a biological function or a foreign body. The pieces of solid matter are not taken out.

Body Part Character 4	Approach Character 5	Device Character 6	Qualifier Character 7

1   Trachea   `NC`
     Cricoid cartilage
2   Carina   `NC`
3   Main Bronchus, Right   `NC`
     Bronchus intermedius
     Intermediate bronchus
4   Upper Lobe Bronchus, Right   `NC`
5   Middle Lobe Bronchus, Right   `NC`
6   Lower Lobe Bronchus, Right   `NC`
7   Main Bronchus, Left   `NC`
8   Upper Lobe Bronchus, Left   `NC`
9   Lingula Bronchus   `NC`
B   Lower Lobe Bronchus, Left   `NC`
	Ø Open
	3 Percutaneous
	4 Percutaneous Endoscopic
	7 Via Natural or Artificial Opening
	8 Via Natural or Artificial Opening
	     Endoscopic
	X External
		Z No Device	Z No Qualifier

Non-OR   ØBF[1,2,3,4,5,6,7,8,9,B]XZZ
Non-OR   ØBF[3,4,5,6,7,8,9,B][7,8]ZZ
`NC`   ØBF[1,2,3,4,5,6,7,8,9,B]XZZ

Ø   Medical and Surgical
B   Respiratory System
H   Insertion   Definition: Putting in a nonbiological appliance that monitors, assists, performs, or prevents a physiological function but does not physically take the place of a body part
Explanation: None

Body Part Character 4	Approach Character 5	Device Character 6	Qualifier Character 7
Ø Tracheobronchial Tree	Ø Open 3 Percutaneous 4 Percutaneous Endoscopic 7 Via Natural or Artificial Opening 8 Via Natural or Artificial Opening Endoscopic	1 Radioactive Element 2 Monitoring Device 3 Infusion Device D Intraluminal Device Y Other Device	Z No Qualifier
1 Trachea Cricoid cartilage	Ø Open	2 Monitoring Device D Intraluminal Device Y Other Device	Z No Qualifier
1 Trachea Cricoid cartilage	3 Percutaneous	D Intraluminal Device E Intraluminal Device, Endotracheal Airway Y Other Device	Z No Qualifier
1 Trachea Cricoid cartilage	4 Percutaneous Endoscopic	D Intraluminal Device Y Other Device	Z No Qualifier
1 Trachea Cricoid cartilage	7 Via Natural or Artificial Opening 8 Via Natural or Artificial Opening Endoscopic	2 Monitoring Device D Intraluminal Device E Intraluminal Device, Endotracheal Airway Y Other Device	Z No Qualifier

3 Main Bronchus, Right
  Bronchus intermedius
  Intermediate bronchus
4 Upper Lobe Bronchus, Right
5 Middle Lobe Bronchus, Right
6 Lower Lobe Bronchus, Right
7 Main Bronchus, Left
8 Upper Lobe Bronchus, Left
9 Lingula Bronchus
B Lower Lobe Bronchus, Left
	Ø Open
	3 Percutaneous
	4 Percutaneous Endoscopic
	7 Via Natural or Artificial Opening
	8 Via Natural or Artificial Opening Endoscopic
		G Intraluminal Device, Endobronchial Valve	Z No Qualifier

K Lung, Right L Lung, Left	Ø Open 3 Percutaneous 4 Percutaneous Endoscopic 7 Via Natural or Artificial Opening 8 Via Natural or Artificial Opening Endoscopic	1 Radioactive Element 2 Monitoring Device 3 Infusion Device Y Other Device	Z No Qualifier
Q Pleura	Ø Open 3 Percutaneous 4 Percutaneous Endoscopic 7 Via Natural or Artificial Opening 8 Via Natural or Artificial Opening Endoscopic	Y Other Device	Z No Qualifier
T Diaphragm	Ø Open 3 Percutaneous 4 Percutaneous Endoscopic	2 Monitoring Device M Diaphragmatic Pacemaker Lead Y Other Device	Z No Qualifier
T Diaphragm	7 Via Natural or Artificial Opening 8 Via Natural or Artificial Opening Endoscopic	Y Other Device	Z No Qualifier

DRG Non-OR	ØBH[3,4,5,6,7,8,9,B]8GZ
Non-OR	ØBHØ3YZ
Non-OR	ØBHØ[7,8][2,3,D,Y]Z
Non-OR	ØBH13[E,Y]Z
Non-OR	ØBH1[7,8][2,D,E,Y]Z
Non-OR	ØBH[K,L]3YZ
Non-OR	ØBH[K,L]7[2,3,Y]Z
Non-OR	ØBH[K,L]8[2,3]Z
Non-OR	ØBHQ[3,7]YZ
Non-OR	ØBHT3YZ
Non-OR	ØBHT[7,8]YZ

Non-OR Procedure   DRG Non-OR Procedure   Valid OR Procedure   HAC Associated Procedure   Combination Only   New/Revised April   New/Revised October

Ø   Medical and Surgical
B   Respiratory System
J   Inspection   Definition: Visually and/or manually exploring a body part

Explanation: Visual exploration may be performed with or without optical instrumentation. Manual exploration may be performed directly or through intervening body layers.

Body Part Character 4	Approach Character 5	Device Character 6	Qualifier Character 7

Ø   Tracheobronchial Tree
1   Trachea
     Cricoid cartilage
K   Lung, Right
L   Lung, Left
Q   Pleura
T   Diaphragm
	Ø Open
	3 Percutaneous
	4 Percutaneous Endoscopic
	7 Via Natural or Artificial Opening
	8 Via Natural or Artificial Opening
	     Endoscopic
	X External
		Z No Device	Z No Qualifier

Non-OR   ØBJ[Ø,K,L,Q,T][3,7,8,X]ZZ
Non-OR   ØBJ1[3,4,7,8,X]ZZ

Ø   Medical and Surgical
B   Respiratory System
L   Occlusion   Definition: Completely closing an orifice or the lumen of a tubular body part

Explanation: The orifice can be a natural orifice or an artificially created orifice

Body Part Character 4	Approach Character 5	Device Character 6	Qualifier Character 7

1   Trachea
     Cricoid cartilage
2   Carina
3   Main Bronchus, Right
     Bronchus intermedius
     Intermediate bronchus
4   Upper Lobe Bronchus, Right
5   Middle Lobe Bronchus, Right
6   Lower Lobe Bronchus, Right
7   Main Bronchus, Left
8   Upper Lobe Bronchus, Left
9   Lingula Bronchus
B   Lower Lobe Bronchus, Left
	Ø Open
	3 Percutaneous
	4 Percutaneous Endoscopic
		C Extraluminal Device
		D Intraluminal Device
		Z No Device
			Z No Qualifier

1   Trachea
     Cricoid cartilage
2   Carina
3   Main Bronchus, Right
     Bronchus intermedius
     Intermediate bronchus
4   Upper Lobe Bronchus, Right
5   Middle Lobe Bronchus, Right
6   Lower Lobe Bronchus, Right
7   Main Bronchus, Left
8   Upper Lobe Bronchus, Left
9   Lingula Bronchus
B   Lower Lobe Bronchus, Left
	7 Via Natural or Artificial Opening
	8 Via Natural or Artificial Opening
	     Endoscopic
		D Intraluminal Device
		Z No Device
			Z No Qualifier

Ø   Medical and Surgical
B   Respiratory System
M   Reattachment   Definition: Putting back in or on all or a portion of a separated body part to its normal location or other suitable location
                         Explanation: Vascular circulation and nervous pathways may or may not be reestablished

Body Part Character 4	Approach Character 5	Device Character 6	Qualifier Character 7

1 Trachea
  Cricoid cartilage
2 Carina
3 Main Bronchus, Right
  Bronchus intermedius
  Intermediate bronchus
4 Upper Lobe Bronchus, Right
5 Middle Lobe Bronchus, Right
6 Lower Lobe Bronchus, Right
7 Main Bronchus, Left
8 Upper Lobe Bronchus, Left
9 Lingula Bronchus
B Lower Lobe Bronchus, Left
C Upper Lung Lobe, Right
D Middle Lung Lobe, Right
F Lower Lung Lobe, Right
G Upper Lung Lobe, Left
H Lung Lingula
J Lower Lung Lobe, Left
K Lung, Right
L Lung, Left
T Diaphragm
	Ø Open	Z No Device	Z No Qualifier

Ø   Medical and Surgical
B   Respiratory System
N   Release   Definition: Freeing a body part from an abnormal physical constraint by cutting or by the use of force
                    Explanation: Some of the restraining tissue may be taken out but none of the body part is taken out

Body Part Character 4	Approach Character 5	Device Character 6	Qualifier Character 7

1 Trachea
  Cricoid cartilage
2 Carina
3 Main Bronchus, Right
  Bronchus intermedius
  Intermediate bronchus
4 Upper Lobe Bronchus, Right
5 Middle Lobe Bronchus, Right
6 Lower Lobe Bronchus, Right
7 Main Bronchus, Left
8 Upper Lobe Bronchus, Left
9 Lingula Bronchus
B Lower Lobe Bronchus, Left
C Upper Lung Lobe, Right
D Middle Lung Lobe, Right
F Lower Lung Lobe, Right
G Upper Lung Lobe, Left
H Lung Lingula
J Lower Lung Lobe, Left
K Lung, Right
L Lung, Left
M Lungs, Bilateral
	Ø Open
	3 Percutaneous
	4 Percutaneous Endoscopic
	7 Via Natural or Artificial Opening
	8 Via Natural or Artificial Opening
	  Endoscopic
		Z No Device	Z No Qualifier

N Pleura, Right P Pleura, Left T Diaphragm	Ø Open 3 Percutaneous 4 Percutaneous Endoscopic	Z No Device	Z No Qualifier

Ø   **Medical and Surgical**
B   **Respiratory System**
P   **Removal**   Definition: Taking out or off a device from a body part

Explanation: If a device is taken out and a similar device put in without cutting or puncturing the skin or mucous membrane, the procedure is coded to the root operation CHANGE. Otherwise, the procedure for taking out a device is coded to the root operation REMOVAL.

Body Part Character 4	Approach Character 5	Device Character 6	Qualifier Character 7
Ø Tracheobronchial Tree	Ø Open 3 Percutaneous 4 Percutaneous Endoscopic 7 Via Natural or Artificial Opening 8 Via Natural or Artificial Opening Endoscopic	Ø Drainage Device 1 Radioactive Element 2 Monitoring Device 3 Infusion Device 7 Autologous Tissue Substitute C Extraluminal Device D Intraluminal Device J Synthetic Substitute K Nonautologous Tissue Substitute Y Other Device	Z No Qualifier
Ø Tracheobronchial Tree	X External	Ø Drainage Device 1 Radioactive Element 2 Monitoring Device 3 Infusion Device D Intraluminal Device	Z No Qualifier
1 Trachea Cricoid cartilage	Ø Open 3 Percutaneous 4 Percutaneous Endoscopic 7 Via Natural or Artificial Opening 8 Via Natural or Artificial Opening Endoscopic	Ø Drainage Device 2 Monitoring Device 7 Autologous Tissue Substitute C Extraluminal Device D Intraluminal Device F Tracheostomy Device J Synthetic Substitute K Nonautologous Tissue Substitute	Z No Qualifier
1 Trachea Cricoid cartilage	X External	Ø Drainage Device 2 Monitoring Device D Intraluminal Device F Tracheostomy Device	Z No Qualifier
K Lung, Right L Lung, Left	Ø Open 3 Percutaneous 4 Percutaneous Endoscopic 7 Via Natural or Artificial Opening 8 Via Natural or Artificial Opening Endoscopic	Ø Drainage Device 1 Radioactive Element 2 Monitoring Device 3 Infusion Device Y Other Device	Z No Qualifier
K Lung, Right L Lung, Left	X External	Ø Drainage Device 1 Radioactive Element 2 Monitoring Device 3 Infusion Device	Z No Qualifier
Q Pleura	Ø Open 3 Percutaneous 4 Percutaneous Endoscopic 7 Via Natural or Artificial Opening 8 Via Natural or Artificial Opening Endoscopic	Ø Drainage Device 1 Radioactive Element 2 Monitoring Device Y Other Device	Z No Qualifier
Q Pleura	X External	Ø Drainage Device 1 Radioactive Element 2 Monitoring Device	Z No Qualifier
T Diaphragm	Ø Open 3 Percutaneous 4 Percutaneous Endoscopic 7 Via Natural or Artificial Opening 8 Via Natural or Artificial Opening Endoscopic	Ø Drainage Device 2 Monitoring Device 7 Autologous Tissue Substitute J Synthetic Substitute K Nonautologous Tissue Substitute M Diaphragmatic Pacemaker Lead Y Other Device	Z No Qualifier
T Diaphragm	X External	Ø Drainage Device 2 Monitoring Device M Diaphragmatic Pacemaker Lead	Z No Qualifier

Non-OR	ØBPØ[3,4]YZ	**Non-OR**	ØBPL7[Ø,2,3,Y]Z
Non-OR	ØBPØ[7,8][Ø,2,3,D,Y]Z	**Non-OR**	ØBPL8[Ø,2,3]Z
Non-OR	ØBPØX[Ø,1,2,3,D]Z	**Non-OR**	ØBP[K,L]X[Ø,1,2,3]Z
Non-OR	ØBP1[Ø,3,4]FZ	**Non-OR**	ØBPQ[Ø,3,4,7,8][Ø,1,2,]Z
Non-OR	ØBP1[7,8][Ø,2,D,F]Z	**Non-OR**	ØBPQ[3,7]YZ
Non-OR	ØBP1X[Ø,2,D,F]Z	**Non-OR**	ØBPQX[Ø,1,2]Z
Non-OR	ØBP[K,L]3YZ	**Non-OR**	ØBPT3YZ
Non-OR	ØBPK7[Ø,1,2,3,Y]Z	**Non-OR**	ØBPT[7,8][Ø,2,Y]Z
Non-OR	ØBPK8[Ø,1,2,3]Z	**Non-OR**	ØBPTX[Ø,2,M]Z

NC Noncovered Procedure   **LC** Limited Coverage   **QA** Questionable OB Admit   **NT** New Tech Add-on   ⊞ Combination Member   ♂ Male   ♀ Female

ICD-10-PCS 2023   349

ØBP–ØBP

Ø   Medical and Surgical
B   Respiratory System
Q   Repair   Definition: Restoring, to the extent possible, a body part to its normal anatomic structure and function
                  Explanation: Used only when the method to accomplish the repair is not one of the other root operations

Body Part Character 4	Approach Character 5	Device Character 6	Qualifier Character 7

1   Trachea
     Cricoid cartilage
2   Carina
3   Main Bronchus, Right
     Bronchus intermedius
     Intermediate bronchus
4   Upper Lobe Bronchus, Right
5   Middle Lobe Bronchus, Right
6   Lower Lobe Bronchus, Right
7   Main Bronchus, Left
8   Upper Lobe Bronchus, Left
9   Lingula Bronchus
B   Lower Lobe Bronchus, Left
C   Upper Lung Lobe, Right
D   Middle Lung Lobe, Right
F   Lower Lung Lobe, Right
G   Upper Lung Lobe, Left
H   Lung Lingula
J   Lower Lung Lobe, Left
K   Lung, Right
L   Lung, Left
M   Lungs, Bilateral
	Ø Open
	3 Percutaneous
	4 Percutaneous Endoscopic
	7 Via Natural or Artificial Opening
	8 Via Natural or Artificial Opening
	     Endoscopic
		Z No Device	Z No Qualifier

N Pleura, Right P Pleura, Left T Diaphragm	Ø Open 3 Percutaneous 4 Percutaneous Endoscopic	Z No Device	Z No Qualifier

Ø   Medical and Surgical
B   Respiratory System
R   Replacement   Definition: Putting in or on biological or synthetic material that physically takes the place and/or function of all or a portion of a body part
                      Explanation: The body part may have been taken out or replaced, or may be taken out, physically eradicated, or rendered nonfunctional during
                      the REPLACEMENT procedure. A REMOVAL procedure is coded for taking out the device used in a previous replacement procedure.

Body Part Character 4	Approach Character 5	Device Character 6	Qualifier Character 7

1   Trachea
     Cricoid cartilage
2   Carina
3   Main Bronchus, Right
     Bronchus intermedius
     Intermediate bronchus
4   Upper Lobe Bronchus, Right
5   Middle Lobe Bronchus, Right
6   Lower Lobe Bronchus, Right
7   Main Bronchus, Left
8   Upper Lobe Bronchus, Left
9   Lingula Bronchus
B   Lower Lobe Bronchus, Left
T   Diaphragm
	Ø Open
	4 Percutaneous Endoscopic
		7 Autologous Tissue Substitute
		J Synthetic Substitute
		K Nonautologous Tissue Substitute
			Z No Qualifier

Ø   **Medical and Surgical**
B   **Respiratory System**
S   **Reposition**   Definition: Moving to its normal location, or other suitable location, all or a portion of a body part

Explanation: The body part is moved to a new location from an abnormal location, or from a normal location where it is not functioning correctly. The body part may or may not be cut out or off to be moved to the new location.

Body Part Character 4	Approach Character 5	Device Character 6	Qualifier Character 7

1   Trachea
    Cricoid cartilage
2   Carina
3   Main Bronchus, Right
    Bronchus intermedius
    Intermediate bronchus
4   Upper Lobe Bronchus, Right
5   Middle Lobe Bronchus, Right
6   Lower Lobe Bronchus, Right
7   Main Bronchus, Left
8   Upper Lobe Bronchus, Left
9   Lingula Bronchus
B   Lower Lobe Bronchus, Left
C   Upper Lung Lobe, Right
D   Middle Lung Lobe, Right
F   Lower Lung Lobe, Right
G   Upper Lung Lobe, Left
H   Lung Lingula
J   Lower Lung Lobe, Left
K   Lung, Right
L   Lung, Left
T   Diaphragm
	Ø Open	Z No Device	Z No Qualifier

Ø   **Medical and Surgical**
B   **Respiratory System**
T   **Resection**   Definition: Cutting out or off, without replacement, all of a body part

Explanation: None

Body Part Character 4	Approach Character 5	Device Character 6	Qualifier Character 7

1   Trachea
    Cricoid cartilage
2   Carina
3   Main Bronchus, Right
    Bronchus intermedius
    Intermediate bronchus
4   Upper Lobe Bronchus, Right
5   Middle Lobe Bronchus, Right
6   Lower Lobe Bronchus, Right
7   Main Bronchus, Left
8   Upper Lobe Bronchus, Left
9   Lingula Bronchus
B   Lower Lobe Bronchus, Left
C   Upper Lung Lobe, Right
D   Middle Lung Lobe, Right
F   Lower Lung Lobe, Right
G   Upper Lung Lobe, Left
H   Lung Lingula
J   Lower Lung Lobe, Left
K   Lung, Right
L   Lung, Left
M   Lungs, Bilateral
T   Diaphragm
	Ø Open
	4 Percutaneous Endoscopic
		Z No Device	Z No Qualifier

NC Noncovered Procedure   LC Limited Coverage   QA Questionable OB Admit   NT New Tech Add-on   ⊞ Combination Member   ♂ Male   ♀ Female

ICD-10-PCS 2023   351

ØBS–ØBT

Ø   **Medical and Surgical**
B   **Respiratory System**
U   **Supplement**   Definition: Putting in or on biological or synthetic material that physically reinforces and/or augments the function of a portion of a body part
       Explanation: The biological material is non-living, or is living and from the same individual. The body part may have been previously replaced, and the SUPPLEMENT procedure is performed to physically reinforce and/or augment the function of the replaced body part.

Body Part Character 4	Approach Character 5	Device Character 6	Qualifier Character 7

1 Trachea
   Cricoid cartilage
2 Carina
3 Main Bronchus, Right
   Bronchus intermedius
   Intermediate bronchus
4 Upper Lobe Bronchus, Right
5 Middle Lobe Bronchus, Right
6 Lower Lobe Bronchus, Right
7 Main Bronchus, Left
8 Upper Lobe Bronchus, Left
9 Lingula Bronchus
B Lower Lobe Bronchus, Left
	Ø Open
	4 Percutaneous Endoscopic
	8 Via Natural or Artificial Opening Endoscopic
		7 Autologous Tissue Substitute
		J Synthetic Substitute
		K Nonautologous Tissue Substitute
			Z No Qualifier

T Diaphragm	**Ø** Open **4** Percutaneous Endoscopic	**7** Autologous Tissue Substitute **J** Synthetic Substitute **K** Nonautologous Tissue Substitute	**Z** No Qualifier

Ø   **Medical and Surgical**
B   **Respiratory System**
V   **Restriction**   Definition: Partially closing an orifice or the lumen of a tubular body part
       Explanation: The orifice can be a natural orifice or an artificially created orifice

Body Part Character 4	Approach Character 5	Device Character 6	Qualifier Character 7

1 Trachea
   Cricoid cartilage
2 Carina
3 Main Bronchus, Right
   Bronchus intermedius
   Intermediate bronchus
4 Upper Lobe Bronchus, Right
5 Middle Lobe Bronchus, Right
6 Lower Lobe Bronchus, Right
7 Main Bronchus, Left
8 Upper Lobe Bronchus, Left
9 Lingula Bronchus
B Lower Lobe Bronchus, Left
	Ø Open
	3 Percutaneous
	4 Percutaneous Endoscopic
		C Extraluminal Device
		D Intraluminal Device
		Z No Device
			Z No Qualifier

1 Trachea
   Cricoid cartilage
2 Carina
3 Main Bronchus, Right
   Bronchus intermedius
   Intermediate bronchus
4 Upper Lobe Bronchus, Right
5 Middle Lobe Bronchus, Right
6 Lower Lobe Bronchus, Right
7 Main Bronchus, Left
8 Upper Lobe Bronchus, Left
9 Lingula Bronchus
B Lower Lobe Bronchus, Left
	7 Via Natural or Artificial Opening
	8 Via Natural or Artificial Opening Endoscopic
		D Intraluminal Device
		Z No Device
			Z No Qualifier

Non-OR Procedure   DRG Non-OR Procedure   Valid OR Procedure   HAC Associated Procedure   Combination Only   New/Revised April   New/Revised October

352   ICD-10-PCS 2023

Ø   Medical and Surgical
B   Respiratory System
W   Revision   Definition: Correcting, to the extent possible, a portion of a malfunctioning device or the position of a displaced device
                     Explanation: Revision can include correcting a malfunctioning or displaced device by taking out or putting in components of the device such as a screw or pin

Body Part Character 4	Approach Character 5	Device Character 6	Qualifier Character 7
Ø Tracheobronchial Tree	Ø Open 3 Percutaneous 4 Percutaneous Endoscopic 7 Via Natural or Artificial Opening 8 Via Natural or Artificial Opening Endoscopic	Ø Drainage Device 2 Monitoring Device 3 Infusion Device 7 Autologous Tissue Substitute C Extraluminal Device D Intraluminal Device J Synthetic Substitute K Nonautologous Tissue Substitute Y Other Device	Z No Qualifier
Ø Tracheobronchial Tree	X External	Ø Drainage Device 2 Monitoring Device 3 Infusion Device 7 Autologous Tissue Substitute C Extraluminal Device D Intraluminal Device J Synthetic Substitute K Nonautologous Tissue Substitute	Z No Qualifier

1   Trachea
     Cricoid cartilage
	Ø Open
	3 Percutaneous
	4 Percutaneous Endoscopic
	7 Via Natural or Artificial Opening
	8 Via Natural or Artificial Opening
	     Endoscopic
	X External
		Ø Drainage Device
		2 Monitoring Device
		7 Autologous Tissue Substitute
		C Extraluminal Device
		D Intraluminal Device
		F Tracheostomy Device
		J Synthetic Substitute
		K Nonautologous Tissue Substitute
			Z No Qualifier

K Lung, Right L Lung, Left	Ø Open 3 Percutaneous 4 Percutaneous Endoscopic 7 Via Natural or Artificial Opening 8 Via Natural or Artificial Opening Endoscopic	Ø Drainage Device 2 Monitoring Device 3 Infusion Device Y Other Device	Z No Qualifier
K Lung, Right L Lung, Left	X External	Ø Drainage Device 2 Monitoring Device 3 Infusion Device	Z No Qualifier
Q Pleura	Ø Open 3 Percutaneous 4 Percutaneous Endoscopic 7 Via Natural or Artificial Opening 8 Via Natural or Artificial Opening Endoscopic	Ø Drainage Device 2 Monitoring Device Y Other Device	Z No Qualifier
Q Pleura	X External	Ø Drainage Device 2 Monitoring Device	Z No Qualifier
T Diaphragm	Ø Open 3 Percutaneous 4 Percutaneous Endoscopic 7 Via Natural or Artificial Opening 8 Via Natural or Artificial Opening Endoscopic	Ø Drainage Device 2 Monitoring Device 7 Autologous Tissue Substitute J Synthetic Substitute K Nonautologous Tissue Substitute M Diaphragmatic Pacemaker Lead Y Other Device	Z No Qualifier
T Diaphragm	X External	Ø Drainage Device 2 Monitoring Device 7 Autologous Tissue Substitute J Synthetic Substitute K Nonautologous Tissue Substitute M Diaphragmatic Pacemaker Lead	Z No Qualifier

Non-OR	ØBWØ[3,4]YZ
Non-OR	ØBWØ[7,8][2,3,D,Y]Z
Non-OR	ØBWØX[Ø,2,3,7,C,D,J,K]Z
Non-OR	ØBW1X[Ø,2,7,C,D,F,J,K]Z
Non-OR	ØBW[K,L]3YZ
Non-OR	ØBW[K,L]7[Ø,2,3,Y]Z
Non-OR	ØBW[K,L]8[Ø,2,3]Z
Non-OR	ØBW[K,L]X[Ø,2,3]Z
Non-OR	ØBWQ[Ø,3,4,7,8][Ø,2]Z
Non-OR	ØBWQ[Ø,3,7]YZ
Non-OR	ØBWQX[Ø,2]Z
Non-OR	ØBWT[3,7,8]YZ
Non-OR	ØBWTX[Ø,2,7,J,K,M]Z

NC Noncovered Procedure   LC Limited Coverage   QA Questionable OB Admit   NT New Tech Add-on   ⊞ Combination Member   ♂ Male   ♀ Female

ICD-10-PCS 2023   353

Ø **Medical and Surgical**
B **Respiratory System**
Y **Transplantation** Definition: Putting in or on all or a portion of a living body part taken from another individual or animal to physically take the place and/or function of all or a portion of a similar body part
Explanation: The native body part may or may not be taken out, and the transplanted body part may take over all or a portion of its function

Body Part Character 4		Approach Character 5	Device Character 6	Qualifier Character 7
C Upper Lung Lobe, Right LC	Ø Open	Z No Device	Ø Allogeneic	
D Middle Lung Lobe, Right LC			1 Syngeneic	
F Lower Lung Lobe, Right LC			2 Zooplastic	
G Upper Lung Lobe, Left LC				
H Lung Lingula LC				
J Lower Lung Lobe, Left LC				
K Lung, Right LC				
L Lung, Left LC				
M Lungs, Bilateral LC				

LC   ØBY[C,D,F,G,H,J,K,L,M]ØZ[Ø,1,2]

Mouth and Throat ØCØ–ØCX

Character Meanings

This Character Meaning table is provided as a guide to assist the user in the identification of character members that may be found in this section of code tables. It **SHOULD NOT** be used to build a PCS code.

Operation–Character 3		Body Part–Character 4		Approach–Character 5		Device–Character 6		Qualifier–Character 7	
Ø	Alteration	Ø	Upper Lip	Ø	Open	Ø	Drainage Device	Ø	Single
2	Change	1	Lower Lip	3	Percutaneous	1	Radioactive Element	1	Multiple
5	Destruction	2	Hard Palate	4	Percutaneous Endoscopic	5	External Fixation Device	2	All
7	Dilation	3	Soft Palate	7	Via Natural or Artificial Opening	7	Autologous Tissue Substitute	X	Diagnostic
9	Drainage	4	Buccal Mucosa	8	Via Natural or Artificial Opening Endoscopic	B	Intraluminal Device, Airway	Z	No Qualifier
B	Excision	5	Upper Gingiva	X	External	C	Extraluminal Device		
C	Extirpation	6	Lower Gingiva			D	Intraluminal Device		
D	Extraction	7	Tongue			J	Synthetic Substitute		
F	Fragmentation	8	Parotid Gland, Right			K	Nonautologous Tissue Substitute		
H	Insertion	9	Parotid Gland, Left			Y	Other Device		
J	Inspection	A	Salivary Gland			Z	No Device		
L	Occlusion	B	Parotid Duct, Right						
M	Reattachment	C	Parotid Duct, Left						
N	Release	D	Sublingual Gland, Right						
P	Removal	F	Sublingual Gland, Left						
Q	Repair	G	Submaxillary Gland, Right						
R	Replacement	H	Submaxillary Gland, Left						
S	Reposition	J	Minor Salivary Gland						
T	Resection	M	Pharynx						
U	Supplement	N	Uvula						
V	Restriction	P	Tonsils						
W	Revision	Q	Adenoids						
X	Transfer	R	Epiglottis						
		S	Larynx						
		T	Vocal Cord, Right						
		V	Vocal Cord, Left						
		W	Upper Tooth						
		X	Lower Tooth						
		Y	Mouth and Throat						

AHA Coding Clinic for table ØC9
2017, 2Q, 16   Incision and drainage of floor of mouth

AHA Coding Clinic for table ØCB
2017, 2Q, 16   Excision of floor of mouth
2016, 3Q, 28   Lingual tonsillectomy, tongue base excision and epiglottopexy
2016, 2Q, 19   Biopsy of the base of tongue
2014, 3Q, 21   Superficial parotidectomy

AHA Coding Clinic for table ØCC
2016, 2Q, 20   Sialendoscopy with stone removal

AHA Coding Clinic for table ØCH
2020, 4Q, 43-44   Insertion of radioactive element

AHA Coding Clinic for table ØCQ
2017, 1Q, 20   Preparatory nasal adhesion repair before definitive cleft palate repair

AHA Coding Clinic for table ØCR
2014, 3Q, 25   Excision of soft palate with placement of surgical obturator
2014, 2Q, 5   Oasis acellular matrix graft
2014, 2Q, 6   Composite grafting (synthetic versus nonautologous tissue substitute)

AHA Coding Clinic for table ØCS
2022, 2Q, 24   Palatoplasty with intravelar veloplasty
2016, 3Q, 28   Lingual tonsillectomy, tongue base excision and epiglottopexy

AHA Coding Clinic for table ØCT
2016, 2Q, 12   Resection of malignant neoplasm of infratemporal fossa
2014, 3Q, 21   Superficial parotidectomy
2014, 3Q, 23   Le Fort I osteotomy

Salivary Glands

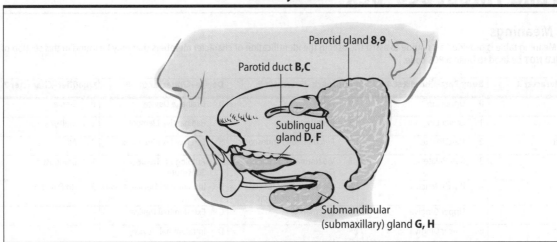

Parotid gland **8,9**

Parotid duct **B,C**

Sublingual gland **D, F**

Submandibular (submaxillary) gland **G, H**

Oral Anatomy

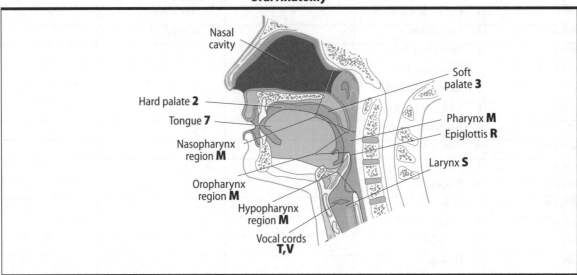

Nasal cavity

Hard palate **2**

Tongue **7**

Nasopharynx region **M**

Oropharynx region **M**

Hypopharynx region **M**

Vocal cords **T,V**

Soft palate **3**

Pharynx **M**

Epiglottis **R**

Larynx **S**

Mouth Frontal View (Upper)

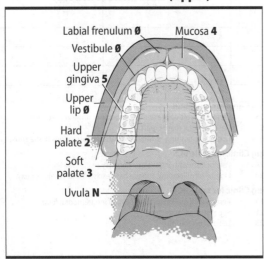

Labial frenulum **Ø**

Mucosa **4**

Vestibule **Ø**

Upper gingiva **5**

Upper lip **Ø**

Hard palate **2**

Soft palate **3**

Uvula **N**

Mouth Frontal View (Lower)

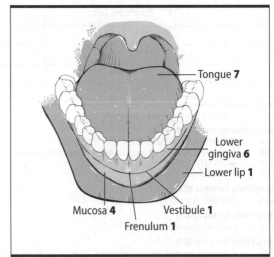

Tongue **7**

Lower gingiva **6**

Lower lip **1**

Mucosa **4**

Vestibule **1**

Frenulum **1**

0   **Medical and Surgical**
C   **Mouth and Throat**
0   **Alteration**   Definition: Modifying the anatomic structure of a body part without affecting the function of the body part
                     Explanation: Principal purpose is to improve appearance

Body Part Character 4	Approach Character 5	Device Character 6	Qualifier Character 7

0 Upper Lip
   Frenulum labii superioris
   Labial gland
   Vermilion border
1 Lower Lip
   Frenulum labii inferioris
   Labial gland
   Vermilion border
	X External	**7** Autologous Tissue Substitute
		J Synthetic Substitute
		K Nonautologous Tissue Substitute
		Z No Device
			Z No Qualifier

0   **Medical and Surgical**
C   **Mouth and Throat**
2   **Change**   Definition: Taking out or off a device from a body part and putting back an identical or similar device in or on the same body part without cutting or puncturing the skin or a mucous membrane
                   Explanation: All CHANGE procedures are coded using the approach EXTERNAL

Body Part Character 4	Approach Character 5	Device Character 6	Qualifier Character 7

A Salivary Gland
S Larynx
   Aryepiglottic fold
   Arytenoid cartilage
   Corniculate cartilage
   Cuneiform cartilage
   False vocal cord
   Glottis
   Rima glottidis
   Thyroid cartilage
   Ventricular fold
Y Mouth and Throat
	X External	**0** Drainage Device
		Y Other Device
			Z No Qualifier

Non-OR   All body part, approach, device, and qualifier values

NC Noncovered Procedure   **LC** Limited Coverage   **QA** Questionable OB Admit   **NT** New Tech Add-on   ⊞ Combination Member   ♂ Male   ♀ Female

ICD-10-PCS 2023   357

0C0–0C2

Mouth and Throat

ØC5–ØC7

Ø　Medical and Surgical
C　Mouth and Throat
5　Destruction　　Definition: Physical eradication of all or a portion of a body part by the direct use of energy, force, or a destructive agent
　　　　　　　　　　Explanation: None of the body part is physically taken out

Body Part Character 4		Approach Character 5	Device Character 6	Qualifier Character 7
Ø　Upper Lip 　　Frenulum labii superioris 　　Labial gland 　　Vermilion border **1　Lower Lip** 　　Frenulum labii inferioris 　　Labial gland 　　Vermilion border **2　Hard Palate** **3　Soft Palate** **4　Buccal Mucosa** 　　Buccal gland 　　Molar gland 　　Palatine gland	**5　Upper Gingiva** **6　Lower Gingiva** **7　Tongue** 　　Frenulum linguae **N　Uvula** 　　Palatine uvula **P　Tonsils** 　　Palatine tonsil **Q　Adenoids** 　　Pharyngeal tonsil	**Ø　Open** **3　Percutaneous** **X　External**	**Z　No Device**	**Z　No Qualifier**
8　Parotid Gland, Right **9　Parotid Gland, Left** **B　Parotid Duct, Right** 　　Stensen's duct **C　Parotid Duct, Left** 　　*See B Parotid Duct, Right* **D　Sublingual Gland, Right**	**F　Sublingual Gland, Left** **G　Submaxillary Gland, Right** 　　Submandibular gland **H　Submaxillary Gland, Left** 　　*See G Submaxillary Gland, Right* **J　Minor Salivary Gland** 　　Anterior lingual gland	**Ø　Open** **3　Percutaneous**	**Z　No Device**	**Z　No Qualifier**
M　Pharynx 　　Base of tongue 　　Hypopharynx 　　Laryngopharynx 　　Lingual tonsil 　　Oropharynx 　　Piriform recess (sinus) 　　Tongue, base of **R　Epiglottis** 　　Glossoepiglottic fold	**S　Larynx** 　　Aryepiglottic fold 　　Arytenoid cartilage 　　Corniculate cartilage 　　Cuneiform cartilage 　　False vocal cord 　　Glottis 　　Rima glottidis 　　Thyroid cartilage 　　Ventricular fold **T　Vocal Cord, Right** 　　Vocal fold **V　Vocal Cord, Left** 　　*See T Vocal Cord, Right*	**Ø　Open** **3　Percutaneous** **4　Percutaneous Endoscopic** **7　Via Natural or Artificial 　　Opening** **8　Via Natural or Artificial 　　Opening Endoscopic**	**Z　No Device**	**Z　No Qualifier**
W　Upper Tooth **X　Lower Tooth**		**Ø　Open** **X　External**	**Z　No Device**	**Ø　Single** **1　Multiple** **2　All**

Non-OR　ØC5[5,6][Ø,3,X]ZZ
Non-OR　ØC5[W,X][Ø,X]Z[Ø,1,2]

Ø　Medical and Surgical
C　Mouth and Throat
7　Dilation　　Definition: Expanding an orifice or the lumen of a tubular body part
　　　　　　　　Explanation: The orifice can be a natural orifice or an artificially created orifice. Accomplished by stretching a tubular body part using
　　　　　　　　intraluminal pressure or by cutting part of the orifice or wall of the tubular body part.

Body Part Character 4	Approach Character 5	Device Character 6	Qualifier Character 7
B　Parotid Duct, Right 　　Stensen's duct **C　Parotid Duct, Left** 　　*See B Parotid Duct, Right*	**Ø　Open** **3　Percutaneous** **7　Via Natural or Artificial 　　Opening**	**D　Intraluminal Device** **Z　No Device**	**Z　No Qualifier**
M　Pharynx 　　Base of tongue 　　Hypopharynx 　　Laryngopharynx 　　Lingual tonsil 　　Oropharynx 　　Piriform recess (sinus) 　　Tongue, base of	**7　Via Natural or Artificial 　　Opening** **8　Via Natural or Artificial 　　Opening Endoscopic**	**D　Intraluminal Device** **Z　No Device**	**Z　No Qualifier**
S　Larynx 　　Aryepiglottic fold 　　Arytenoid cartilage 　　Corniculate cartilage 　　Cuneiform cartilage 　　False vocal cord 　　Glottis 　　Rima glottidis 　　Thyroid cartilage 　　Ventricular fold	**Ø　Open** **3　Percutaneous** **4　Percutaneous Endoscopic** **7　Via Natural or Artificial 　　Opening** **8　Via Natural or Artificial 　　Opening Endoscopic**	**D　Intraluminal Device** **Z　No Device**	**Z　No Qualifier**

Non-OR　ØC7[B,C][Ø,3,7][D,Z]Z
Non-OR　ØC7M[7,8][D,Z]Z

Non-OR Procedure　　　DRG Non-OR Procedure　　　Valid OR Procedure　　　HAC Associated Procedure　　　Combination Only　　　New/Revised April　　　New/Revised October

Ø　**Medical and Surgical**
C　**Mouth and Throat**
9　**Drainage**　　　　Definition: Taking or letting out fluids and/or gases from a body part
　　　　　　　　　　　　Explanation: The qualifier DIAGNOSTIC is used to identify drainage procedures that are biopsies

Body Part Character 4		Approach Character 5	Device Character 6	Qualifier Character 7
Ø　Upper Lip 　　Frenulum labii superioris 　　Labial gland 　　Vermilion border 1　Lower Lip 　　Frenulum labii inferioris 　　Labial gland 　　Vermilion border 2　Hard Palate 3　Soft Palate 4　Buccal Mucosa 　　Buccal gland 　　Molar gland 　　Palatine gland	5　Upper Gingiva 6　Lower Gingiva 7　Tongue 　　Frenulum linguae N　Uvula 　　Palatine uvula P　Tonsils 　　Palatine tonsil Q　Adenoids 　　Pharyngeal tonsil	Ø　Open 3　Percutaneous X　External	Ø　Drainage Device	Z　No Qualifier
Ø　Upper Lip 　　Frenulum labii superioris 　　Labial gland 　　Vermilion border 1　Lower Lip 　　Frenulum labii inferioris 　　Labial gland 　　Vermilion border 2　Hard Palate 3　Soft Palate 4　Buccal Mucosa 　　Buccal gland 　　Molar gland 　　Palatine gland	5　Upper Gingiva 6　Lower Gingiva 7　Tongue 　　Frenulum linguae N　Uvula 　　Palatine uvula P　Tonsils 　　Palatine tonsil Q　Adenoids 　　Pharyngeal tonsil	Ø　Open 3　Percutaneous X　External	Z　No Device	X　Diagnostic Z　No Qualifier
8　Parotid Gland, Right 9　Parotid Gland, Left B　Parotid Duct, Right 　　Stensen's duct C　Parotid Duct, Left 　　*See B Parotid Duct, Right* D　Sublingual Gland, Right	F　Sublingual Gland, Left G　Submaxillary Gland, Right 　　Submandibular gland H　Submaxillary Gland, Left 　　*See G Submaxillary Gland, Right* J　Minor Salivary Gland 　　Anterior lingual gland	Ø　Open 3　Percutaneous	Ø　Drainage Device	Z　No Qualifier
8　Parotid Gland, Right 9　Parotid Gland, Left B　Parotid Duct, Right 　　Stensen's duct C　Parotid Duct, Left 　　*See B Parotid Duct, Right*	D　Sublingual Gland, Right F　Sublingual Gland, Left G　Submaxillary Gland, Right 　　Submandibular gland H　Submaxillary Gland, Left 　　*See G Submaxillary Gland, Right* J　Minor Salivary Gland 　　Anterior lingual gland	Ø　Open 3　Percutaneous	Z　No Device	X　Diagnostic Z　No Qualifier
M　Pharynx 　　Base of tongue 　　Hypopharynx 　　Laryngopharynx 　　Lingual tonsil 　　Oropharynx 　　Piriform recess (sinus) 　　Tongue, base of R　Epiglottis 　　Glossoepiglottic fold	S　Larynx 　　Aryepiglottic fold 　　Arytenoid cartilage 　　Corniculate cartilage 　　Cuneiform cartilage 　　False vocal cord 　　Glottis 　　Rima glottidis 　　Thyroid cartilage 　　Ventricular fold T　Vocal Cord, Right 　　Vocal fold V　Vocal Cord, Left 　　*See T Vocal Cord, Right*	Ø　Open 3　Percutaneous 4　Percutaneous Endoscopic 7　Via Natural or Artificial Opening 8　Via Natural or Artificial Opening Endoscopic	Ø　Drainage Device	Z　No Qualifier

Non-OR　ØC9[Ø,1,2,3,4,7,N,P,Q]3ØZ
Non-OR　ØC9[5,6][Ø,3,X]ØZ
Non-OR　ØC9[Ø,1,4][Ø,3,X]ZX
Non-OR　ØC9[Ø,1,2,3,4,7,N,P,Q]3ZZ
Non-OR　ØC9[5,6][Ø,3,X]Z[X,Z]
Non-OR　ØC97[3,X]ZX
Non-OR　ØC9[8,9,B,C,D,F,G,H,J][Ø,3]ØZ
Non-OR　ØC9[8,9,B,C,D,F,G,H,J]3ZX
Non-OR　ØC9[8,9,G,H]3ZZ
Non-OR　ØC9[B,C,D, F,J][Ø,3]ZZ
Non-OR　ØC9[M,R,S,T,V]3ØZ

ØC9 Continued on next page

ØC9–ØC9

NC Noncovered Procedure　　**LC** Limited Coverage　　**OA** Questionable OB Admit　　**NT** New Tech Add-on　　✚ Combination Member　　♂ Male　　♀ Female

ICD-10-PCS 2023　　　　　　　　　　　　　　　　　　　　　　　　　　　　　　　　　　　　　　　359

Mouth and Throat

Ø	Medical and Surgical
C	Mouth and Throat
9	Drainage

Definition: Taking or letting out fluids and/or gases from a body part

Explanation: The qualifier DIAGNOSTIC is used to identify drainage procedures that are biopsies

Body Part Character 4		Approach Character 5	Device Character 6	Qualifier Character 7
M Pharynx 　Base of tongue 　Hypopharynx 　Laryngopharynx 　Lingual tonsil 　Oropharynx 　Piriform recess (sinus) 　Tongue, base of R Epiglottis 　Glossoepiglottic fold	S Larynx 　Aryepiglottic fold 　Arytenoid cartilage 　Corniculate cartilage 　Cuneiform cartilage 　False vocal cord 　Glottis 　Rima glottidis 　Thyroid cartilage 　Ventricular fold T Vocal Cord, Right 　Vocal fold V Vocal Cord, Left 　*See T Vocal Cord, Right*	Ø Open 3 Percutaneous 4 Percutaneous Endoscopic 7 Via Natural or Artificial Opening 8 Via Natural or Artificial Opening Endoscopic	Z No Device	X Diagnostic Z No Qualifier
W Upper Tooth X Lower Tooth		Ø Open X External	Ø Drainage Device Z No Device	Ø Single 1 Multiple 2 All

Non-OR	ØC9M[Ø,3,4,7,8]ZX
Non-OR	ØC9[M,R,S,T,V]3ZZ
Non-OR	ØC9[R,S,T,V][3,4,7,8]ZX
Non-OR	ØC9[W,X][Ø,X][Ø,Z][Ø,1,2]

Ø	Medical and Surgical
C	Mouth and Throat
B	Excision

Definition: Cutting out or off, without replacement, a portion of a body part

Explanation: The qualifier DIAGNOSTIC is used to identify excision procedures that are biopsies

Body Part Character 4		Approach Character 5	Device Character 6	Qualifier Character 7
Ø Upper Lip 　Frenulum labii superioris 　Labial gland 　Vermilion border 1 Lower Lip 　Frenulum labii inferioris 　Labial gland 　Vermilion border 2 Hard Palate 3 Soft Palate 4 Buccal Mucosa 　Buccal gland 　Molar gland 　Palatine gland	5 Upper Gingiva 6 Lower Gingiva 7 Tongue 　Frenulum linguae N Uvula 　Palatine uvula P Tonsils 　Palatine tonsil Q Adenoids 　Pharyngeal tonsil	Ø Open 3 Percutaneous X External	Z No Device	X Diagnostic Z No Qualifier
8 Parotid Gland, Right 9 Parotid Gland, Left B Parotid Duct, Right 　Stensen's duct C Parotid Duct, Left 　*See B Parotid Duct, Right* D Sublingual Gland, Right	F Sublingual Gland, Left G Submaxillary Gland, Right 　Submandibular gland H Submaxillary Gland, Left 　*See G Submaxillary Gland, Right* J Minor Salivary Gland 　Anterior lingual gland	Ø Open 3 Percutaneous	Z No Device	X Diagnostic Z No Qualifier
M Pharynx 　Base of tongue 　Hypopharynx 　Laryngopharynx 　Lingual tonsil 　Oropharynx 　Piriform recess (sinus) 　Tongue, base of R Epiglottis 　Glossoepiglottic fold	S Larynx 　Aryepiglottic fold 　Arytenoid cartilage 　Corniculate cartilage 　Cuneiform cartilage 　False vocal cord 　Glottis 　Rima glottidis 　Thyroid cartilage 　Ventricular fold T Vocal Cord, Right 　Vocal fold V Vocal Cord, Left 　*See T Vocal Cord, Right*	Ø Open 3 Percutaneous 4 Percutaneous Endoscopic 7 Via Natural or Artificial Opening 8 Via Natural or Artificial Opening Endoscopic	Z No Device	X Diagnostic Z No Qualifier
W Upper Tooth X Lower Tooth		Ø Open X External	Z No Device	Ø Single 1 Multiple 2 All

Non-OR	ØCB[Ø,1,4][Ø,3,X]ZX	Non-OR	ØCBM[Ø,3,4,7,8]ZX
Non-OR	ØCB[5,6][Ø,3,X]Z[X,Z]	Non-OR	ØCB[R,S,T,V][3,4,7,8]ZX
Non-OR	ØCB7[3,X]ZX	Non-OR	ØCB[W,X][Ø,X]Z[Ø,1,2]
Non-OR	ØCB[8,9,B,C,D,F,G,H,J]3ZX		

Ø   **Medical and Surgical**
C   **Mouth and Throat**
C   **Extirpation**   Definition: Taking or cutting out solid matter from a body part

                     Explanation: The solid matter may be an abnormal byproduct of a biological function or a foreign body; it may be imbedded in a body part or in the lumen of a tubular body part. The solid matter may or may not have been previously broken into pieces.

Body Part Character 4		Approach Character 5	Device Character 6	Qualifier Character 7
Ø Upper Lip Frenulum labii superioris Labial gland Vermilion border **1 Lower Lip** Frenulum labii inferioris Labial gland Vermilion border **2 Hard Palate** **3 Soft Palate** **4 Buccal Mucosa** Buccal gland Molar gland Palatine gland	**5 Upper Gingiva** **6 Lower Gingiva** **7 Tongue** Frenulum linguae **N Uvula** Palatine uvula **P Tonsils** Palatine tonsil **Q Adenoids** Pharyngeal tonsil	**Ø Open** **3 Percutaneous** **X External**	**Z No Device**	**Z No Qualifier**
8 Parotid Gland, Right **9 Parotid Gland, Left** **B Parotid Duct, Right** Stensen's duct **C Parotid Duct, Left** *See B Parotid Duct, Right* **D Sublingual Gland, Right**	**F Sublingual Gland, Left** **G Submaxillary Gland, Right** Submandibular gland **H Submaxillary Gland, Left** *See G Submaxillary Gland, Right* **J Minor Salivary Gland** Anterior lingual gland	**Ø Open** **3 Percutaneous**	**Z No Device**	**Z No Qualifier**
M Pharynx Base of tongue Hypopharynx Laryngopharynx Lingual tonsil Oropharynx Piriform recess (sinus) Tongue, base of **R Epiglottis** Glossoepiglottic fold	**S Larynx** Aryepiglottic fold Arytenoid cartilage Corniculate cartilage Cuneiform cartilage False vocal cord Glottis Rima glottidis Thyroid cartilage Ventricular fold **T Vocal Cord, Right** Vocal fold **V Vocal Cord, Left** *See T Vocal Cord, Right*	**Ø Open** **3 Percutaneous** **4 Percutaneous Endoscopic** **7 Via Natural or Artificial Opening** **8 Via Natural or Artificial Opening Endoscopic**	**Z No Device**	**Z No Qualifier**
W Upper Tooth **X Lower Tooth**		**Ø Open** **X External**	**Z No Device**	**Ø Single** **1 Multiple** **2 All**

Non-OR	ØCC[Ø,1,2,3,4,7,N,P,Q]XZZ
Non-OR	ØCC[5,6][Ø,3,X]ZZ
Non-OR	ØCC[8,9,G,H]3ZZ
Non-OR	ØCC[B,C,D,F,J][Ø,3]ZZ
Non-OR	ØCC[M,S][7,8]ZZ
Non-OR	ØCC[W,X][Ø,X]Z[Ø,1,2]

Ø   **Medical and Surgical**
C   **Mouth and Throat**
D   **Extraction**   Definition: Pulling or stripping out or off all or a portion of a body part by the use of force

                     Explanation: The qualifier DIAGNOSTIC is used to identify extraction procedures that are biopsies

Body Part Character 4	Approach Character 5	Device Character 6	Qualifier Character 7
T Vocal Cord, Right Vocal fold **V Vocal Cord, Left** *See T Vocal Cord, Right*	**Ø Open** **3 Percutaneous** **4 Percutaneous Endoscopic** **7 Via Natural or Artificial Opening** **8 Via Natural or Artificial Opening Endoscopic**	**Z No Device**	**Z No Qualifier**
W Upper Tooth **X Lower Tooth**	**X External**	**Z No Device**	**Ø Single** **1 Multiple** **2 All**

Non-OR	ØCD[W,X]XZ[Ø,1,2]

NC Noncovered Procedure   **LC** Limited Coverage   **QA** Questionable OB Admit   **NT** New Tech Add-on   ⊞ Combination Member   ♂ Male   ♀ Female

ICD-10-PCS 2023   361

Mouth and Throat

0   **Medical and Surgical**
C   **Mouth and Throat**
F   **Fragmentation**   Definition: Breaking solid matter in a body part into pieces

Explanation: Physical force (e.g., manual, ultrasonic) applied directly or indirectly is used to break the solid matter into pieces. The solid matter may be an abnormal byproduct of a biological function or a foreign body. The pieces of solid matter are not taken out.

Body Part Character 4	Approach Character 5	Device Character 6	Qualifier Character 7
B Parotid Duct, Right NC Stensen's duct **C** Parotid Duct, Left NC *See B Parotid Duct, Right*	**0** Open **3** Percutaneous **7** Via Natural or Artificial Opening **X** External	**Z** No Device	**Z** No Qualifier

Non-OR   All body part, approach, device, and qualifier values
NC   0CF[B,C]XZZ

0   **Medical and Surgical**
C   **Mouth and Throat**
H   **Insertion**   Definition: Putting in a nonbiological appliance that monitors, assists, performs, or prevents a physiological function but does not physically take the place of a body part

Explanation: None

Body Part Character 4	Approach Character 5	Device Character 6	Qualifier Character 7
7 Tongue Frenulum linguae	**0** Open **3** Percutaneous **X** External	**1** Radioactive Element	**Z** No Qualifier
A Salivary Gland **S** Larynx Aryepiglottic fold Arytenoid cartilage Corniculate cartilage Cuneiform cartilage False vocal cord Glottis Rima glottidis Thyroid cartilage Ventricular fold	**0** Open **3** Percutaneous **7** Via Natural or Artificial Opening **8** Via Natural or Artificial Opening Endoscopic	**1** Radioactive Element **Y** Other Device	**Z** No Qualifier
Y Mouth and Throat	**0** Open **3** Percutaneous	**1** Radioactive Element **Y** Other Device	**Z** No Qualifier
Y Mouth and Throat	**7** Via Natural or Artificial Opening **8** Via Natural or Artificial Opening Endoscopic	**1** Radioactive Element **B** Intraluminal Device, Airway **Y** Other Device	**Z** No Qualifier

Non-OR   0CH[A,S]01Z
Non-OR   0CHS0YZ
Non-OR   0CH[A,S][3,7,8][1,Y]Z
Non-OR   0CHY[0,3][1,Y]Z
Non-OR   0CHY[7,8][1,B,Y]Z

0   **Medical and Surgical**
C   **Mouth and Throat**
J   **Inspection**   Definition: Visually and/or manually exploring a body part

Explanation: Visual exploration may be performed with or without optical instrumentation. Manual exploration may be performed directly or through intervening body layers.

Body Part Character 4	Approach Character 5	Device Character 6	Qualifier Character 7
A Salivary Gland	**0** Open **3** Percutaneous **X** External	**Z** No Device	**Z** No Qualifier
S Larynx Aryepiglottic fold Arytenoid cartilage Corniculate cartilage Cuneiform cartilage False vocal cord Glottis Rima glottidis Thyroid cartilage Ventricular fold **Y** Mouth and Throat	**0** Open **3** Percutaneous **4** Percutaneous Endoscopic **7** Via Natural or Artificial Opening **8** Via Natural or Artificial Opening Endoscopic **X** External	**Z** No Device	**Z** No Qualifier

Non-OR   All body part, approach, device, and qualifier values

Non-OR Procedure   DRG Non-OR Procedure   Valid OR Procedure   HAC Associated Procedure   Combination Only   New/Revised April   New/Revised October

362   ICD-10-PCS 2023

Ø **Medical and Surgical**
C **Mouth and Throat**
L **Occlusion**   Definition: Completely closing an orifice or the lumen of a tubular body part
                   Explanation: The orifice can be a natural orifice or an artificially created orifice

Body Part Character 4	Approach Character 5	Device Character 6	Qualifier Character 7
B Parotid Duct, Right Stensen's duct **C** Parotid Duct, Left *See B Parotid Duct, Right*	**Ø** Open **3** Percutaneous **4** Percutaneous Endoscopic	**C** Extraluminal Device **D** Intraluminal Device **Z** No Device	**Z** No Qualifier
B Parotid Duct, Right Stensen's duct **C** Parotid Duct, Left *See B Parotid Duct, Right*	**7** Via Natural or Artificial Opening **8** Via Natural or Artificial Opening Endoscopic	**D** Intraluminal Device **Z** No Device	**Z** No Qualifier

Ø **Medical and Surgical**
C **Mouth and Throat**
M **Reattachment**   Definition: Putting back in or on all or a portion of a separated body part to its normal location or other suitable location
                      Explanation: Vascular circulation and nervous pathways may or may not be reestablished

Body Part Character 4	Approach Character 5	Device Character 6	Qualifier Character 7
Ø Upper Lip Frenulum labii superioris Labial gland Vermilion border **1** Lower Lip Frenulum labii inferioris Labial gland Vermilion border **3** Soft Palate **7** Tongue Frenulum linguae **N** Uvula Palatine uvula	**Ø** Open	**Z** No Device	**Z** No Qualifier
W Upper Tooth **X** Lower Tooth	**Ø** Open **X** External	**Z** No Device	**Ø** Single **1** Multiple **2** All

Non-OR   ØCM[W,X][Ø,X]Z[Ø,1,2]

NC Noncovered Procedure   **LC** Limited Coverage   **QA** Questionable OB Admit   **NT** New Tech Add-on   ⊞ Combination Member   ♂ Male   ♀ Female

ICD-10-PCS 2023   363

Mouth and Throat

Ø **Medical and Surgical**
C **Mouth and Throat**
N **Release**   Definition: Freeing a body part from an abnormal physical constraint by cutting or by the use of force
Explanation: Some of the restraining tissue may be taken out but none of the body part is taken out

Body Part Character 4	Approach Character 5	Device Character 6	Qualifier Character 7
Ø Upper Lip Frenulum labii superioris Labial gland Vermilion border **1** Lower Lip Frenulum labii inferioris Labial gland Vermilion border **2** Hard Palate **3** Soft Palate **4** Buccal Mucosa Buccal gland Molar gland Palatine gland **5** Upper Gingiva **6** Lower Gingiva **7** Tongue Frenulum linguae **N** Uvula Palatine uvula **P** Tonsils Palatine tonsil **Q** Adenoids Pharyngeal tonsil	**Ø** Open **3** Percutaneous **X** External	**Z** No Device	**Z** No Qualifier
8 Parotid Gland, Right **9** Parotid Gland, Left **B** Parotid Duct, Right Stensen's duct **C** Parotid Duct, Left *See B Parotid Duct, Right* **D** Sublingual Gland, Right **F** Sublingual Gland, Left **G** Submaxillary Gland, Right Submandibular gland **H** Submaxillary Gland, Left *See G Submaxillary Gland, Right* **J** Minor Salivary Gland Anterior lingual gland	**Ø** Open **3** Percutaneous	**Z** No Device	**Z** No Qualifier
M Pharynx Base of tongue Hypopharynx Laryngopharynx Lingual tonsil Oropharynx Piriform recess (sinus) Tongue, base of **R** Epiglottis Glossoepiglottic fold **S** Larynx Aryepiglottic fold Arytenoid cartilage Corniculate cartilage Cuneiform cartilage False vocal cord Glottis Rima glottidis Thyroid cartilage Ventricular fold **T** Vocal Cord, Right Vocal fold **V** Vocal Cord, Left *See T Vocal Cord, Right*	**Ø** Open **3** Percutaneous **4** Percutaneous Endoscopic **7** Via Natural or Artificial Opening **8** Via Natural or Artificial Opening Endoscopic	**Z** No Device	**Z** No Qualifier
W Upper Tooth **X** Lower Tooth	**Ø** Open **X** External	**Z** No Device	**Ø** Single **1** Multiple **2** All

Non-OR   ØCN[Ø,1,5,6,7][Ø,3,X]ZZ
Non-OR   ØCN[W,X][Ø,X]Z[Ø,1,2]

Ø　Medical and Surgical
C　Mouth and Throat
P　Removal　　　Definition: Taking out or off a device from a body part

Explanation: If a device is taken out and a similar device put in without cutting or puncturing the skin or mucous membrane, the procedure is coded to the root operation CHANGE. Otherwise, the procedure for taking out a device is coded to the root operation REMOVAL.

Body Part Character 4	Approach Character 5	Device Character 6	Qualifier Character 7
A　Salivary Gland	**Ø** Open **3** Percutaneous	**Ø** Drainage Device **C** Extraluminal Device **Y** Other Device	**Z** No Qualifier
A　Salivary Gland	**7** Via Natural or Artificial Opening **8** Via Natural or Artificial Opening Endoscopic	**Y** Other Device	**Z** No Qualifier
S　Larynx 　Aryepiglottic fold 　Arytenoid cartilage 　Corniculate cartilage 　Cuneiform cartilage 　False vocal cord 　Glottis 　Rima glottidis 　Thyroid cartilage 　Ventricular fold	**Ø** Open **3** Percutaneous **7** Via Natural or Artificial Opening **8** Via Natural or Artificial Opening Endoscopic	**Ø** Drainage Device **7** Autologous Tissue Substitute **D** Intraluminal Device **J** Synthetic Substitute **K** Nonautologous Tissue Substitute **Y** Other Device	**Z** No Qualifier
S　Larynx 　Aryepiglottic fold 　Arytenoid cartilage 　Corniculate cartilage 　Cuneiform cartilage 　False vocal cord 　Glottis 　Rima glottidis 　Thyroid cartilage 　Ventricular fold	**X** External	**Ø** Drainage Device **7** Autologous Tissue Substitute **D** Intraluminal Device **J** Synthetic Substitute **K** Nonautologous Tissue Substitute	**Z** No Qualifier
Y　Mouth and Throat	**Ø** Open **3** Percutaneous **7** Via Natural or Artificial Opening **8** Via Natural or Artificial Opening Endoscopic	**Ø** Drainage Device **1** Radioactive Element **7** Autologous Tissue Substitute **D** Intraluminal Device **J** Synthetic Substitute **K** Nonautologous Tissue Substitute **Y** Other Device	**Z** No Qualifier
Y　Mouth and Throat	**X** External	**Ø** Drainage Device **1** Radioactive Element **7** Autologous Tissue Substitute **D** Intraluminal Device **J** Synthetic Substitute **K** Nonautologous Tissue Substitute	**Z** No Qualifier

Non-OR　ØCPA[Ø,3][Ø,C,Y]Z
Non-OR　ØCPA[7,8]YZ
Non-OR　ØCPS3YZ
Non-OR　ØCPS[7,8][Ø,D,Y]Z
Non-OR　ØCPSX[Ø,7,D,J,K]Z
Non-OR　ØCPY3YZ
Non-OR　ØCPY[7,8][Ø,D,Y]Z
Non-OR　ØCPYX[Ø,1,7,D,J,K]Z

NC Noncovered Procedure　　LC Limited Coverage　　QA Questionable OB Admit　　NT New Tech Add-on　　⊞ Combination Member　　♂ Male　　♀ Female

ICD-10-PCS 2023　　365

ØCP–ØCP

Ø   Medical and Surgical
C   Mouth and Throat
Q   Repair   Definition: Restoring, to the extent possible, a body part to its normal anatomic structure and function
                         Explanation: Used only when the method to accomplish the repair is not one of the other root operations

Body Part Character 4	Approach Character 5	Device Character 6	Qualifier Character 7
Ø Upper Lip Frenulum labii superioris Labial gland Vermilion border **1 Lower Lip** Frenulum labii inferioris Labial gland Vermilion border **2 Hard Palate** **3 Soft Palate** **4 Buccal Mucosa** Buccal gland Molar gland Palatine gland **5 Upper Gingiva** **6 Lower Gingiva** **7 Tongue** Frenulum linguae **N Uvula** Palatine uvula **P Tonsils** Palatine tonsil **Q Adenoids** Pharyngeal tonsil	**Ø Open** **3 Percutaneous** **X External**	**Z No Device**	**Z No Qualifier**
8 Parotid Gland, Right **9 Parotid Gland, Left** **B Parotid Duct, Right** Stensen's duct **C Parotid Duct, Left** *See B Parotid Duct, Right* **D Sublingual Gland, Right** **F Sublingual Gland, Left** **G Submaxillary Gland, Right** Submandibular gland **H Submaxillary Gland, Left** *See G Submaxillary Gland, Right* **J Minor Salivary Gland** Anterior lingual gland	**Ø Open** **3 Percutaneous**	**Z No Device**	**Z No Qualifier**
M Pharynx Base of tongue Hypopharynx Laryngopharynx Lingual tonsil Oropharynx Piriform recess (sinus) Tongue, base of **R Epiglottis** Glossoepiglottic fold **S Larynx** Aryepiglottic fold Arytenoid cartilage Corniculate cartilage Cuneiform cartilage False vocal cord Glottis Rima glottidis Thyroid cartilage Ventricular fold **T Vocal Cord, Right** Vocal fold **V Vocal Cord, Left** *See T Vocal Cord, Right*	**Ø Open** **3 Percutaneous** **4 Percutaneous Endoscopic** **7 Via Natural or Artificial Opening** **8 Via Natural or Artificial Opening** **Endoscopic**	**Z No Device**	**Z No Qualifier**
W Upper Tooth **X Lower Tooth**	**Ø Open** **X External**	**Z No Device**	**Ø Single** **1 Multiple** **2 All**

Non-OR	ØCQ[Ø,1,4,7]XZZ
Non-OR	ØCQ[5,6][Ø,3,X]ZZ
Non-OR	ØCQ[W,X][Ø,X]Z[Ø,1,2]

ØCQ–ØCQ

Non-OR Procedure   DRG Non-OR Procedure   Valid OR Procedure   HAC Associated Procedure   Combination Only   New/Revised April   New/Revised October

366   ICD-10-PCS 2023

Ø   **Medical and Surgical**
C   **Mouth and Throat**
R   **Replacement**   Definition: Putting in or on biological or synthetic material that physically takes the place and/or function of all or a portion of a body part

Explanation: The body part may have been taken out or replaced, or may be taken out, physically eradicated, or rendered nonfunctional during the REPLACEMENT procedure. A REMOVAL procedure is coded for taking out the device used in a previous replacement procedure.

Body Part Character 4		Approach Character 5		Device Character 6		Qualifier Character 7	
Ø	**Upper Lip** Frenulum labii superioris Labial gland Vermilion border	**Ø**	**Open**	**7**	**Autologous Tissue Substitute**	**Z**	**No Qualifier**
1	**Lower Lip** Frenulum labii inferioris Labial gland Vermilion border	**3**	**Percutaneous**	**J**	**Synthetic Substitute**		
2	**Hard Palate**	**X**	**External**	**K**	**Nonautologous Tissue Substitute**		
3	**Soft Palate**						
4	**Buccal Mucosa** Buccal gland Molar gland Palatine gland						
5	**Upper Gingiva**						
6	**Lower Gingiva**						
7	**Tongue** Frenulum linguae						
N	**Uvula** Palatine uvula						
B	**Parotid Duct, Right** Stensen's duct	**Ø**	**Open**	**7**	**Autologous Tissue Substitute**	**Z**	**No Qualifier**
C	**Parotid Duct, Left** *See B Parotid Duct, Right*	**3**	**Percutaneous**	**J**	**Synthetic Substitute**		
				K	**Nonautologous Tissue Substitute**		
M	**Pharynx** Base of tongue Hypopharynx Laryngopharynx Lingual tonsil Oropharynx Piriform recess (sinus) Tongue, base of	**Ø**	**Open**	**7**	**Autologous Tissue Substitute**	**Z**	**No Qualifier**
R	**Epiglottis** Glossoepiglottic fold	**7**	**Via Natural or Artificial Opening**	**J**	**Synthetic Substitute**		
S	**Larynx** Aryepiglottic fold Arytenoid cartilage Corniculate cartilage Cuneiform cartilage False vocal cord Glottis Rima glottidis Thyroid cartilage Ventricular fold	**8**	**Via Natural or Artificial Opening Endoscopic**	**K**	**Nonautologous Tissue Substitute**		
T	**Vocal Cord, Right** Vocal fold						
V	**Vocal Cord, Left** *See T Vocal Cord, Right*						
W	**Upper Tooth**	**Ø**	**Open**	**7**	**Autologous Tissue Substitute**	**Ø**	**Single**
X	**Lower Tooth**	**X**	**External**	**J**	**Synthetic Substitute**	**1**	**Multiple**
				K	**Nonautologous Tissue Substitute**	**2**	**All**

Non-OR   ØCR[W,X][Ø,X][7,J,K][Ø,1,2]

NC Noncovered Procedure   **LC** Limited Coverage   **QA** Questionable OB Admit   **NT** New Tech Add-on   ⊞ Combination Member   ♂ Male   ♀ Female

ICD-10-PCS 2023   367

Ø   Medical and Surgical
C   Mouth and Throat
S   Reposition   Definition: Moving to its normal location, or other suitable location, all or a portion of a body part

Explanation: The body part is moved to a new location from an abnormal location, or from a normal location where it is not functioning correctly. The body part may or may not be cut out or off to be moved to the new location.

Body Part Character 4	Approach Character 5	Device Character 6	Qualifier Character 7

Ø Upper Lip
   Frenulum labii superioris
   Labial gland
   Vermilion border
1 Lower Lip
   Frenulum labii inferioris
   Labial gland
   Vermilion border
2 Hard Palate
3 Soft Palate
7 Tongue
   Frenulum linguae
N Uvula
   Palatine uvula
	Ø Open
	X External
		Z No Device	**Z** No Qualifier

B Parotid Duct, Right
   Stensen's duct
C Parotid Duct, Left
   See B Parotid Duct, Right
	Ø Open
	3 Percutaneous
		Z No Device	**Z** No Qualifier

R Epiglottis
   Glossoepiglottic fold
T Vocal Cord, Right
   Vocal fold
V Vocal Cord, Left
   See T Vocal Cord, Right
	Ø Open
	7 Via Natural or Artificial Opening
	8 Via Natural or Artificial Opening
	   Endoscopic
		Z No Device	**Z** No Qualifier

W Upper Tooth **X** Lower Tooth	**Ø** Open **X** External	**5** External Fixation Device **Z** No Device	**Ø** Single **1** Multiple **2** All

Non-OR   ØCS[W,X][Ø,X][5,Z][Ø,1,2]

Non-OR Procedure   DRG Non-OR Procedure   Valid OR Procedure   HAC Associated Procedure   Combination Only   New/Revised April   New/Revised October

368   ICD-10-PCS 2023

Ø   **Medical and Surgical**
C   **Mouth and Throat**
T   **Resection**   Definition: Cutting out or off, without replacement, all of a body part
                    Explanation: None

Body Part Character 4	Approach Character 5	Device Character 6	Qualifier Character 7

Ø   **Upper Lip**
    Frenulum labii superioris
    Labial gland
    Vermilion border
1   **Lower Lip**
    Frenulum labii inferioris
    Labial gland
    Vermilion border
2   **Hard Palate**
3   **Soft Palate**
7   **Tongue**
    Frenulum linguae
N   **Uvula**
    Palatine uvula
P   **Tonsils**
    Palatine tonsil
Q   **Adenoids**
    Pharyngeal tonsil
	Ø Open
	X External
		Z No Device	**Z** No Qualifier

8   **Parotid Gland, Right**
9   **Parotid Gland, Left**
B   **Parotid Duct, Right**
    Stensen's duct
C   **Parotid Duct, Left**
    See B Parotid Duct, Right
D   **Sublingual Gland, Right**
F   **Sublingual Gland, Left**
G   **Submaxillary Gland, Right**
    Submandibular gland
H   **Submaxillary Gland, Left**
    See G Submaxillary Gland, Right
J   **Minor Salivary Gland**
    Anterior lingual gland
	Ø Open	**Z** No Device	**Z** No Qualifier

M   **Pharynx**
    Base of tongue
    Hypopharynx
    Laryngopharynx
    Lingual tonsil
    Oropharynx
    Piriform recess (sinus)
    Tongue, base of
R   **Epiglottis**
    Glossoepiglottic fold
S   **Larynx**
    Aryepiglottic fold
    Arytenoid cartilage
    Corniculate cartilage
    Cuneiform cartilage
    False vocal cord
    Glottis
    Rima glottidis
    Thyroid cartilage
    Ventricular fold
T   **Vocal Cord, Right**
    Vocal fold
V   **Vocal Cord, Left**
    See T Vocal Cord, Right
	Ø Open
	4 Percutaneous Endoscopic
	7 Via Natural or Artificial Opening
	8 Via Natural or Artificial Opening
	    Endoscopic
		Z No Device	**Z** No Qualifier

W **Upper Tooth** **X** **Lower Tooth**	**Ø** Open	**Z** No Device	**Ø** Single **1** Multiple **2** All

Non-OR   ØCT[W,X]ØZ[Ø,1,2]

NC Noncovered Procedure   **LC** Limited Coverage   **QA** Questionable OB Admit   **NT** New Tech Add-on   ✚ Combination Member   ♂ Male   ♀ Female

ICD-10-PCS 2023   **369**

Ø **Medical and Surgical**
C **Mouth and Throat**
U **Supplement**　　Definition: Putting in or on biological or synthetic material that physically reinforces and/or augments the function of a portion of a body part

Explanation: The biological material is non-living, or is living and from the same individual. The body part may have been previously replaced, and the SUPPLEMENT procedure is performed to physically reinforce and/or augment the function of the replaced body part.

Body Part Character 4	Approach Character 5	Device Character 6	Qualifier Character 7
Ø Upper Lip 　Frenulum labii superioris 　Labial gland 　Vermilion border **1** Lower Lip 　Frenulum labii inferioris 　Labial gland 　Vermilion border **2** Hard Palate **3** Soft Palate **4** Buccal Mucosa 　Buccal gland 　Molar gland 　Palatine gland **5** Upper Gingiva **6** Lower Gingiva **7** Tongue 　Frenulum linguae **N** Uvula 　Palatine uvula	**Ø** Open **3** Percutaneous **X** External	**7** Autologous Tissue Substitute **J** Synthetic Substitute **K** Nonautologous Tissue Substitute	**Z** No Qualifier
M Pharynx 　Base of tongue 　Hypopharynx 　Laryngopharynx 　Lingual tonsil 　Oropharynx 　Piriform recess (sinus) 　Tongue, base of **R** Epiglottis 　Glossoepiglottic fold **S** Larynx 　Aryepiglottic fold 　Arytenoid cartilage 　Corniculate cartilage 　Cuneiform cartilage 　False vocal cord 　Glottis 　Rima glottidis 　Thyroid cartilage 　Ventricular fold **T** Vocal Cord, Right 　Vocal fold **V** Vocal Cord, Left 　*See T Vocal Cord, Right*	**Ø** Open **7** Via Natural or Artificial Opening **8** Via Natural or Artificial Opening Endoscopic	**7** Autologous Tissue Substitute **J** Synthetic Substitute **K** Nonautologous Tissue Substitute	**Z** No Qualifier

Non-OR　ØCU2[Ø,3]JZ

Ø **Medical and Surgical**
C **Mouth and Throat**
V **Restriction**　　Definition: Partially closing an orifice or the lumen of a tubular body part

Explanation: The orifice can be a natural orifice or an artificially created orifice

Body Part Character 4	Approach Character 5	Device Character 6	Qualifier Character 7
B Parotid Duct, Right 　Stensen's duct **C** Parotid Duct, Left 　*See B Parotid Duct, Right*	**Ø** Open **3** Percutaneous	**C** Extraluminal Device **D** Intraluminal Device **Z** No Device	**Z** No Qualifier
B Parotid Duct, Right 　Stensen's duct **C** Parotid Duct, Left 　*See B Parotid Duct, Right*	**7** Via Natural or Artificial Opening **8** Via Natural or Artificial Opening Endoscopic	**D** Intraluminal Device **Z** No Device	**Z** No Qualifier

Non-OR Procedure　　DRG Non-OR Procedure　　Valid OR Procedure　　HAC Associated Procedure　　Combination Only　　New/Revised April　　New/Revised October

370　　　　　　　　　　　　　　　　　　　　　　　　　　　　　　　　　　　　ICD-10-PCS 2023

0   **Medical and Surgical**
C   **Mouth and Throat**
W   **Revision**   Definition: Correcting, to the extent possible, a portion of a malfunctioning device or the position of a displaced device

                       Explanation: Revision can include correcting a malfunctioning or displaced device by taking out or putting in components of the device such as a screw or pin

Body Part Character 4	Approach Character 5	Device Character 6	Qualifier Character 7
A Salivary Gland	**0** Open **3** Percutaneous	**0** Drainage Device **C** Extraluminal Device **Y** Other Device	**Z** No Qualifier
A Salivary Gland	**7** Via Natural or Artificial Opening **8** Via Natural or Artificial Opening Endoscopic	**Y** Other Device	**Z** No Qualifier
A Salivary Gland	**X** External	**0** Drainage Device **C** Extraluminal Device	**Z** No Qualifier

S   Larynx
     Aryepiglottic fold
     Arytenoid cartilage
     Corniculate cartilage
     Cuneiform cartilage
     False vocal cord
     Glottis
     Rima glottidis
     Thyroid cartilage
     Ventricular fold
	0 Open
	3 Percutaneous
	7 Via Natural or Artificial Opening
	8 Via Natural or Artificial Opening Endoscopic
		0 Drainage Device
		7 Autologous Tissue Substitute
		D Intraluminal Device
		J Synthetic Substitute
		K Nonautologous Tissue Substitute
		Y Other Device
			Z No Qualifier

S   Larynx
     Aryepiglottic fold
     Arytenoid cartilage
     Corniculate cartilage
     Cuneiform cartilage
     False vocal cord
     Glottis
     Rima glottidis
     Thyroid cartilage
     Ventricular fold
	X External	**0** Drainage Device
		7 Autologous Tissue Substitute
		D Intraluminal Device
		J Synthetic Substitute
		K Nonautologous Tissue Substitute
			Z No Qualifier

Y Mouth and Throat	**0** Open **3** Percutaneous **7** Via Natural or Artificial Opening **8** Via Natural or Artificial Opening Endoscopic	**0** Drainage Device **1** Radioactive Element **7** Autologous Tissue Substitute **D** Intraluminal Device **J** Synthetic Substitute **K** Nonautologous Tissue Substitute **Y** Other Device	**Z** No Qualifier
Y Mouth and Throat	**X** External	**0** Drainage Device **1** Radioactive Element **7** Autologous Tissue Substitute **D** Intraluminal Device **J** Synthetic Substitute **K** Nonautologous Tissue Substitute	**Z** No Qualifier

Non-OR	0CWA[0,3][0,C,Y]Z
Non-OR	0CWA[7,8]YZ
Non-OR	0CWAX[0,C]Z
Non-OR	0CWS[3,7,8]YZ
Non-OR	0CWSX[0,7,D,J,K]Z
Non-OR	0CWY07Z
Non-OR	0CWY[3,7,8]YZ
Non-OR	0CWYX[0,1,7,D,J,K]Z

NC Noncovered Procedure   **LC** Limited Coverage   **QA** Questionable OB Admit   **NT** New Tech Add-on   ⊞ Combination Member   ♂ Male   ♀ Female

ICD-10-PCS 2023   **371**

Mouth and Throat

Ø   **Medical and Surgical**
C   **Mouth and Throat**
X   **Transfer**   Definition: Moving, without taking out, all or a portion of a body part to another location to take over the function of all or a portion of a body part
                Explanation: The body part transferred remains connected to its vascular and nervous supply

Body Part Character 4	Approach Character 5	Device Character 6	Qualifier Character 7

Ø   **Upper Lip**
     Frenulum labii superioris
     Labial gland
     Vermilion border
 1   **Lower Lip**
     Frenulum labii inferioris
     Labial gland
     Vermilion border
 3   **Soft Palate**
 4   **Buccal Mucosa**
     Buccal gland
     Molar gland
     Palatine gland
 5   **Upper Gingiva**
 6   **Lower Gingiva**
 7   **Tongue**
     Frenulum linguae
	Ø Open
	 X External
		Z No Device	**Z** No Qualifier

Gastrointestinal System ØD1–ØDY

Character Meanings

This Character Meaning table is provided as a guide to assist the user in the identification of character members that may be found in this section of code tables. It **SHOULD NOT** be used to build a PCS code.

Operation–Character 3		Body Part–Character 4		Approach–Character 5		Device–Character 6		Qualifier–Character 7	
1	Bypass	Ø	Upper Intestinal Tract	Ø	Open	Ø	Drainage Device	Ø	Allogeneic
2	Change	1	Esophagus, Upper	3	Percutaneous	1	Radioactive Element	1	Syngeneic
5	Destruction	2	Esophagus, Middle	4	Percutaneous Endoscopic	2	Monitoring Device	2	Zooplastic
7	Dilation	3	Esophagus, Lower	7	Via Natural or Artificial Opening	3	Infusion Device	3	Vertical OR Laser Interstitial Thermal Therapy
8	Division	4	Esophagogastric Junction	8	Via Natural or Artificial Opening Endoscopic	7	Autologous Tissue Substitute	4	Cutaneous
9	Drainage	5	Esophagus	F	Via Natural or Artificial Opening with Percutaneous Endoscopic Assistance	B	Intraluminal Device, Airway	5	Esophagus
B	Excision	6	Stomach	X	External	C	Extraluminal Device	6	Stomach
C	Extirpation	7	Stomach, Pylorus			D	Intraluminal Device	7	Vagina
D	Extraction	8	Small Intestine			J	Synthetic Substitute	8	Small Intestine
F	Fragmentation	9	Duodenum			K	Nonautologous Tissue Substitute	9	Duodenum
H	Insertion	A	Jejunum			L	Artificial Sphincter	A	Jejunum
J	Inspection	B	Ileum			M	Stimulator Lead	B	Ileum OR Bladder
L	Occlusion	C	Ileocecal Valve			U	Feeding Device	C	Ureter, Right
M	Reattachment	D	Lower Intestinal Tract			Y	Other Device	D	Ureter, Left
N	Release	E	Large Intestine			Z	No Device	E	Large Intestine
P	Removal	F	Large Intestine, Right					F	Ureters, Bilateral
Q	Repair	G	Large Intestine, Left					H	Cecum
R	Replacement	H	Cecum					K	Ascending Colon
S	Reposition	J	Appendix					L	Transverse Colon
T	Resection	K	Ascending Colon					M	Descending Colon
U	Supplement	L	Transverse Colon					N	Sigmoid Colon
V	Restriction	M	Descending Colon					P	Rectum
W	Revision	N	Sigmoid Colon					Q	Anus
X	Transfer	P	Rectum					X	Diagnostic
Y	Transplantation	Q	Anus					Z	No Qualifier
		R	Anal Sphincter						
		U	Omentum						
		V	Mesentery						
		W	Peritoneum						

Gastrointestinal System ØD1–ØDY

AHA Coding Clinic for Gastrointestinal System

2022, 1Q, 11	Procedures performed on a continuous vessel, ICD-10-PCS Guideline B4.1c

AHA Coding Clinic for table ØD1

2021, 1Q, 19	Kock pouch revision surgery
2019, 4Q, 29	Intestinal bypass
2017, 2Q, 17	Billroth II (distal gastrectomy and gastrojejunostomy)
2016, 2Q, 31	Laparoscopic biliopancreatic diversion with duodenal switch
2014, 4Q, 41	Abdominoperineal resection (APR) with flap closure of perineum and colostomy

AHA Coding Clinic for table ØD2

2022, 1Q, 45	Insertion, removal and replacement of endoluminal vacuum application
2019, 1Q, 26	Exchange of clogged gastrojejunostomy tube

AHA Coding Clinic for table ØD5

2017, 1Q, 34	Debulking of tumor and peritoneum ablation

AHA Coding Clinic for table ØD7

2020, 3Q, 45	Dilation versus drainage of perirectal cyst
2017, 3Q, 23	Laparoscopic pyloromyotomy
2014, 4Q, 40	Dilation of gastrojejunostomy anastomosis stricture

AHA Coding Clinic for table ØD8

2019, 2Q, 15	Reversal of Roux-en-Y bypass
2017, 3Q, 22	Laparoscopic esophagomyotomy (Heller type) and Toupet fundoplication
2017, 3Q, 23	Laparoscopic pyloromyotomy

AHA Coding Clinic for table ØD9

2020, 3Q, 45	Dilation versus drainage of perirectal cyst
2015, 2Q, 29	Insertion of nasogastric tube for drainage and feeding

AHA Coding Clinic for table ØDB

2021, 3Q, 28	Retrieval of capsule via small bowel excision
2021, 2Q, 11	Serosal injury with excision of small intestine
2021, 1Q, 20	Rectal suction biopsy
2021, 1Q, 22	Total proctocolectomy with creation of J-pouch
2019, 2Q, 15	Reversal of Roux-en-Y bypass
2019, 1Q, 3-8	Whipple procedure
2019, 1Q, 27	Excision of pelvic sidewall mass
2017, 2Q, 17	Billroth II (distal gastrectomy and gastrojejunostomy)
2017, 1Q, 16	Hepatic flexure versus transverse colon
2016, 3Q, 3-7	Stoma creation & takedown procedures
2016, 2Q, 31	Laparoscopic biliopancreatic diversion with duodenal switch
2016, 1Q, 22	Perineal proctectomy
2016, 1Q, 24	Endoscopic brush biopsy of esophagus
2014, 4Q, 40	Abdominoperineal resection (APR) with flap closure of perineum and colostomy
2014, 3Q, 28	Ileostomy takedown and parastomal hernia repair
2014, 3Q, 32	Pyloric-sparing Whipple procedure

AHA Coding Clinic for table ØDD

2021, 1Q, 20	Rectal suction biopsy
2017, 4Q, 41-42	Extraction procedures

AHA Coding Clinic for table ØDH

2022, 1Q, 44	Insertion, removal and replacement of endoluminal vacuum application
2020, 4Q, 43-44	Insertion of radioactive element
2020, 3Q, 43	Staged laparoscopic gastric conduit and placement of feeding tube
2019, 2Q, 18	Endoscopic wound VAC placement
2016, 3Q, 26	Insertion of gastrostomy tube
2013, 4Q, 117	Percutaneous endoscopic placement of gastrostomy tube

AHA Coding Clinic for table ØDJ

2019, 1Q, 25	Laparoscopic appendectomy converted to open procedure
2019, 1Q, 25	Milking of inspissated material from ileum to colon
2017, 2Q, 15	Low anterior resection with sigmoidoscopy
2016, 2Q, 20	Capsule endoscopy of small intestine
2015, 3Q, 24	Esophagogastroduodenoscopy with epinephrine injection for control of bleeding

AHA Coding Clinic for table ØDL

2013, 4Q, 112	Endoscopic banding of esophageal varices

AHA Coding Clinic for table ØDN

2017, 4Q, 49-50	New and revised body part values - Repositioning of the intestine
2017, 1Q, 35	Lysis of omental and peritoneal adhesions
2015, 3Q, 15	Vascular ring surgery with release of esophagus and trachea
2015, 3Q, 16	Vascular ring surgery and double aortic arch

AHA Coding Clinic for table ØDP

2019, 2Q, 18	Removal of wound VAC

AHA Coding Clinic for table ØDQ

2019, 2Q, 15	Reversal of Roux-en-Y bypass
2018, 2Q, 25	Third and fourth degree obstetric lacerations
2018, 1Q, 11	Repair of internal hernia at Petersen space
2017, 3Q, 17	Posterior sagittal anorectoplasty
2016, 3Q, 3-7	Stoma creation & takedown procedures
2016, 3Q, 26	Insertion of gastrostomy tube
2016, 1Q, 7	Obstetrical perineal laceration repair
2016, 1Q, 8	Obstetrical perineal laceration repair
2014, 4Q, 20	Control of bleeding duodenal ulcer

AHA Coding Clinic for table ØDS

2019, 1Q, 30	Laparoscopic-assisted rectopexy with manual reduction of prolapse
2017, 4Q, 49-50	New and revised body part values - Repositioning of the intestine
2017, 3Q, 9	Ileocolic intussusception reduction via air enema
2017, 3Q, 17	Posterior sagittal anorectoplasty
2016, 3Q, 3-5	Stoma creation & takedown procedures

AHA Coding Clinic for table ØDT

2022, 1Q, 49	Robotic-assisted low anterior resection of colon
2021, 1Q, 22	Total proctocolectomy with creation of J-pouch
2020, 4Q, 100	Robotic-assisted sigmoid colectomy with extension of incision for specimen removal
2019, 1Q, 3-8	Whipple procedure
2019, 1Q, 14	Esophagectomy with colon interposition
2017, 4Q, 49-50	New and revised body part values - Repositioning of the intestine
2014, 4Q, 40	Abdominoperineal resection (APR) with flap closure of perineum and colostomy
2014, 4Q, 42	Right colectomy with side-to-side functional end-to-end anastomosis
2014, 3Q, 6	Ileocecectomy including cecum, terminal ileum and appendix
2014, 3Q, 6	Right colectomy

AHA Coding Clinic for table ØDU

2021, 2Q, 20	Malone antegrade continence enema procedure
2021, 1Q, 22	Total proctocolectomy with creation of J-pouch
2019, 1Q, 30	Laparoscopic-assisted rectopexy with manual reduction of prolapse

AHA Coding Clinic for table ØDV

2017, 3Q, 22	Laparoscopic esophagomyotomy (Heller type) and Toupet fundoplication
2016, 2Q, 22	Esophageal lengthening Collis gastroplasty with Nissen fundoplication and hiatal hernia
2014, 3Q, 28	Laparoscopic Nissen fundoplication and diaphragmatic hernia repair

AHA Coding Clinic for table ØDW

2021, 1Q, 19	Kock pouch revision surgery
2018, 1Q, 20	Adjustment of gastric band

AHA Coding Clinic for table ØDX

2019, 4Q, 29-30	Transfer large intestine to vagina
2019, 1Q, 14	Esophagectomy with colon interposition
2017, 2Q, 18	Esophagectomy and esophagogastrectomy with cervical esophagogastrostomy
2016, 2Q, 22	Esophageal lengthening Collis gastroplasty with Nissen fundoplication and hiatal hernia
2015, 1Q, 28	Repair of bronchopleural fistula using omental pedicle graft

Upper Intestinal Tract (Ø) and Lower Intestinal Tract (D)

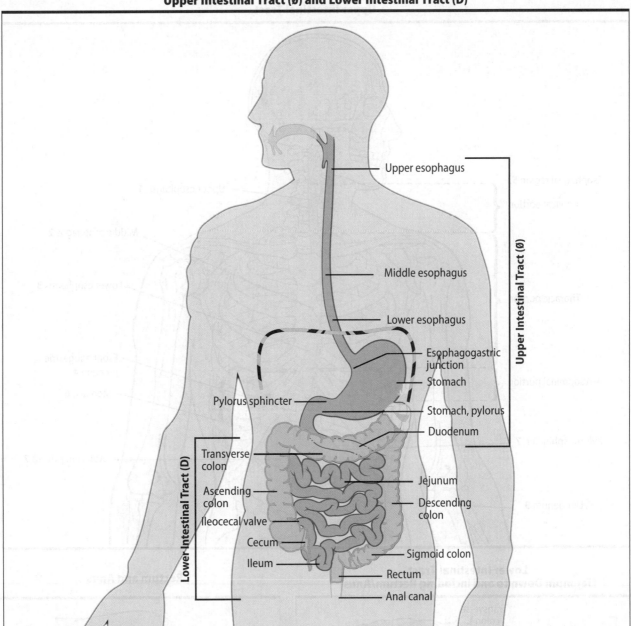

Upper Intestinal Tract

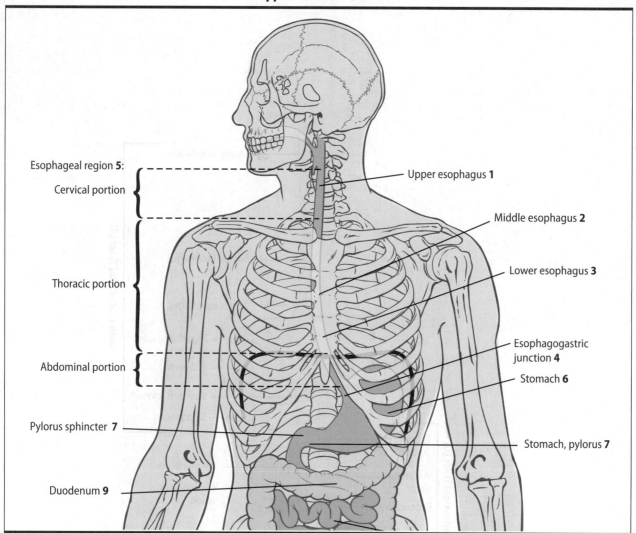

Esophageal region **5**:

Cervical portion

Thoracic portion

Abdominal portion

Pylorus sphincter **7**

Duodenum **9**

Upper esophagus **1**

Middle esophagus **2**

Lower esophagus **3**

Esophagogastric junction **4**

Stomach **6**

Stomach, pylorus **7**

Lower Intestinal Tract
(Jejunum Down to and Including Rectum/Anus)

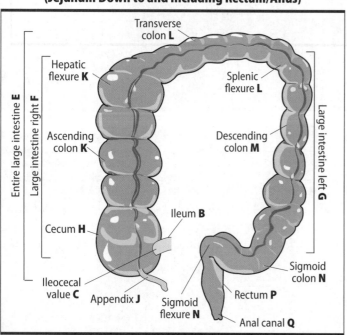

Transverse colon **L**

Hepatic flexure **K**

Splenic flexure **L**

Ascending colon **K**

Descending colon **M**

Entire large intestine **E**

Large intestine right **F**

Large intestine left **G**

Cecum **H**

Ileum **B**

Ileocecal value **C**

Appendix **J**

Sigmoid flexure **N**

Rectum **P**

Sigmoid colon **N**

Anal canal **Q**

Rectum and Anus

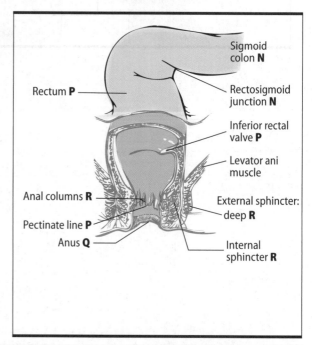

Rectum **P**

Anal columns **R**

Pectinate line **P**

Anus **Q**

Sigmoid colon **N**

Rectosigmoid junction **N**

Inferior rectal valve **P**

Levator ani muscle

External sphincter: deep **R**

Internal sphincter **R**

Ø Medical and Surgical
D Gastrointestinal System
1 Bypass   Definition: Altering the route of passage of the contents of a tubular body part

Explanation: Rerouting contents of a body part to a downstream area of the normal route, to a similar route and body part, or to an abnormal route and dissimilar body part. Includes one or more anastomoses, with or without the use of a device.

Body Part Character 4	Approach Character 5	Device Character 6	Qualifier Character 7
1 Esophagus, Upper Cervical esophagus 2 Esophagus, Middle Thoracic esophagus 3 Esophagus, Lower Abdominal esophagus 5 Esophagus	Ø Open 4 Percutaneous Endoscopic 8 Via Natural or Artificial Opening Endoscopic	7 Autologous Tissue Substitute J Synthetic Substitute K Nonautologous Tissue Substitute Z No Device	4 Cutaneous 6 Stomach 9 Duodenum A Jejunum B Ileum
1 Esophagus, Upper Cervical esophagus 2 Esophagus, Middle Thoracic esophagus 3 Esophagus, Lower Abdominal esophagus 5 Esophagus	3 Percutaneous	J Synthetic Substitute	4 Cutaneous
6 Stomach 9 Duodenum	Ø Open 4 Percutaneous Endoscopic 8 Via Natural or Artificial Opening Endoscopic	7 Autologous Tissue Substitute J Synthetic Substitute K Nonautologous Tissue Substitute Z No Device	4 Cutaneous 9 Duodenum A Jejunum B Ileum L Transverse Colon
6 Stomach 9 Duodenum	3 Percutaneous	J Synthetic Substitute	4 Cutaneous
8 Small Intestine	Ø Open 4 Percutaneous Endoscopic 8 Via Natural or Artificial Opening Endoscopic	7 Autologous Tissue Substitute J Synthetic Substitute K Nonautologous Tissue Substitute Z No Device	4 Cutaneous 8 Small Intestine H Cecum K Ascending Colon L Transverse Colon M Descending Colon N Sigmoid Colon P Rectum Q Anus
A Jejunum Duodenojejunal flexure	Ø Open 4 Percutaneous Endoscopic 8 Via Natural or Artificial Opening Endoscopic	7 Autologous Tissue Substitute J Synthetic Substitute K Nonautologous Tissue Substitute Z No Device	4 Cutaneous A Jejunum B Ileum H Cecum K Ascending Colon L Transverse Colon M Descending Colon N Sigmoid Colon P Rectum Q Anus
A Jejunum Duodenojejunal flexure	3 Percutaneous	J Synthetic Substitute	4 Cutaneous
B Ileum	Ø Open 4 Percutaneous Endoscopic 8 Via Natural or Artificial Opening Endoscopic	7 Autologous Tissue Substitute J Synthetic Substitute K Nonautologous Tissue Substitute Z No Device	4 Cutaneous B Ileum H Cecum K Ascending Colon L Transverse Colon M Descending Colon N Sigmoid Colon P Rectum Q Anus
B Ileum	3 Percutaneous	J Synthetic Substitute	4 Cutaneous
E Large Intestine	Ø Open 4 Percutaneous Endoscopic 8 Via Natural or Artificial Opening Endoscopic	7 Autologous Tissue Substitute J Synthetic Substitute K Nonautologous Tissue Substitute Z No Device	4 Cutaneous E Large Intestine P Rectum
H Cecum	Ø Open 4 Percutaneous Endoscopic 8 Via Natural or Artificial Opening Endoscopic	7 Autologous Tissue Substitute J Synthetic Substitute K Nonautologous Tissue Substitute Z No Device	4 Cutaneous H Cecum K Ascending Colon L Transverse Colon M Descending Colon N Sigmoid Colon P Rectum
H Cecum	3 Percutaneous	J Synthetic Substitute	4 Cutaneous

Non-OR ØD16[Ø,4,8][7,J,K,Z]4
Non-OR ØD163J4
HAC ØD16[Ø,4,8][7,J,K,Z][9,A,B,L] when reported with PDx E66.Ø1 and SDx K68.11, K95.Ø1, K95.81 or T81.4Ø–T81.49 with 7th character A

ØD1 Continued on next page

NC Noncovered Procedure   LC Limited Coverage   QA Questionable OB Admit   NT New Tech Add-on   ⊞ Combination Member   ♂ Male   ♀ Female

ICD-10-PCS 2023   377

ØD1–ØD1

Ø   Medical and Surgical
D   Gastrointestinal System
1   Bypass   Definition: Altering the route of passage of the contents of a tubular body part

ØD1 Continued

Explanation: Rerouting contents of a body part to a downstream area of the normal route, to a similar route and body part, or to an abnormal route and dissimilar body part. Includes one or more anastomoses, with or without the use of a device.

Body Part Character 4	Approach Character 5	Device Character 6	Qualifier Character 7
K Ascending Colon	Ø Open 4 Percutaneous Endoscopic 8 Via Natural or Artificial Opening Endoscopic	7 Autologous Tissue Substitute J Synthetic Substitute K Nonautologous Tissue Substitute Z No Device	4 Cutaneous K Ascending Colon L Transverse Colon M Descending Colon N Sigmoid Colon P Rectum
K Ascending Colon	3 Percutaneous	J Synthetic Substitute	4 Cutaneous

L   Transverse Colon
     Hepatic flexure
     Splenic flexure
	Ø Open
	4 Percutaneous Endoscopic
	8 Via Natural or Artificial Opening
	     Endoscopic
		7 Autologous Tissue Substitute
		J Synthetic Substitute
		K Nonautologous Tissue Substitute
		Z No Device
			4 Cutaneous
			L Transverse Colon
			M Descending Colon
			N Sigmoid Colon
			P Rectum

L   Transverse Colon
     Hepatic flexure
     Splenic flexure
	3 Percutaneous	J Synthetic Substitute	4 Cutaneous

M Descending Colon	Ø Open 4 Percutaneous Endoscopic 8 Via Natural or Artificial Opening Endoscopic	7 Autologous Tissue Substitute J Synthetic Substitute K Nonautologous Tissue Substitute Z No Device	4 Cutaneous M Descending Colon N Sigmoid Colon P Rectum
M Descending Colon	3 Percutaneous	J Synthetic Substitute	4 Cutaneous

N   Sigmoid Colon
     Rectosigmoid junction
     Sigmoid flexure
	Ø Open
	4 Percutaneous Endoscopic
	8 Via Natural or Artificial Opening
	     Endoscopic
		7 Autologous Tissue Substitute
		J Synthetic Substitute
		K Nonautologous Tissue Substitute
		Z No Device
			4 Cutaneous
			N Sigmoid Colon
			P Rectum

N   Sigmoid Colon
     Rectosigmoid junction
     Sigmoid flexure
	3 Percutaneous	J Synthetic Substitute	4 Cutaneous

Ø   Medical and Surgical
D   Gastrointestinal System
2   Change   Definition: Taking out or off a device from a body part and putting back an identical or similar device in or on the same body part without cutting or puncturing the skin or a mucous membrane

Explanation: All CHANGE procedures are coded using the approach EXTERNAL

Body Part Character 4	Approach Character 5	Device Character 6	Qualifier Character 7
Ø Upper Intestinal Tract D Lower Intestinal Tract	X External	Ø Drainage Device U Feeding Device Y Other Device	Z No Qualifier

U   Omentum
     Gastrocolic ligament
     Gastrocolic omentum
     Gastrohepatic omentum
     Gastrophrenic ligament
     Gastrosplenic ligament
     Greater Omentum
     Hepatogastric ligament
     Lesser Omentum
V   Mesentery
     Mesoappendix
     Mesocolon
W   Peritoneum
     Epiploic foramen
	X External	Ø Drainage Device
		Y Other Device
			Z No Qualifier

Non-OR   All body part, approach, device, and qualifier values

Non-OR Procedure   DRG Non-OR Procedure   Valid OR Procedure   HAC Associated Procedure   Combination Only   New/Revised April   New/Revised October

378   ICD-10-PCS 2023

Ø Medical and Surgical
D Gastrointestinal System
5 Destruction   Definition: Physical eradication of all or a portion of a body part by the direct use of energy, force, or a destructive agent
                Explanation: None of the body part is physically taken out

Body Part — Character 4		Approach — Character 5	Device — Character 6	Qualifier — Character 7

1 Esophagus, Upper
   Cervical esophagus
2 Esophagus, Middle
   Thoracic esophagus
3 Esophagus, Lower
   Abdominal esophagus
4 Esophagogastric Junction
   Cardia
   Cardioesophageal junction
   Gastroesophageal (GE)
      junction
5 Esophagus
6 Stomach
7 Stomach, Pylorus
   Pyloric antrum
   Pyloric canal
   Pyloric sphincter
8 Small Intestine
9 Duodenum
	A Jejunum
	   Duodenojejunal flexure
	B Ileum
	C Ileocecal Valve
	E Large Intestine
	F Large Intestine, Right
	G Large Intestine, Left
	H Cecum
	J Appendix
	   Vermiform appendix
	K Ascending Colon
	L Transverse Colon
	   Hepatic flexure
	   Splenic flexure
	M Descending Colon
	N Sigmoid Colon
	   Rectosigmoid junction
	   Sigmoid flexure
	P Rectum
	   Anorectal junction
		Ø Open
		3 Percutaneous
		4 Percutaneous Endoscopic
			Z No Device	**3 Laser Interstitial Thermal Therapy**
				Z No Qualifier

1 Esophagus, Upper
   Cervical esophagus
2 Esophagus, Middle
   Thoracic esophagus
3 Esophagus, Lower
   Abdominal esophagus
4 Esophagogastric Junction
   Cardia
   Cardioesophageal junction
   Gastroesophageal (GE)
      junction
5 Esophagus
6 Stomach
7 Stomach, Pylorus
   Pyloric antrum
   Pyloric canal
   Pyloric sphincter
8 Small Intestine
9 Duodenum
	A Jejunum
	   Duodenojejunal flexure
	B Ileum
	C Ileocecal Valve
	E Large Intestine
	F Large Intestine, Right
	G Large Intestine, Left
	H Cecum
	J Appendix
	   Vermiform appendix
	K Ascending Colon
	L Transverse Colon
	   Hepatic flexure
	   Splenic flexure
	M Descending Colon
	N Sigmoid Colon
	   Rectosigmoid junction
	   Sigmoid flexure
	P Rectum
	   Anorectal junction
		7 Via Natural or Artificial Opening
		8 Via Natural or Artificial Opening Endoscopic
			Z No Device	**Z No Qualifier**

Q Anus Anal orifice		**Ø Open** **3 Percutaneous** **4 Percutaneous Endoscopic**	**Z No Device**	**3 Laser Interstitial Thermal Therapy** **Z No Qualifier**
Q Anus Anal orifice		**7 Via Natural or Artificial Opening** **8 Via Natural or Artificial Opening Endoscopic** **X External**	**Z No Device**	**Z No Qualifier**

R Anal Sphincter
   External anal sphincter
   Internal anal sphincter
U Omentum
   Gastrocolic ligament
   Gastrocolic omentum
   Gastrohepatic omentum
   Gastrophrenic ligament
   Gastrosplenic ligament
   Greater Omentum
   Hepatogastric ligament
   Lesser Omentum
V Mesentery
   Mesoappendix
   Mesocolon
W Peritoneum
   Epiploic foramen
		Ø Open
		3 Percutaneous
		4 Percutaneous Endoscopic
			Z No Device	**Z No Qualifier**

Non-OR	ØD5[1,2,3,4,5,6,7,9,E,F,G,H,K,L,M,N]4ZZ
Non-OR	ØD5P[Ø,3,4]ZZ
Non-OR	ØD5[1,2,3,4,5,6,7,8,9,A,B,C,E,F,G,H,K,L,M,N]8ZZ
Non-OR	ØD5P[7,8]ZZ
Non-OR	ØD5Q4ZZ
Non-OR	ØD5Q8ZZ
Non-OR	ØD5R4ZZ

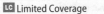 Noncovered Procedure   Limited Coverage   **QA** Questionable OB Admit   **NT** New Tech Add-on   ⊞ Combination Member   ♂ Male   ♀ Female

ICD-10-PCS 2023   **379**

Gastrointestinal System

Ø   Medical and Surgical
D   Gastrointestinal System
7   Dilation   Definition: Expanding an orifice or the lumen of a tubular body part

Explanation: The orifice can be a natural orifice or an artificially created orifice. Accomplished by stretching a tubular body part using intraluminal pressure or by cutting part of the orifice or wall of the tubular body part.

Body Part Character 4	Approach Character 5	Device Character 6	Qualifier Character 7
1 Esophagus, Upper Cervical esophagus **2 Esophagus, Middle** Thoracic esophagus **3 Esophagus, Lower** Abdominal esophagus **4 Esophagogastric Junction** Cardia Cardioesophageal junction Gastroesophageal (GE) junction **5 Esophagus** **6 Stomach** **7 Stomach, Pylorus** Pyloric antrum Pyloric canal Pyloric sphincter **8 Small Intestine** **9 Duodenum** **A Jejunum** Duodenojejunal flexure **B Ileum** **C Ileocecal Valve** **E Large Intestine** **F Large Intestine, Right** **G Large Intestine, Left** **H Cecum** **K Ascending Colon** **L Transverse Colon** Hepatic flexure Splenic flexure **M Descending Colon** **N Sigmoid Colon** Rectosigmoid junction Sigmoid flexure **P Rectum** Anorectal junction **Q Anus** Anal orifice	**Ø Open** **3 Percutaneous** **4 Percutaneous Endoscopic** **7 Via Natural or Artificial Opening** **8 Via Natural or Artificial Opening** **Endoscopic**	**D Intraluminal Device** **Z No Device**	**Z No Qualifier**

Non-OR ØD7[1,2,3,4,5,6,8,9,A,B,C,E,F,G,H,K,L,M,N,P,Q][7,8][D,Z]Z
Non-OR ØD77[4,8]DZ
Non-OR ØD777[D,Z]Z
Non-OR ØD7[8,9,A,B,C,E,F,G,H,K,L,M,N][Ø,3,4]DZ

Ø   Medical and Surgical
D   Gastrointestinal System
8   Division   Definition: Cutting into a body part, without draining fluids and/or gases from the body part, in order to separate or transect a body part

Explanation: All or a portion of the body part is separated into two or more portions

Body Part Character 4	Approach Character 5	Device Character 6	Qualifier Character 7
4 Esophagogastric Junction Cardia Cardioesophageal junction Gastroesophageal (GE) junction **7 Stomach, Pylorus** Pyloric antrum Pyloric canal Pyloric sphincter	**Ø Open** **3 Percutaneous** **4 Percutaneous Endoscopic** **7 Via Natural or Artificial Opening** **8 Via Natural or Artificial Opening** **Endoscopic**	**Z No Device**	**Z No Qualifier**
R Anal Sphincter External anal sphincter Internal anal sphincter	**Ø Open** **3 Percutaneous**	**Z No Device**	**Z No Qualifier**

Ø **Medical and Surgical**
D **Gastrointestinal System**
9 **Drainage**　　　Definition: Taking or letting out fluids and/or gases from a body part
　　　　　　　　　　　Explanation: The qualifier DIAGNOSTIC is used to identify drainage procedures that are biopsies

Body Part Character 4		Approach Character 5	Device Character 6	Qualifier Character 7
1 Esophagus, Upper 　Cervical esophagus **2** Esophagus, Middle 　Thoracic esophagus **3** Esophagus, Lower 　Abdominal esophagus **4** Esophagogastric 　Junction 　Cardia 　Cardioesophageal 　　junction 　Gastroesophageal (GE) 　　junction **5** Esophagus **6** Stomach **7** Stomach, Pylorus 　Pyloric antrum 　Pyloric canal 　Pyloric sphincter **8** Small Intestine **9** Duodenum	**A** Jejunum 　Duodenojejunal flexure **B** Ileum **C** Ileocecal Valve **E** Large Intestine **F** Large Intestine, Right **G** Large Intestine, Left **H** Cecum **J** Appendix 　Vermiform appendix **K** Ascending Colon **L** Transverse Colon 　Hepatic flexure 　Splenic flexure **M** Descending Colon **N** Sigmoid Colon 　Rectosigmoid junction 　Sigmoid flexure **P** Rectum 　Anorectal junction	**Ø** Open **3** Percutaneous **4** Percutaneous Endoscopic **7** Via Natural or Artificial 　Opening **8** Via Natural or Artificial 　Opening Endoscopic	**Ø** Drainage Device	**Z** No Qualifier
1 Esophagus, Upper 　Cervical esophagus **2** Esophagus, Middle 　Thoracic esophagus **3** Esophagus, Lower 　Abdominal esophagus **4** Esophagogastric 　Junction 　Cardia 　Cardioesophageal 　　junction 　Gastroesophageal (GE) 　　junction **5** Esophagus **6** Stomach **7** Stomach, Pylorus 　Pyloric antrum 　Pyloric canal 　Pyloric sphincter **8** Small Intestine **9** Duodenum	**A** Jejunum 　Duodenojejunal flexure **B** Ileum **C** Ileocecal Valve **E** Large Intestine **F** Large Intestine, Right **G** Large Intestine, Left **H** Cecum **J** Appendix 　Vermiform appendix **K** Ascending Colon **L** Transverse Colon 　Hepatic flexure 　Splenic flexure **M** Descending Colon **N** Sigmoid Colon 　Rectosigmoid junction 　Sigmoid flexure **P** Rectum 　Anorectal junction	**Ø** Open **3** Percutaneous **4** Percutaneous Endoscopic **7** Via Natural or Artificial 　Opening **8** Via Natural or Artificial 　Opening Endoscopic	**Z** No Device	**X** Diagnostic **Z** No Qualifier
Q Anus 　Anal orifice		**Ø** Open **3** Percutaneous **4** Percutaneous Endoscopic **7** Via Natural or Artificial 　Opening **8** Via Natural or Artificial 　Opening Endoscopic **X** External	**Ø** Drainage Device	**Z** No Qualifier
Q Anus 　Anal orifice		**Ø** Open **3** Percutaneous **4** Percutaneous Endoscopic **7** Via Natural or Artificial 　Opening **8** Via Natural or Artificial 　Opening Endoscopic **X** External	**Z** No Device	**X** Diagnostic **Z** No Qualifier

Non-OR	ØD9[1,2,3,4,5,C,J]3ØZ
Non-OR	ØD9[6,7,8,9,A,B,E,F,G,H,K,L,M,N,P][3,7,8]ØZ
Non-OR	ØD9[1,2,3,4,5,6,7,8,9,A,B,C,E,F,G,H,K,L,M,N,P][3,4,7,8]ZX
Non-OR	ØD9[1,2,3,4,5,6,7,8,9,A,B,C,E,F,G,H,J,K,L,M,N,P]3ZZ
Non-OR	ØD9Q3ØZ
Non-OR	ØD9Q[Ø,3,4,7,8,X]ZX
Non-OR	ØD9Q3ZZ

ØD9 Continued on next page

NC Noncovered Procedure　　LC Limited Coverage　　QA Questionable OB Admit　　NT New Tech Add-on　　⊞ Combination Member　　♂ Male　　♀ Female

ICD-10-PCS 2023　　　**381**

ØD9–ØD9

Gastrointestinal System

Ø　**Medical and Surgical**
D　**Gastrointestinal System**
9　**Drainage**　　　Definition: Taking or letting out fluids and/or gases from a body part
　　　　　　　　　　　Explanation: The qualifier DIAGNOSTIC is used to identify drainage procedures that are biopsies

Body Part Character 4	Approach Character 5	Device Character 6	Qualifier Character 7
R Anal Sphincter 　External anal sphincter 　Internal anal sphincter **U** Omentum 　Gastrocolic ligament 　Gastrocolic omentum 　Gastrohepatic omentum 　Gastrophrenic ligament 　Gastrosplenic ligament 　Greater Omentum 　Hepatogastric ligament 　Lesser Omentum **V** Mesentery 　Mesoappendix 　Mesocolon **W** Peritoneum 　Epiploic foramen	**Ø** Open **3** Percutaneous **4** Percutaneous Endoscopic	**Ø** Drainage Device	**Z** No Qualifier
R Anal Sphincter 　External anal sphincter 　Internal anal sphincter **U** Omentum 　Gastrocolic ligament 　Gastrocolic omentum 　Gastrohepatic omentum 　Gastrophrenic ligament 　Gastrosplenic ligament 　Greater Omentum 　Hepatogastric ligament 　Lesser Omentum **V** Mesentery 　Mesoappendix 　Mesocolon **W** Peritoneum 　Epiploic foramen	**Ø** Open **3** Percutaneous **4** Percutaneous Endoscopic	**Z** No Device	**X** Diagnostic **Z** No Qualifier

Non-OR	ØD9[R,W]3ØZ
Non-OR	ØD9[U,V][3,4]ØZ
Non-OR	ØD9[R,U,V,W]3Z[X,Z]
Non-OR	ØD9R[Ø,4]ZX
Non-OR	ØD9[U,V]4ZZ

Ø Medical and Surgical
D Gastrointestinal System
B Excision   Definition: Cutting out or off, without replacement, a portion of a body part
                    Explanation: The qualifier DIAGNOSTIC is used to identify excision procedures that are biopsies

Body Part Character 4		Approach Character 5	Device Character 6	Qualifier Character 7

1 **Esophagus, Upper**
  Cervical esophagus
2 **Esophagus, Middle**
  Thoracic esophagus
3 **Esophagus, Lower**
  Abdominal esophagus
4 **Esophagogastric**
Junction
  Cardia
  Cardioesophageal
    junction
  Gastroesophageal (GE)
    junction
5 **Esophagus**
7 **Stomach, Pylorus**
  Pyloric antrum
  Pyloric canal
  Pyloric sphincter
	8 **Small Intestine**
	9 **Duodenum**
	A **Jejunum**
	  Duodenojejunal flexure
	B **Ileum**
	C **Ileocecal Valve**
	E **Large Intestine**
	F **Large Intestine, Right**
	H **Cecum**
	J **Appendix**
	  Vermiform appendix
	K **Ascending Colon**
	P **Rectum**
	  Anorectal junction
		Ø Open
		3 Percutaneous
		4 Percutaneous Endoscopic
		7 Via Natural or Artificial
		  Opening
		8 Via Natural or Artificial
		  Opening Endoscopic
			Z No Device	X Diagnostic
				Z No Qualifier

6 **Stomach**		Ø Open
		3 Percutaneous
		4 Percutaneous Endoscopic
		7 Via Natural or Artificial
		  Opening
		8 Via Natural or Artificial
		  Opening Endoscopic
			Z No Device	3 Vertical
				X Diagnostic
				Z No Qualifier

G **Large Intestine, Left**
L **Transverse Colon**
  Hepatic flexure
  Splenic flexure
M **Descending Colon**
N **Sigmoid Colon**
  Rectosigmoid junction
  Sigmoid flexure
		Ø Open
		3 Percutaneous
		4 Percutaneous Endoscopic
		7 Via Natural or Artificial
		  Opening
		8 Via Natural or Artificial
		  Opening Endoscopic
			Z No Device	X Diagnostic
				Z No Qualifier

G **Large Intestine, Left**
L **Transverse Colon**
  Hepatic flexure
  Splenic flexure
M **Descending Colon**
N **Sigmoid Colon**
  Rectosigmoid junction
  Sigmoid flexure
		F Via Natural or Artificial
		  Opening with Percutaneous
		  Endoscopic Assistance
			Z No Device	Z No Qualifier

Q **Anus**
  Anal orifice
		Ø Open
		3 Percutaneous
		4 Percutaneous Endoscopic
		7 Via Natural or Artificial
		  Opening
		8 Via Natural or Artificial
		  Opening Endoscopic
		X External
			Z No Device	X Diagnostic
				Z No Qualifier

R **Anal Sphincter**
  External anal sphincter
  Internal anal sphincter
U **Omentum**
  Gastrocolic ligament
  Gastrocolic omentum
  Gastrohepatic omentum
  Gastrophrenic ligament
  Gastrosplenic ligament
  Greater Omentum
  Hepatogastric ligament
  Lesser Omentum
V **Mesentery**
  Mesoappendix
  Mesocolon
W **Peritoneum**
  Epiploic foramen
		Ø Open
		3 Percutaneous
		4 Percutaneous Endoscopic
			Z No Device	X Diagnostic
				Z No Qualifier

Non-OR	ØDB[1,2,3,4,5,7,8,9,A,B,C,E,F,H,K,P][3,4,7,8]ZX		**Non-OR**	ØDB[G,L,M,N]8ZZ
Non-OR	ØDB[1,2,3,5,7,9][4,8]ZZ		**Non-OR**	ØDBQ[Ø,3,4,7,8,X]ZX
Non-OR	ØDB[4,E,F,H,K,P]8ZZ		**Non-OR**	ØDBQ8ZZ
Non-OR	ØDB6[3,7]ZX		**Non-OR**	ØDBR[Ø,3,4]ZX
Non-OR	ØDB68Z[X,Z]		**Non-OR**	ØDB[U,V,W][3,4]ZX
Non-OR	ØDB[G,L,M,N][3,4,7,8]ZX			

Ø **Medical and Surgical**
D **Gastrointestinal System**
C **Extirpation**   Definition: Taking or cutting out solid matter from a body part

Explanation: The solid matter may be an abnormal byproduct of a biological function or a foreign body; it may be imbedded in a body part or in the lumen of a tubular body part. The solid matter may or may not have been previously broken into pieces.

Body Part Character 4	Approach Character 5	Device Character 6	Qualifier Character 7

1 **Esophagus, Upper**
  Cervical esophagus
2 **Esophagus, Middle**
  Thoracic esophagus
3 **Esophagus, Lower**
  Abdominal esophagus
4 **Esophagogastric Junction**
  Cardia
  Cardioesophageal junction
  Gastroesophageal (GE) junction
5 **Esophagus**
6 **Stomach**
7 **Stomach, Pylorus**
  Pyloric antrum
  Pyloric canal
  Pyloric sphincter
8 **Small Intestine**
9 **Duodenum**
A **Jejunum**
  Duodenojejunal flexure
B **Ileum**
C **Ileocecal Valve**
E **Large Intestine**
F **Large Intestine, Right**
G **Large Intestine, Left**
H **Cecum**
J **Appendix**
  Vermiform appendix
K **Ascending Colon**
L **Transverse Colon**
  Hepatic flexure
  Splenic flexure
M **Descending Colon**
N **Sigmoid Colon**
  Rectosigmoid junction
  Sigmoid flexure
P **Rectum**
  Anorectal junction
	Ø **Open**
	3 **Percutaneous**
	4 **Percutaneous Endoscopic**
	7 **Via Natural or Artificial Opening**
	8 **Via Natural or Artificial Opening Endoscopic**
		Z **No Device**	Z **No Qualifier**

Q **Anus** Anal orifice	Ø **Open** 3 **Percutaneous** 4 **Percutaneous Endoscopic** 7 **Via Natural or Artificial Opening** 8 **Via Natural or Artificial Opening Endoscopic** X **External**	Z **No Device**	Z **No Qualifier**

R **Anal Sphincter**
  External anal sphincter
  Internal anal sphincter
U **Omentum**
  Gastrocolic ligament
  Gastrocolic omentum
  Gastrohepatic omentum
  Gastrophrenic ligament
  Gastrosplenic ligament
  Greater Omentum
  Hepatogastric ligament
  Lesser Omentum
V **Mesentery**
  Mesoappendix
  Mesocolon
W **Peritoneum**
  Epiploic foramen
	Ø **Open**
	3 **Percutaneous**
	4 **Percutaneous Endoscopic**
		Z **No Device**	Z **No Qualifier**

Non-OR ØDC[1,2,3,4,5,6,7,8,9,A,B,C,E,F,G,H,K,L,M,N,P][7,8]ZZ
Non-OR ØDCQ[7,8,X]ZZ

Ø   **Medical and Surgical**
D   **Gastrointestinal System**
D   **Extraction**   Definition: Pulling or stripping out or off all or a portion of a body part by the use of force
                      Explanation: The qualifier DIAGNOSTIC is used to identify extraction procedures that are biopsies

Body Part Character 4	Approach Character 5	Device Character 6	Qualifier Character 7
1 Esophagus, Upper Cervical esophagus **2 Esophagus, Middle** Thoracic esophagus **3 Esophagus, Lower** Abdominal esophagus **4 Esophagogastric Junction** Cardia Cardioesophageal junction Gastroesophageal (GE) junction **5 Esophagus** **6 Stomach** **7 Stomach, Pylorus** Pyloric antrum Pyloric canal Pyloric sphincter **8 Small Intestine** **9 Duodenum** **A Jejunum** Duodenojejunal flexure **B Ileum** **C Ileocecal Valve** **E Large Intestine** **F Large Intestine, Right** **G Large Intestine, Left** **H Cecum** **J Appendix** Vermiform appendix **K Ascending Colon** **L Transverse Colon** Hepatic flexure Splenic flexure **M Descending Colon** **N Sigmoid Colon** Rectosigmoid junction Sigmoid flexure **P Rectum** Anorectal junction	**3 Percutaneous** **4 Percutaneous Endoscopic** **8 Via Natural or Artificial Opening Endoscopic**	**Z No Device**	**X Diagnostic**
Q Anus Anal orifice	**3 Percutaneous** **4 Percutaneous Endoscopic** **8 Via Natural or Artificial Opening Endoscopic** **X External**	**Z No Device**	**X Diagnostic**

Non-OR   ØDD[1,2,3,4,5,6,7,8,9,A,B,C,E,F,G,H,K,L,M,N,P][3,4,8]ZX
Non-OR   ØDDQ[3,4,8,X]ZX

NC Noncovered Procedure   **LC** Limited Coverage   **QA** Questionable OB Admit   **NT** New Tech Add-on   ⊞ Combination Member   ♂ Male   ♀ Female

ICD-10-PCS 2023   **385**

ØDD–ØDD

Ø **Medical and Surgical**
D **Gastrointestinal System**
F **Fragmentation** Definition: Breaking solid matter in a body part into pieces

Explanation: Physical force (e.g., manual, ultrasonic) applied directly or indirectly is used to break the solid matter into pieces. The solid matter may be an abnormal byproduct of a biological function or a foreign body. The pieces of solid matter are not taken out.

Body Part Character 4	Approach Character 5	Device Character 6	Qualifier Character 7
5 Esophagus `NC` **6** Stomach `NC` **8** Small Intestine `NC` **9** Duodenum `NC` **A** Jejunum `NC` Duodenojejunal flexure **B** Ileum `NC` **E** Large Intestine `NC` **F** Large Intestine, Right `NC` **G** Large Intestine, Left `NC` **H** Cecum `NC` **J** Appendix `NC` Vermiform appendix **K** Ascending Colon `NC` **L** Transverse Colon `NC` Hepatic flexure Splenic flexure **M** Descending Colon `NC` **N** Sigmoid Colon `NC` Rectosigmoid junction Sigmoid flexure **P** Rectum `NC` Anorectal junction **Q** Anus `NC` Anal orifice	**Ø** Open **3** Percutaneous **4** Percutaneous Endoscopic **7** Via Natural or Artificial Opening **8** Via Natural or Artificial Opening Endoscopic **X** External	**Z** No Device	**Z** No Qualifier

Non-OR ØDF[5,6,8,9,A,B,E,F,G,H,J,K,L,M,N,P,Q]XZZ
`NC` ØDF[5,6,8,9,A,B,E,F,G,H,J,K,L,M,N,P,Q]XZZ

Ø	Medical and Surgical
D	Gastrointestinal System
H	Insertion

Definition: Putting in a nonbiological appliance that monitors, assists, performs, or prevents a physiological function but does not physically take the place of a body part

Explanation: None

Body Part Character 4	Approach Character 5	Device Character 6	Qualifier Character 7
Ø Upper Intestinal Tract D Lower Intestinal Tract	Ø Open 3 Percutaneous 4 Percutaneous Endoscopic 7 Via Natural or Artificial Opening 8 Via Natural or Artificial Opening Endoscopic	Y Other Device	Z No Qualifier
5 Esophagus	Ø Open 3 Percutaneous 4 Percutaneous Endoscopic	1 Radioactive Element 2 Monitoring Device 3 Infusion Device D Intraluminal Device U Feeding Device Y Other Device	Z No Qualifier
5 Esophagus	7 Via Natural or Artificial Opening 8 Via Natural or Artificial Opening Endoscopic	1 Radioactive Element 2 Monitoring Device 3 Infusion Device B Intraluminal Device, Airway D Intraluminal Device U Feeding Device Y Other Device	Z No Qualifier
6 Stomach ⊞	Ø Open 3 Percutaneous 4 Percutaneous Endoscopic	1 Radioactive Element 2 Monitoring Device 3 Infusion Device D Intraluminal Device M Stimulator Lead U Feeding Device Y Other Device	Z No Qualifier
6 Stomach	7 Via Natural or Artificial Opening 8 Via Natural or Artificial Opening Endoscopic	1 Radioactive Element 2 Monitoring Device 3 Infusion Device D Intraluminal Device U Feeding Device Y Other Device	Z No Qualifier
8 Small Intestine 9 Duodenum A Jejunum 　Duodenojejunal flexure B Ileum	Ø Open 3 Percutaneous 4 Percutaneous Endoscopic 7 Via Natural or Artificial Opening 8 Via Natural or Artificial Opening Endoscopic	1 Radioactive Element 2 Monitoring Device 3 Infusion Device D Intraluminal Device U Feeding Device	Z No Qualifier
E Large Intestine P Rectum 　Anorectal junction	Ø Open 3 Percutaneous 4 Percutaneous Endoscopic 7 Via Natural or Artificial Opening 8 Via Natural or Artificial Opening Endoscopic	1 Radioactive Element D Intraluminal Device	Z No Qualifier
Q Anus 　Anal orifice	Ø Open 3 Percutaneous 4 Percutaneous Endoscopic	D Intraluminal Device L Artificial Sphincter	Z No Qualifier
Q Anus 　Anal orifice	7 Via Natural or Artificial Opening 8 Via Natural or Artificial Opening Endoscopic	D Intraluminal Device	Z No Qualifier
R Anal Sphincter 　External anal sphincter 　Internal anal sphincter	Ø Open 3 Percutaneous 4 Percutaneous Endoscopic	M Stimulator Lead	Z No Qualifier

Non-OR	ØDH[Ø,D][Ø,3,4,7,8]YZ
Non-OR	ØDH5[Ø,3,4][D,U]Z
Non-OR	ØDH5[3,4]YZ
Non-OR	ØDH5[7,8][2,3,B,D,U,Y]Z
Non-OR	ØDH631Z
Non-OR	ØDH6[Ø,3,4]UZ
Non-OR	ØDH6[3,4]YZ
Non-OR	ØDH6[7,8][1,2,3,D,U,Y]Z
Non-OR	ØDH[8,9,A,B][Ø,3,4,7,8][1,D,U]Z
Non-OR	ØDH[8,9,A,B][7,8][2,3]Z
Non-OR	ØDHE[Ø,3,4,7,8][1,D]Z
Non-OR	ØDHP[Ø,3,4,7,8]DZ

See Appendix L for Procedure Combinations
　⊞　ØDH6[Ø,3,4]MZ

NC Noncovered Procedure　**LC** Limited Coverage　**QA** Questionable OB Admit　**NT** New Tech Add-on　⊞ Combination Member　♂ Male　♀ Female

ICD-10-PCS 2023　　　　　　　　　　　　　　　　　　　　　　　　　　　　　　**387**

ØDH–ØDH

Gastrointestinal System

Ø   **Medical and Surgical**
D   **Gastrointestinal System**
J   **Inspection**   Definition: Visually and/or manually exploring a body part

                         Explanation: Visual exploration may be performed with or without optical instrumentation. Manual exploration may be performed directly or through intervening body layers.

Body Part Character 4	Approach Character 5	Device Character 6	Qualifier Character 7
Ø Upper Intestinal Tract **6** Stomach **D** Lower Intestinal Tract	**Ø** Open **3** Percutaneous **4** Percutaneous Endoscopic **7** Via Natural or Artificial Opening **8** Via Natural or Artificial Opening Endoscopic **X** External	**Z** No Device	**Z** No Qualifier

U Omentum
    Gastrocolic ligament
    Gastrocolic omentum
    Gastrohepatic omentum
    Gastrophrenic ligament
    Gastrosplenic ligament
    Greater Omentum
    Hepatogastric ligament
    Lesser Omentum
V Mesentery
    Mesoappendix
    Mesocolon
W Peritoneum
    Epiploic foramen
	Ø Open
	3 Percutaneous
	4 Percutaneous Endoscopic
	X External
		Z No Device	**Z** No Qualifier

Non-OR	ØDJ[Ø,6,D][3,7,8,X]ZZ
Non-OR	ØDJ[U,V,W][3,X]ZZ

Non-OR Procedure   DRG Non-OR Procedure   Valid OR Procedure   HAC Associated Procedure   Combination Only   New/Revised April   New/Revised October

388   ICD-10-PCS 2023

Gastrointestinal System

Ø   **Medical and Surgical**
D   **Gastrointestinal System**
L   **Occlusion**   Definition: Completely closing an orifice or the lumen of a tubular body part
                 Explanation: The orifice can be a natural orifice or an artificially created orifice

Body Part Character 4		Approach Character 5	Device Character 6	Qualifier Character 7

1 **Esophagus, Upper**
 Cervical esophagus
 2 **Esophagus, Middle**
 Thoracic esophagus
 3 **Esophagus, Lower**
 Abdominal esophagus
 4 **Esophagogastric Junction**
 Cardia
 Cardioesophageal junction
 Gastroesophageal (GE) junction
 5 **Esophagus**
 6 **Stomach**
 7 **Stomach, Pylorus**
 Pyloric antrum
 Pyloric canal
 Pyloric sphincter
 8 **Small Intestine**
	9 **Duodenum**
	 A **Jejunum**
	    Duodenojejunal flexure
	 B **Ileum**
	 C **Ileocecal Valve**
	 E **Large Intestine**
	 F **Large Intestine, Right**
	 G **Large Intestine, Left**
	 H **Cecum**
	 K **Ascending Colon**
	 L **Transverse Colon**
	    Hepatic flexure
	    Splenic flexure
	 M **Descending Colon**
	 N **Sigmoid Colon**
	    Rectosigmoid junction
	    Sigmoid flexure
	 P **Rectum**
	    Anorectal junction
		Ø **Open**
		 3 **Percutaneous**
		 4 **Percutaneous Endoscopic**
			C **Extraluminal Device**
			 D **Intraluminal Device**
			 Z **No Device**
				Z **No Qualifier**

1 **Esophagus, Upper**
 Cervical esophagus
 2 **Esophagus, Middle**
 Thoracic esophagus
 3 **Esophagus, Lower**
 Abdominal esophagus
 4 **Esophagogastric Junction**
 Cardia
 Cardioesophageal junction
 Gastroesophageal (GE) junction
 5 **Esophagus**
 6 **Stomach**
 7 **Stomach, Pylorus**
 Pyloric antrum
 Pyloric canal
 Pyloric sphincter
 8 **Small Intestine**
	9 **Duodenum**
	 A **Jejunum**
	    Duodenojejunal flexure
	 B **Ileum**
	 C **Ileocecal Valve**
	 E **Large Intestine**
	 F **Large Intestine, Right**
	 G **Large Intestine, Left**
	 H **Cecum**
	 K **Ascending Colon**
	 L **Transverse Colon**
	    Hepatic flexure
	    Splenic flexure
	 M **Descending Colon**
	 N **Sigmoid Colon**
	    Rectosigmoid junction
	    Sigmoid flexure
	 P **Rectum**
	    Anorectal junction
		7 **Via Natural or Artificial Opening**
		 8 **Via Natural or Artificial Opening Endoscopic**
			D **Intraluminal Device**
			 Z **No Device**
				Z **No Qualifier**

Q **Anus** Anal orifice		Ø **Open** 3 **Percutaneous** 4 **Percutaneous Endoscopic** X **External**	C **Extraluminal Device** D **Intraluminal Device** Z **No Device**	Z **No Qualifier**
Q **Anus** Anal orifice		7 **Via Natural or Artificial Opening** 8 **Via Natural or Artificial Opening Endoscopic**	D **Intraluminal Device** Z **No Device**	Z **No Qualifier**

Non-OR   ØDL[1,2,3,4,5][Ø,3,4][C,D,Z]Z
Non-OR   ØDL[1,2,3,4,5][7,8][D,Z]Z

Gastrointestinal System

Ø　Medical and Surgical
D　Gastrointestinal System
M　Reattachment　　Definition: Putting back in or on all or a portion of a separated body part to its normal location or other suitable location
　　　　　　　　　　Explanation: Vascular circulation and nervous pathways may or may not be reestablished

Body Part Character 4	Approach Character 5	Device Character 6	Qualifier Character 7
5　Esophagus 6　Stomach 8　Small Intestine 9　Duodenum A　Jejunum 　　Duodenojejunal flexure B　Ileum E　Large Intestine F　Large Intestine, Right G　Large Intestine, Left H　Cecum K　Ascending Colon L　Transverse Colon 　　Hepatic flexure 　　Splenic flexure M　Descending Colon N　Sigmoid Colon 　　Rectosigmoid junction 　　Sigmoid flexure P　Rectum 　　Anorectal junction	Ø　Open 4　Percutaneous Endoscopic	Z　No Device	Z　No Qualifier

Ø　Medical and Surgical
D　Gastrointestinal System
N　Release　　　Definition: Freeing a body part from an abnormal physical constraint by cutting or by the use of force
　　　　　　　　Explanation: Some of the restraining tissue may be taken out but none of the body part is taken out

Body Part Character 4	Approach Character 5	Device Character 6	Qualifier Character 7
1　Esophagus, Upper 　　Cervical esophagus 2　Esophagus, Middle 　　Thoracic esophagus 3　Esophagus, Lower 　　Abdominal esophagus 4　Esophagogastric Junction 　　Cardia 　　Cardioesophageal junction 　　Gastroesophageal (GE) junction 5　Esophagus 6　Stomach 7　Stomach, Pylorus 　　Pyloric antrum 　　Pyloric canal 　　Pyloric sphincter 8　Small Intestine 9　Duodenum A　Jejunum 　　Duodenojejunal flexure B　Ileum C　Ileocecal Valve E　Large Intestine F　Large Intestine, Right G　Large Intestine, Left H　Cecum J　Appendix 　　Vermiform appendix K　Ascending Colon L　Transverse Colon 　　Hepatic flexure 　　Splenic flexure M　Descending Colon N　Sigmoid Colon 　　Rectosigmoid junction 　　Sigmoid flexure P　Rectum 　　Anorectal junction	Ø　Open 3　Percutaneous 4　Percutaneous Endoscopic 7　Via Natural or Artificial Opening 8　Via Natural or Artificial Opening Endoscopic	Z　No Device	Z　No Qualifier
Q　Anus 　　Anal orifice	Ø　Open 3　Percutaneous 4　Percutaneous Endoscopic 7　Via Natural or Artificial Opening 8　Via Natural or Artificial Opening Endoscopic X　External	Z　No Device	Z　No Qualifier
R　Anal Sphincter 　　External anal sphincter 　　Internal anal sphincter U　Omentum 　　Gastrocolic ligament 　　Gastrocolic omentum 　　Gastrohepatic omentum 　　Gastrophrenic ligament 　　Gastrosplenic ligament 　　Greater Omentum 　　Hepatogastric ligament 　　Lesser Omentum V　Mesentery 　　Mesoappendix 　　Mesocolon W　Peritoneum 　　Epiploic foramen	Ø　Open 3　Percutaneous 4　Percutaneous Endoscopic	Z　No Device	Z　No Qualifier

Non-OR　ØDN[8,9,A,B,E,F,G,H,K,L,M,N][7,8]ZZ

Ø   **Medical and Surgical**
D   **Gastrointestinal System**
P   **Removal**   Definition: Taking out or off a device from a body part

           Explanation: If a device is taken out and a similar device put in without cutting or puncturing the skin or mucous membrane, the procedure is coded to the root operation CHANGE. Otherwise, the procedure for taking out a device is coded to the root operation REMOVAL.

Body Part Character 4	Approach Character 5	Device Character 6	Qualifier Character 7
Ø Upper Intestinal Tract D Lower Intestinal Tract	Ø Open 3 Percutaneous 4 Percutaneous Endoscopic 7 Via Natural or Artificial Opening 8 Via Natural or Artificial Opening Endoscopic	Ø Drainage Device 2 Monitoring Device 3 Infusion Device 7 Autologous Tissue Substitute C Extraluminal Device D Intraluminal Device J Synthetic Substitute K Nonautologous Tissue Substitute U Feeding Device Y Other Device	Z No Qualifier
Ø Upper Intestinal Tract D Lower Intestinal Tract	X External	Ø Drainage Device 2 Monitoring Device 3 Infusion Device D Intraluminal Device U Feeding Device	Z No Qualifier
5 Esophagus	Ø Open 3 Percutaneous 4 Percutaneous Endoscopic	1 Radioactive Element 2 Monitoring Device 3 Infusion Device U Feeding Device Y Other Device	Z No Qualifier
5 Esophagus	7 Via Natural or Artificial Opening 8 Via Natural or Artificial Opening Endoscopic	1 Radioactive Element D Intraluminal Device Y Other Device	Z No Qualifier
5 Esophagus	X External	1 Radioactive Element 2 Monitoring Device 3 Infusion Device D Intraluminal Device U Feeding Device	Z No Qualifier
6 Stomach	Ø Open 3 Percutaneous 4 Percutaneous Endoscopic	Ø Drainage Device 2 Monitoring Device 3 Infusion Device 7 Autologous Tissue Substitute C Extraluminal Device D Intraluminal Device J Synthetic Substitute K Nonautologous Tissue Substitute M Stimulator Lead U Feeding Device Y Other Device	Z No Qualifier
6 Stomach	7 Via Natural or Artificial Opening 8 Via Natural or Artificial Opening Endoscopic	Ø Drainage Device 2 Monitoring Device 3 Infusion Device 7 Autologous Tissue Substitute C Extraluminal Device D Intraluminal Device J Synthetic Substitute K Nonautologous Tissue Substitute U Feeding Device Y Other Device	Z No Qualifier
6 Stomach	X External	Ø Drainage Device 2 Monitoring Device 3 Infusion Device D Intraluminal Device U Feeding Device	Z No Qualifier

Non-OR   ØDP[Ø,D][3,4]YZ
Non-OR   ØDP[Ø,D][7,8][Ø,2,3,D,U,Y]Z
Non-OR   ØDP[Ø,D]X[Ø,2,3,D,U]Z
Non-OR   ØDP5[3,4]YZ
Non-OR   ØDP5[7,8][1,D,Y]Z
Non-OR   ØDP5X[1,2,3,D,U]Z
Non-OR   ØDP6[3,4]YZ
Non-OR   ØDP6[7,8][Ø,2,3,D,U,Y]Z
Non-OR   ØDP6X[Ø,2,3,D,U]Z

ØDP Continued on next page

NC Noncovered Procedure   LC Limited Coverage   QA Questionable OB Admit   NT New Tech Add-on   ⊞ Combination Member   ♂ Male   ♀ Female

ICD-10-PCS 2023   **391**

ØDP–ØDP

Gastrointestinal System

Ø   **Medical and Surgical**
D   **Gastrointestinal System**
P   **Removal**   Definition: Taking out or off a device from a body part

Explanation: If a device is taken out and a similar device put in without cutting or puncturing the skin or mucous membrane, the procedure is coded to the root operation CHANGE. Otherwise, the procedure for taking out a device is coded to the root operation REMOVAL.

Body Part Character 4	Approach Character 5	Device Character 6	Qualifier Character 7

P   Rectum
    Anorectal junction
	Ø Open
	3 Percutaneous
	4 Percutaneous Endoscopic
	7 Via Natural or Artificial Opening
	8 Via Natural or Artificial Opening
	    Endoscopic
	X External
		1 Radioactive Element	**Z** No Qualifier

Q   Anus
    Anal orifice
	Ø Open
	3 Percutaneous
	4 Percutaneous Endoscopic
	7 Via Natural or Artificial Opening
	8 Via Natural or Artificial Opening
	    Endoscopic
		L Artificial Sphincter	**Z** No Qualifier

R   Anal Sphincter
    External anal sphincter
    Internal anal sphincter
	Ø Open
	3 Percutaneous
	4 Percutaneous Endoscopic
		M Stimulator Lead	**Z** No Qualifier

U   Omentum
    Gastrocolic ligament
    Gastrocolic omentum
    Gastrohepatic omentum
    Gastrophrenic ligament
    Gastrosplenic ligament
    Greater Omentum
    Hepatogastric ligament
    Lesser Omentum
V   Mesentery
    Mesoappendix
    Mesocolon
W   Peritoneum
    Epiploic foramen
	Ø Open
	3 Percutaneous
	4 Percutaneous Endoscopic
		Ø Drainage Device
		1 Radioactive Element
		7 Autologous Tissue Substitute
		J Synthetic Substitute
		K Nonautologous Tissue Substitute
			Z No Qualifier

Non-OR   ØDPP[7,8,X]1Z

Non-OR Procedure   DRG Non-OR Procedure   Valid OR Procedure   HAC Associated Procedure   Combination Only   New/Revised April   New/Revised October

392   ICD-10-PCS 2023

Ø   **Medical and Surgical**
D   **Gastrointestinal System**
Q   **Repair**   Definition: Restoring, to the extent possible, a body part to its normal anatomic structure and function
                Explanation: Used only when the method to accomplish the repair is not one of the other root operations

Body Part Character 4	Approach Character 5	Device Character 6	Qualifier Character 7

1 Esophagus, Upper
  Cervical esophagus
2 Esophagus, Middle
  Thoracic esophagus
3 Esophagus, Lower
  Abdominal esophagus
4 Esophagogastric Junction
  Cardia
  Cardioesophageal junction
  Gastroesophageal (GE) junction
5 Esophagus
6 Stomach
7 Stomach, Pylorus
  Pyloric antrum
  Pyloric canal
  Pyloric sphincter
8 Small Intestine ⊞
9 Duodenum ⊞
A Jejunum ⊞
  Duodenojejunal flexure
B Ileum ⊞
C Ileocecal Valve
E Large Intestine ⊞
F Large Intestine, Right ⊞
G Large Intestine, Left ⊞
H Cecum ⊞
J Appendix
  Vermiform appendix
K Ascending Colon ⊞
L Transverse Colon ⊞
  Hepatic flexure
  Splenic flexure
M Descending Colon ⊞
N Sigmoid Colon ⊞
  Rectosigmoid junction
  Sigmoid flexure
P Rectum
  Anorectal junction
	Ø Open
	3 Percutaneous
	4 Percutaneous Endoscopic
	7 Via Natural or Artificial Opening
	**8 Via Natural or Artificial Opening
	  Endoscopic**
		Z No Device	**Z No Qualifier**

Q Anus
  Anal orifice
	Ø Open
	3 Percutaneous
	4 Percutaneous Endoscopic
	7 Via Natural or Artificial Opening
	**8 Via Natural or Artificial Opening
	  Endoscopic**
	X External
		Z No Device	**Z No Qualifier**

R Anal Sphincter
  External anal sphincter
  Internal anal sphincter
U Omentum
  Gastrocolic ligament
  Gastrocolic omentum
  Gastrohepatic omentum
  Gastrophrenic ligament
  Gastrosplenic ligament
  Greater Omentum
  Hepatogastric ligament
  Lesser Omentum
V Mesentery
  Mesoappendix
  Mesocolon
W Peritoneum
  Epiploic foramen
	Ø Open
	3 Percutaneous
	4 Percutaneous Endoscopic
		Z No Device	**Z No Qualifier**

Non-OR ØDQU[Ø,3,4]ZZ

See Appendix L for Procedure Combinations
⊞   ØDQ[8,9,A,B,E,F,G,H,K,L,M,N]ØZZ

NC Noncovered Procedure   LC Limited Coverage   QA Questionable OB Admit   NT New Tech Add-on   ⊞ Combination Member   ♂ Male   ♀ Female

ICD-10-PCS 2023   393

ØDQ–ØDQ

Ø   **Medical and Surgical**
D   **Gastrointestinal System**
R   **Replacement**   Definition: Putting in or on biological or synthetic material that physically takes the place and/or function of all or a portion of a body part

                      Explanation: The body part may have been taken out or replaced, or may be taken out, physically eradicated, or rendered nonfunctional during the REPLACEMENT procedure. A REMOVAL procedure is coded for taking out the device used in a previous replacement procedure.

Body Part Character 4	Approach Character 5	Device Character 6	Qualifier Character 7
5 Esophagus	**Ø** Open **4** Percutaneous Endoscopic **7** Via Natural or Artificial Opening **8** Via Natural or Artificial Opening Endoscopic	**7** Autologous Tissue Substitute **J** Synthetic Substitute **K** Nonautologous Tissue Substitute	**Z** No Qualifier

R Anal Sphincter
    External anal sphincter
    Internal anal sphincter
U Omentum
    Gastrocolic ligament
    Gastrocolic omentum
    Gastrohepatic omentum
    Gastrophrenic ligament
    Gastrosplenic ligament
    Greater Omentum
    Hepatogastric ligament
    Lesser Omentum
V Mesentery
    Mesoappendix
    Mesocolon
W Peritoneum
    Epiploic foramen
	Ø Open
	4 Percutaneous Endoscopic
		7 Autologous Tissue Substitute
		J Synthetic Substitute
		K Nonautologous Tissue Substitute
			Z No Qualifier

Ø   **Medical and Surgical**
D   **Gastrointestinal System**
S   **Reposition**   Definition: Moving to its normal location, or other suitable location, all or a portion of a body part

                      Explanation: The body part is moved to a new location from an abnormal location, or from a normal location where it is not functioning correctly. The body part may or may not be cut out or off to be moved to the new location.

Body Part Character 4	Approach Character 5	Device Character 6	Qualifier Character 7

5 Esophagus
6 Stomach
9 Duodenum
A Jejunum
    Duodenojejunal flexure
B Ileum
H Cecum
K Ascending Colon
L Transverse Colon
    Hepatic flexure
    Splenic flexure
M Descending Colon
N Sigmoid Colon
    Rectosigmoid junction
    Sigmoid flexure
P Rectum
    Anorectal junction
Q Anus
    Anal orifice
	Ø Open
	4 Percutaneous Endoscopic
	7 Via Natural or Artificial Opening
	8 Via Natural or Artificial Opening Endoscopic
	X External
		Z No Device	**Z** No Qualifier

8 Small Intestine **E** Large Intestine	**Ø** Open **4** Percutaneous Endoscopic **7** Via Natural or Artificial Opening **8** Via Natural or Artificial Opening Endoscopic	**Z** No Device	**Z** No Qualifier

    Non-OR   ØDS[5,6,9,A,B,H,K,L,M,N,P,Q]XZZ

Non-OR Procedure   DRG Non-OR Procedure   Valid OR Procedure   HAC Associated Procedure   Combination Only   New/Revised April   New/Revised October

394   ICD-10-PCS 2023

0   **Medical and Surgical**
D   **Gastrointestinal System**
T   **Resection**   Definition: Cutting out or off, without replacement, all of a body part
                   Explanation: None

Body Part Character 4	Approach Character 5	Device Character 6	Qualifier Character 7

1   **Esophagus, Upper**
    Cervical esophagus
2   **Esophagus, Middle**
    Thoracic esophagus
3   **Esophagus, Lower**
    Abdominal esophagus
4   **Esophagogastric Junction**
    Cardia
    Cardioesophageal junction
    Gastroesophageal (GE) junction
5   **Esophagus**
6   **Stomach**
7   **Stomach, Pylorus**
    Pyloric antrum
    Pyloric canal
    Pyloric sphincter
8   **Small Intestine**
9   **Duodenum**   ⊞
A   **Jejunum**
    Duodenojejunal flexure
B   **Ileum**
C   **Ileocecal Valve**
E   **Large Intestine**
F   **Large Intestine, Right**
H   **Cecum**
J   **Appendix**
    Vermiform appendix
K   **Ascending Colon**
P   **Rectum**
    Anorectal junction
Q   **Anus**
    Anal orifice
	0 Open
	4 Percutaneous Endoscopic
	7 Via Natural or Artificial Opening
	8 Via Natural or Artificial Opening
	    Endoscopic
		Z No Device	**Z** No Qualifier

G   **Large Intestine, Left**
L   **Transverse Colon**
    Hepatic flexure
    Splenic flexure
M   **Descending Colon**
N   **Sigmoid Colon**
    Rectosigmoid junction
    Sigmoid flexure
	0 Open
	4 Percutaneous Endoscopic
	7 Via Natural or Artificial Opening
	8 Via Natural or Artificial Opening
	    Endoscopic
	F Via Natural or Artificial Opening
	    with Percutaneous Endoscopic
	    Assistance
		Z No Device	**Z** No Qualifier

R   **Anal Sphincter**
    External anal sphincter
    Internal anal sphincter
U   **Omentum**
    Gastrocolic ligament
    Gastrocolic omentum
    Gastrohepatic omentum
    Gastrophrenic ligament
    Gastrosplenic ligament
    Greater Omentum
    Hepatogastric ligament
    Lesser Omentum
	0 Open
	4 Percutaneous Endoscopic
		Z No Device	**Z** No Qualifier

See Appendix L for Procedure Combinations
   ⊞   0DT90ZZ

⊞ Noncoverage Procedure   LC Limited Coverage   QA Questionable OB Admit   NT New Tech Add-on   ⊞ Combination Member   ♂ Male   ♀ Female

ICD-10-PCS 2023   395

Ø   Medical and Surgical
D   Gastrointestinal System
U   Supplement   Definition: Putting in or on biological or synthetic material that physically reinforces and/or augments the function of a portion of a body part
Explanation: The biological material is non-living, or is living and from the same individual. The body part may have been previously replaced, and the SUPPLEMENT procedure is performed to physically reinforce and/or augment the function of the replaced body part.

Body Part Character 4	Approach Character 5	Device Character 6	Qualifier Character 7
1 Esophagus, Upper 　Cervical esophagus **2** Esophagus, Middle 　Thoracic esophagus **3** Esophagus, Lower 　Abdominal esophagus **4** Esophagogastric Junction 　Cardia 　Cardioesophageal junction 　Gastroesophageal (GE) junction **5** Esophagus **6** Stomach **7** Stomach, Pylorus 　Pyloric antrum 　Pyloric canal 　Pyloric sphincter **8** Small Intestine **9** Duodenum **A** Jejunum 　Duodenojejunal flexure **B** Ileum **C** Ileocecal Valve **E** Large Intestine **F** Large Intestine, Right **G** Large Intestine, Left **H** Cecum **K** Ascending Colon **L** Transverse Colon 　Hepatic flexure 　Splenic flexure **M** Descending Colon **N** Sigmoid Colon 　Rectosigmoid junction 　Sigmoid flexure **P** Rectum 　Anorectal junction	**Ø** Open **4** Percutaneous Endoscopic **7** Via Natural or Artificial Opening **8** Via Natural or Artificial Opening 　Endoscopic	**7** Autologous Tissue Substitute **J** Synthetic Substitute **K** Nonautologous Tissue Substitute	**Z** No Qualifier
Q Anus 　Anal orifice	**Ø** Open **4** Percutaneous Endoscopic **7** Via Natural or Artificial Opening **8** Via Natural or Artificial Opening 　Endoscopic **X** External	**7** Autologous Tissue Substitute **J** Synthetic Substitute **K** Nonautologous Tissue Substitute	**Z** No Qualifier
R Anal Sphincter 　External anal sphincter 　Internal anal sphincter **U** Omentum 　Gastrocolic ligament 　Gastrocolic omentum 　Gastrohepatic omentum 　Gastrophrenic ligament 　Gastrosplenic ligament 　Greater Omentum 　Hepatogastric ligament 　Lesser Omentum **V** Mesentery 　Mesoappendix 　Mesocolon **W** Peritoneum 　Epiploic foramen	**Ø** Open **4** Percutaneous Endoscopic	**7** Autologous Tissue Substitute **J** Synthetic Substitute **K** Nonautologous Tissue Substitute	**Z** No Qualifier

Non-OR Procedure　DRG Non-OR Procedure　Valid OR Procedure　HAC Associated Procedure　Combination Only　New/Revised April　New/Revised October

396

ICD-10-PCS 2023

Ø   **Medical and Surgical**
D   **Gastrointestinal System**
V   **Restriction**   Definition: Partially closing an orifice or the lumen of a tubular body part
                         Explanation: The orifice can be a natural orifice or an artificially created orifice

Body Part Character 4		Approach Character 5	Device Character 6	Qualifier Character 7

1 Esophagus, Upper
   Cervical esophagus
2 Esophagus, Middle
   Thoracic esophagus
3 Esophagus, Lower
   Abdominal esophagus
4 Esophagogastric
   Junction
   Cardia
   Cardioesophageal
     junction
   Gastroesophageal (GE)
     junction
5 Esophagus
6 Stomach
7 Stomach, Pylorus
   Pyloric antrum
   Pyloric canal
   Pyloric sphincter
8 Small Intestine
	9 Duodenum
	A Jejunum
	   Duodenojejunal flexure
	B Ileum
	C Ileocecal Valve
	E Large Intestine
	F Large Intestine, Right
	G Large Intestine, Left
	H Cecum
	K Ascending Colon
	L Transverse Colon
	   Hepatic flexure
	   Splenic flexure
	M Descending Colon
	N Sigmoid Colon
	   Rectosigmoid junction
	   Sigmoid flexure
	P Rectum
	   Anorectal junction
		Ø Open
		3 Percutaneous
		4 Percutaneous Endoscopic
			C Extraluminal Device
			D Intraluminal Device
			Z No Device
				Z No Qualifier

1 Esophagus, Upper
   Cervical esophagus
2 Esophagus, Middle
   Thoracic esophagus
3 Esophagus, Lower
   Abdominal esophagus
4 Esophagogastric
   Junction
   Cardia
   Cardioesophageal
     junction
   Gastroesophageal (GE)
     junction
5 Esophagus
6 Stomach NC
7 Stomach, Pylorus
   Pyloric antrum
   Pyloric canal
   Pyloric sphincter
8 Small Intestine
	9 Duodenum
	A Jejunum
	   Duodenojejunal flexure
	B Ileum
	C Ileocecal Valve
	E Large Intestine
	F Large Intestine, Right
	G Large Intestine, Left
	H Cecum
	K Ascending Colon
	L Transverse Colon
	   Hepatic flexure
	   Splenic flexure
	M Descending Colon
	N Sigmoid Colon
	   Rectosigmoid junction
	   Sigmoid flexure
	P Rectum
	   Anorectal junction
		7 Via Natural or Artificial
		   Opening
		8 Via Natural or Artificial
		   Opening Endoscopic
			D Intraluminal Device
			Z No Device
				Z No Qualifier

Q Anus Anal orifice		Ø Open 3 Percutaneous 4 Percutaneous Endoscopic X External	C Extraluminal Device D Intraluminal Device Z No Device	Z No Qualifier

Q Anus
   Anal orifice
		7 Via Natural or Artificial
		   Opening
		8 Via Natural or Artificial
		   Opening Endoscopic
			D Intraluminal Device
			Z No Device
				Z No Qualifier

Non-OR   ØDV6[7,8]DZ
HAC   ØDV64CZ when reported with PDx E66.Ø1 and SDx K68.11, K95.Ø1, K95.81, or T81.4Ø–T81.49 with 7th character A
NC   ØDV6[7,8]DZ

NC Noncovered Procedure   LC Limited Coverage   QA Questionable OB Admit   NT New Tech Add-on   ⊞ Combination Member   ♂ Male   ♀ Female

ICD-10-PCS 2023   397

ØDV–ØDV

Gastrointestinal System

Ø Medical and Surgical
D Gastrointestinal System
W Revision　　Definition: Correcting, to the extent possible, a portion of a malfunctioning device or the position of a displaced device

　　　　　　　Explanation: Revision can include correcting a malfunctioning or displaced device by taking out or putting in components of the device such as a screw or pin

Body Part Character 4	Approach Character 5	Device Character 6	Qualifier Character 7
Ø Upper Intestinal Tract D Lower Intestinal Tract	Ø Open 3 Percutaneous 4 Percutaneous Endoscopic 7 Via Natural or Artificial Opening 8 Via Natural or Artificial Opening Endoscopic	Ø Drainage Device 2 Monitoring Device 3 Infusion Device 7 Autologous Tissue Substitute C Extraluminal Device D Intraluminal Device J Synthetic Substitute K Nonautologous Tissue Substitute U Feeding Device Y Other Device	Z No Qualifier
Ø Upper Intestinal Tract D Lower Intestinal Tract	X External	Ø Drainage Device 2 Monitoring Device 3 Infusion Device 7 Autologous Tissue Substitute C Extraluminal Device D Intraluminal Device J Synthetic Substitute K Nonautologous Tissue Substitute U Feeding Device	Z No Qualifier
5 Esophagus	Ø Open 3 Percutaneous 4 Percutaneous Endoscopic	Y Other Device	Z No Qualifier
5 Esophagus	7 Via Natural or Artificial Opening 8 Via Natural or Artificial Opening Endoscopic	D Intraluminal Device Y Other Device	Z No Qualifier
5 Esophagus	X External	D Intraluminal Device	Z No Qualifier
6 Stomach	Ø Open 3 Percutaneous 4 Percutaneous Endoscopic	Ø Drainage Device 2 Monitoring Device 3 Infusion Device 7 Autologous Tissue Substitute C Extraluminal Device D Intraluminal Device J Synthetic Substitute K Nonautologous Tissue Substitute M Stimulator Lead U Feeding Device Y Other Device	Z No Qualifier
6 Stomach	7 Via Natural or Artificial Opening 8 Via Natural or Artificial Opening Endoscopic	Ø Drainage Device 2 Monitoring Device 3 Infusion Device 7 Autologous Tissue Substitute C Extraluminal Device D Intraluminal Device J Synthetic Substitute K Nonautologous Tissue Substitute U Feeding Device Y Other Device	Z No Qualifier
6 Stomach	X External	Ø Drainage Device 2 Monitoring Device 3 Infusion Device 7 Autologous Tissue Substitute C Extraluminal Device D Intraluminal Device J Synthetic Substitute K Nonautologous Tissue Substitute U Feeding Device	Z No Qualifier

Non-OR　ØDW[Ø,D][3,4,7,8]YZ
Non-OR　ØDW[Ø,D]8UZ
Non-OR　ØDW[Ø,D]X[Ø,2,3,7,C,D,J,K,U]Z
Non-OR　ØDW5[Ø,3,4]YZ
Non-OR　ØDW5[7,8]YZ
Non-OR　ØDW5XDZ
Non-OR　ØDW6[3,4]YZ
Non-OR　ØDW68UZ
Non-OR　ØDW6[7,8]YZ
Non-OR　ØDW6X[Ø,2,3,7,C,D,J,K,U]Z

ØDW Continued on next page

Ø   **Medical and Surgical**
D   **Gastrointestinal System**
W   **Revision**   Definition: Correcting, to the extent possible, a portion of a malfunctioning device or the position of a displaced device

ØDW Continued

                    Explanation: Revision can include correcting a malfunctioning or displaced device by taking out or putting in components of the device such as a screw or pin

Body Part Character 4	Approach Character 5	Device Character 6	Qualifier Character 7
8 Small Intestine E Large Intestine	Ø Open 4 Percutaneous Endoscopic 7 Via Natural or Artificial Opening 8 Via Natural or Artificial Opening Endoscopic	7 Autologous Tissue Substitute J Synthetic Substitute K Nonautologous Tissue Substitute	Z No Qualifier
Q Anus Anal orifice	Ø Open 3 Percutaneous 4 Percutaneous Endoscopic 7 Via Natural or Artificial Opening 8 Via Natural or Artificial Opening Endoscopic	L Artificial Sphincter	Z No Qualifier

R   Anal Sphincter
     External anal sphincter
     Internal anal sphincter
	Ø Open
	3 Percutaneous
	4 Percutaneous Endoscopic
		M Stimulator Lead	Z No Qualifier

U   Omentum
     Gastrocolic ligament
     Gastrocolic omentum
     Gastrohepatic omentum
     Gastrophrenic ligament
     Gastrosplenic ligament
     Greater Omentum
     Hepatogastric ligament
     Lesser Omentum
V   Mesentery
     Mesoappendix
     Mesocolon
W   Peritoneum
     Epiploic foramen
	Ø Open
	3 Percutaneous
	4 Percutaneous Endoscopic
		Ø Drainage Device
		7 Autologous Tissue Substitute
		J Synthetic Substitute
		K Nonautologous Tissue Substitute
			Z No Qualifier

Non-OR   ØDW[U,V,W][Ø,3,4]ØZ

Ø   **Medical and Surgical**
D   **Gastrointestinal System**
X   **Transfer**   Definition: Moving, without taking out, all or a portion of a body part to another location to take over the function of all or a portion of a body part

                    Explanation: The body part transferred remains connected to its vascular and nervous supply

Body Part Character 4	Approach Character 5	Device Character 6	Qualifier Character 7
6 Stomach	Ø Open 4 Percutaneous Endoscopic	Z No Device	5 Esophagus
8 Small Intestine	Ø Open 4 Percutaneous Endoscopic	Z No Device	5 Esophagus B Bladder C Ureter, Right D Ureter, Left F Ureters, Bilateral
E Large Intestine	Ø Open 4 Percutaneous Endoscopic	Z No Device	5 Esophagus 7 Vagina ♀ B Bladder

♀   ØDXE[Ø,4]Z7

Ø   **Medical and Surgical**
D   **Gastrointestinal System**
Y   **Transplantation**   Definition: Putting in or on all or a portion of a living body part taken from another individual or animal to physically take the place and/or function of all or a portion of a similar body part

                    Explanation: The native body part may or may not be taken out, and the transplanted body part may take over all or a portion of its function

Body Part Character 4	Approach Character 5	Device Character 6	Qualifier Character 7
5 Esophagus 6 Stomach 8 Small Intestine LC E Large Intestine LC	Ø Open	Z No Device	Ø Allogeneic 1 Syngeneic 2 Zooplastic

Non-OR   ØDY5ØZ[Ø,1,2]
LC   ØDY[8,E]ØZ[Ø,1,2]

NC Noncovered Procedure   LC Limited Coverage   QA Questionable OB Admit   NT New Tech Add-on   ⊞ Combination Member   ♂ Male   ♀ Female

ICD-10-PCS 2023   399

Hepatobiliary System and Pancreas ØF1–ØFY

Character Meanings

This Character Meaning table is provided as a guide to assist the user in the identification of character members that may be found in this section of code tables. It **SHOULD NOT** be used to build a PCS code.

Operation–Character 3		Body Part–Character 4		Approach–Character 5		Device–Character 6		Qualifier–Character 7	
1	Bypass	Ø	Liver	Ø	Open	Ø	Drainage Device	Ø	Allogeneic
2	Change	1	Liver, Right Lobe	3	Percutaneous	1	Radioactive Element	1	Syngeneic
5	Destruction	2	Liver, Left Lobe	4	Percutaneous Endoscopic	2	Monitoring Device	2	Zooplastic
7	Dilation	4	Gallbladder	7	Via Natural or Artificial Opening	3	Infusion Device	3	Duodenum OR Laser Interstitial Thermal Therapy
8	Division	5	Hepatic Duct, Right	8	Via Natural or Artificial Opening Endoscopic	7	Autologous Tissue Substitute	4	Stomach
9	Drainage	6	Hepatic Duct, Left	X	External	C	Extraluminal Device	5	Hepatic Duct, Right
B	Excision	7	Hepatic Duct, Common			D	Intraluminal Device	6	Hepatic Duct, Left
C	Extirpation	8	Cystic Duct			J	Synthetic Substitute	7	Hepatic Duct, Caudate
D	Extraction	9	Common Bile Duct			K	Nonautologous Tissue Substitute	8	Cystic Duct
F	Fragmentation	B	Hepatobiliary Duct			Y	Other Device	9	Common Bile Duct
H	Insertion	C	Ampulla of Vater			Z	No Device	B	Small Intestine
J	Inspection	D	Pancreatic Duct					C	Large Intestine
L	Occlusion	F	Pancreatic Duct, Accessory					F	Irreversible Electroporation
M	Reattachment	G	Pancreas					X	Diagnostic
N	Release							Z	No Qualifier
P	Removal								
Q	Repair								
R	Replacement								
S	Reposition								
T	Resection								
U	Supplement								
V	Restriction								
W	Revision								
Y	Transplantation								

AHA Coding Clinic for table ØF1
2020, 4Q, 53   Bypass pancreatic duct to stomach

AHA Coding Clinic for table ØF5
2018, 4Q, 39   Irreversible electroporation

AHA Coding Clinic for table ØF7
2016, 3Q, 27   Endoscopic retrograde cholangiopancreatography with sphincterotomy and insertion of pancreatic stent
2016, 1Q, 25   Endoscopic retrograde cholangiopancreatography with brush biopsy of pancreatic and common bile ducts
2015, 1Q, 32   Percutaneous transhepatic biliary drainage catheter placement
2014, 3Q, 15   Drainage of pancreatic pseudocyst

AHA Coding Clinic for table ØF8
2021, 4Q, 48-49   Division of liver for staged hepatectomy

AHA Coding Clinic for table ØF9
2020, 3Q, 34   Cystogastrostomy with stent insertion
2015, 1Q, 32   Percutaneous transhepatic biliary drainage catheter placement
2014, 3Q, 15   Drainage of pancreatic pseudocyst

AHA Coding Clinic for table ØFB
2019, 1Q, 3-8   Whipple procedure
2016, 3Q, 41   Open cholecystectomy with needle biopsy of liver
2016, 1Q, 23   Endoscopic ultrasound with aspiration biopsy of common hepatic duct
2016, 1Q, 25   Endoscopic retrograde cholangiopancreatography with brush biopsy of pancreatic and common bile ducts
2014, 3Q, 32   Pyloric-sparing Whipple procedure

AHA Coding Clinic for table ØFC
2016, 3Q, 27   Endoscopic retrograde cholangiopancreatography with sphincterotomy and insertion of pancreatic stent

AHA Coding Clinic for table ØFH
2022, 2Q, 26   Radioembolization of right hepatic lobe
2020, 4Q, 43-44   Insertion of radioactive element

AHA Coding Clinic for table ØFQ
2016, 3Q, 27   Revision of common bile duct anastomosis
2013, 4Q, 109   Separating conjoined twins

AHA Coding Clinic for table ØFT
2021, 4Q, 49   Division of liver for staged hepatectomy
2019, 1Q, 3-8   Whipple procedure
2012, 4Q, 99   Domino liver transplant

AHA Coding Clinic for table ØFY
2014, 3Q, 13   Orthotopic liver transplant with end to side cavoplasty
2012, 4Q, 99   Domino liver transplant

Liver

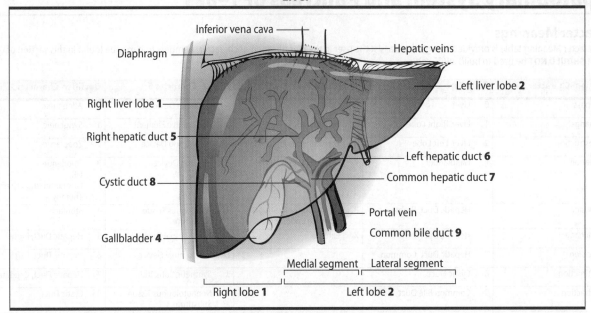

Pancreas

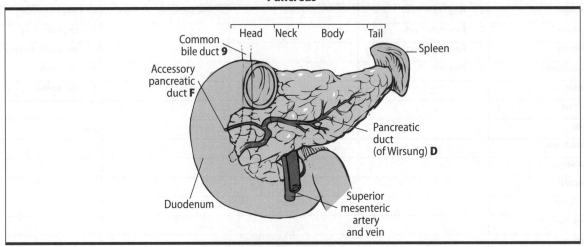

Gallbladder and Ducts

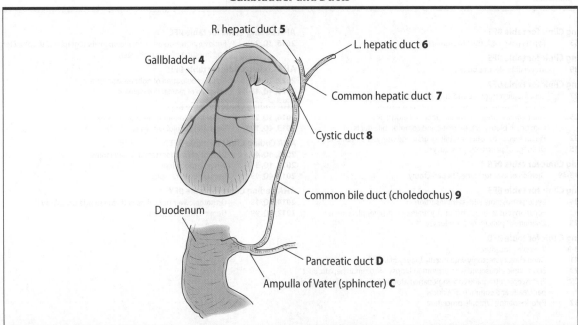

Ø   **Medical and Surgical**
F   **Hepatobiliary System and Pancreas**
1   **Bypass**   Definition: Altering the route of passage of the contents of a tubular body part

                        Explanation: Rerouting contents of a body part to a downstream area of the normal route, to a similar route and body part, or to an abnormal route and dissimilar body part. Includes one or more anastomoses, with or without the use of a device.

Body Part Character 4	Approach Character 5	Device Character 6	Qualifier Character 7
4 Gallbladder **5** Hepatic Duct, Right **6** Hepatic Duct, Left **7** Hepatic Duct, Common **8** Cystic Duct **9** Common Bile Duct	**Ø** Open **4** Percutaneous Endoscopic	**D** Intraluminal Device **Z** No Device	**3** Duodenum **4** Stomach **5** Hepatic Duct, Right **6** Hepatic Duct, Left **7** Hepatic Duct, Caudate **8** Cystic Duct **9** Common Bile Duct **B** Small Intestine
D Pancreatic Duct Duct of Wirsung	**Ø** Open **4** Percutaneous Endoscopic	**D** Intraluminal Device **Z** No Device	**3** Duodenum **4** Stomach **B** Small Intestine **C** Large Intestine
F Pancreatic Duct, Accessory Duct of Santorini **G** Pancreas	**Ø** Open **4** Percutaneous Endoscopic	**D** Intraluminal Device **Z** No Device	**3** Duodenum **B** Small Intestine **C** Large Intestine

Ø   **Medical and Surgical**
F   **Hepatobiliary System and Pancreas**
2   **Change**   Definition: Taking out or off a device from a body part and putting back an identical or similar device in or on the same body part without cutting or puncturing the skin or a mucous membrane

                        Explanation: All CHANGE procedures are coded using the approach EXTERNAL

Body Part Character 4	Approach Character 5	Device Character 6	Qualifier Character 7
Ø Liver Quadrate lobe **4** Gallbladder **B** Hepatobiliary Duct **D** Pancreatic Duct Duct of Wirsung **G** Pancreas	**X** External	**Ø** Drainage Device **Y** Other Device	**Z** No Qualifier

Non-OR   All body part, approach, device, and qualifier values

NC Noncovered Procedure   **LC** Limited Coverage   **QA** Questionable OB Admit   **NT** New Tech Add-on   ⊞ Combination Member   ♂ Male   ♀ Female

ICD-10-PCS 2023   403

Ø   **Medical and Surgical**
F   **Hepatobiliary System and Pancreas**
5   **Destruction**   Definition: Physical eradication of all or a portion of a body part by the direct use of energy, force, or a destructive agent
                            Explanation: None of the body part is physically taken out

Body Part Character 4	Approach Character 5	Device Character 6	Qualifier Character 7
Ø Liver Quadrate lobe 1 Liver, Right Lobe 2 Liver, Left Lobe	Ø Open 3 Percutaneous 4 Percutaneous Endoscopic	Z No Device	3 Laser Interstitial Thermal Therapy F Irreversible Electroporation Z No Qualifier
4 Gallbladder	Ø Open 3 Percutaneous 4 Percutaneous Endoscopic	Z No Device	3 Laser Interstitial Thermal Therapy Z No Qualifier
4 Gallbladder	8 Via Natural or Artificial Opening Endoscopic	Z No Device	Z No Qualifier

5 Hepatic Duct, Right
6 Hepatic Duct, Left
7 Hepatic Duct, Common
8 Cystic Duct
9 Common Bile Duct
C Ampulla of Vater
   Duodenal ampulla
   Hepatopancreatic ampulla
D Pancreatic Duct
   Duct of Wirsung
F Pancreatic Duct, Accessory
   Duct of Santorini
	Ø Open
	3 Percutaneous
	4 Percutaneous Endoscopic
		Z No Device	3 Laser Interstitial Thermal Therapy
			Z No Qualifier

5 Hepatic Duct, Right
6 Hepatic Duct, Left
7 Hepatic Duct, Common
8 Cystic Duct
9 Common Bile Duct
C Ampulla of Vater
   Duodenal ampulla
   Hepatopancreatic ampulla
D Pancreatic Duct
   Duct of Wirsung
F Pancreatic Duct, Accessory
   Duct of Santorini
	7 Via Natural or Artificial Opening
	8 Via Natural or Artificial Opening
	   Endoscopic
		Z No Device	Z No Qualifier

G Pancreas	Ø Open 3 Percutaneous 4 Percutaneous Endoscopic	Z No Device	3 Laser Interstitial Thermal Therapy F Irreversible Electroporation Z No Qualifier
G Pancreas	8 Via Natural or Artificial Opening Endoscopic	Z No Device	Z No Qualifier

Non-OR	ØF5[5,6,7,8,9,C,D,F]4ZZ
Non-OR	ØF5[5,6,7,8,9,C,D,F]8ZZ
Non-OR	ØF5G4Z[F,Z]
Non-OR	ØF5G8ZZ

Ø   **Medical and Surgical**
F   **Hepatobiliary System and Pancreas**
7   **Dilation**   Definition: Expanding an orifice or the lumen of a tubular body part
                        Explanation: The orifice can be a natural orifice or an artificially created orifice. Accomplished by stretching a tubular body part using intraluminal pressure or by cutting part of the orifice or wall of the tubular body part.

Body Part Character 4	Approach Character 5	Device Character 6	Qualifier Character 7

5 Hepatic Duct, Right
6 Hepatic Duct, Left
7 Hepatic Duct, Common
8 Cystic Duct
9 Common Bile Duct
C Ampulla of Vater
   Duodenal ampulla
   Hepatopancreatic ampulla
D Pancreatic Duct
   Duct of Wirsung
F Pancreatic Duct, Accessory
   Duct of Santorini
	Ø Open
	3 Percutaneous
	4 Percutaneous Endoscopic
	7 Via Natural or Artificial Opening
	8 Via Natural or Artificial Opening
	   Endoscopic
		D Intraluminal Device
		Z No Device
			Z No Qualifier

Non-OR	ØF7[5,6,7,8,9][3,4,8][D,Z]Z
Non-OR	ØF7[5,6,7,8,9,D]]7DZ
Non-OR	ØF7C8[D,Z]Z
Non-OR	ØF7[D,F][4,8][D,Z]Z

0   **Medical and Surgical**
F   **Hepatobiliary System and Pancreas**
8   **Division**   Definition: Cutting into a body part, without draining fluids and/or gases from the body part, in order to separate or transect a body part

                          Explanation: All or a portion of the body part is separated into two or more portions

Body Part Character 4	Approach Character 5	Device Character 6	Qualifier Character 7
0 Liver 1 Liver, Right Lobe 2 Liver, Left Lobe G Pancreas	0 Open 3 Percutaneous 4 Percutaneous Endoscopic	Z No Device	Z No Qualifier

Non-OR   0F8[0,1,2]3ZZ

0   **Medical and Surgical**
F   **Hepatobiliary System and Pancreas**
9   **Drainage**   Definition: Taking or letting out fluids and/or gases from a body part

                          Explanation: The qualifier DIAGNOSTIC is used to identify drainage procedures that are biopsies

Body Part Character 4	Approach Character 5	Device Character 6	Qualifier Character 7
0 Liver Quadrate lobe 1 Liver, Right Lobe 2 Liver, Left Lobe	0 Open 3 Percutaneous 4 Percutaneous Endoscopic	0 Drainage Device	Z No Qualifier
0 Liver Quadrate lobe 1 Liver, Right Lobe 2 Liver, Left Lobe	0 Open 3 Percutaneous 4 Percutaneous Endoscopic	Z No Device	X Diagnostic Z No Qualifier
4 Gallbladder G Pancreas	0 Open 3 Percutaneous 4 Percutaneous Endoscopic 8 Via Natural or Artificial Opening Endoscopic	0 Drainage Device	Z No Qualifier
4 Gallbladder G Pancreas	0 Open 3 Percutaneous 4 Percutaneous Endoscopic 8 Via Natural or Artificial Opening Endoscopic	Z No Device	X Diagnostic Z No Qualifier

5 Hepatic Duct, Right
6 Hepatic Duct, Left
7 Hepatic Duct, Common
8 Cystic Duct
9 Common Bile Duct
C Ampulla of Vater
  Duodenal ampulla
  Hepatopancreatic ampulla
D Pancreatic Duct
  Duct of Wirsung
F Pancreatic Duct, Accessory
  Duct of Santorini
	0 Open
	3 Percutaneous
	4 Percutaneous Endoscopic
	7 Via Natural or Artificial Opening
	8 Via Natural or Artificial Opening Endoscopic
		0 Drainage Device	Z No Qualifier

5 Hepatic Duct, Right
6 Hepatic Duct, Left
7 Hepatic Duct, Common
8 Cystic Duct
9 Common Bile Duct
C Ampulla of Vater
  Duodenal ampulla
  Hepatopancreatic ampulla
D Pancreatic Duct
  Duct of Wirsung
F Pancreatic Duct, Accessory
  Duct of Santorini
	0 Open
	3 Percutaneous
	4 Percutaneous Endoscopic
	7 Via Natural or Artificial Opening
	8 Via Natural or Artificial Opening Endoscopic
		Z No Device	X Diagnostic
			Z No Qualifier

Non-OR 0F9[0,1,2][3,4]0Z	Non-OR 0F99[3,8]0Z
Non-OR 0F9[0,1,2][3,4]Z[X,Z]	Non-OR 0F9C[3,4,8]0Z
Non-OR 0F9[4,G]80Z	Non-OR 0F9[D,F][3,8]0Z
Non-OR 0F9G30Z	Non-OR 0F9[5,6,8,9,C,D,F]3Z[X,Z]
Non-OR 0F9[4,G]8Z[X,Z]	Non-OR 0F9[5,6,8,9,C,D,F][4,7,8]ZX
Non-OR 0F9G3Z[XZ]	Non-OR 0F9[5,6,8,D,F]8ZZ
Non-OR 0F9G4ZX	Non-OR 0F97[3,4,7,8]Z[X,Z]
Non-OR 0F9[5,6,8][3,8]0Z	Non-OR 0F99[4,7,8]ZZ
Non-OR 0F97[3,4,7,8]0Z	Non-OR 0F9C[4,8]ZZ

NC Noncovered Procedure   LC Limited Coverage   QA Questionable OB Admit   NT New Tech Add-on   ⊞ Combination Member   ♂ Male   ♀ Female

ICD-10-PCS 2023   405

0F8–0F9

Ø   Medical and Surgical
F   Hepatobiliary System and Pancreas
B   Excision   Definition: Cutting out or off, without replacement, a portion of a body part
                     Explanation: The qualifier DIAGNOSTIC is used to identify excision procedures that are biopsies

Body Part Character 4	Approach Character 5	Device Character 6	Qualifier Character 7
Ø Liver Quadrate lobe 1 Liver, Right Lobe 2 Liver, Left Lobe	Ø Open 3 Percutaneous 4 Percutaneous Endoscopic	Z No Device	X Diagnostic Z No Qualifier
4 Gallbladder G Pancreas	Ø Open 3 Percutaneous 4 Percutaneous Endoscopic 8 Via Natural or Artificial Opening Endoscopic	Z No Device	X Diagnostic Z No Qualifier

5 Hepatic Duct, Right
6 Hepatic Duct, Left
7 Hepatic Duct, Common
8 Cystic Duct
9 Common Bile Duct
C Ampulla of Vater
   Duodenal ampulla
   Hepatopancreatic ampulla
D Pancreatic Duct
   Duct of Wirsung
F Pancreatic Duct, Accessory
   Duct of Santorini
	Ø Open
	3 Percutaneous
	4 Percutaneous Endoscopic
	7 Via Natural or Artificial Opening
	8 Via Natural or Artificial Opening
	   Endoscopic
		Z No Device	X Diagnostic
			Z No Qualifier

Non-OR   ØFB[Ø,1,2]3ZX
Non-OR   ØFB[4,G][3,4,8]ZX
Non-OR   ØFB[5,6,7,8,9,C,D,F][3,4,7,8]ZX
Non-OR   ØFB[5,6,7,8,9,C,D,F][4,8]ZZ

Ø   Medical and Surgical
F   Hepatobiliary System and Pancreas
C   Extirpation   Definition: Taking or cutting out solid matter from a body part
                     Explanation: The solid matter may be an abnormal byproduct of a biological function or a foreign body; it may be imbedded in a body part or in the lumen of a tubular body part. The solid matter may or may not have been previously broken into pieces.

Body Part Character 4	Approach Character 5	Device Character 6	Qualifier Character 7
Ø Liver Quadrate lobe 1 Liver, Right Lobe 2 Liver, Left Lobe	Ø Open 3 Percutaneous 4 Percutaneous Endoscopic	Z No Device	Z No Qualifier
4 Gallbladder G Pancreas	Ø Open 3 Percutaneous 4 Percutaneous Endoscopic 8 Via Natural or Artificial Opening Endoscopic	Z No Device	Z No Qualifier

5 Hepatic Duct, Right
6 Hepatic Duct, Left
7 Hepatic Duct, Common
8 Cystic Duct
9 Common Bile Duct
C Ampulla of Vater
   Duodenal ampulla
   Hepatopancreatic ampulla
D Pancreatic Duct
   Duct of Wirsung
F Pancreatic Duct, Accessory
   Duct of Santorini
	Ø Open
	3 Percutaneous
	4 Percutaneous Endoscopic
	7 Via Natural or Artificial Opening
	8 Via Natural or Artificial Opening
	   Endoscopic
		Z No Device	Z No Qualifier

Non-OR   ØFC[5,6,7,8][3,4,7,8]ZZ
Non-OR   ØFC9[3,7,8]ZZ
Non-OR   ØFCC[4,8]ZZ
Non-OR   ØFC[D,F][3,4,8]ZZ

Non-OR Procedure   DRG Non-OR Procedure   Valid OR Procedure   HAC Associated Procedure   Combination Only   New/Revised April   New/Revised October

406   ICD-10-PCS 2023

Ø   **Medical and Surgical**
F   **Hepatobiliary System and Pancreas**
D   **Extraction**   Definition: Pulling or stripping out or off all or a portion of a body part by the use of force

                   Explanation: The qualifier DIAGNOSTIC is used to identify extraction procedures that are biopsies

Body Part Character 4	Approach Character 5	Device Character 6	Qualifier Character 7
Ø Liver Quadrate lobe 1 Liver, Right Lobe 2 Liver, Left Lobe	3 Percutaneous 4 Percutaneous Endoscopic	Z No Device	X Diagnostic

4 Gallbladder
5 Hepatic Duct, Right
6 Hepatic Duct, Left
7 Hepatic Duct, Common
8 Cystic Duct
9 Common Bile Duct
C Ampulla of Vater
    Duodenal ampulla
    Hepatopancreatic ampulla
D Pancreatic Duct
    Duct of Wirsung
F Pancreatic Duct, Accessory
    Duct of Santorini
G Pancreas
	3 Percutaneous
	4 Percutaneous Endoscopic
	8 Via Natural or Artificial Opening
	    Endoscopic
		Z No Device	X Diagnostic

Non-OR   ØFD[Ø,1,2]3ZX
Non-OR   ØFD[4,5,6,7,8,9,C,D,F,G][3,4,8]ZX

Ø   **Medical and Surgical**
F   **Hepatobiliary System and Pancreas**
F   **Fragmentation**   Definition: Breaking solid matter in a body part into pieces

                   Explanation: Physical force (e.g., manual, ultrasonic) applied directly or indirectly is used to break the solid matter into pieces. The solid matter may be an abnormal byproduct of a biological function or a foreign body. The pieces of solid matter are not taken out.

Body Part Character 4	Approach Character 5	Device Character 6	Qualifier Character 7

4 Gallbladder `NC`
5 Hepatic Duct, Right `NC`
6 Hepatic Duct, Left `NC`
7 Hepatic Duct, Common
8 Cystic Duct `NC`
9 Common Bile Duct `NC`
C Ampulla of Vater `NC`
    Duodenal ampulla
    Hepatopancreatic ampulla
D Pancreatic Duct `NC`
    Duct of Wirsung
F Pancreatic Duct, Accessory `NC`
    Duct of Santorini
	Ø Open
	3 Percutaneous
	4 Percutaneous Endoscopic
	7 Via Natural or Artificial Opening
	8 Via Natural or Artificial Opening
	    Endoscopic
	X External
		Z No Device	Z No Qualifier

Non-OR   ØFF[4,5,6,7,8,9,C,D,F][8,X]ZZ
`NC`   ØFF[4,5,6,8,9,C,D,F]XZZ

Ø   **Medical and Surgical**
F   **Hepatobiliary System and Pancreas**
H   **Insertion**   Definition: Putting in a nonbiological appliance that monitors, assists, performs, or prevents a physiological function but does not physically take the place of a body part

                   Explanation: None

Body Part Character 4	Approach Character 5	Device Character 6	Qualifier Character 7
Ø Liver Quadrate lobe 4 Gallbladder G Pancreas	Ø Open 3 Percutaneous 4 Percutaneous Endoscopic	1 Radioactive Element 2 Monitoring Device 3 Infusion Device Y Other Device	Z No Qualifier
1 Liver, Right Lobe 2 Liver, Left Lobe	Ø Open 3 Percutaneous 4 Percutaneous Endoscopic	2 Monitoring Device 3 Infusion Device	Z No Qualifier

B Hepatobiliary Duct ⊞
D Pancreatic Duct
    Duct of Wirsung
	Ø Open
	3 Percutaneous
	4 Percutaneous Endoscopic
	7 Via Natural or Artificial Opening
	8 Via Natural or Artificial Opening
	    Endoscopic
		1 Radioactive Element
		2 Monitoring Device
		3 Infusion Device
		D Intraluminal Device
		Y Other Device
			Z No Qualifier

Non-OR   ØFH[Ø,4,G]31Z
Non-OR   ØFH[Ø,4,G][Ø,3,4]3Z
Non-OR   ØFH[Ø,4,G][3,4]YZ
Non-OR   ØFH[1,2][Ø,3,4]3Z

Non-OR   ØFH[B,D][Ø,3,4]3Z
Non-OR   ØFH[B,D][4,8]DZ
Non-OR   ØFH[B,D][7,8][2,3]Z
Non-OR   ØFH[B,D][3,4,7,8]YZ

See Appendix L for Procedure Combinations
 ⊞   ØFHB7DZ

`NC` Noncovered Procedure   `LC` Limited Coverage   `OA` Questionable OB Admit   `NT` New Tech Add-on   ⊞ Combination Member   ♂ Male   ♀ Female

ICD-10-PCS 2023   407

Ø **Medical and Surgical**
F **Hepatobiliary System and Pancreas**
J **Inspection** Definition: Visually and/or manually exploring a body part

Explanation: Visual exploration may be performed with or without optical instrumentation. Manual exploration may be performed directly or through intervening body layers.

Body Part Character 4	Approach Character 5	Device Character 6	Qualifier Character 7
Ø Liver Quadrate lobe	Ø Open 3 Percutaneous 4 Percutaneous Endoscopic X External	Z No Device	Z No Qualifier
4 Gallbladder G Pancreas	Ø Open 3 Percutaneous 4 Percutaneous Endoscopic 8 Via Natural or Artificial Opening Endoscopic X External	Z No Device	Z No Qualifier

B Hepatobiliary Duct
D Pancreatic Duct
    Duct of Wirsung
	Ø Open
	3 Percutaneous
	4 Percutaneous Endoscopic
	7 Via Natural or Artificial Opening
	8 Via Natural or Artificial Opening
	    Endoscopic
		Z No Device	Z No Qualifier

Non-OR ØFJØ[3,X]ZZ
Non-OR ØFJ[4,G][3,8,X]ZZ
Non-OR ØFJ[B,D][3,7,8]ZZ

Ø **Medical and Surgical**
F **Hepatobiliary System and Pancreas**
L **Occlusion** Definition: Completely closing an orifice or the lumen of a tubular body part

Explanation: The orifice can be a natural orifice or an artificially created orifice

Body Part Character 4	Approach Character 5	Device Character 6	Qualifier Character 7

5 Hepatic Duct, Right
6 Hepatic Duct, Left
7 Hepatic Duct, Common
8 Cystic Duct
9 Common Bile Duct
C Ampulla of Vater
    Duodenal ampulla
    Hepatopancreatic ampulla
D Pancreatic Duct
    Duct of Wirsung
F Pancreatic Duct, Accessory
    Duct of Santorini
	Ø Open
	3 Percutaneous
	4 Percutaneous Endoscopic
		C Extraluminal Device
		D Intraluminal Device
		Z No Device
			Z No Qualifier

5 Hepatic Duct, Right
6 Hepatic Duct, Left
7 Hepatic Duct, Common
8 Cystic Duct
9 Common Bile Duct
C Ampulla of Vater
    Duodenal ampulla
    Hepatopancreatic ampulla
D Pancreatic Duct
    Duct of Wirsung
F Pancreatic Duct, Accessory
    Duct of Santorini
	7 Via Natural or Artificial Opening
	8 Via Natural or Artificial Opening
	    Endoscopic
		D Intraluminal Device
		Z No Device
			Z No Qualifier

Non-OR ØFL[5,6,7,8,9][3,4][C,D,Z]Z
Non-OR ØFL[5,6,7,8,9][7,8][D,Z]Z

Ø   Medical and Surgical
F   Hepatobiliary System and Pancreas
M   Reattachment   Definition: Putting back in or on all or a portion of a separated body part to its normal location or other suitable location

                     Explanation: Vascular circulation and nervous pathways may or may not be reestablished

Body Part Character 4	Approach Character 5	Device Character 6	Qualifier Character 7

Ø   Liver
     Quadrate lobe
1   Liver, Right Lobe
2   Liver, Left Lobe
4   Gallbladder
5   Hepatic Duct, Right
6   Hepatic Duct, Left
7   Hepatic Duct, Common
8   Cystic Duct
9   Common Bile Duct
C   Ampulla of Vater
     Duodenal ampulla
     Hepatopancreatic ampulla
D   Pancreatic Duct
     Duct of Wirsung
F   Pancreatic Duct, Accessory
     Duct of Santorini
G   Pancreas
	Ø Open
	4 Percutaneous Endoscopic
		Z No Device	Z No Qualifier

Non-OR   ØFM[4,5,6,7,8,9]4ZZ

Ø   Medical and Surgical
F   Hepatobiliary System and Pancreas
N   Release   Definition: Freeing a body part from an abnormal physical constraint by cutting or by the use of force

                   Explanation: Some of the restraining tissue may be taken out but none of the body part is taken out

Body Part Character 4	Approach Character 5	Device Character 6	Qualifier Character 7
Ø Liver Quadrate lobe 1 Liver, Right Lobe 2 Liver, Left Lobe	Ø Open 3 Percutaneous 4 Percutaneous Endoscopic	Z No Device	Z No Qualifier
4 Gallbladder G Pancreas	Ø Open 3 Percutaneous 4 Percutaneous Endoscopic 8 Via Natural or Artificial Opening Endoscopic	Z No Device	Z No Qualifier

5   Hepatic Duct, Right
6   Hepatic Duct, Left
7   Hepatic Duct, Common
8   Cystic Duct
9   Common Bile Duct
C   Ampulla of Vater
     Duodenal ampulla
     Hepatopancreatic ampulla
D   Pancreatic Duct
     Duct of Wirsung
F   Pancreatic Duct, Accessory
     Duct of Santorini
	Ø Open
	3 Percutaneous
	4 Percutaneous Endoscopic
	7 Via Natural or Artificial Opening
	8 Via Natural or Artificial Opening
	     Endoscopic
		Z No Device	Z No Qualifier

Ø **Medical and Surgical**
F **Hepatobiliary System and Pancreas**
P **Removal**   Definition: Taking out or off a device from a body part

Explanation: If a device is taken out and a similar device put in without cutting or puncturing the skin or mucous membrane, the procedure is coded to the root operation CHANGE. Otherwise, the procedure for taking out a device is coded to the root operation REMOVAL.

Body Part Character 4	Approach Character 5	Device Character 6	Qualifier Character 7
Ø Liver Quadrate lobe	Ø Open 3 Percutaneous 4 Percutaneous Endoscopic	Ø Drainage Device 2 Monitoring Device 3 Infusion Device Y Other Device	Z No Qualifier
Ø Liver Quadrate lobe	X External	Ø Drainage Device 2 Monitoring Device 3 Infusion Device	Z No Qualifier
4 Gallbladder G Pancreas	Ø Open 3 Percutaneous 4 Percutaneous Endoscopic	Ø Drainage Device 2 Monitoring Device 3 Infusion Device D Intraluminal Device Y Other Device	Z No Qualifier
4 Gallbladder G Pancreas	X External	Ø Drainage Device 2 Monitoring Device 3 Infusion Device D Intraluminal Device	Z No Qualifier

B Hepatobiliary Duct
D Pancreatic Duct
  Duct of Wirsung
	Ø Open
	3 Percutaneous
	4 Percutaneous Endoscopic
	7 Via Natural or Artificial Opening
	8 Via Natural or Artificial Opening
	  Endoscopic
		Ø Drainage Device
		1 Radioactive Element
		2 Monitoring Device
		3 Infusion Device
		7 Autologous Tissue Substitute
		C Extraluminal Device
		D Intraluminal Device
		J Synthetic Substitute
		K Nonautologous Tissue Substitute
		Y Other Device
			Z No Qualifier

B Hepatobiliary Duct D Pancreatic Duct Duct of Wirsung	X External	Ø Drainage Device 1 Radioactive Element 2 Monitoring Device 3 Infusion Device D Intraluminal Device	Z No Qualifier

Non-OR	ØFPØ[3,4]YZ
Non-OR	ØFPØX[Ø,2,3]Z
Non-OR	ØFPG3ØZ
Non-OR	ØFP[4,G][3,4]YZ
Non-OR	ØFP4X[Ø,2,3,D]Z
Non-OR	ØFPGX[Ø,2,3]Z
Non-OR	ØFP[B,D][3,4]YZ
Non-OR	ØFP[B,D][7,8][Ø,2,3,D,Y]Z
Non-OR	ØFP[B,D]X[Ø,1,2,3,D]Z

See Appendix L for Procedure Combinations

Combo-only	ØFP[B,D][7,8]DZ
Combo-only	ØFP[B,D]XDZ

Ø   **Medical and Surgical**
F   **Hepatobiliary System and Pancreas**
Q   **Repair**   Definition: Restoring, to the extent possible, a body part to its normal anatomic structure and function

               Explanation: Used only when the method to accomplish the repair is not one of the other root operations

Body Part Character 4	Approach Character 5	Device Character 6	Qualifier Character 7
Ø Liver Quadrate lobe 1 Liver, Right Lobe 2 Liver, Left Lobe	Ø Open 3 Percutaneous 4 Percutaneous Endoscopic	Z No Device	Z No Qualifier
4 Gallbladder G Pancreas	Ø Open 3 Percutaneous 4 Percutaneous Endoscopic 8 Via Natural or Artificial Opening Endoscopic	Z No Device	Z No Qualifier

5 Hepatic Duct, Right
6 Hepatic Duct, Left
7 Hepatic Duct, Common
8 Cystic Duct
9 Common Bile Duct
C Ampulla of Vater
   Duodenal ampulla
   Hepatopancreatic ampulla
D Pancreatic Duct
   Duct of Wirsung
F Pancreatic Duct, Accessory
   Duct of Santorini
	Ø Open
	3 Percutaneous
	4 Percutaneous Endoscopic
	7 Via Natural or Artificial Opening
	8 Via Natural or Artificial Opening Endoscopic
		Z No Device	Z No Qualifier

Ø   **Medical and Surgical**
F   **Hepatobiliary System and Pancreas**
R   **Replacement**   Definition: Putting in or on biological or synthetic material that physically takes the place and/or function of all or a portion of a body part

               Explanation: The body part may have been taken out or replaced, or may be taken out, physically eradicated, or rendered nonfunctional during the REPLACEMENT procedure. A REMOVAL procedure is coded for taking out the device used in a previous replacement procedure.

Body Part Character 4	Approach Character 5	Device Character 6	Qualifier Character 7

5 Hepatic Duct, Right
6 Hepatic Duct, Left
7 Hepatic Duct, Common
8 Cystic Duct
9 Common Bile Duct
C Ampulla of Vater
   Duodenal ampulla
   Hepatopancreatic ampulla
D Pancreatic Duct
   Duct of Wirsung
F Pancreatic Duct, Accessory
   Duct of Santorini
	Ø Open
	4 Percutaneous Endoscopic
	8 Via Natural or Artificial Opening Endoscopic
		7 Autologous Tissue Substitute
		J Synthetic Substitute
		K Nonautologous Tissue Substitute
			Z No Qualifier

Ø   **Medical and Surgical**
F   **Hepatobiliary System and Pancreas**
S   **Reposition**   Definition: Moving to its normal location, or other suitable location, all or a portion of a body part

               Explanation: The body part is moved to a new location from an abnormal location, or from a normal where it is not functioning correctly. The body part may or may not be cut out or off to be moved to the new location.

Body Part Character 4	Approach Character 5	Device Character 6	Qualifier Character 7

Ø Liver
   Quadrate lobe
4 Gallbladder
5 Hepatic Duct, Right
6 Hepatic Duct, Left
7 Hepatic Duct, Common
8 Cystic Duct
9 Common Bile Duct
C Ampulla of Vater
   Duodenal ampulla
   Hepatopancreatic ampulla
D Pancreatic Duct
   Duct of Wirsung
F Pancreatic Duct, Accessory
   Duct of Santorini
G Pancreas
	Ø Open
	4 Percutaneous Endoscopic
		Z No Device	Z No Qualifier

NC Noncovered Procedure   **LC** Limited Coverage   **QA** Questionable OB Admit   **NT** New Tech Add-on   ⊞ Combination Member   ♂ Male   ♀ Female

ICD-10-PCS 2023   411

Ø　Medical and Surgical
F　Hepatobiliary System and Pancreas
T　Resection　　Definition: Cutting out or off, without replacement, all of a body part
　　　　　　　　　　　Explanation: None

Body Part Character 4	Approach Character 5	Device Character 6	Qualifier Character 7
Ø　Liver 　　Quadrate lobe 1　Liver, Right Lobe 2　Liver, Left Lobe 4　Gallbladder G　Pancreas　⊞	Ø　Open 4　Percutaneous Endoscopic	Z　No Device	Z　No Qualifier
5　Hepatic Duct, Right 6　Hepatic Duct, Left 7　Hepatic Duct, Common 8　Cystic Duct 9　Common Bile Duct C　Ampulla of Vater 　　Duodenal ampulla 　　Hepatopancreatic ampulla D　Pancreatic Duct 　　Duct of Wirsung F　Pancreatic Duct, Accessory 　　Duct of Santorini	Ø　Open 4　Percutaneous Endoscopic 7　Via Natural or Artificial Opening 8　Via Natural or Artificial Opening 　　Endoscopic	Z　No Device	Z　No Qualifier

Non-OR　ØFT[D,F][4,8]ZZ

See Appendix L for Procedure Combinations
　⊞　　ØFTGØZZ

Ø　Medical and Surgical
F　Hepatobiliary System and Pancreas
U　Supplement　　Definition: Putting in or on biological or synthetic material that physically reinforces and/or augments the function of a portion of a body part
　　　　　　　　　　　Explanation: The biological material is non-living, or is living and from the same individual. The body part may have been previously replaced, and the SUPPLEMENT procedure is performed to physically reinforce and/or augment the function of the replaced body part.

Body Part Character 4	Approach Character 5	Device Character 6	Qualifier Character 7
5　Hepatic Duct, Right 6　Hepatic Duct, Left 7　Hepatic Duct, Common 8　Cystic Duct 9　Common Bile Duct C　Ampulla of Vater 　　Duodenal ampulla 　　Hepatopancreatic ampulla D　Pancreatic Duct 　　Duct of Wirsung F　Pancreatic Duct, Accessory 　　Duct of Santorini	Ø　Open 3　Percutaneous 4　Percutaneous Endoscopic 8　Via Natural or Artificial Opening 　　Endoscopic	7　Autologous Tissue Substitute J　Synthetic Substitute K　Nonautologous Tissue Substitute	Z　No Qualifier

Ø　**Medical and Surgical**
F　**Hepatobiliary System and Pancreas**
V　**Restriction**　　　　Definition: Partially closing an orifice or the lumen of a tubular body part
　　　　　　　　　　　　Explanation: The orifice can be a natural orifice or an artificially created orifice

Body Part Character 4	Approach Character 5	Device Character 6	Qualifier Character 7
5　Hepatic Duct, Right 6　Hepatic Duct, Left 7　Hepatic Duct, Common 8　Cystic Duct 9　Common Bile Duct C　Ampulla of Vater 　　Duodenal ampulla 　　Hepatopancreatic ampulla D　Pancreatic Duct 　　Duct of Wirsung F　Pancreatic Duct, Accessory 　　Duct of Santorini	Ø　Open 3　Percutaneous 4　Percutaneous Endoscopic	C　Extraluminal Device D　Intraluminal Device Z　No Device	Z　No Qualifier
5　Hepatic Duct, Right 6　Hepatic Duct, Left 7　Hepatic Duct, Common 8　Cystic Duct 9　Common Bile Duct C　Ampulla of Vater 　　Duodenal ampulla 　　Hepatopancreatic ampulla D　Pancreatic Duct 　　Duct of Wirsung F　Pancreatic Duct, Accessory 　　Duct of Santorini	7　Via Natural or Artificial Opening 8　Via Natural or Artificial Opening 　　Endoscopic	D　Intraluminal Device Z　No Device	Z　No Qualifier

Non-OR　ØFV[5,6,7,8,9][3,4][C,D,Z]Z
Non-OR　ØFV[5,6,7,8,9][7,8][D,Z]Z

Ø **Medical and Surgical**
F **Hepatobiliary System and Pancreas**
W **Revision**   Definition: Correcting, to the extent possible, a portion of a malfunctioning device or the position of a displaced device

Explanation: Revision can include correcting a malfunctioning or displaced device by taking out or putting in components of the device such as a screw or pin

Body Part Character 4	Approach Character 5	Device Character 6	Qualifier Character 7
Ø Liver Quadrate lobe	**Ø** Open **3** Percutaneous **4** Percutaneous Endoscopic	**Ø** Drainage Device **2** Monitoring Device **3** Infusion Device **Y** Other Device	**Z** No Qualifier
Ø Liver Quadrate lobe	**X** External	**Ø** Drainage Device **2** Monitoring Device **3** Infusion Device	**Z** No Qualifier
4 Gallbladder **G** Pancreas	**Ø** Open **3** Percutaneous **4** Percutaneous Endoscopic	**Ø** Drainage Device **2** Monitoring Device **3** Infusion Device **D** Intraluminal Device **Y** Other Device	**Z** No Qualifier
4 Gallbladder **G** Pancreas	**X** External	**Ø** Drainage Device **2** Monitoring Device **3** Infusion Device **D** Intraluminal Device	**Z** No Qualifier
B Hepatobiliary Duct **D** Pancreatic Duct Duct of Wirsung	**Ø** Open **3** Percutaneous **4** Percutaneous Endoscopic **7** Via Natural or Artificial Opening **8** Via Natural or Artificial Opening Endoscopic	**Ø** Drainage Device **2** Monitoring Device **3** Infusion Device **7** Autologous Tissue Substitute **C** Extraluminal Device **D** Intraluminal Device **J** Synthetic Substitute **K** Nonautologous Tissue Substitute **Y** Other Device	**Z** No Qualifier
B Hepatobiliary Duct **D** Pancreatic Duct Duct of Wirsung	**X** External	**Ø** Drainage Device **2** Monitoring Device **3** Infusion Device **7** Autologous Tissue Substitute **C** Extraluminal Device **D** Intraluminal Device **J** Synthetic Substitute **K** Nonautologous Tissue Substitute	**Z** No Qualifier

Non-OR	ØFWØ[3,4]YZ
Non-OR	ØFWØX[Ø,2,3]Z
Non-OR	ØFW[4,G][3,4]YZ
Non-OR	ØFW[4,G]X[Ø,2,3,D]Z
Non-OR	ØFW[B,D][3,4,7,8]YZ
Non-OR	ØFW[B,D]X[Ø,2,3,7,C,D,J,K]Z

Ø **Medical and Surgical**
F **Hepatobiliary System and Pancreas**
Y **Transplantation**   Definition: Putting in or on all or a portion of a living body part taken from another individual or animal to physically take the place and/or function of all or a portion of a similar body part

Explanation: The native body part may or may not be taken out, and the transplanted body part may take over all or a portion of its function

Body Part Character 4	Approach Character 5	Device Character 6	Qualifier Character 7
Ø Liver `LC` Quadrate lobe **G** Pancreas `LC` `NC` ⊞	**Ø** Open	**Z** No Device	**Ø** Allogeneic **1** Syngeneic **2** Zooplastic

`LC`	ØFYØØZ[Ø,1,2]	**See Appendix L for Procedure Combinations**	
`LC`	ØFYGØZ[Ø,1]	⊞ ØFYGØZ[Ø,1,2]	
`NC`	ØFYGØZ2		
`NC`	ØFYGØZ[Ø,1] If reported alone without one of the following procedures ØTYØØZ[Ø,1,2], ØTY1ØZ[Ø,1,2] and without one of the following diagnoses E1Ø.1Ø-E1Ø.9, E89.1		

Endocrine System 0G2–0GW

Character Meanings

This Character Meaning table is provided as a guide to assist the user in the identification of character members that may be found in this section of code tables. It **SHOULD NOT** be used to build a PCS code.

Operation–Character 3	Body Part–Character 4	Approach–Character 5	Device–Character 6	Qualifier–Character 7
2 Change	0 Pituitary Gland	0 Open	0 Drainage Device	3 Laser Interstitial Thermal Therapy
5 Destruction	1 Pineal Body	3 Percutaneous	1 Radioactive Element	X Diagnostic
8 Division	2 Adrenal Gland, Left	4 Percutaneous Endoscopic	2 Monitoring Device	Z No Qualifier
9 Drainage	3 Adrenal Gland, Right	X External	3 Infusion Device	
B Excision	4 Adrenal Glands, Bilateral		Y Other Device	
C Extirpation	5 Adrenal Gland		Z No Device	
H Insertion	6 Carotid Body, Left			
J Inspection	7 Carotid Body, Right			
M Reattachment	8 Carotid Bodies, Bilateral			
N Release	9 Para-aortic Body			
P Removal	B Coccygeal Glomus			
Q Repair	C Glomus Jugulare			
S Reposition	D Aortic Body			
T Resection	F Paraganglion Extremity			
W Revision	G Thyroid Gland Lobe, Left			
	H Thyroid Gland Lobe, Right			
	J Thyroid Gland Isthmus			
	K Thyroid Gland			
	L Superior Parathyroid Gland, Right			
	M Superior Parathyroid Gland, Left			
	N Inferior Parathyroid Gland, Right			
	P Inferior Parathyroid Gland, Left			
	Q Parathyroid Glands, Multiple			
	R Parathyroid Gland			
	S Endocrine Gland			

AHA Coding Clinic for table 0GB

2021, 2Q, 7	Infrarenal para-aortic paraganglioma with excision
2017, 2Q, 20	Near total thyroidectomy
2014, 3Q, 22	Transsphenoidal removal of pituitary tumor and fat graft placement

AHA Coding Clinic for table 0GH

| 2020, 4Q, 43-44 | Insertion of radioactive element |

AHA Coding Clinic for table 0GT

| 2017, 2Q, 20 | Near total thyroidectomy |

Endocrine System

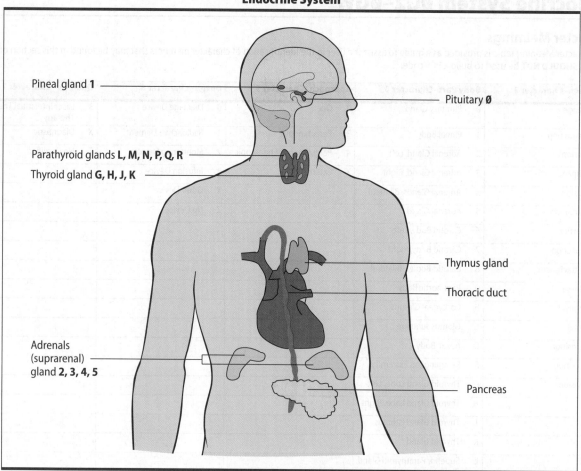

Pineal gland **1**

Pituitary **Ø**

Parathyroid glands **L, M, N, P, Q, R**

Thyroid gland **G, H, J, K**

Thymus gland

Thoracic duct

Adrenals (suprarenal) gland **2, 3, 4, 5**

Pancreas

Left Adrenal Gland

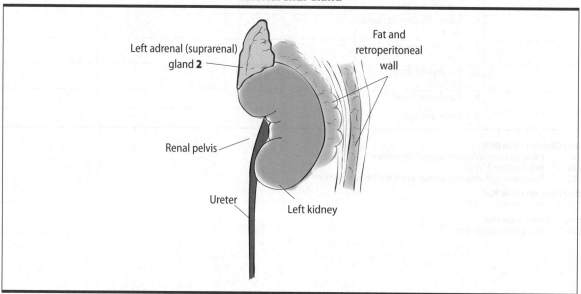

Left adrenal (suprarenal) gland **2**

Fat and retroperitoneal wall

Renal pelvis

Ureter

Left kidney

Thyroid

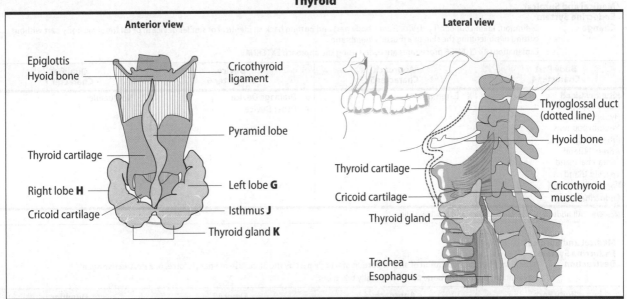

Anterior view

- Epiglottis
- Hyoid bone
- Cricothyroid ligament
- Pyramid lobe
- Thyroid cartilage
- Right lobe **H**
- Left lobe **G**
- Cricoid cartilage
- Isthmus **J**
- Thyroid gland **K**

Lateral view

- Thyroglossal duct (dotted line)
- Hyoid bone
- Thyroid cartilage
- Cricothyroid muscle
- Cricoid cartilage
- Thyroid gland
- Trachea
- Esophagus

Thyroid and Parathyroid Glands

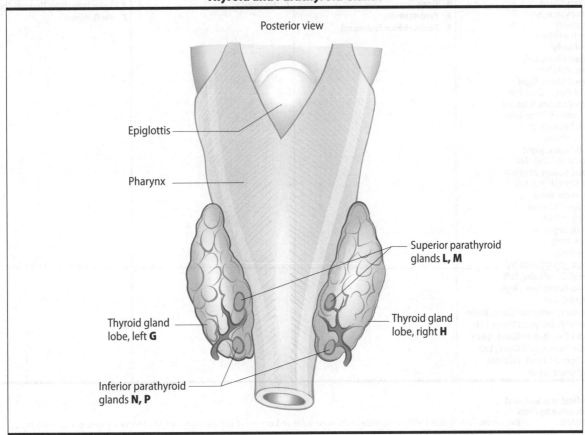

Posterior view

- Epiglottis
- Pharynx
- Superior parathyroid glands **L, M**
- Thyroid gland lobe, left **G**
- Thyroid gland lobe, right **H**
- Inferior parathyroid glands **N, P**

0 **Medical and Surgical**
G **Endocrine System**
2 **Change**   Definition: Taking out or off a device from a body part and putting back an identical or similar device in or on the same body part without cutting or puncturing the skin or a mucous membrane

Explanation: All CHANGE procedures are coded using the approach EXTERNAL

Body Part Character 4	Approach Character 5	Device Character 6	Qualifier Character 7
0 Pituitary Gland Adenohypophysis Hypophysis Neurohypophysis **1** Pineal Body **5** Adrenal Gland Suprarenal gland **K** Thyroid Gland **R** Parathyroid Gland **S** Endocrine Gland	**X** External	**0** Drainage Device **Y** Other Device	**Z** No Qualifier

Non-OR All body part, approach, device, and qualifier values

0 **Medical and Surgical**
G **Endocrine System**
5 **Destruction**   Definition: Physical eradication of all or a portion of a body part by the direct use of energy, force, or a destructive agent

Explanation: None of the body part is physically taken out

Body Part Character 4	Approach Character 5	Device Character 6	Qualifier Character 7
0 Pituitary Gland Adenohypophysis Hypophysis Neurohypophysis **1** Pineal Body **2** Adrenal Gland, Left Suprarenal gland **3** Adrenal Gland, Right See 2 Adrenal Gland, Left **4** Adrenal Glands, Bilateral See 2 Adrenal Gland, Left **6** Carotid Body, Left Carotid glomus **7** Carotid Body, Right See 6 Carotid Body, Left **8** Carotid Bodies, Bilateral See 6 Carotid Body, Left **9** Para-aortic Body **B** Coccygeal Glomus Coccygeal body **C** Glomus Jugulare Jugular body **D** Aortic Body **F** Paraganglion Extremity **G** Thyroid Gland Lobe, Left **H** Thyroid Gland Lobe, Right **K** Thyroid Gland **L** Superior Parathyroid Gland, Right **M** Superior Parathyroid Gland, Left **N** Inferior Parathyroid Gland, Right **P** Inferior Parathyroid Gland, Left **Q** Parathyroid Glands, Multiple **R** Parathyroid Gland	**0** Open **3** Percutaneous **4** Percutaneous Endoscopic	**Z** No Device	**3** Laser Interstitial Thermal Therapy **Z** No Qualifier

0 **Medical and Surgical**
G **Endocrine System**
8 **Division**   Definition: Cutting into a body part, without draining fluids and/or gases from the body part, in order to separate or transect a body part

Explanation: All or a portion of the body part is separated into two or more portions

Body Part Character 4	Approach Character 5	Device Character 6	Qualifier Character 7
0 Pituitary Gland Adenohypophysis Hypophysis Neurohypophysis **J** Thyroid Gland Isthmus	**0** Open **3** Percutaneous **4** Percutaneous Endoscopic	**Z** No Device	**Z** No Qualifier

Endocrine System

0   **Medical and Surgical**
G   **Endocrine System**
9   **Drainage**   Definition: Taking or letting out fluids and/or gases from a body part
                       Explanation: The qualifier DIAGNOSTIC is used to identify drainage procedures that are biopsies

Body Part Character 4	Approach Character 5	Device Character 6	Qualifier Character 7

0 **Pituitary Gland**
     Adenohypophysis
     Hypophysis
     Neurohypophysis
1 **Pineal Body**
2 **Adrenal Gland, Left**
     Suprarenal gland
3 **Adrenal Gland, Right**
     See 2 Adrenal Gland, Left
4 **Adrenal Glands, Bilateral**
     See 2 Adrenal Gland, Left
6 **Carotid Body, Left**
     Carotid glomus
7 **Carotid Body, Right**
     See 6 Carotid Body, Left
8 **Carotid Bodies, Bilateral**
     See 6 Carotid Body, Left
9 **Para-aortic Body**
B **Coccygeal Glomus**
     Coccygeal body
C **Glomus Jugulare**
     Jugular body
D **Aortic Body**
F **Paraganglion Extremity**
G **Thyroid Gland Lobe, Left**
H **Thyroid Gland Lobe, Right**
K **Thyroid Gland**
L **Superior Parathyroid Gland, Right**
M **Superior Parathyroid Gland, Left**
N **Inferior Parathyroid Gland, Right**
P **Inferior Parathyroid Gland, Left**
Q **Parathyroid Glands, Multiple**
R **Parathyroid Gland**
	0 Open
	3 Percutaneous
	4 Percutaneous Endoscopic
		0 Drainage Device	**Z** No Qualifier

0 **Pituitary Gland**
     Adenohypophysis
     Hypophysis
     Neurohypophysis
1 **Pineal Body**
2 **Adrenal Gland, Left**
     Suprarenal gland
3 **Adrenal Gland, Right**
     See 2 Adrenal Gland, Left
4 **Adrenal Glands, Bilateral**
     See 2 Adrenal Gland, Left
6 **Carotid Body, Left**
     Carotid glomus
7 **Carotid Body, Right**
     See 6 Carotid Body, Left
8 **Carotid Bodies, Bilateral**
     See 6 Carotid Body, Left
9 **Para-aortic Body**
B **Coccygeal Glomus**
     Coccygeal body
C **Glomus Jugulare**
     Jugular body
D **Aortic Body**
F **Paraganglion Extremity**
G **Thyroid Gland Lobe, Left**
H **Thyroid Gland Lobe, Right**
K **Thyroid Gland**
L **Superior Parathyroid Gland, Right**
M **Superior Parathyroid Gland, Left**
N **Inferior Parathyroid Gland, Right**
P **Inferior Parathyroid Gland, Left**
Q **Parathyroid Glands, Multiple**
R **Parathyroid Gland**
	0 Open
	3 Percutaneous
	4 Percutaneous Endoscopic
		Z No Device	**X** Diagnostic
			Z No Qualifier

Non-OR   0G9[0,1,2,3,4,6,7,8,9,B,C,D,F,G,H,K,L,M,N,P,Q,R]30Z
Non-OR   0G9[G,H,K,L,M,N,P,Q,R]40Z
Non-OR   0G9[2,3,4,G,H,K][3,4]ZX
Non-OR   0G9[0,1,2,3,4,6,7,8,9,B,C,D,F,G,H,K,L,M,N,P,Q,R]3ZZ
Non-OR   0G9[G,H,K,L,M,N,P,Q,R]4ZZ

NC Noncovered Procedure   **LC** Limited Coverage   **QA** Questionable OB Admit   **NT** New Tech Add-on   ⊞ Combination Member   ♂ Male   ♀ Female

ICD-10-PCS 2023   419

0G9–0G9

Endocrine System (side tab)

Ø Medical and Surgical
G Endocrine System
B Excision Definition: Cutting out or off, without replacement, a portion of a body part

Explanation: The qualifier DIAGNOSTIC is used to identify excision procedures that are biopsies

Body Part Character 4	Approach Character 5	Device Character 6	Qualifier Character 7
Ø Pituitary Gland Adenohypophysis Hypophysis Neurohypophysis 1 Pineal Body 2 Adrenal Gland, Left Suprarenal gland 3 Adrenal Gland, Right See 2 Adrenal Gland, Left 4 Adrenal Glands, Bilateral See 2 Adrenal Gland, Left 6 Carotid Body, Left Carotid glomus 7 Carotid Body, Right See 6 Carotid Body, Left 8 Carotid Bodies, Bilateral See 6 Carotid Body, Left 9 Para-aortic Body B Coccygeal Glomus Coccygeal body C Glomus Jugulare Jugular body D Aortic Body F Paraganglion Extremity G Thyroid Gland Lobe, Left H Thyroid Gland Lobe, Right J Thyroid Gland Isthmus L Superior Parathyroid Gland, Right M Superior Parathyroid Gland, Left N Inferior Parathyroid Gland, Right P Inferior Parathyroid Gland, Left Q Parathyroid Glands, Multiple R Parathyroid Gland	Ø Open 3 Percutaneous 4 Percutaneous Endoscopic	Z No Device	X Diagnostic Z No Qualifier

Non-OR ØGB[2,3,4,G,H,J][3,4]ZX

Ø Medical and Surgical
G Endocrine System
C Extirpation Definition: Taking or cutting out solid matter from a body part

Explanation: The solid matter may be an abnormal byproduct of a biological function or a foreign body; it may be imbedded in a body part or in the lumen of a tubular body part. The solid matter may or may not have been previously broken into pieces.

Body Part Character 4	Approach Character 5	Device Character 6	Qualifier Character 7
Ø Pituitary Gland Adenohypophysis Hypophysis Neurohypophysis 1 Pineal Body 2 Adrenal Gland, Left Suprarenal gland 3 Adrenal Gland, Right See 2 Adrenal Gland, Left 4 Adrenal Glands, Bilateral See 2 Adrenal Gland, Left 6 Carotid Body, Left Carotid glomus 7 Carotid Body, Right See 6 Carotid Body, Left 8 Carotid Bodies, Bilateral See 6 Carotid Body, Left 9 Para-aortic Body B Coccygeal Glomus Coccygeal body C Glomus Jugulare Jugular body D Aortic Body F Paraganglion Extremity G Thyroid Gland Lobe, Left H Thyroid Gland Lobe, Right K Thyroid Gland L Superior Parathyroid Gland, Right M Superior Parathyroid Gland, Left N Inferior Parathyroid Gland, Right P Inferior Parathyroid Gland, Left Q Parathyroid Glands, Multiple R Parathyroid Gland	Ø Open 3 Percutaneous 4 Percutaneous Endoscopic	Z No Device	Z No Qualifier

Non-OR Procedure   DRG Non-OR Procedure   Valid OR Procedure   HAC Associated Procedure   Combination Only   New/Revised April   New/Revised October

420

ØGB–ØGC

ICD-10-PCS 2023

Ø   Medical and Surgical
G   Endocrine System
H   Insertion   Definition: Putting in a nonbiological appliance that monitors, assists, performs, or prevents a physiological function but does not physically take the place of a body part

Explanation: None

Body Part Character 4	Approach Character 5	Device Character 6	Qualifier Character 7
S Endocrine Gland	**Ø** Open **3** Percutaneous **4** Percutaneous Endoscopic	**1** Radioactive Element **2** Monitoring Device **3** Infusion Device **Y** Other Device	**Z** No Qualifier

Non-OR	ØGHS31Z
Non-OR	ØGHS[3,4]YZ

Ø   Medical and Surgical
G   Endocrine System
J   Inspection   Definition: Visually and/or manually exploring a body part

Explanation: Visual exploration may be performed with or without optical instrumentation. Manual exploration may be performed directly or through intervening body layers.

Body Part Character 4	Approach Character 5	Device Character 6	Qualifier Character 7

Ø Pituitary Gland
  Adenohypophysis
  Hypophysis
  Neurohypophysis
1 Pineal Body
5 Adrenal Gland
  Suprarenal gland
K Thyroid Gland
R Parathyroid Gland
S Endocrine Gland
	Ø Open
	3 Percutaneous
	4 Percutaneous Endoscopic
		Z No Device	**Z** No Qualifier

Non-OR	ØGJ[Ø,1,5,K,R,S]3ZZ

Ø   Medical and Surgical
G   Endocrine System
M   Reattachment   Definition: Putting back in or on all or a portion of a separated body part to its normal location or other suitable location

Explanation: Vascular circulation and nervous pathways may or may not be reestablished

Body Part Character 4	Approach Character 5	Device Character 6	Qualifier Character 7

2 Adrenal Gland, Left
  Suprarenal gland
3 Adrenal Gland, Right
  See 2 Adrenal Gland, Left
G Thyroid Gland Lobe, Left
H Thyroid Gland Lobe, Right
L Superior Parathyroid Gland, Right
M Superior Parathyroid Gland, Left
N Inferior Parathyroid Gland, Right
P Inferior Parathyroid Gland, Left
Q Parathyroid Glands, Multiple
R Parathyroid Gland
	Ø Open
	4 Percutaneous Endoscopic
		Z No Device	**Z** No Qualifier

Endocrine System

Ø Medical and Surgical
G Endocrine System
N Release   Definition: Freeing a body part from an abnormal physical constraint by cutting or by the use of force
                 Explanation: Some of the restraining tissue may be taken out but none of the body part is taken out

Body Part Character 4	Approach Character 5	Device Character 6	Qualifier Character 7

Ø Pituitary Gland
   Adenohypophysis
   Hypophysis
   Neurohypophysis
1 Pineal Body
2 Adrenal Gland, Left
   Suprarenal gland
3 Adrenal Gland, Right
   See 2 Adrenal Gland, Left
4 Adrenal Glands, Bilateral
   See 2 Adrenal Gland, Left
6 Carotid Body, Left
   Carotid glomus
7 Carotid Body, Right
   See 6 Carotid Body, Left
8 Carotid Bodies, Bilateral
   See 6 Carotid Body, Left
9 Para-aortic Body
B Coccygeal Glomus
   Coccygeal body
C Glomus Jugulare
   Jugular body
D Aortic Body
F Paraganglion Extremity
G Thyroid Gland Lobe, Left
H Thyroid Gland Lobe, Right
K Thyroid Gland
L Superior Parathyroid Gland, Right
M Superior Parathyroid Gland, Left
N Inferior Parathyroid Gland, Right
P Inferior Parathyroid Gland, Left
Q Parathyroid Glands, Multiple
R Parathyroid Gland
	Ø Open
	3 Percutaneous
	4 Percutaneous Endoscopic
		Z No Device	Z No Qualifier

Non-OR   ØGN[6,7,8,9,B,C,D,F][Ø,3,4]ZZ

Ø Medical and Surgical
G Endocrine System
P Removal   Definition: Taking out or off a device from a body part
                 Explanation: If a device is taken out and a similar device put in without cutting or puncturing the skin or mucous membrane, the procedure is coded to the root operation CHANGE. Otherwise, the procedure for taking out a device is coded to the root operation REMOVAL.

Body Part Character 4	Approach Character 5	Device Character 6	Qualifier Character 7

Ø Pituitary Gland
   Adenohypophysis
   Hypophysis
   Neurohypophysis
1 Pineal Body
5 Adrenal Gland
   Suprarenal gland
K Thyroid Gland
R Parathyroid Gland
	Ø Open
	3 Percutaneous
	4 Percutaneous Endoscopic
	X External
		Ø Drainage Device	Z No Qualifier

S Endocrine Gland	Ø Open 3 Percutaneous 4 Percutaneous Endoscopic	Ø Drainage Device 2 Monitoring Device 3 Infusion Device Y Other Device	Z No Qualifier
S Endocrine Gland	X External	Ø Drainage Device 2 Monitoring Device 3 Infusion Device	Z No Qualifier

Non-OR   ØGP[Ø,1,5,K,R]XØZ
Non-OR   ØGPS[3,4]YZ
Non-OR   ØGPSX[Ø,2,3]Z

Non-OR Procedure   DRG Non-OR Procedure   Valid OR Procedure   HAC Associated Procedure   Combination Only   New/Revised April   New/Revised October

Ø Medical and Surgical
G Endocrine System
Q Repair   Definition: Restoring, to the extent possible, a body part to its normal anatomic structure and function

Explanation: Used only when the method to accomplish the repair is not one of the other root operations

Body Part Character 4	Approach Character 5	Device Character 6	Qualifier Character 7

Ø Pituitary Gland
    Adenohypophysis
    Hypophysis
    Neurohypophysis
1 Pineal Body
2 Adrenal Gland, Left
    Suprarenal gland
3 Adrenal Gland, Right
    See 2 Adrenal Gland, Left
4 Adrenal Glands, Bilateral
    See 2 Adrenal Gland, Left
6 Carotid Body, Left
    Carotid glomus
7 Carotid Body, Right
    See 6 Carotid Body, Left
8 Carotid Bodies, Bilateral
    See 6 Carotid Body, Left
9 Para-aortic Body
B Coccygeal Glomus
    Coccygeal body
C Glomus Jugulare
    Jugular body
D Aortic Body
F Paraganglion Extremity
G Thyroid Gland Lobe, Left
H Thyroid Gland Lobe, Right
J Thyroid Gland Isthmus
K Thyroid Gland
L Superior Parathyroid Gland, Right
M Superior Parathyroid Gland, Left
N Inferior Parathyroid Gland, Right
P Inferior Parathyroid Gland, Left
Q Parathyroid Glands, Multiple
R Parathyroid Gland
	Ø Open
	3 Percutaneous
	4 Percutaneous Endoscopic
		Z No Device	**Z No Qualifier**

Ø Medical and Surgical
G Endocrine System
S Reposition   Definition: Moving to its normal location, or other suitable location, all or a portion of a body part

Explanation: The body part is moved to a new location from an abnormal location, or from a normal location where it is not functioning correctly. The body part may or may not be cut out or off to be moved to the new location.

Body Part Character 4	Approach Character 5	Device Character 6	Qualifier Character 7

2 Adrenal Gland, Left
    Suprarenal gland
3 Adrenal Gland, Right
    See 2 Adrenal Gland, Left
G Thyroid Gland Lobe, Left
H Thyroid Gland Lobe, Right
L Superior Parathyroid Gland, Right
M Superior Parathyroid Gland, Left
N Inferior Parathyroid Gland, Right
P Inferior Parathyroid Gland, Left
Q Parathyroid Glands, Multiple
R Parathyroid Gland
	Ø Open
	4 Percutaneous Endoscopic
		Z No Device	**Z No Qualifier**

NC Noncovered Procedure   **LC** Limited Coverage   **QA** Questionable OB Admit   **NT** New Tech Add-on   ⊞ Combination Member   ♂ Male   ♀ Female

ICD-10-PCS 2023   423

Ø   **Medical and Surgical**
G   **Endocrine System**
T   **Resection**   Definition: Cutting out or off, without replacement, all of a body part
                              Explanation: None

Body Part Character 4	Approach Character 5	Device Character 6	Qualifier Character 7

Ø Pituitary Gland
  Adenohypophysis
  Hypophysis
  Neurohypophysis
1 Pineal Body
2 Adrenal Gland, Left
  Suprarenal gland
3 Adrenal Gland, Right
  See 2 Adrenal Gland, Left
4 Adrenal Glands, Bilateral
  See 2 Adrenal Gland, Left
6 Carotid Body, Left
  Carotid glomus
7 Carotid Body, Right
  See 6 Carotid Body, Left
8 Carotid Bodies, Bilateral
  See 6 Carotid Body, Left
9 Para-aortic Body
B Coccygeal Glomus
  Coccygeal body
C Glomus Jugulare
  Jugular body
D Aortic Body
F Paraganglion Extremity
G Thyroid Gland Lobe, Left
H Thyroid Gland Lobe, Right
J Thyroid Gland Isthmus
K Thyroid Gland
L Superior Parathyroid Gland, Right
M Superior Parathyroid Gland, Left
N Inferior Parathyroid Gland, Right
P Inferior Parathyroid Gland, Left
Q Parathyroid Glands, Multiple
R Parathyroid Gland
	Ø Open
	4 Percutaneous Endoscopic
		Z No Device	**Z** No Qualifier

Non-OR   ØGT[6,7,8,9,B,C,D,F][Ø,4]ZZ

Ø   **Medical and Surgical**
G   **Endocrine System**
W   **Revision**   Definition: Correcting, to the extent possible, a portion of a malfunctioning device or the position of a displaced device
                              Explanation: Revision can include correcting a malfunctioning or displaced device by taking out or putting in components of the device such as a screw or pin

Body Part Character 4	Approach Character 5	Device Character 6	Qualifier Character 7

Ø Pituitary Gland
  Adenohypophysis
  Hypophysis
  Neurohypophysis
1 Pineal Body
5 Adrenal Gland
  Suprarenal gland
K Thyroid Gland
R Parathyroid Gland
	Ø Open
	3 Percutaneous
	4 Percutaneous Endoscopic
	X External
		Ø Drainage Device	**Z** No Qualifier

S Endocrine Gland	**Ø** Open **3** Percutaneous **4** Percutaneous Endoscopic	**Ø** Drainage Device **2** Monitoring Device **3** Infusion Device **Y** Other Device	**Z** No Qualifier
S Endocrine Gland	**X** External	**Ø** Drainage Device **2** Monitoring Device **3** Infusion Device	**Z** No Qualifier

Non-OR   ØGW[Ø,1,5,K,R]XØZ
Non-OR   ØGWS[3,4]YZ
Non-OR   ØGWSX[Ø,2,3]Z

Non-OR Procedure   DRG Non-OR Procedure   Valid OR Procedure   HAC Associated Procedure   Combination Only   New/Revised April   New/Revised October
424   ICD-10-PCS 2023

ØGT–ØGW

Skin and Breast ØHØ–ØHX

Character Meanings*

This Character Meaning table is provided as a guide to assist the user in the identification of character members that may be found in this section of code tables. It **SHOULD NOT** be used to build a PCS code.

Operation–Character 3		Body Part–Character 4		Approach–Character 5		Device–Character 6		Qualifier–Character 7	
Ø	Alteration	Ø	Skin, Scalp	Ø	Open	Ø	Drainage Device	2	Cell Suspension Technique
2	Change	1	Skin, Face	3	Percutaneous	1	Radioactive Element	3	Full Thickness OR Laser Interstitial Thermal Therapy
5	Destruction	2	Skin, Right Ear	7	Via Natural or Artificial Opening	7	Autologous Tissue Substitute	4	Partial Thickness
8	Division	3	Skin, Left Ear	8	Via Natural or Artificial Opening Endoscopic	J	Synthetic Substitute	5	Latissimus Dorsi Myocutaneous Flap
9	Drainage	4	Skin, Neck	X	External	K	Nonautologous Tissue Substitute	6	Transverse Rectus Abdominis Myocutaneous Flap
B	Excision	5	Skin, Chest			N	Tissue Expander	7	Deep Inferior Epigastric Artery Perforator Flap
C	Extirpation	6	Skin, Back			Y	Other Device	8	Superficial Inferior Epigastric Artery Flap
D	Extraction	7	Skin, Abdomen			Z	No Device	9	Gluteal Artery Perforator Flap
H	Insertion	8	Skin, Buttock					D	Multiple
J	Inspection	9	Skin, Perineum					X	Diagnostic
M	Reattachment	A	Skin, Inguinal					Z	No Qualifier
N	Release	B	Skin, Right Upper Arm						
P	Removal	C	Skin, Left Upper Arm						
Q	Repair	D	Skin, Right Lower Arm						
R	Replacement	E	Skin, Left Lower Arm						
S	Reposition	F	Skin, Right Hand						
T	Resection	G	Skin, Left Hand						
U	Supplement	H	Skin, Right Upper Leg						
W	Revision	J	Skin, Left Upper Leg						
X	Transfer	K	Skin, Right Lower Leg						
		L	Skin, Left Lower Leg						
		M	Skin, Right Foot						
		N	Skin, Left Foot						
		P	Skin						
		Q	Finger Nail						
		R	Toe Nail						
		S	Hair						
		T	Breast, Right						
		U	Breast, Left						
		V	Breast, Bilateral						
		W	Nipple, Right						
		X	Nipple, Left						
		Y	Supernumerary Breast						

* Includes skin and breast glands and ducts.

AHA Coding Clinic for table ØHØ

2022, 1Q, 14	Reduction mammoplasty for breast symmetry
2022, 1Q, 15	Nipple reconstruction and breast reduction
2019, 4Q, 30-31	Breast procedures

AHA Coding Clinic for table ØH5

2019, 4Q, 30-31	Breast procedures

AHA Coding Clinic for table ØH9

2019, 4Q, 30-31	Breast procedures

AHA Coding Clinic for table ØHB

2022, 1Q, 14	Reduction mammoplasty for breast symmetry
2020, 1Q, 31	Repair of buried penis
2019, 4Q, 30-31	Breast procedures
2018, 1Q, 14	Excisional debridement of breast tissue and skin
2016, 3Q, 29	Closure of bilateral alveolar clefts
2015, 3Q, 3-8	Excisional and nonexcisional debridement

AHA Coding Clinic for table ØHC

2019, 4Q, 30-31	Breast procedures

AHA Coding Clinic for table ØHD

2019, 4Q, 30-31	Breast procedures
2016, 1Q, 40	Nonexcisional debridement of skin and subcutaneous tissue
2015, 3Q, 3-8	Excisional and nonexcisional debridement

AHA Coding Clinic for table ØHH

2019, 4Q, 30-31	Breast procedures
2017, 4Q, 67	New qualifier values - Pedicle flap procedures
2014, 2Q, 12	Pedicle latissimus myocutaneous flap with placement of breast tissue expanders
2013, 4Q, 107	Breast tissue expander placement using acellular dermal matrix

AHA Coding Clinic for table ØHJ

2019, 4Q, 30-31	Breast procedures

AHA Coding Clinic for table ØHN

2019, 4Q, 30-31	Breast procedures

AHA Coding Clinic for table ØHP

2019, 4Q, 30-31	Breast procedures
2018, 3Q, 13	Deep inferior epigastric artery perforator flap breast reconstruction
2016, 2Q, 27	Removal of nonviable transverse rectus abdominis myocutaneous (TRAM) flaps

AHA Coding Clinic for table ØHQ

2019, 4Q, 30-31	Breast procedures
2018, 2Q, 25	Third and fourth degree obstetric lacerations
2016, 1Q, 7	Obstetrical perineal laceration repair
2014, 4Q, 31	Delayed wound closure following fracture treatment

AHA Coding Clinic for table ØHR

2022, 1Q, 15	Nipple reconstruction and breast reduction
2020, 1Q, 27	Delayed reconstruction following mastectomy using gracilis musculocutaneous free flap
2020, 1Q, 28	Free flap microvascular breast reconstruction
2020, 1Q, 30	Polarity Skin TE™ application
2019, 4Q, 30-31	Breast procedures
2019, 4Q, 32	Cell suspension epithelial autograft
2019, 3Q, 32	Breast reconstruction with neurotization
2018, 3Q, 13	Deep inferior epigastric artery perforator flap breast reconstruction
2017, 1Q, 35	Epifix® allograft
2014, 3Q, 14	Application of TheraSkin® and excisional debridement

AHA Coding Clinic for table ØHT

2021, 2Q, 16	Goldilocks breast reconstruction
2018, 3Q, 13	Deep inferior epigastric artery perforator flap breast reconstruction
2014, 4Q, 34	Skin-sparing mastectomy

AHA Coding Clinic for table ØHU

2019, 4Q, 30-31	Breast procedures

AHA Coding Clinic for table ØHW

2019, 4Q, 30-31	Breast procedures

Integumentary Anatomy

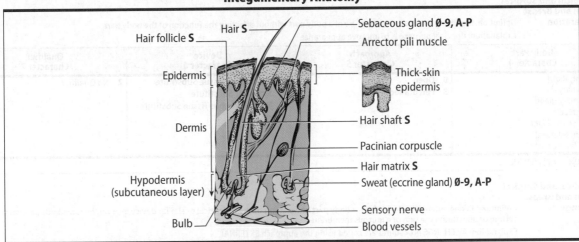

Hair **S**
Hair follicle **S**
Epidermis
Dermis
Hypodermis (subcutaneous layer)
Bulb

Sebaceous gland **Ø-9, A-P**
Arrector pili muscle
Thick-skin epidermis
Hair shaft **S**
Pacinian corpuscle
Hair matrix **S**
Sweat (eccrine gland) **Ø-9, A-P**
Sensory nerve
Blood vessels

Nail Anatomy

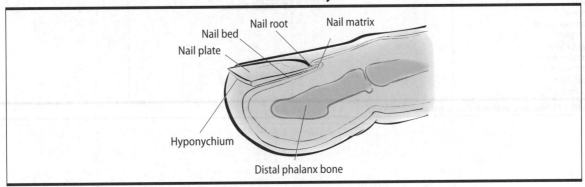

Nail root
Nail bed
Nail matrix
Nail plate
Hyponychium
Distal phalanx bone

Breast

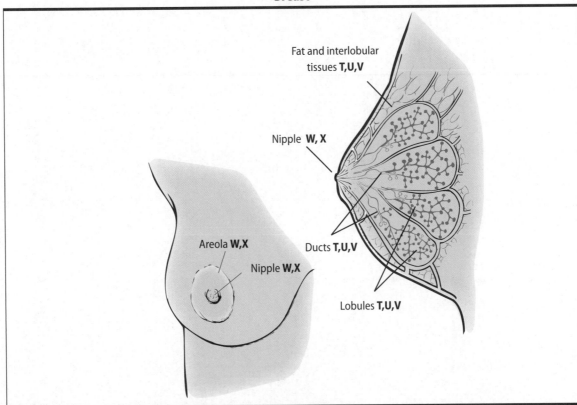

Fat and interlobular tissues **T,U,V**
Nipple **W, X**
Areola **W,X**
Nipple **W,X**
Ducts **T,U,V**
Lobules **T,U,V**

Skin and Breast *(side tab)*

Ø   **Medical and Surgical**
H   **Skin and Breast**
Ø   **Alteration**   Definition: Modifying the anatomic structure of a body part without affecting the function of the body part
                    Explanation: Principal purpose is to improve appearance

Body Part Character 4	Approach Character 5	Device Character 6	Qualifier Character 7

T Breast, Right
    Mammary duct
    Mammary gland
U Breast, Left
    See T Breast, Right
V Breast, Bilateral
    See T Breast, Right
	Ø Open
	3 Percutaneous
		7 Autologous Tissue Substitute
		J Synthetic Substitute
		K Nonautologous Tissue Substitute
		Z No Device
			Z No Qualifier

Non-OR   ØHØ[T,U,V]3JZ

Ø   **Medical and Surgical**
H   **Skin and Breast**
2   **Change**   Definition: Taking out or off a device from a body part and putting back an identical or similar device in or on the same body part without
                    cutting or puncturing the skin or a mucous membrane
                    Explanation: All CHANGE procedures are coded using the approach EXTERNAL

Body Part Character 4	Approach Character 5	Device Character 6	Qualifier Character 7

P Skin
    Dermis
    Epidermis
    Sebaceous gland
    Sweat gland
T Breast, Right
    Mammary duct
    Mammary gland
U Breast, Left
    See T Breast, Right
	X External	**Ø** Drainage Device
		Y Other Device
			Z No Qualifier

Non-OR   All body part, approach, device, and qualifier values

---

Non-OR Procedure   DRG Non-OR Procedure   Valid OR Procedure   HAC Associated Procedure   Combination Only   New/Revised April   New/Revised October

428   ICD-10-PCS 2023

Ø   **Medical and Surgical**
H   **Skin and Breast**
5   **Destruction**   Definition: Physical eradication of all or a portion of a body part by the direct use of energy, force, or a destructive agent

                                   Explanation: None of the body part is physically taken out

Body Part Character 4	Approach Character 5	Device Character 6	Qualifier Character 7

Ø Skin, Scalp
1 Skin, Face
2 Skin, Right Ear
3 Skin, Left Ear
4 Skin, Neck
5 Skin, Chest
    Breast procedures, skin only
6 Skin, Back
7 Skin, Abdomen
8 Skin, Buttock
9 Skin, Perineum
    Perianal skin
A Skin, Inguinal
B Skin, Right Upper Arm
C Skin, Left Upper Arm
D Skin, Right Lower Arm
E Skin, Left Lower Arm
F Skin, Right Hand
G Skin, Left Hand
H Skin, Right Upper Leg
J Skin, Left Upper Leg
K Skin, Right Lower Leg
L Skin, Left Lower Leg
M Skin, Right Foot
N Skin, Left Foot
	X External	**Z** No Device	**D** Multiple
			Z No Qualifier

Q Finger Nail
    Nail bed
    Nail plate
R Toe Nail
    See Q Finger Nail
	X External	**Z** No Device	**Z** No Qualifier

T Breast, Right
    Mammary duct
    Mammary gland
U Breast, Left
    See T Breast, Right
V Breast, Bilateral
    See T Breast, Right
	Ø Open
	3 Percutaneous
		Z No Device	**3** Laser Interstitial Thermal Therapy
			Z No Qualifier

T Breast, Right
    Mammary duct
    Mammary gland
U Breast, Left
    See T Breast, Right
V Breast, Bilateral
    See T Breast, Right
	7 Via Natural or Artificial Opening
	8 Via Natural or Artificial Opening Endoscopic
		Z No Device	**Z** No Qualifier

W Nipple, Right
    Areola
X Nipple, Left
    See W Nipple, Right
	Ø Open
	3 Percutaneous
	7 Via Natural or Artificial Opening
	8 Via Natural or Artificial Opening Endoscopic
	X External
		Z No Device	**Z** No Qualifier

DRG Non-OR	ØH5[Ø,1,4,5,6,7,8,9,A,B,C,D,E,F,G,H,J,K,L,M,N]XZ[D,Z]
DRG Non-OR	ØH5[Q,R]XZZ
Non-OR	ØH5[2,3]XZ[D,Z]

NC Noncovered Procedure   LC Limited Coverage   QA Questionable OB Admit   NT New Tech Add-on   ⊞ Combination Member   ♂ Male   ♀ Female

ICD-10-PCS 2023   429

Ø Medical and Surgical
H Skin and Breast
8 Division   Definition: Cutting into a body part, without draining fluids and/or gases from the body part, in order to separate or transect a body part
                    Explanation: All or a portion of the body part is separated into two or more portions

Body Part Character 4	Approach Character 5	Device Character 6	Qualifier Character 7
Ø Skin, Scalp	X External	Z No Device	Z No Qualifier
1 Skin, Face			
2 Skin, Right Ear			
3 Skin, Left Ear			
4 Skin, Neck			
5 Skin, Chest Breast procedures, skin only			
6 Skin, Back			
7 Skin, Abdomen			
8 Skin, Buttock			
9 Skin, Perineum Perianal skin			
A Skin, Inguinal			
B Skin, Right Upper Arm			
C Skin, Left Upper Arm			
D Skin, Right Lower Arm			
E Skin, Left Lower Arm			
F Skin, Right Hand			
G Skin, Left Hand			
H Skin, Right Upper Leg			
J Skin, Left Upper Leg			
K Skin, Right Lower Leg			
L Skin, Left Lower Leg			
M Skin, Right Foot			
N Skin, Left Foot			

Non-OR	All body part, approach, device, and qualifier values

Ø   **Medical and Surgical**
H   **Skin and Breast**
9   **Drainage**   Definition: Taking or letting out fluids and/or gases from a body part
                    Explanation: The qualifier DIAGNOSTIC is used to identify drainage procedures that are biopsies

Body Part Character 4		Approach Character 5	Device Character 6	Qualifier Character 7

Ø Skin, Scalp
 1 Skin, Face
 2 Skin, Right Ear
 3 Skin, Left Ear
 4 Skin, Neck
 5 Skin, Chest
    Breast procedures, skin
    only
 6 Skin, Back
 7 Skin, Abdomen
 8 Skin, Buttock
 9 Skin, Perineum
    Perianal skin
 A Skin, Inguinal
 B Skin, Right Upper Arm
 C Skin, Left Upper Arm
 D Skin, Right Lower Arm
	E Skin, Left Lower Arm
	 F Skin, Right Hand
	 G Skin, Left Hand
	 H Skin, Right Upper Leg
	 J Skin, Left Upper Leg
	 K Skin, Right Lower Leg
	 L Skin, Left Lower Leg
	 M Skin, Right Foot
	 N Skin, Left Foot
	 Q Finger Nail
	    Nail bed
	    Nail plate
	 R Toe Nail
	    See Q Finger Nail
		X External	Ø Drainage Device	Z No Qualifier

Ø Skin, Scalp
 1 Skin, Face
 2 Skin, Right Ear
 3 Skin, Left Ear
 4 Skin, Neck
 5 Skin, Chest
    Breast procedures, skin
    only
 6 Skin, Back
 7 Skin, Abdomen
 8 Skin, Buttock
 9 Skin, Perineum
    Perianal skin
 A Skin, Inguinal
 B Skin, Right Upper Arm
 C Skin, Left Upper Arm
 D Skin, Right Lower Arm
	E Skin, Left Lower Arm
	 F Skin, Right Hand
	 G Skin, Left Hand
	 H Skin, Right Upper Leg
	 J Skin, Left Upper Leg
	 K Skin, Right Lower Leg
	 L Skin, Left Lower Leg
	 M Skin, Right Foot
	 N Skin, Left Foot
	 Q Finger Nail
	    Nail bed
	    Nail plate
	 R Toe Nail
	    See Q Finger Nail
		X External	Z No Device	X Diagnostic
				 Z No Qualifier

T Breast, Right
    Mammary duct
    Mammary gland
 U Breast, Left
    See T Breast, Right
 V Breast, Bilateral
    See T Breast, Right
		Ø Open
		 3 Percutaneous
		 7 Via Natural or Artificial
		    Opening
		 8 Via Natural or Artificial
		    Opening Endoscopic
			Ø Drainage Device	Z No Qualifier

T Breast, Right
    Mammary duct
    Mammary gland
 U Breast, Left
    See T Breast, Right
 V Breast, Bilateral
    See T Breast, Right
		Ø Open
		 3 Percutaneous
		 7 Via Natural or Artificial
		    Opening
		 8 Via Natural or Artificial
		    Opening Endoscopic
			Z No Device	X Diagnostic
				 Z No Qualifier

W Nipple, Right
    Areola
 X Nipple, Left
    See W Nipple, Right
		Ø Open
		 3 Percutaneous
		 7 Via Natural or Artificial
		    Opening
		 8 Via Natural or Artificial
		    Opening Endoscopic
		 X External
			Ø Drainage Device	Z No Qualifier

W Nipple, Right
    Areola
 X Nipple, Left
    See W Nipple, Right
		Ø Open
		 3 Percutaneous
		 7 Via Natural or Artificial
		    Opening
		 8 Via Natural or Artificial
		    Opening Endoscopic
		 X External
			Z No Device	X Diagnostic
				 Z No Qualifier

Non-OR   ØH9[Ø,1,2,3,4,5,6,7,8,A,B,C,D,E,F,G,H,J,K,L,M,N,Q,R]XØZ
Non-OR   ØH9[Ø,1,2,3,4,5,6,7,8,A,B,C,D,E,F,G,H,J,K,L,M,N,Q,R]XZ[X,Z]
Non-OR   ØH99XZX
Non-OR   ØH9[T,U,V][Ø,3,7,8]ØZ
Non-OR   ØH9[T,U,V][3,7,8]Z[X,Z]
Non-OR   ØH9[W,X][Ø,3,7,8,X]ØZ
Non-OR   ØH9[W,X][3,7,8,X]Z[X,Z]

 NC Noncovered Procedure   LC Limited Coverage   QA Questionable OB Admit   NT New Tech Add-on   ⊞ Combination Member   ♂ Male   ♀ Female

ICD-10-PCS 2023   431

ØH9–ØH9

Skin and Breast

Ø   Medical and Surgical
H   Skin and Breast
B   Excision   Definition: Cutting out or off, without replacement, a portion of a body part
                     Explanation: The qualifier DIAGNOSTIC is used to identify excision procedures that are biopsies

Body Part Character 4	Approach Character 5	Device Character 6	Qualifier Character 7
Ø Skin, Scalp	X External	Z No Device	X Diagnostic
1 Skin, Face			Z No Qualifier
2 Skin, Right Ear			
3 Skin, Left Ear			
4 Skin, Neck			
5 Skin, Chest			
Breast procedures, skin only			
6 Skin, Back			
7 Skin, Abdomen			
8 Skin, Buttock			
9 Skin, Perineum			
Perianal skin			
A Skin, Inguinal			
B Skin, Right Upper Arm			
C Skin, Left Upper Arm			
D Skin, Right Lower Arm			
E Skin, Left Lower Arm			
F Skin, Right Hand			
G Skin, Left Hand			
H Skin, Right Upper Leg			
J Skin, Left Upper Leg			
K Skin, Right Lower Leg			
L Skin, Left Lower Leg			
M Skin, Right Foot			
N Skin, Left Foot			
Q Finger Nail			
Nail bed			
Nail plate			
R Toe Nail			
See Q Finger Nail			
T Breast, Right	Ø Open	Z No Device	X Diagnostic
Mammary duct	3 Percutaneous		Z No Qualifier
Mammary gland	7 Via Natural or Artificial Opening		
U Breast, Left	8 Via Natural or Artificial Opening		
See T Breast, Right	Endoscopic		
V Breast, Bilateral			
See T Breast, Right			
Y Supernumerary Breast			
W Nipple, Right	Ø Open	Z No Device	X Diagnostic
Areola	3 Percutaneous		Z No Qualifier
X Nipple, Left	7 Via Natural or Artificial Opening		
See W Nipple, Right	8 Via Natural or Artificial Opening		
	Endoscopic		
	X External		

DRG Non-OR	ØHB9XZZ
Non-OR	ØHB[Ø,1,2,3,4,5,6,7,8,A,B,C,D,E,F,G,H,J,K,L,M,N,Q,R]XZ[X,Z]
Non-OR	ØHB9XZX
Non-OR	ØHB[T,U,V,Y][3,7,8]ZX
Non-OR	ØHB[W,X][3,7,8,X]ZX

Non-OR Procedure   DRG Non-OR Procedure   Valid OR Procedure   HAC Associated Procedure   Combination Only   New/Revised April   New/Revised October

432

ICD-10-PCS 2023

Skin and Breast

Ø   Medical and Surgical
H   Skin and Breast
C   Extirpation   Definition: Taking or cutting out solid matter from a body part

Explanation: The solid matter may be an abnormal byproduct of a biological function or a foreign body; it may be imbedded in a body part or in the lumen of a tubular body part. The solid matter may or may not have been previously broken into pieces.

Body Part Character 4	Approach Character 5	Device Character 6	Qualifier Character 7

Ø Skin, Scalp
1 Skin, Face
2 Skin, Right Ear
3 Skin, Left Ear
4 Skin, Neck
5 Skin, Chest
    Breast procedures, skin only
6 Skin, Back
7 Skin, Abdomen
8 Skin, Buttock
9 Skin, Perineum
    Perianal skin
A Skin, Inguinal
B Skin, Right Upper Arm
C Skin, Left Upper Arm
D Skin, Right Lower Arm
E Skin, Left Lower Arm
F Skin, Right Hand
G Skin, Left Hand
H Skin, Right Upper Leg
J Skin, Left Upper Leg
K Skin, Right Lower Leg
L Skin, Left Lower Leg
M Skin, Right Foot
N Skin, Left Foot
Q Finger Nail
    Nail bed
    Nail plate
R Toe Nail
    See Q Finger Nail
	X External	**Z** No Device	**Z** No Qualifier

T Breast, Right
    Mammary duct
    Mammary gland
U Breast, Left
    See T Breast, Right
V Breast, Bilateral
    See T Breast, Right
	Ø Open
	3 Percutaneous
	7 Via Natural or Artificial Opening
	8 Via Natural or Artificial Opening
	    Endoscopic
		Z No Device	**Z** No Qualifier

W Nipple, Right
    Areola
X Nipple, Left
    See W Nipple, Right
	Ø Open
	3 Percutaneous
	7 Via Natural or Artificial Opening
	8 Via Natural or Artificial Opening
	    Endoscopic
	X External
		Z No Device	**Z** No Qualifier

Non-OR   ØHC[Ø,1,2,3,4,5,6,7,8,9,A,B,C,D,E,F,G,H,J,K,L,M,N,Q,R]XZZ
Non-OR   ØHC[T,U,V][3,7,8]ZZ
Non-OR   ØHC[W,X][3,7,8,X]ZZ

NC Noncovered Procedure   **LC** Limited Coverage   **QA** Questionable OB Admit   **NT** New Tech Add-on   ⊞ Combination Member   ♂ Male   ♀ Female

ICD-10-PCS 2023   **433**

Ø   **Medical and Surgical**
H   **Skin and Breast**
D   **Extraction**   Definition: Pulling or stripping out or off all or a portion of a body part by the use of force
                        Explanation: The qualifier DIAGNOSTIC is used to identify extraction procedures that are biopsies

Body Part Character 4	Approach Character 5	Device Character 6	Qualifier Character 7
Ø Skin, Scalp	X External	Z No Device	Z No Qualifier
1 Skin, Face			
2 Skin, Right Ear			
3 Skin, Left Ear			
4 Skin, Neck			
5 Skin, Chest Breast procedures, skin only			
6 Skin, Back			
7 Skin, Abdomen			
8 Skin, Buttock			
9 Skin, Perineum Perianal skin			
A Skin, Inguinal			
B Skin, Right Upper Arm			
C Skin, Left Upper Arm			
D Skin, Right Lower Arm			
E Skin, Left Lower Arm			
F Skin, Right Hand			
G Skin, Left Hand			
H Skin, Right Upper Leg			
J Skin, Left Upper Leg			
K Skin, Right Lower Leg			
L Skin, Left Lower Leg			
M Skin, Right Foot			
N Skin, Left Foot			

Q Finger Nail
  Nail bed
  Nail plate			

R Toe Nail *See Q Finger Nail*			
S Hair			

T Breast, Right
  Mammary duct
  Mammary gland
	Ø Open	Z No Device	Z No Qualifier

U Breast, Left *See T Breast, Right*			
V Breast, Bilateral *See T Breast, Right*			
Y Supernumerary Breast			

Non-OR   All body part, approach, device, and qualifier values

Ø   Medical and Surgical
H   Skin and Breast
H   Insertion   Definition: Putting in a nonbiological appliance that monitors, assists, performs, or prevents a physiological function but does not physically take the place of a body part

Explanation: None

Body Part Character 4	Approach Character 5	Device Character 6	Qualifier Character 7
P Skin	**X** External	**Y** Other Device	**Z** No Qualifier
T Breast, Right Mammary duct Mammary gland **U** Breast, Left *See T Breast, Right*	**Ø** Open **3** Percutaneous **7** Via Natural or Artificial Opening **8** Via Natural or Artificial Opening Endoscopic	**1** Radioactive Element **N** Tissue Expander **Y** Other Device	**Z** No Qualifier
V Breast, Bilateral Mammary duct Mammary gland	**Ø** Open **3** Percutaneous **7** Via Natural or Artificial Opening **8** Via Natural or Artificial Opening Endoscopic	**1** Radioactive Element **N** Tissue Expander	**Z** No Qualifier
W Nipple, Right Areola **X** Nipple, Left *See W Nipple, Right*	**Ø** Open **3** Percutaneous **7** Via Natural or Artificial Opening **8** Via Natural or Artificial Opening Endoscopic	**1** Radioactive Element **N** Tissue Expander	**Z** No Qualifier
W Nipple, Right Areola **X** Nipple, Left *See W Nipple, Right*	**X** External	**1** Radioactive Element	**Z** No Qualifier

Non-OR   ØHHPXYZ
Non-OR   ØHH[T,U][3,7,8]YZ

Ø   Medical and Surgical
H   Skin and Breast
J   Inspection   Definition: Visually and/or manually exploring a body part

Explanation: Visual exploration may be performed with or without optical instrumentation. Manual exploration may be performed directly or through intervening body layers.

Body Part Character 4	Approach Character 5	Device Character 6	Qualifier Character 7
P Skin Dermis Epidermis Sebaceous gland Sweat gland **Q** Finger Nail Nail bed Nail plate **R** Toe Nail *See Q Finger Nail*	**X** External	**Z** No Device	**Z** No Qualifier
T Breast, Right Mammary duct Mammary gland **U** Breast, Left *See T Breast, Right*	**Ø** Open **3** Percutaneous **7** Via Natural or Artificial Opening **8** Via Natural or Artificial Opening Endoscopic	**Z** No Device	**Z** No Qualifier

Non-OR   All body part, approach, device and qualifier values

NC Noncovered Procedure   **LC** Limited Coverage   **QA** Questionable OB Admit   **NT** New Tech Add-on   ⊞ Combination Member   ♂ Male   ♀ Female

ICD-10-PCS 2023   **435**

ØHH–ØHJ

Ø   **Medical and Surgical**
H   **Skin and Breast**
M   **Reattachment**   Definition: Putting back in or on all or a portion of a separated body part to its normal location or other suitable location
                          Explanation: Vascular circulation and nervous pathways may or may not be reestablished

Body Part Character 4	Approach Character 5	Device Character 6	Qualifier Character 7
Ø Skin, Scalp	**X** External	**Z** No Device	**Z** No Qualifier
1 Skin, Face			
2 Skin, Right Ear			
3 Skin, Left Ear			
4 Skin, Neck			
5 Skin, Chest Breast procedures, skin only			
6 Skin, Back			
7 Skin, Abdomen			
8 Skin, Buttock			
9 Skin, Perineum Perianal skin			
A Skin, Inguinal			
B Skin, Right Upper Arm			
C Skin, Left Upper Arm			
D Skin, Right Lower Arm			
E Skin, Left Lower Arm			
F Skin, Right Hand			
G Skin, Left Hand			
H Skin, Right Upper Leg			
J Skin, Left Upper Leg			
K Skin, Right Lower Leg			
L Skin, Left Lower Leg			
M Skin, Right Foot			
N Skin, Left Foot			

T Breast, Right
   Mammary duct
   Mammary gland			

U Breast, Left *See T Breast, Right*			
V Breast, Bilateral *See T Breast, Right*			
W Nipple, Right Areola			
X Nipple, Left *See W Nipple, Right*			

Non-OR   ØHMØXZZ

Ø   **Medical and Surgical**
H   **Skin and Breast**
N   **Release**   Definition: Freeing a body part from an abnormal physical constraint by cutting or by the use of force
                              Explanation: Some of the restraining tissue may be taken out but none of the body part is taken out

Body Part Character 4	Approach Character 5	Device Character 6	Qualifier Character 7
Ø **Skin, Scalp**	**X** External	**Z** No Device	**Z** No Qualifier
1 **Skin, Face**			
2 **Skin, Right Ear**			
3 **Skin, Left Ear**			
4 **Skin, Neck**			
5 **Skin, Chest**			
Breast procedures, skin only			
6 **Skin, Back**			
7 **Skin, Abdomen**			
8 **Skin, Buttock**			
9 **Skin, Perineum**			
Perianal skin			
A **Skin, Inguinal**			
B **Skin, Right Upper Arm**			
C **Skin, Left Upper Arm**			
D **Skin, Right Lower Arm**			
E **Skin, Left Lower Arm**			
F **Skin, Right Hand**			
G **Skin, Left Hand**			
H **Skin, Right Upper Leg**			
J **Skin, Left Upper Leg**			
K **Skin, Right Lower Leg**			
L **Skin, Left Lower Leg**			
M **Skin, Right Foot**			
N **Skin, Left Foot**			
Q **Finger Nail**			
Nail bed			
Nail plate			
R **Toe Nail**			
See Q Finger Nail			
T **Breast, Right**	**Ø** Open	**Z** No Device	**Z** No Qualifier
Mammary duct	**3** Percutaneous		
Mammary gland	**7** Via Natural or Artificial Opening		
U **Breast, Left**	**8** Via Natural or Artificial Opening Endoscopic		
See T Breast, Right			
V **Breast, Bilateral**			
See T Breast, Right			
W **Nipple, Right**	**Ø** Open	**Z** No Device	**Z** No Qualifier
Areola	**3** Percutaneous		
X **Nipple, Left**	**7** Via Natural or Artificial Opening		
See W Nipple, Right	**8** Via Natural or Artificial Opening Endoscopic		
	X External		

Ø Medical and Surgical
H Skin and Breast
P Removal

Definition: Taking out or off a device from a body part

Explanation: If a device is taken out and a similar device put in without cutting or puncturing the skin or mucous membrane, the procedure is coded to the root operation CHANGE. Otherwise, the procedure for taking out a device is coded to the root operation REMOVAL.

Body Part Character 4	Approach Character 5	Device Character 6	Qualifier Character 7

P Skin
    Dermis
    Epidermis
    Sebaceous gland
    Sweat gland
	X External	**Ø** Drainage Device
		7 Autologous Tissue Substitute
		J Synthetic Substitute
		K Nonautologous Tissue Substitute
		Y Other Device
			Z No Qualifier

Q Finger Nail
    Nail bed
    Nail plate
R Toe Nail
    See Q Finger Nail
	X External	**Ø** Drainage Device
		7 Autologous Tissue Substitute
		J Synthetic Substitute
		K Nonautologous Tissue Substitute
			Z No Qualifier

S Hair	**X** External	**7** Autologous Tissue Substitute **J** Synthetic Substitute **K** Nonautologous Tissue Substitute	**Z** No Qualifier

T Breast, Right
    Mammary duct
    Mammary gland
U Breast, Left
    See T Breast, Right
	Ø Open
	3 Percutaneous
	7 Via Natural or Artificial Opening
	8 Via Natural or Artificial Opening Endoscopic
		Ø Drainage Device
		1 Radioactive Element
		7 Autologous Tissue Substitute
		J Synthetic Substitute
		K Nonautologous Tissue Substitute
		N Tissue Expander
		Y Other Device
			Z No Qualifier

Non-OR   ØHPPX[Ø,7,J,K,Y]Z
Non-OR   ØHP[Q,R]X[Ø,7,J,K]Z
Non-OR   ØHPSX[7,J,K]Z
Non-OR   ØHP[T,U]Ø[Ø,1,7,K]Z
Non-OR   ØHP[T,U]3[Ø,1,7,K,Y]Z
Non-OR   ØHP[T,U][7,8][Ø,1,7,J,K,N,Y]Z

Ø　Medical and Surgical
H　Skin and Breast
Q　Repair　　　Definition: Restoring, to the extent possible, a body part to its normal anatomic structure and function

Explanation: Used only when the method to accomplish the repair is not one of the other root operations

Body Part Character 4	Approach Character 5	Device Character 6	Qualifier Character 7

Ø Skin, Scalp
1 Skin, Face
2 Skin, Right Ear
3 Skin, Left Ear
4 Skin, Neck
5 Skin, Chest
   Breast procedures, skin only
6 Skin, Back
7 Skin, Abdomen
8 Skin, Buttock
9 Skin, Perineum
   Perianal skin
A Skin, Inguinal
B Skin, Right Upper Arm
C Skin, Left Upper Arm
D Skin, Right Lower Arm
E Skin, Left Lower Arm
F Skin, Right Hand
G Skin, Left Hand
H Skin, Right Upper Leg
J Skin, Left Upper Leg
K Skin, Right Lower Leg
L Skin, Left Lower Leg
M Skin, Right Foot
N Skin, Left Foot
Q Finger Nail
   Nail bed
   Nail plate
R Toe Nail
   See Q Finger Nail
	X External	**Z** No Device	**Z** No Qualifier

T Breast, Right
   Mammary duct
   Mammary gland
U Breast, Left
   See T Breast, Right
V Breast, Bilateral
   See T Breast, Right
Y Supernumerary Breast
	Ø Open
	3 Percutaneous
	7 Via Natural or Artificial Opening
	8 Via Natural or Artificial Opening
	   Endoscopic
		Z No Device	**Z** No Qualifier

W Nipple, Right
   Areola
X Nipple, Left
   See W Nipple, Right
	Ø Open
	3 Percutaneous
	7 Via Natural or Artificial Opening
	8 Via Natural or Artificial Opening
	   Endoscopic
	X External
		Z No Device	**Z** No Qualifier

DRG Non-OR　ØHQ9XZZ
Non-OR　　　ØHQ[Ø,1,2,3,4,5,6,7,8,A,B,C,D,E,F,G,H,J,K,L,M,N]XZZ

NC Noncovered Procedure　　**LC** Limited Coverage　　**QA** Questionable OB Admit　　**NT** New Tech Add-on　　✠ Combination Member　　♂ Male　　♀ Female

ICD-10-PCS 2023　　　　　　　　　　　　　　　　　　　　　　　　　　　　　　　　　　　　　　**439**

ØHQ–ØHQ

Skin and Breast

ØHR–ØHR

Ø Medical and Surgical
H Skin and Breast
R Replacement

Definition: Putting in or on biological or synthetic material that physically takes the place and/or function of all or a portion of a body part

Explanation: The body part may have been taken out or replaced, or may be taken out, physically eradicated, or rendered nonfunctional during the REPLACEMENT procedure. A REMOVAL procedure is coded for taking out the device used in a previous replacement procedure.

Body Part Character 4		Approach Character 5	Device Character 6	Qualifier Character 7

Ø Skin, Scalp
1 Skin, Face
2 Skin, Right Ear
3 Skin, Left Ear
4 Skin, Neck
5 Skin, Chest
   Breast procedures, skin only
6 Skin, Back
7 Skin, Abdomen
8 Skin, Buttock
9 Skin, Perineum
   Perianal skin
A Skin, Inguinal
	B Skin, Right Upper Arm
	C Skin, Left Upper Arm
	D Skin, Right Lower Arm
	E Skin, Left Lower Arm
	F Skin, Right Hand
	G Skin, Left Hand
	H Skin, Right Upper Leg
	J Skin, Left Upper Leg
	K Skin, Right Lower Leg
	L Skin, Left Lower Leg
	M Skin, Right Foot
	N Skin, Left Foot
		X External	7 Autologous Tissue Substitute	2 Cell Suspension Technique
				3 Full Thickness
				4 Partial Thickness

Ø Skin, Scalp
1 Skin, Face
2 Skin, Right Ear
3 Skin, Left Ear
4 Skin, Neck
5 Skin, Chest
   Breast procedures, skin only
6 Skin, Back
7 Skin, Abdomen
8 Skin, Buttock
9 Skin, Perineum
   Perianal skin
A Skin, Inguinal
	B Skin, Right Upper Arm
	C Skin, Left Upper Arm
	D Skin, Right Lower Arm
	E Skin, Left Lower Arm
	F Skin, Right Hand
	G Skin, Left Hand
	H Skin, Right Upper Leg
	J Skin, Left Upper Leg
	K Skin, Right Lower Leg
	L Skin, Left Lower Leg
	M Skin, Right Foot
	N Skin, Left Foot
		X External	J Synthetic Substitute	3 Full Thickness
				4 Partial Thickness
				Z No Qualifier

Ø Skin, Scalp
1 Skin, Face
2 Skin, Right Ear
3 Skin, Left Ear
4 Skin, Neck
5 Skin, Chest
   Breast procedures, skin only
6 Skin, Back
7 Skin, Abdomen
8 Skin Buttock
9 Skin, Perineum
   Perianal skin
A Skin, Inguinal
	B Skin, Right Upper Arm
	C Skin, Left Upper Arm
	D Skin, Right Lower Arm
	E Skin, Left Lower Arm
	F Skin, Right Hand
	G Skin, Left Hand
	H Skin, Right Upper Leg
	J Skin, Left Upper Leg
	K Skin, Right Lower Leg
	L Skin, Left Lower Leg
	M Skin, Right Foot
	N Skin, Left Foot
		X External	K Nonautologous Tissue Substitute	3 Full Thickness
				4 Partial Thickness

Q Finger Nail
   Nail bed
   Nail plate
	R Toe Nail
	   See Q Finger Nail
	S Hair
		X External	7 Autologous Tissue Substitute
			J Synthetic Substitute
			K Nonautologous Tissue Substitute
				Z No Qualifier

T Breast, Right
   Mammary duct
   Mammary gland
	U Breast, Left
	   See T Breast, Right
	V Breast, Bilateral
	   See T Breast, Right
		Ø Open	7 Autologous Tissue Substitute	5 Latissimus Dorsi Myocutaneous Flap
				6 Transverse Rectus Abdominis Myocutaneous Flap
				7 Deep Inferior Epigastric Artery Perforator Flap
				8 Superficial Inferior Epigastric Artery Flap
				9 Gluteal Artery Perforator Flap
				Z No Qualifier

T Breast, Right
   Mammary duct
   Mammary gland
	U Breast, Left
	   See T Breast, Right
	V Breast, Bilateral
	   See T Breast, Right
		Ø Open	J Synthetic Substitute
			K Nonautologous Tissue Substitute
				Z No Qualifier

T Breast, Right ⊞
   Mammary duct
   Mammary gland
U Breast, Left ⊞
   See T Breast, Right
	V Breast, Bilateral ⊞
	   See T Breast, Right
		3 Percutaneous	7 Autologous Tissue Substitute
			J Synthetic Substitute
			K Nonautologous Tissue Substitute
				Z No Qualifier

W Nipple, Right
   Areola
	X Nipple, Left
	   See W Nipple, Right
		Ø Open
		3 Percutaneous
		X External
			7 Autologous Tissue Substitute
			J Synthetic Substitute
			K Nonautologous Tissue Substitute
				Z No Qualifier

Non-OR   ØHRSX7Z

See Appendix L for Procedure Combinations
   ⊞   ØHR[T,U,V]37Z

Non-OR Procedure   DRG Non-OR Procedure   Valid OR Procedure   HAC Associated Procedure   Combination Only   New/Revised April   New/Revised October

Ø   Medical and Surgical
H   Skin and Breast
S   Reposition   Definition: Moving to its normal location, or other suitable location, all or a portion of a body part

       Explanation: The body part is moved to a new location from an abnormal location, or from a normal location where it is not functioning correctly. The body part may or may not be cut out or off to be moved to the new location.

Body Part Character 4	Approach Character 5	Device Character 6	Qualifier Character 7

S Hair
W Nipple, Right
   Areola
X Nipple, Left
   See W Nipple, Right
	X External	**Z** No Device	**Z** No Qualifier

T Breast, Right
   Mammary duct
   Mammary gland
U Breast, Left
   See T Breast, Right
V Breast, Bilateral
   See T Breast, Right
	Ø Open	**Z** No Device	**Z** No Qualifier

    Non-OR   ØHSSXZZ

Ø   Medical and Surgical
H   Skin and Breast
T   Resection   Definition: Cutting out or off, without replacement, all of a body part

       Explanation: None

Body Part Character 4	Approach Character 5	Device Character 6	Qualifier Character 7

Q Finger Nail
   Nail bed
   Nail plate
R Toe Nail
   See Q Finger Nail
W Nipple, Right
   Areola
X Nipple, Left
   See W Nipple, Right
	X External	**Z** No Device	**Z** No Qualifier

T Breast, Right ⊞
   Mammary duct
   Mammary gland
U Breast, Left ⊞
   See T Breast, Right
V Breast, Bilateral ⊞
   See T Breast, Right
Y Supernumerary Breast
	Ø Open	**Z** No Device	**Z** No Qualifier

    Non-OR   ØHT[Q,R]XZZ   **See Appendix L for Procedure Combinations**
                                   ⊞   ØHT[T,U,V]ØZZ

Ø   Medical and Surgical
H   Skin and Breast
U   Supplement   Definition: Putting in or on biological or synthetic material that physically reinforces and/or augments the function of a portion of a body part

       Explanation: The biological material is non-living, or is living and from the same individual. The body part may have been previously replaced, and the SUPPLEMENT procedure is performed to physically reinforce and/or augment the function of the replaced body part.

Body Part Character 4	Approach Character 5	Device Character 6	Qualifier Character 7

T Breast, Right
   Mammary duct
   Mammary gland
U Breast, Left
   See T Breast, Right
V Breast, Bilateral
   See T Breast, Right
	Ø Open
	3 Percutaneous
	7 Via Natural or Artificial Opening
	8 Via Natural or Artificial Opening
	   Endoscopic
		7 Autologous Tissue Substitute
		J Synthetic Substitute
		K Nonautologous Tissue Substitute
			Z No Qualifier

W Nipple, Right
   Areola
X Nipple, Left
   See W Nipple, Right
	Ø Open
	3 Percutaneous
	7 Via Natural or Artificial Opening
	8 Via Natural or Artificial Opening
	   Endoscopic
	X External
		7 Autologous Tissue Substitute
		J Synthetic Substitute
		K Nonautologous Tissue Substitute
			Z No Qualifier

    Non-OR   ØHU[T,U,V]3JZ

Skin and Breast *(left margin)*

Ø   **Medical and Surgical**
H   **Skin and Breast**
W   **Revision**   Definition: Correcting, to the extent possible, a portion of a malfunctioning device or the position of a displaced device

                 Explanation: Revision can include correcting a malfunctioning or displaced device by taking out or putting in components of the device such as a screw or pin

Body Part Character 4	Approach Character 5	Device Character 6	Qualifier Character 7

P   Skin
    Dermis
    Epidermis
    Sebaceous gland
    Sweat gland
	X External	Ø Drainage Device
		7 Autologous Tissue Substitute
		J Synthetic Substitute
		K Nonautologous Tissue Substitute
		Y Other Device
			Z No Qualifier

Q   Finger Nail
    Nail bed
    Nail plate
R   Toe Nail
    See Q Finger Nail
	X External	Ø Drainage Device
		7 Autologous Tissue Substitute
		J Synthetic Substitute
		K Nonautologous Tissue Substitute
			Z No Qualifier

S Hair	X External	7 Autologous Tissue Substitute J Synthetic Substitute K Nonautologous Tissue Substitute	Z No Qualifier

T   Breast, Right
    Mammary duct
    Mammary gland
U   Breast, Left
    See T Breast, Right
	Ø Open
	3 Percutaneous
	7 Via Natural or Artificial Opening
	8 Via Natural or Artificial Opening
	      Endoscopic
		Ø Drainage Device
		7 Autologous Tissue Substitute
		J Synthetic Substitute
		K Nonautologous Tissue Substitute
		N Tissue Expander
		Y Other Device
			Z No Qualifier

Non-OR   ØHWPX[Ø,7,J,K,Y]Z
Non-OR   ØHW[Q,R]X[Ø,7,J,K]Z
Non-OR   ØHWSX[7,J,K]Z
Non-OR   ØHW[T,U]Ø[Ø,7,K,N]Z
Non-OR   ØHW[T,U]3[Ø,7,K,N,Y]Z
Non-OR   ØHW[T,U][7,8][Ø,7,J,K,N,Y]Z

Ø   **Medical and Surgical**
H   **Skin and Breast**
X   **Transfer**   Definition: Moving, without taking out, all or a portion of a body part to another location to take over the function of all or a portion of a body part

                 Explanation: The body part transferred remains connected to its vascular and nervous supply

Body Part Character 4	Approach Character 5	Device Character 6	Qualifier Character 7

Ø   Skin, Scalp
1   Skin, Face
2   Skin, Right Ear
3   Skin, Left Ear
4   Skin, Neck
5   Skin, Chest
    Breast procedures, skin only
6   Skin, Back
7   Skin, Abdomen
8   Skin, Buttock
9   Skin, Perineum
    Perianal skin
A   Skin, Inguinal
B   Skin, Right Upper Arm
C   Skin, Left Upper Arm
D   Skin, Right Lower Arm
E   Skin, Left Lower Arm
F   Skin, Right Hand
G   Skin, Left Hand
H   Skin, Right Upper Leg
J   Skin, Left Upper Leg
K   Skin, Right Lower Leg
L   Skin, Left Lower Leg
M   Skin, Right Foot
N   Skin, Left Foot
	X External	Z No Device	Z No Qualifier

ØHW–ØHX *(left margin)*

Non-OR Procedure   DRG Non-OR Procedure   Valid OR Procedure   HAC Associated Procedure   Combination Only   New/Revised April   New/Revised October

442   ICD-10-PCS 2023

Subcutaneous Tissue and Fascia ØJØ–ØJX

Character Meanings

This Character Meaning table is provided as a guide to assist the user in the identification of character members that may be found in this section of code tables. It **SHOULD NOT** be used to build a PCS code.

Operation–Character 3	Body Part–Character 4	Approach–Character 5	Device–Character 6	Qualifier–Character 7
Ø Alteration	Ø Subcutaneous Tissue and Fascia, Scalp	Ø Open	Ø Drainage Device OR Monitoring Device, Hemodynamic	B Skin and Subcutaneous Tissue
2 Change	1 Subcutaneous Tissue and Fascia, Face	3 Percutaneous	1 Radioactive Element	C Skin, Subcutaneous Tissue and Fascia
5 Destruction	4 Subcutaneous Tissue and Fascia, Right Neck	X External	2 Monitoring Device	X Diagnostic
8 Division	5 Subcutaneous Tissue and Fascia, Left Neck		3 Infusion Device	Z No Qualifier
9 Drainage	6 Subcutaneous Tissue and Fascia, Chest		4 Pacemaker, Single Chamber	
B Excision	7 Subcutaneous Tissue and Fascia, Back		5 Pacemaker, Single Chamber Rate Responsive	
C Extirpation	8 Subcutaneous Tissue and Fascia, Abdomen		6 Pacemaker, Dual Chamber	
D Extraction	9 Subcutaneous Tissue and Fascia, Buttock		7 Autologous Tissue Substitute OR Cardiac Resynchronization Pacemaker Pulse Generator	
H Insertion	B Subcutaneous Tissue and Fascia, Perineum		8 Defibrillator Generator	
J Inspection	C Subcutaneous Tissue and Fascia, Pelvic Region		9 Cardiac Resynchronization Defibrillator Pulse Generator	
N Release	D Subcutaneous Tissue and Fascia, Right Upper Arm		A Contractility Modulation Device	
P Removal	F Subcutaneous Tissue and Fascia, Left Upper Arm		B Stimulator Generator, Single Array	
Q Repair	G Subcutaneous Tissue and Fascia, Right Lower Arm		C Stimulator Generator, Single Array Rechargeable	
R Replacement	H Subcutaneous Tissue and Fascia, Left Lower Arm		D Stimulator Generator, Multiple Array	
U Supplement	J Subcutaneous Tissue and Fascia, Right Hand		E Stimulator Generator, Multiple Array Rechargeable	
W Revision	K Subcutaneous Tissue and Fascia, Left Hand		F Subcutaneous Defibrillator Lead	
X Transfer	L Subcutaneous Tissue and Fascia, Right Upper Leg		H Contraceptive Device	
	M Subcutaneous Tissue and Fascia, Left Upper Leg		J Synthetic Substitute	
	N Subcutaneous Tissue and Fascia, Right Lower Leg		K Nonautologous Tissue Substitute	
	P Subcutaneous Tissue and Fascia, Left Lower Leg		M Stimulator Generator	
	Q Subcutaneous Tissue and Fascia, Right Foot		N Tissue Expander	
	R Subcutaneous Tissue and Fascia, Left Foot		P Cardiac Rhythm Related Device	
	S Subcutaneous Tissue and Fascia, Head and Neck		V Infusion Device, Pump	
	T Subcutaneous Tissue and Fascia, Trunk		W Vascular Access Device, Totally Implantable	
	V Subcutaneous Tissue and Fascia, Upper Extremity		X Vascular Access Device, Tunneled	
	W Subcutaneous Tissue and Fascia, Lower Extremity		Y Other Device	
			Z No Device	

AHA Coding Clinic for table ØJ2

2018, 3Q, 10	Disruption of perma-catheter fibrin sheath via angioplasty of superior vena cava
2017, 2Q, 26	Exchange of tunneled catheter

AHA Coding Clinic for table ØJ5

2019, 3Q, 25	Endoscopic removal of pilonidal sinus and cyst

AHA Coding Clinic for table ØJ8

2017, 3Q, 11	Bilateral escharotomy of leg, thigh and foot

AHA Coding Clinic for table ØJ9

2018, 3Q, 16	Incision and drainage of submandibular space
2018, 3Q, 16	Incision and drainage of neck abscess
2015, 3Q, 23	Incision and drainage of multiple abscess cavities using vessel loop

AHA Coding Clinic for table ØJB

2020, 1Q, 31	Repair of buried penis
2019, 3Q, 25	Endoscopic removal of pilonidal sinus and cyst
2018, 3Q, 17	Excisional debridement of periosteum
2018, 1Q, 7	Placement of fat graft following lumbar decompression surgery
2015, 3Q, 3-8	Excisional and nonexcisional debridement
2015, 2Q, 13	Transfer of free flap to reconstruct orbital defect
2015, 1Q, 29	Fistulectomy with placement of seton
2014, 4Q, 38	Abdominoplasty and abdominal wall plication for hernia repair
2014, 3Q, 22	Transsphenoidal removal of pituitary tumor and fat graft placement

AHA Coding Clinic for table ØJC

2017, 3Q, 22	Replacement of native skull bone flap

AHA Coding Clinic for table ØJD

2016, 3Q, 20	VersaJet™ nonexcisional debridement of leg muscle
2016, 3Q, 21	Nonexcisional debridement of infected lumbar wound
2016, 3Q, 21	Nonexcisional pulsed lavage debridement
2016, 3Q, 22	Debridement of bone and tendon using Tenex ultrasound device
2016, 1Q, 40	Nonexcisional debridement of skin and subcutaneous tissue
2015, 3Q, 3-8	Excisional and nonexcisional debridement
2015, 1Q, 23	Non-Excisional debridement with lavage of wound

AHA Coding Clinic for table ØJH

2020, 4Q, 54	Insertion of other device into subcutaneous tissue and fascia
2020, 4Q, 55	Insertion of subcutaneous pump system for ascites drainage
2020, 2Q, 15	Ommaya reservoir with ventricular catheter placement
2020, 2Q, 16	Ommaya reservoir placement for cerebrospinal fluid infusion therapy
2019, 4Q, 33	Subcutaneous implantable cardioverter defibrillator lead
2017, 4Q, 63-64	Added and revised device values - Vascular access reservoir
2017, 2Q, 24	Tunneled catheter versus totally implantable catheter
2017, 2Q, 26	Exchange of tunneled catheter
2016, 4Q, 97-98	Phrenic neurostimulator
2016, 2Q, 14	Insertion of peritoneal totally implantable venous access device
2016, 2Q, 15	Removal and replacement of tunneled internal jugular catheter
2015, 4Q, 14	New Section X codes—New Technology procedures
2015, 4Q, 30-31	Vascular access devices
2015, 2Q, 33	Totally implantable central venous access device (Port-a-Cath)
2014, 3Q, 19	End of life replacement of Baclofen pump
2013, 4Q, 116	Device character for Port-A-Cath placement
2012, 4Q, 104	Placement of subcutaneous implantable cardioverter defibrillator

AHA Coding Clinic for table ØJN

2017, 3Q, 11	Bilateral escharotomy of leg, thigh and foot

AHA Coding Clinic for table ØJP

2019, 4Q, 33	Subcutaneous implantable cardioverter defibrillator lead
2018, 4Q, 86	Placement of lumboatrial shunt
2018, 3Q, 29	Decommissioning of left ventricular assist device with exploration of mediastinum
2016, 2Q, 15	Removal and replacement of tunneled internal jugular catheter
2015, 4Q, 31	Vascular access devices
2014, 3Q, 19	End of life replacement of Baclofen pump
2013, 4Q, 109	Separating conjoined twins
2012, 4Q, 104	Placement of subcutaneous implantable cardioverter defibrillator

AHA Coding Clinic for table ØJQ

2017, 3Q, 19	Anterior repair of cystocele
2014, 4Q, 44	Posterior colporrhaphy/rectocele repair

AHA Coding Clinic for table ØJR

2015, 2Q, 13	Transfer of free flap to reconstruct orbital defect

AHA Coding Clinic for table ØJU

2018, 2Q, 20	Prelaminated free flap graft using Alloderm™
2018, 1Q, 7	Placement of fat graft following lumbar decompression surgery

AHA Coding Clinic for table ØJW

2019, 4Q, 33	Subcutaneous implantable cardioverter defibrillator lead
2018, 1Q, 8	Ventricular peritoneal shunt ligation
2015, 4Q, 33	Externalization of peritoneal dialysis catheter
2015, 2Q, 9	Revision of ventriculoperitoneal (VP) shunt
2012, 4Q, 104	Placement of subcutaneous implantable cardioverter defibrillator

AHA Coding Clinic for table ØJX

2022, 1Q, 48	Repair of facial fractures of frontal sinus and orbital roof
2021, 3Q, 19	Elbow amputation and targeted muscle reinnervation
2021, 2Q, 16	Goldilocks breast reconstruction
2018, 1Q, 10	Complex wound closure using pericranial flap
2014, 3Q, 18	Placement of reverse sural fasciocutaneous pedicle flap
2013, 4Q, 109	Separating conjoined twins

0　Medical and Surgical
J　Subcutaneous Tissue and Fascia
0　Alteration　　Definition: Modifying the anatomic structure of a body part without affecting the function of the body part
　　　　　　　　Explanation: Principal purpose is to improve appearance

Body Part Character 4		Approach Character 5	Device Character 6	Qualifier Character 7
1 Subcutaneous Tissue and Fascia, Face 　Masseteric fascia 　Orbital fascia 　Submandibular space **4** Subcutaneous Tissue and Fascia, Right Neck 　Deep cervical fascia 　Pretracheal fascia 　Prevertebral fascia **5** Subcutaneous Tissue and Fascia, Left Neck 　*See* 4 Subcutaneous Tissue and Fascia, Right Neck **6** Subcutaneous Tissue and Fascia, Chest 　Pectoral fascia **7** Subcutaneous Tissue and Fascia, Back **8** Subcutaneous Tissue and Fascia, Abdomen **9** Subcutaneous Tissue and Fascia, Buttock **D** Subcutaneous Tissue and Fascia, Right Upper Arm 　Axillary fascia 　Deltoid fascia 　Infraspinatus fascia 　Subscapular aponeurosis 　Supraspinatus fascia	**F** Subcutaneous Tissue and Fascia, Left Upper Arm 　*See* D Subcutaneous Tissue and Fascia, Right Upper Arm **G** Subcutaneous Tissue and Fascia, Right Lower Arm 　Antebrachial fascia 　Bicipital aponeurosis **H** Subcutaneous Tissue and Fascia, Left Lower Arm 　*See* G Subcutaneous Tissue and Fascia, Right Lower Arm **L** Subcutaneous Tissue and Fascia, Right Upper Leg 　Crural fascia 　Fascia lata 　Iliac fascia 　Iliotibial tract (band) **M** Subcutaneous Tissue and Fascia, Left Upper Leg 　*See* L Subcutaneous Tissue and Fascia, Right Upper Leg **N** Subcutaneous Tissue and Fascia, Right Lower Leg **P** Subcutaneous Tissue and Fascia, Left Lower Leg	**0** Open **3** Percutaneous	**Z** No Device	**Z** No Qualifier

0　Medical and Surgical
J　Subcutaneous Tissue and Fascia
2　Change　　Definition: Taking out or off a device from a body part and putting back an identical or similar device in or on the same body part without cutting or puncturing the skin or a mucous membrane
　　　　　　Explanation: All CHANGE procedures are coded using the approach EXTERNAL

Body Part Character 4	Approach Character 5	Device Character 6	Qualifier Character 7
S Subcutaneous Tissue and Fascia, Head and Neck **T** Subcutaneous Tissue and Fascia, Trunk 　External oblique aponeurosis 　Transversalis fascia **V** Subcutaneous Tissue and Fascia, Upper Extremity **W** Subcutaneous Tissue and Fascia, Lower Extremity	**X** External	**0** Drainage Device **Y** Other Device	**Z** No Qualifier

Non-OR　All body part, approach, device, and qualifier values

NC Noncovered Procedure　　**LC** Limited Coverage　　**QA** Questionable OB Admit　　**NT** New Tech Add-on　　⊞ Combination Member　　♂ Male　　♀ Female

ICD-10-PCS 2023　　　　　　　　　　　　　　　　　　　　　　　　　　　　　445

Ø　Medical and Surgical
J　Subcutaneous Tissue and Fascia
5　Destruction　　Definition: Physical eradication of all or a portion of a body part by the direct use of energy, force, or a destructive agent

Explanation: None of the body part is physically taken out

Body Part Character 4		Approach Character 5	Device Character 6	Qualifier Character 7
Ø　Subcutaneous Tissue and Fascia, Scalp　Galea aponeurotica	**G　Subcutaneous Tissue and Fascia, Right Lower Arm**　Antebrachial fascia　Bicipital aponeurosis	**Ø　Open**　**3　Percutaneous**	**Z　No Device**	**Z　No Qualifier**
1　Subcutaneous Tissue and Fascia, Face　Masseteric fascia　Orbital fascia　Submandibular space	**H　Subcutaneous Tissue and Fascia, Left Lower Arm**　*See G Subcutaneous Tissue and Fascia, Right Lower Arm*			
4　Subcutaneous Tissue and Fascia, Right Neck　Deep cervical fascia　Pretracheal fascia　Prevertebral fascia	**J　Subcutaneous Tissue and Fascia, Right Hand**　Palmar fascia (aponeurosis)			
5　Subcutaneous Tissue and Fascia, Left Neck　*See 4 Subcutaneous Tissue and Fascia, Right Neck*	**K　Subcutaneous Tissue and Fascia, Left Hand**　*See J Subcutaneous Tissue and Fascia, Right Hand*			
6　Subcutaneous Tissue and Fascia, Chest　Pectoral fascia	**L　Subcutaneous Tissue and Fascia, Right Upper Leg**　Crural fascia　Fascia lata　Iliac fascia　Iliotibial tract (band)			
7　Subcutaneous Tissue and Fascia, Back	**M　Subcutaneous Tissue and Fascia, Left Upper Leg**　*See L Subcutaneous Tissue and Fascia, Right Upper Leg*			
8　Subcutaneous Tissue and Fascia, Abdomen	**N　Subcutaneous Tissue and Fascia, Right Lower Leg**			
9　Subcutaneous Tissue and Fascia, Buttock	**P　Subcutaneous Tissue and Fascia, Left Lower Leg**			
B　Subcutaneous Tissue and Fascia, Perineum	**Q　Subcutaneous Tissue and Fascia, Right Foot**　Plantar fascia (aponeurosis)			
C　Subcutaneous Tissue and Fascia, Pelvic Region	**R　Subcutaneous Tissue and Fascia, Left Foot**　*See Q Subcutaneous Tissue and Fascia, Right Foot*			
D　Subcutaneous Tissue and Fascia, Right Upper Arm　Axillary fascia　Deltoid fascia　Infraspinatus fascia　Subscapular aponeurosis　Supraspinatus fascia				
F　Subcutaneous Tissue and Fascia, Left Upper Arm　*See D Subcutaneous Tissue and Fascia, Right Upper Arm*				

DRG Non-OR　All body part, approach, device, and qualifier values

Ø Medical and Surgical
J Subcutaneous Tissue and Fascia
8 Division   Definition: Cutting into a body part, without draining fluids and/or gases from the body part, in order to separate or transect a body part
            Explanation: All or a portion of the body part is separated into two or more portions

Body Part Character 4		Approach Character 5	Device Character 6	Qualifier Character 7
Ø Subcutaneous Tissue and Fascia, Scalp Galea aponeurotica	**H Subcutaneous Tissue and Fascia, Left Lower Arm** *See G Subcutaneous Tissue and Fascia, Right Lower Arm*	**Ø Open** **3 Percutaneous**	**Z No Device**	**Z No Qualifier**
1 Subcutaneous Tissue and Fascia, Face Masseteric fascia Orbital fascia Submandibular space	**J Subcutaneous Tissue and Fascia, Right Hand** Palmar fascia (aponeurosis)			
4 Subcutaneous Tissue and Fascia, Right Neck Deep cervical fascia Pretracheal fascia Prevertebral fascia	**K Subcutaneous Tissue and Fascia, Left Hand** *See J Subcutaneous Tissue and Fascia, Right Hand*			
5 Subcutaneous Tissue and Fascia, Left Neck *See 4 Subcutaneous Tissue and Fascia, Right Neck*	**L Subcutaneous Tissue and Fascia, Right Upper Leg** Crural fascia Fascia lata Iliac fascia Iliotibial tract (band)			
6 Subcutaneous Tissue and Fascia, Chest Pectoral fascia	**M Subcutaneous Tissue and Fascia, Left Upper Leg** *See L Subcutaneous Tissue and Fascia, Right Upper Leg*			
7 Subcutaneous Tissue and Fascia, Back	**N Subcutaneous Tissue and Fascia, Right Lower Leg**			
8 Subcutaneous Tissue and Fascia, Abdomen	**P Subcutaneous Tissue and Fascia, Left Lower Leg**			
9 Subcutaneous Tissue and Fascia, Buttock	**Q Subcutaneous Tissue and Fascia, Right Foot** Plantar fascia (aponeurosis)			
B Subcutaneous Tissue and Fascia, Perineum	**R Subcutaneous Tissue and Fascia, Left Foot** *See Q Subcutaneous Tissue and Fascia, Right Foot*			
C Subcutaneous Tissue and Fascia, Pelvic Region	**S Subcutaneous Tissue and Fascia, Head and Neck**			
D Subcutaneous Tissue and Fascia, Right Upper Arm Axillary fascia Deltoid fascia Infraspinatus fascia Subscapular aponeurosis Supraspinatus fascia	**T Subcutaneous Tissue and Fascia, Trunk** External oblique aponeurosis Transversalis fascia			
F Subcutaneous Tissue and Fascia, Left Upper Arm *See D Subcutaneous Tissue and Fascia, Right Upper Arm*	**V Subcutaneous Tissue and Fascia, Upper Extremity**			
G Subcutaneous Tissue and Fascia, Right Lower Arm Antebrachial fascia Bicipital aponeurosis	**W Subcutaneous Tissue and Fascia, Lower Extremity**			

NC Noncovered Procedure   **LC** Limited Coverage   **QA** Questionable OB Admit   **NT** New Tech Add-on   ⊞ Combination Member   ♂ Male   ♀ Female

ICD-10-PCS 2023   447

Subcutaneous Tissue and Fascia

Ø   **Medical and Surgical**
J   **Subcutaneous Tissue and Fascia**
9   **Drainage**   Definition: Taking or letting out fluids and/or gases from a body part
                           Explanation: The qualifier DIAGNOSTIC is used to identify drainage procedures that are biopsies

Body Part Character 4		Approach Character 5	Device Character 6	Qualifier Character 7
Ø **Subcutaneous Tissue and Fascia, Scalp** Galea aponeurotica	G **Subcutaneous Tissue and Fascia, Right Lower Arm** Antebrachial fascia Bicipital aponeurosis	Ø Open 3 Percutaneous	Ø Drainage Device	Z No Qualifier
1 **Subcutaneous Tissue and Fascia, Face** Masseteric fascia Orbital fascia Submandibular space	H **Subcutaneous Tissue and Fascia, Left Lower Arm** *See* G *Subcutaneous Tissue and Fascia, Right Lower Arm*			
4 **Subcutaneous Tissue and Fascia, Right Neck** Deep cervical fascia Pretracheal fascia Prevertebral fascia	J **Subcutaneous Tissue and Fascia, Right Hand** Palmar fascia (aponeurosis)			
5 **Subcutaneous Tissue and Fascia, Left Neck** *See* 4 *Subcutaneous Tissue and Fascia, Right Neck*	K **Subcutaneous Tissue and Fascia, Left Hand** *See* J *Subcutaneous Tissue and Fascia, Right Hand*			
6 **Subcutaneous Tissue and Fascia, Chest** Pectoral fascia	L **Subcutaneous Tissue and Fascia, Right Upper Leg** Crural fascia Fascia lata Iliac fascia Iliotibial tract (band)			
7 **Subcutaneous Tissue and Fascia, Back**	M **Subcutaneous Tissue and Fascia, Left Upper Leg** *See* L *Subcutaneous Tissue and Fascia, Right Upper Leg*			
8 **Subcutaneous Tissue and Fascia, Abdomen**	N **Subcutaneous Tissue and Fascia, Right Lower Leg**			
9 **Subcutaneous Tissue and Fascia, Buttock**	P **Subcutaneous Tissue and Fascia, Left Lower Leg**			
B **Subcutaneous Tissue and Fascia, Perineum**	Q **Subcutaneous Tissue and Fascia, Right Foot** Plantar fascia (aponeurosis)			
C **Subcutaneous Tissue and Fascia, Pelvic Region**	R **Subcutaneous Tissue and Fascia, Left Foot** *See* Q *Subcutaneous Tissue and Fascia, Right Foot*			
D **Subcutaneous Tissue and Fascia, Right Upper Arm** Axillary fascia Deltoid fascia Infraspinatus fascia Subscapular aponeurosis Supraspinatus fascia				
F **Subcutaneous Tissue and Fascia, Left Upper Arm** *See* D *Subcutaneous Tissue and Fascia, Right Upper Arm*				

Non-OR   All body part, approach, device, and qualifier values

ØJ9 Continued on next page

Ø Medical and Surgical
J Subcutaneous Tissue and Fascia
9 Drainage   Definition: Taking or letting out fluids and/or gases from a body part

ØJ9 Continued

Explanation: The qualifier DIAGNOSTIC is used to identify drainage procedures that are biopsies

Body Part Character 4		Approach Character 5	Device Character 6	Qualifier Character 7
Ø Subcutaneous Tissue and Fascia, Scalp	**G Subcutaneous Tissue and Fascia, Right Lower Arm**	**Ø Open**	**Z No Device**	**X Diagnostic**
Galea aponeurotica	Antebrachial fascia	**3 Percutaneous**		**Z No Qualifier**
1 Subcutaneous Tissue and Fascia, Face	Bicipital aponeurosis			
Masseteric fascia	**H Subcutaneous Tissue and Fascia, Left Lower Arm**			
Orbital fascia	*See G Subcutaneous Tissue and Fascia, Right Lower Arm*			
Submandibular space	**J Subcutaneous Tissue and Fascia, Right Hand**			
4 Subcutaneous Tissue and Fascia, Right Neck	Palmar fascia (aponeurosis)			
Deep cervical fascia	**K Subcutaneous Tissue and Fascia, Left Hand**			
Pretracheal fascia	*See J Subcutaneous Tissue and Fascia, Right Hand*			
Prevertebral fascia	**L Subcutaneous Tissue and Fascia, Right Upper Leg**			
5 Subcutaneous Tissue and Fascia, Left Neck	Crural fascia			
See 4 Subcutaneous Tissue and Fascia, Right Neck	Fascia lata			
6 Subcutaneous Tissue and Fascia, Chest	Iliac fascia			
Pectoral fascia	Iliotibial tract (band)			
7 Subcutaneous Tissue and Fascia, Back	**M Subcutaneous Tissue and Fascia, Left Upper Leg**			
8 Subcutaneous Tissue and Fascia, Abdomen	*See L Subcutaneous Tissue and Fascia, Right Upper Leg*			
9 Subcutaneous Tissue and Fascia, Buttock	**N Subcutaneous Tissue and Fascia, Right Lower Leg**			
B Subcutaneous Tissue and Fascia, Perineum	**P Subcutaneous Tissue and Fascia, Left Lower Leg**			
C Subcutaneous Tissue and Fascia, Pelvic Region	**Q Subcutaneous Tissue and Fascia, Right Foot**			
D Subcutaneous Tissue and Fascia, Right Upper Arm	Plantar fascia (aponeurosis)			
Axillary fascia	**R Subcutaneous Tissue and Fascia, Left Foot**			
Deltoid fascia	*See Q Subcutaneous Tissue and Fascia, Right Foot*			
Infraspinatus fascia				
Subscapular aponeurosis				
Supraspinatus fascia				
F Subcutaneous Tissue and Fascia, Left Upper Arm				
See D Subcutaneous Tissue and Fascia, Right Upper Arm				

Non-OR   All body part, approach, device, and qualifier values

NC Noncovered Procedure   **LC** Limited Coverage   **QA** Questionable OB Admit   **NT** New Tech Add-on   ⊞ Combination Member   ♂ Male   ♀ Female

ICD-10-PCS 2023   449

Ø   Medical and Surgical
J   Subcutaneous Tissue and Fascia
B   Excision   Definition: Cutting out or off, without replacement, a portion of a body part
            Explanation: The qualifier DIAGNOSTIC is used to identify excision procedures that are biopsies

Body Part Character 4		Approach Character 5	Device Character 6	Qualifier Character 7

Ø Subcutaneous Tissue and Fascia, Scalp
  Galea aponeurotica
	G Subcutaneous Tissue and Fascia, Right Lower Arm
	  Antebrachial fascia
	  Bicipital aponeurosis
		Ø Open
		3 Percutaneous
			Z No Device	**X** Diagnostic
				Z No Qualifier

1 Subcutaneous Tissue and Fascia, Face
  Masseteric fascia
  Orbital fascia
  Submandibular space
	H Subcutaneous Tissue and Fascia, Left Lower Arm
	  See G Subcutaneous Tissue and Fascia, Right Lower Arm			

4 Subcutaneous Tissue and Fascia, Right Neck
  Deep cervical fascia
  Pretracheal fascia
  Prevertebral fascia
	J Subcutaneous Tissue and Fascia, Right Hand
	  Palmar fascia (aponeurosis)			

5 Subcutaneous Tissue and Fascia, Left Neck
  See 4 Subcutaneous Tissue and Fascia, Right Neck
	K Subcutaneous Tissue and Fascia, Left Hand
	  See J Subcutaneous Tissue and Fascia, Right Hand			

6 Subcutaneous Tissue and Fascia, Chest
  Pectoral fascia
	L Subcutaneous Tissue and Fascia, Right Upper Leg
	  Crural fascia
	  Fascia lata
	  Iliac fascia
	  Iliotibial tract (band)			

7 Subcutaneous Tissue and Fascia, Back	**M** Subcutaneous Tissue and Fascia, Left Upper Leg *See L Subcutaneous Tissue and Fascia, Right Upper Leg*			
8 Subcutaneous Tissue and Fascia, Abdomen	**N** Subcutaneous Tissue and Fascia, Right Lower Leg			
9 Subcutaneous Tissue and Fascia, Buttock	**P** Subcutaneous Tissue and Fascia, Left Lower Leg			
B Subcutaneous Tissue and Fascia, Perineum	**Q** Subcutaneous Tissue and Fascia, Right Foot Plantar fascia (aponeurosis)			
C Subcutaneous Tissue and Fascia, Pelvic Region	**R** Subcutaneous Tissue and Fascia, Left Foot *See Q Subcutaneous Tissue and Fascia, Right Foot*			

D Subcutaneous Tissue and Fascia, Right Upper Arm
  Axillary fascia
  Deltoid fascia
  Infraspinatus fascia
  Subscapular aponeurosis
  Supraspinatus fascia				

F Subcutaneous Tissue and Fascia, Left Upper Arm *See D Subcutaneous Tissue and Fascia, Right Upper Arm*				

DRG Non-OR   ØJB[Ø,4,5,6,7,8,9,B,C,D,F,G,H,L,M,N,P,Q,R]3ZZ
Non-OR   ØJB[Ø,1,4,5,6,7,8,9,B,C,D,F,G,H,J,K,L,M,N,P,Q,R][Ø,3]ZX

Ø   **Medical and Surgical**
J   **Subcutaneous Tissue and Fascia**
C   **Extirpation**   Definition: Taking or cutting out solid matter from a body part

Explanation: The solid matter may be an abnormal byproduct of a biological function or a foreign body; it may be imbedded in a body part or in the lumen of a tubular body part. The solid matter may or may not have been previously broken into pieces.

Body Part Character 4		Approach Character 5	Device Character 6	Qualifier Character 7

Ø **Subcutaneous Tissue and Fascia, Scalp**
   Galea aponeurotica
1 **Subcutaneous Tissue and Fascia, Face**
   Masseteric fascia
   Orbital fascia
   Submandibular space
4 **Subcutaneous Tissue and Fascia, Right Neck**
   Deep cervical fascia
   Pretracheal fascia
   Prevertebral fascia
5 **Subcutaneous Tissue and Fascia, Left Neck**
   See 4 *Subcutaneous Tissue and Fascia, Right Neck*
6 **Subcutaneous Tissue and Fascia, Chest**
   Pectoral fascia
7 **Subcutaneous Tissue and Fascia, Back**
8 **Subcutaneous Tissue and Fascia, Abdomen**
9 **Subcutaneous Tissue and Fascia, Buttock**
B **Subcutaneous Tissue and Fascia, Perineum**
C **Subcutaneous Tissue and Fascia, Pelvic Region**
D **Subcutaneous Tissue and Fascia, Right Upper Arm**
   Axillary fascia
   Deltoid fascia
   Infraspinatus fascia
   Subscapular aponeurosis
   Supraspinatus fascia
F **Subcutaneous Tissue and Fascia, Left Upper Arm**
   See D *Subcutaneous Tissue and Fascia, Right Upper Arm*
	G **Subcutaneous Tissue and Fascia, Right Lower Arm**
	   Antebrachial fascia
	   Bicipital aponeurosis
	H **Subcutaneous Tissue and Fascia, Left Lower Arm**
	   See G *Subcutaneous Tissue and Fascia, Right Lower Arm*
	J **Subcutaneous Tissue and Fascia, Right Hand**
	   Palmar fascia (aponeurosis)
	K **Subcutaneous Tissue and Fascia, Left Hand**
	   See J *Subcutaneous Tissue and Fascia, Right Hand*
	L **Subcutaneous Tissue and Fascia, Right Upper Leg**
	   Crural fascia
	   Fascia lata
	   Iliac fascia
	   Iliotibial tract (band)
	M **Subcutaneous Tissue and Fascia, Left Upper Leg**
	   See L *Subcutaneous Tissue and Fascia, Right Upper Leg*
	N **Subcutaneous Tissue and Fascia, Right Lower Leg**
	P **Subcutaneous Tissue and Fascia, Left Lower Leg**
	Q **Subcutaneous Tissue and Fascia, Right Foot**
	   Plantar fascia (aponeurosis)
	R **Subcutaneous Tissue and Fascia, Left Foot**
	   See Q *Subcutaneous Tissue and Fascia, Right Foot*
		Ø Open
		3 Percutaneous
			Z No Device	**Z** No Qualifier

Non-OR   ØJC[Ø,1,4,5,6,7,8,9,B,C,D,F,G,H,J,K,L,M,N,P,Q,R]3ZZ

NC Noncovered Procedure   LC Limited Coverage   QA Questionable OB Admit   NT New Tech Add-on   ⊞ Combination Member   ♂ Male   ♀ Female

ICD-10-PCS 2023   451

ØJC–ØJC

Ø   **Medical and Surgical**
J   **Subcutaneous Tissue and Fascia**
D   **Extraction**   Definition: Pulling or stripping out or off all or a portion of a body part by the use of force
                            Explanation: The qualifier DIAGNOSTIC is used to identify extraction procedures that are biopsies

Body Part Character 4		Approach Character 5	Device Character 6	Qualifier Character 7
Ø **Subcutaneous Tissue and Fascia, Scalp** Galea aponeurotica **1** **Subcutaneous Tissue and Fascia, Face** Masseteric fascia Orbital fascia Submandibular space **4** **Subcutaneous Tissue and Fascia, Right Neck** Deep cervical fascia Pretracheal fascia Prevertebral fascia **5** **Subcutaneous Tissue and Fascia, Left Neck** *See 4 Subcutaneous Tissue and Fascia, Right Neck* **6** **Subcutaneous Tissue and Fascia, Chest** Pectoral fascia **7** **Subcutaneous Tissue and Fascia, Back** **8** **Subcutaneous Tissue and Fascia, Abdomen** **9** **Subcutaneous Tissue and Fascia, Buttock** **B** **Subcutaneous Tissue and Fascia, Perineum** **C** **Subcutaneous Tissue and Fascia, Pelvic Region** **D** **Subcutaneous Tissue and Fascia, Right Upper Arm** Axillary fascia Deltoid fascia Infraspinatus fascia Subscapular aponeurosis Supraspinatus fascia **F** **Subcutaneous Tissue and Fascia, Left Upper Arm** *See D Subcutaneous Tissue and Fascia, Right Upper Arm*	**G** **Subcutaneous Tissue and Fascia, Right Lower Arm** Antebrachial fascia Bicipital aponeurosis **H** **Subcutaneous Tissue and Fascia, Left Lower Arm** *See G Subcutaneous Tissue and Fascia, Right Lower Arm* **J** **Subcutaneous Tissue and Fascia, Right Hand** Palmar fascia (aponeurosis) **K** **Subcutaneous Tissue and Fascia, Left Hand** *See J Subcutaneous Tissue and Fascia, Right Hand* **L** **Subcutaneous Tissue and Fascia, Right Upper Leg** Crural fascia Fascia lata Iliac fascia Iliotibial tract (band) **M** **Subcutaneous Tissue and Fascia, Left Upper Leg** *See L Subcutaneous Tissue and Fascia, Right Upper Leg* **N** **Subcutaneous Tissue and Fascia, Right Lower Leg** **P** **Subcutaneous Tissue and Fascia, Left Lower Leg** **Q** **Subcutaneous Tissue and Fascia, Right Foot** Plantar fascia (aponeurosis) **R** **Subcutaneous Tissue and Fascia, Left Foot** *See Q Subcutaneous Tissue and Fascia, Right Foot*	**Ø** Open **3** Percutaneous	**Z** No Device	**Z** No Qualifier

Non-OR   ØJD[Ø,1,4,5,B,C,D,F,G,H,J,K,N,P,Q,R]3ZZ
                         See Appendix L for Procedure Combinations
                           Combo-only   ØJD[6,7,8,9,L,M]3ZZ

Non-OR Procedure   DRG Non-OR Procedure   Valid OR Procedure   HAC Associated Procedure   Combination Only   New/Revised April   New/Revised October

452   ICD-10-PCS 2023

Ø   Medical and Surgical
J   Subcutaneous Tissue and Fascia
H   Insertion   Definition: Putting in a nonbiological appliance that monitors, assists, performs, or prevents a physiological function but does not physically take the place of a body part
           Explanation: None

Body Part Character 4		Approach Character 5	Device Character 6	Qualifier Character 7
Ø Subcutaneous Tissue and Fascia, Scalp Galea aponeurotica **1** Subcutaneous Tissue and Fascia, Face Masseteric fascia Orbital fascia Submandibular space **4** Subcutaneous Tissue and Fascia, Right Neck Deep cervical fascia Pretracheal fascia Prevertebral fascia **5** Subcutaneous Tissue and Fascia, Left Neck *See 4 Subcutaneous Tissue and Fascia, Right Neck* **9** Subcutaneous Tissue and Fascia, Buttock **B** Subcutaneous Tissue and Fascia, Perineum	**C** Subcutaneous Tissue and Fascia, Pelvic Region **J** Subcutaneous Tissue and Fascia, Right Hand Palmar fascia (aponeurosis) **K** Subcutaneous Tissue and Fascia, Left Hand *See J Subcutaneous Tissue and Fascia, Right Hand* **Q** Subcutaneous Tissue and Fascia, Right Foot Plantar fascia (aponeurosis) **R** Subcutaneous Tissue and Fascia, Left Foot *See Q Subcutaneous Tissue and Fascia, Right Foot*	**Ø** Open **3** Percutaneous	**N** Tissue Expander	**Z** No Qualifier
6 Subcutaneous Tissue and Fascia, Chest ⊞ Pectoral fascia		**Ø** Open **3** Percutaneous	**Ø** Monitoring Device, Hemodynamic **2** Monitoring Device **4** Pacemaker, Single Chamber **5** Pacemaker, Single Chamber Rate Responsive **6** Pacemaker, Dual Chamber **7** Cardiac Resynchronization Pacemaker Pulse Generator **8** Defibrillator Generator **9** Cardiac Resynchronization Defibrillator Pulse Generator **A** Contractility Modulation Device **B** Stimulator Generator, Single Array **C** Stimulator Generator, Single Array Rechargeable **D** Stimulator Generator, Multiple Array **E** Stimulator Generator, Multiple Array Rechargeable **F** Subcutaneous Defibrillator Lead **H** Contraceptive Device **M** Stimulator Generator **N** Tissue Expander **P** Cardiac Rhythm Related Device **V** Infusion Device, Pump **W** Vascular Access Device, Totally Implantable **X** Vascular Access Device, Tunneled **Y** Other Device	**Z** No Qualifier
7 Subcutaneous Tissue and Fascia, Back NC ⊞		**Ø** Open **3** Percutaneous	**B** Stimulator Generator, Single Array **C** Stimulator Generator, Single Array Rechargeable **D** Stimulator Generator, Multiple Array **E** Stimulator Generator, Multiple Array Rechargeable **M** Stimulator Generator **N** Tissue Expander **V** Infusion Device, Pump **Y** Other Device	**Z** No Qualifier

DRG Non-OR   ØJH6[Ø,3][4,5,6,7,H,P,X]Z
DRG Non-OR   ØJH63WX
Non-OR   ØJH63YZ
Non-OR   ØJH73YZ
HAC   ØJH6[Ø,3][4,5,6,7,8,9,P]Z when reported with SDx K68.11 or T81.4Ø-T81.49, T82.7 with 7th character A
HAC   ØJH63XZ when reported with SDx J95.811

NC   ØJH7[Ø,3]MZ

See Appendix L for Procedure Combinations
⊞   ØJH6[Ø,3][4,5,6,7,8,9,A,B,C,D,E,F,M,P]Z
⊞   ØJH7[Ø,3][B,C,D,E,M]Z

ØJH Continued on next page

Ø Medical and Surgical
J Subcutaneous Tissue and Fascia
H Insertion   Definition: Putting in a nonbiological appliance that monitors, assists, performs, or prevents a physiological function but does not physically take the place of a body part

Explanation: None

ØJH Continued

Body Part — Character 4	Approach — Character 5	Device — Character 6	Qualifier — Character 7
8 Subcutaneous Tissue and Fascia, Abdomen NC ⊞	0 Open 3 Percutaneous	0 Monitoring Device, Hemodynamic 2 Monitoring Device 4 Pacemaker, Single Chamber 5 Pacemaker, Single Chamber Rate Responsive 6 Pacemaker, Dual Chamber 7 Cardiac Resynchronization Pacemaker Pulse Generator 8 Defibrillator Generator 9 Cardiac Resynchronization Defibrillator Pulse Generator A Contractility Modulation Device B Stimulator Generator, Single Array C Stimulator Generator, Single Array Rechargeable D Stimulator Generator, Multiple Array E Stimulator Generator, Multiple Array Rechargeable H Contraceptive Device M Stimulator Generator N Tissue Expander P Cardiac Rhythm Related Device V Infusion Device, Pump W Vascular Access Device, Totally Implantable X Vascular Access Device, Tunneled Y Other Device	Z No Qualifier
D Subcutaneous Tissue and Fascia, Right Upper Arm Axillary fascia Deltoid fascia Infraspinatus fascia Subscapular aponeurosis Supraspinatus fascia **F Subcutaneous Tissue and Fascia, Left Upper Arm** *See D Subcutaneous Tissue and Fascia, Right Upper Arm* **G Subcutaneous Tissue and Fascia, Right Lower Arm** Antebrachial fascia Bicipital aponeurosis **H Subcutaneous Tissue and Fascia, Left Lower Arm** *See G Subcutaneous Tissue and Fascia, Right Lower Arm* **L Subcutaneous Tissue and Fascia, Right Upper Leg** Crural fascia Fascia lata Iliac fascia Iliotibial tract (band) **M Subcutaneous Tissue and Fascia, Left Upper Leg** *See L Subcutaneous Tissue and Fascia, Right Upper Leg* **N Subcutaneous Tissue and Fascia, Right Lower Leg** **P Subcutaneous Tissue and Fascia, Left Lower Leg**	0 Open 3 Percutaneous	H Contraceptive Device N Tissue Expander V Infusion Device, Pump W Vascular Access Device, Totally Implantable X Vascular Access Device, Tunneled	Z No Qualifier
S Subcutaneous Tissue and Fascia, Head and Neck **V Subcutaneous Tissue and Fascia, Upper Extremity** **W Subcutaneous Tissue and Fascia, Lower Extremity**	0 Open 3 Percutaneous	1 Radioactive Element 3 Infusion Device Y Other Device	Z No Qualifier
T Subcutaneous Tissue and Fascia, Trunk External oblique aponeurosis Transversalis fascia	0 Open 3 Percutaneous	1 Radioactive Element 3 Infusion Device V Infusion Device, Pump Y Other Device	Z No Qualifier

DRG Non-OR   ØJH8[0,3][2,4,5,6,7,H,P,X]Z
DRG Non-OR   ØJH83WX
DRG Non-OR   ØJH[D,F,G,H,L,M,N,P]ØXZ
DRG Non-OR   ØJH[D,F,G,H,L,M,N,P]3[W,X]Z
DRG Non-OR   ØJHN3HZ
DRG Non-OR   ØJHP[0,3]HZ

Non-OR   ØJH83YZ
Non-OR   ØJH[D,F,G,H,L,M][0,3]HZ
Non-OR   ØJHNØHZ
Non-OR   ØJH[S,V,W]03Z
Non-OR   ØJH[S,V,W]3[3,Y]Z
Non-OR   ØJHT03Z
Non-OR   ØJHT3[3,Y]Z

HAC   ØJH8[0,3][4,5,6,7,8,9,P]Z when reported with SDx K68.11 or T81.40-T81.49, T82.7 with 7th character A
NC   ØJH8[0,3]MZ

See Appendix L for Procedure Combinations
⊞   ØJH8[0,3][4,5,6,7,8,9,A,B,C,D,E,M,P]Z

Ø   **Medical and Surgical**
J   **Subcutaneous Tissue and Fascia**
J   **Inspection**   Definition: Visually and/or manually exploring a body part

Explanation: Visual exploration may be performed with or without optical instrumentation. Manual exploration may be performed directly or through intervening body layers.

Body Part Character 4	Approach Character 5	Device Character 6	Qualifier Character 7

S   Subcutaneous Tissue and Fascia, Head and Neck
T   Subcutaneous Tissue and Fascia, Trunk
     External oblique aponeurosis
     Transversalis fascia
V   Subcutaneous Tissue and Fascia, Upper Extremity
W   Subcutaneous Tissue and Fascia, Lower Extremity
	Ø Open
	3 Percutaneous
	X External
		Z No Device	**Z** No Qualifier

Non-OR   All body part, approach, device, and qualifier values

---

Ø   **Medical and Surgical**
J   **Subcutaneous Tissue and Fascia**
N   **Release**   Definition: Freeing a body part from an abnormal physical constraint by cutting or by the use of force

Explanation: Some of the restraining tissue may be taken out but none of the body part is taken out

Body Part Character 4	Approach Character 5	Device Character 6	Qualifier Character 7

Ø   Subcutaneous Tissue and Fascia, Scalp
     Galea aponeurotica
1   Subcutaneous Tissue and Fascia, Face
     Masseteric fascia
     Orbital fascia
     Submandibular space
4   Subcutaneous Tissue and Fascia, Right Neck
     Deep cervical fascia
     Pretracheal fascia
     Prevertebral fascia
5   Subcutaneous Tissue and Fascia, Left Neck
     See 4 Subcutaneous Tissue and Fascia, Right Neck
6   Subcutaneous Tissue and Fascia, Chest
     Pectoral fascia
7   Subcutaneous Tissue and Fascia, Back
8   Subcutaneous Tissue and Fascia, Abdomen
9   Subcutaneous Tissue and Fascia, Buttock
B   Subcutaneous Tissue and Fascia, Perineum
C   Subcutaneous Tissue and Fascia, Pelvic Region
D   Subcutaneous Tissue and Fascia, Right Upper Arm
     Axillary fascia
     Deltoid fascia
     Infraspinatus fascia
     Subscapular aponeurosis
     Supraspinatus fascia
F   Subcutaneous Tissue and Fascia, Left Upper Arm
     See D Subcutaneous Tissue and Fascia, Right Upper Arm
 	
G   Subcutaneous Tissue and Fascia, Right Lower Arm
     Antebrachial fascia
     Bicipital aponeurosis
H   Subcutaneous Tissue and Fascia, Left Lower Arm
     See G Subcutaneous Tissue and Fascia, Right Lower Arm
J   Subcutaneous Tissue and Fascia, Right Hand
     Palmar fascia (aponeurosis)
K   Subcutaneous Tissue and Fascia, Left Hand
     See J Subcutaneous Tissue and Fascia, Right Hand
L   Subcutaneous Tissue and Fascia, Right Upper Leg
     Crural fascia
     Fascia lata
     Iliac fascia
     Iliotibial tract (band)
M   Subcutaneous Tissue and Fascia, Left Upper Leg
     See L Subcutaneous Tissue and Fascia, Right Upper Leg
N   Subcutaneous Tissue and Fascia, Right Lower Leg
P   Subcutaneous Tissue and Fascia, Left Lower Leg
Q   Subcutaneous Tissue and Fascia, Right Foot
     Plantar fascia (aponeurosis)
R   Subcutaneous Tissue and Fascia, Left Foot
     See Q Subcutaneous Tissue and Fascia, Right Foot
	Ø Open
	3 Percutaneous
	X External
		Z No Device	**Z** No Qualifier

Non-OR   ØJN[Ø,1,4,5,6,7,8,9,B,C,D,F,G,H,J,K,L,M,N,P,Q,R]XZZ

Ø Medical and Surgical
J Subcutaneous Tissue and Fascia
P Removal — Definition: Taking out or off a device from a body part

Explanation: If a device is taken out and a similar device put in without cutting or puncturing the skin or mucous membrane, the procedure is coded to the root operation CHANGE. Otherwise, the procedure for taking out a device is coded to the root operation REMOVAL.

Body Part Character 4	Approach Character 5	Device Character 6	Qualifier Character 7
S Subcutaneous Tissue and Fascia, Head and Neck	Ø Open 3 Percutaneous	Ø Drainage Device 1 Radioactive Element 3 Infusion Device 7 Autologous Tissue Substitute J Synthetic Substitute K Nonautologous Tissue Substitute N Tissue Expander Y Other Device	Z No Qualifier
S Subcutaneous Tissue and Fascia, Head and Neck	X External	Ø Drainage Device 1 Radioactive Element 3 Infusion Device	Z No Qualifier
T Subcutaneous Tissue and Fascia, Trunk External oblique aponeurosis Transversalis fascia	Ø Open 3 Percutaneous	Ø Drainage Device 1 Radioactive Element 2 Monitoring Device 3 Infusion Device 7 Autologous Tissue Substitute F Subcutaneous Defibrillator Lead H Contraceptive Device J Synthetic Substitute K Nonautologous Tissue Substitute M Stimulator Generator N Tissue Expander P Cardiac Rhythm Related Device V Infusion Device, Pump W Vascular Access Device, Totally Implantable X Vascular Access Device, Tunneled Y Other Device	Z No Qualifier
T Subcutaneous Tissue and Fascia, Trunk External oblique aponeurosis Transversalis fascia	X External	Ø Drainage Device 1 Radioactive Element 2 Monitoring Device 3 Infusion Device H Contraceptive Device V Infusion Device, Pump X Vascular Access Device, Tunneled	Z No Qualifier
V Subcutaneous Tissue and Fascia, Upper Extremity W Subcutaneous Tissue and Fascia, Lower Extremity	Ø Open 3 Percutaneous	Ø Drainage Device 1 Radioactive Element 3 Infusion Device 7 Autologous Tissue Substitute H Contraceptive Device J Synthetic Substitute K Nonautologous Tissue Substitute N Tissue Expander V Infusion Device, Pump W Vascular Access Device, Totally Implantable X Vascular Access Device, Tunneled Y Other Device	Z No Qualifier
V Subcutaneous Tissue and Fascia, Upper Extremity W Subcutaneous Tissue and Fascia, Lower Extremity	X External	Ø Drainage Device 1 Radioactive Element 3 Infusion Device H Contraceptive Device V Infusion Device, Pump X Vascular Access Device, Tunneled	Z No Qualifier

Non-OR ØJPS[Ø,3][Ø,1,3,7,J,K,N,Y]Z
Non-OR ØJPSX[Ø,1,3]Z
Non-OR ØJPT[Ø,3][Ø,1,2,3,7,H,J,K,M,N,V,W,X,Y]Z
Non-OR ØJPTX[Ø,1,2,3,H,V,X]Z
Non-OR ØJP[V,W][Ø,3][Ø,1,3,7,H,J,K,N,V,W,X,Y]Z
Non-OR ØJP[V,W]X[Ø,1,3,H,V,X]Z
HAC ØJPT[Ø,3][F,P]Z when reported with SDx K68.11 or T81.4Ø-T81.49, T82.7 with 7th character A

Ø   Medical and Surgical
J   Subcutaneous Tissue and Fascia
Q   Repair   Definition: Restoring, to the extent possible, a body part to its normal anatomic structure and function
                         Explanation: Used only when the method to accomplish the repair is not one of the other root operations

Body Part Character 4		Approach Character 5	Device Character 6	Qualifier Character 7
Ø Subcutaneous Tissue and Fascia, Scalp Galea aponeurotica **1 Subcutaneous Tissue and Fascia, Face** Masseteric fascia Orbital fascia Submandibular space **4 Subcutaneous Tissue and Fascia, Right Neck** Deep cervical fascia Pretracheal fascia Prevertebral fascia **5 Subcutaneous Tissue and Fascia, Left Neck** *See 4 Subcutaneous Tissue and Fascia, Right Neck* **6 Subcutaneous Tissue and Fascia, Chest** Pectoral fascia **7 Subcutaneous Tissue and Fascia, Back** **8 Subcutaneous Tissue and Fascia, Abdomen** **9 Subcutaneous Tissue and Fascia, Buttock** **B Subcutaneous Tissue and Fascia, Perineum** **C Subcutaneous Tissue and Fascia, Pelvic Region** **D Subcutaneous Tissue and Fascia, Right Upper Arm** Axillary fascia Deltoid fascia Infraspinatus fascia Subscapular aponeurosis Supraspinatus fascia **F Subcutaneous Tissue and Fascia, Left Upper Arm** *See D Subcutaneous Tissue and Fascia, Right Upper Arm*	**G Subcutaneous Tissue and Fascia, Right Lower Arm** Antebrachial fascia Bicipital aponeurosis **H Subcutaneous Tissue and Fascia, Left Lower Arm** *See G Subcutaneous Tissue and Fascia, Right Lower Arm* **J Subcutaneous Tissue and Fascia, Right Hand** Palmar fascia (aponeurosis) **K Subcutaneous Tissue and Fascia, Left Hand** *See J Subcutaneous Tissue and Fascia, Right Hand* **L Subcutaneous Tissue and Fascia, Right Upper Leg** Crural fascia Fascia lata Iliac fascia Iliotibial tract (band) **M Subcutaneous Tissue and Fascia, Left Upper Leg** *See L Subcutaneous Tissue and Fascia, Right Upper Leg* **N Subcutaneous Tissue and Fascia, Right Lower Leg** **P Subcutaneous Tissue and Fascia, Left Lower Leg** **Q Subcutaneous Tissue and Fascia, Right Foot** Plantar fascia (aponeurosis) **R Subcutaneous Tissue and Fascia, Left Foot** *See Q Subcutaneous Tissue and Fascia, Right Foot*	**Ø Open** **3 Percutaneous**	**Z No Device**	**Z No Qualifier**

Non-OR   ØJQ[Ø,1,4,5,6,7,8,9,B,C,D,F,G,H,J,K,L,M,N,P,Q,R]3ZZ

NC Noncovered Procedure   **LC** Limited Coverage   **QA** Questionable OB Admit   **NT** New Tech Add-on   ✚ Combination Member   ♂ Male   ♀ Female

ICD-10-PCS 2023   457

Ø Medical and Surgical
J Subcutaneous Tissue and Fascia
R Replacement   Definition: Putting in or on biological or synthetic material that physically takes the place and/or function of all or a portion of a body part

Explanation: The body part may have been taken out or replaced, or may be taken out, physically eradicated, or rendered nonfunctional during the REPLACEMENT procedure. A REMOVAL procedure is coded for taking out the device used in a previous replacement procedure.

Body Part Character 4		Approach Character 5	Device Character 6	Qualifier Character 7
Ø Subcutaneous Tissue and Fascia, Scalp Galea aponeurotica	**G Subcutaneous Tissue and Fascia, Right Lower Arm** Antebrachial fascia Bicipital aponeurosis	**Ø Open** **3 Percutaneous**	**7 Autologous Tissue Substitute** **J Synthetic Substitute** **K Nonautologous Tissue Substitute**	**Z No Qualifier**
1 Subcutaneous Tissue and Fascia, Face Masseteric fascia Orbital fascia Submandibular space	**H Subcutaneous Tissue and Fascia, Left Lower Arm** *See G Subcutaneous Tissue and Fascia, Right Lower Arm*			
4 Subcutaneous Tissue and Fascia, Right Neck Deep cervical fascia Pretracheal fascia Prevertebral fascia	**J Subcutaneous Tissue and Fascia, Right Hand** Palmar fascia (aponeurosis)			
5 Subcutaneous Tissue and Fascia, Left Neck *See 4 Subcutaneous Tissue and Fascia, Right Neck*	**K Subcutaneous Tissue and Fascia, Left Hand** *See J Subcutaneous Tissue and Fascia, Right Hand*			
6 Subcutaneous Tissue and Fascia, Chest Pectoral fascia	**L Subcutaneous Tissue and Fascia, Right Upper Leg** Crural fascia Fascia lata Iliac fascia Iliotibial tract (band)			
7 Subcutaneous Tissue and Fascia, Back	**M Subcutaneous Tissue and Fascia, Left Upper Leg** *See L Subcutaneous Tissue and Fascia, Right Upper Leg*			
8 Subcutaneous Tissue and Fascia, Abdomen	**N Subcutaneous Tissue and Fascia, Right Lower Leg**			
9 Subcutaneous Tissue and Fascia, Buttock	**P Subcutaneous Tissue and Fascia, Left Lower Leg**			
B Subcutaneous Tissue and Fascia, Perineum	**Q Subcutaneous Tissue and Fascia, Right Foot** Plantar fascia (aponeurosis)			
C Subcutaneous Tissue and Fascia, Pelvic Region	**R Subcutaneous Tissue and Fascia, Left Foot** *See Q Subcutaneous Tissue and Fascia, Right Foot*			
D Subcutaneous Tissue and Fascia, Right Upper Arm Axillary fascia Deltoid fascia Infraspinatus fascia Subscapular aponeurosis Supraspinatus fascia				
F Subcutaneous Tissue and Fascia, Left Upper Arm *See D Subcutaneous Tissue and Fascia, Right Upper Arm*				

Non-OR Procedure   DRG Non-OR Procedure   Valid OR Procedure   HAC Associated Procedure   Combination Only   New/Revised April   New/Revised October

458

ICD-10-PCS 2023

Ø   **Medical and Surgical**
J   **Subcutaneous Tissue and Fascia**
U   **Supplement:**   Definition: Putting in or on biological or synthetic material that physically reinforces and/or augments the function of a portion of a body part
                    Explanation: The biological material is non-living, or is living and from the same individual. The body part may have been previously replaced, and the SUPPLEMENT procedure is performed to physically reinforce and/or augment the function of the replaced body part.

Body Part Character 4		Approach Character 5	Device Character 6	Qualifier Character 7

Ø Subcutaneous Tissue and Fascia, Scalp
  Galea aponeurotica
1 Subcutaneous Tissue and Fascia, Face
  Masseteric fascia
  Orbital fascia
  Submandibular space
4 Subcutaneous Tissue and Fascia, Right Neck
  Deep cervical fascia
  Pretracheal fascia
  Prevertebral fascia
5 Subcutaneous Tissue and Fascia, Left Neck
  See 4 Subcutaneous Tissue and Fascia, Right Neck
6 Subcutaneous Tissue and Fascia, Chest
  Pectoral fascia
7 Subcutaneous Tissue and Fascia, Back
8 Subcutaneous Tissue and Fascia, Abdomen
9 Subcutaneous Tissue and Fascia, Buttock
B Subcutaneous Tissue and Fascia, Perineum
C Subcutaneous Tissue and Fascia, Pelvic Region
D Subcutaneous Tissue and Fascia, Right Upper Arm
  Axillary fascia
  Deltoid fascia
  Infraspinatus fascia
  Subscapular aponeurosis
  Supraspinatus fascia
F Subcutaneous Tissue and Fascia, Left Upper Arm
  See D Subcutaneous Tissue and Fascia, Right Upper Arm
	G Subcutaneous Tissue and Fascia, Right Lower Arm
	  Antebrachial fascia
	  Bicipital aponeurosis
	H Subcutaneous Tissue and Fascia, Left Lower Arm
	  See G Subcutaneous Tissue and Fascia, Right Lower Arm
	J Subcutaneous Tissue and Fascia, Right Hand
	  Palmar fascia (aponeurosis)
	K Subcutaneous Tissue and Fascia, Left Hand
	  See J Subcutaneous Tissue and Fascia, Right Hand
	L Subcutaneous Tissue and Fascia, Right Upper Leg
	  Crural fascia
	  Fascia lata
	  Iliac fascia
	  Iliotibial tract (band)
	M Subcutaneous Tissue and Fascia, Left Upper Leg
	  See L Subcutaneous Tissue and Fascia, Right Upper Leg
	N Subcutaneous Tissue and Fascia, Right Lower Leg
	P Subcutaneous Tissue and Fascia, Left Lower Leg
	Q Subcutaneous Tissue and Fascia, Right Foot
	  Plantar fascia (aponeurosis)
	R Subcutaneous Tissue and Fascia, Left Foot
	  See Q Subcutaneous Tissue and Fascia, Right Foot
		Ø Open
		3 Percutaneous
			7 Autologous Tissue Substitute
			J Synthetic Substitute
			K Nonautologous Tissue Substitute
				Z No Qualifier

Ø Medical and Surgical
J Subcutaneous Tissue and Fascia
W Revision Definition: Correcting, to the extent possible, a portion of a malfunctioning device or the position of a displaced device

Explanation: Revision can include correcting a malfunctioning or displaced device by taking out or putting in components of the device such as a screw or pin

Body Part Character 4	Approach Character 5	Device Character 6	Qualifier Character 7
S Subcutaneous Tissue and Fascia, Head and Neck	**Ø** Open **3** Percutaneous	**Ø** Drainage Device **3** Infusion Device **7** Autologous Tissue Substitute **J** Synthetic Substitute **K** Nonautologous Tissue Substitute **N** Tissue Expander **Y** Other Device	**Z** No Qualifier
S Subcutaneous Tissue and Fascia, Head and Neck	**X** External	**Ø** Drainage Device **3** Infusion Device **7** Autologous Tissue Substitute **J** Synthetic Substitute **K** Nonautologous Tissue Substitute **N** Tissue Expander	**Z** No Qualifier
T Subcutaneous Tissue and Fascia, Trunk External oblique aponeurosis Transversalis fascia	**Ø** Open **3** Percutaneous	**Ø** Drainage Device **2** Monitoring Device **3** Infusion Device **7** Autologous Tissue Substitute **F** Subcutaneous Defibrillator Lead **H** Contraceptive Device **J** Synthetic Substitute **K** Nonautologous Tissue Substitute **M** Stimulator Generator **N** Tissue Expander **P** Cardiac Rhythm Related Device **V** Infusion Device, Pump **W** Vascular Access Device, Totally Implantable **X** Vascular Access Device, Tunneled **Y** Other Device	**Z** No Qualifier
T Subcutaneous Tissue and Fascia, Trunk External oblique aponeurosis Transversalis fascia	**X** External	**Ø** Drainage Device **2** Monitoring Device **3** Infusion Device **7** Autologous Tissue Substitute **F** Subcutaneous Defibrillator Lead **H** Contraceptive Device **J** Synthetic Substitute **K** Nonautologous Tissue Substitute **M** Stimulator Generator **N** Tissue Expander **P** Cardiac Rhythm Related Device **V** Infusion Device, Pump **W** Vascular Access Device, Totally Implantable **X** Vascular Access Device, Tunneled	**Z** No Qualifier
V Subcutaneous Tissue and Fascia, Upper Extremity **W** Subcutaneous Tissue and Fascia, Lower Extremity	**Ø** Open **3** Percutaneous	**Ø** Drainage Device **3** Infusion Device **7** Autologous Tissue Substitute **H** Contraceptive Device **J** Synthetic Substitute **K** Nonautologous Tissue Substitute **N** Tissue Expander **V** Infusion Device, Pump **W** Vascular Access Device, Totally Implantable **X** Vascular Access Device, Tunneled **Y** Other Device	**Z** No Qualifier
V Subcutaneous Tissue and Fascia, Upper Extremity **W** Subcutaneous Tissue and Fascia, Lower Extremity	**X** External	**Ø** Drainage Device **3** Infusion Device **7** Autologous Tissue Substitute **H** Contraceptive Device **J** Synthetic Substitute **K** Nonautologous Tissue Substitute **N** Tissue Expander **V** Infusion Device, Pump **W** Vascular Access Device, Totally Implantable **X** Vascular Access Device, Tunneled	**Z** No Qualifier

DRG Non-OR	ØJWS[Ø,3][Ø,3,7,J,K,N,Y]Z	**HAC**	ØJWT[Ø,3][F,P]Z when reported with SDx K68.11 or T81.4Ø-T81.49, T82.7 with 7th character A
DRG Non-OR	ØJWT[Ø,3][Ø,3,7,H,J,K,M,N,V,W,X]Z		
DRG Non-OR	ØJWTXMZ		
DRG Non-OR	ØJW[V,W][Ø,3][Ø,3,7,H,J,K,N,V,W,X,Y]Z		
Non-OR	ØJWSX[Ø,3,7,J,K,N]Z		
Non-OR	ØJWT3YZ		
Non-OR	ØJWTX[Ø,2,3,7,F,H,J,K,N,P,V,W,X]Z		
Non-OR	ØJW[V,W]X[Ø,3,7,H,J,K,N,V,W,X]Z		

Non-OR Procedure   DRG Non-OR Procedure   Valid OR Procedure   HAC Associated Procedure   Combination Only   New/Revised April   New/Revised October

Ø   Medical and Surgical
J   Subcutaneous Tissue and Fascia
X   Transfer   Definition: Moving, without taking out, all or a portion of a body part to another location to take over the function of all or a portion of a body part
                         Explanation: The body part transferred remains connected to its vascular and nervous supply

Body Part Character 4		Approach Character 5	Device Character 6	Qualifier Character 7
Ø **Subcutaneous Tissue and Fascia, Scalp** Galea aponeurotica	**G** **Subcutaneous Tissue and Fascia, Right Lower Arm** Antebrachial fascia Bicipital aponeurosis	**Ø** Open **3** Percutaneous	**Z** No Device	**B** Skin and Subcutaneous Tissue **C** Skin, Subcutaneous Tissue and Fascia **Z** No Qualifier
1 **Subcutaneous Tissue and Fascia, Face** Masseteric fascia Orbital fascia Submandibular space	**H** **Subcutaneous Tissue and Fascia, Left Lower Arm** *See G Subcutaneous Tissue and Fascia, Right Lower Arm*			
4 **Subcutaneous Tissue and Fascia, Right Neck** Deep cervical fascia Pretracheal fascia Prevertebral fascia	**J** **Subcutaneous Tissue and Fascia, Right Hand** Palmar fascia (aponeurosis)			
5 **Subcutaneous Tissue and Fascia, Left Neck** *See 4 Subcutaneous Tissue and Fascia, Right Neck*	**K** **Subcutaneous Tissue and Fascia, Left Hand** *See J Subcutaneous Tissue and Fascia, Right Hand*			
6 **Subcutaneous Tissue and Fascia, Chest** Pectoral fascia	**L** **Subcutaneous Tissue and Fascia, Right Upper Leg** Crural fascia Fascia lata Iliac fascia Iliotibial tract (band)			
7 **Subcutaneous Tissue and Fascia, Back**	**M** **Subcutaneous Tissue and Fascia, Left Upper Leg** *See L Subcutaneous Tissue and Fascia, Right Upper Leg*			
8 **Subcutaneous Tissue and Fascia, Abdomen**	**N** **Subcutaneous Tissue and Fascia, Right Lower Leg**			
9 **Subcutaneous Tissue and Fascia, Buttock**	**P** **Subcutaneous Tissue and Fascia, Left Lower Leg**			
B **Subcutaneous Tissue and Fascia, Perineum**	**Q** **Subcutaneous Tissue and Fascia, Right Foot** Plantar fascia (aponeurosis)			
C **Subcutaneous Tissue and Fascia, Pelvic Region**	**R** **Subcutaneous Tissue and Fascia, Left Foot** *See Q Subcutaneous Tissue and Fascia, Right Foot*			
D **Subcutaneous Tissue and Fascia, Right Upper Arm** Axillary fascia Deltoid fascia Infraspinatus fascia Subscapular aponeurosis Supraspinatus fascia				
F **Subcutaneous Tissue and Fascia, Left Upper Arm** *See D Subcutaneous Tissue and Fascia, Right Upper Arm*				

Muscles ØK2–ØKX

Character Meanings

This Character Meaning table is provided as a guide to assist the user in the identification of character members that may be found in this section of code tables. It **SHOULD NOT** be used to build a PCS code.

Operation–Character 3	Body Part–Character 4	Approach–Character 5	Device–Character 6	Qualifier–Character 7
2 Change	Ø Head Muscle	Ø Open	Ø Drainage Device	Ø Skin
5 Destruction	1 Facial Muscle	3 Percutaneous	7 Autologous Tissue Substitute	1 Subcutaneous Tissue
8 Division	2 Neck Muscle, Right	4 Percutaneous Endoscopic	J Synthetic Substitute	2 Skin and Subcutaneous Tissue
9 Drainage	3 Neck Muscle, Left	7 Via Natural or Artificial Opening	K Nonautologous Tissue Substitute	5 Latissimus Dorsi Myocutaneous Flap
B Excision	4 Tongue, Palate, Pharynx Muscle	8 Via Natural or Artificial Opening Endoscopic	M Stimulator Lead	6 Transverse Rectus Abdominis Myocutaneous Flap
C Extirpation	5 Shoulder Muscle, Right	X External	Y Other Device	7 Deep Inferior Epigastric Artery Perforator Flap
D Extraction	6 Shoulder Muscle, Left		Z No Device	8 Superficial Inferior Epigastric Artery Flap
H Insertion	7 Upper Arm Muscle, Right			9 Gluteal Artery Perforator Flap
J Inspection	8 Upper Arm Muscle, Left			X Diagnostic
M Reattachment	9 Lower Arm and Wrist Muscle, Right			Z No Qualifier
N Release	B Lower Arm and Wrist Muscle, Left			
P Removal	C Hand Muscle, Right			
Q Repair	D Hand Muscle, Left			
R Replacement	F Trunk Muscle, Right			
S Reposition	G Trunk Muscle, Left			
T Resection	H Thorax Muscle, Right			
U Supplement	J Thorax Muscle, Left			
W Revision	K Abdomen Muscle, Right			
X Transfer	L Abdomen Muscle, Left			
	M Perineum Muscle			
	N Hip Muscle, Right			
	P Hip Muscle, Left			
	Q Upper Leg Muscle, Right			
	R Upper Leg Muscle, Left			
	S Lower Leg Muscle, Right			
	T Lower Leg Muscle, Left			
	V Foot Muscle, Right			
	W Foot Muscle, Left			
	X Upper Muscle			
	Y Lower Muscle			

AHA Coding Clinic for table ØK8
2021, 4Q, 50   Endoscopic division of tongue, palate and pharynx muscle
2020, 2Q, 25   Endoscopic stapling of Zenker's diverticulum

AHA Coding Clinic for table ØKB
2020, 1Q, 27   Delayed reconstruction following mastectomy using gracilis musculocutaneous free flap
2016, 3Q, 20   Excisional debridement of sacrum
2015, 3Q, 3-8   Excisional and nonexcisional debridement

AHA Coding Clinic for table ØKD
2017, 4Q, 41-42   Extraction procedures

AHA Coding Clinic for table ØKH
2020, 4Q, 63   Intercompartmental pressure measurement

AHA Coding Clinic for table ØKN
2017, 2Q, 12   Compartment syndrome and fasciotomy of foot
2017, 2Q, 13   Compartment syndrome and fasciotomy of leg
2015, 2Q, 22   Arthroscopic subacromial decompression
2014, 4Q, 39   Abdominal component release with placement of mesh for hernia repair

AHA Coding Clinic for table ØKQ
2018, 2Q, 25   Third and fourth degree obstetric lacerations
2016, 2Q, 34   Assisted vaginal delivery
2016, 1Q, 7   Obstetrical perineal laceration repair
2014, 4Q, 43   Second degree obstetric perineal laceration
2013, 4Q, 120   Repair of second degree perineum obstetric laceration

AHA Coding Clinic for table ØKS
2017, 1Q, 41   Manual reduction of hernia

AHA Coding Clinic for table ØKT
2016, 2Q, 12   Resection of malignant neoplasm of infratemporal fossa
2015, 1Q, 38   Abdominoperineal resection with flap closure of the perineum and colostomy

AHA Coding Clinic for table ØKX
2018, 2Q, 18   Transverse rectus abdominis myocutaneous (TRAM) delay
2017, 4Q, 67   New qualifier values - Pedicle flap procedures
2016, 3Q, 30   Resection of femur with interposition arthroplasty
2015, 3Q, 33   Cleft lip repair using Millard rotation advancement
2015, 2Q, 26   Pharyngeal flap to soft palate
2014, 4Q, 41   Abdominoperineal resection (APR) with flap closure of perineum and colostomy
2014, 2Q, 10   Transverse abdominomyocutaneous (TRAM) breast reconstruction
2014, 2Q, 12   Pedicle latissimus myocutaneous flap with placement of breast tissue expanders

Muscles

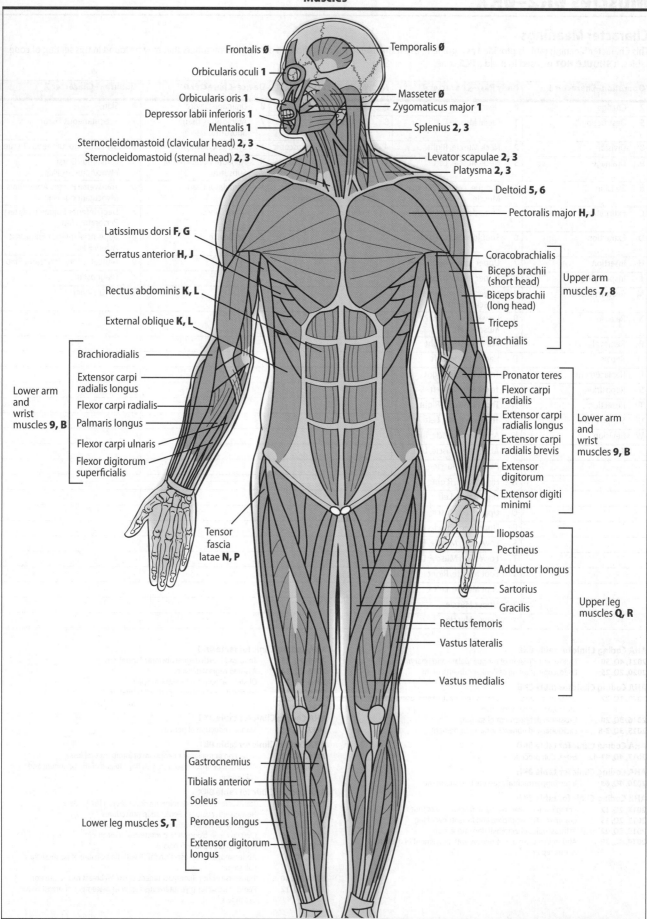

Frontalis **Ø**

Orbicularis oculi **1**

Orbicularis oris **1**

Depressor labii inferioris **1**

Mentalis **1**

Sternocleidomastoid (clavicular head) **2, 3**

Sternocleidomastoid (sternal head) **2, 3**

Temporalis **Ø**

Masseter **Ø**

Zygomaticus major **1**

Splenius **2, 3**

Levator scapulae **2, 3**

Platysma **2, 3**

Deltoid **5, 6**

Pectoralis major **H, J**

Latissimus dorsi **F, G**

Serratus anterior **H, J**

Rectus abdominis **K, L**

External oblique **K, L**

Coracobrachialis

Biceps brachii (short head)

Biceps brachii (long head)

Triceps

Brachialis

Upper arm muscles **7, 8**

Lower arm and wrist muscles **9, B**

Brachioradialis

Extensor carpi radialis longus

Flexor carpi radialis

Palmaris longus

Flexor carpi ulnaris

Flexor digitorum superficialis

Pronator teres

Flexor carpi radialis

Extensor carpi radialis longus

Extensor carpi radialis brevis

Extensor digitorum

Extensor digiti minimi

Lower arm and wrist muscles **9, B**

Tensor fascia latae **N, P**

Iliopsoas

Pectineus

Adductor longus

Sartorius

Gracilis

Rectus femoris

Vastus lateralis

Vastus medialis

Upper leg muscles **Q, R**

Gastrocnemius

Tibialis anterior

Soleus

Peroneus longus

Extensor digitorum longus

Lower leg muscles **S, T**

0   Medical and Surgical
K   Muscles
2   Change   Definition: Taking out or off a device from a body part and putting back an identical or similar device in or on the same body part without cutting or puncturing the skin or a mucous membrane

         Explanation: All CHANGE procedures are coded using the approach EXTERNAL

Body Part Character 4	Approach Character 5	Device Character 6	Qualifier Character 7
X Upper Muscle Y Lower Muscle	X External	0 Drainage Device Y Other Device	Z No Qualifier

Non-OR   All body part, approach, device, and qualifier values

0   Medical and Surgical
K   Muscles
5   Destruction   Definition: Physical eradication of all or a portion of a body part by the direct use of energy, force, or a destructive agent

         Explanation: None of the body part is physically taken out

Body Part Character 4			Approach Character 5	Device Character 6	Qualifier Character 7
0 Head Muscle Auricularis muscle Masseter muscle Pterygoid muscle Splenius capitis muscle Temporalis muscle Temporoparietalis muscle **1 Facial Muscle** Buccinator muscle Corrugator supercilii muscle Depressor anguli oris muscle Depressor labii inferioris muscle Depressor septi nasi muscle Depressor supercilii muscle Levator anguli oris muscle Levator labii superioris alaeque nasi muscle Levator labii superioris muscle Mentalis muscle Nasalis muscle Occipitofrontalis muscle Orbicularis oris muscle Procerus muscle Risorius muscle Zygomaticus muscle **2 Neck Muscle, Right** Anterior vertebral muscle Arytenoid muscle Cricothyroid muscle Infrahyoid muscle Levator scapulae muscle Platysma muscle Scalene muscle Splenius cervicis muscle Sternocleidomastoid muscle Suprahyoid muscle Thyroarytenoid muscle **3 Neck Muscle, Left** *See 2 Neck Muscle, Right* **4 Tongue, Palate, Pharynx Muscle** Chondroglossus muscle Genioglossus muscle Hyoglossus muscle Inferior longitudinal muscle Levator veli palatini muscle Palatoglossal muscle Palatopharyngeal muscle Pharyngeal constrictor muscle Salpingopharyngeus muscle Styloglossus muscle Stylopharyngeus muscle Superior longitudinal muscle Tensor veli palatini muscle **5 Shoulder Muscle, Right** Deltoid muscle Infraspinatus muscle Subscapularis muscle Supraspinatus muscle Teres major muscle Teres minor muscle **6 Shoulder Muscle, Left** *See 5 Shoulder Muscle, Right*	**7 Upper Arm Muscle, Right** Biceps brachii muscle Brachialis muscle Coracobrachialis muscle Triceps brachii muscle **8 Upper Arm Muscle, Left** *See 7 Upper Arm Muscle, Right* **9 Lower Arm and Wrist Muscle, Right** Anatomical snuffbox Brachioradialis muscle Extensor carpi radialis muscle Extensor carpi ulnaris muscle Flexor carpi radialis muscle Flexor carpi ulnaris muscle Flexor pollicis longus muscle Palmaris longus muscle Pronator quadratus muscle Pronator teres muscle **B Lower Arm and Wrist Muscle, Left** *See 9 Lower Arm and Wrist Muscle, Right* **C Hand Muscle, Right** Hypothenar muscle Palmar interosseous muscle Thenar muscle **D Hand Muscle, Left** *See C Hand Muscle, Right* **F Trunk Muscle, Right** Coccygeus muscle Erector spinae muscle Interspinalis muscle Intertransversarius muscle Latissimus dorsi muscle Quadratus lumborum muscle Rhomboid major muscle Rhomboid minor muscle Serratus posterior muscle Transversospinalis muscle Trapezius muscle **G Trunk Muscle, Left** *See F Trunk Muscle, Right* **H Thorax Muscle, Right** Intercostal muscle Levatores costarum muscle Pectoralis major muscle Pectoralis minor muscle Serratus anterior muscle Subclavius muscle Subcostal muscle Transverse thoracis muscle **J Thorax Muscle, Left** *See H Thorax Muscle, Right* **K Abdomen Muscle, Right** External oblique muscle Internal oblique muscle Pyramidalis muscle Rectus abdominis muscle Transversus abdominis muscle **L Abdomen Muscle, Left** *See K Abdomen Muscle, Right*	**M Perineum Muscle** Bulbospongiosus muscle Cremaster muscle Deep transverse perineal muscle Ischiocavernosus muscle Levator ani muscle Superficial transverse perineal muscle **N Hip Muscle, Right** Gemellus muscle Gluteus maximus muscle Gluteus medius muscle Gluteus minimus muscle Iliacus muscle Obturator muscle Piriformis muscle Psoas muscle Quadratus femoris muscle Tensor fasciae latae muscle **P Hip Muscle, Left** *See N Hip Muscle, Right* **Q Upper Leg Muscle, Right** Adductor brevis muscle Adductor longus muscle Adductor magnus muscle Biceps femoris muscle Gracilis muscle Pectineus muscle Quadriceps (femoris) Rectus femoris muscle Sartorius muscle Semimembranosus muscle Semitendinosus muscle Vastus intermedius muscle Vastus lateralis muscle Vastus medialis muscle **R Upper Leg Muscle, Left** *See Q Upper Leg Muscle, Right* **S Lower Leg Muscle, Right** Extensor digitorum longus muscle Extensor hallucis longus muscle Fibularis brevis muscle Fibularis longus muscle Flexor digitorum longus muscle Flexor hallucis longus muscle Gastrocnemius muscle Peroneus brevis muscle Peroneus longus muscle Popliteus muscle Soleus muscle Tibialis anterior muscle Tibialis posterior muscle **T Lower Leg Muscle, Left** *See S Lower Leg Muscle, Right* **V Foot Muscle, Right** Abductor hallucis muscle Adductor hallucis muscle Extensor digitorum brevis muscle Extensor hallucis brevis muscle Flexor digitorum brevis muscle Flexor hallucis brevis muscle Quadratus plantae muscle **W Foot Muscle, Left** *See V Foot Muscle, Right*	**0 Open** **3 Percutaneous** **4 Percutaneous Endoscopic**	**Z No Device**	**Z No Qualifier**

NC Noncovered Procedure   **LC** Limited Coverage   **UA** Questionable OB Admit   **NT** New Tech Add-on   ⊞ Combination Member   ♂ Male   ♀ Female

ICD-10-PCS 2023   465

Ø   Medical and Surgical
K   Muscles
8   Division   Definition: Cutting into a body part, without draining fluids and/or gases from the body part, in order to separate or transect a body part

           Explanation: All or a portion of the body part is separated into two or more portions

Body Part Character 4			Approach Character 5	Device Character 6	Qualifier Character 7
Ø Head Muscle Auricularis muscle Masseter muscle Pterygoid muscle Splenius capitis muscle Temporalis muscle Temporoparietalis muscle **1 Facial Muscle** Buccinator muscle Corrugator supercilii muscle Depressor anguli oris muscle Depressor labii inferioris muscle Depressor septi nasi muscle Depressor supercilii muscle Levator anguli oris muscle Levator labii superioris alaeque nasi muscle Levator labii superioris muscle Mentalis muscle Nasalis muscle Occipitofrontalis muscle Orbicularis oris muscle Procerus muscle Risorius muscle Zygomaticus muscle **2 Neck Muscle, Right** Anterior vertebral muscle Arytenoid muscle Cricothyroid muscle Infrahyoid muscle Levator scapulae muscle Platysma muscle Scalene muscle Splenius cervicis muscle Sternocleidomastoid muscle Suprahyoid muscle Thyroarytenoid muscle **3 Neck Muscle, Left** *See 2 Neck Muscle, Right* Tensor veli palatini muscle **5 Shoulder Muscle, Right** Deltoid muscle Infraspinatus muscle Subscapularis muscle Supraspinatus muscle Teres major muscle Teres minor muscle **6 Shoulder Muscle, Left** *See 5 Shoulder Muscle, Right* **7 Upper Arm Muscle, Right** Biceps brachii muscle Brachialis muscle Coracobrachialis muscle Triceps brachii muscle **8 Upper Arm Muscle, Left** *See 7 Upper Arm Muscle, Right*	**9 Lower Arm and Wrist Muscle, Right** Anatomical snuffbox Brachioradialis muscle Extensor carpi radialis muscle Extensor carpi ulnaris muscle Flexor carpi radialis muscle Flexor carpi ulnaris muscle Flexor pollicis longus muscle Palmaris longus muscle Pronator quadratus muscle Pronator teres muscle **B Lower Arm and Wrist Muscle, Left** *See 9 Lower Arm and Wrist Muscle, Right* **C Hand Muscle, Right** Hypothenar muscle Palmar interosseous muscle Thenar muscle **D Hand Muscle, Left** *See C Hand Muscle, Right* **F Trunk Muscle, Right** Coccygeus muscle Erector spinae muscle Interspinalis muscle Intertransversarius muscle Latissimus dorsi muscle Quadratus lumborum muscle Rhomboid major muscle Rhomboid minor muscle Serratus posterior muscle Transversospinalis muscle Trapezius muscle **G Trunk Muscle, Left** *See F Trunk Muscle, Right* **H Thorax Muscle, Right** Intercostal muscle Levatores costarum muscle Pectoralis major muscle Pectoralis minor muscle Serratus anterior muscle Subclavius muscle Subcostal muscle Transverse thoracis muscle **J Thorax Muscle, Left** *See H Thorax Muscle, Right* **K Abdomen Muscle, Right** External oblique muscle Internal oblique muscle Pyramidalis muscle Rectus abdominis muscle Transversus abdominis muscle **L Abdomen Muscle, Left** *See K Abdomen Muscle, Right* **M Perineum Muscle** Bulbospongiosus muscle Cremaster muscle Deep transverse perineal muscle Ischiocavernosus muscle Levator ani muscle Superficial transverse perineal muscle	**N Hip Muscle, Right** Gemellus muscle Gluteus maximus muscle Gluteus medius muscle Gluteus minimus muscle Iliacus muscle Obturator muscle Piriformis muscle Psoas muscle Quadratus femoris muscle Tensor fasciae latae muscle **P Hip Muscle, Left** *See N Hip Muscle, Right* **Q Upper Leg Muscle, Right** Adductor brevis muscle Adductor longus muscle Adductor magnus muscle Biceps femoris muscle Gracilis muscle Pectineus muscle Quadriceps (femoris) Rectus femoris muscle Sartorius muscle Semimembranosus muscle Semitendinosus muscle Vastus intermedius muscle Vastus lateralis muscle Vastus medialis muscle **R Upper Leg Muscle, Left** *See Q Upper Leg Muscle, Right* **S Lower Leg Muscle, Right** Extensor digitorum longus muscle Extensor hallucis longus muscle Fibularis brevis muscle Fibularis longus muscle Flexor digitorum longus muscle Flexor hallucis longus muscle Gastrocnemius muscle Peroneus brevis muscle Peroneus longus muscle Popliteus muscle Soleus muscle Tibialis anterior muscle Tibialis posterior muscle **T Lower Leg Muscle, Left** *See S Lower Leg Muscle, Right* **V Foot Muscle, Right** Abductor hallucis muscle Adductor hallucis muscle Extensor digitorum brevis muscle Extensor hallucis brevis muscle Flexor digitorum brevis muscle Flexor hallucis brevis muscle Quadratus plantae muscle **W Foot Muscle, Left** *See V Foot Muscle, Right*	**Ø Open** **3 Percutaneous** **4 Percutaneous Endoscopic**	**Z No Device**	**Z No Qualifier**
4 Tongue, Palate, Pharynx Muscle Chondroglossus muscle Genioglossus muscle Hyoglossus muscle Inferior longitudinal muscle Levator veli palatini muscle Palatoglossal muscle Palatopharyngeal muscle Pharyngeal constrictor muscle Salpingopharyngeus muscle Styloglossus muscle Stylopharyngeus muscle Superior longitudinal muscle Tensor veli palatini muscle			**Ø Open** **3 Percutaneous** **4 Percutaneous Endoscopic** **7 Via Natural or Artificial Opening** **8 Via Natural or Artificial Opening Endoscopic**	**Z No Device**	**Z No Qualifier**

Non-OR Procedure   DRG Non-OR Procedure   Valid OR Procedure   HAC Associated Procedure   Combination Only   New/Revised April   New/Revised October

466   ICD-10-PCS 2023

ØK8–ØK8

Ø　Medical and Surgical
K　Muscles
9　Drainage　　Definition: Taking or letting out fluids and/or gases from a body part
　　　　　　　　　Explanation: The qualifier DIAGNOSTIC is used to identify drainage procedures that are biopsies

Body Part — Character 4			Approach — Character 5	Device — Character 6	Qualifier — Character 7
Ø Head Muscle	**7 Upper Arm Muscle, Right**	**M Perineum Muscle**	**Ø Open**	**Ø Drainage Device**	**Z No Qualifier**
Auricularis muscle	Biceps brachii muscle	Bulbospongiosus muscle	**3 Percutaneous**		
Masseter muscle	Brachialis muscle	Cremaster muscle	**4 Percutaneous Endoscopic**		
Pterygoid muscle	Coracobrachialis muscle	Deep transverse perineal muscle			
Splenius capitis muscle	Triceps brachii muscle	Ischiocavernosus muscle			
Temporalis muscle	**8 Upper Arm Muscle, Left**	Levator ani muscle			
Temporoparietalis muscle	*See 7 Upper Arm Muscle, Right*	Superficial transverse perineal muscle			
1 Facial Muscle	**9 Lower Arm and Wrist Muscle, Right**	**N Hip Muscle, Right**			
Buccinator muscle	Anatomical snuffbox	Gemellus muscle			
Corrugator supercilii muscle	Brachioradialis muscle	Gluteus maximus muscle			
Depressor anguli oris muscle	Extensor carpi radialis muscle	Gluteus medius muscle			
Depressor labii inferioris muscle	Extensor carpi ulnaris muscle	Gluteus minimus muscle			
Depressor septi nasi muscle	Flexor carpi radialis muscle	Iliacus muscle			
Depressor supercilii muscle	Flexor carpi ulnaris muscle	Obturator muscle			
Levator anguli oris muscle	Flexor pollicis longus muscle	Piriformis muscle			
Levator labii superioris alaeque nasi muscle	Palmaris longus muscle	Psoas muscle			
Levator labii superioris muscle	Pronator quadratus muscle	Quadratus femoris muscle			
Mentalis muscle	Pronator teres muscle	Tensor fasciae latae muscle			
Nasalis muscle	**B Lower Arm and Wrist Muscle, Left**	**P Hip Muscle, Left**			
Occipitofrontalis muscle	*See 9 Lower Arm and Wrist Muscle, Right*	*See N Hip Muscle, Right*			
Orbicularis oris muscle	**C Hand Muscle, Right**	**Q Upper Leg Muscle, Right**			
Procerus muscle	Hypothenar muscle	Adductor brevis muscle			
Risorius muscle	Palmar interosseous muscle	Adductor longus muscle			
Zygomaticus muscle	Thenar muscle	Adductor magnus muscle			
2 Neck Muscle, Right	**D Hand Muscle, Left**	Biceps femoris muscle			
Anterior vertebral muscle	*See C Hand Muscle, Right*	Gracilis muscle			
Arytenoid muscle	**F Trunk Muscle, Right**	Pectineus muscle			
Cricothyroid muscle	Coccygeus muscle	Quadriceps (femoris)			
Infrahyoid muscle	Erector spinae muscle	Rectus femoris muscle			
Levator scapulae muscle	Interspinalis muscle	Sartorius muscle			
Platysma muscle	Intertransversarius muscle	Semimembranosus muscle			
Scalene muscle	Latissimus dorsi muscle	Semitendinosus muscle			
Splenius cervicis muscle	Quadratus lumborum muscle	Vastus intermedius muscle			
Sternocleidomastoid muscle	Rhomboid major muscle	Vastus lateralis muscle			
Suprahyoid muscle	Rhomboid minor muscle	Vastus medialis muscle			
Thyroarytenoid muscle	Serratus posterior muscle	**R Upper Leg Muscle, Left**			
3 Neck Muscle, Left	Transversospinalis muscle	*See Q Upper Leg Muscle, Right*			
See 2 Neck Muscle, Right	Trapezius muscle	**S Lower Leg Muscle, Right**			
4 Tongue, Palate, Pharynx Muscle	**G Trunk Muscle, Left**	Extensor digitorum longus muscle			
Chondroglossus muscle	*See F Trunk Muscle, Right*	Extensor hallucis longus muscle			
Genioglossus muscle	**H Thorax Muscle, Right**	Fibularis brevis muscle			
Hyoglossus muscle	Intercostal muscle	Fibularis longus muscle			
Inferior longitudinal muscle	Levatores costarum muscle	Flexor digitorum longus muscle			
Levator veli palatini muscle	Pectoralis major muscle	Flexor hallucis longus muscle			
Palatoglossal muscle	Pectoralis minor muscle	Gastrocnemius muscle			
Palatopharyngeal muscle	Serratus anterior muscle	Peroneus brevis muscle			
Pharyngeal constrictor muscle	Subclavius muscle	Peroneus longus muscle			
Salpingopharyngeus muscle	Subcostal muscle	Popliteus muscle			
Styloglossus muscle	Transverse thoracis muscle	Soleus muscle			
Stylopharyngeus muscle	**J Thorax Muscle, Left**	Tibialis anterior muscle			
Superior longitudinal muscle	*See H Thorax Muscle, Right*	Tibialis posterior muscle			
Tensor veli palatini muscle	**K Abdomen Muscle, Right**	**T Lower Leg Muscle, Left**			
5 Shoulder Muscle, Right	External oblique muscle	*See S Lower Leg Muscle, Right*			
Deltoid muscle	Internal oblique muscle	**V Foot Muscle, Right**			
Infraspinatus muscle	Pyramidalis muscle	Abductor hallucis muscle			
Subscapularis muscle	Rectus abdominis muscle	Adductor hallucis muscle			
Supraspinatus muscle	Transversus abdominis muscle	Extensor digitorum brevis muscle			
Teres major muscle	**L Abdomen Muscle, Left**	Extensor hallucis brevis muscle			
Teres minor muscle	*See K Abdomen Muscle, Right*	Flexor digitorum brevis muscle			
6 Shoulder Muscle, Left		Flexor hallucis brevis muscle			
See 5 Shoulder Muscle, Right		Quadratus plantae muscle			
		W Foot Muscle, Left			
		See V Foot Muscle, Right			

Non-OR　ØK9[Ø,1,2,3,4,5,6,7,8,9,B,C,D,F,G,H,J,K,L,M,N,P,Q,R,S,T,V,W]3ØZ

ØK9 Continued on next page

Ø   **Medical and Surgical**   *ØK9 Continued*
K   **Muscles**
9   **Drainage**   Definition: Taking or letting out fluids and/or gases from a body part
                           Explanation: The qualifier DIAGNOSTIC is used to identify drainage procedures that are biopsies

Body Part Character 4			Approach Character 5	Device Character 6	Qualifier Character 7
Ø Head Muscle Auricularis muscle Masseter muscle Pterygoid muscle Splenius capitis muscle Temporalis muscle Temporoparietalis muscle	**7 Upper Arm Muscle, Right** Biceps brachii muscle Brachialis muscle Coracobrachialis muscle Triceps brachii muscle	**M Perineum Muscle** Bulbospongiosus muscle Cremaster muscle Deep transverse perineal muscle Ischiocavernosus muscle	**Ø Open** **3 Percutaneous** **4 Percutaneous Endoscopic**	**Z No Device**	**X Diagnostic** **Z No Qualifier**
1 Facial Muscle Buccinator muscle Corrugator supercilii muscle Depressor anguli oris muscle Depressor labii inferioris muscle Depressor septi nasi muscle Depressor supercilii muscle Levator anguli oris muscle Levator labii superioris alaeque nasi muscle Levator labii superioris muscle Mentalis muscle Nasalis muscle Occipitofrontalis muscle Orbicularis oris muscle Procerus muscle Risorius muscle Zygomaticus muscle	**8 Upper Arm Muscle, Left** *See 7 Upper Arm Muscle, Right* **9 Lower Arm and Wrist Muscle, Right** Anatomical snuffbox Brachioradialis muscle Extensor carpi radialis muscle Extensor carpi ulnaris muscle Flexor carpi radialis muscle Flexor carpi ulnaris muscle Flexor pollicis longus muscle Palmaris longus muscle Pronator quadratus muscle Pronator teres muscle	Levator ani muscle Superficial transverse perineal muscle **N Hip Muscle, Right** Gemellus muscle Gluteus maximus muscle Gluteus medius muscle Gluteus minimus muscle Iliacus muscle Obturator muscle Piriformis muscle Psoas muscle Quadratus femoris muscle Tensor fasciae latae muscle			
2 Neck Muscle, Right Anterior vertebral muscle Arytenoid muscle Cricothyroid muscle Infrahyoid muscle Levator scapulae muscle Platysma muscle Scalene muscle Splenius cervicis muscle Sternocleidomastoid muscle Suprahyoid muscle Thyroarytenoid muscle	**B Lower Arm and Wrist Muscle, Left** *See 9 Lower Arm and Wrist Muscle, Right* **C Hand Muscle, Right** Hypothenar muscle Palmar interosseous muscle Thenar muscle	**P Hip Muscle, Left** *See N Hip Muscle, Right* **Q Upper Leg Muscle, Right** Adductor brevis muscle Adductor longus muscle Adductor magnus muscle Biceps femoris muscle Gracilis muscle Pectineus muscle Quadriceps (femoris) Rectus femoris muscle Sartorius muscle Semimembranosus muscle			
3 Neck Muscle, Left *See 2 Neck Muscle, Right* **4 Tongue, Palate, Pharynx Muscle** Chondroglossus muscle Genioglossus muscle Hyoglossus muscle Inferior longitudinal muscle Levator veli palatini muscle Palatoglossal muscle Palatopharyngeal muscle Pharyngeal constrictor muscle Salpingopharyngeus muscle Styloglossus muscle Stylopharyngeus muscle Superior longitudinal muscle Tensor veli palatini muscle	**D Hand Muscle, Left** *See C Hand Muscle, Right* **F Trunk Muscle, Right** Coccygeus muscle Erector spinae muscle Interspinalis muscle Intertransversarius muscle Latissimus dorsi muscle Quadratus lumborum muscle Rhomboid major muscle Rhomboid minor muscle Serratus posterior muscle Transversospinalis muscle Trapezius muscle **G Trunk Muscle, Left** *See F Trunk Muscle, Right*	Semitendinosus muscle Vastus intermedius muscle Vastus lateralis muscle Vastus medialis muscle **R Upper Leg Muscle, Left** *See Q Upper Leg Muscle, Right* **S Lower Leg Muscle, Right** Extensor digitorum longus muscle Extensor hallucis longus muscle Fibularis brevis muscle Fibularis longus muscle Flexor digitorum longus muscle Flexor hallucis longus muscle Gastrocnemius muscle Peroneus brevis muscle			
5 Shoulder Muscle, Right Deltoid muscle Infraspinatus muscle Subscapularis muscle Supraspinatus muscle Teres major muscle Teres minor muscle **6 Shoulder Muscle, Left** *See 5 Shoulder Muscle, Right*	**H Thorax Muscle, Right** Intercostal muscle Levatores costarum muscle Pectoralis major muscle Pectoralis minor muscle Serratus anterior muscle Subclavius muscle Subcostal muscle Transverse thoracis muscle **J Thorax Muscle, Left** *See H Thorax Muscle, Right* **K Abdomen Muscle, Right** External oblique muscle Internal oblique muscle Pyramidalis muscle Rectus abdominis muscle Transversus abdominis muscle **L Abdomen Muscle, Left** *See K Abdomen Muscle, Right*	Peroneus longus muscle Popliteus muscle Soleus muscle Tibialis anterior muscle Tibialis posterior muscle **T Lower Leg Muscle, Left** *See S Lower Leg Muscle, Right* **V Foot Muscle, Right** Abductor hallucis muscle Adductor hallucis muscle Extensor digitorum brevis muscle Extensor hallucis brevis muscle Flexor digitorum brevis muscle Flexor hallucis brevis muscle Quadratus plantae muscle **W Foot Muscle, Left** *See V Foot Muscle, Right*			

Non-OR   ØK9[Ø,1,2,3,4,5,6,7,8,9,B,F,G,H,J,K,L,M,N,P,Q,R,S,T,V,W]3ZZ
Non-OR   ØK9[C,D][3,4]ZZ

Non-OR Procedure   DRG Non-OR Procedure   Valid OR Procedure   HAC Associated Procedure   Combination Only   New/Revised April   New/Revised October

Ø   Medical and Surgical
K   Muscles
B   Excision   Definition: Cutting out or off, without replacement, a portion of a body part
                       Explanation: The qualifier DIAGNOSTIC is used to identify excision procedures that are biopsies

Body Part Character 4			Approach Character 5	Device Character 6	Qualifier Character 7
Ø Head Muscle Auricularis muscle Masseter muscle Pterygoid muscle Splenius capitis muscle Temporalis muscle Temporoparietalis muscle **1 Facial Muscle** Buccinator muscle Corrugator supercilii muscle Depressor anguli oris muscle Depressor labii inferioris muscle Depressor septi nasi muscle Depressor supercilii muscle Levator anguli oris muscle Levator labii superioris alaeque nasi muscle Levator labii superioris muscle Mentalis muscle Nasalis muscle Occipitofrontalis muscle Orbicularis oris muscle Procerus muscle Risorius muscle Zygomaticus muscle **2 Neck Muscle, Right** Anterior vertebral muscle Arytenoid muscle Cricothyroid muscle Infrahyoid muscle Levator scapulae muscle Platysma muscle Scalene muscle Splenius cervicis muscle Sternocleidomastoid muscle Suprahyoid muscle Thyroarytenoid muscle **3 Neck Muscle, Left** *See 2 Neck Muscle, Right* **4 Tongue, Palate, Pharynx Muscle** Chondroglossus muscle Genioglossus muscle Hyoglossus muscle Inferior longitudinal muscle Levator veli palatini muscle Palatoglossal muscle Palatopharyngeal muscle Pharyngeal constrictor muscle Salpingopharyngeus muscle Styloglossus muscle Stylopharyngeus muscle Superior longitudinal muscle Tensor veli palatini muscle **5 Shoulder Muscle, Right** Deltoid muscle Infraspinatus muscle Subscapularis muscle Supraspinatus muscle Teres major muscle Teres minor muscle **6 Shoulder Muscle, Left** *See 5 Shoulder Muscle, Right*	**7 Upper Arm Muscle, Right** Biceps brachii muscle Brachialis muscle Coracobrachialis muscle Triceps brachii muscle **8 Upper Arm Muscle, Left** *See 7 Upper Arm Muscle, Right* **9 Lower Arm and Wrist Muscle, Right** Anatomical snuffbox Brachioradialis muscle Extensor carpi radialis muscle Extensor carpi ulnaris muscle Flexor carpi radialis muscle Flexor carpi ulnaris muscle Flexor pollicis longus muscle Palmaris longus muscle Pronator quadratus muscle Pronator teres muscle **B Lower Arm and Wrist Muscle, Left** *See 9 Lower Arm and Wrist Muscle, Right* **C Hand Muscle, Right** Hypothenar muscle Palmar interosseous muscle Thenar muscle **D Hand Muscle, Left** *See C Hand Muscle, Right* **F Trunk Muscle, Right** Coccygeus muscle Erector spinae muscle Interspinalis muscle Intertransversarius muscle Latissimus dorsi muscle Quadratus lumborum muscle Rhomboid major muscle Rhomboid minor muscle Serratus posterior muscle Transversospinalis muscle Trapezius muscle **G Trunk Muscle, Left** *See F Trunk Muscle, Right* **H Thorax Muscle, Right** Intercostal muscle Levatores costarum muscle Pectoralis major muscle Pectoralis minor muscle Serratus anterior muscle Subclavius muscle Subcostal muscle Transverse thoracis muscle **J Thorax Muscle, Left** *See H Thorax Muscle, Right* **K Abdomen Muscle, Right** External oblique muscle Internal oblique muscle Pyramidalis muscle Rectus abdominis muscle Transversus abdominis muscle **L Abdomen Muscle, Left** *See K Abdomen Muscle, Right*	**M Perineum Muscle** Bulbospongiosus muscle Cremaster muscle Deep transverse perineal muscle Ischiocavernosus muscle Levator ani muscle Superficial transverse perineal muscle **N Hip Muscle, Right** Gemellus muscle Gluteus maximus muscle Gluteus medius muscle Gluteus minimus muscle Iliacus muscle Obturator muscle Piriformis muscle Psoas muscle Quadratus femoris muscle Tensor fasciae latae muscle **P Hip Muscle, Left** *See N Hip Muscle, Right* **Q Upper Leg Muscle, Right** Adductor brevis muscle Adductor longus muscle Adductor magnus muscle Biceps femoris muscle Gracilis muscle Pectineus muscle Quadriceps (femoris) Rectus femoris muscle Sartorius muscle Semimembranosus muscle Semitendinosus muscle Vastus intermedius muscle Vastus lateralis muscle Vastus medialis muscle **R Upper Leg Muscle, Left** *See Q Upper Leg Muscle, Right* **S Lower Leg Muscle, Right** Extensor digitorum longus muscle Extensor hallucis longus muscle Fibularis brevis muscle Fibularis longus muscle Flexor digitorum longus muscle Flexor hallucis longus muscle Gastrocnemius muscle Peroneus brevis muscle Peroneus longus muscle Popliteus muscle Soleus muscle Tibialis anterior muscle Tibialis posterior muscle **T Lower Leg Muscle, Left** *See S Lower Leg Muscle, Right* **V Foot Muscle, Right** Abductor hallucis muscle Adductor hallucis muscle Extensor digitorum brevis muscle Extensor hallucis brevis muscle Flexor digitorum brevis muscle Flexor hallucis brevis muscle Quadratus plantae muscle **W Foot Muscle, Left** *See V Foot Muscle, Right*	**Ø Open** **3 Percutaneous** **4 Percutaneous Endoscopic**	**Z No Device**	**X Diagnostic** **Z No Qualifier**

Non-OR   ØKB[N,P]3Z[X,Z]

NC Noncovered Procedure   **LC** Limited Coverage   **QA** Questionable OB Admit   **NT** New Tech Add-on   ✚ Combination Member   ♂ Male   ♀ Female
ICD-10-PCS 2023   **469**

Ø   **Medical and Surgical**
K   **Muscles**
C   **Extirpation**   Definition: Taking or cutting out solid matter from a body part

Explanation: The solid matter may be an abnormal byproduct of a biological function or a foreign body; it may be imbedded in a body part or in the lumen of a tubular body part. The solid matter may or may not have been previously broken into pieces.

Body Part Character 4		Approach Character 5	Device Character 6	Qualifier Character 7

Ø **Head Muscle**
   Auricularis muscle
   Masseter muscle
   Pterygoid muscle
   Splenius capitis muscle
   Temporalis muscle
   Temporoparietalis muscle
1 **Facial Muscle**
   Buccinator muscle
   Corrugator supercilii
     muscle
   Depressor anguli oris
     muscle
   Depressor labii inferioris
     muscle
   Depressor septi nasi
     muscle
   Depressor supercilii
     muscle
   Levator anguli oris muscle
   Levator labii superioris
     alaeque nasi muscle
   Levator labii superioris
     muscle
   Mentalis muscle
   Nasalis muscle
   Occipitofrontalis muscle
   Orbicularis oris muscle
   Procerus muscle
   Risorius muscle
   Zygomaticus muscle
2 **Neck Muscle, Right**
   Anterior vertebral muscle
   Arytenoid muscle
   Cricothyroid muscle
   Infrahyoid muscle
   Levator scapulae muscle
   Platysma muscle
   Scalene muscle
   Splenius cervicis muscle
   Sternocleidomastoid
     muscle
   Suprahyoid muscle
   Thyroarytenoid muscle
3 **Neck Muscle, Left**
   See 2 Neck Muscle, Right
4 **Tongue, Palate, Pharynx**
   Muscle
   Chondroglossus muscle
   Genioglossus muscle
   Hyoglossus muscle
   Inferior longitudinal
     muscle
   Levator veli palatini
     muscle
   Palatoglossal muscle
   Palatopharyngeal muscle
   Pharyngeal constrictor
     muscle
   Salpingopharyngeus
     muscle
   Styloglossus muscle
   Stylopharyngeus muscle
   Superior longitudinal
     muscle
   Tensor veli palatini muscle
5 **Shoulder Muscle, Right**
   Deltoid muscle
   Infraspinatus muscle
   Subscapularis muscle
   Supraspinatus muscle
   Teres major muscle
   Teres minor muscle
6 **Shoulder Muscle, Left**
   See 5 Shoulder Muscle,
   Right
	7 **Upper Arm Muscle, Right**
	   Biceps brachii muscle
	   Brachialis muscle
	   Coracobrachialis muscle
	   Triceps brachii muscle
	8 **Upper Arm Muscle, Left**
	   See 7 Upper Arm Muscle,
	   Right
	9 **Lower Arm and Wrist**
	   Muscle, Right
	   Anatomical snuffbox
	   Brachioradialis muscle
	   Extensor carpi radialis
	     muscle
	   Extensor carpi ulnaris
	     muscle
	   Flexor carpi radialis
	     muscle
	   Flexor carpi ulnaris muscle
	   Flexor pollicis longus
	     muscle
	   Palmaris longus muscle
	   Pronator quadratus
	     muscle
	   Pronator teres muscle
	B **Lower Arm and Wrist**
	   Muscle, Left
	   See 9 Lower Arm and Wrist
	   Muscle, Right
	C **Hand Muscle, Right**
	   Hypothenar muscle
	   Palmar interosseous
	     muscle
	   Thenar muscle
	D **Hand Muscle, Left**
	   See C Hand Muscle, Right
	F **Trunk Muscle, Right**
	   Coccygeus muscle
	   Erector spinae muscle
	   Interspinalis muscle
	   Intertransversarius muscle
	   Latissimus dorsi muscle
	   Quadratus lumborum
	     muscle
	   Rhomboid major muscle
	   Rhomboid minor muscle
	   Serratus posterior muscle
	   Transversospinalis muscle
	   Trapezius muscle
	G **Trunk Muscle, Left**
	   See F Trunk Muscle, Right
	H **Thorax Muscle, Right**
	   Intercostal muscle
	   Levatores costarum
	     muscle
	   Pectoralis major muscle
	   Pectoralis minor muscle
	   Serratus anterior muscle
	   Subclavius muscle
	   Subcostal muscle
	   Transverse thoracis
	     muscle
	J **Thorax Muscle, Left**
	   See H Thorax Muscle, Right
	K **Abdomen Muscle, Right**
	   External oblique muscle
	   Internal oblique muscle
	   Pyramidalis muscle
	   Rectus abdominis muscle
	   Transversus abdominis
	     muscle
	L **Abdomen Muscle, Left**
	   See K Abdomen Muscle,
	   Right
		M **Perineum Muscle**
		   Bulbospongiosus muscle
		   Cremaster muscle
		   Deep transverse perineal
		     muscle
		   Ischiocavernosus muscle
		   Levator ani muscle
		   Superficial transverse
		     perineal muscle
		N **Hip Muscle, Right**
		   Gemellus muscle
		   Gluteus maximus muscle
		   Gluteus medius muscle
		   Gluteus minimus muscle
		   Iliacus muscle
		   Obturator muscle
		   Piriformis muscle
		   Psoas muscle
		   Quadratus femoris muscle
		   Tensor fasciae latae
		     muscle
		P **Hip Muscle, Left**
		   See N Hip Muscle, Right
		Q **Upper Leg Muscle, Right**
		   Adductor brevis muscle
		   Adductor longus muscle
		   Adductor magnus muscle
		   Biceps femoris muscle
		   Gracilis muscle
		   Pectineus muscle
		   Quadriceps (femoris)
		   Rectus femoris muscle
		   Sartorius muscle
		   Semimembranosus
		     muscle
		   Semitendinosus muscle
		   Vastus intermedius muscle
		   Vastus lateralis muscle
		   Vastus medialis muscle
		R **Upper Leg Muscle, Left**
		   See Q Upper Leg Muscle,
		   Right
		S **Lower Leg Muscle, Right**
		   Extensor digitorum longus
		     muscle
		   Extensor hallucis longus
		     muscle
		   Fibularis brevis muscle
		   Fibularis longus muscle
		   Flexor digitorum longus
		     muscle
		   Flexor hallucis longus
		     muscle
		   Gastrocnemius muscle
		   Peroneus brevis muscle
		   Peroneus longus muscle
		   Popliteus muscle
		   Soleus muscle
		   Tibialis anterior muscle
		   Tibialis posterior muscle
		T **Lower Leg Muscle, Left**
		   See S Lower Leg Muscle,
		   Right
		V **Foot Muscle, Right**
		   Abductor hallucis muscle
		   Adductor hallucis muscle
		   Extensor digitorum brevis
		     muscle
		   Extensor hallucis brevis
		     muscle
		   Flexor digitorum brevis
		     muscle
		   Flexor hallucis brevis
		     muscle
		   Quadratus plantae muscle
		W **Foot Muscle, Left**
		   See V Foot Muscle, Right
			Ø Open
			3 Percutaneous
			4 Percutaneous
			   Endoscopic
				Z No Device	**Z** No Qualifier

Non-OR Procedure   DRG Non-OR Procedure   Valid OR Procedure   HAC Associated Procedure   Combination Only   New/Revised April   New/Revised October

470   ICD-10-PCS 2023

ØKC–ØKC

Ø   **Medical and Surgical**
K   **Muscles**
D   **Extraction**   Definition: Pulling or stripping out or off all or a portion of a body part by the use of force
                  Explanation: The qualifier DIAGNOSTIC is used to identify extraction procedures that are biopsies

Body Part Character 4		Approach Character 5	Device Character 6	Qualifier Character 7
Ø **Head Muscle** Auricularis muscle Masseter muscle Pterygoid muscle Splenius capitis muscle Temporalis muscle Temporoparietalis muscle **1** **Facial Muscle** Buccinator muscle Corrugator supercilii muscle Depressor anguli oris muscle Depressor labii inferioris muscle Depressor septi nasi muscle Depressor supercilii muscle Levator anguli oris muscle Levator labii superioris alaeque nasi muscle Levator labii superioris muscle Mentalis muscle Nasalis muscle Occipitofrontalis muscle Orbicularis oris muscle Procerus muscle Risorius muscle Zygomaticus muscle **2** **Neck Muscle, Right** Anterior vertebral muscle Arytenoid muscle Cricothyroid muscle Infrahyoid muscle Levator scapulae muscle Platysma muscle Scalene muscle Splenius cervicis muscle Sternocleidomastoid muscle Suprahyoid muscle Thyroarytenoid muscle **3** **Neck Muscle, Left** *See 2 Neck Muscle, Right* **4** **Tongue, Palate, Pharynx Muscle** Chondroglossus muscle Genioglossus muscle Hyoglossus muscle Inferior longitudinal muscle Levator veli palatini muscle Palatoglossal muscle Palatopharyngeal muscle Pharyngeal constrictor muscle Salpingopharyngeus muscle Styloglossus muscle Stylopharyngeus muscle Superior longitudinal muscle Tensor veli palatini muscle **5** **Shoulder Muscle, Right** Deltoid muscle Infraspinatus muscle Subscapularis muscle Supraspinatus muscle Teres major muscle Teres minor muscle **6** **Shoulder Muscle, Left** *See 5 Shoulder Muscle, Right*	**7** **Upper Arm Muscle, Right** Biceps brachii muscle Brachialis muscle Coracobrachialis muscle Triceps brachii muscle **8** **Upper Arm Muscle, Left** *See 7 Upper Arm Muscle, Right* **9** **Lower Arm and Wrist Muscle, Right** Anatomical snuffbox Brachioradialis muscle Extensor carpi radialis muscle Extensor carpi ulnaris muscle Flexor carpi radialis muscle Flexor carpi ulnaris muscle Flexor pollicis longus muscle Palmaris longus muscle Pronator quadratus muscle Pronator teres muscle **B** **Lower Arm and Wrist Muscle, Left** *See 9 Lower Arm and Wrist Muscle, Right* **C** **Hand Muscle, Right** Hypothenar muscle Palmar interosseous muscle Thenar muscle **D** **Hand Muscle, Left** *See C Hand Muscle, Right* **F** **Trunk Muscle, Right** Coccygeus muscle Erector spinae muscle Interspinalis muscle Intertransversarius muscle Latissimus dorsi muscle Quadratus lumborum muscle Rhomboid major muscle Rhomboid minor muscle Serratus posterior muscle Transversospinalis muscle Trapezius muscle **G** **Trunk Muscle, Left** *See F Trunk Muscle, Right* **H** **Thorax Muscle, Right** Intercostal muscle Levatores costarum muscle Pectoralis major muscle Pectoralis minor muscle Serratus anterior muscle Subclavius muscle Subcostal muscle Transverse thoracis muscle **J** **Thorax Muscle, Left** *See H Thorax Muscle, Right* **K** **Abdomen Muscle, Right** External oblique muscle Internal oblique muscle Pyramidalis muscle Rectus abdominis muscle Transversus abdominis muscle **L** **Abdomen Muscle, Left** *See K Abdomen Muscle, Right*	**M** **Perineum Muscle** Bulbospongiosus muscle Cremaster muscle Deep transverse perineal muscle Ischiocavernosus muscle Levator ani muscle Superficial transverse perineal muscle **N** **Hip Muscle, Right** Gemellus muscle Gluteus maximus muscle Gluteus medius muscle Gluteus minimus muscle Iliacus muscle Obturator muscle Piriformis muscle Psoas muscle Quadratus femoris muscle Tensor fasciae latae muscle **P** **Hip Muscle, Left** *See N Hip Muscle, Right* **Q** **Upper Leg Muscle, Right** Adductor brevis muscle Adductor longus muscle Adductor magnus muscle Biceps femoris muscle Gracilis muscle Pectineus muscle Quadriceps (femoris) Rectus femoris muscle Sartorius muscle Semimembranosus muscle Semitendinosus muscle Vastus intermedius muscle Vastus lateralis muscle Vastus medialis muscle **R** **Upper Leg Muscle, Left** *See Q Upper Leg Muscle, Right* **S** **Lower Leg Muscle, Right** Extensor digitorum longus muscle Extensor hallucis longus muscle Fibularis brevis muscle Fibularis longus muscle Flexor digitorum longus muscle Flexor hallucis longus muscle Gastrocnemius muscle Peroneus brevis muscle Peroneus longus muscle Popliteus muscle Soleus muscle Tibialis anterior muscle Tibialis posterior muscle **T** **Lower Leg Muscle, Left** *See S Lower Leg Muscle, Right* **V** **Foot Muscle, Right** Abductor hallucis muscle Adductor hallucis muscle Extensor digitorum brevis muscle Extensor hallucis brevis muscle Flexor digitorum brevis muscle Flexor hallucis brevis muscle Quadratus plantae muscle **W** **Foot Muscle, Left** *See V Foot Muscle, Right*	**Ø** Open	**Z** No Device	**Z** No Qualifier

NC Noncovered Procedure   LC Limited Coverage   QA Questionable OB Admit   NT New Tech Add-on   ✚ Combination Member   ♂ Male   ♀ Female

ICD-10-PCS 2023   471

ØKD–ØKD

Ø   Medical and Surgical
K   Muscles
H   Insertion   Definition: Putting in a nonbiological appliance that monitors, assists, performs, or prevents a physiological function but does not physically take the place of a body part
Explanation: None

Body Part Character 4	Approach Character 5	Device Character 6	Qualifier Character 7
X Upper Muscle Y Lower Muscle	Ø Open 3 Percutaneous 4 Percutaneous Endoscopic	M Stimulator Lead Y Other Device	Z No Qualifier

Non-OR   ØKH[X,Y][3,4]YZ

Ø   Medical and Surgical
K   Muscles
J   Inspection   Definition: Visually and/or manually exploring a body part
Explanation: Visual exploration may be performed with or without optical instrumentation. Manual exploration may be performed directly or through intervening body layers.

Body Part Character 4	Approach Character 5	Device Character 6	Qualifier Character 7
X Upper Muscle Y Lower Muscle	Ø Open 3 Percutaneous 4 Percutaneous Endoscopic X External	Z No Device	Z No Qualifier

Non-OR   ØKJ[X,Y][3,X]ZZ

Non-OR Procedure   DRG Non-OR Procedure   Valid OR Procedure   HAC Associated Procedure   Combination Only   New/Revised April   New/Revised October

472

ØKH–ØKJ

ICD-10-PCS 2023

Ø   **Medical and Surgical**
K   **Muscles**
M   **Reattachment**   Definition: Putting back in or on all or a portion of a separated body part to its normal location or other suitable location
                            Explanation: Vascular circulation and nervous pathways may or may not be reestablished

Body Part Character 4			Approach Character 5	Device Character 6	Qualifier Character 7
Ø **Head Muscle**	**7** **Upper Arm Muscle, Right**	**M** **Perineum Muscle**	**Ø** Open	**Z** No Device	**Z** No Qualifier
Auricularis muscle	Biceps brachii muscle	Bulbospongiosus muscle	**4** Percutaneous		
Masseter muscle	Brachialis muscle	Cremaster muscle	Endoscopic		
Pterygoid muscle	Coracobrachialis muscle	Deep transverse perineal			
Splenius capitis muscle	Triceps brachii muscle	muscle			
Temporalis muscle	**8** **Upper Arm Muscle, Left**	Ischiocavernosus muscle			
Temporoparietalis muscle	*See 7 Upper Arm Muscle,*	Levator ani muscle			
1 **Facial Muscle**	*Right*	Superficial transverse			
Buccinator muscle	**9** **Lower Arm and Wrist**	perineal muscle			
Corrugator supercilii	**Muscle, Right**	**N** **Hip Muscle, Right**			
muscle	Anatomical snuffbox	Gemellus muscle			
Depressor anguli oris	Brachioradialis muscle	Gluteus maximus muscle			
muscle	Extensor carpi radialis	Gluteus medius muscle			
Depressor labii inferioris	muscle	Gluteus minimus muscle			
muscle	Extensor carpi ulnaris	Iliacus muscle			
Depressor septi nasi	muscle	Obturator muscle			
muscle	Flexor carpi radialis	Piriformis muscle			
Depressor supercilii	muscle	Psoas muscle			
muscle	Flexor carpi ulnaris muscle	Quadratus femoris muscle			
Levator anguli oris muscle	Flexor pollicis longus	Tensor fasciae latae			
Levator labii superioris	muscle	muscle			
alaeque nasi muscle	Palmaris longus muscle	**P** **Hip Muscle, Left**			
Levator labii superioris	Pronator quadratus	*See N Hip Muscle, Right*			
muscle	muscle	**Q** **Upper Leg Muscle, Right**			
Mentalis muscle	Pronator teres muscle	Adductor brevis muscle			
Nasalis muscle	**B** **Lower Arm and Wrist**	Adductor longus muscle			
Occipitofrontalis muscle	**Muscle, Left**	Adductor magnus muscle			
Orbicularis oris muscle	*See 9 Lower Arm and Wrist*	Biceps femoris muscle			
Procerus muscle	*Muscle, Right*	Gracilis muscle			
Risorius muscle	**C** **Hand Muscle, Right**	Pectineus muscle			
Zygomaticus muscle	Hypothenar muscle	Quadriceps (femoris)			
2 **Neck Muscle, Right**	Palmar interosseous	Rectus femoris muscle			
Anterior vertebral muscle	muscle	Sartorius muscle			
Arytenoid muscle	Thenar muscle	Semimembranosus			
Cricothyroid muscle	**D** **Hand Muscle, Left**	muscle			
Infrahyoid muscle	*See C Hand Muscle, Right*	Semitendinosus muscle			
Levator scapulae muscle	**F** **Trunk Muscle, Right**	Vastus intermedius muscle			
Platysma muscle	Coccygeus muscle	Vastus lateralis muscle			
Scalene muscle	Erector spinae muscle	Vastus medialis muscle			
Splenius cervicis muscle	Interspinalis muscle	**R** **Upper Leg Muscle, Left**			
Sternocleidomastoid	Intertransversarius muscle	*See Q Upper Leg Muscle,*			
muscle	Latissimus dorsi muscle	*Right*			
Suprahyoid muscle	Quadratus lumborum	**S** **Lower Leg Muscle, Right**			
Thyroarytenoid muscle	muscle	Extensor digitorum longus			
3 **Neck Muscle, Left**	Rhomboid major muscle	muscle			
See 2 Neck Muscle, Right	Rhomboid minor muscle	Extensor hallucis longus			
4 **Tongue, Palate, Pharynx**	Serratus posterior muscle	muscle			
Muscle	Transversospinalis muscle	Fibularis brevis muscle			
Chondroglossus muscle	Trapezius muscle	Fibularis longus muscle			
Genioglossus muscle	**G** **Trunk Muscle, Left**	Flexor digitorum longus			
Hyoglossus muscle	*See F Trunk Muscle, Right*	muscle			
Inferior longitudinal	**H** **Thorax Muscle, Right**	Flexor hallucis longus			
muscle	Intercostal muscle	muscle			
Levator veli palatini	Levatores costarum	Gastrocnemius muscle			
muscle	muscle	Peroneus brevis muscle			
Palatoglossal muscle	Pectoralis major muscle	Peroneus longus muscle			
Palatopharyngeal muscle	Pectoralis minor muscle	Popliteus muscle			
Pharyngeal constrictor	Serratus anterior muscle	Soleus muscle			
muscle	Subclavius muscle	Tibialis anterior muscle			
Salpingopharyngeus	Subcostal muscle	Tibialis posterior muscle			
muscle	Transverse thoracis	**T** **Lower Leg Muscle, Left**			
Styloglossus muscle	muscle	*See S Lower Leg Muscle,*			
Stylopharyngeus muscle	**J** **Thorax Muscle, Left**	*Right*			
Superior longitudinal	*See H Thorax Muscle, Right*	**V** **Foot Muscle, Right**			
muscle	**K** **Abdomen Muscle, Right**	Abductor hallucis muscle			
Tensor veli palatini muscle	External oblique muscle	Adductor hallucis muscle			
5 **Shoulder Muscle, Right**	Internal oblique muscle	Extensor digitorum brevis			
Deltoid muscle	Pyramidalis muscle	muscle			
Infraspinatus muscle	Rectus abdominis muscle	Extensor hallucis brevis			
Subscapularis muscle	Transversus abdominis	muscle			
Supraspinatus muscle	muscle	Flexor digitorum brevis			
Teres major muscle	**L** **Abdomen Muscle, Left**	muscle			
Teres minor muscle	*See K Abdomen Muscle,*	Flexor hallucis brevis			
6 **Shoulder Muscle, Left**	*Right*	muscle			
See 5 Shoulder Muscle,		Quadratus plantae muscle			
Right		**W** **Foot Muscle, Left**			
		See V Foot Muscle, Right			

NC Noncovered Procedure   **LC** Limited Coverage   **QA** Questionable OB Admit   **NT** New Tech Add-on   ✚ Combination Member   ♂ Male   ♀ Female

ICD-10-PCS 2023   **473**

ØKM–ØKM

Ø **Medical and Surgical**
K **Muscles**
N **Release**

Definition: Freeing a body part from an abnormal physical constraint by cutting or by the use of force
Explanation: Some of the restraining tissue may be taken out but none of the body part is taken out

Body Part Character 4			Approach Character 5	Device Character 6	Qualifier Character 7
Ø Head Muscle	**7 Upper Arm Muscle, Right**	**M Perineum Muscle**	**Ø** Open	**Z** No Device	**Z** No Qualifier
Auricularis muscle	Biceps brachii muscle	Bulbospongiosus muscle	**3** Percutaneous		
Masseter muscle	Brachialis muscle	Cremaster muscle	**4** Percutaneous		
Pterygoid muscle	Coracobrachialis muscle	Deep transverse perineal	Endoscopic		
Splenius capitis muscle	Triceps brachii muscle	muscle	**X** External		
Temporalis muscle	**8 Upper Arm Muscle, Left**	Ischiocavernosus muscle			
Temporoparietalis muscle	*See 7 Upper Arm Muscle,*	Levator ani muscle			
1 Facial Muscle	*Right*	Superficial transverse			
Buccinator muscle	**9 Lower Arm and Wrist**	perineal muscle			
Corrugator supercilii	**Muscle, Right**	**N Hip Muscle, Right**			
muscle	Anatomical snuffbox	Gemellus muscle			
Depressor anguli oris	Brachioradialis muscle	Gluteus maximus muscle			
muscle	Extensor carpi radialis	Gluteus medius muscle			
Depressor labii inferioris	muscle	Gluteus minimus muscle			
muscle	Extensor carpi ulnaris	Iliacus muscle			
Depressor septi nasi	muscle	Obturator muscle			
muscle	Flexor carpi radialis	Piriformis muscle			
Depressor supercilii	muscle	Psoas muscle			
muscle	Flexor carpi ulnaris muscle	Quadratus femoris muscle			
Levator anguli oris muscle	Flexor pollicis longus	Tensor fasciae latae			
Levator labii superioris	muscle	muscle			
alaeque nasi muscle	Palmaris longus muscle	**P Hip Muscle, Left**			
Levator labii superioris	Pronator quadratus	*See N Hip Muscle, Right*			
muscle	muscle	**Q Upper Leg Muscle, Right**			
Mentalis muscle	Pronator teres muscle	Adductor brevis muscle			
Nasalis muscle	**B Lower Arm and Wrist**	Adductor longus muscle			
Occipitofrontalis muscle	**Muscle, Left**	Adductor magnus muscle			
Orbicularis oris muscle	*See 9 Lower Arm and Wrist*	Biceps femoris muscle			
Procerus muscle	*Muscle, Right*	Gracilis muscle			
Risorius muscle	**C Hand Muscle, Right**	Pectineus muscle			
Zygomaticus muscle	Hypothenar muscle	Quadriceps (femoris)			
2 Neck Muscle, Right	Palmar interosseous	Rectus femoris muscle			
Anterior vertebral muscle	muscle	Sartorius muscle			
Arytenoid muscle	Thenar muscle	Semimembranosus			
Cricothyroid muscle	**D Hand Muscle, Left**	muscle			
Infrahyoid muscle	*See C Hand Muscle, Right*	Semitendinosus muscle			
Levator scapulae muscle	**F Trunk Muscle, Right**	Vastus intermedius muscle			
Platysma muscle	Coccygeus muscle	Vastus lateralis muscle			
Scalene muscle	Erector spinae muscle	Vastus medialis muscle			
Splenius cervicis muscle	Interspinalis muscle	**R Upper Leg Muscle, Left**			
Sternocleidomastoid	Intertransversarius muscle	*See Q Upper Leg Muscle,*			
muscle	Latissimus dorsi muscle	*Right*			
Suprahyoid muscle	Quadratus lumborum	**S Lower Leg Muscle, Right**			
Thyroarytenoid muscle	muscle	Extensor digitorum longus			
3 Neck Muscle, Left	Rhomboid major muscle	muscle			
See 2 Neck Muscle, Right	Rhomboid minor muscle	Extensor hallucis longus			
4 Tongue, Palate, Pharynx	Serratus posterior muscle	muscle			
Muscle	Transversospinalis muscle	Fibularis brevis muscle			
Chondroglossus muscle	Trapezius muscle	Fibularis longus muscle			
Genioglossus muscle	**G Trunk Muscle, Left**	Flexor digitorum longus			
Hyoglossus muscle	*See F Trunk Muscle, Right*	muscle			
Inferior longitudinal	**H Thorax Muscle, Right**	Flexor hallucis longus			
muscle	Intercostal muscle	muscle			
Levator veli palatini	Levatores costarum	Gastrocnemius muscle			
muscle	muscle	Peroneus brevis muscle			
Palatoglossal muscle	Pectoralis major muscle	Peroneus longus muscle			
Palatopharyngeal muscle	Pectoralis minor muscle	Popliteus muscle			
Pharyngeal constrictor	Serratus anterior muscle	Soleus muscle			
muscle	Subclavius muscle	Tibialis anterior muscle			
Salpingopharyngeus	Subcostal muscle	Tibialis posterior muscle			
muscle	Transverse thoracis	**T Lower Leg Muscle, Left**			
Styloglossus muscle	muscle	*See S Lower Leg Muscle,*			
Stylopharyngeus muscle	**J Thorax Muscle, Left**	*Right*			
Superior longitudinal	*See H Thorax Muscle, Right*	**V Foot Muscle, Right**			
muscle	**K Abdomen Muscle, Right**	Abductor hallucis muscle			
Tensor veli palatini muscle	External oblique muscle	Adductor hallucis muscle			
5 Shoulder Muscle, Right	Internal oblique muscle	Extensor digitorum brevis			
Deltoid muscle	Pyramidalis muscle	muscle			
Infraspinatus muscle	Rectus abdominis muscle	Extensor hallucis brevis			
Subscapularis muscle	Transversus abdominis	muscle			
Supraspinatus muscle	muscle	Flexor digitorum brevis			
Teres major muscle	**L Abdomen Muscle, Left**	muscle			
Teres minor muscle	*See K Abdomen Muscle,*	Flexor hallucis brevis			
6 Shoulder Muscle, Left	*Right*	muscle			
See 5 Shoulder Muscle,		Quadratus plantae muscle			
Right		**W Foot Muscle, Left**			
		See V Foot Muscle, Right			

Non-OR ØKN[Ø,1,2,3,4,5,6,7,8,9,B,C,D,F,G,H,J,K,L,M,N,P,Q,R,S,T,V,W]XZZ

Non-OR Procedure   DRG Non-OR Procedure   Valid OR Procedure   HAC Associated Procedure   Combination Only   New/Revised April   New/Revised October

Ø   **Medical and Surgical**
K   **Muscles**
P   **Removal**   Definition: Taking out or off a device from a body part

Explanation: If a device is taken out and a similar device put in without cutting or puncturing the skin or mucous membrane, the procedure is coded to the root operation CHANGE. Otherwise, the procedure for taking out a device is coded to the root operation REMOVAL.

Body Part Character 4	Approach Character 5	Device Character 6	Qualifier Character 7
X Upper Muscle Y Lower Muscle	Ø Open 3 Percutaneous 4 Percutaneous Endoscopic	Ø Drainage Device 7 Autologous Tissue Substitute J Synthetic Substitute K Nonautologous Tissue Substitute M Stimulator Lead Y Other Device	Z No Qualifier
X Upper Muscle Y Lower Muscle	X External	Ø Drainage Device M Stimulator Lead	Z No Qualifier

Non-OR	ØKP[X,Y][3,4]YZ
Non-OR	ØKP[X,Y]X[Ø,M]Z

NC Noncovered Procedure   LC Limited Coverage   QA Questionable OB Admit   NT New Tech Add-on   ⊞ Combination Member   ♂ Male   ♀ Female

ICD-10-PCS 2023   475

Ø   **Medical and Surgical**
K   **Muscles**
Q   **Repair**   Definition: Restoring, to the extent possible, a body part to its normal anatomic structure and function
           Explanation: Used only when the method to accomplish the repair is not one of the other root operations

Body Part Character 4		Approach Character 5	Device Character 6	Qualifier Character 7
Ø Head Muscle	**7 Upper Arm Muscle, Right**	**Ø Open**	**Z No Device**	**Z No Qualifier**
Auricularis muscle	Biceps brachii muscle	**3 Percutaneous**		
Masseter muscle	Brachialis muscle	**4 Percutaneous**		
Pterygoid muscle	Coracobrachialis muscle	**Endoscopic**		
Splenius capitis muscle	Triceps brachii muscle			
Temporalis muscle	**8 Upper Arm Muscle, Left**			
Temporoparietalis muscle	*See 7 Upper Arm Muscle,*			
1 Facial Muscle	*Right*			
Buccinator muscle	**9 Lower Arm and Wrist**	**N Hip Muscle, Right**		
Corrugator supercilii	**Muscle, Right**	Gemellus muscle		
muscle	Anatomical snuffbox	Gluteus maximus muscle		
Depressor anguli oris	Brachioradialis muscle	Gluteus medius muscle		
muscle	Extensor carpi radialis	Gluteus minimus muscle		
Depressor labii inferioris	muscle	Iliacus muscle		
muscle	Extensor carpi ulnaris	Obturator muscle		
Depressor septi nasi	muscle	Piriformis muscle		
muscle	Flexor carpi radialis	Psoas muscle		
Depressor supercilii	muscle	Quadratus femoris muscle		
muscle	Flexor carpi ulnaris muscle	Tensor fasciae latae		
Levator anguli oris muscle	Flexor pollicis longus	muscle		
Levator labii superioris	muscle	**P Hip Muscle, Left**		
alaeque nasi muscle	Palmaris longus muscle	*See N Hip Muscle, Right*		
Levator labii superioris	Pronator quadratus	**Q Upper Leg Muscle, Right**		
muscle	muscle	Adductor brevis muscle		
Mentalis muscle	Pronator teres muscle	Adductor longus muscle		
Nasalis muscle	**B Lower Arm and Wrist**	Adductor magnus muscle		
Occipitofrontalis muscle	**Muscle, Left**	Biceps femoris muscle		
Orbicularis oris muscle	*See 9 Lower Arm and Wrist*	Gracilis muscle		
Procerus muscle	*Muscle, Right*	Pectineus muscle		
Risorius muscle	**C Hand Muscle, Right**	Quadriceps (femoris)		
Zygomaticus muscle	Hypothenar muscle	Rectus femoris muscle		
2 Neck Muscle, Right	Palmar interosseous	Sartorius muscle		
Anterior vertebral muscle	muscle	Semimembranosus		
Arytenoid muscle	Thenar muscle	muscle		
Cricothyroid muscle	**D Hand Muscle, Left**	Semitendinosus muscle		
Infrahyoid muscle	*See C Hand Muscle, Right*	Vastus intermedius muscle		
Levator scapulae muscle	**F Trunk Muscle, Right**	Vastus lateralis muscle		
Platysma muscle	Coccygeus muscle	Vastus medialis muscle		
Scalene muscle	Erector spinae muscle	**R Upper Leg Muscle, Left**		
Splenius cervicis muscle	Interspinalis muscle	*See Q Upper Leg Muscle,*		
Sternocleidomastoid	Intertransversarius muscle	*Right*		
muscle	Latissimus dorsi muscle	**S Lower Leg Muscle, Right**		
Suprahyoid muscle	Quadratus lumborum	Extensor digitorum longus		
Thyroarytenoid muscle	muscle	muscle		
3 Neck Muscle, Left	Rhomboid major muscle	Extensor hallucis longus		
See 2 Neck Muscle, Right	Rhomboid minor muscle	muscle		
4 Tongue, Palate, Pharynx	Serratus posterior muscle	Fibularis brevis muscle		
Muscle	Transversospinalis muscle	Fibularis longus muscle		
Chondroglossus muscle	Trapezius muscle	Flexor digitorum longus		
Genioglossus muscle	**G Trunk Muscle, Left**	muscle		
Hyoglossus muscle	*See F Trunk Muscle, Right*	Flexor hallucis longus		
Inferior longitudinal	**H Thorax Muscle, Right**	muscle		
muscle	Intercostal muscle	Gastrocnemius muscle		
Levator veli palatini	Levatores costarum	Peroneus brevis muscle		
muscle	muscle	Peroneus longus muscle		
Palatoglossal muscle	Pectoralis major muscle	Popliteus muscle		
Palatopharyngeal muscle	Pectoralis minor muscle	Soleus muscle		
Pharyngeal constrictor	Serratus anterior muscle	Tibialis anterior muscle		
muscle	Subclavius muscle	Tibialis posterior muscle		
Salpingopharyngeus	Subcostal muscle	**T Lower Leg Muscle, Left**		
muscle	Transverse thoracis	*See S Lower Leg Muscle,*		
Styloglossus muscle	muscle	*Right*		
Stylopharyngeus muscle	**J Thorax Muscle, Left**	**V Foot Muscle, Right**		
Superior longitudinal	*See H Thorax Muscle, Right*	Abductor hallucis muscle		
muscle	**K Abdomen Muscle, Right**	Adductor hallucis muscle		
Tensor veli palatini muscle	External oblique muscle	Extensor digitorum brevis		
5 Shoulder Muscle, Right	Internal oblique muscle	muscle		
Deltoid muscle	Pyramidalis muscle	Extensor hallucis brevis		
Infraspinatus muscle	Rectus abdominis muscle	muscle		
Subscapularis muscle	Transversus abdominis	Flexor digitorum brevis		
Supraspinatus muscle	muscle	muscle		
Teres major muscle	**L Abdomen Muscle, Left**	Flexor hallucis brevis		
Teres minor muscle	*See K Abdomen Muscle,*	muscle		
6 Shoulder Muscle, Left	*Right*	Quadratus plantae muscle		
See 5 Shoulder Muscle,		**W Foot Muscle, Left**		
Right		*See V Foot Muscle, Right*		
M Perineum Muscle				
Bulbospongiosus muscle				
Cremaster muscle				
Deep transverse perineal				
muscle				
Ischiocavernosus muscle				
Levator ani muscle				
Superficial transverse				
perineal muscle				

Non-OR Procedure   DRG Non-OR Procedure   Valid OR Procedure   HAC Associated Procedure   Combination Only   New/Revised April   New/Revised October

476   ICD-10-PCS 2023

ØKQ–ØKQ

Ø　Medical and Surgical
K　Muscles
R　Replacement Definition: Putting in or on biological or synthetic material that physically takes the place and/or function of all or a portion of a body part
　　　　Explanation: The body part may have been taken out or replaced, or may be taken out, physically eradicated, or rendered nonfunctional during the REPLACEMENT procedure. A REMOVAL procedure is coded for taking out the device used in a previous replacement procedure.

Body Part — Character 4			Approach Character 5	Device Character 6	Qualifier Character 7
Ø　Head Muscle	**7　Upper Arm Muscle, Right**	**M　Perineum Muscle**	**Ø　Open**	**7　Autologous Tissue Substitute**	**Z　No Qualifier**
Auricularis muscle	Biceps brachii muscle	Bulbospongiosus muscle	**4　Percutaneous**	**J　Synthetic Substitute**	
Masseter muscle	Brachialis muscle	Cremaster muscle	Endoscopic	**K　Nonautologous Tissue Substitute**	
Pterygoid muscle	Coracobrachialis muscle	Deep transverse perineal muscle			
Splenius capitis muscle	Triceps brachii muscle	Ischiocavernosus muscle			
Temporalis muscle	**8　Upper Arm Muscle, Left**	Levator ani muscle			
Temporoparietalis muscle	*See 7 Upper Arm Muscle, Right*	Superficial transverse perineal muscle			
1　Facial Muscle	**9　Lower Arm and Wrist Muscle, Right**	**N　Hip Muscle, Right**			
Buccinator muscle	Anatomical snuffbox	Gemellus muscle			
Corrugator supercilii muscle	Brachioradialis muscle	Gluteus maximus muscle			
Depressor anguli oris muscle	Extensor carpi radialis muscle	Gluteus medius muscle			
Depressor labii inferioris muscle	Extensor carpi ulnaris muscle	Gluteus minimus muscle			
Depressor septi nasi muscle	Flexor carpi radialis muscle	Iliacus muscle			
Depressor supercilii muscle	Flexor carpi ulnaris muscle	Obturator muscle			
Levator anguli oris muscle	Flexor pollicis longus muscle	Piriformis muscle			
Levator labii superioris alaeque nasi muscle	Palmaris longus muscle	Psoas muscle			
Levator labii superioris muscle	Pronator quadratus muscle	Quadratus femoris muscle			
Mentalis muscle	Pronator teres muscle	Tensor fasciae latae muscle			
Nasalis muscle	**B　Lower Arm and Wrist Muscle, Left**	**P　Hip Muscle, Left**			
Occipitofrontalis muscle	*See 9 Lower Arm and Wrist Muscle, Right*	*See N Hip Muscle, Right*			
Orbicularis oris muscle	**C　Hand Muscle, Right**	**Q　Upper Leg Muscle, Right**			
Procerus muscle	Hypothenar muscle	Adductor brevis muscle			
Risorius muscle	Palmar interosseous muscle	Adductor longus muscle			
Zygomaticus muscle	Thenar muscle	Adductor magnus muscle			
2　Neck Muscle, Right	**D　Hand Muscle, Left**	Biceps femoris muscle			
Anterior vertebral muscle	*See C Hand Muscle, Right*	Gracilis muscle			
Arytenoid muscle	**F　Trunk Muscle, Right**	Pectineus muscle			
Cricothyroid muscle	Coccygeus muscle	Quadriceps (femoris)			
Infrahyoid muscle	Erector spinae muscle	Rectus femoris muscle			
Levator scapulae muscle	Interspinalis muscle	Sartorius muscle			
Platysma muscle	Intertransversarius muscle	Semimembranosus muscle			
Scalene muscle	Latissimus dorsi muscle	Semitendinosus muscle			
Splenius cervicis muscle	Quadratus lumborum muscle	Vastus intermedius muscle			
Sternocleidomastoid muscle	Rhomboid major muscle	Vastus lateralis muscle			
Suprahyoid muscle	Rhomboid minor muscle	Vastus medialis muscle			
Thyroarytenoid muscle	Serratus posterior muscle	**R　Upper Leg Muscle, Left**			
3　Neck Muscle, Left	Transversospinalis muscle	*See Q Upper Leg Muscle, Right*			
See 2 Neck Muscle, Right	Trapezius muscle	**S　Lower Leg Muscle, Right**			
4　Tongue, Palate, Pharynx Muscle	**G　Trunk Muscle, Left**	Extensor digitorum longus muscle			
Chondroglossus muscle	*See F Trunk Muscle, Right*	Extensor hallucis longus muscle			
Genioglossus muscle	**H　Thorax Muscle, Right**	Fibularis brevis muscle			
Hyoglossus muscle	Intercostal muscle	Fibularis longus muscle			
Inferior longitudinal muscle	Levatores costarum muscle	Flexor digitorum longus muscle			
Levator veli palatini muscle	Pectoralis major muscle	Flexor hallucis longus muscle			
Palatoglossal muscle	Pectoralis minor muscle	Gastrocnemius muscle			
Palatopharyngeal muscle	Serratus anterior muscle	Peroneus brevis muscle			
Pharyngeal constrictor muscle	Subclavius muscle	Peroneus longus muscle			
Salpingopharyngeus muscle	Subcostal muscle	Popliteus muscle			
Styloglossus muscle	Transverse thoracis muscle	Soleus muscle			
Stylopharyngeus muscle	**J　Thorax Muscle, Left**	Tibialis anterior muscle			
Superior longitudinal muscle	*See H Thorax Muscle, Right*	Tibialis posterior muscle			
Tensor veli palatini muscle	**K　Abdomen Muscle, Right**	**T　Lower Leg Muscle, Left**			
5　Shoulder Muscle, Right	External oblique muscle	*See S Lower Leg Muscle, Right*			
Deltoid muscle	Internal oblique muscle	**V　Foot Muscle, Right**			
Infraspinatus muscle	Pyramidalis muscle	Abductor hallucis muscle			
Subscapularis muscle	Rectus abdominis muscle	Adductor hallucis muscle			
Supraspinatus muscle	Transversus abdominis muscle	Extensor digitorum brevis muscle			
Teres major muscle	**L　Abdomen Muscle, Left**	Extensor hallucis brevis muscle			
Teres minor muscle	*See K Abdomen Muscle, Right*	Flexor digitorum brevis muscle			
6　Shoulder Muscle, Left		Flexor hallucis brevis muscle			
See 5 Shoulder Muscle, Right		Quadratus plantae muscle			
		W　Foot Muscle, Left			
		See V Foot Muscle, Right			

NC Noncovered Procedure　　**LC** Limited Coverage　　**OA** Questionable OB Admit　　**NT** New Tech Add-on　　✚ Combination Member　　♂ Male　　♀ Female

ICD-10-PCS 2023　　　　　　　　　　　　　　　　　　　　　　　　　　　　　　477

ØKR–ØKR

Ø   Medical and Surgical
K   Muscles
S   Reposition   Definition: Moving to its normal location, or other suitable location, all or a portion of a body part

Explanation: The body part is moved to a new location from an abnormal location, or from a normal location where it is not functioning correctly. The body part may or may not be cut out or off to be moved to the new location.

Body Part Character 4		Approach Character 5	Device Character 6	Qualifier Character 7
Ø Head Muscle Auricularis muscle Masseter muscle Pterygoid muscle Splenius capitis muscle Temporalis muscle Temporoparietalis muscle **1 Facial Muscle** Buccinator muscle Corrugator supercilii muscle Depressor anguli oris muscle Depressor labii inferioris muscle Depressor septi nasi muscle Depressor supercilii muscle Levator anguli oris muscle Levator labii superioris alaeque nasi muscle Levator labii superioris muscle Mentalis muscle Nasalis muscle Occipitofrontalis muscle Orbicularis oris muscle Procerus muscle Risorius muscle Zygomaticus muscle **2 Neck Muscle, Right** Anterior vertebral muscle Arytenoid muscle Cricothyroid muscle Infrahyoid muscle Levator scapulae muscle Platysma muscle Scalene muscle Splenius cervicis muscle Sternocleidomastoid muscle Suprahyoid muscle Thyroarytenoid muscle **3 Neck Muscle, Left** *See 2 Neck Muscle, Right* **4 Tongue, Palate, Pharynx Muscle** Chondroglossus muscle Genioglossus muscle Hyoglossus muscle Inferior longitudinal muscle Levator veli palatini muscle Palatoglossal muscle Palatopharyngeal muscle Pharyngeal constrictor muscle Salpingopharyngeus muscle Styloglossus muscle Stylopharyngeus muscle Superior longitudinal muscle Tensor veli palatini muscle **5 Shoulder Muscle, Right** Deltoid muscle Infraspinatus muscle Subscapularis muscle Supraspinatus muscle Teres major muscle Teres minor muscle **6 Shoulder Muscle, Left** *See 5 Shoulder Muscle, Right*	**7 Upper Arm Muscle, Right** Biceps brachii muscle Brachialis muscle Coracobrachialis muscle Triceps brachii muscle **8 Upper Arm Muscle, Left** *See 7 Upper Arm Muscle, Right* **9 Lower Arm and Wrist Muscle, Right** Anatomical snuffbox Brachioradialis muscle Extensor carpi radialis muscle Extensor carpi ulnaris muscle Flexor carpi radialis muscle Flexor carpi ulnaris muscle Flexor pollicis longus muscle Palmaris longus muscle Pronator quadratus muscle Pronator teres muscle **B Lower Arm and Wrist Muscle, Left** *See 9 Lower Arm and Wrist Muscle, Right* **C Hand Muscle, Right** Hypothenar muscle Palmar interosseous muscle Thenar muscle **D Hand Muscle, Left** *See C Hand Muscle, Right* **F Trunk Muscle, Right** Coccygeus muscle Erector spinae muscle Interspinalis muscle Intertransversarius muscle Latissimus dorsi muscle Quadratus lumborum muscle Rhomboid major muscle Rhomboid minor muscle Serratus posterior muscle Transversospinalis muscle Trapezius muscle **G Trunk Muscle, Left** *See F Trunk Muscle, Right* **H Thorax Muscle, Right** Intercostal muscle Levatores costarum muscle Pectoralis major muscle Pectoralis minor muscle Serratus anterior muscle Subclavius muscle Subcostal muscle Transverse thoracis muscle **J Thorax Muscle, Left** *See H Thorax Muscle, Right* **K Abdomen Muscle, Right** External oblique muscle Internal oblique muscle Pyramidalis muscle Rectus abdominis muscle Transversus abdominis muscle **L Abdomen Muscle, Left** *See K Abdomen Muscle, Right*	**M Perineum Muscle** Bulbospongiosus muscle Cremaster muscle Deep transverse perineal muscle Ischiocavernosus muscle Levator ani muscle Superficial transverse perineal muscle **N Hip Muscle, Right** Gemellus muscle Gluteus maximus muscle Gluteus medius muscle Gluteus minimus muscle Iliacus muscle Obturator muscle Piriformis muscle Psoas muscle Quadratus femoris muscle Tensor fasciae latae muscle **P Hip Muscle, Left** *See N Hip Muscle, Right* **Q Upper Leg Muscle, Right** Adductor brevis muscle Adductor longus muscle Adductor magnus muscle Biceps femoris muscle Gracilis muscle Pectineus muscle Quadriceps (femoris) Rectus femoris muscle Sartorius muscle Semimembranosus muscle Semitendinosus muscle Vastus intermedius muscle Vastus lateralis muscle Vastus medialis muscle **R Upper Leg Muscle, Left** *See Q Upper Leg Muscle, Right* **S Lower Leg Muscle, Right** Extensor digitorum longus muscle Extensor hallucis longus muscle Fibularis brevis muscle Fibularis longus muscle Flexor digitorum longus muscle Flexor hallucis longus muscle Gastrocnemius muscle Peroneus brevis muscle Peroneus longus muscle Popliteus muscle Soleus muscle Tibialis anterior muscle Tibialis posterior muscle **T Lower Leg Muscle, Left** *See S Lower Leg Muscle, Right* **V Foot Muscle, Right** Abductor hallucis muscle Adductor hallucis muscle Extensor digitorum brevis muscle Extensor hallucis brevis muscle Flexor digitorum brevis muscle Flexor hallucis brevis muscle Quadratus plantae muscle **W Foot Muscle, Left** *See V Foot Muscle, Right*	**Ø Open** **4 Percutaneous Endoscopic**	**Z No Device**	**Z No Qualifier**

Non-OR Procedure   DRG Non-OR Procedure   Valid OR Procedure   HAC Associated Procedure   Combination Only   New/Revised April   New/Revised October

478   ICD-10-PCS 2023

ØKS–ØKS

Ø Medical and Surgical
K Muscles
T Resection   Definition: Cutting out or off, without replacement, all of a body part
                 Explanation: None

Body Part Character 4		Approach Character 5	Device Character 6	Qualifier Character 7
Ø Head Muscle Auricularis muscle Masseter muscle Pterygoid muscle Splenius capitis muscle Temporalis muscle Temporoparietalis muscle **1 Facial Muscle** Buccinator muscle Corrugator supercilii muscle Depressor anguli oris muscle Depressor labii inferioris muscle Depressor septi nasi muscle Depressor supercilii muscle Levator anguli oris muscle Levator labii superioris alaeque nasi muscle Levator labii superioris muscle Mentalis muscle Nasalis muscle Occipitofrontalis muscle Orbicularis oris muscle Procerus muscle Risorius muscle Zygomaticus muscle **2 Neck Muscle, Right** Anterior vertebral muscle Arytenoid muscle Cricothyroid muscle Infrahyoid muscle Levator scapulae muscle Platysma muscle Scalene muscle Splenius cervicis muscle Sternocleidomastoid muscle Suprahyoid muscle Thyroarytenoid muscle **3 Neck Muscle, Left** *See 2 Neck Muscle, Right* **4 Tongue, Palate, Pharynx Muscle** Chondroglossus muscle Genioglossus muscle Hyoglossus muscle Inferior longitudinal muscle Levator veli palatini muscle Palatoglossal muscle Palatopharyngeal muscle Pharyngeal constrictor muscle Salpingopharyngeus muscle Styloglossus muscle Stylopharyngeus muscle Superior longitudinal muscle Tensor veli palatini muscle **5 Shoulder Muscle, Right** Deltoid muscle Infraspinatus muscle Subscapularis muscle Supraspinatus muscle Teres major muscle Teres minor muscle **6 Shoulder Muscle, Left** *See 5 Shoulder Muscle, Right*	**7 Upper Arm Muscle, Right** Biceps brachii muscle Brachialis muscle Coracobrachialis muscle Triceps brachii muscle **8 Upper Arm Muscle, Left** *See 7 Upper Arm Muscle, Right* **9 Lower Arm and Wrist Muscle, Right** Anatomical snuffbox Brachioradialis muscle Extensor carpi radialis muscle Extensor carpi ulnaris muscle Flexor carpi radialis muscle Flexor carpi ulnaris muscle Flexor pollicis longus muscle Palmaris longus muscle Pronator quadratus muscle Pronator teres muscle **B Lower Arm and Wrist Muscle, Left** *See 9 Lower Arm and Wrist Muscle, Right* **C Hand Muscle, Right** Hypothenar muscle Palmar interosseous muscle Thenar muscle **D Hand Muscle, Left** *See C Hand Muscle, Right* **F Trunk Muscle, Right** Coccygeus muscle Erector spinae muscle Interspinalis muscle Intertransversarius muscle Latissimus dorsi muscle Quadratus lumborum muscle Rhomboid major muscle Rhomboid minor muscle Serratus posterior muscle Transversospinalis muscle Trapezius muscle **G Trunk Muscle, Left** *See F Trunk Muscle, Right* **H Thorax Muscle, Right** ⊞ Intercostal muscle Levatores costarum muscle Pectoralis major muscle Pectoralis minor muscle Serratus anterior muscle Subclavius muscle Subcostal muscle Transverse thoracis muscle **J Thorax Muscle, Left** ⊞ *See H Thorax Muscle, Right* **K Abdomen Muscle, Right** External oblique muscle Internal oblique muscle Pyramidalis muscle Rectus abdominis muscle Transversus abdominis muscle **L Abdomen Muscle, Left** *See K Abdomen Muscle, Right* **W Foot Muscle, Left** *See V Foot Muscle, Right*	**M Perineum Muscle** Bulbospongiosus muscle Cremaster muscle Deep transverse perineal muscle Ischiocavernosus muscle Levator ani muscle Superficial transverse perineal muscle **N Hip Muscle, Right** Gemellus muscle Gluteus maximus muscle Gluteus medius muscle Gluteus minimus muscle Iliacus muscle Obturator muscle Piriformis muscle Psoas muscle Quadratus femoris muscle Tensor fasciae latae muscle **P Hip Muscle, Left** *See N Hip Muscle, Right* **Q Upper Leg Muscle, Right** Adductor brevis muscle Adductor longus muscle Adductor magnus muscle Biceps femoris muscle Gracilis muscle Pectineus muscle Quadriceps (femoris) Rectus femoris muscle Sartorius muscle Semimembranosus muscle Semitendinosus muscle Vastus intermedius muscle Vastus lateralis muscle Vastus medialis muscle **R Upper Leg Muscle, Left** *See Q Upper Leg Muscle, Right* **S Lower Leg Muscle, Right** Extensor digitorum longus muscle Extensor hallucis longus muscle Fibularis brevis muscle Fibularis longus muscle Flexor digitorum longus muscle Flexor hallucis longus muscle Gastrocnemius muscle Peroneus brevis muscle Peroneus longus muscle Popliteus muscle Soleus muscle Tibialis anterior muscle Tibialis posterior muscle **T Lower Leg Muscle, Left** *See S Lower Leg Muscle, Right* **V Foot Muscle, Right** Abductor hallucis muscle Adductor hallucis muscle Extensor digitorum brevis muscle Extensor hallucis brevis muscle Flexor digitorum brevis muscle Flexor hallucis brevis muscle Quadratus plantae muscle	**Ø Open** **4 Percutaneous Endoscopic**	**Z No Device**	**Z No Qualifier**

See Appendix L for Procedure Combinations
⊞   ØKT[H,J]ØZZ

NC Noncovered Procedure   **LC** Limited Coverage   **QA** Questionable OB Admit   **NT** New Tech Add-on   ⊞ Combination Member   ♂ Male   ♀ Female

Muscles

ØKU–ØKU

Ø   Medical and Surgical
K   Muscles
U   Supplement   Definition: Putting in or on biological or synthetic material that physically reinforces and/or augments the function of a portion of a body part
Explanation: The biological material is non-living, or is living and from the same individual. The body part may have been previously replaced, and the SUPPLEMENT procedure is performed to physically reinforce and/or augment the function of the replaced body part.

Body Part Character 4			Approach Character 5	Device Character 6	Qualifier Character 7

Ø Head Muscle
     Auricularis muscle
     Masseter muscle
     Pterygoid muscle
     Splenius capitis muscle
     Temporalis muscle
     Temporoparietalis muscle
1 Facial Muscle
     Buccinator muscle
     Corrugator supercilii
        muscle
     Depressor anguli oris
        muscle
     Depressor labii inferioris
        muscle
     Depressor septi nasi
        muscle
     Depressor supercilii
        muscle
     Levator anguli oris muscle
     Levator labii superioris
        alaeque nasi muscle
     Levator labii superioris
        muscle
     Mentalis muscle
     Nasalis muscle
     Occipitofrontalis muscle
     Orbicularis oris muscle
     Procerus muscle
     Risorius muscle
     Zygomaticus muscle
2 Neck Muscle, Right
     Anterior vertebral muscle
     Arytenoid muscle
     Cricothyroid muscle
     Infrahyoid muscle
     Levator scapulae muscle
     Platysma muscle
     Scalene muscle
     Splenius cervicis muscle
     Sternocleidomastoid
        muscle
     Suprahyoid muscle
     Thyroarytenoid muscle
3 Neck Muscle, Left
     See 2 Neck Muscle, Right
4 Tongue, Palate, Pharynx
     Muscle
     Chondroglossus muscle
     Genioglossus muscle
     Hyoglossus muscle
     Inferior longitudinal
        muscle
     Levator veli palatini
        muscle
     Palatoglossal muscle
     Palatopharyngeal muscle
     Pharyngeal constrictor
        muscle
     Salpingopharyngeus
        muscle
     Styloglossus muscle
     Stylopharyngeus muscle
     Superior longitudinal
        muscle
     Tensor veli palatini muscle
5 Shoulder Muscle, Right
     Deltoid muscle
     Infraspinatus muscle
     Subscapularis muscle
     Supraspinatus muscle
     Teres major muscle
     Teres minor muscle
6 Shoulder Muscle, Left
     *See 5 Shoulder Muscle,
        Right*
	7 Upper Arm Muscle, Right
	     Biceps brachii muscle
	     Brachialis muscle
	     Coracobrachialis muscle
	     Triceps brachii muscle
	8 Upper Arm Muscle, Left
	     *See 7 Upper Arm Muscle,
	        Right*
	9 Lower Arm and Wrist
	     Muscle, Right
	     Anatomical snuffbox
	     Brachioradialis muscle
	     Extensor carpi radialis
	        muscle
	     Extensor carpi ulnaris
	        muscle
	     Flexor carpi radialis
	        muscle
	     Flexor carpi ulnaris muscle
	     Flexor pollicis longus
	        muscle
	     Palmaris longus muscle
	     Pronator quadratus
	        muscle
	     Pronator teres muscle
	B Lower Arm and Wrist
	     Muscle, Left
	     *See 9 Lower Arm and Wrist
	        Muscle, Right*
	C Hand Muscle, Right
	     Hypothenar muscle
	     Palmar interosseous
	        muscle
	     Thenar muscle
	D Hand Muscle, Left
	     See C Hand Muscle, Right
	F Trunk Muscle, Right
	     Coccygeus muscle
	     Erector spinae muscle
	     Interspinalis muscle
	     Intertransversarius muscle
	     Latissimus dorsi muscle
	     Quadratus lumborum
	        muscle
	     Rhomboid major muscle
	     Rhomboid minor muscle
	     Serratus posterior muscle
	     Transversospinalis muscle
	     Trapezius muscle
	G Trunk Muscle, Left
	     See F Trunk Muscle, Right
	H Thorax Muscle, Right
	     Intercostal muscle
	     Levatores costarum
	        muscle
	     Pectoralis major muscle
	     Pectoralis minor muscle
	     Serratus anterior muscle
	     Subclavius muscle
	     Subcostal muscle
	     Transverse thoracis
	        muscle
	J Thorax Muscle, Left
	     See H Thorax Muscle, Right
	K Abdomen Muscle, Right
	     External oblique muscle
	     Internal oblique muscle
	     Pyramidalis muscle
	     Rectus abdominis muscle
	     Transversus abdominis
	        muscle
	L Abdomen Muscle, Left
	     *See K Abdomen Muscle,
	        Right*
		M Perineum Muscle
		     Bulbospongiosus muscle
		     Cremaster muscle
		     Deep transverse perineal
		        muscle
		     Ischiocavernosus muscle
		     Levator ani muscle
		     Superficial transverse
		        perineal muscle
		N Hip Muscle, Right
		     Gemellus muscle
		     Gluteus maximus muscle
		     Gluteus medius muscle
		     Gluteus minimus muscle
		     Iliacus muscle
		     Obturator muscle
		     Piriformis muscle
		     Psoas muscle
		     Quadratus femoris muscle
		     Tensor fasciae latae
		        muscle
		P Hip Muscle, Left
		     See N Hip Muscle, Right
		Q Upper Leg Muscle, Right
		     Adductor brevis muscle
		     Adductor longus muscle
		     Adductor magnus muscle
		     Biceps femoris muscle
		     Gracilis muscle
		     Pectineus muscle
		     Quadriceps (femoris)
		     Rectus femoris muscle
		     Sartorius muscle
		     Semimembranosus
		        muscle
		     Semitendinosus muscle
		     Vastus intermedius muscle
		     Vastus lateralis muscle
		     Vastus medialis muscle
		R Upper Leg Muscle, Left
		     *See Q Upper Leg Muscle,
		        Right*
		S Lower Leg Muscle, Right
		     Extensor digitorum longus
		        muscle
		     Extensor hallucis longus
		        muscle
		     Fibularis brevis muscle
		     Fibularis longus muscle
		     Flexor digitorum longus
		        muscle
		     Flexor hallucis longus
		        muscle
		     Gastrocnemius muscle
		     Peroneus brevis muscle
		     Peroneus longus muscle
		     Popliteus muscle
		     Soleus muscle
		     Tibialis anterior muscle
		     Tibialis posterior muscle
		T Lower Leg Muscle, Left
		     *See S Lower Leg Muscle,
		        Right*
		V Foot Muscle, Right
		     Abductor hallucis muscle
		     Adductor hallucis muscle
		     Extensor digitorum brevis
		        muscle
		     Extensor hallucis brevis
		        muscle
		     Flexor digitorum brevis
		        muscle
		     Flexor hallucis brevis
		        muscle
		     Quadratus plantae muscle
		W Foot Muscle, Left
		     See V Foot Muscle, Right
			Ø Open
			4 Percutaneous
			     Endoscopic
				7 Autologous Tissue
				     Substitute
				J Synthetic
				     Substitute
				K Nonautologous
				     Tissue Substitute
					Z No Qualifier

Non-OR Procedure   DRG Non-OR Procedure   Valid OR Procedure   HAC Associated Procedure   Combination Only   New/Revised April   New/Revised October

480   ICD-10-PCS 2023

Ø   Medical and Surgical
K   Muscles
W   Revision

Definition: Correcting, to the extent possible, a portion of a malfunctioning device or the position of a displaced device

Explanation: Revision can include correcting a malfunctioning or displaced device by taking out or putting in components of the device such as a screw or pin

Body Part Character 4	Approach Character 5	Device Character 6	Qualifier Character 7
X Upper Muscle Y Lower Muscle	Ø Open 3 Percutaneous 4 Percutaneous Endoscopic	Ø Drainage Device 7 Autologous Tissue Substitute J Synthetic Substitute K Nonautologous Tissue Substitute M Stimulator Lead Y Other Device	Z No Qualifier
X Upper Muscle Y Lower Muscle	X External	Ø Drainage Device 7 Autologous Tissue Substitute J Synthetic Substitute K Nonautologous Tissue Substitute M Stimulator Lead	Z No Qualifier

Non-OR   ØKW[X,Y][3,4]YZ
Non-OR   ØKW[X,Y]X[Ø,7,J,K,M]Z

NC Noncovered Procedure   LC Limited Coverage   QA Questionable OB Admit   NT New Tech Add-on   ⊞ Combination Member   ♂ Male   ♀ Female

ICD-10-PCS 2023   481

Ø   Medical and Surgical
K   Muscles
X   Transfer   Definition: Moving, without taking out, all or a portion of a body part to another location to take over the function of all or a portion of a body part
                Explanation: The body part transferred remains connected to its vascular and nervous supply

Body Part Character 4			Approach Character 5	Device Character 6	Qualifier Character 7
Ø Head Muscle	**6 Shoulder Muscle, Left**	**P Hip Muscle, Left**	**Ø Open**	**Z No Device**	**Ø Skin**
Auricularis muscle	*See 5 Shoulder Muscle,*	*See N Hip Muscle, Right*	**4 Percutaneous**		**1 Subcutaneous**
Masseter muscle	*Right*	**Q Upper Leg Muscle, Right**	**Endoscopic**		**Tissue**
Pterygoid muscle	**7 Upper Arm Muscle, Right**	Adductor brevis muscle			**2 Skin and**
Splenius capitis muscle	Biceps brachii muscle	Adductor longus muscle			**Subcutaneous**
Temporalis muscle	Brachialis muscle	Adductor magnus muscle			**Tissue**
Temporoparietalis muscle	Coracobrachialis muscle	Biceps femoris muscle			**Z No Qualifier**
1 Facial Muscle	Triceps brachii muscle	Gracilis muscle			
Buccinator muscle	**8 Upper Arm Muscle, Left**	Pectineus muscle			
Corrugator supercilii muscle	*See 7 Upper Arm Muscle,*	Quadriceps (femoris)			
Depressor anguli oris	*Right*	Rectus femoris muscle			
muscle	**9 Lower Arm and Wrist**	Sartorius muscle			
Depressor labii inferioris	**Muscle, Right**	Semimembranosus muscle			
muscle	Anatomical snuffbox	Semitendinosus muscle			
Depressor septi nasi	Brachioradialis muscle	Vastus intermedius muscle			
muscle	Extensor carpi radialis	Vastus lateralis muscle			
Depressor supercilii	muscle	Vastus medialis muscle			
muscle	Extensor carpi ulnaris	**R Upper Leg Muscle, Left**			
Levator anguli oris muscle	muscle	*See Q Upper Leg Muscle,*			
Levator labii superioris	Flexor carpi radialis	*Right*			
alaeque nasi muscle	muscle	**S Lower Leg Muscle,**			
Levator labii superioris	Flexor carpi ulnaris muscle	**Right**			
muscle	Flexor pollicis longus	Extensor digitorum longus			
Mentalis muscle	muscle	muscle			
Nasalis muscle	Palmaris longus muscle	Extensor hallucis longus			
Occipitofrontalis muscle	Pronator quadratus	muscle			
Orbicularis oris muscle	muscle	Fibularis brevis muscle			
Procerus muscle	Pronator teres muscle	Fibularis longus muscle			
Risorius muscle	**B Lower Arm and Wrist**	Flexor digitorum longus			
Zygomaticus muscle	**Muscle, Left**	muscle			
2 Neck Muscle, Right	*See 9 Lower Arm and Wrist*	Flexor hallucis longus			
Anterior vertebral muscle	*Muscle, Right*	muscle			
Arytenoid muscle	**C Hand Muscle, Right**	Gastrocnemius muscle			
Cricothyroid muscle	Hypothenar muscle	Peroneus brevis muscle			
Infrahyoid muscle	Palmar interosseous	Peroneus longus muscle			
Levator scapulae muscle	muscle	Popliteus muscle			
Platysma muscle	Thenar muscle	Soleus muscle			
Scalene muscle	**D Hand Muscle, Left**	Tibialis anterior muscle			
Splenius cervicis muscle	*See C Hand Muscle, Right*	Tibialis posterior muscle			
Sternocleidomastoid	**H Thorax Muscle, Right**	**T Lower Leg Muscle, Left**			
muscle	Intercostal muscle	*See S Lower Leg Muscle,*			
Suprahyoid muscle	Levatores costarum	*Right*			
Thyroarytenoid muscle	muscle	**V Foot Muscle, Right**			
3 Neck Muscle, Left	Pectoralis major muscle	Abductor hallucis muscle			
See 2 Neck Muscle, Right	Pectoralis minor muscle	Adductor hallucis muscle			
4 Tongue, Palate, Pharynx	Serratus anterior muscle	Extensor digitorum brevis			
Muscle	Subclavius muscle	muscle			
Chondroglossus muscle	Subcostal muscle	Extensor hallucis brevis			
Genioglossus muscle	Transverse thoracis	muscle			
Hyoglossus muscle	muscle	Flexor digitorum brevis			
Inferior longitudinal muscle	**J Thorax Muscle, Left**	muscle			
Levator veli palatini muscle	*See H Thorax Muscle, Right*	Flexor hallucis brevis			
Palatoglossal muscle	**M Perineum Muscle**	muscle			
Palatopharyngeal muscle	Bulbospongiosus muscle	Quadratus plantae muscle			
Pharyngeal constrictor	Cremaster muscle	**W Foot Muscle, Left**			
muscle	Deep transverse perineal	*See V Foot Muscle, Right*			
Salpingopharyngeus	muscle				
muscle	Ischiocavernosus muscle				
Styloglossus muscle	Levator ani muscle				
Stylopharyngeus muscle	Superficial transverse				
Superior longitudinal	perineal muscle				
muscle	**N Hip Muscle, Right**				
Tensor veli palatini muscle	Gemellus muscle				
5 Shoulder Muscle, Right	Gluteus maximus muscle				
Deltoid muscle	Gluteus medius muscle				
Infraspinatus muscle	Gluteus minimus muscle				
Subscapularis muscle	Iliacus muscle				
Supraspinatus muscle	Obturator muscle				
Teres major muscle	Piriformis muscle				
Teres minor muscle	Psoas muscle				
	Quadratus femoris muscle				
	Tensor fasciae latae muscle				

ØKX Continued on next page

Ø   **Medical and Surgical**   *ØKX Continued*
K   **Muscles**
X   **Transfer**   Definition: Moving, without taking out, all or a portion of a body part to another location to take over the function of all or a portion of a body part
                          Explanation: The body part transferred remains connected to its vascular and nervous supply

Body Part Character 4	Approach Character 5	Device Character 6	Qualifier Character 7
F Trunk Muscle, Right Coccygeus muscle Erector spinae muscle Interspinalis muscle Intertransversarius muscle Latissimus dorsi muscle Quadratus lumborum muscle Rhomboid major muscle Rhomboid minor muscle Serratus posterior muscle Transversospinalis muscle Trapezius muscle **G Trunk Muscle, Left** *See F Trunk Muscle, Right*	**Ø Open** **4 Percutaneous Endoscopic**	**Z No Device**	**Ø Skin** **1 Subcutaneous Tissue** **2 Skin and Subcutaneous Tissue** **5 Latissimus Dorsi Myocutaneous Flap** **7 Deep Inferior Epigastric Artery Perforator Flap** **8 Superficial Inferior Epigastric Artery Flap** **9 Gluteal Artery Perforator Flap** **Z No Qualifier**
K Abdomen Muscle, Right External oblique muscle Internal oblique muscle Pyramidalis muscle Rectus abdominis muscle Transversus abdominis muscle **L Abdomen Muscle, Left** *See K Abdomen Muscle, Right*	**Ø Open** **4 Percutaneous Endoscopic**	**Z No Device**	**Ø Skin** **1 Subcutaneous Tissue** **2 Skin and Subcutaneous Tissue** **6 Transverse Rectus Abdominis Myocutaneous Flap** **Z No Qualifier**

Tendons ØL2–ØLX

Character Meanings*

This Character Meaning table is provided as a guide to assist the user in the identification of character members that may be found in this section of code tables. It **SHOULD NOT** be used to build a PCS code.

Operation–Character 3	Body Part–Character 4	Approach–Character 5	Device–Character 6	Qualifier–Character 7
2 Change	Ø Head and Neck Tendon	Ø Open	Ø Drainage Device	X Diagnostic
5 Destruction	1 Shoulder Tendon, Right	3 Percutaneous	7 Autologous Tissue Substitute	Z No Qualifier
8 Division	2 Shoulder Tendon, Left	4 Percutaneous Endoscopic	J Synthetic Substitute	
9 Drainage	3 Upper Arm Tendon, Right	X External	K Nonautologous Tissue Substitute	
B Excision	4 Upper Arm Tendon, Left		Y Other Device	
C Extirpation	5 Lower Arm and Wrist Tendon, Right		Z No Device	
D Extraction	6 Lower Arm and Wrist Tendon, Left			
H Insertion	7 Hand Tendon, Right			
J Inspection	8 Hand Tendon, Left			
M Reattachment	9 Trunk Tendon, Right			
N Release	B Trunk Tendon, Left			
P Removal	C Thorax Tendon, Right			
Q Repair	D Thorax Tendon, Left			
R Replacement	F Abdomen Tendon, Right			
S Reposition	G Abdomen Tendon, Left			
T Resection	H Perineum Tendon			
U Supplement	J Hip Tendon, Right			
W Revision	K Hip Tendon, Left			
X Transfer	L Upper Leg Tendon, Right			
	M Upper Leg Tendon, Left			
	N Lower Leg Tendon, Right			
	P Lower Leg Tendon, Left			
	Q Knee Tendon, Right			
	R Knee Tendon, Left			
	S Ankle Tendon, Right			
	T Ankle Tendon, Left			
	V Foot Tendon, Right			
	W Foot Tendon, Left			
	X Upper Tendon			
	Y Lower Tendon			

* Includes synovial membrane.

AHA Coding Clinic for table ØL8
2016, 3Q, 30   Resection of femur with interposition arthroplasty

AHA Coding Clinic for table ØLB
2017, 2Q, 21   Arthroscopic anterior cruciate ligament revision using autograft with anterolateral ligament reconstruction
2015, 3Q, 26   Thumb arthroplasty with resection of trapezium
2014, 3Q, 14   Application of TheraSkin® and excisional debridement
2014, 3Q, 18   Placement of reverse sural fasciocutaneous pedicle flap

AHA Coding Clinic for table ØLD
2017, 4Q, 41   Extraction procedures

AHA Coding Clinic for table ØLQ
2016, 3Q, 32   Rotator cuff repair, tenodesis, decompression, acromioplasty and coracoplasty
2015, 2Q, 11   Repair of patellar and quadriceps tendons with allograft
2013, 3Q, 20   Superior labrum anterior posterior (SLAP) repair and subacromial decompression

AHA Coding Clinic for table ØLS
2016, 3Q, 32   Rotator cuff repair, tenodesis, decompression, acromioplasty and coracoplasty
2015, 3Q, 14   Endoprosthetic replacement of humerus and tendon reattachment

AHA Coding Clinic for table ØLU
2015, 2Q, 11   Repair of patellar and quadriceps tendons with allograft

Foot Tendons

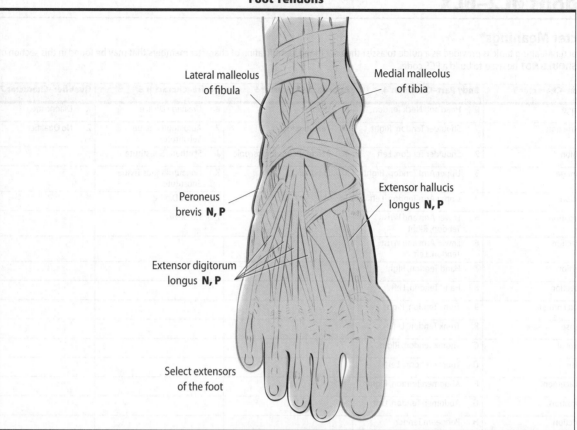

Lateral malleolus
of fibula

Medial malleolus
of tibia

Peroneus
brevis **N, P**

Extensor hallucis
longus **N, P**

Extensor digitorum
longus **N, P**

Select extensors
of the foot

Shoulder Tendons

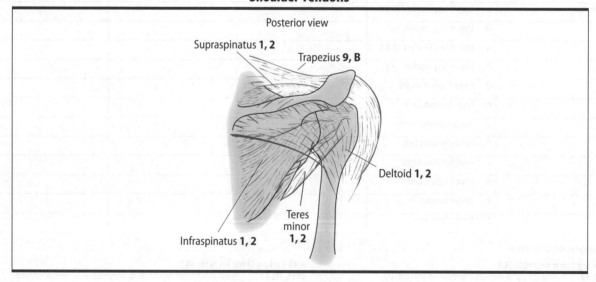

Posterior view

Supraspinatus **1, 2**

Trapezius **9, B**

Deltoid **1, 2**

Teres
minor
1, 2

Infraspinatus **1, 2**

Tendons of Wrist and Hand

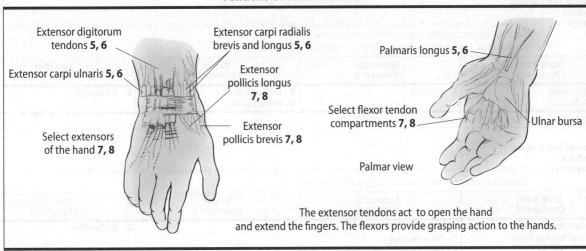

Extensor digitorum tendons **5, 6**

Extensor carpi ulnaris **5, 6**

Select extensors of the hand **7, 8**

Extensor carpi radialis brevis and longus **5, 6**

Extensor pollicis longus **7, 8**

Extensor pollicis brevis **7, 8**

Palmaris longus **5, 6**

Select flexor tendon compartments **7, 8**

Ulnar bursa

Palmar view

The extensor tendons act to open the hand and extend the fingers. The flexors provide grasping action to the hands.

Leg Muscles and Tendons

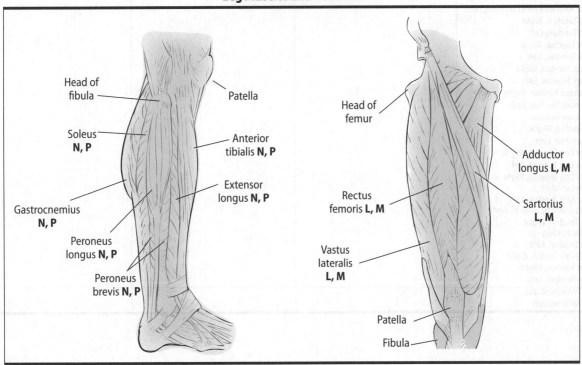

Head of fibula

Soleus **N, P**

Gastrocnemius **N, P**

Peroneus longus **N, P**

Peroneus brevis **N, P**

Patella

Anterior tibialis **N, P**

Extensor longus **N, P**

Head of femur

Rectus femoris **L, M**

Vastus lateralis **L, M**

Adductor longus **L, M**

Sartorius **L, M**

Patella

Fibula

Ø Medical and Surgical
L Tendons
2 Change

Definition: Taking out or off a device from a body part and putting back an identical or similar device in or on the same body part without cutting or puncturing the skin or a mucous membrane

Explanation: All CHANGE procedures are coded using the approach EXTERNAL

Body Part Character 4	Approach Character 5	Device Character 6	Qualifier Character 7
X Upper Tendon Y Lower Tendon	X External	Ø Drainage Device Y Other Device	Z No Qualifier

Non-OR	All body part, approach, device, and qualifier values

Ø Medical and Surgical
L Tendons
5 Destruction

Definition: Physical eradication of all or a portion of a body part by the direct use of energy, force, or a destructive agent

Explanation: None of the body part is physically taken out

Body Part Character 4	Approach Character 5	Device Character 6	Qualifier Character 7

Ø Head and Neck Tendon
1 Shoulder Tendon, Right
2 Shoulder Tendon, Left
3 Upper Arm Tendon, Right
4 Upper Arm Tendon, Left
5 Lower Arm and Wrist Tendon, Right
6 Lower Arm and Wrist Tendon, Left
7 Hand Tendon, Right
8 Hand Tendon, Left
9 Trunk Tendon, Right
B Trunk Tendon, Left
C Thorax Tendon, Right
D Thorax Tendon, Left
F Abdomen Tendon, Right
G Abdomen Tendon, Left
H Perineum Tendon
J Hip Tendon, Right
K Hip Tendon, Left
L Upper Leg Tendon, Right
M Upper Leg Tendon, Left
N Lower Leg Tendon, Right
   Achilles tendon
P Lower Leg Tendon, Left
   See N Lower Leg Tendon, Right
Q Knee Tendon, Right
   Patellar tendon
R Knee Tendon, Left
   See Q Knee Tendon, Right
S Ankle Tendon, Right
T Ankle Tendon, Left
V Foot Tendon, Right
W Foot Tendon, Left
	Ø Open
	3 Percutaneous
	4 Percutaneous Endoscopic
		Z No Device	Z No Qualifier

Ø **Medical and Surgical**
L **Tendons**
8 **Division**　　Definition: Cutting into a body part, without draining fluids and/or gases from the body part, in order to separate or transect a body part
　　　　　　　　　Explanation: All or a portion of the body part is separated into two or more portions

Body Part Character 4	Approach Character 5	Device Character 6	Qualifier Character 7
Ø Head and Neck Tendon	**Ø** Open	**Z** No Device	**Z** No Qualifier
1 Shoulder Tendon, Right	**3** Percutaneous		
2 Shoulder Tendon, Left	**4** Percutaneous Endoscopic		
3 Upper Arm Tendon, Right			
4 Upper Arm Tendon, Left			
5 Lower Arm and Wrist Tendon, Right			
6 Lower Arm and Wrist Tendon, Left			
7 Hand Tendon, Right			
8 Hand Tendon, Left			
9 Trunk Tendon, Right			
B Trunk Tendon, Left			
C Thorax Tendon, Right			
D Thorax Tendon, Left			
F Abdomen Tendon, Right			
G Abdomen Tendon, Left			
H Perineum Tendon			
J Hip Tendon, Right			
K Hip Tendon, Left			
L Upper Leg Tendon, Right			
M Upper Leg Tendon, Left			
N Lower Leg Tendon, Right 　　Achilles tendon			
P Lower Leg Tendon, Left 　　See N Lower Leg Tendon, Right			
Q Knee Tendon, Right 　　Patellar tendon			
R Knee Tendon, Left 　　See Q Knee Tendon, Right			
S Ankle Tendon, Right			
T Ankle Tendon, Left			
V Foot Tendon, Right			
W Foot Tendon, Left			

Ø   **Medical and Surgical**
L   **Tendons**
9   **Drainage**   Definition: Taking or letting out fluids and/or gases from a body part

               Explanation: The qualifier DIAGNOSTIC is used to identify drainage procedures that are biopsies

Body Part Character 4	Approach Character 5	Device Character 6	Qualifier Character 7
Ø Head and Neck Tendon	**Ø** Open	**Ø** Drainage Device	**Z** No Qualifier
1 Shoulder Tendon, Right	**3** Percutaneous		
2 Shoulder Tendon, Left	**4** Percutaneous Endoscopic		
3 Upper Arm Tendon, Right			
4 Upper Arm Tendon, Left			
5 Lower Arm and Wrist Tendon, Right			
6 Lower Arm and Wrist Tendon, Left			
7 Hand Tendon, Right			
8 Hand Tendon, Left			
9 Trunk Tendon, Right			
B Trunk Tendon, Left			
C Thorax Tendon, Right			
D Thorax Tendon, Left			
F Abdomen Tendon, Right			
G Abdomen Tendon, Left			
H Perineum Tendon			
J Hip Tendon, Right			
K Hip Tendon, Left			
L Upper Leg Tendon, Right			
M Upper Leg Tendon, Left			
N Lower Leg Tendon, Right Achilles tendon			
P Lower Leg Tendon, Left *See N Lower Leg Tendon, Right*			
Q Knee Tendon, Right Patellar tendon			
R Knee Tendon, Left *See Q Knee Tendon, Right*			
S Ankle Tendon, Right			
T Ankle Tendon, Left			
V Foot Tendon, Right			
W Foot Tendon, Left			
Ø Head and Neck Tendon	**Ø** Open	**Z** No Device	**X** Diagnostic
1 Shoulder Tendon, Right	**3** Percutaneous		**Z** No Qualifier
2 Shoulder Tendon, Left	**4** Percutaneous Endoscopic		
3 Upper Arm Tendon, Right			
4 Upper Arm Tendon, Left			
5 Lower Arm and Wrist Tendon, Right			
6 Lower Arm and Wrist Tendon, Left			
7 Hand Tendon, Right			
8 Hand Tendon, Left			
9 Trunk Tendon, Right			
B Trunk Tendon, Left			
C Thorax Tendon, Right			
D Thorax Tendon, Left			
F Abdomen Tendon, Right			
G Abdomen Tendon, Left			
H Perineum Tendon			
J Hip Tendon, Right			
K Hip Tendon, Left			
L Upper Leg Tendon, Right			
M Upper Leg Tendon, Left			
N Lower Leg Tendon, Right Achilles tendon			
P Lower Leg Tendon, Left *See N Lower Leg Tendon, Right*			
Q Knee Tendon, Right Patellar tendon			
R Knee Tendon, Left *See Q Knee Tendon, Right*			
S Ankle Tendon, Right			
T Ankle Tendon, Left			
V Foot Tendon, Right			
W Foot Tendon, Left			

Non-OR   ØL9[Ø,1,2,3,4,5,6,7,8,9,B,C,D,F,G,H,J,K,L,M,N,P,Q,R,S,T,V,W]3ØZ   **Non-OR**   ØL9[7,8]4ZZ
Non-OR   ØL9[Ø,1,2,3,4,5,6,7,8,9,B,C,D,F,G,H,J,K,L,M,N,P,Q,R,S,T,V,W]3ZZ

Non-OR Procedure   DRG Non-OR Procedure   Valid OR Procedure   HAC Associated Procedure   Combination Only   New/Revised April   New/Revised October

490   ICD-10-PCS 2023

Ø Medical and Surgical
L Tendons
B Excision Definition: Cutting out or off, without replacement, a portion of a body part

Explanation: The qualifier DIAGNOSTIC is used to identify excision procedures that are biopsies

Body Part Character 4	Approach Character 5	Device Character 6	Qualifier Character 7
Ø Head and Neck Tendon	Ø Open	Z No Device	X Diagnostic
1 Shoulder Tendon, Right	3 Percutaneous		Z No Qualifier
2 Shoulder Tendon, Left	4 Percutaneous Endoscopic		
3 Upper Arm Tendon, Right			
4 Upper Arm Tendon, Left			
5 Lower Arm and Wrist Tendon, Right			
6 Lower Arm and Wrist Tendon, Left			
7 Hand Tendon, Right			
8 Hand Tendon, Left			
9 Trunk Tendon, Right			
B Trunk Tendon, Left			
C Thorax Tendon, Right			
D Thorax Tendon, Left			
F Abdomen Tendon, Right			
G Abdomen Tendon, Left			
H Perineum Tendon			
J Hip Tendon, Right			
K Hip Tendon, Left			
L Upper Leg Tendon, Right			
M Upper Leg Tendon, Left			
N Lower Leg Tendon, Right Achilles tendon			
P Lower Leg Tendon, Left See N Lower Leg Tendon, Right			
Q Knee Tendon, Right Patellar tendon			
R Knee Tendon, Left See Q Knee Tendon, Right			
S Ankle Tendon, Right			
T Ankle Tendon, Left			
V Foot Tendon, Right			
W Foot Tendon, Left			

Ø   Medical and Surgical
L   Tendons
C   Extirpation   Definition: Taking or cutting out solid matter from a body part

Explanation: The solid matter may be an abnormal byproduct of a biological function or a foreign body; it may be imbedded in a body part or in the lumen of a tubular body part. The solid matter may or may not have been previously broken into pieces.

Body Part Character 4	Approach Character 5	Device Character 6	Qualifier Character 7
Ø Head and Neck Tendon	Ø Open	Z No Device	Z No Qualifier
1 Shoulder Tendon, Right	3 Percutaneous		
2 Shoulder Tendon, Left	4 Percutaneous Endoscopic		
3 Upper Arm Tendon, Right			
4 Upper Arm Tendon, Left			
5 Lower Arm and Wrist Tendon, Right			
6 Lower Arm and Wrist Tendon, Left			
7 Hand Tendon, Right			
8 Hand Tendon, Left			
9 Trunk Tendon, Right			
B Trunk Tendon, Left			
C Thorax Tendon, Right			
D Thorax Tendon, Left			
F Abdomen Tendon, Right			
G Abdomen Tendon, Left			
H Perineum Tendon			
J Hip Tendon, Right			
K Hip Tendon, Left			
L Upper Leg Tendon, Right			
M Upper Leg Tendon, Left			
N Lower Leg Tendon, Right Achilles tendon			
P Lower Leg Tendon, Left *See N Lower Leg Tendon, Right*			
Q Knee Tendon, Right Patellar tendon			
R Knee Tendon, Left *See Q Knee Tendon, Right*			
S Ankle Tendon, Right			
T Ankle Tendon, Left			
V Foot Tendon, Right			
W Foot Tendon, Left			

Ø   **Medical and Surgical**
L   **Tendons**
D   **Extraction**   Definition: Pulling or stripping out or off all or a portion of a body part by the use of force
                       Explanation: The qualifier DIAGNOSTIC is used to identify extraction procedures that are biopsies

Body Part Character 4	Approach Character 5	Device Character 6	Qualifier Character 7

Ø Head and Neck Tendon
1 Shoulder Tendon, Right
2 Shoulder Tendon, Left
3 Upper Arm Tendon, Right
4 Upper Arm Tendon, Left
5 Lower Arm and Wrist Tendon, Right
6 Lower Arm and Wrist Tendon, Left
7 Hand Tendon, Right
8 Hand Tendon, Left
9 Trunk Tendon, Right
B Trunk Tendon, Left
C Thorax Tendon, Right
D Thorax Tendon, Left
F Abdomen Tendon, Right
G Abdomen Tendon, Left
H Perineum Tendon
J Hip Tendon, Right
K Hip Tendon, Left
L Upper Leg Tendon, Right
M Upper Leg Tendon, Left
N Lower Leg Tendon, Right
    Achilles tendon
P Lower Leg Tendon, Left
    See N Lower Leg Tendon, Right
Q Knee Tendon, Right
    Patellar tendon
R Knee Tendon, Left
    See Q Knee Tendon, Right
S Ankle Tendon, Right
T Ankle Tendon, Left
V Foot Tendon, Right
W Foot Tendon, Left
	Ø Open	**Z** No Device	**Z** No Qualifier

Ø   **Medical and Surgical**
L   **Tendons**
H   **Insertion**   Definition: Putting in a nonbiological appliance that monitors, assists, performs, or prevents a physiological function but does not physically
                       take the place of a body part
                       Explanation: None

Body Part Character 4	Approach Character 5	Device Character 6	Qualifier Character 7
X Upper Tendon **Y** Lower Tendon	**Ø** Open **3** Percutaneous **4** Percutaneous Endoscopic	**Y** Other Device	**Z** No Qualifier

Non-OR   ØLH[X,Y][3,4]YZ

Ø   **Medical and Surgical**
L   **Tendons**
J   **Inspection**   Definition: Visually and/or manually exploring a body part
                       Explanation: Visual exploration may be performed with or without optical instrumentation. Manual exploration may be performed directly or
                       through intervening body layers.

Body Part Character 4	Approach Character 5	Device Character 6	Qualifier Character 7
X Upper Tendon **Y** Lower Tendon	**Ø** Open **3** Percutaneous **4** Percutaneous Endoscopic **X** External	**Z** No Device	**Z** No Qualifier

Non-OR   ØLJ[X,Y][3,X]ZZ

NC Noncovered Procedure   LC Limited Coverage   QA Questionable OB Admit   NT New Tech Add-on   ⊞ Combination Member   ♂ Male   ♀ Female

ICD-10-PCS 2023   493

Ø   **Medical and Surgical**
L   **Tendons**
M   **Reattachment**   Definition: Putting back in or on all or a portion of a separated body part to its normal location or other suitable location
                            Explanation: Vascular circulation and nervous pathways may or may not be reestablished

Body Part Character 4	Approach Character 5	Device Character 6	Qualifier Character 7
Ø Head and Neck Tendon	**Ø** Open	**Z** No Device	**Z** No Qualifier
1 Shoulder Tendon, Right	**4** Percutaneous Endoscopic		
2 Shoulder Tendon, Left			
3 Upper Arm Tendon, Right			
4 Upper Arm Tendon, Left			
5 Lower Arm and Wrist Tendon, Right			
6 Lower Arm and Wrist Tendon, Left			
7 Hand Tendon, Right			
8 Hand Tendon, Left			
9 Trunk Tendon, Right			
B Trunk Tendon, Left			
C Thorax Tendon, Right			
D Thorax Tendon, Left			
F Abdomen Tendon, Right			
G Abdomen Tendon, Left			
H Perineum Tendon			
J Hip Tendon, Right			
K Hip Tendon, Left			
L Upper Leg Tendon, Right			
M Upper Leg Tendon, Left			
N Lower Leg Tendon, Right Achilles tendon			
P Lower Leg Tendon, Left See N Lower Leg Tendon, Right			
Q Knee Tendon, Right Patellar tendon			
R Knee Tendon, Left See Q Knee Tendon, Right			
S Ankle Tendon, Right			
T Ankle Tendon, Left			
V Foot Tendon, Right			
W Foot Tendon, Left			

Ø   **Medical and Surgical**
L   **Tendons**
N   **Release**   Definition: Freeing a body part from an abnormal physical constraint by cutting or by the use of force
                      Explanation: Some of the restraining tissue may be taken out but none of the body part is taken out

Body Part Character 4	Approach Character 5	Device Character 6	Qualifier Character 7
Ø Head and Neck Tendon	**Ø** Open	**Z** No Device	**Z** No Qualifier
1 Shoulder Tendon, Right	**3** Percutaneous		
2 Shoulder Tendon, Left	**4** Percutaneous Endoscopic		
3 Upper Arm Tendon, Right	**X** External		
4 Upper Arm Tendon, Left			
5 Lower Arm and Wrist Tendon, Right			
6 Lower Arm and Wrist Tendon, Left			
7 Hand Tendon, Right			
8 Hand Tendon, Left			
9 Trunk Tendon, Right			
B Trunk Tendon, Left			
C Thorax Tendon, Right			
D Thorax Tendon, Left			
F Abdomen Tendon, Right			
G Abdomen Tendon, Left			
H Perineum Tendon			
J Hip Tendon, Right			
K Hip Tendon, Left			
L Upper Leg Tendon, Right			
M Upper Leg Tendon, Left			
N Lower Leg Tendon, Right Achilles tendon			
P Lower Leg Tendon, Left See N Lower Leg Tendon, Right			
Q Knee Tendon, Right Patellar tendon			
R Knee Tendon, Left See Q Knee Tendon, Right			
S Ankle Tendon, Right			
T Ankle Tendon, Left			
V Foot Tendon, Right			
W Foot Tendon, Left			

Non-OR	ØLN[Ø,1,2,3,4,5,6,7,8,9,B,C,D,F,G,H,J,K,L,M,N,P,Q,R,S,T,V,W]XZZ

Non-OR Procedure   DRG Non-OR Procedure   Valid OR Procedure   HAC Associated Procedure   Combination Only   New/Revised April   New/Revised October

Ø   **Medical and Surgical**
L   **Tendons**
P   **Removal**   Definition: Taking out or off a device from a body part

                      Explanation: If a device is taken out and a similar device put in without cutting or puncturing the skin or mucous membrane, the procedure is coded to the root operation CHANGE. Otherwise, the procedure for taking out a device is coded to the root operation REMOVAL.

Body Part Character 4	Approach Character 5	Device Character 6	Qualifier Character 7
X Upper Tendon **Y** Lower Tendon	**Ø** Open **3** Percutaneous **4** Percutaneous Endoscopic	**Ø** Drainage Device **7** Autologous Tissue Substitute **J** Synthetic Substitute **K** Nonautologous Tissue Substitute **Y** Other Device	**Z** No Qualifier
X Upper Tendon **Y** Lower Tendon	**X** External	**Ø** Drainage Device	**Z** No Qualifier

Non-OR	ØLP[X,Y]3ØZ
Non-OR	ØLP[X,Y][3,4]YZ
Non-OR	ØLP[X,Y]XØZ

Ø   **Medical and Surgical**
L   **Tendons**
Q   **Repair**   Definition: Restoring, to the extent possible, a body part to its normal anatomic structure and function

                      Explanation: Used only when the method to accomplish the repair is not one of the other root operations

Body Part Character 4	Approach Character 5	Device Character 6	Qualifier Character 7

Ø Head and Neck Tendon
1 Shoulder Tendon, Right
2 Shoulder Tendon, Left
3 Upper Arm Tendon, Right
4 Upper Arm Tendon, Left
5 Lower Arm and Wrist Tendon, Right
6 Lower Arm and Wrist Tendon, Left
7 Hand Tendon, Right
8 Hand Tendon, Left
9 Trunk Tendon, Right
B Trunk Tendon, Left
C Thorax Tendon, Right
D Thorax Tendon, Left
F Abdomen Tendon, Right
G Abdomen Tendon, Left
H Perineum Tendon
J Hip Tendon, Right
K Hip Tendon, Left
L Upper Leg Tendon, Right
M Upper Leg Tendon, Left
N Lower Leg Tendon, Right
    Achilles tendon
P Lower Leg Tendon, Left
    See N Lower Leg Tendon, Right
Q Knee Tendon, Right
    Patellar tendon
R Knee Tendon, Left
    See Q Knee Tendon, Right
S Ankle Tendon, Right
T Ankle Tendon, Left
V Foot Tendon, Right
W Foot Tendon, Left
	Ø Open
	3 Percutaneous
	4 Percutaneous Endoscopic
		Z No Device	**Z** No Qualifier

Ø   **Medical and Surgical**
L   **Tendons**
R   **Replacement**   Definition: Putting in or on biological or synthetic material that physically takes the place and/or function of all or a portion of a body part

           Explanation: The body part may have been taken out or replaced, or may be taken out, physically eradicated, or rendered nonfunctional during the REPLACEMENT procedure. A REMOVAL procedure is coded for taking out the device used in a previous replacement procedure.

Body Part Character 4	Approach Character 5	Device Character 6	Qualifier Character 7

Ø   Head and Neck Tendon
1   Shoulder Tendon, Right
2   Shoulder Tendon, Left
3   Upper Arm Tendon, Right
4   Upper Arm Tendon, Left
5   Lower Arm and Wrist Tendon, Right
6   Lower Arm and Wrist Tendon, Left
7   Hand Tendon, Right
8   Hand Tendon, Left
9   Trunk Tendon, Right
B   Trunk Tendon, Left
C   Thorax Tendon, Right
D   Thorax Tendon, Left
F   Abdomen Tendon, Right
G   Abdomen Tendon, Left
H   Perineum Tendon
J   Hip Tendon, Right
K   Hip Tendon, Left
L   Upper Leg Tendon, Right
M   Upper Leg Tendon, Left
N   Lower Leg Tendon, Right
     Achilles tendon
P   Lower Leg Tendon, Left
     See N Lower Leg Tendon, Right
Q   Knee Tendon, Right
     Patellar tendon
R   Knee Tendon, Left
     See Q Knee Tendon, Right
S   Ankle Tendon, Right
T   Ankle Tendon, Left
V   Foot Tendon, Right
W   Foot Tendon, Left
	Ø Open
	4 Percutaneous Endoscopic
		7 Autologous Tissue Substitute
		J Synthetic Substitute
		K Nonautologous Tissue Substitute
			Z No Qualifier

Ø   **Medical and Surgical**
L   **Tendons**
S   **Reposition**   Definition: Moving to its normal location, or other suitable location, all or a portion of a body part

           Explanation: The body part is moved to a new location from an abnormal location, or from a normal location where it is not functioning correctly. The body part may or may not be cut out or off to be moved to the new location.

Body Part Character 4	Approach Character 5	Device Character 6	Qualifier Character 7

Ø   Head and Neck Tendon
1   Shoulder Tendon, Right
2   Shoulder Tendon, Left
3   Upper Arm Tendon, Right
4   Upper Arm Tendon, Left
5   Lower Arm and Wrist Tendon, Right
6   Lower Arm and Wrist Tendon, Left
7   Hand Tendon, Right
8   Hand Tendon, Left
9   Trunk Tendon, Right
B   Trunk Tendon, Left
C   Thorax Tendon, Right
D   Thorax Tendon, Left
F   Abdomen Tendon, Right
G   Abdomen Tendon, Left
H   Perineum Tendon
J   Hip Tendon, Right
K   Hip Tendon, Left
L   Upper Leg Tendon, Right
M   Upper Leg Tendon, Left
N   Lower Leg Tendon, Right
     Achilles tendon
P   Lower Leg Tendon, Left
     See N Lower Leg Tendon, Right
Q   Knee Tendon, Right
     Patellar tendon
R   Knee Tendon, Left
     See Q Knee Tendon, Right
S   Ankle Tendon, Right
T   Ankle Tendon, Left
V   Foot Tendon, Right
W   Foot Tendon, Left
	Ø Open
	4 Percutaneous Endoscopic
		Z No Device	Z No Qualifier

Non-OR Procedure   DRG Non-OR Procedure   Valid OR Procedure   HAC Associated Procedure   Combination Only   New/Revised April   New/Revised October

496   ICD-10-PCS 2023

Ø   Medical and Surgical
L   Tendons
T   Resection   Definition: Cutting out or off, without replacement, all of a body part
                      Explanation: None

Body Part Character 4	Approach Character 5	Device Character 6	Qualifier Character 7

Ø   Head and Neck Tendon
1   Shoulder Tendon, Right
2   Shoulder Tendon, Left
3   Upper Arm Tendon, Right
4   Upper Arm Tendon, Left
5   Lower Arm and Wrist Tendon, Right
6   Lower Arm and Wrist Tendon, Left
7   Hand Tendon, Right
8   Hand Tendon, Left
9   Trunk Tendon, Right
B   Trunk Tendon, Left
C   Thorax Tendon, Right
D   Thorax Tendon, Left
F   Abdomen Tendon, Right
G   Abdomen Tendon, Left
H   Perineum Tendon
J   Hip Tendon, Right
K   Hip Tendon, Left
L   Upper Leg Tendon, Right
M   Upper Leg Tendon, Left
N   Lower Leg Tendon, Right
      Achilles tendon
P   Lower Leg Tendon, Left
      See N Lower Leg Tendon, Right
Q   Knee Tendon, Right
      Patellar tendon
R   Knee Tendon, Left
      See Q Knee Tendon, Right
S   Ankle Tendon, Right
T   Ankle Tendon, Left
V   Foot Tendon, Right
W   Foot Tendon, Left
	Ø Open
	4 Percutaneous Endoscopic
		Z No Device	Z No Qualifier

Ø   Medical and Surgical
L   Tendons
U   Supplement   Definition: Putting in or on biological or synthetic material that physically reinforces and/or augments the function of a portion of a body part
                      Explanation: The biological material is non-living, or is living and from the same individual. The body part may have been previously replaced, and the SUPPLEMENT procedure is performed to physically reinforce and/or augment the function of the replaced body part.

Body Part Character 4	Approach Character 5	Device Character 6	Qualifier Character 7

Ø   Head and Neck Tendon
1   Shoulder Tendon, Right
2   Shoulder Tendon, Left
3   Upper Arm Tendon, Right
4   Upper Arm Tendon, Left
5   Lower Arm and Wrist Tendon, Right
6   Lower Arm and Wrist Tendon, Left
7   Hand Tendon, Right
8   Hand Tendon, Left
9   Trunk Tendon, Right
B   Trunk Tendon, Left
C   Thorax Tendon, Right
D   Thorax Tendon, Left
F   Abdomen Tendon, Right
G   Abdomen Tendon, Left
H   Perineum Tendon
J   Hip Tendon, Right
K   Hip Tendon, Left
L   Upper Leg Tendon, Right
M   Upper Leg Tendon, Left
N   Lower Leg Tendon, Right
      Achilles tendon
P   Lower Leg Tendon, Left
      See N Lower Leg Tendon, Right
Q   Knee Tendon, Right
      Patellar tendon
R   Knee Tendon, Left
      See Q Knee Tendon, Right
S   Ankle Tendon, Right
T   Ankle Tendon, Left
V   Foot Tendon, Right
W   Foot Tendon, Left
	Ø Open
	4 Percutaneous Endoscopic
		7 Autologous Tissue Substitute
		J Synthetic Substitute
		K Nonautologous Tissue Substitute
			Z No Qualifier

Ø   Medical and Surgical
L   Tendons
W   Revision   Definition: Correcting, to the extent possible, a portion of a malfunctioning device or the position of a displaced device

Explanation: Revision can include correcting a malfunctioning or displaced device by taking out or putting in components of the device such as a screw or pin

Body Part Character 4	Approach Character 5	Device Character 6	Qualifier Character 7
X Upper Tendon Y Lower Tendon	Ø Open 3 Percutaneous 4 Percutaneous Endoscopic	Ø Drainage Device 7 Autologous Tissue Substitute J Synthetic Substitute K Nonautologous Tissue Substitute Y Other Device	Z No Qualifier
X Upper Tendon Y Lower Tendon	X External	Ø Drainage Device 7 Autologous Tissue Substitute J Synthetic Substitute K Nonautologous Tissue Substitute	Z No Qualifier

Non-OR   ØLW[X,Y][3,4]YZ
Non-OR   ØLW[X,Y]X[Ø,7,J,K]Z

Ø   Medical and Surgical
L   Tendons
X   Transfer   Definition: Moving, without taking out, all or a portion of a body part to another location to take over the function of all or a portion of a body part

Explanation: The body part transferred remains connected to its vascular and nervous supply

Body Part Character 4	Approach Character 5	Device Character 6	Qualifier Character 7

Ø Head and Neck Tendon
1 Shoulder Tendon, Right
2 Shoulder Tendon, Left
3 Upper Arm Tendon, Right
4 Upper Arm Tendon, Left
5 Lower Arm and Wrist Tendon, Right
6 Lower Arm and Wrist Tendon, Left
7 Hand Tendon, Right
8 Hand Tendon, Left
9 Trunk Tendon, Right
B Trunk Tendon, Left
C Thorax Tendon, Right
D Thorax Tendon, Left
F Abdomen Tendon, Right
G Abdomen Tendon, Left
H Perineum Tendon
J Hip Tendon, Right
K Hip Tendon, Left
L Upper Leg Tendon, Right
M Upper Leg Tendon, Left
N Lower Leg Tendon, Right
    Achilles tendon
P Lower Leg Tendon, Left
    See N Lower Leg Tendon, Right
Q Knee Tendon, Right
    Patellar tendon
R Knee Tendon, Left
    See Q Knee Tendon, Right
S Ankle Tendon, Right
T Ankle Tendon, Left
V Foot Tendon, Right
W Foot Tendon, Left
	Ø Open
	4 Percutaneous Endoscopic
		Z No Device	Z No Qualifier

Non-OR Procedure   DRG Non-OR Procedure   Valid OR Procedure   HAC Associated Procedure   Combination Only   New/Revised April   New/Revised October

498   ICD-10-PCS 2023

Bursae and Ligaments ØM2–ØMX

Character Meanings*

This Character Meaning table is provided as a guide to assist the user in the identification of character members that may be found in this section of code tables. It **SHOULD NOT** be used to build a PCS code.

Operation–Character 3		Body Part–Character 4		Approach–Character 5		Device–Character 6		Qualifier–Character 7	
2	Change	Ø	Head and Neck Bursa and Ligament	Ø	Open	Ø	Drainage Device	X	Diagnostic
5	Destruction	1	Shoulder Bursa and Ligament, Right	3	Percutaneous	7	Autologous Tissue Substitute	Z	No Qualifier
8	Division	2	Shoulder Bursa and Ligament, Left	4	Percutaneous Endoscopic	J	Synthetic Substitute		
9	Drainage	3	Elbow Bursa and Ligament, Right	X	External	K	Nonautologous Tissue Substitute		
B	Excision	4	Elbow Bursa and Ligament, Left			Y	Other Device		
C	Extirpation	5	Wrist Bursa and Ligament, Right			Z	No Device		
D	Extraction	6	Wrist Bursa and Ligament, Left						
H	Insertion	7	Hand Bursa and Ligament, Right						
J	Inspection	8	Hand Bursa and Ligament, Left						
M	Reattachment	9	Upper Extremity Bursa and Ligament, Right						
N	Release	B	Upper Extremity Bursa and Ligament, Left						
P	Removal	C	Upper Spine Bursa and Ligament						
Q	Repair	D	Lower Spine Bursa and Ligament						
R	Replacement	F	Sternum Bursa and Ligament						
S	Reposition	G	Rib(s) Bursa and Ligament						
T	Resection	H	Abdomen Bursa and Ligament, Right						
U	Supplement	J	Abdomen Bursa and Ligament, Left						
W	Revision	K	Perineum Bursa and Ligament						
X	Transfer	L	Hip Bursa and Ligament, Right						
		M	Hip Bursa and Ligament, Left						
		N	Knee Bursa and Ligament, Right						
		P	Knee Bursa and Ligament, Left						
		Q	Ankle Bursa and Ligament, Right						
		R	Ankle Bursa and Ligament, Left						
		S	Foot Bursa and Ligament, Right						
		T	Foot Bursa and Ligament, Left						
		V	Lower Extremity Bursa and Ligament, Right						
		W	Lower Extremity Bursa and Ligament, Left						
		X	Upper Bursa and Ligament						
		Y	Lower Bursa and Ligament						

* Includes synovial membrane.

AHA Coding Clinic for table ØMB
2018, 3Q, 17   Excisional debridement of periosteum

AHA Coding Clinic for table ØMM
2013, 3Q, 20   Superior labrum anterior posterior (SLAP) repair and subacromial decompression

AHA Coding Clinic for table ØMQ
2014, 3Q, 9   Interspinous ligamentoplasty

AHA Coding Clinic for table ØMT
2017, 2Q, 21   Arthroscopic anterior cruciate ligament revision using autograft with anterolateral ligament reconstruction

AHA Coding Clinic for table ØMU
2017, 2Q, 21   Arthroscopic anterior cruciate ligament revision using autograft with anterolateral ligament reconstruction

Shoulder Ligaments

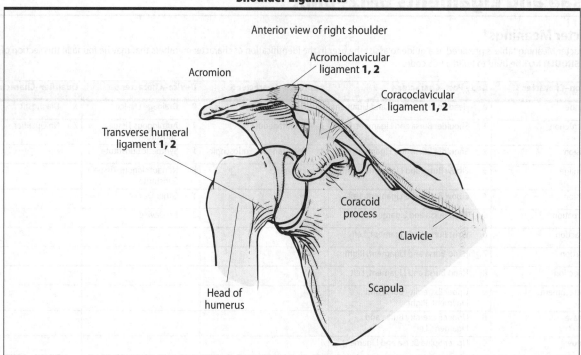

Anterior view of right shoulder

Acromion

Acromioclavicular ligament **1, 2**

Coracoclavicular ligament **1, 2**

Transverse humeral ligament **1, 2**

Coracoid process

Clavicle

Head of humerus

Scapula

Knee Bursae

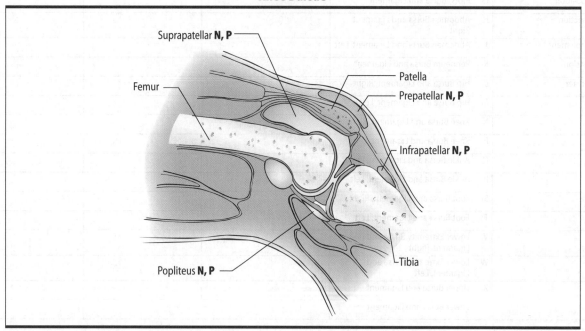

Suprapatellar **N, P**

Femur

Patella

Prepatellar **N, P**

Infrapatellar **N, P**

Popliteus **N, P**

Tibia

Knee Ligaments

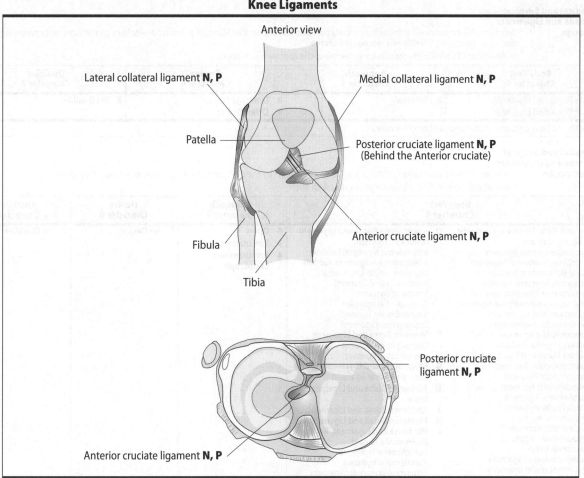

Anterior view

Lateral collateral ligament **N, P**

Medial collateral ligament **N, P**

Patella

Posterior cruciate ligament **N, P**
(Behind the Anterior cruciate)

Anterior cruciate ligament **N, P**

Fibula

Tibia

Posterior cruciate ligament **N, P**

Anterior cruciate ligament **N, P**

Wrist Ligaments

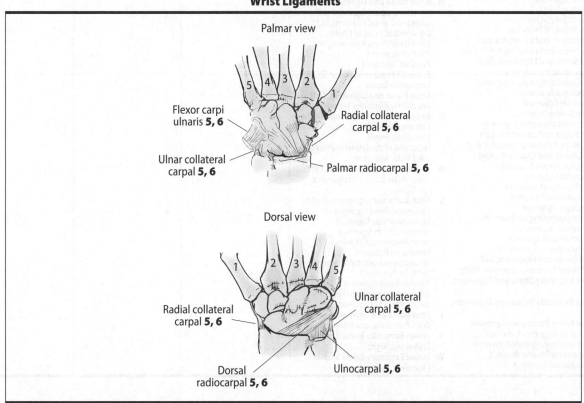

Palmar view

Flexor carpi ulnaris **5, 6**

Radial collateral carpal **5, 6**

Ulnar collateral carpal **5, 6**

Palmar radiocarpal **5, 6**

Dorsal view

Radial collateral carpal **5, 6**

Ulnar collateral carpal **5, 6**

Dorsal radiocarpal **5, 6**

Ulnocarpal **5, 6**

Ø   Medical and Surgical
M   Bursae and Ligaments
2   Change   Definition: Taking out or off a device from a body part and putting back an identical or similar device in or on the same body part without cutting or puncturing the skin or a mucous membrane

Explanation: All CHANGE procedures are coded using the approach EXTERNAL

Body Part Character 4	Approach Character 5	Device Character 6	Qualifier Character 7
X Upper Bursa and Ligament Y Lower Bursa and Ligament	X External	Ø Drainage Device Y Other Device	Z No Qualifier

Non-OR   All body part, approach, device, and qualifier values

Ø   Medical and Surgical
M   Bursae and Ligaments
5   Destruction   Definition: Physical eradication of all or a portion of a body part by the direct use of energy, force, or a destructive agent

Explanation: None of the body part is physically taken out

Body Part Character 4		Approach Character 5	Device Character 6	Qualifier Character 7
Ø Head and Neck Bursa and Ligament Alar ligament of axis Cervical interspinous ligament Cervical intertransverse ligament Cervical ligamentum flavum Interspinous ligament, cervical Intertransverse ligament, cervical Lateral temporomandibular ligament Ligamentum flavum, cervical Sphenomandibular ligament Stylomandibular ligament Transverse ligament of atlas **1 Shoulder Bursa and Ligament, Right** Acromioclavicular ligament Coracoacromial ligament Coracoclavicular ligament Coracohumeral ligament Costoclavicular ligament Glenohumeral ligament Interclavicular ligament Sternoclavicular ligament Subacromial bursa Transverse humeral ligament Transverse scapular ligament **2 Shoulder Bursa and Ligament, Left** *See 1 Shoulder Bursa and Ligament, Right* **3 Elbow Bursa and Ligament, Right** Annular ligament Olecranon bursa Radial collateral ligament Ulnar collateral ligament **4 Elbow Bursa and Ligament, Left** *See 3 Elbow Bursa and Ligament, Right* **5 Wrist Bursa and Ligament, Right** Palmar ulnocarpal ligament Radial collateral carpal ligament Radiocarpal ligament Radioulnar ligament Scapholunate ligament Ulnar collateral carpal ligament **6 Wrist Bursa and Ligament, Left** *See 5 Wrist Bursa and Ligament, Right* **7 Hand Bursa and Ligament, Right** Carpometacarpal ligament Intercarpal ligament Interphalangeal ligament Lunotriquetral ligament Metacarpal ligament Metacarpophalangeal ligament Pisohamate ligament Pisometacarpal ligament Scaphotrapezium ligament **8 Hand Bursa and Ligament, Left** *See 7 Hand Bursa and Ligament, Right* **9 Upper Extremity Bursa and Ligament, Right** **B Upper Extremity Bursa and Ligament, Left** **C Upper Spine Bursa and Ligament** Interspinous ligament, thoracic Intertransverse ligament, thoracic Ligamentum flavum, thoracic Supraspinous ligament	**D Lower Spine Bursa and Ligament** Iliolumbar ligament Interspinous ligament, lumbar Intertransverse ligament, lumbar Ligamentum flavum, lumbar Sacrococcygeal ligament Sacroiliac ligament Sacrospinous ligament Sacrotuberous ligament Supraspinous ligament **F Sternum Bursa and Ligament** Costoxiphoid ligament Sternocostal ligament **G Rib(s) Bursa and Ligament** Costotransverse ligament **H Abdomen Bursa and Ligament, Right** **J Abdomen Bursa and Ligament, Left** **K Perineum Bursa and Ligament** **L Hip Bursa and Ligament, Right** Iliofemoral ligament Ischiofemoral ligament Pubofemoral ligament Transverse acetabular ligament Trochanteric bursa **M Hip Bursa and Ligament, Left** *See L Hip Bursa and Ligament, Right* **N Knee Bursa and Ligament, Right** Anterior cruciate ligament (ACL) Lateral collateral ligament (LCL) Ligament of head of fibula Medial collateral ligament (MCL) Patellar ligament Popliteal ligament Posterior cruciate ligament (PCL) Prepatellar bursa **P Knee Bursa and Ligament, Left** *See N Knee Bursa and Ligament, Right* **Q Ankle Bursa and Ligament, Right** Calcaneofibular ligament Deltoid ligament Ligament of the lateral malleolus Talofibular ligament **R Ankle Bursa and Ligament, Left** *See Q Ankle Bursa and Ligament, Right* **S Foot Bursa and Ligament, Right** Calcaneocuboid ligament Cuneonavicular ligament Intercuneiform ligament Interphalangeal ligament Metatarsal ligament Metatarsophalangeal ligament Subtalar ligament Talocalcaneal ligament Talocalcaneonavicular ligament Tarsometatarsal ligament **T Foot Bursa and Ligament, Left** *See S Foot Bursa and Ligament, Right* **V Lower Extremity Bursa and Ligament, Right** **W Lower Extremity Bursa and Ligament, Left**	Ø Open 3 Percutaneous 4 Percutaneous Endoscopic	Z No Device	Z No Qualifier

Ø   **Medical and Surgical**
M   **Bursae and Ligaments**
8   **Division**   Definition: Cutting into a body part, without draining fluids and/or gases from the body part, in order to separate or transect a body part
                              Explanation: All or a portion of the body part is separated into two or more portions

Body Part Character 4		Approach Character 5	Device Character 6	Qualifier Character 7
Ø **Head and Neck Bursa and Ligament** Alar ligament of axis Cervical interspinous ligament Cervical intertransverse ligament Cervical ligamentum flavum Interspinous ligament, cervical Intertransverse ligament, cervical Lateral temporomandibular ligament Ligamentum flavum, cervical Sphenomandibular ligament Stylomandibular ligament Transverse ligament of atlas **1** **Shoulder Bursa and Ligament, Right** Acromioclavicular ligament Coracoacromial ligament Coracoclavicular ligament Coracohumeral ligament Costoclavicular ligament Glenohumeral ligament Interclavicular ligament Sternoclavicular ligament Subacromial bursa Transverse humeral ligament Transverse scapular ligament **2** **Shoulder Bursa and Ligament, Left** *See 1 Shoulder Bursa and Ligament, Right* **3** **Elbow Bursa and Ligament, Right** Annular ligament Olecranon bursa Radial collateral ligament Ulnar collateral ligament **4** **Elbow Bursa and Ligament, Left** *See 3 Elbow Bursa and Ligament, Right* **5** **Wrist Bursa and Ligament, Right** Palmar ulnocarpal ligament Radial collateral carpal ligament Radiocarpal ligament Radioulnar ligament Scapholunate ligament Ulnar collateral carpal ligament **6** **Wrist Bursa and Ligament, Left** *See 5 Wrist Bursa and Ligament, Right* **7** **Hand Bursa and Ligament, Right** Carpometacarpal ligament Intercarpal ligament Interphalangeal ligament Lunotriquetral ligament Metacarpal ligament Metacarpophalangeal ligament Pisohamate ligament Pisometacarpal ligament Scaphotrapezium ligament **8** **Hand Bursa and Ligament, Left** *See 7 Hand Bursa and Ligament, Right* **9** **Upper Extremity Bursa and Ligament, Right** **B** **Upper Extremity Bursa and Ligament, Left** **C** **Upper Spine Bursa and Ligament** Interspinous ligament, thoracic Intertransverse ligament, thoracic Ligamentum flavum, thoracic Supraspinous ligament	**D** **Lower Spine Bursa and Ligament** Iliolumbar ligament Interspinous ligament, lumbar Intertransverse ligament, lumbar Ligamentum flavum, lumbar Sacrococcygeal ligament Sacroiliac ligament Sacrospinous ligament Sacrotuberous ligament Supraspinous ligament **F** **Sternum Bursa and Ligament** Costoxiphoid ligament Sternocostal ligament **G** **Rib(s) Bursa and Ligament** Costotransverse ligament **H** **Abdomen Bursa and Ligament, Right** **J** **Abdomen Bursa and Ligament, Left** **K** **Perineum Bursa and Ligament** **L** **Hip Bursa and Ligament, Right** Iliofemoral ligament Ischiofemoral ligament Pubofemoral ligament Transverse acetabular ligament Trochanteric bursa **M** **Hip Bursa and Ligament, Left** *See L Hip Bursa and Ligament, Right* **N** **Knee Bursa and Ligament, Right** Anterior cruciate ligament (ACL) Lateral collateral ligament (LCL) Ligament of head of fibula Medial collateral ligament (MCL) Patellar ligament Popliteal ligament Posterior cruciate ligament (PCL) Prepatellar bursa **P** **Knee Bursa and Ligament, Left** *See N Knee Bursa and Ligament, Right* **Q** **Ankle Bursa and Ligament, Right** Calcaneofibular ligament Deltoid ligament Ligament of the lateral malleolus Talofibular ligament **R** **Ankle Bursa and Ligament, Left** *See Q Ankle Bursa and Ligament, Right* **S** **Foot Bursa and Ligament, Right** Calcaneocuboid ligament Cuneonavicular ligament Intercuneiform ligament Interphalangeal ligament Metatarsal ligament Metatarsophalangeal ligament Subtalar ligament Talocalcaneal ligament Talocalcaneonavicular ligament Tarsometatarsal ligament **T** **Foot Bursa and Ligament, Left** *See S Foot Bursa and Ligament, Right* **V** **Lower Extremity Bursa and Ligament, Right** **W** **Lower Extremity Bursa and Ligament, Left**	**Ø** Open **3** Percutaneous **4** Percutaneous Endoscopic	**Z** No Device	**Z** No Qualifier

ØM8 Continued on next page

NC Noncovered Procedure   LC Limited Coverage   QA Questionable OB Admit   NT New Tech Add-on   ⊞ Combination Member   ♂ Male   ♀ Female

ICD-10-PCS 2023   503

Ø Medical and Surgical
M Bursae and Ligaments
9 Drainage   Definition: Taking or letting out fluids and/or gases from a body part
                 Explanation: The qualifier DIAGNOSTIC is used to identify drainage procedures that are biopsies

Body Part Character 4		Approach Character 5	Device Character 6	Qualifier Character 7
Ø Head and Neck Bursa and Ligament Alar ligament of axis Cervical interspinous ligament Cervical intertransverse ligament Cervical ligamentum flavum Interspinous ligament, cervical Intertransverse ligament, cervical Lateral temporomandibular ligament Ligamentum flavum, cervical Sphenomandibular ligament Stylomandibular ligament Transverse ligament of atlas	**D Lower Spine Bursa and Ligament** Iliolumbar ligament Interspinous ligament, lumbar Intertransverse ligament, lumbar Ligamentum flavum, lumbar Sacrococcygeal ligament Sacroiliac ligament Sacrospinous ligament Sacrotuberous ligament Supraspinous ligament	**Ø Open** **3 Percutaneous** **4 Percutaneous Endoscopic**	**Ø Drainage Device**	**Z No Qualifier**
1 Shoulder Bursa and Ligament, Right Acromioclavicular ligament Coracoacromial ligament Coracoclavicular ligament Coracohumeral ligament Costoclavicular ligament Glenohumeral ligament Interclavicular ligament Sternoclavicular ligament Subacromial bursa Transverse humeral ligament Transverse scapular ligament	**F Sternum Bursa and Ligament** Costoxiphoid ligament Sternocostal ligament **G Rib(s) Bursa and Ligament** Costotransverse ligament **H Abdomen Bursa and Ligament, Right** **J Abdomen Bursa and Ligament, Left** **K Perineum Bursa and Ligament**			
2 Shoulder Bursa and Ligament, Left *See* 1 Shoulder Bursa and Ligament, Right	**L Hip Bursa and Ligament, Right** Iliofemoral ligament Ischiofemoral ligament Pubofemoral ligament Transverse acetabular ligament Trochanteric bursa			
3 Elbow Bursa and Ligament, Right Annular ligament Olecranon bursa Radial collateral ligament Ulnar collateral ligament	**M Hip Bursa and Ligament, Left** *See* L Hip Bursa and Ligament, Right			
4 Elbow Bursa and Ligament, Left *See* 3 Elbow Bursa and Ligament, Right	**N Knee Bursa and Ligament, Right** Anterior cruciate ligament (ACL) Lateral collateral ligament (LCL) Ligament of head of fibula Medial collateral ligament (MCL) Patellar ligament Popliteal ligament Posterior cruciate ligament (PCL) Prepatellar bursa			
5 Wrist Bursa and Ligament, Right Palmar ulnocarpal ligament Radial collateral carpal ligament Radiocarpal ligament Radioulnar ligament Scapholunate ligament Ulnar collateral carpal ligament	**P Knee Bursa and Ligament, Left** *See* N Knee Bursa and Ligament, Right			
6 Wrist Bursa and Ligament, Left *See* 5 Wrist Bursa and Ligament, Right	**Q Ankle Bursa and Ligament, Right** Calcaneofibular ligament Deltoid ligament Ligament of the lateral malleolus Talofibular ligament			
7 Hand Bursa and Ligament, Right Carpometacarpal ligament Intercarpal ligament Interphalangeal ligament Lunotriquetral ligament Metacarpal ligament Metacarpophalangeal ligament Pisohamate ligament Pisometacarpal ligament Scaphotrapezium ligament	**R Ankle Bursa and Ligament, Left** *See* Q Ankle Bursa and Ligament, Right			
8 Hand Bursa and Ligament, Left *See* 7 Hand Bursa and Ligament, Right	**S Foot Bursa and Ligament, Right** Calcaneocuboid ligament Cuneonavicular ligament Intercuneiform ligament Interphalangeal ligament Metatarsal ligament Metatarsophalangeal ligament Subtalar ligament Talocalcaneal ligament Talocalcaneonavicular ligament Tarsometatarsal ligament			
9 Upper Extremity Bursa and Ligament, Right	**T Foot Bursa and Ligament, Left** *See* S Foot Bursa and Ligament, Right			
B Upper Extremity Bursa and Ligament, Left	**V Lower Extremity Bursa and Ligament, Right**			
C Upper Spine Bursa and Ligament Interspinous ligament, thoracic Intertransverse ligament, thoracic Ligamentum flavum, thoracic Supraspinous ligament	**W Lower Extremity Bursa and Ligament, Left**			

Non-OR   ØM9[Ø,1,2,3,4,5,6,7,8,9,B,C,D,F,G,H,J,K,L,M,N,P,Q,R,S,T,V,W]3ØZ
Non-OR   ØM9[1,2,3,4,7,8,9,B,C,D,F,G,H,J,K,L,M,V,W]4ØZ

ØM9 Continued on next page

Non-OR Procedure   DRG Non-OR Procedure   Valid OR Procedure   HAC Associated Procedure   Combination Only   New/Revised April   New/Revised October

Ø   **Medical and Surgical**   *ØM9 Continued*
M   **Bursae and Ligaments**
9   **Drainage**   Definition: Taking or letting out fluids and/or gases from a body part

                               Explanation: The qualifier DIAGNOSTIC is used to identify drainage procedures that are biopsies

Body Part Character 4		Approach Character 5	Device Character 6	Qualifier Character 7
Ø Head and Neck Bursa and Ligament Alar ligament of axis Cervical interspinous ligament Cervical intertransverse ligament Cervical ligamentum flavum Interspinous ligament, cervical Intertransverse ligament, cervical Lateral temporomandibular ligament Ligamentum flavum, cervical Sphenomandibular ligament Stylomandibular ligament Transverse ligament of atlas	**D Lower Spine Bursa and Ligament** Iliolumbar ligament Interspinous ligament, lumbar Intertransverse ligament, lumbar Ligamentum flavum, lumbar Sacrococcygeal ligament Sacroiliac ligament Sacrospinous ligament Sacrotuberous ligament Supraspinous ligament	**Ø Open** **3 Percutaneous** **4 Percutaneous Endoscopic**	**Z No Device**	**X Diagnostic** **Z No Qualifier**
1 Shoulder Bursa and Ligament, Right Acromioclavicular ligament Coracoacromial ligament Coracoclavicular ligament Coracohumeral ligament Costoclavicular ligament Glenohumeral ligament Interclavicular ligament Sternoclavicular ligament Subacromial bursa Transverse humeral ligament Transverse scapular ligament	**F Sternum Bursa and Ligament** Costoxiphoid ligament Sternocostal ligament **G Rib(s) Bursa and Ligament** Costotransverse ligament **H Abdomen Bursa and Ligament, Right** **J Abdomen Bursa and Ligament, Left** **K Perineum Bursa and Ligament**			
2 Shoulder Bursa and Ligament, Left *See 1 Shoulder Bursa and Ligament, Right*	**L Hip Bursa and Ligament, Right** Iliofemoral ligament Ischiofemoral ligament Pubofemoral ligament Transverse acetabular ligament Trochanteric bursa			
3 Elbow Bursa and Ligament, Right Annular ligament Olecranon bursa Radial collateral ligament Ulnar collateral ligament	**M Hip Bursa and Ligament, Left** *See L Hip Bursa and Ligament, Right* **N Knee Bursa and Ligament, Right** Anterior cruciate ligament (ACL) Lateral collateral ligament (LCL) Ligament of head of fibula Medial collateral ligament (MCL) Patellar ligament Popliteal ligament Posterior cruciate ligament (PCL) Prepatellar bursa			
4 Elbow Bursa and Ligament, Left *See 3 Elbow Bursa and Ligament, Right*				
5 Wrist Bursa and Ligament, Right Palmar ulnocarpal ligament Radial collateral carpal ligament Radiocarpal ligament Radioulnar ligament Scapholunate ligament Ulnar collateral carpal ligament	**P Knee Bursa and Ligament, Left** *See N Knee Bursa and Ligament, Right* **Q Ankle Bursa and Ligament, Right** Calcaneofibular ligament Deltoid ligament Ligament of the lateral malleolus Talofibular ligament			
6 Wrist Bursa and Ligament, Left *See 5 Wrist Bursa and Ligament, Right*	**R Ankle Bursa and Ligament, Left** *See Q Ankle Bursa and Ligament, Right*			
7 Hand Bursa and Ligament, Right Carpometacarpal ligament Intercarpal ligament Interphalangeal ligament Lunotriquetral ligament Metacarpal ligament Metacarpophalangeal ligament Pisohamate ligament Pisometacarpal ligament Scaphotrapezium ligament	**S Foot Bursa and Ligament, Right** Calcaneocuboid ligament Cuneonavicular ligament Intercuneiform ligament Interphalangeal ligament Metatarsal ligament Metatarsophalangeal ligament Subtalar ligament Talocalcaneal ligament Talocalcaneonavicular ligament Tarsometatarsal ligament			
8 Hand Bursa and Ligament, Left *See 7 Hand Bursa and Ligament, Right*	**T Foot Bursa and Ligament, Left** *See S Foot Bursa and Ligament, Right*			
9 Upper Extremity Bursa and Ligament, Right **B Upper Extremity Bursa and Ligament, Left** **C Upper Spine Bursa and Ligament** Interspinous ligament, thoracic Intertransverse ligament, thoracic Ligamentum flavum, thoracic Supraspinous ligament	**V Lower Extremity Bursa and Ligament, Right** **W Lower Extremity Bursa and Ligament, Left**			

Non-OR	ØM9[Ø,1,2,3,4,5,6,7,8,C,D,F,G,L,M,N,P,Q,R,S,T][Ø,3,4]ZX
Non-OR	ØM9[Ø,1,2,3,4,5,6,7,8,9,B,C,D,F,G,H,J,K,L,M,N,P,Q,R,S,T,V,W]3ZZ
Non-OR	ØM9[Ø,5,6,7,8,9,B,C,D,F,G,H,J,K,N,P,Q,R,S,T,V,W]4ZZ

NC Noncovered Procedure   **LC** Limited Coverage   **QA** Questionable OB Admit   **NT** New Tech Add-on   ⊞ Combination Member   ♂ Male   ♀ Female

ICD-10-PCS 2023   **505**

Ø Medical and Surgical
M Bursae and Ligaments
B Excision   Definition: Cutting out or off, without replacement, a portion of a body part
                      Explanation: The qualifier DIAGNOSTIC is used to identify excision procedures that are biopsies

Body Part Character 4	Approach Character 5	Device Character 6	Qualifier Character 7
Ø Head and Neck Bursa and Ligament Alar ligament of axis Cervical interspinous ligament Cervical intertransverse ligament Cervical ligamentum flavum Interspinous ligament, cervical Intertransverse ligament, cervical Lateral temporomandibular ligament Ligamentum flavum, cervical Sphenomandibular ligament Stylomandibular ligament Transverse ligament of atlas **1 Shoulder Bursa and Ligament, Right** Acromioclavicular ligament Coracoacromial ligament Coracoclavicular ligament Coracohumeral ligament Costoclavicular ligament Glenohumeral ligament Interclavicular ligament Sternoclavicular ligament Subacromial bursa Transverse humeral ligament Transverse scapular ligament **2 Shoulder Bursa and Ligament, Left** *See 1 Shoulder Bursa and Ligament, Right* **3 Elbow Bursa and Ligament, Right** Annular ligament Olecranon bursa Radial collateral ligament Ulnar collateral ligament **4 Elbow Bursa and Ligament, Left** *See 3 Elbow Bursa and Ligament, Right* **5 Wrist Bursa and Ligament, Right** Palmar ulnocarpal ligament Radial collateral carpal ligament Radiocarpal ligament Radioulnar ligament Scapholunate ligament Ulnar collateral carpal ligament **6 Wrist Bursa and Ligament, Left** *See 5 Wrist Bursa and Ligament, Right* **7 Hand Bursa and Ligament, Right** Carpometacarpal ligament Intercarpal ligament Interphalangeal ligament Lunotriquetral ligament Metacarpal ligament Metacarpophalangeal ligament Pisohamate ligament Pisometacarpal ligament Scaphotrapezium ligament **8 Hand Bursa and Ligament, Left** *See 7 Hand Bursa and Ligament, Right* **9 Upper Extremity Bursa and Ligament, Right** **B Upper Extremity Bursa and Ligament, Left** **C Upper Spine Bursa and Ligament** Interspinous ligament, thoracic Intertransverse ligament, thoracic Ligamentum flavum, thoracic Supraspinous ligament	**Ø Open** **3 Percutaneous** **4 Percutaneous Endoscopic**	**Z No Device**	**X Diagnostic** **Z No Qualifier**

D Lower Spine Bursa and Ligament
Iliolumbar ligament
Interspinous ligament, lumbar
Intertransverse ligament, lumbar
Ligamentum flavum, lumbar
Sacrococcygeal ligament
Sacroiliac ligament
Sacrospinous ligament
Sacrotuberous ligament
Supraspinous ligament
F Sternum Bursa and Ligament
Costoxiphoid ligament
Sternocostal ligament
G Rib(s) Bursa and Ligament
Costotransverse ligament
H Abdomen Bursa and Ligament, Right
J Abdomen Bursa and Ligament, Left
K Perineum Bursa and Ligament
L Hip Bursa and Ligament, Right
Iliofemoral ligament
Ischiofemoral ligament
Pubofemoral ligament
Transverse acetabular ligament
Trochanteric bursa
M Hip Bursa and Ligament, Left
See L Hip Bursa and Ligament, Right
N Knee Bursa and Ligament, Right
Anterior cruciate ligament (ACL)
Lateral collateral ligament (LCL)
Ligament of head of fibula
Medial collateral ligament (MCL)
Patellar ligament
Popliteal ligament
Posterior cruciate ligament (PCL)
Prepatellar bursa
P Knee Bursa and Ligament, Left
See N Knee Bursa and Ligament, Right
Q Ankle Bursa and Ligament, Right
Calcaneofibular ligament
Deltoid ligament
Ligament of the lateral malleolus
Talofibular ligament
R Ankle Bursa and Ligament, Left
See Q Ankle Bursa and Ligament, Right
S Foot Bursa and Ligament, Right
Calcaneocuboid ligament
Cuneonavicular ligament
Intercuneiform ligament
Interphalangeal ligament
Metatarsal ligament
Metatarsophalangeal ligament
Subtalar ligament
Talocalcaneal ligament
Talocalcaneonavicular ligament
Tarsometatarsal ligament
T Foot Bursa and Ligament, Left
See S Foot Bursa and Ligament, Right
V Lower Extremity Bursa and Ligament, Right
W Lower Extremity Bursa and Ligament, Left

Non-OR   ØMB[Ø,1,2,3,4,5,6,7,8,B,C,D,F,G,L,M,N,P,Q,R,S,T][Ø,3,4]ZX
Non-OR   ØMB94ZX

Ø **Medical and Surgical**
M **Bursae and Ligaments**
C **Extirpation**   Definition: Taking or cutting out solid matter from a body part
Explanation: The solid matter may be an abnormal byproduct of a biological function or a foreign body; it may be imbedded in a body part or in the lumen of a tubular body part. The solid matter may or may not have been previously broken into pieces.

Body Part Character 4		Approach Character 5	Device Character 6	Qualifier Character 7

Ø Head and Neck Bursa and Ligament
   Alar ligament of axis
   Cervical interspinous ligament
   Cervical intertransverse ligament
   Cervical ligamentum flavum
   Interspinous ligament, cervical
   Intertransverse ligament, cervical
   Lateral temporomandibular ligament
   Ligamentum flavum, cervical
   Sphenomandibular ligament
   Stylomandibular ligament
   Transverse ligament of atlas
1 Shoulder Bursa and Ligament, Right
   Acromioclavicular ligament
   Coracoacromial ligament
   Coracoclavicular ligament
   Coracohumeral ligament
   Costoclavicular ligament
   Glenohumeral ligament
   Interclavicular ligament
   Sternoclavicular ligament
   Subacromial bursa
   Transverse humeral ligament
   Transverse scapular ligament
2 Shoulder Bursa and Ligament, Left
   See 1 Shoulder Bursa and Ligament, Right
3 Elbow Bursa and Ligament, Right
   Annular ligament
   Olecranon bursa
   Radial collateral ligament
   Ulnar collateral ligament
4 Elbow Bursa and Ligament, Left
   See 3 Elbow Bursa and Ligament, Right
5 Wrist Bursa and Ligament, Right
   Palmar ulnocarpal ligament
   Radial collateral carpal ligament
   Radiocarpal ligament
   Radioulnar ligament
   Scapholunate ligament
   Ulnar collateral carpal ligament
6 Wrist Bursa and Ligament, Left
   See 5 Wrist Bursa and Ligament, Right
7 Hand Bursa and Ligament, Right
   Carpometacarpal ligament
   Intercarpal ligament
   Interphalangeal ligament
   Lunotriquetral ligament
   Metacarpal ligament
   Metacarpophalangeal ligament
   Pisohamate ligament
   Pisometacarpal ligament
   Scaphotrapezium ligament
8 Hand Bursa and Ligament, Left
   See 7 Hand Bursa and Ligament, Right
9 Upper Extremity Bursa and Ligament, Right
B Upper Extremity Bursa and Ligament, Left
C Upper Spine Bursa and Ligament
   Interspinous ligament, thoracic
   Intertransverse ligament, thoracic
   Ligamentum flavum, thoracic
   Supraspinous ligament
	D Lower Spine Bursa and Ligament
	   Iliolumbar ligament
	   Interspinous ligament, lumbar
	   Intertransverse ligament, lumbar
	   Ligamentum flavum, lumbar
	   Sacrococcygeal ligament
	   Sacroiliac ligament
	   Sacrospinous ligament
	   Sacrotuberous ligament
	   Supraspinous ligament
	F Sternum Bursa and Ligament
	   Costoxiphoid ligament
	   Sternocostal ligament
	G Rib(s) Bursa and Ligament
	   Costotransverse ligament
	H Abdomen Bursa and Ligament, Right
	J Abdomen Bursa and Ligament, Left
	K Perineum Bursa and Ligament
	L Hip Bursa and Ligament, Right
	   Iliofemoral ligament
	   Ischiofemoral ligament
	   Pubofemoral ligament
	   Transverse acetabular ligament
	   Trochanteric bursa
	M Hip Bursa and Ligament, Left
	   See L Hip Bursa and Ligament, Right
	N Knee Bursa and Ligament, Right
	   Anterior cruciate ligament (ACL)
	   Lateral collateral ligament (LCL)
	   Ligament of head of fibula
	   Medial collateral ligament (MCL)
	   Patellar ligament
	   Popliteal ligament
	   Posterior cruciate ligament (PCL)
	   Prepatellar bursa
	P Knee Bursa and Ligament, Left
	   See N Knee Bursa and Ligament, Right
	Q Ankle Bursa and Ligament, Right
	   Calcaneofibular ligament
	   Deltoid ligament
	   Ligament of the lateral malleolus
	   Talofibular ligament
	R Ankle Bursa and Ligament, Left
	   See Q Ankle Bursa and Ligament, Right
	S Foot Bursa and Ligament, Right
	   Calcaneocuboid ligament
	   Cuneonavicular ligament
	   Intercuneiform ligament
	   Interphalangeal ligament
	   Metatarsal ligament
	   Metatarsophalangeal ligament
	   Subtalar ligament
	   Talocalcaneal ligament
	   Talocalcaneonavicular ligament
	   Tarsometatarsal ligament
	T Foot Bursa and Ligament, Left
	   See S Foot Bursa and Ligament, Right
	V Lower Extremity Bursa and Ligament, Right
	W Lower Extremity Bursa and Ligament, Left
		Ø Open
		3 Percutaneous
		4 Percutaneous Endoscopic
			Z No Device	**Z No Qualifier**

NC Noncovered Procedure   **LC** Limited Coverage   **QA** Questionable OB Admit   **NT** New Tech Add-on   ⊞ Combination Member   ♂ Male   ♀ Female

ICD-10-PCS 2023   507

Bursae and Ligaments

Ø	Medical and Surgical
M	Bursae and Ligaments
D	Extraction

Definition: Pulling or stripping out or off all or a portion of a body part by the use of force

Explanation: The qualifier DIAGNOSTIC is used to identify extraction procedures that are biopsies

Body Part Character 4		Approach Character 5	Device Character 6	Qualifier Character 7
Ø Head and Neck Bursa and Ligament Alar ligament of axis Cervical interspinous ligament Cervical intertransverse ligament Cervical ligamentum flavum Interspinous ligament, cervical Intertransverse ligament, cervical Lateral temporomandibular ligament Ligamentum flavum, cervical Sphenomandibular ligament Stylomandibular ligament Transverse ligament of atlas	**D Lower Spine Bursa and Ligament** Iliolumbar ligament Interspinous ligament, lumbar Intertransverse ligament, lumbar Ligamentum flavum, lumbar Sacrococcygeal ligament Sacroiliac ligament Sacrospinous ligament Sacrotuberous ligament Supraspinous ligament	**Ø Open** **3 Percutaneous** **4 Percutaneous Endoscopic**	**Z No Device**	**Z No Qualifier**
1 Shoulder Bursa and Ligament, Right Acromioclavicular ligament Coracoacromial ligament Coracoclavicular ligament Coracohumeral ligament Costoclavicular ligament Glenohumeral ligament Interclavicular ligament Sternoclavicular ligament Subacromial bursa Transverse humeral ligament Transverse scapular ligament	**F Sternum Bursa and Ligament** Costoxiphoid ligament Sternocostal ligament **G Rib(s) Bursa and Ligament** Costotransverse ligament **H Abdomen Bursa and Ligament, Right** **J Abdomen Bursa and Ligament, Left** **K Perineum Bursa and Ligament** **L Hip Bursa and Ligament, Right** Iliofemoral ligament Ischiofemoral ligament Pubofemoral ligament Transverse acetabular ligament Trochanteric bursa			
2 Shoulder Bursa and Ligament, Left *See 1 Shoulder Bursa and Ligament, Right*	**M Hip Bursa and Ligament, Left** *See L Hip Bursa and Ligament, Right*			
3 Elbow Bursa and Ligament, Right Annular ligament Olecranon bursa Radial collateral ligament Ulnar collateral ligament	**N Knee Bursa and Ligament, Right** Anterior cruciate ligament (ACL) Lateral collateral ligament (LCL) Ligament of head of fibula Medial collateral ligament (MCL) Patellar ligament Popliteal ligament Posterior cruciate ligament (PCL) Prepatellar bursa			
4 Elbow Bursa and Ligament, Left *See 3 Elbow Bursa and Ligament, Right*	**P Knee Bursa and Ligament, Left** *See N Knee Bursa and Ligament, Right*			
5 Wrist Bursa and Ligament, Right Palmar ulnocarpal ligament Radial collateral carpal ligament Radiocarpal ligament Radioulnar ligament Scapholunate ligament Ulnar collateral carpal ligament	**Q Ankle Bursa and Ligament, Right** Calcaneofibular ligament Deltoid ligament Ligament of the lateral malleolus Talofibular ligament			
6 Wrist Bursa and Ligament, Left *See 5 Wrist Bursa and Ligament, Right*	**R Ankle Bursa and Ligament, Left** *See Q Ankle Bursa and Ligament, Right*			
7 Hand Bursa and Ligament, Right Carpometacarpal ligament Intercarpal ligament Interphalangeal ligament Lunotriquetral ligament Metacarpal ligament Metacarpophalangeal ligament Pisohamate ligament Pisometacarpal ligament Scaphotrapezium ligament	**S Foot Bursa and Ligament, Right** Calcaneocuboid ligament Cuneonavicular ligament Intercuneiform ligament Interphalangeal ligament Metatarsal ligament Metatarsophalangeal ligament Subtalar ligament Talocalcaneal ligament Talocalcaneonavicular ligament Tarsometatarsal ligament			
8 Hand Bursa and Ligament, Left *See 7 Hand Bursa and Ligament, Right*	**T Foot Bursa and Ligament, Left** *See S Foot Bursa and Ligament, Right*			
9 Upper Extremity Bursa and Ligament, Right **B Upper Extremity Bursa and Ligament, Left** **C Upper Spine Bursa and Ligament** Interspinous ligament, thoracic Intertransverse ligament, thoracic Ligamentum flavum, thoracic Supraspinous ligament	**V Lower Extremity Bursa and Ligament, Right** **W Lower Extremity Bursa and Ligament, Left**			

Non-OR Procedure   DRG Non-OR Procedure   Valid OR Procedure   HAC Associated Procedure   Combination Only   New/Revised April   New/Revised October

508

ICD-10-PCS 2023

Ø   **Medical and Surgical**
M   **Bursae and Ligaments**
H   **Insertion**   Definition: Putting in a nonbiological appliance that monitors, assists, performs, or prevents a physiological function but does not physically take the place of a body part
                     Explanation: None

Body Part Character 4	Approach Character 5	Device Character 6	Qualifier Character 7
X Upper Bursa and Ligament Y Lower Bursa and Ligament	Ø Open 3 Percutaneous 4 Percutaneous Endoscopic	Y Other Device	Z No Qualifier

Non-OR   ØMH[X,Y][3,4]YZ

Ø   **Medical and Surgical**
M   **Bursae and Ligaments**
J   **Inspection**   Definition: Visually and/or manually exploring a body part
                     Explanation: Visual exploration may be performed with or without optical instrumentation. Manual exploration may be performed directly or through intervening body layers.

Body Part Character 4	Approach Character 5	Device Character 6	Qualifier Character 7
X Upper Bursa and Ligament Y Lower Bursa and Ligament	Ø Open 3 Percutaneous 4 Percutaneous Endoscopic X External	Z No Device	Z No Qualifier

Non-OR   ØMJ[X,Y][3,X]ZZ

NC Noncovered Procedure   LC Limited Coverage   QA Questionable OB Admit   NT New Tech Add-on   ⊞ Combination Member   ♂ Male   ♀ Female

ICD-10-PCS 2023   509

Ø   Medical and Surgical
M   Bursae and Ligaments
M   Reattachment   Definition: Putting back in or on all or a portion of a separated body part to its normal location or other suitable location
                    Explanation: Vascular circulation and nervous pathways may or may not be reestablished

Body Part Character 4		Approach Character 5	Device Character 6	Qualifier Character 7
Ø Head and Neck Bursa and Ligament	**D Lower Spine Bursa and Ligament**	**Ø Open**	**Z No Device**	**Z No Qualifier**
Alar ligament of axis	Iliolumbar ligament	**4 Percutaneous Endoscopic**		
Cervical interspinous ligament	Interspinous ligament, lumbar			
Cervical intertransverse ligament	Intertransverse ligament, lumbar			
Cervical ligamentum flavum	Ligamentum flavum, lumbar			
Interspinous ligament, cervical	Sacrococcygeal ligament			
Intertransverse ligament, cervical	Sacroiliac ligament			
Lateral temporomandibular ligament	Sacrospinous ligament			
	Sacrotuberous ligament			
Ligamentum flavum, cervical	Supraspinous ligament			
Sphenomandibular ligament	**F Sternum Bursa and Ligament**			
Stylomandibular ligament	Costoxiphoid ligament			
Transverse ligament of atlas	Sternocostal ligament			
1 Shoulder Bursa and Ligament, Right	**G Rib(s) Bursa and Ligament**			
Acromioclavicular ligament	Costotransverse ligament			
Coracoacromial ligament	**H Abdomen Bursa and Ligament, Right**			
Coracoclavicular ligament	**J Abdomen Bursa and Ligament, Left**			
Coracohumeral ligament				
Costoclavicular ligament	**K Perineum Bursa and Ligament**			
Glenohumeral ligament	**L Hip Bursa and Ligament, Right**			
Interclavicular ligament	Iliofemoral ligament			
Sternoclavicular ligament	Ischiofemoral ligament			
Subacromial bursa	Pubofemoral ligament			
Transverse humeral ligament	Transverse acetabular ligament			
Transverse scapular ligament	Trochanteric bursa			
2 Shoulder Bursa and Ligament, Left	**M Hip Bursa and Ligament, Left**			
See 1 Shoulder Bursa and Ligament, Right	*See L Hip Bursa and Ligament, Right*			
3 Elbow Bursa and Ligament, Right	**N Knee Bursa and Ligament, Right**			
Annular ligament	Anterior cruciate ligament (ACL)			
Olecranon bursa	Lateral collateral ligament (LCL)			
Radial collateral ligament	Ligament of head of fibula			
Ulnar collateral ligament	Medial collateral ligament (MCL)			
4 Elbow Bursa and Ligament, Left	Patellar ligament			
See 3 Elbow Bursa and Ligament, Right	Popliteal ligament			
	Posterior cruciate ligament (PCL)			
	Prepatellar bursa			
5 Wrist Bursa and Ligament, Right	**P Knee Bursa and Ligament, Left**			
Palmar ulnocarpal ligament	*See N Knee Bursa and Ligament, Right*			
Radial collateral carpal ligament				
Radiocarpal ligament	**Q Ankle Bursa and Ligament, Right**			
Radioulnar ligament	Calcaneofibular ligament			
Scapholunate ligament	Deltoid ligament			
Ulnar collateral carpal ligament	Ligament of the lateral malleolus			
6 Wrist Bursa and Ligament, Left	Talofibular ligament			
See 5 Wrist Bursa and Ligament, Right	**R Ankle Bursa and Ligament, Left**			
	See Q Ankle Bursa and Ligament, Right			
7 Hand Bursa and Ligament, Right	**S Foot Bursa and Ligament, Right**			
Carpometacarpal ligament	Calcaneocuboid ligament			
Intercarpal ligament	Cuneonavicular ligament			
Interphalangeal ligament	Intercuneiform ligament			
Lunotriquetral ligament	Interphalangeal ligament			
Metacarpal ligament	Metatarsal ligament			
Metacarpophalangeal ligament	Metatarsophalangeal ligament			
Pisohamate ligament	Subtalar ligament			
Pisometacarpal ligament	Talocalcaneal ligament			
Scaphotrapezium ligament	Talocalcaneonavicular ligament			
8 Hand Bursa and Ligament, Left	Tarsometatarsal ligament			
See 7 Hand Bursa and Ligament, Right	**T Foot Bursa and Ligament, Left**			
	See S Foot Bursa and Ligament, Right			
9 Upper Extremity Bursa and Ligament, Right	**V Lower Extremity Bursa and Ligament, Right**			
B Upper Extremity Bursa and Ligament, Left	**W Lower Extremity Bursa and Ligament, Left**			
C Upper Spine Bursa and Ligament				
Interspinous ligament, thoracic				
Intertransverse ligament, thoracic				
Ligamentum flavum, thoracic				
Supraspinous ligament				

Ø   Medical and Surgical
M   Bursae and Ligaments
N   Release   Definition: Freeing a body part from an abnormal physical constraint by cutting or by the use of force
              Explanation: Some of the restraining tissue may be taken out but none of the body part is taken out

Body Part Character 4		Approach Character 5	Device Character 6	Qualifier Character 7

Ø Head and Neck Bursa and Ligament
  Alar ligament of axis
  Cervical interspinous ligament
  Cervical intertransverse ligament
  Cervical ligamentum flavum
  Interspinous ligament, cervical
  Intertransverse ligament, cervical
  Lateral temporomandibular ligament
  Ligamentum flavum, cervical
  Sphenomandibular ligament
  Stylomandibular ligament
  Transverse ligament of atlas
 	
1 Shoulder Bursa and Ligament, Right
  Acromioclavicular ligament
  Coracoacromial ligament
  Coracoclavicular ligament
  Coracohumeral ligament
  Costoclavicular ligament
  Glenohumeral ligament
  Interclavicular ligament
  Sternoclavicular ligament
  Subacromial bursa
  Transverse humeral ligament
  Transverse scapular ligament
 	
2 Shoulder Bursa and Ligament, Left
  See 1 Shoulder Bursa and Ligament, Right
 	
3 Elbow Bursa and Ligament, Right
  Annular ligament
  Olecranon bursa
  Radial collateral ligament
  Ulnar collateral ligament
 	
4 Elbow Bursa and Ligament, Left
  See 3 Elbow Bursa and Ligament, Right
 	
5 Wrist Bursa and Ligament, Right
  Palmar ulnocarpal ligament
  Radial collateral carpal ligament
  Radiocarpal ligament
  Radioulnar ligament
  Scapholunate ligament
  Ulnar collateral carpal ligament
 	
6 Wrist Bursa and Ligament, Left
  See 5 Wrist Bursa and Ligament, Right
 	
7 Hand Bursa and Ligament, Right
  Carpometacarpal ligament
  Intercarpal ligament
  Interphalangeal ligament
  Lunotriquetral ligament
  Metacarpal ligament
  Metacarpophalangeal ligament
  Pisohamate ligament
  Pisometacarpal ligament
  Scaphotrapezium ligament
 	
8 Hand Bursa and Ligament, Left
  See 7 Hand Bursa and Ligament, Right
 	
9 Upper Extremity Bursa and Ligament, Right
 	
B Upper Extremity Bursa and Ligament, Left
 	
C Upper Spine Bursa and Ligament
  Interspinous ligament, thoracic
  Intertransverse ligament, thoracic
  Ligamentum flavum, thoracic
  Supraspinous ligament
	D Lower Spine Bursa and Ligament
	  Iliolumbar ligament
	  Interspinous ligament, lumbar
	  Intertransverse ligament, lumbar
	  Ligamentum flavum, lumbar
	  Sacrococcygeal ligament
	  Sacroiliac ligament
	  Sacrospinous ligament
	  Sacrotuberous ligament
	  Supraspinous ligament
	
	F Sternum Bursa and Ligament
	  Costoxiphoid ligament
	  Sternocostal ligament
	
	G Rib(s) Bursa and Ligament
	  Costotransverse ligament
	
	H Abdomen Bursa and Ligament, Right
	
	J Abdomen Bursa and Ligament, Left
	
	K Perineum Bursa and Ligament
	
	L Hip Bursa and Ligament, Right
	  Iliofemoral ligament
	  Ischiofemoral ligament
	  Pubofemoral ligament
	  Transverse acetabular ligament
	  Trochanteric bursa
	
	M Hip Bursa and Ligament, Left
	  See L Hip Bursa and Ligament, Right
	
	N Knee Bursa and Ligament, Right
	  Anterior cruciate ligament (ACL)
	  Lateral collateral ligament (LCL)
	  Ligament of head of fibula
	  Medial collateral ligament (MCL)
	  Patellar ligament
	  Popliteal ligament
	  Posterior cruciate ligament (PCL)
	  Prepatellar bursa
	
	P Knee Bursa and Ligament, Left
	  See N Knee Bursa and Ligament, Right
	
	Q Ankle Bursa and Ligament, Right
	  Calcaneofibular ligament
	  Deltoid ligament
	  Ligament of the lateral malleolus
	  Talofibular ligament
	
	R Ankle Bursa and Ligament, Left
	  See Q Ankle Bursa and Ligament, Right
	
	S Foot Bursa and Ligament, Right
	  Calcaneocuboid ligament
	  Cuneonavicular ligament
	  Intercuneiform ligament
	  Interphalangeal ligament
	  Metatarsal ligament
	  Metatarsophalangeal ligament
	  Subtalar ligament
	  Talocalcaneal ligament
	  Talocalcaneonavicular ligament
	  Tarsometatarsal ligament
	
	T Foot Bursa and Ligament, Left
	  See S Foot Bursa and Ligament, Right
	
	V Lower Extremity Bursa and Ligament, Right
	
	W Lower Extremity Bursa and Ligament, Left
		Ø Open
		3 Percutaneous
		4 Percutaneous Endoscopic
		X External
			Z No Device	**Z** No Qualifier

Non-OR   ØMN[Ø,1,2,3,4,5,6,7,8,9,B,C,D,F,G,H,J,K,L,M,N,P,Q,R,S,T,V,W]XZZ

NC Noncovered Procedure   **LC** Limited Coverage   **QA** Questionable OB Admit   **NT** New Tech Add-on   ⊞ Combination Member   ♂ Male   ♀ Female

ICD-10-PCS 2023   511

ØMN–ØMN

Ø   Medical and Surgical
M   Bursae and Ligaments
P   Removal   Definition: Taking out or off a device from a body part

Explanation: If a device is taken out and a similar device put in without cutting or puncturing the skin or mucous membrane, the procedure is coded to the root operation CHANGE. Otherwise, the procedure for taking out a device is coded to the root operation REMOVAL.

Body Part Character 4	Approach Character 5	Device Character 6	Qualifier Character 7
X Upper Bursa and Ligament **Y** Lower Bursa and Ligament	**Ø** Open **3** Percutaneous **4** Percutaneous Endoscopic	**Ø** Drainage Device **7** Autologous Tissue Substitute **J** Synthetic Substitute **K** Nonautologous Tissue Substitute **Y** Other Device	**Z** No Qualifier
X Upper Bursa and Ligament **Y** Lower Bursa and Ligament	**X** External	**Ø** Drainage Device	**Z** No Qualifier

Non-OR   ØMP[X,Y]3ØZ
Non-OR   ØMP[X,Y][3,4]YZ
Non-OR   ØMP[X,Y]XØZ

Ø   **Medical and Surgical**
M   **Bursae and Ligaments**
Q   **Repair**   Definition: Restoring, to the extent possible, a body part to its normal anatomic structure and function
                         Explanation: Used only when the method to accomplish the repair is not one of the other root operations

Body Part Character 4		Approach Character 5	Device Character 6	Qualifier Character 7

Ø   **Head and Neck Bursa and Ligament**
    Alar ligament of axis
    Cervical interspinous ligament
    Cervical intertransverse ligament
    Cervical ligamentum flavum
    Interspinous ligament, cervical
    Intertransverse ligament, cervical
    Lateral temporomandibular ligament
    Ligamentum flavum, cervical
    Sphenomandibular ligament
    Stylomandibular ligament
    Transverse ligament of atlas
1   **Shoulder Bursa and Ligament, Right**
    Acromioclavicular ligament
    Coracoacromial ligament
    Coracoclavicular ligament
    Coracohumeral ligament
    Costoclavicular ligament
    Glenohumeral ligament
    Interclavicular ligament
    Sternoclavicular ligament
    Subacromial bursa
    Transverse humeral ligament
    Transverse scapular ligament
2   **Shoulder Bursa and Ligament, Left**
    See 1 Shoulder Bursa and Ligament, Right
3   **Elbow Bursa and Ligament, Right**
    Annular ligament
    Olecranon bursa
    Radial collateral ligament
    Ulnar collateral ligament
4   **Elbow Bursa and Ligament, Left**
    See 3 Elbow Bursa and Ligament, Right
5   **Wrist Bursa and Ligament, Right**
    Palmar ulnocarpal ligament
    Radial collateral carpal ligament
    Radiocarpal ligament
    Radioulnar ligament
    Scapholunate ligament
    Ulnar collateral carpal ligament
6   **Wrist Bursa and Ligament, Left**
    See 5 Wrist Bursa and Ligament, Right
7   **Hand Bursa and Ligament, Right**
    Carpometacarpal ligament
    Intercarpal ligament
    Interphalangeal ligament
    Lunotriquetral ligament
    Metacarpal ligament
    Metacarpophalangeal ligament
    Pisohamate ligament
    Pisometacarpal ligament
    Scaphotrapezium ligament
8   **Hand Bursa and Ligament, Left**
    See 7 Hand Bursa and Ligament, Right
9   **Upper Extremity Bursa and Ligament, Right**
B   **Upper Extremity Bursa and Ligament, Left**
C   **Upper Spine Bursa and Ligament**
    Interspinous ligament, thoracic
    Intertransverse ligament, thoracic
    Ligamentum flavum, thoracic
    Supraspinous ligament
	D **Lower Spine Bursa and Ligament**
	    Iliolumbar ligament
	    Interspinous ligament, lumbar
	    Intertransverse ligament, lumbar
	    Ligamentum flavum, lumbar
	    Sacrococcygeal ligament
	    Sacroiliac ligament
	    Sacrospinous ligament
	    Sacrotuberous ligament
	    Supraspinous ligament
	F **Sternum Bursa and Ligament**
	    Costoxiphoid ligament
	    Sternocostal ligament
	G **Rib(s) Bursa and Ligament**
	    Costotransverse ligament
	H **Abdomen Bursa and Ligament, Right**
	J **Abdomen Bursa and Ligament, Left**
	K **Perineum Bursa and Ligament**
	L **Hip Bursa and Ligament, Right**
	    Iliofemoral ligament
	    Ischiofemoral ligament
	    Pubofemoral ligament
	    Transverse acetabular ligament
	    Trochanteric bursa
	M **Hip Bursa and Ligament, Left**
	    See L Hip Bursa and Ligament, Right
	N **Knee Bursa and Ligament, Right**
	    Anterior cruciate ligament (ACL)
	    Lateral collateral ligament (LCL)
	    Ligament of head of fibula
	    Medial collateral ligament (MCL)
	    Patellar ligament
	    Popliteal ligament
	    Posterior cruciate ligament (PCL)
	    Prepatellar bursa
	P **Knee Bursa and Ligament, Left**
	    See N Knee Bursa and Ligament, Right
	Q **Ankle Bursa and Ligament, Right**
	    Calcaneofibular ligament
	    Deltoid ligament
	    Ligament of the lateral malleolus
	    Talofibular ligament
	R **Ankle Bursa and Ligament, Left**
	    See Q Ankle Bursa and Ligament, Right
	S **Foot Bursa and Ligament, Right**
	    Calcaneocuboid ligament
	    Cuneonavicular ligament
	    Intercuneiform ligament
	    Interphalangeal ligament
	    Metatarsal ligament
	    Metatarsophalangeal ligament
	    Subtalar ligament
	    Talocalcaneal ligament
	    Talocalcaneonavicular ligament
	    Tarsometatarsal ligament
	T **Foot Bursa and Ligament, Left**
	    See S Foot Bursa and Ligament, Right
	V **Lower Extremity Bursa and Ligament, Right**
	W **Lower Extremity Bursa and Ligament, Left**
		Ø Open
		3 Percutaneous
		4 Percutaneous Endoscopic
			Z No Device	**Z** No Qualifier

NC Noncovered Procedure   **LC** Limited Coverage   **QA** Questionable OB Admit   **NT** New Tech Add-on   ⊞ Combination Member   ♂ Male   ♀ Female

ICD-10-PCS 2023   513

Bursae and Ligaments *(side tab)*

Ø   **Medical and Surgical**
M   **Bursae and Ligaments**
R   **Replacement**   Definition: Putting in or on biological or synthetic material that physically takes the place and/or function of all or a portion of a body part
               Explanation: The body part may have been taken out or replaced, or may be taken out, physically eradicated, or rendered nonfunctional during the REPLACEMENT procedure. A REMOVAL procedure is coded for taking out the device used in a previous replacement procedure.

Body Part Character 4		Approach Character 5	Device Character 6	Qualifier Character 7
Ø Head and Neck Bursa and Ligament Alar ligament of axis Cervical interspinous ligament Cervical intertransverse ligament Cervical ligamentum flavum Interspinous ligament, cervical Intertransverse ligament, cervical Lateral temporomandibular ligament Ligamentum flavum, cervical Sphenomandibular ligament Stylomandibular ligament Transverse ligament of atlas	**D** Lower Spine Bursa and Ligament Iliolumbar ligament Interspinous ligament, lumbar Intertransverse ligament, lumbar Ligamentum flavum, lumbar Sacrococcygeal ligament Sacroiliac ligament Sacrospinous ligament Sacrotuberous ligament Supraspinous ligament	**Ø** Open **4** Percutaneous Endoscopic	**7** Autologous Tissue Substitute **J** Synthetic Substitute **K** Nonautologous Tissue Substitute	**Z** No Qualifier
1 Shoulder Bursa and Ligament, Right Acromioclavicular ligament Coracoacromial ligament Coracoclavicular ligament Coracohumeral ligament Costoclavicular ligament Glenohumeral ligament Interclavicular ligament Sternoclavicular ligament Subacromial bursa Transverse humeral ligament Transverse scapular ligament	**F** Sternum Bursa and Ligament Costoxiphoid ligament Sternocostal ligament **G** Rib(s) Bursa and Ligament Costotransverse ligament **H** Abdomen Bursa and Ligament, Right **J** Abdomen Bursa and Ligament, Left **K** Perineum Bursa and Ligament			
2 Shoulder Bursa and Ligament, Left *See 1 Shoulder Bursa and Ligament, Right*	**L** Hip Bursa and Ligament, Right Iliofemoral ligament Ischiofemoral ligament Pubofemoral ligament Transverse acetabular ligament Trochanteric bursa			
3 Elbow Bursa and Ligament, Right Annular ligament Olecranon bursa Radial collateral ligament Ulnar collateral ligament	**M** Hip Bursa and Ligament, Left *See L Hip Bursa and Ligament, Right*			
4 Elbow Bursa and Ligament, Left *See 3 Elbow Bursa and Ligament, Right*	**N** Knee Bursa and Ligament, Right Anterior cruciate ligament (ACL) Lateral collateral ligament (LCL) Ligament of head of fibula Medial collateral ligament (MCL) Patellar ligament Popliteal ligament Posterior cruciate ligament (PCL) Prepatellar bursa			
5 Wrist Bursa and Ligament, Right Palmar ulnocarpal ligament Radial collateral carpal ligament Radiocarpal ligament Radioulnar ligament Scapholunate ligament Ulnar collateral carpal ligament	**P** Knee Bursa and Ligament, Left *See N Knee Bursa and Ligament, Right*			
6 Wrist Bursa and Ligament, Left *See 5 Wrist Bursa and Ligament, Right*	**Q** Ankle Bursa and Ligament, Right Calcaneofibular ligament Deltoid ligament Ligament of the lateral malleolus Talofibular ligament			
7 Hand Bursa and Ligament, Right Carpometacarpal ligament Intercarpal ligament Interphalangeal ligament Lunotriquetral ligament Metacarpal ligament Metacarpophalangeal ligament Pisohamate ligament Pisometacarpal ligament Scaphotrapezium ligament	**R** Ankle Bursa and Ligament, Left *See Q Ankle Bursa and Ligament, Right* **S** Foot Bursa and Ligament, Right Calcaneocuboid ligament Cuneonavicular ligament Intercuneiform ligament Interphalangeal ligament Metatarsal ligament Metatarsophalangeal ligament Subtalar ligament Talocalcaneal ligament Talocalcaneonavicular ligament Tarsometatarsal ligament			
8 Hand Bursa and Ligament, Left *See 7 Hand Bursa and Ligament, Right*				
9 Upper Extremity Bursa and Ligament, Right **B** Upper Extremity Bursa and Ligament, Left	**T** Foot Bursa and Ligament, Left *See S Foot Bursa and Ligament, Right* **V** Lower Extremity Bursa and Ligament, Right			
C Upper Spine Bursa and Ligament Interspinous ligament, thoracic Intertransverse ligament, thoracic Ligamentum flavum, thoracic Supraspinous ligament	**W** Lower Extremity Bursa and Ligament, Left			

Ø   **Medical and Surgical**
M   **Bursae and Ligaments**
S   **Reposition**   Definition: Moving to its normal location, or other suitable location, all or a portion of a body part

                       Explanation: The body part is moved to a new location from an abnormal location, or from a normal location where it is not functioning correctly. The body part may or may not be cut out or off to be moved to the new location.

Body Part Character 4		Approach Character 5	Device Character 6	Qualifier Character 7

Ø Head and Neck Bursa and Ligament
  Alar ligament of axis
  Cervical interspinous ligament
  Cervical intertransverse ligament
  Cervical ligamentum flavum
  Interspinous ligament, cervical
  Intertransverse ligament, cervical
  Lateral temporomandibular ligament
  Ligamentum flavum, cervical
  Sphenomandibular ligament
  Stylomandibular ligament
  Transverse ligament of atlas
1 Shoulder Bursa and Ligament, Right
  Acromioclavicular ligament
  Coracoacromial ligament
  Coracoclavicular ligament
  Coracohumeral ligament
  Costoclavicular ligament
  Glenohumeral ligament
  Interclavicular ligament
  Sternoclavicular ligament
  Subacromial bursa
  Transverse humeral ligament
  Transverse scapular ligament
2 Shoulder Bursa and Ligament, Left
  See 1 Shoulder Bursa and Ligament, Right
3 Elbow Bursa and Ligament, Right
  Annular ligament
  Olecranon bursa
  Radial collateral ligament
  Ulnar collateral ligament
4 Elbow Bursa and Ligament, Left
  See 3 Elbow Bursa and Ligament, Right
5 Wrist Bursa and Ligament, Right
  Palmar ulnocarpal ligament
  Radial collateral carpal ligament
  Radiocarpal ligament
  Radioulnar ligament
  Scapholunate ligament
  Ulnar collateral carpal ligament
6 Wrist Bursa and Ligament, Left
  See 5 Wrist Bursa and Ligament, Right
7 Hand Bursa and Ligament, Right
  Carpometacarpal ligament
  Intercarpal ligament
  Interphalangeal ligament
  Lunotriquetral ligament
  Metacarpal ligament
  Metacarpophalangeal ligament
  Pisohamate ligament
  Pisometacarpal ligament
  Scaphotrapezium ligament
8 Hand Bursa and Ligament, Left
  See 7 Hand Bursa and Ligament, Right
9 Upper Extremity Bursa and Ligament, Right
B Upper Extremity Bursa and Ligament, Left
C Upper Spine Bursa and Ligament
  Interspinous ligament, thoracic
  Intertransverse ligament, thoracic
  Ligamentum flavum, thoracic
  Supraspinous ligament
	D Lower Spine Bursa and Ligament
	  Iliolumbar ligament
	  Interspinous ligament, lumbar
	  Intertransverse ligament, lumbar
	  Ligamentum flavum, lumbar
	  Sacrococcygeal ligament
	  Sacroiliac ligament
	  Sacrospinous ligament
	  Sacrotuberous ligament
	  Supraspinous ligament
	F Sternum Bursa and Ligament
	  Costoxiphoid ligament
	  Sternocostal ligament
	G Rib(s) Bursa and Ligament
	  Costotransverse ligament
	H Abdomen Bursa and Ligament, Right
	J Abdomen Bursa and Ligament, Left
	K Perineum Bursa and Ligament
	L Hip Bursa and Ligament, Right
	  Iliofemoral ligament
	  Ischiofemoral ligament
	  Pubofemoral ligament
	  Transverse acetabular ligament
	  Trochanteric bursa
	M Hip Bursa and Ligament, Left
	  See L Hip Bursa and Ligament, Right
	N Knee Bursa and Ligament, Right
	  Anterior cruciate ligament (ACL)
	  Lateral collateral ligament (LCL)
	  Ligament of head of fibula
	  Medial collateral ligament (MCL)
	  Patellar ligament
	  Popliteal ligament
	  Posterior cruciate ligament (PCL)
	  Prepatellar bursa
	P Knee Bursa and Ligament, Left
	  See N Knee Bursa and Ligament, Right
	Q Ankle Bursa and Ligament, Right
	  Calcaneofibular ligament
	  Deltoid ligament
	  Ligament of the lateral malleolus
	  Talofibular ligament
	R Ankle Bursa and Ligament, Left
	  See Q Ankle Bursa and Ligament, Right
	S Foot Bursa and Ligament, Right
	  Calcaneocuboid ligament
	  Cuneonavicular ligament
	  Intercuneiform ligament
	  Interphalangeal ligament
	  Metatarsal ligament
	  Metatarsophalangeal ligament
	  Subtalar ligament
	  Talocalcaneal ligament
	  Talocalcaneonavicular ligament
	  Tarsometatarsal ligament
	T Foot Bursa and Ligament, Left
	  See S Foot Bursa and Ligament, Right
	V Lower Extremity Bursa and Ligament, Right
	W Lower Extremity Bursa and Ligament, Left
		Ø Open
		4 Percutaneous Endoscopic
			Z No Device	**Z** No Qualifier

Ø   Medical and Surgical
M   Bursae and Ligaments
T   Resection   Definition: Cutting out or off, without replacement, all of a body part
                       Explanation: None

Body Part Character 4		Approach Character 5	Device Character 6	Qualifier Character 7
Ø Head and Neck Bursa and Ligament Alar ligament of axis Cervical interspinous ligament Cervical intertransverse ligament Cervical ligamentum flavum Interspinous ligament, cervical Intertransverse ligament, cervical Lateral temporomandibular ligament Ligamentum flavum, cervical Sphenomandibular ligament Stylomandibular ligament Transverse ligament of atlas	**D Lower Spine Bursa and Ligament** Iliolumbar ligament Interspinous ligament, lumbar Intertransverse ligament, lumbar Ligamentum flavum, lumbar Sacrococcygeal ligament Sacroiliac ligament Sacrospinous ligament Sacrotuberous ligament Supraspinous ligament	**Ø Open** **4 Percutaneous Endoscopic**	**Z No Device**	**Z No Qualifier**
1 Shoulder Bursa and Ligament, Right Acromioclavicular ligament Coracoacromial ligament Coracoclavicular ligament Coracohumeral ligament Costoclavicular ligament Glenohumeral ligament Interclavicular ligament Sternoclavicular ligament Subacromial bursa Transverse humeral ligament Transverse scapular ligament	**F Sternum Bursa and Ligament** Costoxiphoid ligament Sternocostal ligament **G Rib(s) Bursa and Ligament** Costotransverse ligament **H Abdomen Bursa and Ligament, Right** **J Abdomen Bursa and Ligament, Left** **K Perineum Bursa and Ligament**			
2 Shoulder Bursa and Ligament, Left *See 1 Shoulder Bursa and Ligament, Right*	**L Hip Bursa and Ligament, Right** Iliofemoral ligament Ischiofemoral ligament Pubofemoral ligament Transverse acetabular ligament Trochanteric bursa			
3 Elbow Bursa and Ligament, Right Annular ligament Olecranon bursa Radial collateral ligament Ulnar collateral ligament	**M Hip Bursa and Ligament, Left** *See L Hip Bursa and Ligament, Right*			
4 Elbow Bursa and Ligament, Left *See 3 Elbow Bursa and Ligament, Right*	**N Knee Bursa and Ligament, Right** Anterior cruciate ligament (ACL) Lateral collateral ligament (LCL) Ligament of head of fibula Medial collateral ligament (MCL) Patellar ligament Popliteal ligament Posterior cruciate ligament (PCL) Prepatellar bursa			
5 Wrist Bursa and Ligament, Right Palmar ulnocarpal ligament Radial collateral carpal ligament Radiocarpal ligament Radioulnar ligament Scapholunate ligament Ulnar collateral carpal ligament	**P Knee Bursa and Ligament, Left** *See N Knee Bursa and Ligament, Right*			
6 Wrist Bursa and Ligament, Left *See 5 Wrist Bursa and Ligament, Right*	**Q Ankle Bursa and Ligament, Right** Calcaneofibular ligament Deltoid ligament Ligament of the lateral malleolus Talofibular ligament			
7 Hand Bursa and Ligament, Right Carpometacarpal ligament Intercarpal ligament Interphalangeal ligament Lunotriquetral ligament Metacarpal ligament Metacarpophalangeal ligament Pisohamate ligament Pisometacarpal ligament Scaphotrapezium ligament	**R Ankle Bursa and Ligament, Left** *See Q Ankle Bursa and Ligament, Right* **S Foot Bursa and Ligament, Right** Calcaneocuboid ligament Cuneonavicular ligament Intercuneiform ligament Interphalangeal ligament Metatarsal ligament Metatarsophalangeal ligament Subtalar ligament Talocalcaneal ligament Talocalcaneonavicular ligament Tarsometatarsal ligament			
8 Hand Bursa and Ligament, Left *See 7 Hand Bursa and Ligament, Right*	**T Foot Bursa and Ligament, Left** *See S Foot Bursa and Ligament, Right*			
9 Upper Extremity Bursa and Ligament, Right **B Upper Extremity Bursa and Ligament, Left**	**V Lower Extremity Bursa and Ligament, Right**			
C Upper Spine Bursa and Ligament Interspinous ligament, thoracic Intertransverse ligament, thoracic Ligamentum flavum, thoracic Supraspinous ligament	**W Lower Extremity Bursa and Ligament, Left**			

Non-OR Procedure   DRG Non-OR Procedure   Valid OR Procedure   HAC Associated Procedure   Combination Only   New/Revised April   New/Revised October

Bursae and Ligaments

Ø   **Medical and Surgical**
M   **Bursae and Ligaments**
U   **Supplement**   Definition: Putting in or on biological or synthetic material that physically reinforces and/or augments the function of a portion of a body part
                Explanation: The biological material is non-living, or is living and from the same individual. The body part may have been previously replaced, and the SUPPLEMENT procedure is performed to physically reinforce and/or augment the function of the replaced body part.

Body Part Character 4		Approach Character 5	Device Character 6	Qualifier Character 7
Ø Head and Neck Bursa and Ligament Alar ligament of axis Cervical interspinous ligament Cervical intertransverse ligament Cervical ligamentum flavum Interspinous ligament, cervical Intertransverse ligament, cervical Lateral temporomandibular ligament Ligamentum flavum, cervical Sphenomandibular ligament Stylomandibular ligament Transverse ligament of atlas **1 Shoulder Bursa and Ligament, Right** Acromioclavicular ligament Coracoacromial ligament Coracoclavicular ligament Coracohumeral ligament Costoclavicular ligament Glenohumeral ligament Interclavicular ligament Sternoclavicular ligament Subacromial bursa Transverse humeral ligament Transverse scapular ligament **2 Shoulder Bursa and Ligament, Left** *See 1 Shoulder Bursa and Ligament, Right* **3 Elbow Bursa and Ligament, Right** Annular ligament Olecranon bursa Radial collateral ligament Ulnar collateral ligament **4 Elbow Bursa and Ligament, Left** *See 3 Elbow Bursa and Ligament, Right* **5 Wrist Bursa and Ligament, Right** Palmar ulnocarpal ligament Radial collateral carpal ligament Radiocarpal ligament Radioulnar ligament Scapholunate ligament Ulnar collateral carpal ligament **6 Wrist Bursa and Ligament, Left** *See 5 Wrist Bursa and Ligament, Right* **7 Hand Bursa and Ligament, Right** Carpometacarpal ligament Intercarpal ligament Interphalangeal ligament Lunotriquetral ligament Metacarpal ligament Metacarpophalangeal ligament Pisohamate ligament Pisometacarpal ligament Scaphotrapezium ligament **8 Hand Bursa and Ligament, Left** *See 7 Hand Bursa and Ligament, Right* **9 Upper Extremity Bursa and Ligament, Right** **B Upper Extremity Bursa and Ligament, Left** **C Upper Spine Bursa and Ligament** Interspinous ligament, thoracic Intertransverse ligament, thoracic Ligamentum flavum, thoracic Supraspinous ligament	**D Lower Spine Bursa and Ligament** Iliolumbar ligament Interspinous ligament, lumbar Intertransverse ligament, lumbar Ligamentum flavum, lumbar Sacrococcygeal ligament Sacroiliac ligament Sacrospinous ligament Sacrotuberous ligament Supraspinous ligament **F Sternum Bursa and Ligament** Costoxiphoid ligament Sternocostal ligament **G Rib(s) Bursa and Ligament** Costotransverse ligament **H Abdomen Bursa and Ligament, Right** **J Abdomen Bursa and Ligament, Left** **K Perineum Bursa and Ligament** **L Hip Bursa and Ligament, Right** Iliofemoral ligament Ischiofemoral ligament Pubofemoral ligament Transverse acetabular ligament Trochanteric bursa **M Hip Bursa and Ligament, Left** *See L Hip Bursa and Ligament, Right* **N Knee Bursa and Ligament, Right** Anterior cruciate ligament (ACL) Lateral collateral ligament (LCL) Ligament of head of fibula Medial collateral ligament (MCL) Patellar ligament Popliteal ligament Posterior cruciate ligament (PCL) Prepatellar bursa **P Knee Bursa and Ligament, Left** *See N Knee Bursa and Ligament, Right* **Q Ankle Bursa and Ligament, Right** Calcaneofibular ligament Deltoid ligament Ligament of the lateral malleolus Talofibular ligament **R Ankle Bursa and Ligament, Left** *See Q Ankle Bursa and Ligament, Right* **S Foot Bursa and Ligament, Right** Calcaneocuboid ligament Cuneonavicular ligament Intercuneiform ligament Interphalangeal ligament Metatarsal ligament Metatarsophalangeal ligament Subtalar ligament Talocalcaneal ligament Talocalcaneonavicular ligament Tarsometatarsal ligament **T Foot Bursa and Ligament, Left** *See S Foot Bursa and Ligament, Right* **V Lower Extremity Bursa and Ligament, Right** **W Lower Extremity Bursa and Ligament, Left**	**Ø Open** **4 Percutaneous Endoscopic**	**7 Autologous Tissue Substitute** **J Synthetic Substitute** **K Nonautologous Tissue Substitute**	**Z No Qualifier**

NC Noncovered Procedure   LC Limited Coverage   QA Questionable OB Admit   NT New Tech Add-on   ⊞ Combination Member   ♂ Male   ♀ Female

ICD-10-PCS 2023   517

Ø   Medical and Surgical
M   Bursae and Ligaments
W   Revision   Definition: Correcting, to the extent possible, a portion of a malfunctioning device or the position of a displaced device
                       Explanation: Revision can include correcting a malfunctioning or displaced device by taking out or putting in components of the device such as
                       a screw or pin

Body Part Character 4	Approach Character 5	Device Character 6	Qualifier Character 7
X Upper Bursa and Ligament Y Lower Bursa and Ligament	Ø Open 3 Percutaneous 4 Percutaneous Endoscopic	Ø Drainage Device 7 Autologous Tissue Substitute J Synthetic Substitute K Nonautologous Tissue Substitute Y Other Device	Z No Qualifier
X Upper Bursa and Ligament Y Lower Bursa and Ligament	X External	Ø Drainage Device 7 Autologous Tissue Substitute J Synthetic Substitute K Nonautologous Tissue Substitute	Z No Qualifier

Non-OR   ØMW[X,Y][3,4]YZ
Non-OR   ØMW[X,Y]X[Ø,7,J,K]Z

Ø　Medical and Surgical
M　Bursae and Ligaments
X　Transfer　　Definition: Moving, without taking out, all or a portion of a body part to another location to take over the function of all or a portion of a body part
　　　　　　　　Explanation: The body part transferred remains connected to its vascular and nervous supply

Body Part Character 4		Approach Character 5	Device Character 6	Qualifier Character 7
Ø Head and Neck Bursa and Ligament Alar ligament of axis Cervical interspinous ligament Cervical intertransverse ligament Cervical ligamentum flavum Interspinous ligament, cervical Intertransverse ligament, cervical Lateral temporomandibular ligament Ligamentum flavum, cervical Sphenomandibular ligament Stylomandibular ligament Transverse ligament of atlas **1 Shoulder Bursa and Ligament, Right** Acromioclavicular ligament Coracoacromial ligament Coracoclavicular ligament Coracohumeral ligament Costoclavicular ligament Glenohumeral ligament Interclavicular ligament Sternoclavicular ligament Subacromial bursa Transverse humeral ligament Transverse scapular ligament **2 Shoulder Bursa and Ligament, Left** *See 1 Shoulder Bursa and Ligament, Right* **3 Elbow Bursa and Ligament, Right** Annular ligament Olecranon bursa Radial collateral ligament Ulnar collateral ligament **4 Elbow Bursa and Ligament, Left** *See 3 Elbow Bursa and Ligament, Right* **5 Wrist Bursa and Ligament, Right** Palmar ulnocarpal ligament Radial collateral carpal ligament Radiocarpal ligament Radioulnar ligament Scapholunate ligament Ulnar collateral carpal ligament **6 Wrist Bursa and Ligament, Left** *See 5 Wrist Bursa and Ligament, Right* **7 Hand Bursa and Ligament, Right** Carpometacarpal ligament Intercarpal ligament Interphalangeal ligament Lunotriquetral ligament Metacarpal ligament Metacarpophalangeal ligament Pisohamate ligament Pisometacarpal ligament Scaphotrapezium ligament **8 Hand Bursa and Ligament, Left** *See 7 Hand Bursa and Ligament, Right* **9 Upper Extremity Bursa and Ligament, Right** **B Upper Extremity Bursa and Ligament, Left** **C Upper Spine Bursa and Ligament** Interspinous ligament, thoracic Intertransverse ligament, thoracic Ligamentum flavum, thoracic Supraspinous ligament	**D Lower Spine Bursa and Ligament** Iliolumbar ligament Interspinous ligament, lumbar Intertransverse ligament, lumbar Ligamentum flavum, lumbar Sacrococcygeal ligament Sacroiliac ligament Sacrospinous ligament Sacrotuberous ligament Supraspinous ligament **F Sternum Bursa and Ligament** Costoxiphoid ligament Sternocostal ligament **G Rib(s) Bursa and Ligament** Costotransverse ligament **H Abdomen Bursa and Ligament, Right** **J Abdomen Bursa and Ligament, Left** **K Perineum Bursa and Ligament** **L Hip Bursa and Ligament, Right** Iliofemoral ligament Ischiofemoral ligament Pubofemoral ligament Transverse acetabular ligament Trochanteric bursa **M Hip Bursa and Ligament, Left** *See L Hip Bursa and Ligament, Right* **N Knee Bursa and Ligament, Right** Anterior cruciate ligament (ACL) Lateral collateral ligament (LCL) Ligament of head of fibula Medial collateral ligament (MCL) Patellar ligament Popliteal ligament Posterior cruciate ligament (PCL) Prepatellar bursa **P Knee Bursa and Ligament, Left** *See N Knee Bursa and Ligament, Right* **Q Ankle Bursa and Ligament, Right** Calcaneofibular ligament Deltoid ligament Ligament of the lateral malleolus Talofibular ligament **R Ankle Bursa and Ligament, Left** *See Q Ankle Bursa and Ligament, Right* **S Foot Bursa and Ligament, Right** Calcaneocuboid ligament Cuneonavicular ligament Intercuneiform ligament Interphalangeal ligament Metatarsal ligament Metatarsophalangeal ligament Subtalar ligament Talocalcaneal ligament Talocalcaneonavicular ligament Tarsometatarsal ligament **T Foot Bursa and Ligament, Left** *See S Foot Bursa and Ligament, Right* **V Lower Extremity Bursa and Ligament, Right** **W Lower Extremity Bursa and Ligament, Left**	**Ø Open** **4 Percutaneous Endoscopic**	**Z No Device**	**Z No Qualifier**

Head and Facial Bones ØN2–ØNW

Character Meanings

This Character Meaning table is provided as a guide to assist the user in the identification of character members that may be found in this section of code tables. It **SHOULD NOT** be used to build a PCS code.

Operation–Character 3	Body Part–Character 4	Approach–Character 5	Device–Character 6	Qualifier–Character 7
2 Change	Ø Skull	Ø Open	Ø Drainage Device	X Diagnostic
5 Destruction	1 Frontal Bone	3 Percutaneous	3 Infusion Device	Z No Qualifier
8 Division	3 Parietal Bone, Right	4 Percutaneous Endoscopic	4 Internal Fixation Device	
9 Drainage	4 Parietal Bone, Left	X External	5 External Fixation Device	
B Excision	5 Temporal Bone, Right		7 Autologous Tissue Substitute	
C Extirpation	6 Temporal Bone, Left		J Synthetic Substitute	
D Extraction	7 Occipital Bone		K Nonautologous Tissue Substitute	
H Insertion	B Nasal Bone		M Bone Growth Stimulator	
J Inspection	C Sphenoid Bone		N Neurostimulator Generator	
N Release	F Ethmoid Bone, Right		S Hearing Device	
P Removal	G Ethmoid Bone, Left		Y Other Device	
Q Repair	H Lacrimal Bone, Right		Z No Device	
R Replacement	J Lacrimal Bone, Left			
S Reposition	K Palatine Bone, Right			
T Resection	L Palatine Bone, Left			
U Supplement	M Zygomatic Bone, Right			
W Revision	N Zygomatic Bone, Left			
	P Orbit, Right			
	Q Orbit, Left			
	R Maxilla			
	T Mandible, Right			
	V Mandible, Left			
	W Facial Bone			
	X Hyoid Bone			

AHA Coding Clinic for table ØNB
2022, 2Q, 17   Congenital nasal pyriform aperture stenosis and repair
2021, 3Q, 21   Excision of thyroglossal duct cyst
2021, 1Q, 21   Maxillectomy with reconstruction of maxilla
2017, 1Q, 20   Preparatory nasal adhesion repair before definitive cleft palate repair
2015, 3Q, 3-8   Excisional and nonexcisional debridement
2015, 2Q, 12   Orbital exenteration

AHA Coding Clinic for table ØND
2017, 4Q, 41   Extraction procedures

AHA Coding Clinic for table ØNH
2021, 4Q, 51   Insertion of infusion device in skull
2015, 3Q, 13   Nonexcisional debridement of cranial wound with removal and replacement of hardware

AHA Coding Clinic for table ØNP
2015, 3Q, 13   Nonexcisional debridement of cranial wound with removal and replacement of hardware

AHA Coding Clinic for table ØNQ
2016, 3Q, 29   Closure of bilateral alveolar clefts

AHA Coding Clinic for table ØNR
2021, 3Q, 29   Repair of superior semicircular canal dehiscence
2021, 1Q, 21   Maxillectomy with reconstruction of maxilla
2017, 3Q, 17   Resection of schwannoma and placement of DuraGen and Lorenz cranial plating system
2017, 3Q, 22   Replacement of native skull bone flap
2017, 1Q, 23   Reconstruction of mandible using titanium and bone
2014, 3Q, 7   Hemi-cranioplasty for repair of cranial defect

AHA Coding Clinic for table ØNS
2022, 1Q, 48   Repair of facial fractures of frontal sinus and orbital roof
2017, 3Q, 22   Replacement of native skull bone flap
2017, 1Q, 20   Preparatory nasal adhesion repair before definitive cleft palate repair
2016, 2Q, 30   Clipping (occlusion) of cerebral artery, decompressive craniectomy and storage of bone flap in abdominal wall
2015, 3Q, 17   Craniosynostosis with cranial vault reconstruction
2015, 3Q, 27   Moyamoya disease and hemispheric pial synangiosis with craniotomy
2014, 3Q, 23   Le Fort I osteotomy
2013, 3Q, 24   Distraction osteogenesis
2013, 3Q, 25   Fracture of frontal bone with repair and coagulation for hemostasis

AHA Coding Clinic for table ØNU
2021, 3Q, 29   Repair of superior semicircular canal dehiscence
2016, 3Q, 29   Closure of bilateral alveolar clefts
2013, 3Q, 24   Distraction osteogenesis

Head and Facial Bones

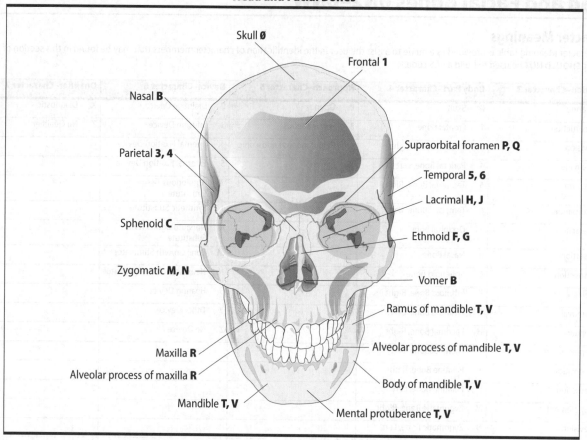

Skull Bones

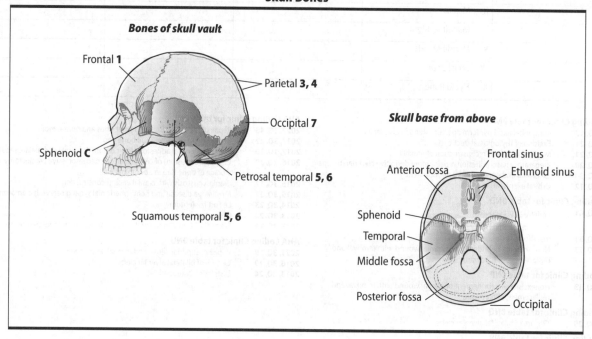

Ø   **Medical and Surgical**
N   **Head and Facial Bones**
2   **Change**   Definition: Taking out or off a device from a body part and putting back an identical or similar device in or on the same body part without cutting or puncturing the skin or a mucous membrane
                 Explanation: All CHANGE procedures are coded using the approach EXTERNAL

Body Part Character 4	Approach Character 5	Device Character 6	Qualifier Character 7
Ø Skull B Nasal Bone Vomer of nasal septum W Facial Bone	X External	Ø Drainage Device Y Other Device	Z No Qualifier

Non-OR   All body part, approach, device, and qualifier values

Ø   **Medical and Surgical**
N   **Head and Facial Bones**
5   **Destruction**   Definition: Physical eradication of all or a portion of a body part by the direct use of energy, force, or a destructive agent
                      Explanation: None of the body part is physically taken out

Body Part Character 4	Approach Character 5	Device Character 6	Qualifier Character 7

Ø   Skull
1   Frontal Bone
     Zygomatic process of frontal bone
3   Parietal Bone, Right
4   Parietal Bone, Left
5   Temporal Bone, Right
     Mastoid process
     Petrous part of temporal bone
     Tympanic part of temporal bone
     Zygomatic process of temporal bone
6   Temporal Bone, Left
     See 5 Temporal Bone, Right
7   Occipital Bone
     Foramen magnum
B   Nasal Bone
     Vomer of nasal septum
C   Sphenoid Bone
     Greater wing
     Lesser wing
     Optic foramen
     Pterygoid process
     Sella turcica
F   Ethmoid Bone, Right
     Cribriform plate
G   Ethmoid Bone, Left
     See F Ethmoid Bone, Right
H   Lacrimal Bone, Right
J   Lacrimal Bone, Left
K   Palatine Bone, Right
L   Palatine Bone, Left
M   Zygomatic Bone, Right
N   Zygomatic Bone, Left
P   Orbit, Right
     Bony orbit
     Orbital portion of ethmoid bone
     Orbital portion of frontal bone
     Orbital portion of lacrimal bone
     Orbital portion of maxilla
     Orbital portion of palatine bone
     Orbital portion of sphenoid bone
     Orbital portion of zygomatic bone
Q   Orbit, Left
     See P Orbit, Right
R   Maxilla
     Alveolar process of maxilla
T   Mandible, Right
     Alveolar process of mandible
     Condyloid process
     Mandibular notch
     Mental foramen
V   Mandible, Left
     See T Mandible, Right
X   Hyoid Bone
	Ø Open
	3 Percutaneous
	4 Percutaneous Endoscopic
		Z No Device	Z No Qualifier

NC Noncovered Procedure   **LC** Limited Coverage   **QA** Questionable OB Admit   **NT** New Tech Add-on   ⊞ Combination Member   ♂ Male   ♀ Female

ICD-10-PCS 2023   523

ØN2–ØN5

Ø Medical and Surgical
N Head and Facial Bones
8 Division Definition: Cutting into a body part, without draining fluids and/or gases from the body part, in order to separate or transect a body part
Explanation: All or a portion of the body part is separated into two or more portions

Body Part Character 4	Approach Character 5	Device Character 6	Qualifier Character 7
Ø Skull **1 Frontal Bone** Zygomatic process of frontal bone **3 Parietal Bone, Right** **4 Parietal Bone, Left** **5 Temporal Bone, Right** Mastoid process Petrous part of temporal bone Tympanic part of temporal bone Zygomatic process of temporal bone **6 Temporal Bone, Left** *See 5 Temporal Bone, Right* **7 Occipital Bone** Foramen magnum **B Nasal Bone** Vomer of nasal septum **C Sphenoid Bone** Greater wing Lesser wing Optic foramen Pterygoid process Sella turcica **F Ethmoid Bone, Right** Cribriform plate **G Ethmoid Bone, Left** *See F Ethmoid Bone, Right* **H Lacrimal Bone, Right** **J Lacrimal Bone, Left** **K Palatine Bone, Right** **L Palatine Bone, Left** **M Zygomatic Bone, Right** **N Zygomatic Bone, Left** **P Orbit, Right** Bony orbit Orbital portion of ethmoid bone Orbital portion of frontal bone Orbital portion of lacrimal bone Orbital portion of maxilla Orbital portion of palatine bone Orbital portion of sphenoid bone Orbital portion of zygomatic bone **Q Orbit, Left** *See P Orbit, Right* **R Maxilla** Alveolar process of maxilla **T Mandible, Right** Alveolar process of mandible Condyloid process Mandibular notch Mental foramen **V Mandible, Left** *See T Mandible, Right* **X Hyoid Bone**	**Ø Open** **3 Percutaneous** **4 Percutaneous Endoscopic**	**Z No Device**	**Z No Qualifier**

Non-OR ØN8B[Ø,3,4]ZZ

Ø   **Medical and Surgical**
N   **Head and Facial Bones**
9   **Drainage**   Definition: Taking or letting out fluids and/or gases from a body part
                       Explanation: The qualifier DIAGNOSTIC is used to identify drainage procedures that are biopsies

Body Part Character 4	Approach Character 5	Device Character 6	Qualifier Character 7
Ø Skull	Ø Open	Ø Drainage Device	Z No Qualifier
1 Frontal Bone Zygomatic process of frontal bone	3 Percutaneous 4 Percutaneous Endoscopic		
3 Parietal Bone, Right			
4 Parietal Bone, Left			

5   Temporal Bone, Right
     Mastoid process
     Petrous part of temporal bone
     Tympanic part of temporal bone
     Zygomatic process of temporal bone			

6 Temporal Bone, Left *See 5 Temporal Bone, Right*			
7 Occipital Bone Foramen magnum			
B Nasal Bone Vomer of nasal septum			

C   Sphenoid Bone
     Greater wing
     Lesser wing
     Optic foramen
     Pterygoid process
     Sella turcica			

F Ethmoid Bone, Right Cribriform plate			
G Ethmoid Bone, Left *See F Ethmoid Bone, Right*			
H Lacrimal Bone, Right			
J Lacrimal Bone, Left			
K Palatine Bone, Right			
L Palatine Bone, Left			
M Zygomatic Bone, Right			
N Zygomatic Bone, Left			

P   Orbit, Right
     Bony orbit
     Orbital portion of ethmoid bone
     Orbital portion of frontal bone
     Orbital portion of lacrimal bone
     Orbital portion of maxilla
     Orbital portion of palatine bone
     Orbital portion of sphenoid bone
     Orbital portion of zygomatic bone			

Q Orbit, Left *See P Orbit, Right*			
R Maxilla Alveolar process of maxilla			

T   Mandible, Right
     Alveolar process of mandible
     Condyloid process
     Mandibular notch
     Mental foramen			

V Mandible, Left *See T Mandible, Right*			
X Hyoid Bone			

Non-OR   ØN9[Ø,1,3,4,5,6,7,C,F,G,H,J,K,L,M,N,P,Q,X]3ØZ
Non-OR   ØN9[B,R,T,V][Ø,3,4]ØZ

ØN9 Continued on next page

Head and Facial Bones

Ø	**Medical and Surgical**
N	**Head and Facial Bones**
9	**Drainage**

Definition: Taking or letting out fluids and/or gases from a body part

Explanation: The qualifier DIAGNOSTIC is used to identify drainage procedures that are biopsies

ØN9 Continued

Body Part Character 4	Approach Character 5	Device Character 6	Qualifier Character 7
Ø **Skull**	Ø Open	Z No Device	X Diagnostic
1 **Frontal Bone**	3 Percutaneous		Z No Qualifier
Zygomatic process of frontal bone	4 Percutaneous Endoscopic		
3 **Parietal Bone, Right**			
4 **Parietal Bone, Left**			
5 **Temporal Bone, Right**			
Mastoid process			
Petrous part of temporal bone			
Tympanic part of temporal bone			
Zygomatic process of temporal bone			
6 **Temporal Bone, Left**			
See 5 Temporal Bone, Right			
7 **Occipital Bone**			
Foramen magnum			
B **Nasal Bone**			
Vomer of nasal septum			
C **Sphenoid Bone**			
Greater wing			
Lesser wing			
Optic foramen			
Pterygoid process			
Sella turcica			
F **Ethmoid Bone, Right**			
Cribriform plate			
G **Ethmoid Bone, Left**			
See F Ethmoid Bone, Right			
H **Lacrimal Bone, Right**			
J **Lacrimal Bone, Left**			
K **Palatine Bone, Right**			
L **Palatine Bone, Left**			
M **Zygomatic Bone, Right**			
N **Zygomatic Bone, Left**			
P **Orbit, Right**			
Bony orbit			
Orbital portion of ethmoid bone			
Orbital portion of frontal bone			
Orbital portion of lacrimal bone			
Orbital portion of maxilla			
Orbital portion of palatine bone			
Orbital portion of sphenoid bone			
Orbital portion of zygomatic bone			
Q **Orbit, Left**			
See P Orbit, Right			
R **Maxilla**			
Alveolar process of maxilla			
T **Mandible, Right**			
Alveolar process of mandible			
Condyloid process			
Mandibular notch			
Mental foramen			
V **Mandible, Left**			
See T Mandible, Right			
X **Hyoid Bone**			

Non-OR	ØN9[Ø,1,3,4,5,6,7,C,F,G,H,J,K,L,M,N,P,Q,X]3ZZ
Non-OR	ØN9B[Ø,3,4]Z[X,Z]
Non-OR	ØN9[R,T,V][Ø,3,4]ZZ

Non-OR Procedure   DRG Non-OR Procedure   Valid OR Procedure   HAC Associated Procedure   Combination Only   New/Revised April   New/Revised October

526   ICD-10-PCS 2023

Ø   **Medical and Surgical**
N   **Head and Facial Bones**
B   **Excision**   Definition: Cutting out or off, without replacement, a portion of a body part
                         Explanation: The qualifier DIAGNOSTIC is used to identify excision procedures that are biopsies

Body Part Character 4	Approach Character 5	Device Character 6	Qualifier Character 7
Ø **Skull**	**Ø** **Open**	**Z** **No Device**	**X** **Diagnostic**
1 **Frontal Bone**	**3** **Percutaneous**		**Z** **No Qualifier**
Zygomatic process of frontal bone	**4** **Percutaneous Endoscopic**		
3 **Parietal Bone, Right**			
4 **Parietal Bone, Left**			
5 **Temporal Bone, Right**			
Mastoid process			
Petrous part of temporal bone			
Tympanic part of temporal bone			
Zygomatic process of temporal bone			
6 **Temporal Bone, Left**			
See 5 Temporal Bone, Right			
7 **Occipital Bone**			
Foramen magnum			
B **Nasal Bone**			
Vomer of nasal septum			
C **Sphenoid Bone**			
Greater wing			
Lesser wing			
Optic foramen			
Pterygoid process			
Sella turcica			
F **Ethmoid Bone, Right**			
Cribriform plate			
G **Ethmoid Bone, Left**			
See F Ethmoid Bone, Right			
H **Lacrimal Bone, Right**			
J **Lacrimal Bone, Left**			
K **Palatine Bone, Right**			
L **Palatine Bone, Left**			
M **Zygomatic Bone, Right**			
N **Zygomatic Bone, Left**			
P **Orbit, Right**			
Bony orbit			
Orbital portion of ethmoid bone			
Orbital portion of frontal bone			
Orbital portion of lacrimal bone			
Orbital portion of maxilla			
Orbital portion of palatine bone			
Orbital portion of sphenoid bone			
Orbital portion of zygomatic bone			
Q **Orbit, Left**			
See P Orbit, Right			
R **Maxilla**			
Alveolar process of maxilla ·			
T **Mandible, Right**			
Alveolar process of mandible			
Condyloid process			
Mandibular notch			
Mental foramen			
V **Mandible, Left**			
See T Mandible, Right			
X **Hyoid Bone**			

Non-OR   ØNB[B,R,T,V][Ø,3,4]ZX

Ø   Medical and Surgical
N   Head and Facial Bones
C   Extirpation   Definition: Taking or cutting out solid matter from a body part

Explanation: The solid matter may be an abnormal byproduct of a biological function or a foreign body; it may be imbedded in a body part or in the lumen of a tubular body part. The solid matter may or may not have been previously broken into pieces.

Body Part Character 4	Approach Character 5	Device Character 6	Qualifier Character 7

1 Frontal Bone
    Zygomatic process of frontal bone
3 Parietal Bone, Right
4 Parietal Bone, Left
5 Temporal Bone, Right
    Mastoid process
    Petrous part of temporal bone
    Tympanic part of temporal bone
    Zygomatic process of temporal bone
6 Temporal Bone, Left
    See 5 Temporal Bone, Right
7 Occipital Bone
    Foramen magnum
B Nasal Bone
    Vomer of nasal septum
C Sphenoid Bone
    Greater wing
    Lesser wing
    Optic foramen
    Pterygoid process
    Sella turcica
F Ethmoid Bone, Right
    Cribriform plate
G Ethmoid Bone, Left
    See F Ethmoid Bone, Right
H Lacrimal Bone, Right
J Lacrimal Bone, Left
K Palatine Bone, Right
L Palatine Bone, Left
M Zygomatic Bone, Right
N Zygomatic Bone, Left
P Orbit, Right
    Bony orbit
    Orbital portion of ethmoid bone
    Orbital portion of frontal bone
    Orbital portion of lacrimal bone
    Orbital portion of maxilla
    Orbital portion of palatine bone
    Orbital portion of sphenoid bone
    Orbital portion of zygomatic bone
Q Orbit, Left
    See P Orbit, Right
R Maxilla
    Alveolar process of maxilla
T Mandible, Right
    Alveolar process of mandible
    Condyloid process
    Mandibular notch
    Mental foramen
V Mandible, Left
    See T Mandible, Right
X Hyoid Bone
	Ø Open
	3 Percutaneous
	4 Percutaneous Endoscopic
		Z No Device	**Z No Qualifier**

Non-OR   ØNC[B,R,T,V][Ø,3,4]ZZ

Non-OR Procedure   DRG Non-OR Procedure   Valid OR Procedure   HAC Associated Procedure   Combination Only   New/Revised April   New/Revised October

528   ICD-10-PCS 2023

0   **Medical and Surgical**
N   **Head and Facial Bones**
D   **Extraction**   Definition: Pulling or stripping out or off all or a portion of a body part by the use of force
                        Explanation: The qualifier DIAGNOSTIC is used to identify extraction procedures that are biopsies

Body Part Character 4	Approach Character 5	Device Character 6	Qualifier Character 7
0 Skull	**0** Open	**Z** No Device	**Z** No Qualifier
1 Frontal Bone Zygomatic process of frontal bone			
3 Parietal Bone, Right			
4 Parietal Bone, Left			

5   Temporal Bone, Right
     Mastoid process
     Petrous part of temporal bone
     Tympanic part of temporal bone
     Zygomatic process of temporal bone			

6 Temporal Bone, Left *See 5 Temporal Bone, Right*			
7 Occipital Bone Foramen magnum			
B Nasal Bone Vomer of nasal septum			

C   Sphenoid Bone
     Greater wing
     Lesser wing
     Optic foramen
     Pterygoid process
     Sella turcica			

F Ethmoid Bone, Right Cribriform plate			
G Ethmoid Bone, Left *See F Ethmoid Bone, Right*			
H Lacrimal Bone, Right			
J Lacrimal Bone, Left			
K Palatine Bone, Right			
L Palatine Bone, Left			
M Zygomatic Bone, Right			
N Zygomatic Bone, Left			

P   Orbit, Right
     Bony orbit
     Orbital portion of ethmoid bone
     Orbital portion of frontal bone
     Orbital portion of lacrimal bone
     Orbital portion of maxilla
     Orbital portion of palatine bone
     Orbital portion of sphenoid bone
     Orbital portion of zygomatic bone			

Q Orbit, Left *See P Orbit, Right*			
R Maxilla Alveolar process of maxilla			

T   Mandible, Right
     Alveolar process of mandible
     Condyloid process
     Mandibular notch
     Mental foramen			

V Mandible, Left *See T Mandible, Right*			
X Hyoid Bone			

NC Noncovered Procedure   **LC** Limited Coverage   **QA** Questionable OB Admit   **NT** New Tech Add-on   ⊞ Combination Member   ♂ Male   ♀ Female

ICD-10-PCS 2023   529

Head and Facial Bones

Ø **Medical and Surgical**
N **Head and Facial Bones**
H **Insertion** Definition: Putting in a nonbiological appliance that monitors, assists, performs, or prevents a physiological function but does not physically take the place of a body part
  Explanation: None

Body Part Character 4	Approach Character 5	Device Character 6	Qualifier Character 7
Ø Skull ⊞	Ø Open	3 Infusion Device 4 Internal Fixation Device 5 External Fixation Device M Bone Growth Stimulator N Neurostimulator Generator	Z No Qualifier
Ø Skull	3 Percutaneous 4 Percutaneous Endoscopic	3 Infusion Device 4 Internal Fixation Device 5 External Fixation Device M Bone Growth Stimulator	Z No Qualifier

1 Frontal Bone
  Zygomatic process of frontal bone
3 Parietal Bone, Right
4 Parietal Bone, Left
7 Occipital Bone
  Foramen magnum
C Sphenoid Bone
  Greater wing
  Lesser wing
  Optic foramen
  Pterygoid process
  Sella turcica
F Ethmoid Bone, Right
  Cribriform plate
G Ethmoid Bone, Left
  See F Ethmoid Bone, Right
H Lacrimal Bone, Right
J Lacrimal Bone, Left
K Palatine Bone, Right
L Palatine Bone, Left
M Zygomatic Bone, Right
N Zygomatic Bone, Left
P Orbit, Right
  Bony orbit
  Orbital portion of ethmoid bone
  Orbital portion of frontal bone
  Orbital portion of lacrimal bone
  Orbital portion of maxilla
  Orbital portion of palatine bone
  Orbital portion of sphenoid bone
  Orbital portion of zygomatic bone
Q Orbit, Left
  See P Orbit, Right
X Hyoid Bone
	Ø Open
	3 Percutaneous
	4 Percutaneous Endoscopic
		4 Internal Fixation Device	Z No Qualifier

5 Temporal Bone, Right
  Mastoid process
  Petrous part of temporal bone
  Tympanic part of temporal bone
  Zygomatic process of temporal bone
6 Temporal Bone, Left
  See 5 Temporal Bone, Right
	Ø Open
	3 Percutaneous
	4 Percutaneous Endoscopic
		4 Internal Fixation Device
		S Hearing Device
			Z No Qualifier

B Nasal Bone Vomer of nasal septum	Ø Open 3 Percutaneous 4 Percutaneous Endoscopic	4 Internal Fixation Device M Bone Growth Stimulator	Z No Qualifier

R Maxilla
  Alveolar process of maxilla
T Mandible, Right
  Alveolar process of mandible
  Condyloid process
  Mandibular notch
  Mental foramen
V Mandible, Left
  See T Mandible, Right
	Ø Open
	3 Percutaneous
	4 Percutaneous Endoscopic
		4 Internal Fixation Device
		5 External Fixation Device
			Z No Qualifier

W Facial Bone	Ø Open 3 Percutaneous 4 Percutaneous Endoscopic	M Bone Growth Stimulator	Z No Qualifier

Non-OR	ØNHØØ5Z
Non-OR	ØNHØ[3,4]5Z
Non-OR	ØNHB[Ø,3,4][4,M]Z

See Appendix L for Procedure Combinations
⊞ ØNHØØNZ

Ø **Medical and Surgical**
N **Head and Facial Bones**
J **Inspection**   Definition: Visually and/or manually exploring a body part

Explanation: Visual exploration may be performed with or without optical instrumentation. Manual exploration may be performed directly or through intervening body layers.

Body Part Character 4	Approach Character 5	Device Character 6	Qualifier Character 7
Ø Skull B Nasal Bone Vomer of nasal septum W Facial Bone	Ø Open 3 Percutaneous 4 Percutaneous Endoscopic X External	Z No Device	Z No Qualifier

Non-OR   ØNJ[Ø,B,W][3,X]ZZ

Ø **Medical and Surgical**
N **Head and Facial Bones**
N **Release**   Definition: Freeing a body part from an abnormal physical constraint by cutting or by the use of force

Explanation: Some of the restraining tissue may be taken out but none of the body part is taken out

Body Part Character 4	Approach Character 5	Device Character 6	Qualifier Character 7

1 Frontal Bone
    Zygomatic process of frontal bone
3 Parietal Bone, Right
4 Parietal Bone, Left
5 Temporal Bone, Right
    Mastoid process
    Petrous part of temporal bone
    Tympanic part of temporal bone
    Zygomatic process of temporal bone
6 Temporal Bone, Left
    See 5 Temporal Bone, Right
7 Occipital Bone
    Foramen magnum
B Nasal Bone
    Vomer of nasal septum
C Sphenoid Bone
    Greater wing
    Lesser wing
    Optic foramen
    Pterygoid process
    Sella turcica
F Ethmoid Bone, Right
    Cribriform plate
G Ethmoid Bone, Left
    See F Ethmoid Bone, Right
H Lacrimal Bone, Right
J Lacrimal Bone, Left
K Palatine Bone, Right
L Palatine Bone, Left
M Zygomatic Bone, Right
N Zygomatic Bone, Left
P Orbit, Right
    Bony orbit
    Orbital portion of ethmoid bone
    Orbital portion of frontal bone
    Orbital portion of lacrimal bone
    Orbital portion of maxilla
    Orbital portion of palatine bone
    Orbital portion of sphenoid bone
    Orbital portion of zygomatic bone
Q Orbit, Left
    See P Orbit, Right
R Maxilla
    Alveolar process of maxilla
T Mandible, Right
    Alveolar process of mandible
    Condyloid process
    Mandibular notch
    Mental foramen
V Mandible, Left
    See T Mandible, Right
X Hyoid Bone
	Ø Open
	3 Percutaneous
	4 Percutaneous Endoscopic
		Z No Device	Z No Qualifier

Non-OR   ØNNB[Ø,3,4]ZZ

NC Noncovered Procedure   **LC** Limited Coverage   **QA** Questionable OB Admit   **NT** New Tech Add-on   ⊞ Combination Member   ♂ Male   ♀ Female

ICD-10-PCS 2023   531

Head and Facial Bones

Ø   Medical and Surgical
N   Head and Facial Bones
P   Removal   Definition: Taking out or off a device from a body part

Explanation: If a device is taken out and a similar device put in without cutting or puncturing the skin or mucous membrane, the procedure is coded to the root operation CHANGE. Otherwise, the procedure for taking out a device is coded to the root operation REMOVAL.

Body Part Character 4	Approach Character 5	Device Character 6	Qualifier Character 7
Ø Skull	Ø Open	Ø Drainage Device 3 Infusion Device 4 Internal Fixation Device 5 External Fixation Device 7 Autologous Tissue Substitute J Synthetic Substitute K Nonautologous Tissue Substitute M Bone Growth Stimulator N Neurostimulator Generator S Hearing Device	Z No Qualifier
Ø Skull	3 Percutaneous 4 Percutaneous Endoscopic	Ø Drainage Device 3 Infusion Device 4 Internal Fixation Device 5 External Fixation Device 7 Autologous Tissue Substitute J Synthetic Substitute K Nonautologous Tissue Substitute M Bone Growth Stimulator S Hearing Device	Z No Qualifier
Ø Skull	X External	Ø Drainage Device 3 Infusion Device 4 Internal Fixation Device 5 External Fixation Device M Bone Growth Stimulator S Hearing Device	Z No Qualifier
B Nasal Bone Vomer of nasal septum W Facial Bone	Ø Open 3 Percutaneous 4 Percutaneous Endoscopic	Ø Drainage Device 4 Internal Fixation Device 7 Autologous Tissue Substitute J Synthetic Substitute K Nonautologous Tissue Substitute M Bone Growth Stimulator	Z No Qualifier
B Nasal Bone Vomer of nasal septum W Facial Bone	X External	Ø Drainage Device 4 Internal Fixation Device M Bone Growth Stimulator	Z No Qualifier

Non-OR	ØNPØ[3,4]5Z
Non-OR	ØNPØX[Ø,3,5]Z
Non-OR	ØNPB[Ø,3,4][Ø,4,7,J,K,M]Z
Non-OR	ØNPBX[Ø,4,M]Z
Non-OR	ØNPWX[Ø,M]Z

Non-OR Procedure   DRG Non-OR Procedure   Valid OR Procedure   HAC Associated Procedure   Combination Only   New/Revised April   New/Revised October

532   ICD-10-PCS 2023

Ø   **Medical and Surgical**
N   **Head and Facial Bones**
Q   **Repair**   Definition: Restoring, to the extent possible, a body part to its normal anatomic structure and function
                           Explanation: Used only when the method to accomplish the repair is not one of the other root operations

Body Part Character 4	Approach Character 5	Device Character 6	Qualifier Character 7
Ø Skull	**Ø** Open	**Z** No Device	**Z** No Qualifier
1 Frontal Bone Zygomatic process of frontal bone	**3** Percutaneous		
3 Parietal Bone, Right	**4** Percutaneous Endoscopic		
4 Parietal Bone, Left	**X** External		

5   Temporal Bone, Right
     Mastoid process
     Petrous part of temporal bone
     Tympanic part of temporal bone
     Zygomatic process of temporal bone			

6 Temporal Bone, Left *See 5 Temporal Bone, Right*			
7 Occipital Bone Foramen magnum			
B Nasal Bone Vomer of nasal septum			

C   Sphenoid Bone
     Greater wing
     Lesser wing
     Optic foramen
     Pterygoid process
     Sella turcica			

F Ethmoid Bone, Right Cribriform plate			
G Ethmoid Bone, Left *See F Ethmoid Bone, Right*			
H Lacrimal Bone, Right			
J Lacrimal Bone, Left			
K Palatine Bone, Right			
L Palatine Bone, Left			
M Zygomatic Bone, Right			
N Zygomatic Bone, Left			

P   Orbit, Right
     Bony orbit
     Orbital portion of ethmoid bone
     Orbital portion of frontal bone
     Orbital portion of lacrimal bone
     Orbital portion of maxilla
     Orbital portion of palatine bone
     Orbital portion of sphenoid bone
     Orbital portion of zygomatic bone			

Q Orbit, Left *See P Orbit, Right*			
R Maxilla Alveolar process of maxilla			

T   Mandible, Right
     Alveolar process of mandible
     Condyloid process
     Mandibular notch
     Mental foramen			

V Mandible, Left *See T Mandible, Right*			
X Hyoid Bone			

Non-OR   ØNQ[Ø,1,3,4,5,6,7,B,C,F,G,H,J,K,L,M,N,P,Q,R,T,V,X]XZZ

NC Noncovered Procedure   **LC** Limited Coverage   **QA** Questionable OB Admit   **NT** New Tech Add-on   ⊞ Combination Member   ♂ Male   ♀ Female

ICD-10-PCS 2023   **533**

ØNQ–ØNQ

Head and Facial Bones

Ø   Medical and Surgical
N   Head and Facial Bones
R   Replacement   Definition: Putting in or on biological or synthetic material that physically takes the place and/or function of all or a portion of a body part

                 Explanation: The body part may have been taken out or replaced, or may be taken out, physically eradicated, or rendered nonfunctional during the REPLACEMENT procedure. A REMOVAL procedure is coded for taking out the device used in a previous replacement procedure.

Body Part Character 4	Approach Character 5	Device Character 6	Qualifier Character 7
Ø Skull	**Ø Open**	**7 Autologous Tissue Substitute**	**Z No Qualifier**
1 Frontal Bone	**3 Percutaneous**	**J Synthetic Substitute**	
Zygomatic process of frontal bone	**4 Percutaneous Endoscopic**	**K Nonautologous Tissue Substitute**	
3 Parietal Bone, Right			
4 Parietal Bone, Left			
5 Temporal Bone, Right			
Mastoid process			
Petrous part of temporal bone			
Tympanic part of temporal bone			
Zygomatic process of temporal bone			
6 Temporal Bone, Left			
See 5 Temporal Bone, Right			
7 Occipital Bone			
Foramen magnum			
B Nasal Bone			
Vomer of nasal septum			
C Sphenoid Bone			
Greater wing			
Lesser wing			
Optic foramen			
Pterygoid process			
Sella turcica			
F Ethmoid Bone, Right			
Cribriform plate			
G Ethmoid Bone, Left			
See F Ethmoid Bone, Right			
H Lacrimal Bone, Right			
J Lacrimal Bone, Left			
K Palatine Bone, Right			
L Palatine Bone, Left			
M Zygomatic Bone, Right			
N Zygomatic Bone, Left			
P Orbit, Right			
Bony orbit			
Orbital portion of ethmoid bone			
Orbital portion of frontal bone			
Orbital portion of lacrimal bone			
Orbital portion of maxilla			
Orbital portion of palatine bone			
Orbital portion of sphenoid bone			
Orbital portion of zygomatic bone			
Q Orbit, Left			
See P Orbit, Right			
R Maxilla			
Alveolar process of maxilla			
T Mandible, Right			
Alveolar process of mandible			
Condyloid process			
Mandibular notch			
Mental foramen			
V Mandible, Left			
See T Mandible, Right			
X Hyoid Bone			

Non-OR Procedure   DRG Non-OR Procedure   Valid OR Procedure   HAC Associated Procedure   Combination Only   New/Revised April   New/Revised October

534   ICD-10-PCS 2023

Ø   Medical and Surgical
N   Head and Facial Bones
S   Reposition   Definition: Moving to its normal location, or other suitable location, all or a portion of a body part

Explanation: The body part is moved to a new location from an abnormal location, or from a normal location where it is not functioning correctly. The body part may or may not be cut out or off to be moved to the new location.

Body Part Character 4	Approach Character 5	Device Character 6	Qualifier Character 7

Ø Skull
R Maxilla
   Alveolar process of maxilla
T Mandible, Right
   Alveolar process of mandible
   Condyloid process
   Mandibular notch
   Mental foramen
V Mandible, Left
   See T Mandible, Right
	Ø Open
	3 Percutaneous
	4 Percutaneous Endoscopic
		4 Internal Fixation Device
		5 External Fixation Device
		Z No Device
			Z No Qualifier

Ø Skull
R Maxilla
   Alveolar process of maxilla
T Mandible, Right
   Alveolar process of mandible
   Condyloid process
   Mandibular notch
   Mental foramen
V Mandible, Left
   See T Mandible, Right
	X External	**Z** No Device	**Z** No Qualifier

1 Frontal Bone
   Zygomatic process of frontal bone
3 Parietal Bone, Right
4 Parietal Bone, Left
5 Temporal Bone, Right
   Mastoid process
   Petrous part of temporal bone
   Tympanic part of temporal bone
   Zygomatic process of temporal bone
6 Temporal Bone, Left
   See 5 Temporal Bone, Right
7 Occipital Bone
   Foramen magnum
B Nasal Bone
   Vomer of nasal septum
C Sphenoid Bone
   Greater wing
   Lesser wing
   Optic foramen
   Pterygoid process
   Sella turcica
F Ethmoid Bone, Right
   Cribriform plate
G Ethmoid Bone, Left
   See F Ethmoid Bone, Right
H Lacrimal Bone, Right
J Lacrimal Bone, Left
K Palatine Bone, Right
L Palatine Bone, Left
M Zygomatic Bone, Right
N Zygomatic Bone, Left
P Orbit, Right
   Bony orbit
   Orbital portion of ethmoid bone
   Orbital portion of frontal bone
   Orbital portion of lacrimal bone
   Orbital portion of maxilla
   Orbital portion of palatine bone
   Orbital portion of sphenoid bone
   Orbital portion of zygomatic bone
Q Orbit, Left
   See P Orbit, Right
X Hyoid Bone
	Ø Open
	3 Percutaneous
	4 Percutaneous Endoscopic
		4 Internal Fixation Device
		Z No Device
			Z No Qualifier

Non-OR	ØNS[R,T,V][3,4][4,5,Z]Z
Non-OR	ØNS[Ø,R,T,V]XZZ
Non-OR	ØNS[B,C,F,G,H,J,K,L,M,N,P,Q,X][3,4][4,Z]Z

ØNS Continued on next page

Head and Facial Bones

Ø   **Medical and Surgical**
N   **Head and Facial Bones**
S   **Reposition**   Definition: Moving to its normal location, or other suitable location, all or a portion of a body part

Explanation: The body part is moved to a new location from an abnormal location, or from a normal location where it is not functioning correctly. The body part may or may not be cut out or off to be moved to the new location.

Body Part Character 4	Approach Character 5	Device Character 6	Qualifier Character 7

1 Frontal Bone
     Zygomatic process of frontal bone
3 Parietal Bone, Right
4 Parietal Bone, Left
5 Temporal Bone, Right
     Mastoid process
     Petrous part of temporal bone
     Tympanic part of temporal bone
     Zygomatic process of temporal bone
6 Temporal Bone, Left
     See 5 Temporal Bone, Right
7 Occipital Bone
     Foramen magnum
B Nasal Bone
     Vomer of nasal septum
C Sphenoid Bone
     Greater wing
     Lesser wing
     Optic foramen
     Pterygoid process
     Sella turcica
F Ethmoid Bone, Right
     Cribriform plate
G Ethmoid Bone, Left
     See F Ethmoid Bone, Right
H Lacrimal Bone, Right
J Lacrimal Bone, Left
K Palatine Bone, Right
L Palatine Bone, Left
M Zygomatic Bone, Right
N Zygomatic Bone, Left
P Orbit, Right
     Bony orbit
     Orbital portion of ethmoid bone
     Orbital portion of frontal bone
     Orbital portion of lacrimal bone
     Orbital portion of maxilla
     Orbital portion of palatine bone
     Orbital portion of sphenoid bone
     Orbital portion of zygomatic bone
Q Orbit, Left
     See P Orbit, Right
X Hyoid Bone
	X External	**Z No Device**	**Z No Qualifier**

Non-OR   ØNS[1,3,4,5,6,7,B,C,F,G,H,J,K,L,M,N,P,Q,X]XZZ

Ø   **Medical and Surgical**
N   **Head and Facial Bones**
T   **Resection**   Definition: Cutting out or off, without replacement, all of a body part
                   Explanation: None

Body Part Character 4	Approach Character 5	Device Character 6	Qualifier Character 7

1 **Frontal Bone**
   Zygomatic process of frontal bone
3 **Parietal Bone, Right**
4 **Parietal Bone, Left**
5 **Temporal Bone, Right**
   Mastoid process
   Petrous part of temporal bone
   Tympanic part of temporal bone
   Zygomatic process of temporal bone
6 **Temporal Bone, Left**
   See 5 Temporal Bone, Right
7 **Occipital Bone**
   Foramen magnum
B **Nasal Bone**
   Vomer of nasal septum
C **Sphenoid Bone**
   Greater wing
   Lesser wing
   Optic foramen
   Pterygoid process
   Sella turcica
F **Ethmoid Bone, Right**
   Cribriform plate
G **Ethmoid Bone, Left**
   See F Ethmoid Bone, Right
H **Lacrimal Bone, Right**
J **Lacrimal Bone, Left**
K **Palatine Bone, Right**
L **Palatine Bone, Left**
M **Zygomatic Bone, Right**
N **Zygomatic Bone, Left**
P **Orbit, Right**
   Bony orbit
   Orbital portion of ethmoid bone
   Orbital portion of frontal bone
   Orbital portion of lacrimal bone
   Orbital portion of maxilla
   Orbital portion of palatine bone
   Orbital portion of sphenoid bone
   Orbital portion of zygomatic bone
Q **Orbit, Left**
   See P Orbit, Right
R **Maxilla**
   Alveolar process of maxilla
T **Mandible, Right**
   Alveolar process of mandible
   Condyloid process
   Mandibular notch
   Mental foramen
V **Mandible, Left**
   See T Mandible, Right
X **Hyoid Bone**
	Ø Open	**Z** No Device	**Z** No Qualifier

NC Noncovered Procedure   **LC** Limited Coverage   **QA** Questionable OB Admit   **NT** New Tech Add-on   ⊞ Combination Member   ♂ Male   ♀ Female

ICD-10-PCS 2023   **537**

Head and Facial Bones

Ø   **Medical and Surgical**
N   **Head and Facial Bones**
U   **Supplement**   Definition: Putting in or on biological or synthetic material that physically reinforces and/or augments the function of a portion of a body part
                      Explanation: The biological material is non-living, or is living and from the same individual. The body part may have been previously replaced, and the SUPPLEMENT procedure is performed to physically reinforce and/or augment the function of the replaced body part.

Body Part Character 4	Approach Character 5	Device Character 6	Qualifier Character 7
Ø **Skull**	**Ø** **Open**	**7** **Autologous Tissue Substitute**	**Z** **No Qualifier**
1 **Frontal Bone**	**3** **Percutaneous**	**J** **Synthetic Substitute**	
Zygomatic process of frontal bone	**4** **Percutaneous Endoscopic**	**K** **Nonautologous Tissue Substitute**	
3 **Parietal Bone, Right**			
4 **Parietal Bone, Left**			
5 **Temporal Bone, Right**			
Mastoid process			
Petrous part of temporal bone			
Tympanic part of temporal bone			
Zygomatic process of temporal bone			
6 **Temporal Bone, Left**			
See 5 Temporal Bone, Right			
7 **Occipital Bone**			
Foramen magnum			
B **Nasal Bone**			
Vomer of nasal septum			
C **Sphenoid Bone**			
Greater wing			
Lesser wing			
Optic foramen			
Pterygoid process			
Sella turcica			
F **Ethmoid Bone, Right**			
Cribriform plate			
G **Ethmoid Bone, Left**			
See F Ethmoid Bone, Right			
H **Lacrimal Bone, Right**			
J **Lacrimal Bone, Left**			
K **Palatine Bone, Right**			
L **Palatine Bone, Left**			
M **Zygomatic Bone, Right**			
N **Zygomatic Bone, Left**			
P **Orbit, Right**			
Bony orbit			
Orbital portion of ethmoid bone			
Orbital portion of frontal bone			
Orbital portion of lacrimal bone			
Orbital portion of maxilla			
Orbital portion of palatine bone			
Orbital portion of sphenoid bone			
Orbital portion of zygomatic bone			
Q **Orbit, Left**			
See P Orbit, Right			
R **Maxilla**			
Alveolar process of maxilla			
T **Mandible, Right**			
Alveolar process of mandible			
Condyloid process			
Mandibular notch			
Mental foramen			
V **Mandible, Left**			
See T Mandible, Right			
X **Hyoid Bone**			

Non-OR Procedure   DRG Non-OR Procedure   Valid OR Procedure   HAC Associated Procedure   Combination Only   New/Revised April   New/Revised October

538

ICD-10-PCS 2023

Ø   Medical and Surgical
N   Head and Facial Bones
W   Revision   Definition: Correcting, to the extent possible, a portion of a malfunctioning device or the position of a displaced device

                  Explanation: Revision can include correcting a malfunctioning or displaced device by taking out or putting in components of the device such as a screw or pin

Body Part Character 4	Approach Character 5	Device Character 6	Qualifier Character 7
Ø Skull	Ø Open	Ø Drainage Device 3 Infusion Device 4 Internal Fixation Device 5 External Fixation Device 7 Autologous Tissue Substitute J Synthetic Substitute K Nonautologous Tissue Substitute M Bone Growth Stimulator N Neurostimulator Generator S Hearing Device	Z No Qualifier
Ø Skull	3 Percutaneous 4 Percutaneous Endoscopic X External	Ø Drainage Device 3 Infusion Device 4 Internal Fixation Device 5 External Fixation Device 7 Autologous Tissue Substitute J Synthetic Substitute K Nonautologous Tissue Substitute M Bone Growth Stimulator S Hearing Device	Z No Qualifier
B Nasal Bone Vomer of nasal septum W Facial Bone	Ø Open 3 Percutaneous 4 Percutaneous Endoscopic X External	Ø Drainage Device 4 Internal Fixation Device 7 Autologous Tissue Substitute J Synthetic Substitute K Nonautologous Tissue Substitute M Bone Growth Stimulator	Z No Qualifier

Non-OR   ØNWØX[Ø,3,4,5,7,J,K,M,S]Z
Non-OR   ØNWB[Ø,3,4,X][Ø,4,7,J,K,M]Z
Non-OR   ØNWWX[Ø,4,7,J,K,M]Z

NC Noncovered Procedure   LC Limited Coverage   QA Questionable OB Admit   NT New Tech Add-on   ⊞ Combination Member   ♂ Male   ♀ Female

ICD-10-PCS 2023   539

Upper Bones 0P2–0PW

Character Meanings

This Character Meaning table is provided as a guide to assist the user in the identification of character members that may be found in this section of code tables. It **SHOULD NOT** be used to build a PCS code.

Operation–Character 3	Body Part–Character 4	Approach–Character 5	Device–Character 6	Qualifier–Character 7
2 Change	0 Sternum	0 Open	0 Drainage Device OR Internal Fixation Device, Rigid Plate	X Diagnostic
5 Destruction	1 Ribs, 1 to 2	3 Percutaneous	3 Spinal Stabilization Device, Vertebral Body Tether	Z No Qualifier
8 Division	2 Ribs, 3 or more	4 Percutaneous Endoscopic	4 Internal Fixation Device	
9 Drainage	3 Cervical Vertebra	X External	5 External Fixation Device	
B Excision	4 Thoracic Vertebra		6 Internal Fixation Device, Intramedullary	
C Extirpation	5 Scapula, Right		7 Autologous Tissue Substitute OR Internal Fixation Device, Intramedullary Limb Lengthening	
D Extraction	6 Scapula, Left		8 External Fixation Device, Limb Lengthening	
H Insertion	7 Glenoid Cavity, Right		B External Fixation Device, Monoplanar	
J Inspection	8 Glenoid Cavity, Left		C External Fixation Device, Ring	
N Release	9 Clavicle, Right		D External Fixation Device, Hybrid	
P Removal	B Clavicle, Left		J Synthetic Substitute	
Q Repair	C Humeral Head, Right		K Nonautologous Tissue Substitute	
R Replacement	D Humeral Head, Left		M Bone Growth Stimulator	
S Reposition	F Humeral Shaft, Right		Y Other Device	
T Resection	G Humeral Shaft, Left		Z No Device	
U Supplement	H Radius, Right			
W Revision	J Radius, Left			
	K Ulna, Right			
	L Ulna, Left			
	M Carpal, Right			
	N Carpal, Left			
	P Metacarpal, Right			
	Q Metacarpal, Left			
	R Thumb Phalanx, Right			
	S Thumb Phalanx, Left			
	T Finger Phalanx, Right			
	V Finger Phalanx, Left			
	Y Upper Bone			

AHA Coding Clinic for table 0PB
2015, 3Q, 3-8   Excisional and nonexcisional debridement
2015, 2Q, 34   Decompressive laminectomy
2013, 4Q, 109   Separating conjoined twins
2013, 4Q, 116   Spinal decompression
2013, 3Q, 20   Superior labrum anterior posterior (SLAP) repair and subacromial decompression
2012, 4Q, 101   Rib resection with reconstruction of anterior chest wall
2012, 2Q, 19   Multiple decompressive cervical laminectomies

AHA Coding Clinic for table 0PC
2021, 3Q, 15   Curettage of bilateral humeral head and bone graft placement
2019, 3Q, 19   Removal of sternal wire

AHA Coding Clinic for table 0PD
2017, 4Q, 41   Extraction procedures

AHA Coding Clinic for table 0PH
2020, 1Q, 29   Repair of sternal dehiscence using Sternal Talon® device
2019, 4Q, 34   Intramedullary limb lengthening internal fixation device
2019, 2Q, 40   Decompression of spinal cord and placement of instrumentation
2018, 3Q, 26   Anterior vertebral tethering using Dynesys Tethering System
2017, 2Q, 20   Exchange of intramedullary antibiotic impregnated spacer
2016, 4Q, 117   Placement of magnetic growth rods
2014, 4Q, 28   Removal and replacement of displaced growing rods

AHA Coding Clinic for table 0PP
2019, 3Q, 19   Removal of sternal wire
2017, 2Q, 20   Exchange of intramedullary antibiotic impregnated spacer
2016, 4Q, 117   Placement of magnetic growth rods
2014, 4Q, 28   Removal and replacement of displaced growing rods

AHA Coding Clinic for table 0PR
2018, 4Q, 92   Radial head arthroplasty

AHA Coding Clinic for table 0PS
2021, 4Q, 51-52   Vertebral body tethering
2020, 1Q, 33   Spinal fusion without use of bone graft
2018, 3Q, 26   Anterior vertebral tethering using Dynesys Tethering System
2017, 4Q, 53   New and revised body part values - Ribs
2016, 1Q, 21   Elongation derotation flexion casting
2015, 4Q, 33   Ravitch operation
2015, 2Q, 35   Application of tongs to reduce and stabilize cervical fracture
2014, 4Q, 26   Placement of vertical expandable prosthetic titanium rib (VEPTR)
2014, 4Q, 32   Open reduction internal fixation of fracture with debridement
2014, 3Q, 33   Radial fracture treatment with open reduction internal fixation, and release of carpal ligament

AHA Coding Clinic for table 0PT
2015, 3Q, 26   Thumb arthroplasty with resection of trapezium

AHA Coding Clinic for table 0PU
2021, 3Q, 15   Curettage of bilateral humeral head and bone graft placement
2015, 2Q, 20   Cervical laminoplasty
2013, 4Q, 109   Separating conjoined twins

AHA Coding Clinic for table 0PW
2014, 4Q, 26   Adjustment of VEPTR lengthening mechanism
2014, 4Q, 27   Bilateral lengthening of growing rods

Upper Bones

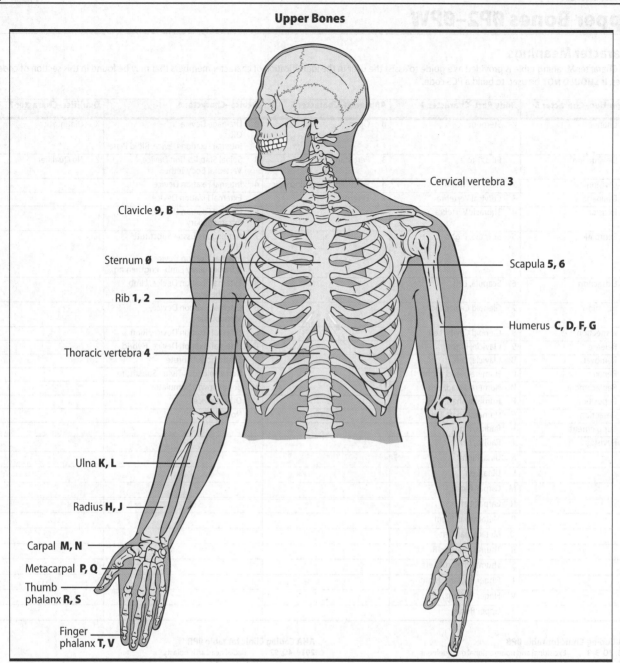

Cervical vertebra **3**

Clavicle **9, B**

Sternum **Ø**

Rib **1, 2**

Thoracic vertebra **4**

Scapula **5, 6**

Humerus **C, D, F, G**

Ulna **K, L**

Radius **H, J**

Carpal **M, N**

Metacarpal **P, Q**

Thumb phalanx **R, S**

Finger phalanx **T, V**

Humerus and Scapula

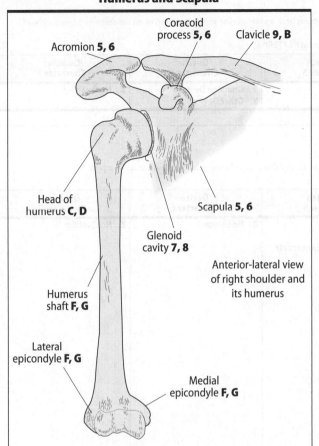

Acromion **5, 6**
Coracoid process **5, 6**
Clavicle **9, B**
Head of humerus **C, D**
Glenoid cavity **7, 8**
Scapula **5, 6**
Humerus shaft **F, G**
Lateral epicondyle **F, G**
Medial epicondyle **F, G**

Anterior-lateral view of right shoulder and its humerus

Radius and Ulna

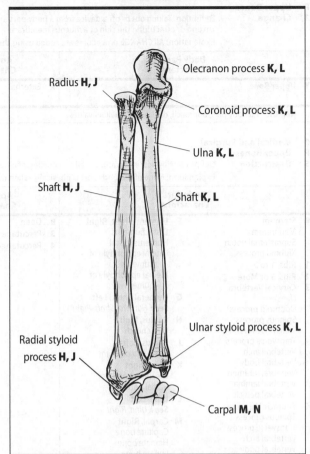

Olecranon process **K, L**
Radius **H, J**
Coronoid process **K, L**
Ulna **K, L**
Shaft **H, J**
Shaft **K, L**
Ulnar styloid process **K, L**
Radial styloid process **H, J**
Carpal **M, N**

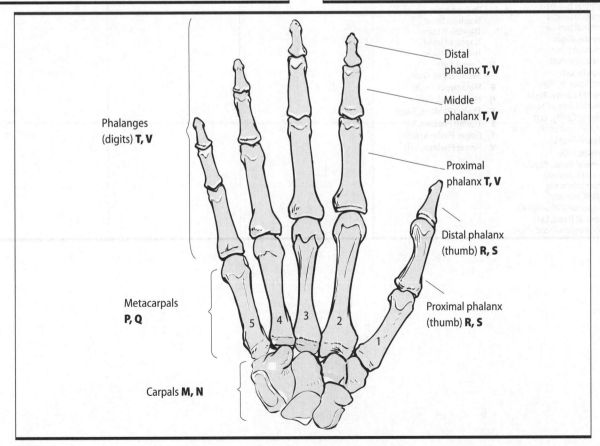

Phalanges (digits) **T, V**
Distal phalanx **T, V**
Middle phalanx **T, V**
Proximal phalanx **T, V**
Distal phalanx (thumb) **R, S**
Proximal phalanx (thumb) **R, S**
Metacarpals **P, Q**
Carpals **M, N**

5 4 3 2 1

Upper Bones *(left margin)*

0   **Medical and Surgical**
P   **Upper Bones**
2   **Change**   Definition: Taking out or off a device from a body part and putting back an identical or similar device in or on the same body part without cutting or puncturing the skin or a mucous membrane

                            Explanation: All CHANGE procedures are coded using the approach EXTERNAL

Body Part Character 4	Approach Character 5	Device Character 6	Qualifier Character 7
Y Upper Bone	X External	0 Drainage Device Y Other Device	Z No Qualifier

Non-OR	All body part, approach, device, and qualifier values

0   **Medical and Surgical**
P   **Upper Bones**
5   **Destruction**   Definition: Physical eradication of all or a portion of a body part by the direct use of energy, force, or a destructive agent

                            Explanation: None of the body part is physically taken out

Body Part Character 4		Approach Character 5	Device Character 6	Qualifier Character 7

0   **Sternum**
     Manubrium
     Suprasternal notch
     Xiphoid process
1   **Ribs, 1 to 2**
2   **Ribs, 3 or More**
3   **Cervical Vertebra**
     Dens
     Odontoid process
     Spinous process
     Transverse foramen
     Transverse process
     Vertebral arch
     Vertebral body
     Vertebral foramen
     Vertebral lamina
     Vertebral pedicle
4   **Thoracic Vertebra**
     Spinous process
     Transverse process
     Vertebral arch
     Vertebral body
     Vertebral foramen
     Vertebral lamina
     Vertebral pedicle
5   **Scapula, Right**
     Acromion (process)
     Coracoid process
6   **Scapula, Left**
     See 5 Scapula, Right
7   **Glenoid Cavity, Right**
     Glenoid fossa (of scapula)
8   **Glenoid Cavity, Left**
     See 7 Glenoid Cavity, Right
9   **Clavicle, Right**
B   **Clavicle, Left**
C   **Humeral Head, Right**
     Greater tuberosity
     Lesser tuberosity
     Neck of humerus
        (anatomical)(surgical)
D   **Humeral Head, Left**
     See C Humeral Head, Right
	F **Humeral Shaft, Right**
	     Distal humerus
	     Humerus, distal
	     Lateral epicondyle of
	        humerus
	     Medial epicondyle of
	        humerus
	G **Humeral Shaft, Left**
	     See F Humeral Shaft, Right
	H **Radius, Right**
	     Ulnar notch
	J **Radius, Left**
	     See H Radius, Right
	K **Ulna, Right**
	     Olecranon process
	     Radial notch
	L **Ulna, Left**
	     See K Ulna, Right
	M **Carpal, Right**
	     Capitate bone
	     Hamate bone
	     Lunate bone
	     Pisiform bone
	     Scaphoid bone
	     Trapezium bone
	     Trapezoid bone
	     Triquetral bone
	N **Carpal, Left**
	     See M Carpal, Right
	P **Metacarpal, Right**
	Q **Metacarpal, Left**
	R **Thumb Phalanx, Right**
	S **Thumb Phalanx, Left**
	T **Finger Phalanx, Right**
	V **Finger Phalanx, Left**
		0 **Open**
		3 **Percutaneous**
		4 **Percutaneous Endoscopic**
			Z No Device	Z No Qualifier

Non-OR Procedure   DRG Non-OR Procedure   Valid OR Procedure   HAC Associated Procedure   Combination Only   *New/Revised April*   *New/Revised October*

544   ICD-10-PCS 2023

Ø	**Medical and Surgical**
P	**Upper Bones**
8	**Division**

Definition: Cutting into a body part, without draining fluids and/or gases from the body part, in order to separate or transect a body part
Explanation: All or a portion of the body part is separated into two or more portions

Body Part Character 4	Approach Character 5	Device Character 6	Qualifier Character 7

Ø   **Sternum**
    Manubrium
    Suprasternal notch
    Xiphoid process
	Ø Open
	3 Percutaneous
	4 Percutaneous Endoscopic
		Z No Device	**Z** No Qualifier

1 **Ribs, 1 to 2**			
2 **Ribs, 3 or More**			

3   **Cervical Vertebra**
    Dens
    Odontoid process
    Spinous process
    Transverse foramen
    Transverse process
    Vertebral arch
    Vertebral body
    Vertebral foramen
    Vertebral lamina
    Vertebral pedicle			

4   **Thoracic Vertebra**
    Spinous process
    Transverse process
    Vertebral arch
    Vertebral body
    Vertebral foramen
    Vertebral lamina
    Vertebral pedicle			

5   **Scapula, Right**
    Acromion (process)
    Coracoid process			

6 **Scapula, Left** *See 5 Scapula, Right*			
7 **Glenoid Cavity, Right** Glenoid fossa (of scapula)			
8 **Glenoid Cavity, Left** *See 7 Glenoid Cavity, Right*			
9 **Clavicle, Right**			
B **Clavicle, Left**			

C   **Humeral Head, Right**
    Greater tuberosity
    Lesser tuberosity
    Neck of humerus (anatomical)(surgical)			

D **Humeral Head, Left** *See C Humeral Head, Right*			

F   **Humeral Shaft, Right**
    Distal humerus
    Humerus, distal
    Lateral epicondyle of humerus
    Medial epicondyle of humerus			

G **Humeral Shaft, Left** *See F Humeral Shaft, Right*			
H **Radius, Right** Ulnar notch			
J **Radius, Left** *See H Radius, Right*			

K   **Ulna, Right**
    Olecranon process
    Radial notch			

L **Ulna, Left** *See K Ulna, Right*			

M   **Carpal, Right**
    Capitate bone
    Hamate bone
    Lunate bone
    Pisiform bone
    Scaphoid bone
    Trapezium bone
    Trapezoid bone
    Triquetral bone			

N **Carpal, Left** *See M Carpal, Right*			
P **Metacarpal, Right**			
Q **Metacarpal, Left**			
R **Thumb Phalanx, Right**			
S **Thumb Phalanx, Left**			
T **Finger Phalanx, Right**			
V **Finger Phalanx, Left**			

NC Noncovered Procedure   **LC** Limited Coverage   **QA** Questionable OB Admit   **NT** New Tech Add-on   ⊞ Combination Member   ♂ Male   ♀ Female

ICD-10-PCS 2023   **545**

ØP8–ØP8

Ø   Medical and Surgical
P   Upper Bones
9   Drainage   Definition: Taking or letting out fluids and/or gases from a body part
                          Explanation: The qualifier DIAGNOSTIC is used to identify drainage procedures that are biopsies

Body Part Character 4		Approach Character 5	Device Character 6	Qualifier Character 7

Ø Sternum
    Manubrium
    Suprasternal notch
    Xiphoid process
1 Ribs, 1 to 2
2 Ribs, 3 or More
3 Cervical Vertebra
    Dens
    Odontoid process
    Spinous process
    Transverse foramen
    Transverse process
    Vertebral arch
    Vertebral body
    Vertebral foramen
    Vertebral lamina
    Vertebral pedicle
4 Thoracic Vertebra
    Spinous process
    Transverse process
    Vertebral arch
    Vertebral body
    Vertebral foramen
    Vertebral lamina
    Vertebral pedicle
5 Scapula, Right
    Acromion (process)
    Coracoid process
6 Scapula, Left
    See 5 Scapula, Right
7 Glenoid Cavity, Right
    Glenoid fossa (of scapula)
8 Glenoid Cavity, Left
    See 7 Glenoid Cavity, Right
9 Clavicle, Right
B Clavicle, Left
C Humeral Head, Right
    Greater tuberosity
    Lesser tuberosity
    Neck of humerus
        (anatomical)(surgical)
	D Humeral Head, Left
	    See C Humeral Head, Right
	F Humeral Shaft, Right
	    Distal humerus
	    Humerus, distal
	    Lateral epicondyle of
	        humerus
	    Medial epicondyle of
	        humerus
	G Humeral Shaft, Left
	    See F Humeral Shaft, Right
	H Radius, Right
	    Ulnar notch
	J Radius, Left
	    See H Radius, Right
	K Ulna, Right
	    Olecranon process
	    Radial notch
	L Ulna, Left
	    See K Ulna, Right
	M Carpal, Right
	    Capitate bone
	    Hamate bone
	    Lunate bone
	    Pisiform bone
	    Scaphoid bone
	    Trapezium bone
	    Trapezoid bone
	    Triquetral bone
	N Carpal, Left
	    See M Carpal, Right
	P Metacarpal, Right
	Q Metacarpal, Left
	R Thumb Phalanx, Right
	S Thumb Phalanx, Left
	T Finger Phalanx, Right
	V Finger Phalanx, Left
		Ø Open
		3 Percutaneous
		4 Percutaneous Endoscopic
			Ø Drainage Device	**Z No Qualifier**

Non-OR   ØP9[Ø,1,2,3,4,5,6,7,8,9,B,C,D,F,G,H,J,K,L,M,N,P,Q,R,S,T,V]3ØZ

ØP9 Continued on next page

Ø	Medical and Surgical		
P	Upper Bones		
9	Drainage		

ØP9 Continued

Definition: Taking or letting out fluids and/or gases from a body part

Explanation: The qualifier DIAGNOSTIC is used to identify drainage procedures that are biopsies

Body Part Character 4		Approach Character 5	Device Character 6	Qualifier Character 7

Ø Sternum
  Manubrium
  Suprasternal notch
  Xiphoid process
1 Ribs, 1 to 2
2 Ribs, 3 or More
3 Cervical Vertebra
  Dens
  Odontoid process
  Spinous process
  Transverse foramen
  Transverse process
  Vertebral arch
  Vertebral body
  Vertebral foramen
  Vertebral lamina
  Vertebral pedicle
4 Thoracic Vertebra
  Spinous process
  Transverse process
  Vertebral arch
  Vertebral body
  Vertebral foramen
  Vertebral lamina
  Vertebral pedicle
5 Scapula, Right
  Acromion (process)
  Coracoid process
6 Scapula, Left
  See 5 Scapula, Right
7 Glenoid Cavity, Right
  Glenoid fossa (of scapula)
8 Glenoid Cavity, Left
  See 7 Glenoid Cavity, Right
9 Clavicle, Right
B Clavicle, Left
C Humeral Head, Right
  Greater tuberosity
  Lesser tuberosity
  Neck of humerus
    (anatomical)(surgical)
	D Humeral Head, Left
	  See C Humeral Head, Right
	F Humeral Shaft, Right
	  Distal humerus
	  Humerus, distal
	  Lateral epicondyle of
	    humerus
	  Medial epicondyle of
	    humerus
	G Humeral Shaft, Left
	  See F Humeral Shaft, Right
	H Radius, Right
	  Ulnar notch
	J Radius, Left
	  See H Radius, Right
	K Ulna, Right
	  Olecranon process
	  Radial notch
	L Ulna, Left
	  See K Ulna, Right
	M Carpal, Right
	  Capitate bone
	  Hamate bone
	  Lunate bone
	  Pisiform bone
	  Scaphoid bone
	  Trapezium bone
	  Trapezoid bone
	  Triquetral bone
	N Carpal, Left
	  See M Carpal, Right
	P Metacarpal, Right
	Q Metacarpal, Left
	R Thumb Phalanx, Right
	S Thumb Phalanx, Left
	T Finger Phalanx, Right
	V Finger Phalanx, Left
		Ø Open
		3 Percutaneous
		4 Percutaneous Endoscopic
			Z No Device	**X Diagnostic**
				Z No Qualifier

Non-OR   ØP9[Ø,1,2,3,4,5,6,7,8,9,B,C,D,F,G,H,J,K,L,M,N,P,Q,R,S,T,V]3ZZ

NC Noncovered Procedure   **LC** Limited Coverage   **QA** Questionable OB Admit   **NT** New Tech Add-on   ⊞ Combination Member   ♂ Male   ♀ Female

ICD-10-PCS 2023   547

Ø   **Medical and Surgical**
P   **Upper Bones**
B   **Excision**   Definition: Cutting out or off, without replacement, a portion of a body part
                        Explanation: The qualifier DIAGNOSTIC is used to identify excision procedures that are biopsies

Body Part Character 4	Approach Character 5	Device Character 6	Qualifier Character 7

Ø   **Sternum**
    Manubrium
    Suprasternal notch
    Xiphoid process
	Ø Open
	3 Percutaneous
	4 Percutaneous Endoscopic
		Z No Device	**X** Diagnostic
			Z No Qualifier

1 **Ribs, 1 to 2**			
2 **Ribs, 3 or More**			

3   **Cervical Vertebra**
    Dens
    Odontoid process
    Spinous process
    Transverse foramen
    Transverse process
    Vertebral arch
    Vertebral body
    Vertebral foramen
    Vertebral lamina
    Vertebral pedicle			

4   **Thoracic Vertebra**
    Spinous process
    Transverse process
    Vertebral arch
    Vertebral body
    Vertebral foramen
    Vertebral lamina
    Vertebral pedicle			

5   **Scapula, Right**
    Acromion (process)
    Coracoid process			

6 **Scapula, Left** *See 5 Scapula, Right*			
7 **Glenoid Cavity, Right** Glenoid fossa (of scapula)			
8 **Glenoid Cavity, Left** *See 7 Glenoid Cavity, Right*			
9 **Clavicle, Right**			
B **Clavicle, Left**			

C   **Humeral Head, Right**
    Greater tuberosity
    Lesser tuberosity
    Neck of humerus (anatomical)(surgical)			

D **Humeral Head, Left** *See C Humeral Head, Right*			

F   **Humeral Shaft, Right**
    Distal humerus
    Humerus, distal
    Lateral epicondyle of humerus
    Medial epicondyle of humerus			

G **Humeral Shaft, Left** *See F Humeral Shaft, Right*			
H **Radius, Right** Ulnar notch			
J **Radius, Left** *See H Radius, Right*			

K   **Ulna, Right**
    Olecranon process
    Radial notch			

L **Ulna, Left** *See K Ulna, Right*			

M   **Carpal, Right**
    Capitate bone
    Hamate bone
    Lunate bone
    Pisiform bone
    Scaphoid bone
    Trapezium bone
    Trapezoid bone
    Triquetral bone			

N **Carpal, Left** *See M Carpal, Right*			
P **Metacarpal, Right**			
Q **Metacarpal, Left**			
R **Thumb Phalanx, Right**			
S **Thumb Phalanx, Left**			
T **Finger Phalanx, Right**			
V **Finger Phalanx, Left**			

Non-OR Procedure   DRG Non-OR Procedure   Valid OR Procedure   HAC Associated Procedure   Combination Only   New/Revised April   New/Revised October

548   **ICD-10-PCS 2023**

Ø   **Medical and Surgical**
P   **Upper Bones**
C   **Extirpation**   Definition: Taking or cutting out solid matter from a body part

Explanation: The solid matter may be an abnormal byproduct of a biological function or a foreign body; it may be imbedded in a body part or in the lumen of a tubular body part. The solid matter may or may not have been previously broken into pieces.

Body Part Character 4	Approach Character 5	Device Character 6	Qualifier Character 7

Ø   **Sternum**
     Manubrium
     Suprasternal notch
     Xiphoid process
1   **Ribs, 1 to 2**
2   **Ribs, 3 or More**
3   **Cervical Vertebra**
     Dens
     Odontoid process
     Spinous process
     Transverse foramen
     Transverse process
     Vertebral arch
     Vertebral body
     Vertebral foramen
     Vertebral lamina
     Vertebral pedicle
4   **Thoracic Vertebra**
     Spinous process
     Transverse process
     Vertebral arch
     Vertebral body
     Vertebral foramen
     Vertebral lamina
     Vertebral pedicle
5   **Scapula, Right**
     Acromion (process)
     Coracoid process
6   **Scapula, Left**
     See 5 Scapula, Right
7   **Glenoid Cavity, Right**
     Glenoid fossa (of scapula)
8   **Glenoid Cavity, Left**
     See 7 Glenoid Cavity, Right
9   **Clavicle, Right**
B   **Clavicle, Left**
C   **Humeral Head, Right**
     Greater tuberosity
     Lesser tuberosity
     Neck of humerus (anatomical)(surgical)
D   **Humeral Head, Left**
     See C Humeral Head, Right
F   **Humeral Shaft, Right**
     Distal humerus
     Humerus, distal
     Lateral epicondyle of humerus
     Medial epicondyle of humerus
G   **Humeral Shaft, Left**
     See F Humeral Shaft, Right
H   **Radius, Right**
     Ulnar notch
J   **Radius, Left**
     See H Radius, Right
K   **Ulna, Right**
     Olecranon process
     Radial notch
L   **Ulna, Left**
     See K Ulna, Right
M   **Carpal, Right**
     Capitate bone
     Hamate bone
     Lunate bone
     Pisiform bone
     Scaphoid bone
     Trapezium bone
     Trapezoid bone
     Triquetral bone
N   **Carpal, Left**
     See M Carpal, Right
P   **Metacarpal, Right**
Q   **Metacarpal, Left**
R   **Thumb Phalanx, Right**
S   **Thumb Phalanx, Left**
T   **Finger Phalanx, Right**
V   **Finger Phalanx, Left**
	Ø Open
	3 Percutaneous
	4 Percutaneous Endoscopic
		Z No Device	**Z** No Qualifier

NC Noncovered Procedure   **LC** Limited Coverage   **QA** Questionable OB Admit   **NT** New Tech Add-on   ⊞ Combination Member   ♂ Male   ♀ Female

Ø Medical and Surgical
P Upper Bones
D Extraction   Definition: Pulling or stripping out or off all or a portion of a body part by the use of force

                     Explanation: The qualifier DIAGNOSTIC is used to identify extraction procedures that are biopsies

Body Part Character 4	Approach Character 5	Device Character 6	Qualifier Character 7

Ø Sternum
    Manubrium
    Suprasternal notch
    Xiphoid process
	Ø Open	**Z No Device**	**Z No Qualifier**

1 Ribs, 1 to 2			
2 Ribs, 3 or More			

3 Cervical Vertebra
    Dens
    Odontoid process
    Spinous process
    Transverse foramen
    Transverse process
    Vertebral arch
    Vertebral body
    Vertebral foramen
    Vertebral lamina
    Vertebral pedicle			

4 Thoracic Vertebra
    Spinous process
    Transverse process
    Vertebral arch
    Vertebral body
    Vertebral foramen
    Vertebral lamina
    Vertebral pedicle			

5 Scapula, Right
    Acromion (process)
    Coracoid process			

6 Scapula, Left *See 5 Scapula, Right*			
7 Glenoid Cavity, Right Glenoid fossa (of scapula)			
8 Glenoid Cavity, Left *See 7 Glenoid Cavity, Right*			
9 Clavicle, Right			
B Clavicle, Left			

C Humeral Head, Right
    Greater tuberosity
    Lesser tuberosity
    Neck of humerus (anatomical)(surgical)			

D Humeral Head, Left *See C Humeral Head, Right*			

F Humeral Shaft, Right
    Distal humerus
    Humerus, distal
    Lateral epicondyle of humerus
    Medial epicondyle of humerus			

G Humeral Shaft, Left *See F Humeral Shaft, Right*			
H Radius, Right Ulnar notch			
J Radius, Left *See H Radius, Right*			

K Ulna, Right
    Olecranon process
    Radial notch			

L Ulna, Left *See K Ulna, Right*			

M Carpal, Right
    Capitate bone
    Hamate bone
    Lunate bone
    Pisiform bone
    Scaphoid bone
    Trapezium bone
    Trapezoid bone
    Triquetral bone			

N Carpal, Left *See M Carpal, Right*			
P Metacarpal, Right			
Q Metacarpal, Left			
R Thumb Phalanx, Right			
S Thumb Phalanx, Left			
T Finger Phalanx, Right			
V Finger Phalanx, Left			

Non-OR Procedure   DRG Non-OR Procedure   Valid OR Procedure   HAC Associated Procedure   Combination Only   New/Revised April   New/Revised October

550   ICD-10-PCS 2023

Ø **Medical and Surgical**
P **Upper Bones**
H **Insertion**　　Definition: Putting in a nonbiological appliance that monitors, assists, performs, or prevents a physiological function but does not physically take the place of a body part
　　Explanation: None

Body Part Character 4		Approach Character 5	Device Character 6	Qualifier Character 7
Ø Sternum Manubrium Suprasternal notch Xiphoid process		**Ø** Open **3** Percutaneous **4** Percutaneous Endoscopic	**Ø** Internal Fixation Device, Rigid Plate **4** Internal Fixation Device	**Z** No Qualifier
1 Ribs, 1 to 2 **2** Ribs, 3 or More **3** Cervical Vertebra 　Dens 　Odontoid process 　Spinous process 　Transverse foramen 　Transverse process 　Vertebral arch 　Vertebral body 　Vertebral foramen 　Vertebral lamina 　Vertebral pedicle **4** Thoracic Vertebra 　Spinous process 　Transverse process 　Vertebral arch 　Vertebral body 　Vertebral foramen 　Vertebral lamina 　Vertebral pedicle	**5** Scapula, Right 　Acromion (process) 　Coracoid process **6** Scapula, Left 　*See 5 Scapula, Right* **7** Glenoid Cavity, Right 　Glenoid fossa (of scapula) **8** Glenoid Cavity, Left 　*See 7 Glenoid Cavity, Right* **9** Clavicle, Right **B** Clavicle, Left	**Ø** Open **3** Percutaneous **4** Percutaneous Endoscopic	**4** Internal Fixation Device	**Z** No Qualifier
C Humeral Head, Right 　Greater tuberosity 　Lesser tuberosity 　Neck of humerus 　　(anatomical)(surgical) **D** Humeral Head, Left 　*See C Humeral Head, Right*	**H** Radius, Right 　Ulnar notch **J** Radius, Left 　*See H Radius, Right* **K** Ulna, Right 　Olecranon process 　Radial notch **L** Ulna, Left 　*See K Ulna, Right*	**Ø** Open **3** Percutaneous **4** Percutaneous Endoscopic	**4** Internal Fixation Device **5** External Fixation Device **6** Internal Fixation Device, Intramedullary **8** External Fixation Device, Limb Lengthening **B** External Fixation Device, Monoplanar **C** External Fixation Device, Ring **D** External Fixation Device, Hybrid	**Z** No Qualifier
F Humeral Shaft, Right 　Distal humerus 　Humerus, distal 　Lateral epicondyle of 　　humerus 　Medial epicondyle of 　　humerus	**G** Humeral Shaft, Left 　*See F Humeral Shaft, Right*	**Ø** Open **3** Percutaneous **4** Percutaneous Endoscopic	**4** Internal Fixation Device **5** External Fixation Device **6** Internal Fixation Device, Intramedullary **7** Internal Fixation Device, Intramedullary Limb Lengthening **8** External Fixation Device, Limb Lengthening **B** External Fixation Device, Monoplanar **C** External Fixation Device, Ring **D** External Fixation Device, Hybrid	**Z** No Qualifier
M Carpal, Right 　Capitate bone 　Hamate bone 　Lunate bone 　Pisiform bone 　Scaphoid bone 　Trapezium bone 　Trapezoid bone 　Triquetral bone **N** Carpal, Left 　*See M Carpal, Right*	**P** Metacarpal, Right **Q** Metacarpal, Left **R** Thumb Phalanx, Right **S** Thumb Phalanx, Left **T** Finger Phalanx, Right **V** Finger Phalanx, Left	**Ø** Open **3** Percutaneous **4** Percutaneous Endoscopic	**4** Internal Fixation Device **5** External Fixation Device	**Z** No Qualifier
Y Upper Bone		**Ø** Open **3** Percutaneous **4** Percutaneous Endoscopic	**M** Bone Growth Stimulator	**Z** No Qualifier

Non-OR　ØPH[C,D,H,J,K,L][Ø,3,4]8Z
Non-OR　ØPH[F,G][Ø,3,4]8Z

NC Noncovered Procedure　　**LC** Limited Coverage　　**QA** Questionable OB Admit　　**NT** New Tech Add-on　　**⊞** Combination Member　　♂Male　　♀Female

ICD-10-PCS 2023　　　**551**

ØPH–ØPH

Ø **Medical and Surgical**
P **Upper Bones**
J **Inspection**   Definition: Visually and/or manually exploring a body part

Explanation: Visual exploration may be performed with or without optical instrumentation. Manual exploration may be performed directly or through intervening body layers.

Body Part Character 4	Approach Character 5	Device Character 6	Qualifier Character 7
Y Upper Bone	Ø Open 3 Percutaneous 4 Percutaneous Endoscopic X External	Z No Device	Z No Qualifier

Non-OR   ØPJY[3,X]ZZ

Ø **Medical and Surgical**
P **Upper Bones**
N **Release**   Definition: Freeing a body part from an abnormal physical constraint by cutting or by the use of force

Explanation: Some of the restraining tissue may be taken out but none of the body part is taken out

Body Part Character 4		Approach Character 5	Device Character 6	Qualifier Character 7
Ø Sternum Manubrium Suprasternal notch Xiphoid process **1 Ribs, 1 to 2** **2 Ribs, 3 or More** **3 Cervical Vertebra** Dens Odontoid process Spinous process Transverse foramen Transverse process Vertebral arch Vertebral body Vertebral foramen Vertebral lamina Vertebral pedicle **4 Thoracic Vertebra** Spinous process Transverse process Vertebral arch Vertebral body Vertebral foramen Vertebral lamina Vertebral pedicle **5 Scapula, Right** Acromion (process) Coracoid process **6 Scapula, Left** *See 5 Scapula, Right* **7 Glenoid Cavity, Right** Glenoid fossa (of scapula) **8 Glenoid Cavity, Left** *See 7 Glenoid Cavity, Right* **9 Clavicle, Right** **B Clavicle, Left** **C Humeral Head, Right** Greater tuberosity Lesser tuberosity Neck of humerus (anatomical) (surgical) **D Humeral Head, Left** *See C Humeral Head, Right*	**F Humeral Shaft, Right** Distal humerus Humerus, distal Lateral epicondyle of humerus Medial epicondyle of humerus **G Humeral Shaft, Left** *See F Humeral Shaft, Right* **H Radius, Right** Ulnar notch **J Radius, Left** *See H Radius, Right* **K Ulna, Right** Olecranon process Radial notch **L Ulna, Left** *See K Ulna, Right* **M Carpal, Right** Capitate bone Hamate bone Lunate bone Pisiform bone Scaphoid bone Trapezium bone Trapezoid bone Triquetral bone **N Carpal, Left** *See M Carpal, Right* **P Metacarpal, Right** **Q Metacarpal, Left** **R Thumb Phalanx, Right** **S Thumb Phalanx, Left** **T Finger Phalanx, Right** **V Finger Phalanx, Left**	Ø Open 3 Percutaneous 4 Percutaneous Endoscopic	Z No Device	Z No Qualifier

Ø   **Medical and Surgical**
P   **Upper Bones**
P   **Removal**   Definition: Taking out or off a device from a body part

Explanation: If a device is taken out and a similar device put in without cutting or puncturing the skin or mucous membrane, the procedure is coded to the root operation CHANGE. Otherwise, the procedure for taking out a device is coded to the root operation REMOVAL.

Body Part Character 4		Approach Character 5	Device Character 6	Qualifier Character 7

Ø **Sternum**
  Manubrium
  Suprasternal notch
  Xiphoid process
1 **Ribs, 1 to 2**
2 **Ribs, 3 or More**
3 **Cervical Vertebra**
  Dens
  Odontoid process
  Spinous process
  Transverse foramen
  Transverse process
  Vertebral arch
  Vertebral body
  Vertebral foramen
  Vertebral lamina
  Vertebral pedicle
	4 **Thoracic Vertebra**
	  Spinous process
	  Transverse process
	  Vertebral arch
	  Vertebral body
	  Vertebral foramen
	  Vertebral lamina
	  Vertebral pedicle
	5 **Scapula, Right**
	  Acromion (process)
	  Coracoid process
	6 **Scapula, Left**
	  See 5 Scapula, Right
	7 **Glenoid Cavity, Right**
	  Glenoid fossa (of scapula)
	8 **Glenoid Cavity, Left**
	  See 7 Glenoid Cavity, Right
	9 **Clavicle, Right**
	B **Clavicle, Left**
		Ø Open
		3 Percutaneous
		4 Percutaneous Endoscopic
			4 Internal Fixation Device
			7 Autologous Tissue
			  Substitute
			J Synthetic Substitute
			K Nonautologous Tissue
			  Substitute
				Z No Qualifier

Ø **Sternum**
  Manubrium
  Suprasternal notch
  Xiphoid process
1 **Ribs, 1 to 2**
2 **Ribs, 3 or More**
3 **Cervical Vertebra**
  Dens
  Odontoid process
  Spinous process
  Transverse foramen
  Transverse process
  Vertebral arch
  Vertebral body
  Vertebral foramen
  Vertebral lamina
  Vertebral pedicle
	4 **Thoracic Vertebra**
	  Spinous process
	  Transverse process
	  Vertebral arch
	  Vertebral body
	  Vertebral foramen
	  Vertebral lamina
	  Vertebral pedicle
	5 **Scapula, Right**
	  Acromion (process)
	  Coracoid process
	6 **Scapula, Left**
	  See 5 Scapula, Right
	7 **Glenoid Cavity, Right**
	  Glenoid fossa (of scapula)
	8 **Glenoid Cavity, Left**
	  See 7 Glenoid Cavity, Right
	9 **Clavicle, Right**
	B **Clavicle, Left**
		X External	**4** Internal Fixation Device	**Z** No Qualifier

C **Humeral Head, Right**
  Greater tuberosity
  Lesser tuberosity
  Neck of humerus
    (anatomical) (surgical)
D **Humeral Head, Left**
  See C Humeral Head, Right
F **Humeral Shaft, Right**
  Distal humerus
  Humerus, distal
  Lateral epicondyle of
    humerus
  Medial epicondyle of
    humerus
G **Humeral Shaft, Left**
  See F Humeral Shaft, Right
H **Radius, Right**
  Ulnar notch
J **Radius, Left**
  See H Radius, Right
K **Ulna, Right**
  Olecranon process
  Radial notch
	L **Ulna, Left**
	  See K Ulna, Right
	M **Carpal, Right**
	  Capitate bone
	  Hamate bone
	  Lunate bone
	  Pisiform bone
	  Scaphoid bone
	  Trapezium bone
	  Trapezoid bone
	  Triquetral bone
	N **Carpal, Left**
	  See M Carpal, Right
	P **Metacarpal, Right**
	Q **Metacarpal, Left**
	R **Thumb Phalanx, Right**
	S **Thumb Phalanx, Left**
	T **Finger Phalanx, Right**
	V **Finger Phalanx, Left**
		Ø Open
		3 Percutaneous
		4 Percutaneous Endoscopic
			4 Internal Fixation Device
			5 External Fixation Device
			7 Autologous Tissue
			  Substitute
			J Synthetic Substitute
			K Nonautologous Tissue
			  Substitute
				Z No Qualifier

Non-OR   ØPP[Ø,1,2,3,4,5,6,7,8,9,B]X4Z

ØPP Continued on next page

NC Noncovered Procedure   **LC** Limited Coverage   **QA** Questionable OB Admit   **NT** New Tech Add-on   ⊞ Combination Member   ♂ Male   ♀ Female

ICD-10-PCS 2023   553

ØPP–ØPP

ØPP Continued

Ø   **Medical and Surgical**
P   **Upper Bones**
P   **Removal**   Definition: Taking out or off a device from a body part

Explanation: If a device is taken out and a similar device put in without cutting or puncturing the skin or mucous membrane, the procedure is coded to the root operation CHANGE. Otherwise, the procedure for taking out a device is coded to the root operation REMOVAL.

Body Part Character 4		Approach Character 5	Device Character 6	Qualifier Character 7

C   **Humeral Head, Right**
     Greater tuberosity
     Lesser tuberosity
     Neck of humerus
         (anatomical) (surgical)
D   **Humeral Head, Left**
     See C Humeral Head, Right
F   **Humeral Shaft, Right**
     Distal humerus
     Humerus, distal
     Lateral epicondyle of
         humerus
     Medial epicondyle of
         humerus
G   **Humeral Shaft, Left**
     See F Humeral Shaft, Right
H   **Radius, Right**
     Ulnar notch
J   **Radius, Left**
     See H Radius, Right
K   **Ulna, Right**
     Olecranon process
Radial notch
	L **Ulna, Left**
	     See K Ulna, Right
	M **Carpal, Right**
	     Capitate bone
	     Hamate bone
	     Lunate bone
	     Pisiform bone
	     Scaphoid bone
	     Trapezium bone
	     Trapezoid bone
	     Triquetral bone
	N **Carpal, Left**
	     See M Carpal, Right
	P **Metacarpal, Right**
	Q **Metacarpal, Left**
	R **Thumb Phalanx, Right**
	S **Thumb Phalanx, Left**
	T **Finger Phalanx, Right**
	V **Finger Phalanx, Left**
		X External	**4** Internal Fixation Device
			5 External Fixation Device
				Z No Qualifier

Y **Upper Bone**		**Ø** Open **3** Percutaneous **4** Percutaneous Endoscopic **X** External	**Ø** Drainage Device **M** Bone Growth Stimulator	**Z** No Qualifier

Non-OR   ØPP[C,D,F,G,H,J,K,L,M,N,P,Q,R,S,T,V]X[4,5]Z
Non-OR   ØPPY3ØZ
Non-OR   ØPPYX[Ø,M]Z

Ø   **Medical and Surgical**
P   **Upper Bones**
Q   **Repair**   Definition: Restoring, to the extent possible, a body part to its normal anatomic structure and function

Explanation: Used only when the method to accomplish the repair is not one of the other root operations

Body Part Character 4		Approach Character 5	Device Character 6	Qualifier Character 7
Ø **Sternum**	**F** **Humeral Shaft, Right**	**Ø** Open	**Z** No Device	**Z** No Qualifier
Manubrium	Distal humerus	**3** Percutaneous		
Suprasternal notch	Humerus, distal	**4** Percutaneous Endoscopic		
Xiphoid process	Lateral epicondyle of	**X** External		
1 **Ribs, 1 to 2**	humerus			
2 **Ribs, 3 or More**	Medial epicondyle of			
3 **Cervical Vertebra**	humerus			
Dens	**G** **Humeral Shaft, Left**			
Odontoid process	*See F Humeral Shaft, Right*			
Spinous process	**H** **Radius, Right**			
Transverse foramen	Ulnar notch			
Transverse process	**J** **Radius, Left**			
Vertebral arch	*See H Radius, Right*			
Vertebral body	**K** **Ulna, Right**			
Vertebral foramen	Olecranon process			
Vertebral lamina	Radial notch			
Vertebral pedicle	**L** **Ulna, Left**			
4 **Thoracic Vertebra**	*See K Ulna, Right*			
Spinous process	**M** **Carpal, Right**			
Transverse process	Capitate bone			
Vertebral arch	Hamate bone			
Vertebral body	Lunate bone			
Vertebral foramen	Pisiform bone			
Vertebral lamina	Scaphoid bone			
Vertebral pedicle	Trapezium bone			
5 **Scapula, Right**	Trapezoid bone			
Acromion (process)	Triquetral bone			
Coracoid process	**N** **Carpal, Left**			
6 **Scapula, Left**	*See M Carpal, Right*			
See 5 Scapula, Right	**P** **Metacarpal, Right**			
7 **Glenoid Cavity, Right**	**Q** **Metacarpal, Left**			
Glenoid fossa (of scapula)	**R** **Thumb Phalanx, Right**			
8 **Glenoid Cavity, Left**	**S** **Thumb Phalanx, Left**			
See 7 Glenoid Cavity, Right	**T** **Finger Phalanx, Right**			
9 **Clavicle, Right**	**V** **Finger Phalanx, Left**			
B **Clavicle, Left**				
C **Humeral Head, Right**				
Greater tuberosity				
Lesser tuberosity				
Neck of humerus				
(anatomical)(surgical)				
D **Humeral Head, Left**				
See C Humeral Head, Right				

Non-OR   ØPQ[Ø,1,2,3,4,5,6,7,8,9,B,C,D,F,G,H,J,K,L,M,N,P,Q,R,S,T,V]XZZ

Upper Bones

ØPR–ØPR

Ø   Medical and Surgical
P   Upper Bones
R   Replacement   Definition: Putting in or on biological or synthetic material that physically takes the place and/or function of all or a portion of a body part

Explanation: The body part may have been taken out or replaced, or may be taken out, physically eradicated, or rendered nonfunctional during the REPLACEMENT procedure. A REMOVAL procedure is coded for taking out the device used in a previous replacement procedure.

Body Part Character 4		Approach Character 5	Device Character 6	Qualifier Character 7

Ø **Sternum**
   Manubrium
   Suprasternal notch
   Xiphoid process
1 **Ribs, 1 to 2**
2 **Ribs, 3 or More**
3 **Cervical Vertebra**
   Dens
   Odontoid process
   Spinous process
   Transverse foramen
   Transverse process
   Vertebral arch
   Vertebral body
   Vertebral foramen
   Vertebral lamina
   Vertebral pedicle
4 **Thoracic Vertebra**
   Spinous process
   Transverse process
   Vertebral arch
   Vertebral body
   Vertebral foramen
   Vertebral lamina
   Vertebral pedicle
5 **Scapula, Right**
   Acromion (process)
   Coracoid process
6 **Scapula, Left**
   See 5 Scapula, Right
7 **Glenoid Cavity, Right**
   Glenoid fossa (of scapula)
8 **Glenoid Cavity, Left**
   See 7 Glenoid Cavity, Right
9 **Clavicle, Right**
B **Clavicle, Left**
C **Humeral Head, Right**
   Greater tuberosity
   Lesser tuberosity
   Neck of humerus
     (anatomical)(surgical)
D **Humeral Head, Left**
   See C Humeral Head, Right
	F **Humeral Shaft, Right**
	   Distal humerus
	   Humerus, distal
	   Lateral epicondyle of
	     humerus
	   Medial epicondyle of
	     humerus
	G **Humeral Shaft, Left**
	   See F Humeral Shaft, Right
	H **Radius, Right**
	   Ulnar notch
	J **Radius, Left**
	   See H Radius, Right
	K **Ulna, Right**
	   Olecranon process
	   Radial notch
	L **Ulna, Left**
	   See K Ulna, Right
	M **Carpal, Right**
	   Capitate bone
	   Hamate bone
	   Lunate bone
	   Pisiform bone
	   Scaphoid bone
	   Trapezium bone
	   Trapezoid bone
	   Triquetral bone
	N **Carpal, Left**
	   See M Carpal, Right
	P **Metacarpal, Right**
	Q **Metacarpal, Left**
	R **Thumb Phalanx, Right**
	S **Thumb Phalanx, Left**
	T **Finger Phalanx, Right**
	V **Finger Phalanx, Left**
		Ø **Open**
		3 **Percutaneous**
		4 **Percutaneous Endoscopic**
			7 **Autologous Tissue**
			   Substitute
			J **Synthetic Substitute**
			K **Nonautologous Tissue**
			   Substitute
				Z **No Qualifier**

Ø   **Medical and Surgical**
P   **Upper Bones**
S   **Reposition**   Definition: Moving to its normal location, or other suitable location, all or a portion of a body part

Explanation: The body part is moved to a new location from an abnormal location, or from a normal location where it is not functioning correctly. The body part may or may not be cut out or off to be moved to the new location.

Body Part — Character 4		Approach — Character 5	Device — Character 6	Qualifier — Character 7
Ø **Sternum** Manubrium Suprasternal notch Xiphoid process		**Ø** Open **3** Percutaneous **4** Percutaneous Endoscopic	**Ø** Internal Fixation Device, Rigid Plate **4** Internal Fixation Device **Z** No Device	**Z** No Qualifier
Ø **Sternum** Manubrium Suprasternal notch Xiphoid process		**X** External	**Z** No Device	**Z** No Qualifier
1 **Ribs, 1 to 2** **2** **Ribs, 3 or More** **3** **Cervical Vertebra** ⊞ Dens Odontoid process Spinous process Transverse foramen Transverse process Vertebral arch Vertebral body Vertebral foramen Vertebral lamina Vertebral pedicle	**5** **Scapula, Right** Acromion (process) Coracoid process **6** **Scapula, Left** *See 5 Scapula, Right* **7** **Glenoid Cavity, Right** Glenoid fossa (of scapula) **8** **Glenoid Cavity, Left** *See 7 Glenoid Cavity, Right* **9** **Clavicle, Right** **B** **Clavicle, Left**	**Ø** Open **3** Percutaneous **4** Percutaneous Endoscopic	**4** Internal Fixation Device **Z** No Device	**Z** No Qualifier
1 **Ribs, 1 to 2** **2** **Ribs, 3 or More** **3** **Cervical Vertebra** Dens Odontoid process Spinous process Transverse foramen Transverse process Vertebral arch Vertebral body Vertebral foramen Vertebral lamina Vertebral pedicle	**5** **Scapula, Right** Acromion (process) Coracoid process **6** **Scapula, Left** *See 5 Scapula, Right* **7** **Glenoid Cavity, Right** Glenoid fossa (of scapula) **8** **Glenoid Cavity, Left** *See 7 Glenoid Cavity, Right* **9** **Clavicle, Right** **B** **Clavicle, Left**	**X** External	**Z** No Device	**Z** No Qualifier
4 **Thoracic Vertebra** Spinous process Transverse process Vertebral arch Vertebral body Vertebral foramen Vertebral lamina Vertebral pedicle		**Ø** Open **4** Percutaneous Endoscopic	**3** Spinal Stabilization Device, Vertebral Body Tether **4** Internal Fixation Device **Z** No Device	**Z** No Qualifier
4 **Thoracic Vertebra** ⊞ Spinous process Transverse process Vertebral arch Vertebral body Vertebral foramen Vertebral lamina Vertebral pedicle		**3** Percutaneous	**4** Internal Fixation Device **Z** No Device	**Z** No Qualifier
4 **Thoracic Vertebra** Spinous process Transverse process Vertebral arch Vertebral body Vertebral foramen Vertebral lamina Vertebral pedicle		**X** External	**Z** No Device	**Z** No Qualifier
C **Humeral Head, Right** Greater tuberosity Lesser tuberosity Neck of humerus (anatomical)(surgical) **D** **Humeral Head, Left** *See C Humeral Head, Right* **F** **Humeral Shaft, Right** Distal humerus Humerus, distal Lateral epicondyle of humerus Medial epicondyle of humerus	**G** **Humeral Shaft, Left** *See F Humeral Shaft, Right* **H** **Radius, Right** Ulnar notch **J** **Radius, Left** *See H Radius, Right* **K** **Ulna, Right** Olecranon process Radial notch **L** **Ulna, Left** *See K Ulna, Right*	**Ø** Open **3** Percutaneous **4** Percutaneous Endoscopic	**4** Internal Fixation Device **5** External Fixation Device **6** Internal Fixation Device, Intramedullary **B** External Fixation Device, Monoplanar **C** External Fixation Device, Ring **D** External Fixation Device, Hybrid **Z** No Device	**Z** No Qualifier

Non-OR ØPSØ[3,4]ZZ	Non-OR ØPS[1,2,3,5,6,7,8,9,B]XZZ	**See Appendix L for Procedure Combinations**	
Non-OR ØPSØXZZ	Non-OR ØPS4XZZ	⊞ ØPS33ZZ	
Non-OR ØPS[1,2,5,6,7,8,9,B][3,4]ZZ	Non-OR ØPS[C,D,F,G,H,J,K,L][3,4]ZZ	⊞ ØPS43ZZ	

ØPS Continued on next page

NC Noncovered Procedure   **LC** Limited Coverage   **QA** Questionable OB Admit   **NT** New Tech Add-on   ⊞ Combination Member   ♂ Male   ♀ Female

Upper Bones *(left margin)*

Ø Medical and Surgical   *ØPS Continued*
P Upper Bones
S Reposition   Definition: Moving to its normal location, or other suitable location, all or a portion of a body part

Explanation: The body part is moved to a new location from an abnormal location, or from a normal location where it is not functioning correctly. The body part may or may not be cut out or off to be moved to the new location.

Body Part Character 4		Approach Character 5	Device Character 6	Qualifier Character 7
C Humeral Head, Right Greater tuberosity Lesser tuberosity Neck of humerus (anatomical)(surgical) **D Humeral Head, Left** *See C Humeral Head, Right* **F Humeral Shaft, Right** Distal humerus Humerus, distal Lateral epicondyle of humerus Medial epicondyle of humerus	**G Humeral Shaft, Left** *See F Humeral Shaft, Right* **H Radius, Right** Ulnar notch **J Radius, Left** *See H Radius, Right* **K Ulna, Right** Olecranon process Radial notch **L Ulna, Left** *See K Ulna, Right*	**X** External	**Z** No Device	**Z** No Qualifier
M Carpal, Right Capitate bone Hamate bone Lunate bone Pisiform bone Scaphoid bone Trapezium bone Trapezoid bone Triquetral bone	**N Carpal, Left** *See M Carpal, Right* **P Metacarpal, Right** **Q Metacarpal, Left** **R Thumb Phalanx, Right** **S Thumb Phalanx, Left** **T Finger Phalanx, Right** **V Finger Phalanx, Left**	**Ø** Open **3** Percutaneous **4** Percutaneous Endoscopic	**4** Internal Fixation Device **5** External Fixation Device **Z** No Device	**Z** No Qualifier
M Carpal, Right Capitate bone Hamate bone Lunate bone Pisiform bone Scaphoid bone Trapezium bone Trapezoid bone Triquetral bone	**N Carpal, Left** *See M Carpal, Right* **P Metacarpal, Right** **Q Metacarpal, Left** **R Thumb Phalanx, Right** **S Thumb Phalanx, Left** **T Finger Phalanx, Right** **V Finger Phalanx, Left**	**X** External	**Z** No Device	**Z** No Qualifier

Non-OR	ØPS[C,D,F,G,H,J,K,L]XZZ
Non-OR	ØPS[M,N,P,Q,R,S,T,V][3,4]ZZ
Non-OR	ØPS[M,N,P,Q,R,S,T,V]XZZ

Ø Medical and Surgical
P Upper Bones
T Resection   Definition: Cutting out or off, without replacement, all of a body part

Explanation: None

Body Part Character 4		Approach Character 5	Device Character 6	Qualifier Character 7
Ø Sternum Manubrium Suprasternal notch Xiphoid process **1 Ribs, 1 to 2** **2 Ribs, 3 or More** **5 Scapula, Right** Acromion (process) Coracoid process **6 Scapula, Left** *See 5 Scapula, Right* **7 Glenoid Cavity, Right** Glenoid fossa (of scapula) **8 Glenoid Cavity, Left** *See 7 Glenoid Cavity, Right* **9 Clavicle, Right** **B Clavicle, Left** **C Humeral Head, Right** Greater tuberosity Lesser tuberosity Neck of humerus (anatomical) (surgical) **D Humeral Head, Left** *See C Humeral Head, Right* **F Humeral Shaft, Right** Distal humerus Humerus, distal Lateral epicondyle of humerus Medial epicondyle of humerus	**G Humeral Shaft, Left** *See F Humeral Shaft, Right* **H Radius, Right** Ulnar notch **J Radius, Left** *See H Radius, Right* **K Ulna, Right** Olecranon process Radial notch **L Ulna, Left** *See K Ulna, Right* **M Carpal, Right** Capitate bone Hamate bone Lunate bone Pisiform bone Scaphoid bone Trapezium bone Trapezoid bone Triquetral bone **N Carpal, Left** *See M Carpal, Right* **P Metacarpal, Right** **Q Metacarpal, Left** **R Thumb Phalanx, Right** **S Thumb Phalanx, Left** **T Finger Phalanx, Right** **V Finger Phalanx, Left**	**Ø** Open	**Z** No Device	**Z** No Qualifier

Non-OR Procedure   DRG Non-OR Procedure   Valid OR Procedure   HAC Associated Procedure   Combination Only   New/Revised April   New/Revised October

558   ICD-10-PCS 2023

Ø   Medical and Surgical
P   Upper Bones
U   Supplement

Definition: Putting in or on biological or synthetic material that physically reinforces and/or augments the function of a portion of a body part

Explanation: The biological material is non-living, or is living and from the same individual. The body part may have been previously replaced, and the SUPPLEMENT procedure is performed to physically reinforce and/or augment the function of the replaced body part.

Body Part Character 4		Approach Character 5	Device Character 6	Qualifier Character 7
Ø Sternum Manubrium Suprasternal notch Xiphoid process **1 Ribs, 1 to 2** **2 Ribs, 3 or More** **3 Cervical Vertebra** ⊞ Dens Odontoid process Spinous process Transverse foramen Transverse process Vertebral arch Vertebral body Vertebral foramen Vertebral lamina Vertebral pedicle **4 Thoracic Vertebra** ⊞ Spinous process Transverse process Vertebral arch Vertebral body Vertebral foramen Vertebral lamina Vertebral pedicle **5 Scapula, Right** Acromion (process) Coracoid process **6 Scapula, Left** *See 5 Scapula, Right* **7 Glenoid Cavity, Right** Glenoid fossa (of scapula) **8 Glenoid Cavity, Left** *See 7 Glenoid Cavity, Right* **9 Clavicle, Right** **B Clavicle, Left** **C Humeral Head, Right** Greater tuberosity Lesser tuberosity Neck of humerus (anatomical) (surgical)	**D Humeral Head, Left** *See C Humeral Head, Right* **F Humeral Shaft, Right** Distal humerus Humerus, distal Lateral epicondyle of humerus Medial epicondyle of humerus **G Humeral Shaft, Left** *See F Humeral Shaft, Right* **H Radius, Right** Ulnar notch **J Radius, Left** *See H Radius, Right* **K Ulna, Right** Olecranon process Radial notch **L Ulna, Left** *See K Ulna, Right* **M Carpal, Right** Capitate bone Hamate bone Lunate bone Pisiform bone Scaphoid bone Trapezium bone Trapezoid bone Triquetral bone **N Carpal, Left** *See M Carpal, Right* **P Metacarpal, Right** **Q Metacarpal, Left** **R Thumb Phalanx, Right** **S Thumb Phalanx, Left** **T Finger Phalanx, Right** **V Finger Phalanx, Left**	**Ø Open** **3 Percutaneous** **4 Percutaneous Endoscopic**	**7 Autologous Tissue Substitute** **J Synthetic Substitute** **K Nonautologous Tissue Substitute**	**Z No Qualifier**

See Appendix L for Procedure Combinations
  ⊞ ØPU[3,4]3JZ

NC Noncovered Procedure   **LC** Limited Coverage   **QA** Questionable OB Admit   **NT** New Tech Add-on   ⊞ Combination Member   ♂ Male   ♀ Female

ICD-10-PCS 2023   ØPU–ØPU   559

Ø   Medical and Surgical
P   Upper Bones
W   Revision   Definition: Correcting, to the extent possible, a portion of a malfunctioning device or the position of a displaced device

Explanation: Revision can include correcting a malfunctioning or displaced device by taking out or putting in components of the device such as a screw or pin

Body Part Character 4		Approach Character 5	Device Character 6	Qualifier Character 7
Ø Sternum Manubrium Suprasternal notch Xiphoid process **1 Ribs, 1 to 2** **2 Ribs, 3 or More** **3 Cervical Vertebra** Dens Odontoid process Spinous process Transverse foramen Transverse process Vertebral arch Vertebral body Vertebral foramen Vertebral lamina Vertebral pedicle **4 Thoracic Vertebra** Spinous process Transverse process Vertebral arch Vertebral body Vertebral foramen Vertebral lamina Vertebral pedicle	**5 Scapula, Right** Acromion (process) Coracoid process **6 Scapula, Left** *See 5 Scapula, Right* **7 Glenoid Cavity, Right** Glenoid fossa (of scapula) **8 Glenoid Cavity, Left** *See 7 Glenoid Cavity, Right* **9 Clavicle, Right** **B Clavicle, Left**	**Ø Open** **3 Percutaneous** **4 Percutaneous Endoscopic** **X External**	**4 Internal Fixation Device** **7 Autologous Tissue Substitute** **J Synthetic Substitute** **K Nonautologous Tissue Substitute**	**Z No Qualifier**

C Humeral Head, Right
Greater tuberosity
Lesser tuberosity
Neck of humerus
  (anatomical)(surgical)
D Humeral Head, Left
See C Humeral Head, Right
F Humeral Shaft, Right
Distal humerus
Humerus, distal
Lateral epicondyle of
  humerus
Medial epicondyle of
  humerus
G Humeral Shaft, Left
See F Humeral Shaft, Right
H Radius, Right
Ulnar notch
J Radius, Left
See H Radius, Right
K Ulna, Right
Olecranon process
Radial notch
	L Ulna, Left
	See K Ulna, Right
	M Carpal, Right
	Capitate bone
	Hamate bone
	Lunate bone
	Pisiform bone
	Scaphoid bone
	Trapezium bone
	Trapezoid bone
	Triquetral bone
	N Carpal, Left
	See M Carpal, Right
	P Metacarpal, Right
	Q Metacarpal, Left
	R Thumb Phalanx, Right
	S Thumb Phalanx, Left
	T Finger Phalanx, Right
	V Finger Phalanx, Left
		Ø Open
		3 Percutaneous
		4 Percutaneous Endoscopic
		X External
			4 Internal Fixation Device
			5 External Fixation Device
			7 Autologous Tissue Substitute
			J Synthetic Substitute
			K Nonautologous Tissue Substitute
				Z No Qualifier

Y Upper Bone		**Ø Open** **3 Percutaneous** **4 Percutaneous Endoscopic** **X External**	**Ø Drainage Device** **M Bone Growth Stimulator**	**Z No Qualifier**

Non-OR	ØPW[Ø,1,2,3,4,5,6,7,8,9,B]X[4,7,J,K]Z
Non-OR	ØPW[C,D,F,G,H,J,K,L,M,N,P,Q,R,S,T,V]X[4,5,7,J,K]Z
Non-OR	ØPWYX[Ø,M]Z

Non-OR Procedure   DRG Non-OR Procedure   Valid OR Procedure   HAC Associated Procedure   Combination Only   New/Revised April   New/Revised October

560   ICD-10-PCS 2023

ØPW–ØPW

Lower Bones 0Q2–0QW

Character Meanings

This Character Meaning table is provided as a guide to assist the user in the identification of character members that may be found in this section of code tables. It **SHOULD NOT** be used to build a PCS code.

Operation–Character 3	Body Part–Character 4	Approach–Character 5	Device–Character 6	Qualifier–Character 7
2 Change	0 Lumbar Vertebra	0 Open	0 Drainage Device	2 Sesamoid Bone(s) 1st Toe
5 Destruction	1 Sacrum	3 Percutaneous	3 Spinal Stabilization Device, Vertebral Body Tether	X Diagnostic
8 Division	2 Pelvic Bone, Right	4 Percutaneous Endoscopic	4 Internal Fixation Device	Z No Qualifier
9 Drainage	3 Pelvic Bone, Left	X External	5 External Fixation Device	
B Excision	4 Acetabulum, Right		6 Internal Fixation Device, Intramedullary	
C Extirpation	5 Acetabulum, Left		7 Autologous Tissue Substitute OR Internal Fixation Device, Intramedullary Limb Lengthening	
D Extraction	6 Upper Femur, Right		8 External Fixation Device, Limb Lengthening	
H Insertion	7 Upper Femur, Left		B External Fixation Device, Monoplanar	
J Inspection	8 Femoral Shaft, Right		C External Fixation Device, Ring	
N Release	9 Femoral Shaft, Left		D External Fixation Device, Hybrid	
P Removal	B Lower Femur, Right		J Synthetic Substitute	
Q Repair	C Lower Femur, Left		K Nonautologous Tissue Substitute	
R Replacement	D Patella, Right		M Bone Growth Stimulator	
S Reposition	F Patella, Left		Y Other Device	
T Resection	G Tibia, Right		Z No Device	
U Supplement	H Tibia, Left			
W Revision	J Fibula, Right			
	K Fibula, Left			
	L Tarsal, Right			
	M Tarsal, Left			
	N Metatarsal, Right			
	P Metatarsal, Left			
	Q Toe Phalanx, Right			
	R Toe Phalanx, Left			
	S Coccyx			
	Y Lower Bone			

AHA Coding Clinic for table 0Q8
2018, 1Q, 25   Periacetabular osteotomy for repair of congenital hip dysplasia
2016, 2Q, 31   Periacetabular osteotomy for repair of congenital hip dysplasia

AHA Coding Clinic for table 0Q9
2022, 1Q, 31   Septic arthritis/osteomyelitis of pubic symphysis and aspiration biopsy

AHA Coding Clinic for table 0QB
2021, 4Q, 52-53   Sesamoidectomy of great toe
2021, 2Q, 18   Excision of tibial sesamoid
2020, 2Q, 26   Sacral pressure ulcer with excisional and nonexcisional debridement of same site
2019, 2Q, 19   Cervical spinal fusion, decompression and placement of interfacet stabilization device
2018, 3Q, 17   Excisional debridement of periosteum
2017, 1Q, 23   Reconstruction of mandible using titanium and bone
2016, 3Q, 30   Resection of femur with interposition arthroplasty
2015, 3Q, 3-8   Excisional and nonexcisional debridement
2015, 3Q, 26   Femoral head resection
2015, 2Q, 34   Decompressive laminectomy
2014, 4Q, 25   Femoroacetabular impingement and labral tear with repair
2014, 2Q, 6   Posterior lumbar fusion with discectomy
2013, 4Q, 116   Spinal decompression
2013, 2Q, 39   Ankle fusion, osteotomy, and removal of hardware
2012, 2Q, 19   Multiple decompressive cervical laminectomies

AHA Coding Clinic for table 0QD
2017, 4Q, 41   Extraction procedures

AHA Coding Clinic for table 0QH
2022, 2Q, 19   Limb lengthening surgery
2019, 4Q, 34   Intramedullary limb lengthening internal fixation device
2017, 1Q, 21   Staged scoliosis surgery with iliac fixation and spinal fusion
2016, 3Q, 34   Tibial/fibula epiphysiodesis

AHA Coding Clinic for table 0QP
2020, 4Q, 56   Removal of external fixation device
2017, 4Q, 74-75   Magnetic growth rods
2015, 2Q, 6   Planned implant break

AHA Coding Clinic for table 0QQ
2018, 1Q, 15   Pubic symphysis fusion
2014, 3Q, 24   Repair of lipomyelomeningocele and tethered cord

AHA Coding Clinic for table 0QR
2017, 1Q, 22   Total knee replacement and patellar component
2016, 3Q, 30   Resection of femur with interposition arthroplasty

AHA Coding Clinic for table 0QS
2022, 2Q, 19   Limb lengthening surgery
2021, 4Q, 51-52   Vertebral body tethering
2020, 1Q, 33   Spinal fusion without use of bone graft
2019, 3Q, 26   Open reduction with internal fixation and placement of strut allograft
2018, 1Q, 13   Bilateral cuboid osteotomy for repair of congenital talipes equinovarus
2018, 1Q, 25   Periacetabular osteotomy for repair of congenital hip dysplasia
2016, 3Q, 34   Tibial/fibula epiphysiodesis
2014, 4Q, 29   Rotational osteosynthesis
2014, 4Q, 31   Reposition of femur for correction of valgus and recurvatum deformities

AHA Coding Clinic for table 0QT
2017, 1Q, 22   Chopart amputation of foot
2016, 3Q, 30   Resection of femur with interposition arthroplasty
2015, 3Q, 26   Femoral head resection
2014, 4Q, 29   Rotational osteosynthesis

AHA Coding Clinic for table 0QU
2019, 3Q, 26   Open reduction with internal fixation and placement of strut allograft
2019, 2Q, 35   Kiva® kyphoplasty
2015, 3Q, 18   Total hip replacement with acetabular reconstruction
2014, 4Q, 31   Reposition of femur for correction of valgus and recurvatum deformities
2014, 2Q, 12   Percutaneous vertebroplasty using cement
2013, 2Q, 35   Use of bone void filler in grafting

AHA Coding Clinic for table 0QW
2017, 4Q, 74-75   Magnetic growth rods

Lower Bones

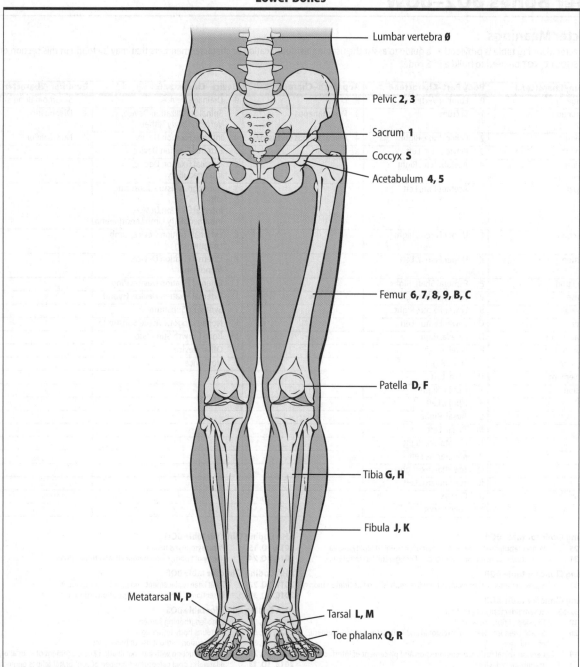

Lumbar vertebra **Ø**

Pelvic **2, 3**

Sacrum **1**

Coccyx **S**

Acetabulum **4, 5**

Femur **6, 7, 8, 9, B, C**

Patella **D, F**

Tibia **G, H**

Fibula **J, K**

Metatarsal **N, P**

Tarsal **L, M**

Toe phalanx **Q, R**

Hip Bone Anatomy

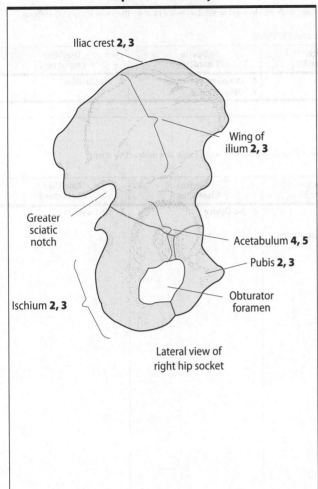

Iliac crest **2, 3**

Wing of ilium **2, 3**

Greater sciatic notch

Acetabulum **4, 5**

Pubis **2, 3**

Obturator foramen

Ischium **2, 3**

Lateral view of right hip socket

Pelvic and Lower Extremity Bones

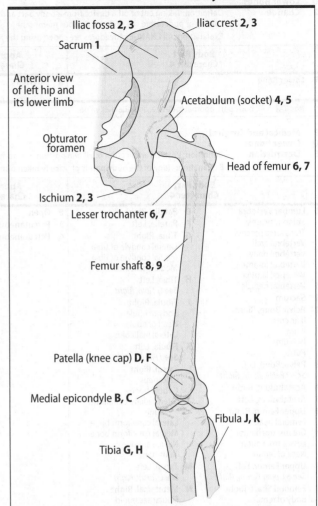

Iliac fossa **2, 3**

Sacrum **1**

Iliac crest **2, 3**

Anterior view of left hip and its lower limb

Obturator foramen

Acetabulum (socket) **4, 5**

Head of femur **6, 7**

Ischium **2, 3**

Lesser trochanter **6, 7**

Femur shaft **8, 9**

Patella (knee cap) **D, F**

Medial epicondyle **B, C**

Fibula **J, K**

Tibia **G, H**

Foot Bones

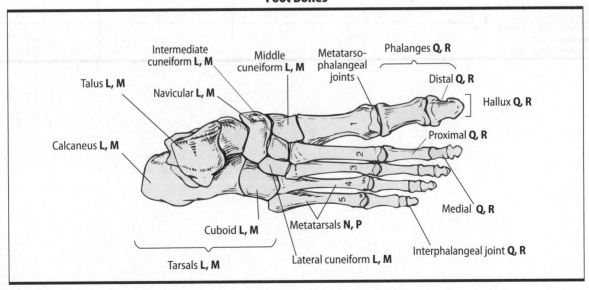

Intermediate cuneiform **L, M**

Middle cuneiform **L, M**

Metatarso-phalangeal joints

Phalanges **Q, R**

Talus **L, M**

Navicular **L, M**

Distal **Q, R**

Hallux **Q, R**

Calcaneus **L, M**

Proximal **Q, R**

Cuboid **L, M**

Metatarsals **N, P**

Medial **Q, R**

Tarsals **L, M**

Lateral cuneiform **L, M**

Interphalangeal joint **Q, R**

Ø   Medical and Surgical
Q   Lower Bones
2   Change   Definition: Taking out or off a device from a body part and putting back an identical or similar device in or on the same body part without cutting or puncturing the skin or a mucous membrane

                       Explanation: All CHANGE procedures are coded using the approach EXTERNAL

Body Part Character 4	Approach Character 5	Device Character 6	Qualifier Character 7
Y Lower Bone	X External	Ø Drainage Device Y Other Device	Z No Qualifier

> **Non-OR**   All body part, approach, device, and qualifier values

Ø   Medical and Surgical
Q   Lower Bones
5   Destruction   Definition: Physical eradication of all or a portion of a body part by the direct use of energy, force, or a destructive agent

                           Explanation: None of the body part is physically taken out

Body Part Character 4	Approach Character 5	Device Character 6	Qualifier Character 7

Ø   **Lumbar Vertebra**
    Spinous process
    Transverse process
    Vertebral arch
    Vertebral body
    Vertebral foramen
    Vertebral lamina
    Vertebral pedicle
1   **Sacrum**
2   **Pelvic Bone, Right**
    Iliac crest
    Ilium
    Ischium
    Pubis
3   **Pelvic Bone, Left**
    See 2 Pelvic Bone, Right
4   **Acetabulum, Right**
5   **Acetabulum, Left**
6   **Upper Femur, Right**
    Femoral head
    Greater trochanter
    Lesser trochanter
    Neck of femur
7   **Upper Femur, Left**
    See 6 Upper Femur, Right
8   **Femoral Shaft, Right**
    Body of femur
9   **Femoral Shaft, Left**
    See 8 Femoral Shaft, Right
B   **Lower Femur, Right**
    Lateral condyle of femur
    Lateral epicondyle of femur
    Medial condyle of femur
    Medial epicondyle of femur
C   **Lower Femur, Left**
    See B Lower Femur, Right
	D **Patella, Right**
	F **Patella, Left**
	G **Tibia, Right**
	    Lateral condyle of tibia
	    Medial condyle of tibia
	    Medial malleolus
	H **Tibia, Left**
	    See G Tibia, Right
	J **Fibula, Right**
	    Body of fibula
	    Head of fibula
	    Lateral malleolus
	K **Fibula, Left**
	    See J Fibula, Right
	L **Tarsal, Right**
	    Calcaneus
	    Cuboid bone
	    Intermediate cuneiform
	      bone
	    Lateral cuneiform bone
	    Medial cuneiform bone
	    Navicular bone
	    Talus bone
	M **Tarsal, Left**
	    See L Tarsal, Right
	N **Metatarsal, Right**
	    Fibular sesamoid
	    Tibial sesamoid
	P **Metatarsal, Left**
	    See N Metatarsal, Right
	Q **Toe Phalanx, Right**
	R **Toe Phalanx, Left**
	S **Coccyx**
		Ø Open
		3 Percutaneous
		4 Percutaneous Endoscopic
			Z No Device	Z No Qualifier

Non-OR Procedure   DRG Non-OR Procedure   Valid OR Procedure   HAC Associated Procedure   Combination Only   New/Revised April   New/Revised October

564   ICD-10-PCS 2023

ØQ2–ØQ5

Ø   **Medical and Surgical**
Q   **Lower Bones**
8   **Division**   Definition: Cutting into a body part, without draining fluids and/or gases from the body part, in order to separate or transect a body part
                       Explanation: All or a portion of the body part is separated into two or more portions

Body Part Character 4	Approach Character 5	Device Character 6	Qualifier Character 7

Ø   **Lumbar Vertebra**
    Spinous process
    Transverse process
    Vertebral arch
    Vertebral body
    Vertebral foramen
    Vertebral lamina
    Vertebral pedicle
	Ø Open
	3 Percutaneous
	4 Percutaneous Endoscopic
		Z No Device	**Z** No Qualifier

1 **Sacrum**			

2   **Pelvic Bone, Right**
    Iliac crest
    Ilium
    Ischium
    Pubis			

3 **Pelvic Bone, Left** *See 2 Pelvic Bone, Right*			
4 **Acetabulum, Right**			
5 **Acetabulum, Left**			

6   **Upper Femur, Right**
    Femoral head
    Greater trochanter
    Lesser trochanter
    Neck of femur			

7 **Upper Femur, Left** *See 6 Upper Femur, Right*			
8 **Femoral Shaft, Right** Body of femur			
9 **Femoral Shaft, Left** *See 8 Femoral Shaft, Right*			

B   **Lower Femur, Right**
    Lateral condyle of femur
    Lateral epicondyle of femur
    Medial condyle of femur
    Medial epicondyle of femur			

C **Lower Femur, Left** *See B Lower Femur, Right*			
D **Patella, Right**			
F **Patella, Left**			

G   **Tibia, Right**
    Lateral condyle of tibia
    Medial condyle of tibia
    Medial malleolus			

H **Tibia, Left** *See G Tibia, Right*			

J   **Fibula, Right**
    Body of fibula
    Head of fibula
    Lateral malleolus			

K **Fibula, Left** *See J Fibula, Right*			

L   **Tarsal, Right**
    Calcaneus
    Cuboid bone
    Intermediate cuneiform bone
    Lateral cuneiform bone
    Medial cuneiform bone
    Navicular bone
    Talus bone			

M **Tarsal, Left** *See L Tarsal, Right*			

N   **Metatarsal, Right**
    Fibular sesamoid
    Tibial sesamoid			

P **Metatarsal, Left** *See N Metatarsal, Right*			
Q **Toe Phalanx, Right**			
R **Toe Phalanx, Left**			
S **Coccyx**			

NC Noncovered Procedure   **LC** Limited Coverage   **QA** Questionable OB Admit   **NT** New Tech Add-on   ✛ Combination Member   ♂ Male   ♀ Female

ICD-10-PCS 2023   **565**

ØQ8–ØQ8

Ø   **Medical and Surgical**
Q   **Lower Bones**
9   **Drainage**   Definition: Taking or letting out fluids and/or gases from a body part
                      Explanation: The qualifier DIAGNOSTIC is used to identify drainage procedures that are biopsies

Body Part Character 4		Approach Character 5	Device Character 6	Qualifier Character 7

Ø Lumbar Vertebra
  Spinous process
  Transverse process
  Vertebral arch
  Vertebral body
  Vertebral foramen
  Vertebral lamina
  Vertebral pedicle
1 Sacrum
2 Pelvic Bone, Right
  Iliac crest
  Ilium
  Ischium
  Pubis
3 Pelvic Bone, Left
  See 2 Pelvic Bone, Right
4 Acetabulum, Right
5 Acetabulum, Left
6 Upper Femur, Right
  Femoral head
  Greater trochanter
  Lesser trochanter
  Neck of femur
7 Upper Femur, Left
  See 6 Upper Femur, Right
8 Femoral Shaft, Right
  Body of femur
9 Femoral Shaft, Left
  See 8 Femoral Shaft, Right
B Lower Femur, Right
  Lateral condyle of femur
  Lateral epicondyle of femur
  Medial condyle of femur
  Medial epicondyle of femur
	C Lower Femur, Left
	  See B Lower Femur, Right
	D Patella, Right
	F Patella, Left
	G Tibia, Right
	  Lateral condyle of tibia
	  Medial condyle of tibia
	  Medial malleolus
	H Tibia, Left
	  See G Tibia, Right
	J Fibula, Right
	  Body of fibula
	  Head of fibula
	  Lateral malleolus
	K Fibula, Left
	  See J Fibula, Right
	L Tarsal, Right
	  Calcaneus
	  Cuboid bone
	  Intermediate cuneiform bone
	  Lateral cuneiform bone
	  Medial cuneiform bone
	  Navicular bone
	  Talus bone
	M Tarsal, Left
	  See L Tarsal, Right
	N Metatarsal, Right
	  Fibular sesamoid
	  Tibial sesamoid
	P Metatarsal, Left
	  See N Metatarsal, Right
	Q Toe Phalanx, Right
	R Toe Phalanx, Left
	S Coccyx
		Ø Open
		3 Percutaneous
		4 Percutaneous Endoscopic
			Ø Drainage Device	**Z** No Qualifier

Ø Lumbar Vertebra
  Spinous process
  Transverse process
  Vertebral arch
  Vertebral body
  Vertebral foramen
  Vertebral lamina
  Vertebral pedicle
1 Sacrum
2 Pelvic Bone, Right
  Iliac crest
  Ilium
  Ischium
  Pubis
3 Pelvic Bone, Left
  See 2 Pelvic Bone, Right
4 Acetabulum, Right
5 Acetabulum, Left
6 Upper Femur, Right
  Femoral head
  Greater trochanter
  Lesser trochanter
  Neck of femur
7 Upper Femur, Left
  See 6 Upper Femur, Right
8 Femoral Shaft, Right
  Body of femur
9 Femoral Shaft, Left
  See 8 Femoral Shaft, Right
B Lower Femur, Right
  Lateral condyle of femur
  Lateral epicondyle of femur
  Medial condyle of femur
  Medial epicondyle of femur
	C Lower Femur, Left
	  See B Lower Femur, Right
	D Patella, Right
	F Patella, Left
	G Tibia, Right
	  Lateral condyle of tibia
	  Medial condyle of tibia
	  Medial malleolus
	H Tibia, Left
	  See G Tibia, Right
	J Fibula, Right
	  Body of fibula
	  Head of fibula
	  Lateral malleolus
	K Fibula, Left
	  See J Fibula, Right
	L Tarsal, Right
	  Calcaneus
	  Cuboid bone
	  Intermediate cuneiform bone
	  Lateral cuneiform bone
	  Medial cuneiform bone
	  Navicular bone
	  Talus bone
	M Tarsal, Left
	  See L Tarsal, Right
	N Metatarsal, Right
	  Fibular sesamoid
	  Tibial sesamoid
	P Metatarsal, Left
	  See N Metatarsal, Right
	Q Toe Phalanx, Right
	R Toe Phalanx, Left
	S Coccyx
		Ø Open
		3 Percutaneous
		4 Percutaneous Endoscopic
			Z No Device	**X** Diagnostic
				Z No Qualifier

Non-OR	ØQ9[Ø,1,2,3,4,5,6,7,8,9,B,C,D,F,G,H,J,K,L,M,P,Q,R,S]3ØZ
Non-OR	ØQ9[Ø,1,2,3,4,5,6,7,8,9,B,C,D,F,G,H,J,K,L,M,P,Q,R,S]3ZZ

Non-OR Procedure   DRG Non-OR Procedure   Valid OR Procedure   HAC Associated Procedure   Combination Only   New/Revised April   New/Revised October

566   ICD-10-PCS 2023

Ø   Medical and Surgical
Q   Lower Bones
B   Excision   Definition: Cutting out or off, without replacement, a portion of a body part
                       Explanation: The qualifier DIAGNOSTIC is used to identify excision procedures that are biopsies

Body Part Character 4	Approach Character 5	Device Character 6	Qualifier Character 7

Ø   Lumbar Vertebra
    Spinous process
    Transverse process
    Vertebral arch
    Vertebral body
    Vertebral foramen
    Vertebral lamina
    Vertebral pedicle
1   Sacrum
2   Pelvic Bone, Right
    Iliac crest
    Ilium
    Ischium
    Pubis
3   Pelvic Bone, Left
    See 2 Pelvic Bone, Right
4   Acetabulum, Right
5   Acetabulum, Left
6   Upper Femur, Right
    Femoral head
    Greater trochanter
    Lesser trochanter
    Neck of femur
7   Upper Femur, Left
    See 6 Upper Femur, Right
8   Femoral Shaft, Right
    Body of femur
9   Femoral Shaft, Left
    See 8 Femoral Shaft, Right
B   Lower Femur, Right
    Lateral condyle of femur
    Lateral epicondyle of femur
    Medial condyle of femur
    Medial epicondyle of femur
C   Lower Femur, Left
    See B Lower Femur, Right
D   Patella, Right
F   Patella, Left
G   Tibia, Right
    Lateral condyle of tibia
    Medial condyle of tibia
    Medial malleolus
H   Tibia, Left
    See G Tibia, Right
J   Fibula, Right
    Body of fibula
    Head of fibula
    Lateral malleolus
K   Fibula, Left
    See J Fibula, Right
L   Tarsal, Right
    Calcaneus
    Cuboid bone
    Intermediate cuneiform bone
    Lateral cuneiform bone
    Medial cuneiform bone
    Navicular bone
    Talus bone
M   Tarsal, Left
    See L Tarsal, Right
Q   Toe Phalanx, Right
R   Toe Phalanx, Left
S   Coccyx
	Ø Open
	3 Percutaneous
	4 Percutaneous Endoscopic
		Z No Device	**X Diagnostic**
			Z No Qualifier

N   Metatarsal, Right
    Fibular sesamoid
    Tibial sesamoid
P   Metatarsal, Left
    See N Metatarsal, Right
	Ø Open
	3 Percutaneous
	4 Percutaneous Endoscopic
		Z No Device	**2 Sesamoid Bone(s) 1st Toe**
			X Diagnostic
			Z No Qualifier

NC Noncovered Procedure   **LC** Limited Coverage   **UA** Questionable OB Admit   **NT** New Tech Add-on   ⊞ Combination Member   ♂ Male   ♀ Female

ICD-10-PCS 2023   567

Lower Bones

Ø   **Medical and Surgical**
Q   **Lower Bones**
C   **Extirpation**   Definition: Taking or cutting out solid matter from a body part

Explanation: The solid matter may be an abnormal byproduct of a biological function or a foreign body; it may be imbedded in a body part or in the lumen of a tubular body part. The solid matter may or may not have been previously broken into pieces.

Body Part Character 4	Approach Character 5	Device Character 6	Qualifier Character 7

Ø   **Lumbar Vertebra**
     Spinous process
     Transverse process
     Vertebral arch
     Vertebral body
     Vertebral foramen
     Vertebral lamina
     Vertebral pedicle
1   **Sacrum**
2   **Pelvic Bone, Right**
     Iliac crest
     Ilium
     Ischium
     Pubis
3   **Pelvic Bone, Left**
     See 2 Pelvic Bone, Right
4   **Acetabulum, Right**
5   **Acetabulum, Left**
6   **Upper Femur, Right**
     Femoral head
     Greater trochanter
     Lesser trochanter
     Neck of femur
7   **Upper Femur, Left**
     See 6 Upper Femur, Right
8   **Femoral Shaft, Right**
     Body of femur
9   **Femoral Shaft, Left**
     See 8 Femoral Shaft, Right
B   **Lower Femur, Right**
     Lateral condyle of femur
     Lateral epicondyle of femur
     Medial condyle of femur
     Medial epicondyle of femur
C   **Lower Femur, Left**
     See B Lower Femur, Right
D   **Patella, Right**
F   **Patella, Left**
G   **Tibia, Right**
     Lateral condyle of tibia
     Medial condyle of tibia
     Medial malleolus
H   **Tibia, Left**
     See G Tibia, Right
J   **Fibula, Right**
     Body of fibula
     Head of fibula
     Lateral malleolus
K   **Fibula, Left**
     See J Fibula, Right
L   **Tarsal, Right**
     Calcaneus
     Cuboid bone
     Intermediate cuneiform bone
     Lateral cuneiform bone
     Medial cuneiform bone
     Navicular bone
     Talus bone
M   **Tarsal, Left**
     See L Tarsal, Right
N   **Metatarsal, Right**
     Fibular sesamoid
     Tibial sesamoid
P   **Metatarsal, Left**
     See N Metatarsal, Right
Q   **Toe Phalanx, Right**
R   **Toe Phalanx, Left**
S   **Coccyx**
	Ø Open
	3 Percutaneous
	4 Percutaneous Endoscopic
		Z No Device	**Z** No Qualifier

Non-OR Procedure   DRG Non-OR Procedure   Valid OR Procedure   HAC Associated Procedure   Combination Only   New/Revised April   New/Revised October

568

ICD-10-PCS 2023

Ø   Medical and Surgical
Q   Lower Bones
D   Extraction   Definition: Pulling or stripping out or off all or a portion of a body part by the use of force
           Explanation: The qualifier DIAGNOSTIC is used to identify extraction procedures that are biopsies

Body Part Character 4	Approach Character 5	Device Character 6	Qualifier Character 7

Ø   **Lumbar Vertebra**
    Spinous process
    Transverse process
    Vertebral arch
    Vertebral body
    Vertebral foramen
    Vertebral lamina
    Vertebral pedicle
	Ø Open	**Z** No Device	**Z** No Qualifier

1 **Sacrum**			

2   **Pelvic Bone, Right**
    Iliac crest
    Ilium
    Ischium
    Pubis			

3 **Pelvic Bone, Left** *See 2 Pelvic Bone, Right*			
4 **Acetabulum, Right**			
5 **Acetabulum, Left**			

6   **Upper Femur, Right**
    Femoral head
    Greater trochanter
    Lesser trochanter
    Neck of femur			

7 **Upper Femur, Left** *See 6 Upper Femur, Right*			
8 **Femoral Shaft, Right** Body of femur			
9 **Femoral Shaft, Left** *See 8 Femoral Shaft, Right*			

B   **Lower Femur, Right**
    Lateral condyle of femur
    Lateral epicondyle of femur
    Medial condyle of femur
    Medial epicondyle of femur			

C **Lower Femur, Left** *See B Lower Femur, Right*			
D **Patella, Right**			
F **Patella, Left**			

G   **Tibia, Right**
    Lateral condyle of tibia
    Medial condyle of tibia
    Medial malleolus			

H **Tibia, Left** *See G Tibia, Right*			

J   **Fibula, Right**
    Body of fibula
    Head of fibula
    Lateral malleolus			

K **Fibula, Left** *See J Fibula, Right*			

L   **Tarsal, Right**
    Calcaneus
    Cuboid bone
    Intermediate cuneiform bone
    Lateral cuneiform bone
    Medial cuneiform bone
    Navicular bone
    Talus bone			

M **Tarsal, Left** *See L Tarsal, Right*			

N   **Metatarsal, Right**
    Fibular sesamoid
    Tibial sesamoid			

P **Metatarsal, Left** *See N Metatarsal, Right*			
Q **Toe Phalanx, Right**			
R **Toe Phalanx, Left**			
S **Coccyx**			

NC Noncovered Procedure   **LC** Limited Coverage   **QA** Questionable OB Admit   **NT** New Tech Add-on   ⊞ Combination Member   ♂ Male   ♀ Female

ICD-10-PCS 2023   569

Lower Bones (side tab)

Ø　**Medical and Surgical**
Q　**Lower Bones**
H　**Insertion**　　Definition: Putting in a nonbiological appliance that monitors, assists, performs, or prevents a physiological function but does not physically take the place of a body part
　　　　　　　　　　Explanation: None

Body Part Character 4		Approach Character 5	Device Character 6	Qualifier Character 7
Ø Lumbar Vertebra 　Spinous process 　Transverse process 　Vertebral arch 　Vertebral body 　Vertebral foramen 　Vertebral lamina 　Vertebral pedicle 1 Sacrum 2 Pelvic Bone, Right 　Iliac crest 　Ilium 　Ischium 　Pubis 3 Pelvic Bone, Left 　See 2 Pelvic Bone, Right 4 Acetabulum, Right 5 Acetabulum, Left	D Patella, Right F Patella, Left L Tarsal, Right 　Calcaneus 　Cuboid bone 　Intermediate cuneiform bone 　Lateral cuneiform bone 　Medial cuneiform bone 　Navicular bone 　Talus bone M Tarsal, Left 　See L Tarsal, Right N Metatarsal, Right 　Fibular sesamoid 　Tibial sesamoid P Metatarsal, Left 　See N Metatarsal, Right Q Toe Phalanx, Right R Toe Phalanx, Left S Coccyx	Ø Open 3 Percutaneous 4 Percutaneous Endoscopic	4 Internal Fixation Device 5 External Fixation Device	Z No Qualifier
6 Upper Femur, Right 　Femoral head 　Greater trochanter 　Lesser trochanter 　Neck of femur 7 Upper Femur, Left 　See 6 Upper Femur, Right B Lower Femur, Right 　Lateral condyle of femur 　Lateral epicondyle of femur 　Medial condyle of femur 　Medial epicondyle of femur	C Lower Femur, Left 　See B Lower Femur, Right J Fibula, Right 　Body of fibula 　Head of fibula 　Lateral malleolus K Fibula, Left 　See J Fibula, Right	Ø Open 3 Percutaneous 4 Percutaneous Endoscopic	4 Internal Fixation Device 5 External Fixation Device 6 Internal Fixation Device, Intramedullary 8 External Fixation Device, Limb Lengthening B External Fixation Device, Monoplanar C External Fixation Device, Ring D External Fixation Device, Hybrid	Z No Qualifier
8 Femoral Shaft, Right 　Body of femur 9 Femoral Shaft, Left 　See 8 Femoral Shaft, Right	G Tibia, Right 　Lateral condyle of tibia 　Medial condyle of tibia 　Medial malleolus H Tibia, Left 　See G Tibia, Right	Ø Open 3 Percutaneous 4 Percutaneous Endoscopic	4 Internal Fixation Device 5 External Fixation Device 6 Internal Fixation Device, Intramedullary 7 Internal Fixation Device, Intramedullary Limb Lengthening 8 External Fixation Device, Limb Lengthening B External Fixation Device, Monoplanar C External Fixation Device, Ring D External Fixation Device, Hybrid	Z No Qualifier
Y Lower Bone		Ø Open 3 Percutaneous 4 Percutaneous Endoscopic	M Bone Growth Stimulator	Z No Qualifier

Non-OR	ØQH[6,7,B,C,J,K][Ø,3,4]8Z
Non-OR	ØQH[8,9,G,H][Ø,3,4]8Z

Ø　**Medical and Surgical**
Q　**Lower Bones**
J　**Inspection**　　Definition: Visually and/or manually exploring a body part
　　　　　　　　　　Explanation: Visual exploration may be performed with or without optical instrumentation. Manual exploration may be performed directly or through intervening body layers.

Body Part Character 4	Approach Character 5	Device Character 6	Qualifier Character 7
Y Lower Bone	Ø Open 3 Percutaneous 4 Percutaneous Endoscopic X External	Z No Device	Z No Qualifier

Non-OR	ØQJY[3,X]ZZ

Ø   **Medical and Surgical**
Q   **Lower Bones**
N   **Release**   Definition: Freeing a body part from an abnormal physical constraint by cutting or by the use of force
                    Explanation: Some of the restraining tissue may be taken out but none of the body part is taken out

Body Part Character 4	Approach Character 5	Device Character 6	Qualifier Character 7

Ø   **Lumbar Vertebra**
     Spinous process
     Transverse process
     Vertebral arch
     Vertebral body
     Vertebral foramen
     Vertebral lamina
     Vertebral pedicle
1   **Sacrum**
2   **Pelvic Bone, Right**
     Iliac crest
     Ilium
     Ischium
     Pubis
3   **Pelvic Bone, Left**
     See 2 Pelvic Bone, Right
4   **Acetabulum, Right**
5   **Acetabulum, Left**
6   **Upper Femur, Right**
     Femoral head
     Greater trochanter
     Lesser trochanter
     Neck of femur
7   **Upper Femur, Left**
     See 6 Upper Femur, Right
8   **Femoral Shaft, Right**
     Body of femur
9   **Femoral Shaft, Left**
     See 8 Femoral Shaft, Right
B   **Lower Femur, Right**
     Lateral condyle of femur
     Lateral epicondyle of femur
     Medial condyle of femur
     Medial epicondyle of femur
C   **Lower Femur, Left**
     See B Lower Femur, Right
D   **Patella, Right**
F   **Patella, Left**
G   **Tibia, Right**
     Lateral condyle of tibia
     Medial condyle of tibia
     Medial malleolus
H   **Tibia, Left**
     See G Tibia, Right
J   **Fibula, Right**
     Body of fibula
     Head of fibula
     Lateral malleolus
K   **Fibula, Left**
     See J Fibula, Right
L   **Tarsal, Right**
     Calcaneus
     Cuboid bone
     Intermediate cuneiform bone
     Lateral cuneiform bone
     Medial cuneiform bone
     Navicular bone
     Talus bone
M   **Tarsal, Left**
     See L Tarsal, Right
N   **Metatarsal, Right**
     Fibular sesamoid
     Tibial sesamoid
P   **Metatarsal, Left**
     See N Metatarsal, Right
Q   **Toe Phalanx, Right**
R   **Toe Phalanx, Left**
S   **Coccyx**
	Ø **Open**
	3 **Percutaneous**
	4 **Percutaneous Endoscopic**
		Z **No Device**	**Z** **No Qualifier**

NC Noncovered Procedure   LC Limited Coverage   QA Questionable OB Admit   NT New Tech Add-on   ⊞ Combination Member   ♂ Male   ♀ Female

ICD-10-PCS 2023   571

Lower Bones *(side tab)*

Ø **Medical and Surgical**
Q **Lower Bones**
P **Removal**

Definition: Taking out or off a device from a body part

Explanation: If a device is taken out and a similar device put in without cutting or puncturing the skin or mucous membrane, the procedure is coded to the root operation CHANGE. Otherwise, the procedure for taking out a device is coded to the root operation REMOVAL.

Body Part Character 4		Approach Character 5	Device Character 6	Qualifier Character 7
Ø **Lumbar Vertebra** Spinous process Transverse process Vertebral arch Vertebral body Vertebral foramen Vertebral lamina Vertebral pedicle 1 **Sacrum** 2 **Pelvic Bone, Right** Iliac crest Ilium Ischium Pubis 3 **Pelvic Bone, Left** *See 2 Pelvic Bone, Right* 4 **Acetabulum, Right** 5 **Acetabulum, Left** 6 **Upper Femur, Right** Femoral head Greater trochanter Lesser trochanter Neck of femur 7 **Upper Femur, Left** *See 6 Upper Femur, Right* 8 **Femoral Shaft, Right** Body of femur 9 **Femoral Shaft, Left** *See 8 Femoral Shaft, Right* B **Lower Femur, Right** Lateral condyle of femur Lateral epicondyle of femur Medial condyle of femur Medial epicondyle of femur	C **Lower Femur, Left** *See B Lower Femur, Right* D **Patella, Right** F **Patella, Left** G **Tibia, Right** Lateral condyle of tibia Medial condyle of tibia Medial malleolus H **Tibia, Left** *See G Tibia, Right* J **Fibula, Right** Body of fibula Head of fibula Lateral malleolus K **Fibula, Left** *See J Fibula, Right* L **Tarsal, Right** Calcaneus Cuboid bone Intermediate cuneiform bone Lateral cuneiform bone Medial cuneiform bone Navicular bone Talus bone M **Tarsal, Left** *See L Tarsal, Right* N **Metatarsal, Right** Fibular sesamoid Tibial sesamoid P **Metatarsal, Left** *See N Metatarsal, Right* Q **Toe Phalanx, Right** R **Toe Phalanx, Left** S **Coccyx**	Ø **Open** 3 **Percutaneous** 4 **Percutaneous Endoscopic**	4 **Internal Fixation Device** 5 **External Fixation Device** 7 **Autologous Tissue Substitute** J **Synthetic Substitute** K **Nonautologous Tissue Substitute**	Z **No Qualifier**
Ø **Lumbar Vertebra** Spinous process Transverse process Vertebral arch Vertebral body Vertebral foramen Vertebral lamina Vertebral pedicle 1 **Sacrum** 2 **Pelvic Bone, Right** Iliac crest Ilium Ischium Pubis 3 **Pelvic Bone, Left** *See 2 Pelvic Bone, Right* 4 **Acetabulum, Right** 5 **Acetabulum, Left** 6 **Upper Femur, Right** Femoral head Greater trochanter Lesser trochanter Neck of femur 7 **Upper Femur, Left** *See 6 Upper Femur, Right* 8 **Femoral Shaft, Right** Body of femur 9 **Femoral Shaft, Left** *See 8 Femoral Shaft, Right* B **Lower Femur, Right** Lateral condyle of femur Lateral epicondyle of femur Medial condyle of femur Medial epicondyle of femur	C **Lower Femur, Left** *See B Lower Femur, Right* D **Patella, Right** F **Patella, Left** G **Tibia, Right** Lateral condyle of tibia Medial condyle of tibia Medial malleolus H **Tibia, Left** *See G Tibia, Right* J **Fibula, Right** Body of fibula Head of fibula Lateral malleolus K **Fibula, Left** *See J Fibula, Right* L **Tarsal, Right** Calcaneus Cuboid bone Intermediate cuneiform bone Lateral cuneiform bone Medial cuneiform bone Navicular bone Talus bone M **Tarsal, Left** *See L Tarsal, Right* N **Metatarsal, Right** Fibular sesamoid Tibial sesamoid P **Metatarsal, Left** *See N Metatarsal, Right* Q **Toe Phalanx, Right** R **Toe Phalanx, Left** S **Coccyx**	X **External**	4 **Internal Fixation Device** 5 **External Fixation Device**	Z **No Qualifier**
Y **Lower Bone**		Ø **Open** 3 **Percutaneous** 4 **Percutaneous Endoscopic** X **External**	Ø **Drainage Device** M **Bone Growth Stimulator**	Z **No Qualifier**

Non-OR ØQPYX[Ø,M]Z   **Non-OR** ØQPY3ØZ   **Non-OR** ØQP[Ø,1,2,3,4,5,6,7,8,9,B,C,D,F,G,H,J,K,L,M,N,P,Q,R,S]X[4,5]Z

Non-OR Procedure   DRG Non-OR Procedure   Valid OR Procedure   HAC Associated Procedure   Combination Only   New/Revised April   New/Revised October

Ø Medical and Surgical
Q Lower Bones
Q Repair   Definition: Restoring, to the extent possible, a body part to its normal anatomic structure and function

Explanation: Used only when the method to accomplish the repair is not one of the other root operations

Body Part Character 4	Approach Character 5	Device Character 6	Qualifier Character 7

Ø Lumbar Vertebra
  Spinous process
  Transverse process
  Vertebral arch
  Vertebral body
  Vertebral foramen
  Vertebral lamina
  Vertebral pedicle
	Ø Open
	3 Percutaneous
	4 Percutaneous Endoscopic
	X External
		Z No Device	**Z No Qualifier**

1 Sacrum			

2 Pelvic Bone, Right
  Iliac crest
  Ilium
  Ischium
  Pubis			

3 Pelvic Bone, Left *See 2 Pelvic Bone, Right*			
4 Acetabulum, Right			
5 Acetabulum, Left			

6 Upper Femur, Right
  Femoral head
  Greater trochanter
  Lesser trochanter
  Neck of femur			

7 Upper Femur, Left *See 6 Upper Femur, Right*			
8 Femoral Shaft, Right Body of femur			
9 Femoral Shaft, Left *See 8 Femoral Shaft, Right*			

B Lower Femur, Right
  Lateral condyle of femur
  Lateral epicondyle of femur
  Medial condyle of femur
  Medial epicondyle of femur			

C Lower Femur, Left *See B Lower Femur, Right*			
D Patella, Right			
F Patella, Left			

G Tibia, Right
  Lateral condyle of tibia
  Medial condyle of tibia
  Medial malleolus			

H Tibia, Left *See G Tibia, Right*			

J Fibula, Right
  Body of fibula
  Head of fibula
  Lateral malleolus			

K Fibula, Left *See J Fibula, Right*			

L Tarsal, Right
  Calcaneus
  Cuboid bone
  Intermediate cuneiform bone
  Lateral cuneiform bone
  Medial cuneiform bone
  Navicular bone
  Talus bone			

M Tarsal, Left *See L Tarsal, Right*			

N Metatarsal, Right
  Fibular sesamoid
  Tibial sesamoid			

P Metatarsal, Left *See N Metatarsal, Right*			
Q Toe Phalanx, Right			
R Toe Phalanx, Left			
S Coccyx			

Non-OR   ØQQ[Ø,1,2,3,4,5,6,7,8,9,B,C,D,F,G,H,J,K,L,M,N,P,Q,R,S]XZZ

NC Noncovered Procedure   LC Limited Coverage   QA Questionable OB Admit   NT New Tech Add-on   ⊞ Combination Member   ♂ Male   ♀ Female

ICD-10-PCS 2023   573

ØQQ–ØQQ

Lower Bones

Ø **Medical and Surgical**
Q **Lower Bones**
R **Replacement** Definition: Putting in or on biological or synthetic material that physically takes the place and/or function of all or a portion of a body part
Explanation: The body part may have been taken out or replaced, or may be taken out, physically eradicated, or rendered nonfunctional during the REPLACEMENT procedure. A REMOVAL procedure is coded for taking out the device used in a previous replacement procedure.

Body Part Character 4	Approach Character 5	Device Character 6	Qualifier Character 7
Ø **Lumbar Vertebra** Spinous process Transverse process Vertebral arch Vertebral body Vertebral foramen Vertebral lamina Vertebral pedicle 1 **Sacrum** 2 **Pelvic Bone, Right** Iliac crest Ilium Ischium Pubis 3 **Pelvic Bone, Left** *See 2 Pelvic Bone, Right* 4 **Acetabulum, Right** 5 **Acetabulum, Left** 6 **Upper Femur, Right** Femoral head Greater trochanter Lesser trochanter Neck of femur 7 **Upper Femur, Left** *See 6 Upper Femur, Right* 8 **Femoral Shaft, Right** Body of femur 9 **Femoral Shaft, Left** *See 8 Femoral Shaft, Right* B **Lower Femur, Right** Lateral condyle of femur Lateral epicondyle of femur Medial condyle of femur Medial epicondyle of femur C **Lower Femur, Left** *See B Lower Femur, Right* D **Patella, Right** F **Patella, Left** G **Tibia, Right** Lateral condyle of tibia Medial condyle of tibia Medial malleolus H **Tibia, Left** *See G Tibia, Right* J **Fibula, Right** Body of fibula Head of fibula Lateral malleolus K **Fibula, Left** *See J Fibula, Right* L **Tarsal, Right** Calcaneus Cuboid bone Intermediate cuneiform bone Lateral cuneiform bone Medial cuneiform bone Navicular bone Talus bone M **Tarsal, Left** *See L Tarsal, Right* N **Metatarsal, Right** Fibular sesamoid Tibial sesamoid P **Metatarsal, Left** *See N Metatarsal, Right* Q **Toe Phalanx, Right** R **Toe Phalanx, Left** S **Coccyx**	Ø **Open** 3 **Percutaneous** 4 **Percutaneous Endoscopic**	7 **Autologous Tissue Substitute** J **Synthetic Substitute** K **Nonautologous Tissue Substitute**	Z **No Qualifier**

Non-OR Procedure   DRG Non-OR Procedure   Valid OR Procedure   HAC Associated Procedure   Combination Only   New/Revised April   New/Revised October

574   ICD-10-PCS 2023

Ø   **Medical and Surgical**
Q   **Lower Bones**
S   **Reposition**   Definition: Moving to its normal location, or other suitable location, all or a portion of a body part

Explanation: The body part is moved to a new location from an abnormal location, or from a normal location where it is not functioning correctly. The body part may or may not be cut out or off to be moved to the new location.

Body Part Character 4		Approach Character 5	Device Character 6	Qualifier Character 7
Ø **Lumbar Vertebra** Spinous process Transverse process Vertebral arch Vertebral body Vertebral foramen Vertebral lamina Vertebral pedicle		**Ø** Open **4** Percutaneous Endoscopic	**3** Spinal Stabilization Device, Vertebral Body Tether **4** Internal Fixation Device **Z** No Device	**Z** No Qualifier
Ø **Lumbar Vertebra** ⊞ Spinous process Transverse process Vertebral arch Vertebral body Vertebral foramen Vertebral lamina Vertebral pedicle		**3** Percutaneous	**4** Internal Fixation Device **Z** No Device	**Z** No Qualifier
Ø **Lumbar Vertebra** Spinous process Transverse process Vertebral arch Vertebral body Vertebral foramen Vertebral lamina Vertebral pedicle		**X** External	**Z** No Device	**Z** No Qualifier
1 **Sacrum** ⊞ **4** **Acetabulum, Right** **5** **Acetabulum, Left** **S** **Coccyx** ⊞		**Ø** Open **3** Percutaneous **4** Percutaneous Endoscopic	**4** Internal Fixation Device **Z** No Device	**Z** No Qualifier
1 **Sacrum** **4** **Acetabulum, Right** **5** **Acetabulum, Left** **S** **Coccyx**		**X** External	**Z** No Device	**Z** No Qualifier
2 **Pelvic Bone, Right** Iliac crest Ilium Ischium Pubis **3** **Pelvic Bone, Left** *See 2 Pelvic Bone, Right* **D** **Patella, Right** **F** **Patella, Left** **L** **Tarsal, Right** Calcaneus Cuboid bone Intermediate cuneiform bone Lateral cuneiform bone Medial cuneiform bone Navicular bone Talus bone	**M** **Tarsal, Left** *See L Tarsal, Right* **Q** **Toe Phalanx, Right** **R** **Toe Phalanx, Left**	**Ø** Open **3** Percutaneous **4** Percutaneous Endoscopic	**4** Internal Fixation Device **5** External Fixation Device **Z** No Device	**Z** No Qualifier
2 **Pelvic Bone, Right** Iliac crest Ilium Ischium Pubis **3** **Pelvic Bone, Left** *See 2 Pelvic Bone, Right* **D** **Patella, Right** **F** **Patella, Left** **L** **Tarsal, Right** Calcaneus Cuboid bone Intermediate cuneiform bone Lateral cuneiform bone Medial cuneiform bone Navicular bone Talus bone	**M** **Tarsal, Left** *See L Tarsal, Right* **Q** **Toe Phalanx, Right** **R** **Toe Phalanx, Left**	**X** External	**Z** No Device	**Z** No Qualifier

Non-OR	ØQSØXZZ
Non-OR	ØQS[4,5][3,4]ZZ
Non-OR	ØQS[1,4,5,S]XZZ
Non-OR	ØQS[2,3,D,F,L,M,Q,R][3,4]ZZ
Non-OR	ØQS[2,3,D,F,L,M,Q,R]XZZ

See Appendix L for Procedure Combinations
⊞   ØQSØ3ZZ
⊞   ØQS[1,S]3ZZ

ØQS Continued on next page

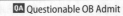

NC Noncovered Procedure   **LC** Limited Coverage   **QA** Questionable OB Admit   **NT** New Tech Add-on   ⊞ Combination Member   ♂ Male   ♀ Female

ICD-10-PCS 2023   **575**

Lower Bones

Ø   **Medical and Surgical**
Q   **Lower Bones**
S   **Reposition**

ØQS Continued

Definition: Moving to its normal location, or other suitable location, all or a portion of a body part

Explanation: The body part is moved to a new location from an abnormal location, or from a normal location where it is not functioning correctly. The body part may or may not be cut out or off to be moved to the new location.

Body Part Character 4	Approach Character 5	Device Character 6	Qualifier Character 7
6 Upper Femur, Right Femoral head Greater trochanter Lesser trochanter Neck of femur **7 Upper Femur, Left** *See 6 Upper Femur, Right* **8 Femoral Shaft, Right** Body of femur **9 Femoral Shaft, Left** *See 8 Femoral Shaft, Right* **B Lower Femur, Right** Lateral condyle of femur Lateral epicondyle of femur Medial condyle of femur Medial epicondyle of femur **C Lower Femur, Left** *See B Lower Femur, Right* **G Tibia, Right** Lateral condyle of tibia Medial condyle of tibia Medial malleolus **H Tibia, Left** *See G Tibia, Right* **J Fibula, Right** Body of fibula Head of fibula Lateral malleolus **K Fibula, Left** *See J Fibula, Right*	**Ø Open** **3 Percutaneous** **4 Percutaneous Endoscopic**	**4 Internal Fixation Device** **5 External Fixation Device** **6 Internal Fixation Device, Intramedullary** **B External Fixation Device, Monoplanar** **C External Fixation Device, Ring** **D External Fixation Device, Hybrid** **Z No Device**	**Z No Qualifier**
6 Upper Femur, Right Femoral head Greater trochanter Lesser trochanter Neck of femur **7 Upper Femur, Left** *See 6 Upper Femur, Right* **8 Femoral Shaft, Right** Body of femur **9 Femoral Shaft, Left** *See 8 Femoral Shaft, Right* **B Lower Femur, Right** Lateral condyle of femur Lateral epicondyle of femur Medial condyle of femur Medial epicondyle of femur **C Lower Femur, Left** *See B Lower Femur, Right* **G Tibia, Right** Lateral condyle of tibia Medial condyle of tibia Medial malleolus **H Tibia, Left** *See G Tibia, Right* **J Fibula, Right** Body of fibula Head of fibula Lateral malleolus **K Fibula, Left** *See J Fibula, Right*	**X External**	**Z No Device**	**Z No Qualifier**
N Metatarsal, Right Fibular sesamoid Tibial sesamoid **P Metatarsal, Left** *See N Metatarsal, Right*	**Ø Open** **3 Percutaneous** **4 Percutaneous Endoscopic**	**4 Internal Fixation Device** **5 External Fixation Device** **Z No Device**	**2 Sesamoid Bone(s) 1st Toe** **Z No Qualifier**
N Metatarsal, Right Fibular sesamoid Tibial sesamoid **P Metatarsal, Left** *See N Metatarsal, Right*	**X External**	**Z No Device**	**2 Sesamoid Bone(s) 1st Toe** **Z No Qualifier**

Non-OR	ØQS[6,7,8,9,B,C,G,H,J,K][3,4]ZZ
Non-OR	ØQS[6,7,8,9,B,C,G,H,J,K]XZZ
Non-OR	ØQS[N,P][3,4]Z[2,Z]
Non-OR	ØQS[N,P]XZ[2,Z]

Non-OR Procedure   DRG Non-OR Procedure   Valid OR Procedure   HAC Associated Procedure   Combination Only   New/Revised April   New/Revised October

Ø **Medical and Surgical**
Q **Lower Bones**
T **Resection**　　Definition: Cutting out or off, without replacement, all of a body part
　　　　　　　　　　Explanation: None

Body Part Character 4		Approach Character 5	Device Character 6	Qualifier Character 7
2 **Pelvic Bone, Right** 　Iliac crest 　Ilium 　Ischium 　Pubis **3** **Pelvic Bone, Left** 　*See 2 Pelvic Bone, Right* **4** **Acetabulum, Right** **5** **Acetabulum, Left** **6** **Upper Femur, Right** 　Femoral head 　Greater trochanter 　Lesser trochanter 　Neck of femur **7** **Upper Femur, Left** 　*See 6 Upper Femur, Right* **8** **Femoral Shaft, Right** 　Body of femur **9** **Femoral Shaft, Left** 　*See 8 Femoral Shaft, Right* **B** **Lower Femur, Right** 　Lateral condyle of femur 　Lateral epicondyle of femur 　Medial condyle of femur 　Medial epicondyle of femur **C** **Lower Femur, Left** 　*See B Lower Femur, Right* **D** **Patella, Right**	**F** **Patella, Left** **G** **Tibia, Right** 　Lateral condyle of tibia 　Medial condyle of tibia 　Medial malleolus **H** **Tibia, Left** 　*See G Tibia, Right* **J** **Fibula, Right** 　Body of fibula 　Head of fibula 　Lateral malleolus **K** **Fibula, Left** 　*See J Fibula, Right* **L** **Tarsal, Right** 　Calcaneus 　Cuboid bone 　Intermediate cuneiform bone 　Lateral cuneiform bone 　Medial cuneiform bone 　Navicular bone 　Talus bone **M** **Tarsal, Left** 　*See L Tarsal, Right* **N** **Metatarsal, Right** 　Fibular sesamoid 　Tibial sesamoid **P** **Metatarsal, Left** 　*See N Metatarsal, Right* **Q** **Toe Phalanx, Right** **R** **Toe Phalanx, Left** **S** **Coccyx**	**Ø** Open	**Z** No Device	**Z** No Qualifier

Ø **Medical and Surgical**
Q **Lower Bones**
U **Supplement**　　Definition: Putting in or on biological or synthetic material that physically reinforces and/or augments the function of a portion of a body part
　　　　　　　　　　Explanation: The biological material is non-living, or is living and from the same individual. The body part may have been previously replaced, and the SUPPLEMENT procedure is performed to physically reinforce and/or augment the function of the replaced body part.

Body Part Character 4		Approach Character 5	Device Character 6	Qualifier Character 7
Ø **Lumbar Vertebra** ⊞ 　Spinous process 　Transverse process 　Vertebral arch 　Vertebral body 　Vertebral foramen 　Vertebral lamina 　Vertebral pedicle **1** **Sacrum** ⊞ **2** **Pelvic Bone, Right** 　Iliac crest 　Ilium 　Ischium 　Pubis **3** **Pelvic Bone, Left** 　*See 2 Pelvic Bone, Right* **4** **Acetabulum, Right** **5** **Acetabulum, Left** **6** **Upper Femur, Right** 　Femoral head 　Greater trochanter 　Lesser trochanter 　Neck of femur **7** **Upper Femur, Left** 　*See 6 Upper Femur, Right* **8** **Femoral Shaft, Right** 　Body of femur **9** **Femoral Shaft, Left** 　*See 8 Femoral Shaft, Right* **B** **Lower Femur, Right** 　Lateral condyle of femur 　Lateral epicondyle of femur 　Medial condyle of femur 　Medial epicondyle of femur	**C** **Lower Femur, Left** 　*See B Lower Femur, Right* **D** **Patella, Right** **F** **Patella, Left** **G** **Tibia, Right** 　Lateral condyle of tibia 　Medial condyle of tibia 　Medial malleolus **H** **Tibia, Left** 　*See G Tibia, Right* **J** **Fibula, Right** 　Body of fibula 　Head of fibula 　Lateral malleolus **K** **Fibula, Left** 　*See J Fibula, Right* **L** **Tarsal, Right** 　Calcaneus 　Cuboid bone 　Intermediate cuneiform bone 　Lateral cuneiform bone 　Medial cuneiform bone 　Navicular bone 　Talus bone **M** **Tarsal, Left** 　*See L Tarsal, Right* **N** **Metatarsal, Right** 　Fibular sesamoid 　Tibial sesamoid **P** **Metatarsal, Left** 　*See N Metatarsal, Right* **Q** **Toe Phalanx, Right** **R** **Toe Phalanx, Left** **S** **Coccyx** ⊞	**Ø** Open **3** Percutaneous **4** Percutaneous Endoscopic	**7** Autologous Tissue 　Substitute **J** Synthetic Substitute **K** Nonautologous Tissue 　Substitute	**Z** No Qualifier

See Appendix L for Procedure Combinations
　⊞　ØQU[Ø,1,S]3JZ

NC Noncovered Procedure　　**LC** Limited Coverage　　**QA** Questionable OB Admit　　**NT** New Tech Add-on　　⊞ Combination Member　　♂ Male　　♀ Female

ICD-10-PCS 2023　　　　　　　　　　　　　　　　　　　　　　　　　　　　　　　　　**577**

Lower Bones

Ø   Medical and Surgical
Q   Lower Bones
W   Revision

Definition: Correcting, to the extent possible, a portion of a malfunctioning device or the position of a displaced device

Explanation: Revision can include correcting a malfunctioning or displaced device by taking out or putting in components of the device such as a screw or pin

Body Part Character 4	Approach Character 5	Device Character 6	Qualifier Character 7
Ø Lumbar Vertebra Spinous process Transverse process Vertebral arch Vertebral body Vertebral foramen Vertebral lamina Vertebral pedicle **1 Sacrum** **4 Acetabulum, Right** **5 Acetabulum, Left** **S Coccyx**	**Ø** Open **3** Percutaneous **4** Percutaneous Endoscopic **X** External	**4** Internal Fixation Device **7** Autologous Tissue Substitute **J** Synthetic Substitute **K** Nonautologous Tissue Substitute	**Z** No Qualifier
2 Pelvic Bone, Right Iliac crest Ilium Ischium Pubis **3 Pelvic Bone, Left** *See 2 Pelvic Bone, Right* **6 Upper Femur, Right** Femoral head Greater trochanter Lesser trochanter Neck of femur **7 Upper Femur, Left** *See 6 Upper Femur, Right* **8 Femoral Shaft, Right** Body of femur **9 Femoral Shaft, Left** *See 8 Femoral Shaft, Right* **B Lower Femur, Right** Lateral condyle of femur Lateral epicondyle of femur Medial condyle of femur Medial epicondyle of femur **C Lower Femur, Left** *See B Lower Femur, Right* **D Patella, Right** **F Patella, Left** **G Tibia, Right** Lateral condyle of tibia Medial condyle of tibia Medial malleolus **H Tibia, Left** *See G Tibia, Right* **J Fibula, Right** Body of fibula Head of fibula Lateral malleolus **K Fibula, Left** *See J Fibula, Right* **L Tarsal, Right** Calcaneus Cuboid bone Intermediate cuneiform bone Lateral cuneiform bone Medial cuneiform bone Navicular bone Talus bone **M Tarsal, Left** *See L Tarsal, Right* **N Metatarsal, Right** Fibular sesamoid Tibial sesamoid **P Metatarsal, Left** *See N Metatarsal, Right* **Q Toe Phalanx, Right** **R Toe Phalanx, Left**	**Ø** Open **3** Percutaneous **4** Percutaneous Endoscopic **X** External	**4** Internal Fixation Device **5** External Fixation Device **7** Autologous Tissue Substitute **J** Synthetic Substitute **K** Nonautologous Tissue Substitute	**Z** No Qualifier
Y Lower Bone	**Ø** Open **3** Percutaneous **4** Percutaneous Endoscopic **X** External	**Ø** Drainage Device **M** Bone Growth Stimulator	**Z** No Qualifier

Non-OR	ØQW[Ø,1,4,5,S]X[4,7,J,K]Z	Non-OR	ØQWYX[Ø,M]Z
Non-OR	ØQW[2,3,6,7,8,9,B,C,D,F,G,H,J,K,L,M,N,P,Q,R]X[4,5,7,J,K]Z		

Non-OR Procedure   DRG Non-OR Procedure   Valid OR Procedure   HAC Associated Procedure   Combination Only   New/Revised April   New/Revised October

Upper Joints ØR2–ØRW

Character Meanings*

This Character Meaning table is provided as a guide to assist the user in the identification of character members that may be found in this section of code tables. It **SHOULD NOT** be used to build a PCS code.

Operation–Character 3	Body Part–Character 4	Approach–Character 5	Device–Character 6	Qualifier–Character 7
2 Change	Ø Occipital-cervical Joint	Ø Open	Ø Drainage Device OR Synthetic Substitute, Reverse Ball and Socket	Ø Anterior Approach, Anterior Column
5 Destruction	1 Cervical Vertebral Joint	3 Percutaneous	3 Infusion Device OR Internal Fixation Device, Sustained Compression	1 Posterior Approach, Posterior Column
9 Drainage	2 Cervical Vertebral Joint, 2 or more	4 Percutaneous Endoscopic	4 Internal Fixation Device	6 Humeral Surface
B Excision	3 Cervical Vertebral Disc	X External	5 External Fixation Device	7 Glenoid Surface
C Extirpation	4 Cervicothoracic Vertebral Joint		7 Autologous Tissue Substitute	J Posterior Approach, Anterior Column
G Fusion	5 Cervicothoracic Vertebral Disc		8 Spacer	X Diagnostic
H Insertion	6 Thoracic Vertebral Joint		A Interbody Fusion Device	Z No Qualifier
J Inspection	7 Thoracic Vertebral Joint, 2 to 7		B Spinal Stabilization Device, Interspinous Process	
N Release	8 Thoracic Vertebral Joint, 8 or more		C Spinal Stabilization Device, Pedicle-Based	
P Removal	9 Thoracic Vertebral Disc		D Spinal Stabilization Device, Facet Replacement	
Q Repair	A Thoracolumbar Vertebral Joint		J Synthetic Substitute	
R Replacement	B Thoracolumbar Vertebral Disc		K Nonautologous Tissue Substitute	
S Reposition	C Temporomandibular Joint, Right		Y Other Device	
T Resection	D Temporomandibular Joint, Left		Z No Device	
U Supplement	E Sternoclavicular Joint, Right			
W Revision	F Sternoclavicular Joint, Left			
	G Acromioclavicular Joint, Right			
	H Acromioclavicular Joint, Left			
	J Shoulder Joint, Right			
	K Shoulder Joint, Left			
	L Elbow Joint, Right			
	M Elbow Joint, Left			
	N Wrist Joint, Right			
	P Wrist Joint, Left			
	Q Carpal Joint, Right			
	R Carpal Joint, Left			
	S Carpometacarpal Joint, Right			
	T Carpometacarpal Joint, Left			
	U Metacarpophalangeal Joint, Right			
	V Metacarpophalangeal Joint, Left			
	W Finger Phalangeal Joint, Right			
	X Finger Phalangeal Joint, Left			
	Y Upper Joint			

* Includes synovial membrane.

AHA Coding Clinic for table ØRB

2019, 3Q, 26	Acromioclavicular joint reconstruction using allograft

AHA Coding Clinic for table ØRG

2021, 4Q, 67	Posterior dynamic distraction
2021, 1Q, 18	Placement of interspinous distraction device (spacer) for decompression
2021, 1Q, 53	Official guidelines for coding and reporting for interbody fusion device B3.10c
2020, 4Q, 56-58	Intramedullary sustained compression joint fusion
2020, 2Q, 27	Spinal fusion with NuVasive® VersaTie®
2020, 1Q, 33	Spinal fusion without use of bone graft
2019, 3Q, 28	Use of VERTE-STACK™ implant with fusion
2019, 3Q, 35	Fusion procedures of the spine (guideline B3.10c)
2019, 2Q, 19	Cervical spinal fusion, decompression and placement of interfacet stabilization device
2019, 1Q, 30	Spinal fusion performed at same level as decompressive laminectomy
2018, 4Q, 43	Joint fusion device value
2018, 1Q, 22	Spinal fusion procedures without bone graft
2017, 4Q, 62	Added and revised device values - Nerve substitutes
2017, 4Q, 76	Radiolucent porous interbody fusion device
2017, 2Q, 23	Decompression of spinal cord and placement of instrumentation
2014, 3Q, 30	Spinal fusion and fixation instrumentation
2014, 2Q, 7	Anterior cervical thoracic fusion with total discectomy
2013, 1Q, 21-23	Spinal fusion of thoracic and lumbar vertebrae
2013, 1Q, 29	Cervical and thoracic spinal fusion

AHA Coding Clinic for table ØRH

2021, 1Q, 18	Placement of interspinous distraction device (spacer) for decompression
2019, 2Q, 40	Decompression of spinal cord and placement of instrumentation
2018, 3Q, 26	Anterior vertebral tethering using Dynesys Tethering System
2017, 2Q, 23	Decompression of spinal cord and placement of instrumentation
2016, 3Q, 32	Rotator cuff repair, tenodesis, decompression, acromioplasty and coracoplasty

AHA Coding Clinic for table ØRN

2019, 1Q, 30	Spinal fusion performed at same level as decompressive laminectomy
2016, 3Q, 32	Rotator cuff repair, tenodesis, decompression, acromioplasty and coracoplasty
2015, 2Q, 22	Arthroscopic subacromial decompression
2015, 2Q, 23	Arthroscopic release of shoulder joint

AHA Coding Clinic for table ØRP

2021, 4Q, 53	Shoulder hemiarthroplasty
2017, 4Q, 107	Total ankle replacement versus revision

AHA Coding Clinic for table ØRQ

2016, 1Q, 30	Thermal capsulorrhaphy of shoulder

AHA Coding Clinic for table ØRR

2018, 4Q, 92	Radial head arthroplasty
2017, 4Q, 107	Total ankle replacement versus revision
2015, 3Q, 14	Endoprosthetic replacement of humerus and tendon reattachment
2015, 1Q, 27	Reverse total shoulder arthroplasty

AHA Coding Clinic for table ØRS

2019, 3Q, 26	Acromioclavicular joint reconstruction using allograft
2018, 3Q, 26	Anterior vertebral tethering using Dynesys Tethering System
2015, 2Q, 35	Application of tongs to reduce and stabilize cervical fracture
2014, 4Q, 32	Open reduction internal fixation of fracture with debridement
2014, 3Q, 33	Radial fracture treatment with open reduction internal fixation, and release of carpal ligament
2013, 2Q, 39	Application of cervical tongs for reduction of cervical fracture

AHA Coding Clinic for table ØRT

2019, 3Q, 26	Acromioclavicular joint reconstruction using allograft
2014, 2Q, 7	Anterior cervical thoracic fusion with total discectomy

AHA Coding Clinic for table ØRU

2019, 3Q, 26	Acromioclavicular joint reconstruction using allograft
2015, 3Q, 26	Thumb arthroplasty with resection of trapezium

AHA Coding Clinic for table ØRW

2021, 4Q, 53	Shoulder hemiarthroplasty
2017, 4Q, 107	Total ankle replacement versus revision

Upper Joints

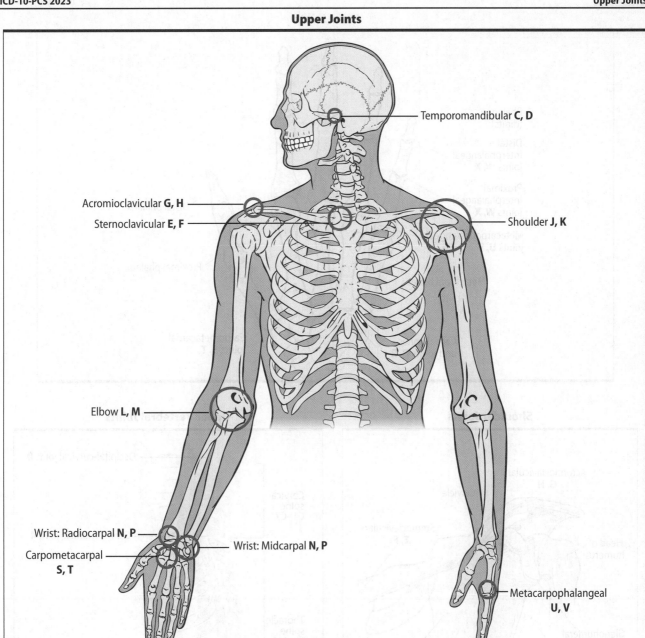

Temporomandibular **C, D**

Acromioclavicular **G, H**

Sternoclavicular **E, F**

Shoulder **J, K**

Elbow **L, M**

Wrist: Radiocarpal **N, P**

Wrist: Midcarpal **N, P**

Carpometacarpal
S, T

Metacarpophalangeal
U, V

Hand Joints

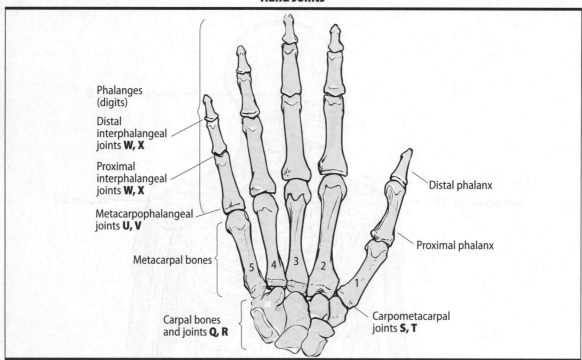

Phalanges (digits)

Distal interphalangeal joints **W, X**

Proximal interphalangeal joints **W, X**

Metacarpophalangeal joints **U, V**

Metacarpal bones

Carpal bones and joints **Q, R**

Distal phalanx

Proximal phalanx

Carpometacarpal joints **S, T**

Shoulder Joints

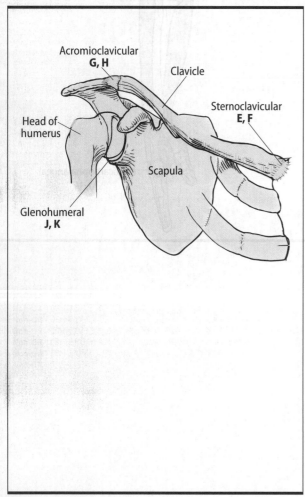

Acromioclavicular **G, H**

Clavicle

Head of humerus

Sternoclavicular **E, F**

Glenohumeral **J, K**

Scapula

Upper Vertebral Joints

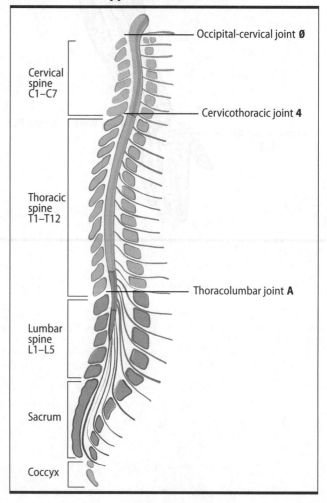

Cervical spine C1–C7

Thoracic spine T1–T12

Lumbar spine L1–L5

Sacrum

Coccyx

Occipital-cervical joint **Ø**

Cervicothoracic joint **4**

Thoracolumbar joint **A**

Ø	Medical and Surgical
R	Upper Joints
2	Change

Definition: Taking out or off a device from a body part and putting back an identical or similar device in or on the same body part without cutting or puncturing the skin or a mucous membrane

Explanation: All CHANGE procedures are coded using the approach EXTERNAL

Body Part Character 4	Approach Character 5	Device Character 6	Qualifier Character 7
Y Upper Joint	X External	Ø Drainage Device Y Other Device	Z No Qualifier

Non-OR	All body part, approach, device, and qualifier values

Ø	Medical and Surgical
R	Upper Joints
5	Destruction

Definition: Physical eradication of all or a portion of a body part by the direct use of energy, force, or a destructive agent

Explanation: None of the body part is physically taken out

Body Part Character 4	Approach Character 5	Device Character 6	Qualifier Character 7
Ø Occipital-cervical Joint	Ø Open	Z No Device	Z No Qualifier

1   Cervical Vertebral Joint
     Atlantoaxial joint
     Cervical facet joint
	3 Percutaneous
	4 Percutaneous Endoscopic		

3 Cervical Vertebral Disc			
4 Cervicothoracic Vertebral Joint Cervicothoracic facet joint			
5 Cervicothoracic Vertebral Disc			

6   Thoracic Vertebral Joint
     Costotransverse joint
     Costovertebral joint
     Thoracic facet joint			

9 Thoracic Vertebral Disc			
A Thoracolumbar Vertebral Joint Thoracolumbar facet joint			
B Thoracolumbar Vertebral Disc			
C Temporomandibular Joint, Right			
D Temporomandibular Joint, Left			
E Sternoclavicular Joint, Right			
F Sternoclavicular Joint, Left			
G Acromioclavicular Joint, Right			
H Acromioclavicular Joint, Left			

J   Shoulder Joint, Right
     Glenohumeral joint
     Glenoid ligament (labrum)			

K Shoulder Joint, Left *See J Shoulder Joint, Right*			

L   Elbow Joint, Right
     Distal humerus, involving joint
     Humeroradial joint
     Humeroulnar joint
     Proximal radioulnar joint			

M Elbow Joint, Left *See L Elbow Joint, Right*			

N   Wrist Joint, Right
     Distal radioulnar joint
     Radiocarpal joint			

P Wrist Joint, Left *See N Wrist Joint, Right*			

Q   Carpal Joint, Right
     Intercarpal joint
     Midcarpal joint			

R Carpal Joint, Left *See Q Carpal Joint, Right*			
S Carpometacarpal Joint, Right			
T Carpometacarpal Joint, Left			
U Metacarpophalangeal Joint, Right			
V Metacarpophalangeal Joint, Left			
W Finger Phalangeal Joint, Right Interphalangeal (IP) joint			
X Finger Phalangeal Joint, Left *See W Finger Phalangeal Joint, Right*			

Non-OR	ØR5[3,5,9,B][3,4]ZZ

NC Noncovered Procedure   LC Limited Coverage   QA Questionable OB Admit   NT New Tech Add-on   ⊞ Combination Member   ♂ Male   ♀ Female

ICD-10-PCS 2023   583

ØR2–ØR5

Upper Joints

Ø   **Medical and Surgical**
R   **Upper Joints**
9   **Drainage**   Definition: Taking or letting out fluids and/or gases from a body part
                    Explanation: The qualifier DIAGNOSTIC is used to identify drainage procedures that are biopsies

Body Part Character 4		Approach Character 5	Device Character 6	Qualifier Character 7

Ø Occipital-cervical Joint
1 Cervical Vertebral Joint
  Atlantoaxial joint
  Cervical facet joint
3 Cervical Vertebral Disc
4 Cervicothoracic Vertebral Joint
  Cervicothoracic facet joint
5 Cervicothoracic Vertebral Disc
6 Thoracic Vertebral Joint
  Costotransverse joint
  Costovertebral joint
  Thoracic facet joint
9 Thoracic Vertebral Disc
A Thoracolumbar Vertebral Joint
  Thoracolumbar facet joint
B Thoracolumbar Vertebral Disc
C Temporomandibular Joint, Right
D Temporomandibular Joint, Left
E Sternoclavicular Joint, Right
F Sternoclavicular Joint, Left
G Acromioclavicular Joint, Right
H Acromioclavicular Joint, Left
J Shoulder Joint, Right
  Glenohumeral joint
  Glenoid ligament (labrum)
K Shoulder Joint, Left
  See J Shoulder Joint, Right
	L Elbow Joint, Right
	  Distal humerus, involving joint
	  Humeroradial joint
	  Humeroulnar joint
	  Proximal radioulnar joint
	M Elbow Joint, Left
	  See L Elbow Joint, Right
	N Wrist Joint, Right
	  Distal radioulnar joint
	  Radiocarpal joint
	P Wrist Joint, Left
	  See N Wrist Joint, Right
	Q Carpal Joint, Right
	  Intercarpal joint
	  Midcarpal joint
	R Carpal Joint, Left
	  See Q Carpal Joint, Right
	S Carpometacarpal Joint, Right
	T Carpometacarpal Joint, Left
	U Metacarpophalangeal Joint, Right
	V Metacarpophalangeal Joint, Left
	W Finger Phalangeal Joint, Right
	  Interphalangeal (IP) joint
	X Finger Phalangeal Joint, Left
	  See W Finger Phalangeal Joint, Right
		Ø Open
		3 Percutaneous
		4 Percutaneous Endoscopic
			Ø Drainage Device	Z No Qualifier

Ø Occipital-cervical Joint
1 Cervical Vertebral Joint
  Atlantoaxial joint
  Cervical facet joint
3 Cervical Vertebral Disc
4 Cervicothoracic Vertebral Joint
  Cervicothoracic facet joint
5 Cervicothoracic Vertebral Disc
6 Thoracic Vertebral Joint
  Costotransverse joint
  Costovertebral joint
  Thoracic facet joint
9 Thoracic Vertebral Disc
A Thoracolumbar Vertebral Joint
  Thoracolumbar facet joint
B Thoracolumbar Vertebral Disc
C Temporomandibular Joint, Right
D Temporomandibular Joint, Left
E Sternoclavicular Joint, Right
F Sternoclavicular Joint, Left
G Acromioclavicular Joint, Right
H Acromioclavicular Joint, Left
J Shoulder Joint, Right
  Glenohumeral joint
  Glenoid ligament (labrum)
K Shoulder Joint, Left
  See J Shoulder Joint, Right
	L Elbow Joint, Right
	  Distal humerus, involving joint
	  Humeroradial joint
	  Humeroulnar joint
	  Proximal radioulnar joint
	M Elbow Joint, Left
	  See L Elbow Joint, Right
	N Wrist Joint, Right
	  Distal radioulnar joint
	  Radiocarpal joint
	P Wrist Joint, Left
	  See N Wrist Joint, Right
	Q Carpal Joint, Right
	  Intercarpal joint
	  Midcarpal joint
	R Carpal Joint, Left
	  See Q Carpal Joint, Right
	S Carpometacarpal Joint, Right
	T Carpometacarpal Joint, Left
	U Metacarpophalangeal Joint, Right
	V Metacarpophalangeal Joint, Left
	W Finger Phalangeal Joint, Right
	  Interphalangeal (IP) joint
	X Finger Phalangeal Joint, Left
	  See W Finger Phalangeal Joint, Right
		Ø Open
		3 Percutaneous
		4 Percutaneous Endoscopic
			Z No Device	X Diagnostic
				Z No Qualifier

Non-OR	ØR9[Ø,1,3,4,5,6,9,A,B,E,F,G,H,J,K,L,M,N,P,Q,R,S,T,U,V,W,X][3,4]ØZ
Non-OR	ØR9[C,D]3ØZ
Non-OR	ØR9[Ø,1,3,4,5,6,9,A,B,E,F,G,H,J,K,L,M,N,P,Q,R,S,T,U,V,W,X][Ø,3,4]ZX
Non-OR	ØR9[Ø,1,3,4,5,6,9,A,B,E,F,G,H,J,K,L,M,N,P,Q,R,S,T,U,V,W,X][3,4]ZZ
Non-OR	ØR9[C,D]3ZZ

Non-OR Procedure   DRG Non-OR Procedure   Valid OR Procedure   HAC Associated Procedure   Combination Only   New/Revised April   New/Revised October

584   ICD-10-PCS 2023

Ø   **Medical and Surgical**
R   **Upper Joints**
B   **Excision**   Definition: Cutting out or off, without replacement, a portion of a body part

                      Explanation: The qualifier DIAGNOSTIC is used to identify excision procedures that are biopsies

Body Part Character 4	Approach Character 5	Device Character 6	Qualifier Character 7
Ø **Occipital-cervical Joint**	**Ø** Open	**Z** No Device	**X** Diagnostic
1 **Cervical Vertebral Joint**	**3** Percutaneous		**Z** No Qualifier
Atlantoaxial joint	**4** Percutaneous Endoscopic		
Cervical facet joint			
3 **Cervical Vertebral Disc**			
4 **Cervicothoracic Vertebral Joint**			
Cervicothoracic facet joint			
5 **Cervicothoracic Vertebral Disc**			
6 **Thoracic Vertebral Joint**			
Costotransverse joint			
Costovertebral joint			
Thoracic facet joint			
9 **Thoracic Vertebral Disc**			
A **Thoracolumbar Vertebral Joint**			
Thoracolumbar facet joint			
B **Thoracolumbar Vertebral Disc**			
C **Temporomandibular Joint, Right**			
D **Temporomandibular Joint, Left**			
E **Sternoclavicular Joint, Right**			
F **Sternoclavicular Joint, Left**			
G **Acromioclavicular Joint, Right**			
H **Acromioclavicular Joint, Left**			
J **Shoulder Joint, Right**			
Glenohumeral joint			
Glenoid ligament (labrum)			
K **Shoulder Joint, Left**			
See J Shoulder Joint, Right			
L **Elbow Joint, Right**			
Distal humerus, involving joint			
Humeroradial joint			
Humeroulnar joint			
Proximal radioulnar joint			
M **Elbow Joint, Left**			
See L Elbow Joint, Right			
N **Wrist Joint, Right**			
Distal radioulnar joint			
Radiocarpal joint			
P **Wrist Joint, Left**			
See N Wrist Joint, Right			
Q **Carpal Joint, Right**			
Intercarpal joint			
Midcarpal joint			
R **Carpal Joint, Left**			
See Q Carpal Joint, Right			
S **Carpometacarpal Joint, Right**			
T **Carpometacarpal Joint, Left**			
U **Metacarpophalangeal Joint, Right**			
V **Metacarpophalangeal Joint, Left**			
W **Finger Phalangeal Joint, Right**			
Interphalangeal (IP) joint			
X **Finger Phalangeal Joint, Left**			
See W Finger Phalangeal Joint, Right			

Non-OR   ØRB[Ø,1,3,4,5,6,9,A,B,E,F,G,H,J,K,L,M,N,P,Q,R,S,T,U,V,W,X][Ø,3,4]ZX

NC Noncovered Procedure   **LC** Limited Coverage   **QA** Questionable OB Admit   **NT** New Tech Add-on   ✚ Combination Member   ♂Male   ♀Female

ICD-10-PCS 2023   585

ØRB–ØRB

Upper Joints

Ø **Medical and Surgical**
R **Upper Joints**
C **Extirpation**　　Definition: Taking or cutting out solid matter from a body part

Explanation: The solid matter may be an abnormal byproduct of a biological function or a foreign body; it may be imbedded in a body part or in the lumen of a tubular body part. The solid matter may or may not have been previously broken into pieces.

Body Part Character 4	Approach Character 5	Device Character 6	Qualifier Character 7
Ø Occipital-cervical Joint	Ø Open	Z No Device	Z No Qualifier
1 Cervical Vertebral Joint	3 Percutaneous		
Atlantoaxial joint	4 Percutaneous Endoscopic		
Cervical facet joint			
3 Cervical Vertebral Disc			
4 Cervicothoracic Vertebral Joint			
Cervicothoracic facet joint			
5 Cervicothoracic Vertebral Disc			
6 Thoracic Vertebral Joint			
Costotransverse joint			
Costovertebral joint			
Thoracic facet joint			
9 Thoracic Vertebral Disc			
A Thoracolumbar Vertebral Joint			
Thoracolumbar facet joint			
B Thoracolumbar Vertebral Disc			
C Temporomandibular Joint, Right			
D Temporomandibular Joint, Left			
E Sternoclavicular Joint, Right			
F Sternoclavicular Joint, Left			
G Acromioclavicular Joint, Right			
H Acromioclavicular Joint, Left			
J Shoulder Joint, Right			
Glenohumeral joint			
Glenoid ligament (labrum)			
K Shoulder Joint, Left			
See J Shoulder Joint, Right			
L Elbow Joint, Right			
Distal humerus, involving joint			
Humeroradial joint			
Humeroulnar joint			
Proximal radioulnar joint			
M Elbow Joint, Left			
See L Elbow Joint, Right			
N Wrist Joint, Right			
Distal radioulnar joint			
Radiocarpal joint			
P Wrist Joint, Left			
See N Wrist Joint, Right			
Q Carpal Joint, Right			
Intercarpal joint			
Midcarpal joint			
R Carpal Joint, Left			
See Q Carpal Joint, Right			
S Carpometacarpal Joint, Right			
T Carpometacarpal Joint, Left			
U Metacarpophalangeal Joint, Right			
V Metacarpophalangeal Joint, Left			
W Finger Phalangeal Joint, Right			
Interphalangeal (IP) joint			
X Finger Phalangeal Joint, Left			
See W Finger Phalangeal Joint, Right			

Non-OR Procedure　　DRG Non-OR Procedure　　Valid OR Procedure　　HAC Associated Procedure　　Combination Only　　New/Revised April　　New/Revised October

586　　　　　　　　　　　　　　　　　　　　　　　　　　　　　　　　　　　　　　ICD-10-PCS 2023

Ø	Medical and Surgical
R	Upper Joints
G	Fusion

Definition: Joining together portions of an articular body part rendering the articular body part immobile

Explanation: The body part is joined together by fixation device, bone graft, or other means

Body Part — Character 4	Approach — Character 5	Device — Character 6	Qualifier — Character 7
Ø **Occipital-cervical Joint** **1** **Cervical Vertebral Joint** Atlantoaxial joint Cervical facet joint **2** **Cervical Vertebral Joints, 2 or more** Cervical facet joint **4** **Cervicothoracic Vertebral Joint** Cervicothoracic facet joint **6** **Thoracic Vertebral Joint** Costotransverse joint Costovertebral joint Thoracic facet joint **7** **Thoracic Vertebral Joints, 2 to 7** ⊞ **8** **Thoracic Vertebral Joints, 8 or more** **A** **Thoracolumbar Vertebral Joint** Thoracolumbar facet joint	**Ø** Open **3** Percutaneous **4** Percutaneous Endoscopic	**7** Autologous Tissue Substitute **J** Synthetic Substitute **K** Nonautologous Tissue Substitute	**Ø** Anterior Approach, Anterior Column **1** Posterior Approach, Posterior Column **J** Posterior Approach, Anterior Column
Ø **Occipital-cervical Joint** **1** **Cervical Vertebral Joint** Atlantoaxial joint Cervical facet joint **2** **Cervical Vertebral Joints, 2 or more** Cervical facet joint **4** **Cervicothoracic Vertebral Joint** Cervicothoracic facet joint **6** **Thoracic Vertebral Joint** Costotransverse joint Costovertebral joint Thoracic facet joint **7** **Thoracic Vertebral Joints, 2 to 7** ⊞ **8** **Thoracic Vertebral Joints, 8 or more** **A** **Thoracolumbar Vertebral Joint** Thoracolumbar facet joint	**Ø** Open **3** Percutaneous **4** Percutaneous Endoscopic	**A** Interbody Fusion Device	**Ø** Anterior Approach, Anterior Column **J** Posterior Approach, Anterior Column
C **Temporomandibular Joint, Right** **D** **Temporomandibular Joint, Left** **E** **Sternoclavicular Joint, Right** **F** **Sternoclavicular Joint, Left** **G** **Acromioclavicular Joint, Right** **H** **Acromioclavicular Joint, Left** **J** **Shoulder Joint, Right** Glenohumeral joint Glenoid ligament (labrum) **K** **Shoulder Joint, Left** *See J Shoulder Joint, Right*	**Ø** Open **3** Percutaneous **4** Percutaneous Endoscopic	**4** Internal Fixation Device **7** Autologous Tissue Substitute **J** Synthetic Substitute **K** Nonautologous Tissue Substitute	**Z** No Qualifier
L **Elbow Joint, Right** Distal humerus, involving joint Humeroradial joint Humeroulnar joint Proximal radioulnar joint **M** **Elbow Joint, Left** *See L Elbow Joint, Right* **N** **Wrist Joint, Right** Distal radioulnar joint Radiocarpal joint **P** **Wrist Joint, Left** *See N Wrist Joint, Right* **Q** **Carpal Joint, Right** Intercarpal joint Midcarpal joint **R** **Carpal Joint, Left** *See Q Carpal Joint, Right* **S** **Carpometacarpal Joint, Right** **T** **Carpometacarpal Joint, Left** **U** **Metacarpophalangeal Joint, Right** **V** **Metacarpophalangeal Joint, Left** **W** **Finger Phalangeal Joint, Right** Interphalangeal (IP) joint **X** **Finger Phalangeal Joint, Left** *See W Finger Phalangeal Joint, Right*	**Ø** Open **3** Percutaneous **4** Percutaneous Endoscopic	**3** Internal Fixation Device, Sustained Compression **4** Internal Fixation Device **5** External Fixation Device **7** Autologous Tissue Substitute **J** Synthetic Substitute **K** Nonautologous Tissue Substitute	**Z** No Qualifier

HAC	ØRG[Ø,1,2,4,6,7,8,A][Ø,3,4][7,J,K][Ø,1,J] when reported with SDx K68.11 or T81.4Ø–T81.49, T84.6Ø-T84.619, T84.63-T84.7 with 7th character A
HAC	ØRG[Ø,1,2,4,6,7,8,A][Ø,3,4]A[Ø,J] when reported with SDx K68.11 or T81.4Ø–T81.49, T84.6Ø-T84.619, T84.63-T84.7 with 7th character A
HAC	ØRG[E,F,G,H,J,K][Ø,3,4][4,7,J,K]Z when reported with SDx K68.11 or T81.4Ø–T81.49, T84.6Ø-T84.619, T84.63-T84.7 with 7th character A
HAC	ØRG[L,M][Ø,3,4][3,4,5,7,J,K]Z when reported with SDx K68.11 or T81.4Ø–T81.49, T84.6Ø-T84.619, T84.63-T84.7 with 7th character A

See Appendix L for Procedure Combinations
⊞ ØRG7[Ø,3,4][7,J,K][Ø,1,J]
⊞ ØRG7[Ø,3,4]A[Ø,J]

NC Noncovered Procedure　　**LC** Limited Coverage　　**QA** Questionable OB Admit　　**NT** New Tech Add-on　　⊞ Combination Member　　♂ Male　　♀ Female

ICD-10-PCS 2023　　　　　　　　　　　　　　　　　　　　　　　　　　　　587

ØRG–ØRG

Upper Joints

Ø   **Medical and Surgical**
R   **Upper Joints**
H   **Insertion**   Definition: Putting in a nonbiological appliance that monitors, assists, performs, or prevents a physiological function but does not physically take the place of a body part
               Explanation: None

Body Part Character 4	Approach Character 5	Device Character 6	Qualifier Character 7

Ø Occipital-cervical Joint
1 Cervical Vertebral Joint
   Atlantoaxial joint
   Cervical facet joint
4 Cervicothoracic Vertebral Joint
   Cervicothoracic facet joint
6 Thoracic Vertebral Joint
   Costotransverse joint
   Costovertebral joint
   Thoracic facet joint
A Thoracolumbar Vertebral Joint
   Thoracolumbar facet joint
	Ø Open
	3 Percutaneous
	4 Percutaneous Endoscopic
		3 Infusion Device
		4 Internal Fixation Device
		8 Spacer
		B Spinal Stabilization Device,
		   Interspinous Process
		C Spinal Stabilization Device,
		   Pedicle-Based
		D Spinal Stabilization Device,
		   Facet Replacement
			Z No Qualifier

3 Cervical Vertebral Disc **5** Cervicothoracic Vertebral Disc **9** Thoracic Vertebral Disc **B** Thoracolumbar Vertebral Disc	**Ø** Open **3** Percutaneous **4** Percutaneous Endoscopic	**3** Infusion Device	**Z** No Qualifier

C Temporomandibular Joint, Right
D Temporomandibular Joint, Left
E Sternoclavicular Joint, Right
F Sternoclavicular Joint, Left
G Acromioclavicular Joint, Right
H Acromioclavicular Joint, Left
J Shoulder Joint, Right
   Glenohumeral joint
   Glenoid ligament (labrum)
K Shoulder Joint, Left
   See J Shoulder Joint, Right
	Ø Open
	3 Percutaneous
	4 Percutaneous Endoscopic
		3 Infusion Device
		4 Internal Fixation Device
		8 Spacer
			Z No Qualifier

L Elbow Joint, Right
   Distal humerus, involving joint
   Humeroradial joint
   Humeroulnar joint
   Proximal radioulnar joint
M Elbow Joint, Left
   See L Elbow Joint, Right
N Wrist Joint, Right
   Distal radioulnar joint
   Radiocarpal joint
P Wrist Joint, Left
   See N Wrist Joint, Right
Q Carpal Joint, Right
   Intercarpal joint
   Midcarpal joint
R Carpal Joint, Left
   See Q Carpal Joint, Right
S Carpometacarpal Joint, Right
T Carpometacarpal Joint, Left
U Metacarpophalangeal Joint, Right
V Metacarpophalangeal Joint, Left
W Finger Phalangeal Joint, Right
   Interphalangeal (IP) joint
X Finger Phalangeal Joint, Left
   See W Finger Phalangeal Joint, Right
	Ø Open
	3 Percutaneous
	4 Percutaneous Endoscopic
		3 Infusion Device
		4 Internal Fixation Device
		5 External Fixation Device
		8 Spacer
			Z No Qualifier

Non-OR	ØRH[Ø,1,4,6,A][Ø,3,4][3,8]Z
Non-OR	ØRH[3,5,9,B][Ø,3,4]3Z
Non-OR	ØRH[C,D][Ø,4]8Z
Non-OR	ØRH[C,D]3[3,8]Z
Non-OR	ØRH[E,F,G,H][Ø,3,4][3,8]Z
Non-OR	ØRH[J,K][Ø,3,4]3Z
Non-OR	ØRH[J,K]38Z
Non-OR	ØRH[L,M,N,P,Q,R,S,T,U,V,W,X][Ø,3,4][3,8]Z

Non-OR Procedure   DRG Non-OR Procedure   Valid OR Procedure   HAC Associated Procedure   Combination Only   New/Revised April   New/Revised October

588   ICD-10-PCS 2023

Ø   Medical and Surgical
R   Upper Joints
J   Inspection   Definition: Visually and/or manually exploring a body part

Explanation: Visual exploration may be performed with or without optical instrumentation. Manual exploration may be performed directly or through intervening body layers.

Body Part Character 4	Approach Character 5	Device Character 6	Qualifier Character 7
Ø Occipital-cervical Joint	**Ø Open**	**Z No Device**	**Z No Qualifier**
1 Cervical Vertebral Joint	**3 Percutaneous**		
Atlantoaxial joint	**4 Percutaneous Endoscopic**		
Cervical facet joint	**X External**		
3 Cervical Vertebral Disc			
4 Cervicothoracic Vertebral Joint			
Cervicothoracic facet joint			
5 Cervicothoracic Vertebral Disc			
6 Thoracic Vertebral Joint			
Costotransverse joint			
Costovertebral joint			
Thoracic facet joint			
9 Thoracic Vertebral Disc			
A Thoracolumbar Vertebral Joint			
Thoracolumbar facet joint			
B Thoracolumbar Vertebral Disc			
C Temporomandibular Joint, Right			
D Temporomandibular Joint, Left			
E Sternoclavicular Joint, Right			
F Sternoclavicular Joint, Left			
G Acromioclavicular Joint, Right			
H Acromioclavicular Joint, Left			
J Shoulder Joint, Right			
Glenohumeral joint			
Glenoid ligament (labrum)			
K Shoulder Joint, Left			
See J Shoulder Joint, Right			
L Elbow Joint, Right			
Distal humerus, involving joint			
Humeroradial joint			
Humeroulnar joint			
Proximal radioulnar joint			
M Elbow Joint, Left			
See L Elbow Joint, Right			
N Wrist Joint, Right			
Distal radioulnar joint			
Radiocarpal joint			
P Wrist Joint, Left			
See N Wrist Joint, Right			
Q Carpal Joint, Right			
Intercarpal joint			
Midcarpal joint			
R Carpal Joint, Left			
See Q Carpal Joint, Right			
S Carpometacarpal Joint, Right			
T Carpometacarpal Joint, Left			
U Metacarpophalangeal Joint, Right			
V Metacarpophalangeal Joint, Left			
W Finger Phalangeal Joint, Right			
Interphalangeal (IP) joint			
X Finger Phalangeal Joint, Left			
See W Finger Phalangeal Joint, Right			

Non-OR   ØRJ[Ø,1,3,4,5,6,9,A,B,C,D,E,F,G,H,J,K,L,M,N,P,Q,R,S,T,U,V,W,X][3,X]ZZ

NC Noncovered Procedure   LC Limited Coverage   QA Questionable OB Admit   NT New Tech Add-on   ⊞ Combination Member   ♂ Male   ♀ Female

ICD-10-PCS 2023   589

ØRJ–ØRJ

Ø   Medical and Surgical
R   Upper Joints
N   Release   Definition: Freeing a body part from an abnormal physical constraint by cutting or by the use of force
                    Explanation: Some of the restraining tissue may be taken out but none of the body part is taken out

Body Part Character 4	Approach Character 5	Device Character 6	Qualifier Character 7
Ø Occipital-cervical Joint	**Ø** Open	**Z** No Device	**Z** No Qualifier
1 Cervical Vertebral Joint	**3** Percutaneous		
Atlantoaxial joint	**4** Percutaneous Endoscopic		
Cervical facet joint	**X** External		
3 Cervical Vertebral Disc			
4 Cervicothoracic Vertebral Joint			
Cervicothoracic facet joint			
5 Cervicothoracic Vertebral Disc			
6 Thoracic Vertebral Joint			
Costotransverse joint			
Costovertebral joint			
Thoracic facet joint			
9 Thoracic Vertebral Disc			
A Thoracolumbar Vertebral Joint			
Thoracolumbar facet joint			
B Thoracolumbar Vertebral Disc			
C Temporomandibular Joint, Right			
D Temporomandibular Joint, Left			
E Sternoclavicular Joint, Right			
F Sternoclavicular Joint, Left			
G Acromioclavicular Joint, Right			
H Acromioclavicular Joint, Left			
J Shoulder Joint, Right			
Glenohumeral joint			
Glenoid ligament (labrum)			
K Shoulder Joint, Left			
See J Shoulder Joint, Right			
L Elbow Joint, Right			
Distal humerus, involving joint			
Humeroradial joint			
Humeroulnar joint			
Proximal radioulnar joint			
M Elbow Joint, Left			
See L Elbow Joint, Right			
N Wrist Joint, Right			
Distal radioulnar joint			
Radiocarpal joint			
P Wrist Joint, Left			
See N Wrist Joint, Right			
Q Carpal Joint, Right			
Intercarpal joint			
Midcarpal joint			
R Carpal Joint, Left			
See Q Carpal Joint, Right			
S Carpometacarpal Joint, Right			
T Carpometacarpal Joint, Left			
U Metacarpophalangeal Joint, Right			
V Metacarpophalangeal Joint, Left			
W Finger Phalangeal Joint, Right			
Interphalangeal (IP) joint			
X Finger Phalangeal Joint, Left			
See W Finger Phalangeal Joint, Right			

Non-OR   ØRN[Ø,1,3,4,5,6,9,A,B,C,D,E,F,G,H,J,K,L,M,N,P,Q,R,S,T,U,V,W,X]XZZ

Ø   **Medical and Surgical**
R   **Upper Joints**
P   **Removal**   Definition: Taking out or off a device from a body part

Explanation: If a device is taken out and a similar device put in without cutting or puncturing the skin or mucous membrane, the procedure is coded to the root operation CHANGE. Otherwise, the procedure for taking out the device is coded to the root operation REMOVAL.

Body Part Character 4	Approach Character 5	Device Character 6	Qualifier Character 7

Ø   Occipital-cervical Joint
1   Cervical Vertebral Joint
    Atlantoaxial joint
    Cervical facet joint
4   Cervicothoracic Vertebral Joint
    Cervicothoracic facet joint
6   Thoracic Vertebral Joint
    Costotransverse joint
    Costovertebral joint
    Thoracic facet joint
A   Thoracolumbar Vertebral Joint
    Thoracolumbar facet joint
	Ø Open
	3 Percutaneous
	4 Percutaneous Endoscopic
		Ø Drainage Device
		3 Infusion Device
		4 Internal Fixation Device
		7 Autologous Tissue Substitute
		8 Spacer
		A Interbody Fusion Device
		J Synthetic Substitute
		K Nonautologous Tissue Substitute
			Z No Qualifier

Ø   Occipital-cervical Joint
1   Cervical Vertebral Joint
    Atlantoaxial joint
    Cervical facet joint
4   Cervicothoracic Vertebral Joint
    Cervicothoracic facet joint
6   Thoracic Vertebral Joint
    Costotransverse joint
    Costovertebral joint
    Thoracic facet joint
A   Thoracolumbar Vertebral Joint
    Thoracolumbar facet joint
	X External	Ø Drainage Device
		3 Infusion Device
		4 Internal Fixation Device
			Z No Qualifier

3 Cervical Vertebral Disc 5 Cervicothoracic Vertebral Disc 9 Thoracic Vertebral Disc B Thoracolumbar Vertebral Disc	Ø Open 3 Percutaneous 4 Percutaneous Endoscopic	Ø Drainage Device 3 Infusion Device 7 Autologous Tissue Substitute J Synthetic Substitute K Nonautologous Tissue Substitute	Z No Qualifier
3 Cervical Vertebral Disc 5 Cervicothoracic Vertebral Disc 9 Thoracic Vertebral Disc B Thoracolumbar Vertebral Disc	X External	Ø Drainage Device 3 Infusion Device	Z No Qualifier
C Temporomandibular Joint, Right D Temporomandibular Joint, Left E Sternoclavicular Joint, Right F Sternoclavicular Joint, Left G Acromioclavicular Joint, Right H Acromioclavicular Joint, Left	Ø Open 3 Percutaneous 4 Percutaneous Endoscopic	Ø Drainage Device 3 Infusion Device 4 Internal Fixation Device 7 Autologous Tissue Substitute 8 Spacer J Synthetic Substitute K Nonautologous Tissue Substitute	Z No Qualifier
C Temporomandibular Joint, Right D Temporomandibular Joint, Left E Sternoclavicular Joint, Right F Sternoclavicular Joint, Left G Acromioclavicular Joint, Right H Acromioclavicular Joint, Left	X External	Ø Drainage Device 3 Infusion Device 4 Internal Fixation Device	Z No Qualifier

J   Shoulder Joint, Right
    Glenohumeral joint
    Glenoid ligament (labrum)
K   Shoulder Joint, Left
    See J Shoulder Joint, Right
	Ø Open
	3 Percutaneous
	4 Percutaneous Endoscopic
		Ø Drainage Device
		3 Infusion Device
		4 Internal Fixation Device
		7 Autologous Tissue Substitute
		8 Spacer
		K Nonautologous Tissue Substitute
			Z No Qualifier

J   Shoulder Joint, Right
    Glenohumeral joint
    Glenoid ligament (labrum)
K   Shoulder Joint, Left
    See J Shoulder Joint, Right
	Ø Open
	3 Percutaneous
	4 Percutaneous Endoscopic
		J Synthetic Substitute	6 Humeral Surface
			7 Glenoid Surface
			Z No Qualifier

J   Shoulder Joint, Right
    Glenohumeral joint
    Glenoid ligament (labrum)
K   Shoulder Joint, Left
    See J Shoulder Joint, Right
	X External	Ø Drainage Device
		3 Infusion Device
		4 Internal Fixation Device
			Z No Qualifier

Non-OR ØRP[Ø,1,4,6,A]3[Ø,3,8]Z	**Non-OR** ØRP[C,D,E,F,G,H][Ø,4]8Z
Non-OR ØRP[Ø,1,4,6,A][Ø,4]8Z	**Non-OR** ØRP[C,D]X[Ø,3]Z
Non-OR ØRP[Ø,1,4,6,A]X[Ø,3,4]Z	**Non-OR** ØRP[E,F,G,H,J,K]X[Ø,3,4]Z
Non-OR ØRP[3,5,9,B]3[Ø,3]Z	**Non-OR** ØRP[J,K]3[Ø,3,8]Z
Non-OR ØRP[3,5,9,B]X[Ø,3]Z	**Non-OR** ØRP[J,K]X[Ø,3,4]Z
Non-OR ØRP[C,D,E,F,G,H]3[Ø,3,8]Z	

ØRP Continued on next page

NC Noncovered Procedure   **LC** Limited Coverage   **QA** Questionable OB Admit   **NT** New Tech Add-on   ⊞ Combination Member   ♂ Male   ♀ Female

Upper Joints

Ø   **Medical and Surgical**   *ØRP Continued*
R   **Upper Joints**
P   **Removal**   Definition: Taking out or off a device from a body part

            Explanation: If a device is taken out and a similar device put in without cutting or puncturing the skin or mucous membrane, the procedure is coded to the root operation CHANGE. Otherwise, the procedure for taking out the device is coded to the root operation REMOVAL.

Body Part Character 4	Approach Character 5	Device Character 6	Qualifier Character 7

L   Elbow Joint, Right
    Distal humerus, involving joint
    Humeroradial joint
    Humeroulnar joint
    Proximal radioulnar joint
M   Elbow Joint, Left
    See L Elbow Joint, Right
N   Wrist Joint, Right
    Distal radioulnar joint
    Radiocarpal joint
P   Wrist Joint, Left
    See N Wrist Joint, Right
Q   Carpal Joint, Right
    Intercarpal joint
    Midcarpal joint
R   Carpal Joint, Left
    See Q Carpal Joint, Right
S   Carpometacarpal Joint, Right
T   Carpometacarpal Joint, Left
U   Metacarpophalangeal Joint, Right
V   Metacarpophalangeal Joint, Left
W   Finger Phalangeal Joint, Right
    Interphalangeal (IP) joint
X   Finger Phalangeal Joint, Left
    See W Finger Phalangeal Joint, Right
	Ø Open
	3 Percutaneous
	4 Percutaneous Endoscopic
		Ø Drainage Device
		3 Infusion Device
		4 Internal Fixation Device
		5 External Fixation Device
		7 Autologous Tissue Substitute
		8 Spacer
		J Synthetic Substitute
		K Nonautologous Tissue Substitute
			Z No Qualifier

L   Elbow Joint, Right
    Distal humerus, involving joint
    Humeroradial joint
    Humeroulnar joint
    Proximal radioulnar joint
M   Elbow Joint, Left
    See L Elbow Joint, Right
N   Wrist Joint, Right
    Distal radioulnar joint
    Radiocarpal joint
P   Wrist Joint, Left
    See N Wrist Joint, Right
Q   Carpal Joint, Right
    Intercarpal joint
    Midcarpal joint
R   Carpal Joint, Left
    See Q Carpal Joint, Right
S   Carpometacarpal Joint, Right
T   Carpometacarpal Joint, Left
U   Metacarpophalangeal Joint, Right
V   Metacarpophalangeal Joint, Left
W   Finger Phalangeal Joint, Right
    Interphalangeal (IP) joint
X   Finger Phalangeal Joint, Left
    See W Finger Phalangeal Joint, Right
	X External	Ø Drainage Device
		3 Infusion Device
		4 Internal Fixation Device
		5 External Fixation Device
			Z No Qualifier

Non-OR	ØRP[L,M,N,P,Q,R,S,T,U,V,W,X]3[Ø,3,8]Z
Non-OR	ØRP[L,M,N,P,Q,R,S,T,U,V,W,X][Ø,4]8Z
Non-OR	ØRP[L,M,N,P,Q,R,S,T,U,V,W,X]X[Ø,3,4,5]Z

Non-OR Procedure   DRG Non-OR Procedure   Valid OR Procedure   HAC Associated Procedure   Combination Only   New/Revised April   New/Revised October

592   ICD-10-PCS 2023

Ø **Medical and Surgical**
R **Upper Joints**
Q **Repair**　　　Definition: Restoring, to the extent possible, a body part to its normal anatomic structure and function
　　　　　　　　　　Explanation: Used only when the method to accomplish the repair is not one of the other root operations

Body Part Character 4	Approach Character 5	Device Character 6	Qualifier Character 7
Ø **Occipital-cervical Joint**	**Ø** Open	**Z** No Device	**Z** No Qualifier
1 **Cervical Vertebral Joint**	**3** Percutaneous		
Atlantoaxial joint	**4** Percutaneous Endoscopic		
Cervical facet joint	**X** External		
3 **Cervical Vertebral Disc**			
4 **Cervicothoracic Vertebral Joint**			
Cervicothoracic facet joint			
5 **Cervicothoracic Vertebral Disc**			
6 **Thoracic Vertebral Joint**			
Costotransverse joint			
Costovertebral joint			
Thoracic facet joint			
9 **Thoracic Vertebral Disc**			
A **Thoracolumbar Vertebral Joint**			
Thoracolumbar facet joint			
B **Thoracolumbar Vertebral Disc**			
C **Temporomandibular Joint, Right**			
D **Temporomandibular Joint, Left**			
E **Sternoclavicular Joint, Right**			
F **Sternoclavicular Joint, Left**			
G **Acromioclavicular Joint, Right**			
H **Acromioclavicular Joint, Left**			
J **Shoulder Joint, Right**			
Glenohumeral joint			
Glenoid ligament (labrum)			
K **Shoulder Joint, Left**			
See J Shoulder Joint, Right			
L **Elbow Joint, Right**			
Distal humerus, involving joint			
Humeroradial joint			
Humeroulnar joint			
Proximal radioulnar joint			
M **Elbow Joint, Left**			
See L Elbow Joint, Right			
N **Wrist Joint, Right**			
Distal radioulnar joint			
Radiocarpal joint			
P **Wrist Joint, Left**			
See N Wrist Joint, Right			
Q **Carpal Joint, Right**			
Intercarpal joint			
Midcarpal joint			
R **Carpal Joint, Left**			
See Q Carpal Joint, Right			
S **Carpometacarpal Joint, Right**			
T **Carpometacarpal Joint, Left**			
U **Metacarpophalangeal Joint, Right**			
V **Metacarpophalangeal Joint, Left**			
W **Finger Phalangeal Joint, Right**			
Interphalangeal (IP) joint			
X **Finger Phalangeal Joint, Left**			
See W Finger Phalangeal Joint, Right			

Non-OR　ØRQ[Ø,1,3,4,5,6,9,A,B,C,D,E,F,G,H,J,K,L,M,N,P,Q,R,S,T,U,V,W,X]XZZ
HAC　　ØRQ[E,F,G,H,J,K,L,M][Ø,3,4]ZZ when reported with SDx K68.11 or T81.4Ø–T81.49, T84.6Ø-T84.619, T84.63-T84.7 with 7th character A

NC Noncovered Procedure　**LC** Limited Coverage　**QA** Questionable OB Admit　**NT** New Tech Add-on　⊞ Combination Member　♂ Male　♀ Female
ICD-10-PCS 2023　　　　　　　　　　　　　　　　　　　　　　　　　　　　　　　　　　　　　　593

ØRQ–ØRQ

Ø　Medical and Surgical
R　Upper Joints
R　Replacement　　Definition: Putting in or on biological or synthetic material that physically takes the place and/or function of all or a portion of a body part

Explanation: The body part may have been taken out or replaced, or may be taken out, physically eradicated, or rendered nonfunctional during the REPLACEMENT procedure. A REMOVAL procedure is coded for taking out the device used in a previous replacement procedure.

Body Part Character 4	Approach Character 5	Device Character 6	Qualifier Character 7
Ø **Occipital-cervical Joint** **1** **Cervical Vertebral Joint** 　Atlantoaxial joint 　Cervical facet joint **3** **Cervical Vertebral Disc** **4** **Cervicothoracic Vertebral Joint** 　Cervicothoracic facet joint **5** **Cervicothoracic Vertebral Disc** **6** **Thoracic Vertebral Joint** 　Costotransverse joint 　Costovertebral joint 　Thoracic facet joint **9** **Thoracic Vertebral Disc** **A** **Thoracolumbar Vertebral Joint** 　Thoracolumbar facet joint **B** **Thoracolumbar Vertebral Disc** **C** **Temporomandibular Joint, Right** **D** **Temporomandibular Joint, Left** **E** **Sternoclavicular Joint, Right** **F** **Sternoclavicular Joint, Left** **G** **Acromioclavicular Joint, Right** **H** **Acromioclavicular Joint, Left** **L** **Elbow Joint, Right** 　Distal humerus, involving joint 　Humeroradial joint 　Humeroulnar joint 　Proximal radioulnar joint **M** **Elbow Joint, Left** 　*See L Elbow Joint, Right* **N** **Wrist Joint, Right** 　Distal radioulnar joint 　Radiocarpal joint **P** **Wrist Joint, Left** 　*See N Wrist Joint, Right* **Q** **Carpal Joint, Right** 　Intercarpal joint 　Midcarpal joint **R** **Carpal Joint, Left** 　*See Q Carpal Joint, Right* **S** **Carpometacarpal Joint, Right** **T** **Carpometacarpal Joint, Left** **U** **Metacarpophalangeal Joint, Right** **V** **Metacarpophalangeal Joint, Left** **W** **Finger Phalangeal Joint, Right** 　Interphalangeal (IP) joint **X** **Finger Phalangeal Joint, Left** 　*See W Finger Phalangeal Joint, Right*	**Ø** Open	**7** Autologous Tissue 　Substitute **J** Synthetic Substitute **K** Nonautologous Tissue 　Substitute	**Z** No Qualifier
J **Shoulder Joint, Right** 　Glenohumeral joint 　Glenoid ligament (labrum) **K** **Shoulder Joint, Left** 　*See J Shoulder Joint, Right*	**Ø** Open	**Ø** Synthetic Substitute, 　Reverse Ball and Socket **7** Autologous Tissue 　Substitute **K** Nonautologous Tissue 　Substitute	**Z** No Qualifier
J **Shoulder Joint, Right** 　Glenohumeral joint 　Glenoid ligament (labrum) **K** **Shoulder Joint, Left** 　*See J Shoulder Joint, Right*	**Ø** Open	**J** Synthetic Substitute	**6** Humeral Surface **7** Glenoid Surface **Z** No Qualifier

Ø   **Medical and Surgical**
R   **Upper Joints**
S   **Reposition**   Definition: Moving to its normal location, or other suitable location, all or a portion of a body part

Explanation: The body part is moved to a new location from an abnormal location, or from a normal location where it is not functioning correctly. The body part may or may not be cut out or off to be moved to the new location.

Body Part Character 4	Approach Character 5	Device Character 6	Qualifier Character 7

Ø   **Occipital-cervical Joint**
1   **Cervical Vertebral Joint**
     Atlantoaxial joint
     Cervical facet joint
4   **Cervicothoracic Vertebral Joint**
     Cervicothoracic facet joint
6   **Thoracic Vertebral Joint**
     Costotransverse joint
     Costovertebral joint
     Thoracic facet joint
A   **Thoracolumbar Vertebral Joint**
     Thoracolumbar facet Joint
C   **Temporomandibular Joint, Right**
D   **Temporomandibular Joint, Left**
E   **Sternoclavicular Joint, Right**
F   **Sternoclavicular Joint, Left**
G   **Acromioclavicular Joint, Right**
H   **Acromioclavicular Joint, Left**
J   **Shoulder Joint, Right**
     Glenohumeral joint
     Glenoid ligament (labrum)
K   **Shoulder Joint, Left**
     See J Shoulder Joint, Right
	Ø Open
	3 Percutaneous
	4 Percutaneous Endoscopic
	X External
		4 Internal Fixation Device
		Z No Device
			Z No Qualifier

L   **Elbow Joint, Right**
     Distal humerus, involving joint
     Humeroradial joint
     Humeroulnar joint
     Proximal radioulnar joint
M   **Elbow Joint, Left**
     See L Elbow Joint, Right
N   **Wrist Joint, Right**
     Distal radioulnar joint
     Radiocarpal joint
P   **Wrist Joint, Left**
     See N Wrist Joint, Right
Q   **Carpal Joint, Right**
     Intercarpal joint
     Midcarpal joint
R   **Carpal Joint, Left**
     See Q Carpal Joint, Right
S   **Carpometacarpal Joint, Right**
T   **Carpometacarpal Joint, Left**
U   **Metacarpophalangeal Joint, Right**
V   **Metacarpophalangeal Joint, Left**
W   **Finger Phalangeal Joint, Right**
     Interphalangeal (IP) joint
X   **Finger Phalangeal Joint, Left**
     See W Finger Phalangeal Joint, Right
	Ø Open
	3 Percutaneous
	4 Percutaneous Endoscopic
	X External
		4 Internal Fixation Device
		5 External Fixation Device
		Z No Device
			Z No Qualifier

Non-OR   ØRS[Ø,1,4,6,A,C,D,E,F,G,H,J,K][3,4,X][4,Z]Z
Non-OR   ØRS[L,M,N,P,Q,R,S,T,U,V,W,X][3,4,X][4,5,Z]Z

NC Noncovered Procedure   **LC** Limited Coverage   **QA** Questionable OB Admit   **NT** New Tech Add-on   ⊞ Combination Member   ♂ Male   ♀ Female

ICD-10-PCS 2023   595

Upper Joints

Ø   **Medical and Surgical**
R   **Upper Joints**
T   **Resection**   Definition: Cutting out or off, without replacement, all of a body part
                      Explanation: None

Body Part Character 4	Approach Character 5	Device Character 6	Qualifier Character 7
3 **Cervical Vertebral Disc**	**Ø** Open	**Z** No Device	**Z** No Qualifier
4 **Cervicothoracic Vertebral Joint** Cervicothoracic facet joint			
5 **Cervicothoracic Vertebral Disc**			
9 **Thoracic Vertebral Disc**			
B **Thoracolumbar Vertebral Disc**			
C **Temporomandibular Joint, Right**			
D **Temporomandibular Joint, Left**			
E **Sternoclavicular Joint, Right**			
F **Sternoclavicular Joint, Left**			
G **Acromioclavicular Joint, Right**			
H **Acromioclavicular Joint, Left**			

J **Shoulder Joint, Right**
    Glenohumeral joint
    Glenoid ligament (labrum)			

K **Shoulder Joint, Left** *See J Shoulder Joint, Right*			

L **Elbow Joint, Right**
    Distal humerus, involving joint
    Humeroradial joint
    Humeroulnar joint
    Proximal radioulnar joint			

M **Elbow Joint, Left** *See L Elbow Joint, Right*			

N **Wrist Joint, Right**
    Distal radioulnar joint
    Radiocarpal joint			

P **Wrist Joint, Left** *See N Wrist Joint, Right*			

Q **Carpal Joint, Right**
    Intercarpal joint
    Midcarpal joint			

R **Carpal Joint, Left** *See Q Carpal Joint, Right*			
S **Carpometacarpal Joint, Right**			
T **Carpometacarpal Joint, Left**			
U **Metacarpophalangeal Joint, Right**			
V **Metacarpophalangeal Joint, Left**			
W **Finger Phalangeal Joint, Right** Interphalangeal (IP) joint			
X **Finger Phalangeal Joint, Left** *See W Finger Phalangeal Joint, Right*			

Non-OR Procedure   DRG Non-OR Procedure   Valid OR Procedure   HAC Associated Procedure   Combination Only   New/Revised April   New/Revised October

596   ICD-10-PCS 2023

Ø	**Medical and Surgical**
R	**Upper Joints**
U	**Supplement**

Definition: Putting in or on biological or synthetic material that physically reinforces and/or augments the function of a portion of a body part

Explanation: The biological material is non-living, or is living and from the same individual. The body part may have been previously replaced, and the SUPPLEMENT procedure is performed to physically reinforce and/or augment the function of the replaced body part.

Body Part Character 4	Approach Character 5	Device Character 6	Qualifier Character 7
Ø Occipital-cervical Joint	**Ø Open**	**7 Autologous Tissue**	**Z No Qualifier**
1 Cervical Vertebral Joint	**3 Percutaneous**	**Substitute**	
Atlantoaxial joint	**4 Percutaneous Endoscopic**	**J Synthetic Substitute**	
Cervical facet joint		**K Nonautologous Tissue**	
3 Cervical Vertebral Disc		**Substitute**	
4 Cervicothoracic Vertebral Joint			
Cervicothoracic facet joint			
5 Cervicothoracic Vertebral Disc			
6 Thoracic Vertebral Joint			
Costotransverse joint			
Costovertebral joint			
Thoracic facet joint			
9 Thoracic Vertebral Disc			
A Thoracolumbar Vertebral Joint			
Thoracolumbar facet joint			
B Thoracolumbar Vertebral Disc			
C Temporomandibular Joint, Right			
D Temporomandibular Joint, Left			
E Sternoclavicular Joint, Right			
F Sternoclavicular Joint, Left			
G Acromioclavicular Joint, Right			
H Acromioclavicular Joint, Left			
J Shoulder Joint, Right			
Glenohumeral joint			
Glenoid ligament (labrum)			
K Shoulder Joint, Left			
See J Shoulder Joint, Right			
L Elbow Joint, Right			
Distal humerus, involving joint			
Humeroradial joint			
Humeroulnar joint			
Proximal radioulnar joint			
M Elbow Joint, Left			
See L Elbow Joint, Right			
N Wrist Joint, Right			
Distal radioulnar joint			
Radiocarpal joint			
P Wrist Joint, Left			
See N Wrist Joint, Right			
Q Carpal Joint, Right			
Intercarpal joint			
Midcarpal joint			
R Carpal Joint, Left			
See Q Carpal Joint, Right			
S Carpometacarpal Joint, Right			
T Carpometacarpal Joint, Left			
U Metacarpophalangeal Joint, Right			
V Metacarpophalangeal Joint, Left			
W Finger Phalangeal Joint, Right			
Interphalangeal (IP) joint			
X Finger Phalangeal Joint, Left			
See W Finger Phalangeal Joint, Right			

HAC   ØRU[E,F,G,H,J,K,L,M][Ø,3,4][7,J,K]Z when reported with SDx K68.11 or T81.4Ø–T81.49, T84.6Ø-T84.619, T84.63-T84.7 with 7th character A

NC Noncovered Procedure   **LC** Limited Coverage   **QA** Questionable OB Admit   **NT** New Tech Add-on   ⊞ Combination Member   ♂ Male   ♀ Female

ICD-10-PCS 2023   597

Ø Medical and Surgical
R Upper Joints
W Revision

Definition: Correcting, to the extent possible, a portion of a malfunctioning device or the position of a displaced device

Explanation: Revision can include correcting a malfunctioning or displaced device by taking out or putting in components of the device such as a screw or pin

Body Part Character 4	Approach Character 5	Device Character 6	Qualifier Character 7

Ø Occipital-cervical Joint
1 Cervical Vertebral Joint
  Atlantoaxial joint
  Cervical facet joint
4 Cervicothoracic Vertebral Joint
  Cervicothoracic facet joint
6 Thoracic Vertebral Joint
  Costotransverse joint
  Costovertebral joint
  Thoracic facet joint
A Thoracolumbar Vertebral Joint
  Thoracolumbar facet joint
	Ø Open
	3 Percutaneous
	4 Percutaneous Endoscopic
	X External
		Ø Drainage Device
		3 Infusion Device
		4 Internal Fixation Device
		7 Autologous Tissue Substitute
		8 Spacer
		A Interbody Fusion Device
		J Synthetic Substitute
		K Nonautologous Tissue Substitute
			Z No Qualifier

3 Cervical Vertebral Disc 5 Cervicothoracic Vertebral Disc 9 Thoracic Vertebral Disc B Thoracolumbar Vertebral Disc	Ø Open 3 Percutaneous 4 Percutaneous Endoscopic X External	Ø Drainage Device 3 Infusion Device 7 Autologous Tissue Substitute J Synthetic Substitute K Nonautologous Tissue Substitute	Z No Qualifier
C Temporomandibular Joint, Right D Temporomandibular Joint, Left E Sternoclavicular Joint, Right F Sternoclavicular Joint, Left G Acromioclavicular Joint, Right H Acromioclavicular Joint, Left	Ø Open 3 Percutaneous 4 Percutaneous Endoscopic X External	Ø Drainage Device 3 Infusion Device 4 Internal Fixation Device 7 Autologous Tissue Substitute 8 Spacer J Synthetic Substitute K Nonautologous Tissue Substitute	Z No Qualifier

J Shoulder Joint, Right
  Glenohumeral joint
  Glenoid ligament (labrum)
K Shoulder Joint, Left
  See J Shoulder Joint, Right
	Ø Open
	3 Percutaneous
	4 Percutaneous Endoscopic
	X External
		Ø Drainage Device
		3 Infusion Device
		4 Internal Fixation Device
		7 Autologous Tissue Substitute
		8 Spacer
		J Synthetic Substitute
		K Nonautologous Tissue Substitute
			Z No Qualifier

J Shoulder Joint, Right
  Glenohumeral joint
  Glenoid ligament (labrum)
K Shoulder Joint, Left
  See J Shoulder Joint, Right
	Ø Open
	3 Percutaneous
	4 Percutaneous Endoscopic
	X External
		J Synthetic Substitute	6 Humeral Surface
			7 Glenoid Surface
			Z No Qualifier

L Elbow Joint, Right
  Distal humerus, involving joint
  Humeroradial joint
  Humeroulnar joint
  Proximal radioulnar joint
M Elbow Joint, Left
  See L Elbow Joint, Right
N Wrist Joint, Right
  Distal radioulnar joint
  Radiocarpal joint
P Wrist Joint, Left
  See N Wrist Joint, Right
Q Carpal Joint, Right
  Intercarpal joint
  Midcarpal joint
R Carpal Joint, Left
  See Q Carpal Joint, Right
S Carpometacarpal Joint, Right
T Carpometacarpal Joint, Left
U Metacarpophalangeal Joint, Right
V Metacarpophalangeal Joint, Left
W Finger Phalangeal Joint, Right
  Interphalangeal (IP) joint
X Finger Phalangeal Joint, Left
  See W Finger Phalangeal Joint, Right
	Ø Open
	3 Percutaneous
	4 Percutaneous Endoscopic
	X External
		Ø Drainage Device
		3 Infusion Device
		4 Internal Fixation Device
		5 External Fixation Device
		7 Autologous Tissue Substitute
		8 Spacer
		J Synthetic Substitute
		K Nonautologous Tissue Substitute
			Z No Qualifier

Non-OR ØRW[Ø,1,4,6,A]X[Ø,3,4,7,8,A,J,K]Z
Non-OR ØRW[3,5,9,B]X[Ø,3,7,J,K]Z
Non-OR ØRW[C,D,E,F,G,H]X[Ø,3,4,7,8,J,K]Z
Non-OR ØRW[J,K]X[Ø,3,4,7,8,J,K]Z
Non-OR ØRW[J,K]XJ[6,7,Z]
Non-OR ØRW[L,M,N,P,Q,R,S,T,U,V,W,X]X[Ø,3,4,5,7,8,J,K]Z

Non-OR Procedure   DRG Non-OR Procedure   Valid OR Procedure   HAC Associated Procedure   Combination Only   New/Revised April   New/Revised October

Lower Joints ØS2–ØSW

Character Meanings*

This Character Meaning table is provided as a guide to assist the user in the identification of character members that may be found in this section of code tables. It **SHOULD NOT** be used to build a PCS code.

Operation–Character 3	Body Part–Character 4	Approach–Character 5	Device–Character 6	Qualifier–Character 7
2 Change	Ø Lumbar Vertebral Joint	Ø Open	Ø Drainage Device OR Synthetic Substitute, Polyethylene	Ø Anterior Approach, Anterior Column
5 Destruction	1 Lumbar Vertebral Joint, 2 or more	3 Percutaneous	1 Synthetic Substitute, Metal	1 Posterior Approach, Posterior Column
9 Drainage	2 Lumbar Vertebral Disc	4 Percutaneous Endoscopic	2 Synthetic Substitute, Metal on Polyethylene	9 Cemented
B Excision	3 Lumbosacral Joint	X External	3 Infusion Device OR Internal Fixation Device, Sustained Compression OR Synthetic Substitute, Ceramic	A Uncemented
C Extirpation	4 Lumbosacral Disc		4 Internal Fixation Device OR Synthetic Substitute, Ceramic on Polyethylene	C Patellar Surface
G Fusion	5 Sacrococcygeal Joint		5 External Fixation Device	J Posterior Approach, Anterior Column
H Insertion	6 Coccygeal Joint		6 Synthetic Substitute, Oxidized Zirconium on Polyethylene	X Diagnostic
J Inspection	7 Sacroiliac Joint, Right		7 Autologous Tissue Substitute	Z No Qualifier
N Release	8 Sacroiliac Joint, Left		8 Spacer	
P Removal	9 Hip Joint, Right		9 Liner	
Q Repair	A Hip Joint, Acetabular Surface, Right		A Interbody Fusion Device	
R Replacement	B Hip Joint, Left		B Resurfacing Device OR Spinal Stabilization Device, Interspinous Process	
S Reposition	C Knee Joint, Right		C Spinal Stabilization Device, Pedicle-Based	
T Resection	D Knee Joint, Left		D Spinal Stabilization Device, Facet Replacement	
U Supplement	E Hip Joint, Acetabular Surface, Left		E Articulating Spacer	
W Revision	F Ankle Joint, Right		J Synthetic Substitute	
	G Ankle Joint, Left		K Nonautologous Tissue Substitute	
	H Tarsal Joint, Right		L Synthetic Substitute, Unicondylar Medial	
	J Tarsal Joint, Left		M Synthetic Substitute, Unicondylar Lateral	
	K Tarsometatarsal Joint, Right		N Synthetic Substitute, Patellofemoral	
	L Tarsometatarsal Joint, Left		Y Other Device	
	M Metatarsal-Phalangeal Joint, Right		Z No Device	
	N Metatarsal-Phalangeal Joint, Left			
	P Toe Phalangeal Joint, Right			
	Q Toe Phalangeal Joint, Left			
	R Hip Joint, Femoral Surface, Right			
	S Hip Joint, Femoral Surface, Left			
	T Knee Joint, Femoral Surface, Right			
	U Knee Joint, Femoral Surface, Left			
	V Knee Joint, Tibial Surface, Right			
	W Knee Joint, Tibial Surface, Left			
	Y Lower Joint			

* Includes synovial membrane.

AHA Coding Clinic for table ØS9

2018, 2Q, 17	Arthroscopic drainage of knee and nonexcisional debridement
2017, 1Q, 50	Dry aspiration of ankle joint

AHA Coding Clinic for table ØSB

2017, 4Q, 76	Radiolucent porous interbody fusion device
2016, 2Q, 16	Decompressive laminectomy/foraminotomy and lumbar discectomy
2016, 1Q, 20	Metatarsophalangeal joint resection arthroplasty
2015, 1Q, 34	Arthroscopic meniscectomy with debridement and abrasion chondroplasty
2014, 2Q, 6	Posterior lumbar fusion with discectomy

AHA Coding Clinic for table ØSG

2022, 2Q, 23	Sacroiliac joint fusion
2021, 4Q, 67	Posterior dynamic distraction
2021, 3Q, 24	Mid-foot fusion with bone graft
2021, 3Q, 25	Placement of X-Spine Axle Cage
2021, 1Q, 18	Placement of interspinous distraction device (spacer) for decompression
2021, 1Q, 53	Official guidelines for coding and reporting for interbody fusion device B3.10c
2020, 4Q, 56-58	Intramedullary sustained compression joint fusion
2020, 2Q, 27	Spinal fusion with NuVasive® VersaTie®
2020, 1Q, 33	Spinal fusion without use of bone graft
2019, 3Q, 35	Fusion procedures of the spine (guideline B3.10c)
2019, 1Q, 30	Spinal fusion performed at same level as decompressive laminectomy
2018, 4Q, 43	Joint fusion device value
2018, 1Q, 22	Spinal fusion procedures without bone graft
2017, 4Q, 76	Radiolucent porous interbody fusion device
2017, 2Q, 23	Decompression of spinal cord and placement of instrumentation
2014, 3Q, 30	Spinal fusion and fixation instrumentation
2014, 3Q, 36	Lumbar interbody fusion of two vertebral levels
2014, 2Q, 6	Posterior lumbar fusion with discectomy
2013, 3Q, 25	360-degree spinal fusion
2013, 2Q, 39	Ankle fusion, osteotomy, and removal of hardware
2013, 1Q, 21-23	Spinal fusion of thoracic and lumbar vertebrae

AHA Coding Clinic for table ØSH

2021, 3Q, 25	Placement of X-Spine Axle Cage
2021, 1Q, 18	Placement of interspinous distraction device (spacer) for decompression
2017, 2Q, 23	Decompression of spinal cord and placement of instrumentation

AHA Coding Clinic for table ØSJ

2017, 1Q, 50	Dry aspiration of ankle joint

AHA Coding Clinic for table ØSN

2020, 2Q, 26	Arthroscopic manipulation and nonexcisional debridement of knee joint
2019, 1Q, 30	Spinal fusion performed at same level as decompressive laminectomy

AHA Coding Clinic for table ØSP

2021, 3Q, 25	Revision total knee arthroplasty
2021, 1Q, 17	Revision of ankle arthroplasty with placement of tibial insert
2018, 4Q, 43	Articulating spacer for hip and knee joint
2018, 2Q, 16	Exchange of tibial polyethylene component with stabilizing insert (tibial tray)
2017, 4Q, 107	Total ankle replacement versus revision
2016, 4Q, 110-112	Removal and revision of hip and knee devices
2015, 2Q, 18	Total knee revision
2015, 2Q, 19	Revision of femoral head and acetabular liner
2013, 2Q, 39	Ankle fusion, osteotomy, and removal of hardware

AHA Coding Clinic for table ØSQ

2014, 4Q, 25	Femoroacetabular impingement and labral tear with repair

AHA Coding Clinic for table ØSR

2022, 1Q, 39	Provisional total hip arthroplasty
2021, 3Q, 25	Revision total knee arthroplasty
2021, 1Q, 17	Revision of ankle arthroplasty with placement of tibial insert
2020, 3Q, 33	Total hip arthroplasty using dual mobility components
2018, 4Q, 43	Articulating spacer for hip and knee joint
2018, 2Q, 16	Exchange of tibial polyethylene component with stabilizing insert (tibial tray)
2017, 4Q, 38-39	Oxidized zirconium on polyethylene bearing surface
2017, 4Q, 107	Total ankle replacement versus revision
2017, 1Q, 22	Total knee replacement and patellar component
2016, 4Q, 110-111	Partial (unicondylar) knee replacement
2016, 4Q, 111-112	Removal and revision of hip and knee devices
2016, 3Q, 35	Use of cemented versus uncemented qualifier for joint replacement
2015, 3Q, 18	Total hip replacement with acetabular reconstruction
2015, 2Q, 18	Total knee revision
2015, 2Q, 19	Revision of femoral head and acetabular liner

AHA Coding Clinic for table ØSS

2022, 2Q, 22	Ankle distraction procedure
2016, 2Q, 31	Periacetabular ostectomy for repair of congenital hip dysplasia

AHA Coding Clinic for table ØST

2016, 1Q, 20	Metatarsophalangeal joint resection arthroplasty
2014, 4Q, 29	Rotational osteosynthesis

AHA Coding Clinic for table ØSU

2022, 1Q, 47	Matrix-induced autologous chondrocyte implantation
2021, 1Q, 17	Revision of ankle arthroplasty with placement of tibial insert
2018, 2Q, 16	Exchange of tibial polyethylene component with stabilizing insert (tibial tray)
2016, 4Q, 111	Removal and revision of hip and knee devices
2015, 2Q, 19	Revision of femoral head and acetabular liner

AHA Coding Clinic for table ØSW

2017, 4Q, 107	Total ankle replacement versus revision
2016, 4Q, 110-112	Removal and revision of hip and knee devices
2015, 2Q, 18	Total knee revision
2015, 2Q, 19	Revision of femoral head and acetabular liner

Lower Joints

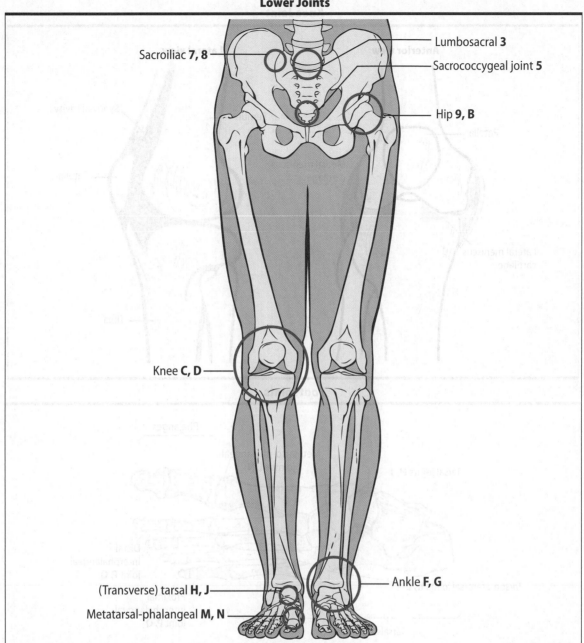

Sacroiliac **7, 8**

Lumbosacral **3**

Sacrococcygeal joint **5**

Hip **9, B**

Knee **C, D**

(Transverse) tarsal **H, J**

Metatarsal-phalangeal **M, N**

Ankle **F, G**

Hip Joint

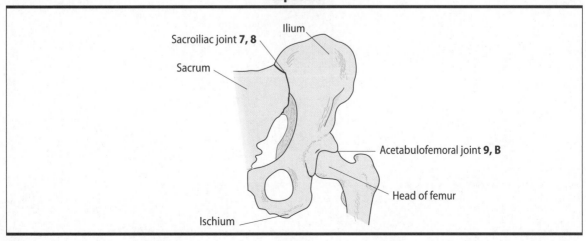

Sacroiliac joint **7, 8**

Ilium

Sacrum

Acetabulofemoral joint **9, B**

Head of femur

Ischium

Knee Joint

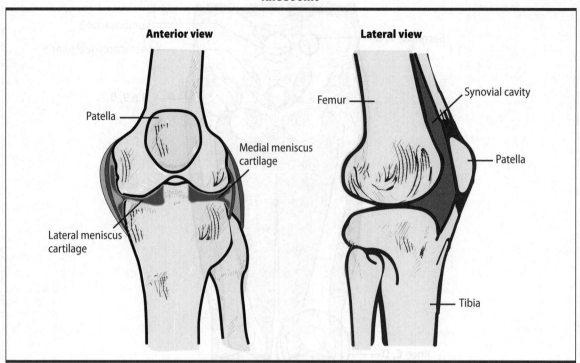

Anterior view

Patella

Medial meniscus cartilage

Lateral meniscus cartilage

Lateral view

Femur

Synovial cavity

Patella

Tibia

Foot Joints

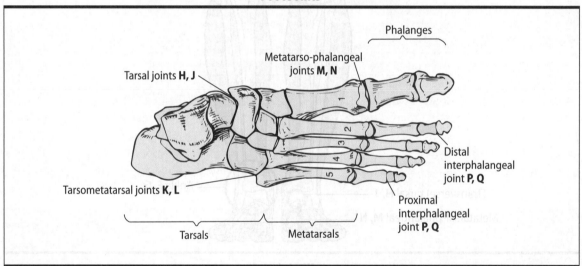

Phalanges

Metatarso-phalangeal joints **M, N**

Tarsal joints **H, J**

Distal interphalangeal joint **P, Q**

Tarsometatarsal joints **K, L**

Proximal interphalangeal joint **P, Q**

Tarsals

Metatarsals

Ø   Medical and Surgical
S   Lower Joints
2   Change   Definition: Taking out or off a device from a body part and putting back an identical or similar device in or on the same body part without cutting or puncturing the skin or a mucous membrane

           Explanation: All CHANGE procedures are coded using the approach EXTERNAL

Body Part Character 4	Approach Character 5	Device Character 6	Qualifier Character 7
Y Lower Joint	X External	Ø Drainage Device Y Other Device	Z No Qualifier

Non-OR	All body part, approach, device, and qualifier values

Ø   Medical and Surgical
S   Lower Joints
5   Destruction   Definition: Physical eradication of all or a portion of a body part by the direct use of energy, force, or a destructive agent

           Explanation: None of the body part is physically taken out

Body Part Character 4	Approach Character 5	Device Character 6	Qualifier Character 7

Ø   **Lumbar Vertebral Joint**
     Lumbar facet joint
2   **Lumbar Vertebral Disc**
3   **Lumbosacral Joint**
     Lumbosacral facet joint
4   **Lumbosacral Disc**
5   **Sacrococcygeal Joint**
     Sacrococcygeal symphysis
6   **Coccygeal Joint**
7   **Sacroiliac Joint, Right**
8   **Sacroiliac Joint, Left**
9   **Hip Joint, Right**
     Acetabulofemoral joint
B   **Hip Joint, Left**
     See 9 Hip Joint, Right
C   **Knee Joint, Right**
     Femoropatellar joint
     Femorotibial joint
     Lateral meniscus
     Medial meniscus
     Patellofemoral joint
     Tibiofemoral joint
D   **Knee Joint, Left**
     See C Knee Joint, Right
F   **Ankle Joint, Right**
     Inferior tibiofibular joint
     Talocrural joint
G   **Ankle Joint, Left**
     See F Ankle Joint, Right
H   **Tarsal Joint, Right**
     Calcaneocuboid joint
     Cuboideonavicular joint
     Cuneonavicular joint
     Intercuneiform joint
     Subtalar (talocalcaneal) joint
     Talocalcaneal (subtalar) joint
     Talocalcaneonavicular joint
J   **Tarsal Joint, Left**
     See H Tarsal Joint, Right
K   **Tarsometatarsal Joint, Right**
L   **Tarsometatarsal Joint, Left**
M   **Metatarsal-Phalangeal Joint, Right**
     Metatarsophalangeal (MTP) joint
N   **Metatarsal-Phalangeal Joint, Left**
     See M Metatarsal-Phalangeal Joint, Right
P   **Toe Phalangeal Joint, Right**
     Interphalangeal (IP) joint
Q   **Toe Phalangeal Joint, Left**
     See P Toe Phalangeal Joint, Right
	Ø Open
	3 Percutaneous
	4 Percutaneous Endoscopic
		Z No Device	Z No Qualifier

NC Noncovered Procedure   LC Limited Coverage   QA Questionable OB Admit   NT New Tech Add-on   ⊞ Combination Member   ♂ Male   ♀ Female

ICD-10-PCS 2023   603

Ø　Medical and Surgical
S　Lower Joints
9　Drainage　　Definition: Taking or letting out fluids and/or gases from a body part

Explanation: The qualifier DIAGNOSTIC is used to identify drainage procedures that are biopsies

Body Part Character 4		Approach Character 5	Device Character 6	Qualifier Character 7
Ø Lumbar Vertebral Joint 　Lumbar facet joint 2 Lumbar Vertebral Disc 3 Lumbosacral Joint 　Lumbosacral facet joint 4 Lumbosacral Disc 5 Sacrococcygeal Joint 　Sacrococcygeal symphysis 6 Coccygeal Joint 7 Sacroiliac Joint, Right 8 Sacroiliac Joint, Left 9 Hip Joint, Right 　Acetabulofemoral joint B Hip Joint, Left 　See 9 Hip Joint, Right C Knee Joint, Right 　Femoropatellar joint 　Femorotibial joint 　Lateral meniscus 　Medial meniscus 　Patellofemoral joint 　Tibiofemoral joint D Knee Joint, Left 　See C Knee Joint, Right F Ankle Joint, Right 　Inferior tibiofibular joint 　Talocrural joint G Ankle Joint, Left 　See F Ankle Joint, Right	H Tarsal Joint, Right 　Calcaneocuboid joint 　Cuboideonavicular joint 　Cuneonavicular joint 　Intercuneiform joint 　Subtalar (talocalcaneal) joint 　Talocalcaneal (subtalar) 　　joint 　Talocalcaneonavicular joint J Tarsal Joint, Left 　See H Tarsal Joint, Right K Tarsometatarsal Joint, 　Right L Tarsometatarsal Joint, Left M Metatarsal-Phalangeal 　Joint, Right 　Metatarsophalangeal (MTP) 　　joint N Metatarsal-Phalangeal 　Joint, Left 　See M Metatarsal-Phalangeal 　　Joint, Right P Toe Phalangeal Joint, Right 　Interphalangeal (IP) joint Q Toe Phalangeal Joint, Left 　See P Toe Phalangeal Joint, 　　Right	Ø Open 3 Percutaneous 4 Percutaneous Endoscopic	Ø Drainage Device	Z No Qualifier
Ø Lumbar Vertebral Joint 　Lumbar facet joint 2 Lumbar Vertebral Disc 3 Lumbosacral Joint 　Lumbosacral facet joint 4 Lumbosacral Disc 5 Sacrococcygeal Joint 　Sacrococcygeal symphysis 6 Coccygeal Joint 7 Sacroiliac Joint, Right 8 Sacroiliac Joint, Left 9 Hip Joint, Right 　Acetabulofemoral joint B Hip Joint, Left 　See 9 Hip Joint, Right C Knee Joint, Right 　Femoropatellar joint 　Femorotibial joint 　Lateral meniscus 　Medial meniscus 　Patellofemoral joint 　Tibiofemoral joint D Knee Joint, Left 　See C Knee Joint, Right F Ankle Joint, Right 　Inferior tibiofibular joint 　Talocrural joint G Ankle Joint, Left 　See F Ankle Joint, Right	H Tarsal Joint, Right 　Calcaneocuboid joint 　Cuboideonavicular joint 　Cuneonavicular joint 　Intercuneiform joint 　Subtalar (talocalcaneal) joint 　Talocalcaneal (subtalar) 　　joint 　Talocalcaneonavicular joint J Tarsal Joint, Left 　See H Tarsal Joint, Right K Tarsometatarsal Joint, 　Right L Tarsometatarsal Joint, Left M Metatarsal-Phalangeal 　Joint, Right 　Metatarsophalangeal (MTP) 　　joint N Metatarsal-Phalangeal 　Joint, Left 　See M Metatarsal-Phalangeal 　　Joint, Right P Toe Phalangeal Joint, Right 　Interphalangeal (IP) joint Q Toe Phalangeal Joint, Left 　See P Toe Phalangeal Joint, 　　Right	Ø Open 3 Percutaneous 4 Percutaneous Endoscopic	Z No Device	X Diagnostic Z No Qualifier

Non-OR　ØS9[Ø,2,3,4,5,6,7,8,9,B,C,D,F,G,H,J,K,L,M,N,P,Q][3,4]ØZ
Non-OR　ØS9[Ø,2,3,4,5,6,7,8,9,B,C,D,F,G,H,J,K,L,M,N,P,Q][Ø,3,4]ZX
Non-OR　ØS9[Ø,2,3,4,5,6,7,8,9,B,C,D,F,G,H,J,K,L,M,N,P,Q][3,4]ZZ

Non-OR Procedure　　DRG Non-OR Procedure　　Valid OR Procedure　　HAC Associated Procedure　　Combination Only　　New/Revised April　　New/Revised October

604　　　　　　　　　　　　　　　　　　　　　　　　　　ICD-10-PCS 2023

ØS9–ØS9

Ø   **Medical and Surgical**
S   **Lower Joints**
B   **Excision**   Definition: Cutting out or off, without replacement, a portion of a body part
                     Explanation: The qualifier DIAGNOSTIC is used to identify excision procedures that are biopsies

Body Part Character 4	Approach Character 5	Device Character 6	Qualifier Character 7

Ø **Lumbar Vertebral Joint**
    Lumbar facet joint
2 **Lumbar Vertebral Disc**
3 **Lumbosacral Joint**
    Lumbosacral facet joint
4 **Lumbosacral Disc**
5 **Sacrococcygeal Joint**
    Sacrococcygeal symphysis
6 **Coccygeal Joint**
7 **Sacroiliac Joint, Right**
8 **Sacroiliac Joint, Left**
9 **Hip Joint, Right**
    Acetabulofemoral joint
B **Hip Joint, Left**
    See 9 Hip Joint, Right
C **Knee Joint, Right**
    Femoropatellar joint
    Femorotibial joint
    Lateral meniscus
    Medial meniscus
    Patellofemoral joint
    Tibiofemoral joint
D **Knee Joint, Left**
    See C Knee Joint, Right
F **Ankle Joint, Right**
    Inferior tibiofibular joint
    Talocrural joint
G **Ankle Joint, Left**
    See F Ankle Joint, Right
H **Tarsal Joint, Right**
    Calcaneocuboid joint
    Cuboideonavicular joint
    Cuneonavicular joint
    Intercuneiform joint
    Subtalar (talocalcaneal) joint
    Talocalcaneal (subtalar) joint
    Talocalcaneonavicular joint
J **Tarsal Joint, Left**
    See H Tarsal Joint, Right
K **Tarsometatarsal Joint, Right**
L **Tarsometatarsal Joint, Left**
M **Metatarsal-Phalangeal Joint, Right**
    Metatarsophalangeal (MTP) joint
N **Metatarsal-Phalangeal Joint, Left**
    See M Metatarsal-Phalangeal Joint, Right
P **Toe Phalangeal Joint, Right**
    Interphalangeal (IP) joint
Q **Toe Phalangeal Joint, Left**
    See P Toe Phalangeal Joint, Right
	Ø Open
	3 Percutaneous
	4 Percutaneous Endoscopic
		Z No Device	**X** Diagnostic
			Z No Qualifier

Non-OR   ØSB[Ø,2,3,4,5,6,7,8,9,B,C,D,F,G,H,J,K,L,M,N,P,Q][Ø,3,4]ZX

Ø   Medical and Surgical
S   Lower Joints
C   Extirpation   Definition: Taking or cutting out solid matter from a body part

                Explanation: The solid matter may be an abnormal byproduct of a biological function or a foreign body; it may be imbedded in a body part or in the lumen of a tubular body part. The solid matter may or may not have been previously broken into pieces.

Body Part Character 4	Approach Character 5	Device Character 6	Qualifier Character 7

Ø   **Lumbar Vertebral Joint**
     Lumbar facet joint
2   **Lumbar Vertebral Disc**
3   **Lumbosacral Joint**
     Lumbosacral facet joint
4   **Lumbosacral Disc**
5   **Sacrococcygeal Joint**
     Sacrococcygeal symphysis
6   **Coccygeal Joint**
7   **Sacroiliac Joint, Right**
8   **Sacroiliac Joint, Left**
9   **Hip Joint, Right**
     Acetabulofemoral joint
B   **Hip Joint, Left**
     See 9 Hip Joint, Right
C   **Knee Joint, Right**
     Femoropatellar joint
     Femorotibial joint
     Lateral meniscus
     Medial meniscus
     Patellofemoral joint
     Tibiofemoral joint
D   **Knee Joint, Left**
     See C Knee Joint, Right
F   **Ankle Joint, Right**
     Inferior tibiofibular joint
     Talocrural joint
G   **Ankle Joint, Left**
     See F Ankle Joint, Right
H   **Tarsal Joint, Right**
     Calcaneocuboid joint
     Cuboideonavicular joint
     Cuneonavicular joint
     Intercuneiform joint
     Subtalar (talocalcaneal) joint
     Talocalcaneal (subtalar) joint
     Talocalcaneonavicular joint
J   **Tarsal Joint, Left**
     See H Tarsal Joint, Right
K   **Tarsometatarsal Joint, Right**
L   **Tarsometatarsal Joint, Left**
M   **Metatarsal-Phalangeal Joint, Right**
     Metatarsophalangeal (MTP) joint
N   **Metatarsal-Phalangeal Joint, Left**
     See M Metatarsal-Phalangeal Joint, Right
P   **Toe Phalangeal Joint, Right**
     Interphalangeal (IP) joint
Q   **Toe Phalangeal Joint, Left**
     See P Toe Phalangeal Joint, Right
	Ø Open
	3 Percutaneous
	4 Percutaneous Endoscopic
		Z No Device	**Z** No Qualifier

Non-OR Procedure   DRG Non-OR Procedure   Valid OR Procedure   HAC Associated Procedure   Combination Only   New/Revised April   New/Revised October

606   ICD-10-PCS 2023

Ø Medical and Surgical
S Lower Joints
G Fusion　　Definition: Joining together portions of an articular body part rendering the articular body part immobile
　　　　　　Explanation: The body part is joined together by fixation device, bone graft, or other means

Body Part Character 4	Approach Character 5	Device Character 6	Qualifier Character 7
Ø Lumbar Vertebral Joint 　Lumbar facet joint **1** Lumbar Vertebral Joints, 2 or more ⊞ **3** Lumbosacral Joint 　Lumbosacral facet joint	**Ø** Open **3** Percutaneous **4** Percutaneous Endoscopic	**7** Autologous Tissue Substitute **J** Synthetic Substitute **K** Nonautologous Tissue Substitute	**Ø** Anterior Approach, Anterior Column **1** Posterior Approach, Posterior Column **J** Posterior Approach, Anterior Column
Ø Lumbar Vertebral Joint 　Lumbar facet joint **1** Lumbar Vertebral Joints, 2 or more ⊞ **3** Lumbosacral Joint 　Lumbosacral facet joint	**Ø** Open **3** Percutaneous **4** Percutaneous Endoscopic	**A** Interbody Fusion Device	**Ø** Anterior Approach, Anterior Column **J** Posterior Approach, Anterior Column
5 Sacrococcygeal Joint 　Sacrococcygeal symphysis **6** Coccygeal Joint **7** Sacroiliac Joint, Right **8** Sacroiliac Joint, Left	**Ø** Open **3** Percutaneous **4** Percutaneous Endoscopic	**4** Internal Fixation Device **7** Autologous Tissue Substitute **J** Synthetic Substitute **K** Nonautologous Tissue Substitute	**Z** No Qualifier
9 Hip Joint, Right 　Acetabulofemoral joint **B** Hip Joint, Left 　*See 9 Hip Joint, Right* **C** Knee Joint, Right 　Femoropatellar joint 　Femorotibial joint 　Lateral meniscus 　Medial meniscus 　Patellofemoral joint 　Tibiofemoral joint **D** Knee Joint, Left 　*See C Knee Joint, Right* **F** Ankle Joint, Right 　Inferior tibiofibular joint 　Talocrural joint **G** Ankle Joint, Left 　*See F Ankle Joint, Right* **H** Tarsal Joint, Right 　Calcaneocuboid joint 　Cuboideonavicular joint 　Cuneonavicular joint 　Intercuneiform joint 　Subtalar (talocalcaneal) joint 　Talocalcaneal (subtalar) joint 　Talocalcaneonavicular joint **J** Tarsal Joint, Left 　*See H Tarsal Joint, Right* **K** Tarsometatarsal Joint, Right **L** Tarsometatarsal Joint, Left **M** Metatarsal-Phalangeal Joint, Right 　Metatarsophalangeal (MTP) joint **N** Metatarsal-Phalangeal Joint, Left 　*See M Metatarsal-Phalangeal Joint, Right* **P** Toe Phalangeal Joint, Right 　Interphalangeal (IP) joint **Q** Toe Phalangeal Joint, Left 　*See P Toe Phalangeal Joint, Right*	**Ø** Open **3** Percutaneous **4** Percutaneous Endoscopic	**3** Internal Fixation Device, Sustained Compression **4** Internal Fixation Device **5** External Fixation Device **7** Autologous Tissue Substitute **J** Synthetic Substitute **K** Nonautologous Tissue Substitute	**Z** No Qualifier

HAC　ØSG[Ø,1,3][Ø,3,4][7,J,K][Ø,1,J] when reported with SDx K68.11 or T81.40–T81.49, T84.60-T84.619, T84.63-T84.7 with 7th character A

HAC　ØSG[Ø,1,3][Ø,3,4]A[Ø,J] when reported with SDx K68.11 or T81.40–T81.49, T84.60-T84.619, T84.63-T84.7 with 7th character A

HAC　ØSG[7,8][Ø,3,4][4,7,J,K]Z when reported with SDx K68.11 or T81.40–T81.49, T84.60-T84.619, T84.63-T84.7 with 7th character A

See Appendix L for Procedure Combinations
⊞　ØSG1[Ø,3,4][7,J,K][Ø,1,J]
⊞　ØSG1[Ø,3,4]A[Ø,J]

NC Noncovered Procedure　　LC Limited Coverage　　QA Questionable OB Admit　　NT New Tech Add-on　　⊞ Combination Member　　♂ Male　　♀ Female

ICD-10-PCS 2023　　　　　　　　　　　　　　　　　　　　　　　　　　　　　　　　607

ØSG–ØSG

Ø Medical and Surgical
S Lower Joints
H Insertion　　Definition: Putting in a nonbiological appliance that monitors, assists, performs, or prevents a physiological function but does not physically take the place of a body part

Explanation: None

Body Part Character 4	Approach Character 5	Device Character 6	Qualifier Character 7
Ø Lumbar Vertebral Joint Lumbar facet joint **3 Lumbosacral Joint** Lumbosacral facet joint	**Ø** Open **3** Percutaneous **4** Percutaneous Endoscopic	**3** Infusion Device **4** Internal Fixation Device **8** Spacer **B** Spinal Stabilization Device, Interspinous Process **C** Spinal Stabilization Device, Pedicle-Based **D** Spinal Stabilization Device, Facet Replacement	**Z** No Qualifier
2 Lumbar Vertebral Disc **4 Lumbosacral Disc**	**Ø** Open **3** Percutaneous **4** Percutaneous Endoscopic	**3** Infusion Device **8** Spacer	**Z** No Qualifier
5 Sacrococcygeal Joint Sacrococcygeal symphysis **6 Coccygeal Joint** **7 Sacroiliac Joint, Right** **8 Sacroiliac Joint, Left**	**Ø** Open **3** Percutaneous **4** Percutaneous Endoscopic	**3** Infusion Device **4** Internal Fixation Device **8** Spacer	**Z** No Qualifier
9 Hip Joint, Right Acetabulofemoral joint **B Hip Joint, Left** *See 9 Hip Joint, Right* **C Knee Joint, Right** Femoropatellar joint Femorotibial joint Lateral meniscus Medial meniscus Patellofemoral joint Tibiofemoral joint **D Knee Joint, Left** *See C Knee Joint, Right* **F Ankle Joint, Right** Inferior tibiofibular joint Talocrural joint **G Ankle Joint, Left** *See F Ankle Joint, Right* **H Tarsal Joint, Right** Calcaneocuboid joint Cuboideonavicular joint Cuneonavicular joint Intercuneiform joint Subtalar (talocalcaneal) joint Talocalcaneal (subtalar) joint Talocalcaneonavicular joint **J Tarsal Joint, Left** *See H Tarsal Joint, Right* **K Tarsometatarsal Joint, Right** **L Tarsometatarsal Joint, Left** **M Metatarsal-Phalangeal Joint, Right** Metatarsophalangeal (MTP) joint **N Metatarsal-Phalangeal Joint, Left** *See M Metatarsal-Phalangeal Joint, Right* **P Toe Phalangeal Joint, Right** Interphalangeal (IP) joint **Q Toe Phalangeal Joint, Left** *See P Toe Phalangeal Joint, Right*	**Ø** Open **3** Percutaneous **4** Percutaneous Endoscopic	**3** Infusion Device **4** Internal Fixation Device **5** External Fixation Device **8** Spacer	**Z** No Qualifier

Non-OR　ØSH[Ø,3][Ø,3,4][3,8]Z
Non-OR　ØSH[2,4][Ø,3,4][3,8]Z
Non-OR　ØSH[5,6,7,8][Ø,3,4][3,8]Z
Non-OR　ØSH[9,B,C,D][Ø,3,4]3Z
Non-OR　ØSH[9,B,C,D][3,4]8Z
Non-OR　ØSH[F,G,H,J,K,L,M,N,P,Q][Ø,3,4][3,8]Z

Non-OR Procedure　　DRG Non-OR Procedure　　Valid OR Procedure　　HAC Associated Procedure　　Combination Only　　New/Revised April　　New/Revised October

608　　　　　　　　　　　　　　　　　　　　　　　　　　　　　　　　　　　ICD-10-PCS 2023

ØSH–ØSH

Ø　Medical and Surgical
S　Lower Joints
J　Inspection　　Definition: Visually and/or manually exploring a body part

Explanation: Visual exploration may be performed with or without optical instrumentation. Manual exploration may be performed directly or through intervening body layers.

Body Part Character 4		Approach Character 5	Device Character 6	Qualifier Character 7
Ø Lumbar Vertebral Joint 　Lumbar facet joint 2 Lumbar Vertebral Disc 3 Lumbosacral Joint 　Lumbosacral facet joint 4 Lumbosacral Disc 5 Sacrococcygeal Joint 　Sacrococcygeal symphysis 6 Coccygeal Joint 7 Sacroiliac Joint, Right 8 Sacroiliac Joint, Left 9 Hip Joint, Right 　Acetabulofemoral joint B Hip Joint, Left 　See 9 Hip Joint, Right C Knee Joint, Right 　Femoropatellar joint 　Femorotibial joint 　Lateral meniscus 　Medial meniscus 　Patellofemoral joint 　Tibiofemoral joint D Knee Joint, Left 　See C Knee Joint, Right F Ankle Joint, Right 　Inferior tibiofibular joint 　Talocrural joint G Ankle Joint, Left 　See F Ankle Joint, Right	H Tarsal Joint, Right 　Calcaneocuboid joint 　Cuboideonavicular joint 　Cuneonavicular joint 　Intercuneiform joint 　Subtalar (talocalcaneal) joint 　Talocalcaneal (subtalar) 　　joint 　Talocalcaneonavicular joint J Tarsal Joint, Left 　See H Tarsal Joint, Right K Tarsometatarsal Joint, 　Right L Tarsometatarsal Joint, Left M Metatarsal-Phalangeal 　Joint, Right 　Metatarsophalangeal (MTP) 　　joint N Metatarsal-Phalangeal 　Joint, Left 　See M Metatarsal-Phalangeal 　　Joint, Right P Toe Phalangeal Joint, Right 　Interphalangeal (IP) joint Q Toe Phalangeal Joint, Left 　See P Toe Phalangeal Joint, 　　Right	Ø Open 3 Percutaneous 4 Percutaneous Endoscopic X External	Z No Device	Z No Qualifier

Non-OR　ØSJ[Ø,2,3,4,5,6,7,8,9,B,C,D,F,G,H,J,K,L,M,N,P,Q][3,X]ZZ

Ø　Medical and Surgical
S　Lower Joints
N　Release　　Definition: Freeing a body part from an abnormal physical constraint by cutting or by the use of force

Explanation: Some of the restraining tissue may be taken out but none of the body part is taken out

Body Part Character 4		Approach Character 5	Device Character 6	Qualifier Character 7
Ø Lumbar Vertebral Joint 　Lumbar facet joint 2 Lumbar Vertebral Disc 3 Lumbosacral Joint 　Lumbosacral facet joint 4 Lumbosacral Disc 5 Sacrococcygeal Joint 　Sacrococcygeal symphysis 6 Coccygeal Joint 7 Sacroiliac Joint, Right 8 Sacroiliac Joint, Left 9 Hip Joint, Right 　Acetabulofemoral joint B Hip Joint, Left 　See 9 Hip Joint, Right C Knee Joint, Right 　Femoropatellar joint 　Femorotibial joint 　Lateral meniscus 　Medial meniscus 　Patellofemoral joint 　Tibiofemoral joint D Knee Joint, Left 　See C Knee Joint, Right F Ankle Joint, Right 　Inferior tibiofibular joint 　Talocrural joint G Ankle Joint, Left 　See F Ankle Joint, Right	H Tarsal Joint, Right 　Calcaneocuboid joint 　Cuboideonavicular joint 　Cuneonavicular joint 　Intercuneiform joint 　Subtalar (talocalcaneal) joint 　Talocalcaneal (subtalar) 　　joint 　Talocalcaneonavicular joint J Tarsal Joint, Left 　See H Tarsal Joint, Right K Tarsometatarsal Joint, 　Right L Tarsometatarsal Joint, Left M Metatarsal-Phalangeal 　Joint, Right 　Metatarsophalangeal (MTP) 　　joint N Metatarsal-Phalangeal 　Joint, Left 　See M Metatarsal-Phalangeal 　　Joint, Right P Toe Phalangeal Joint, Right 　Interphalangeal (IP) joint Q Toe Phalangeal Joint, Left 　See P Toe Phalangeal Joint, 　　Right	Ø Open 3 Percutaneous 4 Percutaneous Endoscopic X External	Z No Device	Z No Qualifier

Non-OR　ØSN[Ø,2,3,4,5,6,7,8,9,B,C,D,F,G,H,J,K,L,M,N,P,Q]XZZ

NC Noncovered Procedure　　**LC** Limited Coverage　　**QA** Questionable OB Admit　　**NT** New Tech Add-on　　⊞ Combination Member　　♂ Male　　♀ Female

ICD-10-PCS 2023　　　　　　　　　　　　　　　　　　　　　　　　　　　　　　　　　　　　　**609**

ØSJ–ØSN

Lower Joints (side tab)

Ø	Medical and Surgical
S	Lower Joints
P	Removal

Definition: Taking out or off a device from a body part

Explanation: If a device is taken out and a similar device put in without cutting or puncturing the skin or mucous membrane, the procedure is coded to the root operation CHANGE. Otherwise, the procedure for taking out the device is coded to the root operation REMOVAL.

Body Part — Character 4	Approach — Character 5	Device — Character 6	Qualifier — Character 7

Ø Lumbar Vertebral Joint
   Lumbar facet joint
3 Lumbosacral Joint
   Lumbosacral facet joint
	Ø Open
	3 Percutaneous
	4 Percutaneous Endoscopic
		Ø Drainage Device
		3 Infusion Device
		4 Internal Fixation Device
		7 Autologous Tissue Substitute
		8 Spacer
		A Interbody Fusion Device
		J Synthetic Substitute
		K Nonautologous Tissue Substitute
			Z No Qualifier

Ø Lumbar Vertebral Joint
   Lumbar facet joint
3 Lumbosacral Joint
   Lumbosacral facet joint
	X External	Ø Drainage Device
		3 Infusion Device
		4 Internal Fixation Device
			Z No Qualifier

2 Lumbar Vertebral Disc 4 Lumbosacral Disc	Ø Open 3 Percutaneous 4 Percutaneous Endoscopic	Ø Drainage Device 3 Infusion Device 7 Autologous Tissue Substitute J Synthetic Substitute K Nonautologous Tissue Substitute	Z No Qualifier
2 Lumbar Vertebral Disc 4 Lumbosacral Disc	X External	Ø Drainage Device 3 Infusion Device	Z No Qualifier
5 Sacrococcygeal Joint Sacrococcygeal symphysis 6 Coccygeal Joint 7 Sacroiliac Joint, Right 8 Sacroiliac Joint, Left	Ø Open 3 Percutaneous 4 Percutaneous Endoscopic	Ø Drainage Device 3 Infusion Device 4 Internal Fixation Device 7 Autologous Tissue Substitute 8 Spacer J Synthetic Substitute K Nonautologous Tissue Substitute	Z No Qualifier
5 Sacrococcygeal Joint Sacrococcygeal symphysis 6 Coccygeal Joint 7 Sacroiliac Joint, Right 8 Sacroiliac Joint, Left	X External	Ø Drainage Device 3 Infusion Device 4 Internal Fixation Device	Z No Qualifier

9 Hip Joint, Right ⊞
   Acetabulofemoral joint
B Hip Joint, Left ⊞
   See 9 Hip Joint, Right
	Ø Open	Ø Drainage Device
		3 Infusion Device
		4 Internal Fixation Device
		5 External Fixation Device
		7 Autologous Tissue Substitute
		8 Spacer
		9 Liner
		B Resurfacing Device
		E Articulating Spacer
		J Synthetic Substitute
		K Nonautologous Tissue Substitute
			Z No Qualifier

9 Hip Joint, Right ⊞
   Acetabulofemoral joint
B Hip Joint, Left ⊞
   See 9 Hip Joint, Right
	3 Percutaneous
	4 Percutaneous Endoscopic
		Ø Drainage Device
		3 Infusion Device
		4 Internal Fixation Device
		5 External Fixation Device
		7 Autologous Tissue Substitute
		8 Spacer
		J Synthetic Substitute
		K Nonautologous Tissue Substitute
			Z No Qualifier

9 Hip Joint, Right ⊞
   Acetabulofemoral joint
B Hip Joint, Left ⊞
   See 9 Hip Joint, Right
	X External	Ø Drainage Device
		3 Infusion Device
		4 Internal Fixation Device
		5 External Fixation Device
			Z No Qualifier

Non-OR	ØSP[Ø,3][Ø,3,4]8Z	
Non-OR	ØSP[Ø,3]3[Ø,3]Z	
Non-OR	ØSP[Ø,3]X[Ø,3,4]Z	
Non-OR	ØSP[2,4]3[Ø,3]Z	
Non-OR	ØSP[2,4]X[Ø,3]Z	
Non-OR	ØSP[5,6,7,8][Ø,3,4]8Z	
Non-OR	ØSP[5,6,7,8]3[Ø,3]Z	
Non-OR	ØSP[5,6,7,8]X[Ø,3,4]Z	
Non-OR	ØSP[9,B]3[Ø,3,8]Z	
Non-OR	ØSP[9,B]X[Ø,3,4,5]Z	

See Appendix L for Procedure Combinations

Combo-only	ØSP[9,B]48Z
⊞	ØSP[9,B]Ø[8,9,B,E,J]Z
⊞	ØSP[9,B]4JZ

ØSP Continued on next page

Non-OR Procedure   DRG Non-OR Procedure   Valid OR Procedure   HAC Associated Procedure   Combination Only   New/Revised April   New/Revised October

610   ICD-10-PCS 2023

ØSP Continued

Ø   **Medical and Surgical**
S   **Lower Joints**
P   **Removal**   Definition: Taking out or off a device from a body part

Explanation: If a device is taken out and a similar device put in without cutting or puncturing the skin or mucous membrane, the procedure is coded to the root operation CHANGE. Otherwise, the procedure for taking out the device is coded to the root operation REMOVAL.

Body Part Character 4	Approach Character 5	Device Character 6	Qualifier Character 7

A Hip Joint, Acetabular Surface, Right ⊞
E Hip Joint, Acetabular Surface, Left ⊞
R Hip Joint, Femoral Surface, Right ⊞
S Hip Joint, Femoral Surface, Left ⊞
T Knee Joint, Femoral Surface, Right ⊞
   Femoropatellar joint
   Patellofemoral joint
U Knee Joint, Femoral Surface, Left ⊞
   See T Knee Joint, Femoral Surface, Right
V Knee Joint, Tibial Surface, Right ⊞
   Femorotibial joint
   Tibiofemoral joint
W Knee Joint, Tibial Surface, Left ⊞
   See V Knee Joint, Tibial Surface, Right
	Ø Open
	3 Percutaneous
	4 Percutaneous Endoscopic
		J Synthetic Substitute	Z No Qualifier

C Knee Joint, Right ⊞
   Femoropatellar joint
   Femorotibial joint
   Lateral meniscus
   Medial meniscus
   Patellofemoral joint
   Tibiofemoral joint
D Knee Joint, Left ⊞
   See C Knee Joint, Right
	Ø Open	Ø Drainage Device
		3 Infusion Device
		4 Internal Fixation Device
		5 External Fixation Device
		7 Autologous Tissue Substitute
		8 Spacer
		9 Liner
		E Articulating Spacer
		K Nonautologous Tissue Substitute
		L Synthetic Substitute, Unicondylar Medial
		M Synthetic Substitute, Unicondylar Lateral
		N Synthetic Substitute, Patellofemoral
			Z No Qualifier

C Knee Joint, Right ⊞
   Femoropatellar joint
   Femorotibial joint
   Lateral meniscus
   Medial meniscus
   Patellofemoral joint
   Tibiofemoral joint
D Knee Joint, Left ⊞
   See C Knee Joint, Right
	Ø Open	J Synthetic Substitute	C Patellar Surface
			Z No Qualifier

C Knee Joint, Right ⊞
   Femoropatellar joint
   Femorotibial joint
   Lateral meniscus
   Medial meniscus
   Patellofemoral joint
   Tibiofemoral joint
D Knee Joint, Left ⊞
   See C Knee Joint, Right
	3 Percutaneous
	4 Percutaneous Endoscopic
		Ø Drainage Device
		3 Infusion Device
		4 Internal Fixation Device
		5 External Fixation Device
		7 Autologous Tissue Substitute
		8 Spacer
		K Nonautologous Tissue Substitute
		L Synthetic Substitute, Unicondylar Medial
		M Synthetic Substitute, Unicondylar Lateral
		N Synthetic Substitute, Patellofemoral
			Z No Qualifier

C Knee Joint, Right ⊞
   Femoropatellar joint
   Femorotibial joint
   Lateral meniscus
   Medial meniscus
   Patellofemoral joint
   Tibiofemoral joint
D Knee Joint, Left ⊞
   See C Knee Joint, Right
	3 Percutaneous
	4 Percutaneous Endoscopic
		J Synthetic Substitute	C Patellar Surface
			Z No Qualifier

Non-OR   ØSP[C,D]3[Ø,3]Z

See Appendix L for Procedure Combinations
Combo-only   ØSP[C,D][3,4]8Z
⊞ ØSP[A,E,R,S,T,U,V,W][Ø,4]JZ
⊞ ØSP[C,D]Ø[8,9,E,L,M,N]Z
⊞ ØSP[C,D]ØJ[C,Z]
⊞ ØSP[C,D]4[L,M,N]Z
⊞ ØSP[C,D]4J[C,Z]

ØSP Continued on next page

NC Noncovered Procedure   LC Limited Coverage   QA Questionable OB Admit   NT New Tech Add-on   ⊞ Combination Member   ♂ Male   ♀ Female

Lower Joints (side tab)

Ø	Medical and Surgical
S	Lower Joints
P	Removal

Definition: Taking out or off a device from a body part

Explanation: If a device is taken out and a similar device put in without cutting or puncturing the skin or mucous membrane, the procedure is coded to the root operation CHANGE. Otherwise, the procedure for taking out the device is coded to the root operation REMOVAL.

Body Part Character 4	Approach Character 5	Device Character 6	Qualifier Character 7

C **Knee Joint, Right**
  Femoropatellar joint
  Femorotibial joint
  Lateral meniscus
  Medial meniscus
  Patellofemoral joint
  Tibiofemoral joint
D **Knee Joint, Left**
  See C Knee Joint, Right
	X External	**Ø** Drainage Device
		3 Infusion Device
		4 Internal Fixation Device
		5 External Fixation Device
			Z No Qualifier

F **Ankle Joint, Right**
  Inferior tibiofibular joint
  Talocrural joint
G **Ankle Joint, Left**
  See F Ankle Joint, Right
H **Tarsal Joint, Right**
  Calcaneocuboid joint
  Cuboideonavicular joint
  Cuneonavicular joint
  Intercuneiform joint
  Subtalar (talocalcaneal) joint
  Talocalcaneal (subtalar) joint
  Talocalcaneonavicular joint
J **Tarsal Joint, Left**
  See H Tarsal Joint, Right
K **Tarsometatarsal Joint, Right**
L **Tarsometatarsal Joint, Left**
M **Metatarsal-Phalangeal Joint, Right**
  Metatarsophalangeal (MTP) joint
N **Metatarsal-Phalangeal Joint, Left**
  See M Metatarsal-Phalangeal Joint,
  Right
P **Toe Phalangeal Joint, Right**
  Interphalangeal (IP) joint
Q **Toe Phalangeal Joint, Left**
  See P Toe Phalangeal Joint, Right
	Ø Open
	3 Percutaneous
	4 Percutaneous Endoscopic
		Ø Drainage Device
		3 Infusion Device
		4 Internal Fixation Device
		5 External Fixation Device
		7 Autologous Tissue Substitute
		8 Spacer
		J Synthetic Substitute
		K Nonautologous Tissue Substitute
			Z No Qualifier

F **Ankle Joint, Right**
  Inferior tibiofibular joint
  Talocrural joint
G **Ankle Joint, Left**
  See F Ankle Joint, Right
H **Tarsal Joint, Right**
  Calcaneocuboid joint
  Cuboideonavicular joint
  Cuneonavicular joint
  Intercuneiform joint
  Subtalar (talocalcaneal) joint
  Talocalcaneal (subtalar) joint
  Talocalcaneonavicular joint
J **Tarsal Joint, Left**
  See H Tarsal Joint, Right
K **Tarsometatarsal Joint, Right**
L **Tarsometatarsal Joint, Left**
M **Metatarsal-Phalangeal Joint, Right**
  Metatarsophalangeal (MTP) joint
N **Metatarsal-Phalangeal Joint, Left**
  See M Metatarsal-Phalangeal Joint,
  Right
P **Toe Phalangeal Joint, Right**
  Interphalangeal (IP) joint
Q **Toe Phalangeal Joint, Left**
  See P Toe Phalangeal Joint, Right
	X External	**Ø** Drainage Device
		3 Infusion Device
		4 Internal Fixation Device
		5 External Fixation Device
			Z No Qualifier

Non-OR	0SP[C,D]X[Ø,3,4,5]Z
Non-OR	0SP[F,G,H,J,K,L,M,N,P,Q]3[Ø,3,8]Z
Non-OR	0SP[F,G,H,J,K,L,M,N,P,Q][Ø,4]8Z
Non-OR	0SP[F,G,H,J,K,L,M,N,P,Q]X[Ø,3,4,5]Z

Non-OR Procedure   DRG Non-OR Procedure   Valid OR Procedure   HAC Associated Procedure   Combination Only   New/Revised April   New/Revised October

612   ICD-10-PCS 2023

Ø   **Medical and Surgical**
S   **Lower Joints**
Q   **Repair**   Definition: Restoring, to the extent possible, a body part to its normal anatomic structure and function
                   Explanation: Used only when the method to accomplish the repair is not one of the other root operations

Body Part Character 4	Approach Character 5	Device Character 6	Qualifier Character 7

Ø   **Lumbar Vertebral Joint**
     Lumbar facet joint
2   **Lumbar Vertebral Disc**
3   **Lumbosacral Joint**
     Lumbosacral facet joint
4   **Lumbosacral Disc**
5   **Sacrococcygeal Joint**
     Sacrococcygeal symphysis
6   **Coccygeal Joint**
7   **Sacroiliac Joint, Right**
8   **Sacroiliac Joint, Left**
9   **Hip Joint, Right**
     Acetabulofemoral joint
B   **Hip Joint, Left**
     See 9 Hip Joint, Right
C   **Knee Joint, Right**
     Femoropatellar joint
     Femorotibial joint
     Lateral meniscus
     Medial meniscus
     Patellofemoral joint
     Tibiofemoral joint
D   **Knee Joint, Left**
     See C Knee Joint, Right
F   **Ankle Joint, Right**
     Inferior tibiofibular joint
     Talocrural joint
G   **Ankle Joint, Left**
     See F Ankle Joint, Right
H   **Tarsal Joint, Right**
     Calcaneocuboid joint
     Cuboideonavicular joint
     Cuneonavicular joint
     Intercuneiform joint
     Subtalar (talocalcaneal) joint
     Talocalcaneal (subtalar) joint
     Talocalcaneonavicular joint
J   **Tarsal Joint, Left**
     See H Tarsal Joint, Right
K   **Tarsometatarsal Joint, Right**
L   **Tarsometatarsal Joint, Left**
M   **Metatarsal-Phalangeal Joint, Right**
     Metatarsophalangeal (MTP) joint
N   **Metatarsal-Phalangeal Joint, Left**
     See M Metatarsal-Phalangeal Joint, Right
P   **Toe Phalangeal Joint, Right**
     Interphalangeal (IP) joint
Q   **Toe Phalangeal Joint, Left**
     See P Toe Phalangeal Joint, Right
	Ø Open
	3 Percutaneous
	4 Percutaneous Endoscopic
	X External
		Z No Device	**Z** No Qualifier

Non-OR   ØSQ[Ø,2,3,4,5,6,7,8,9,B,C,D,F,G,H,J,K,L,M,N,P,Q]XZZ

NC Noncovered Procedure   LC Limited Coverage   QA Questionable OB Admit   NT New Tech Add-on   ⊞ Combination Member   ♂ Male   ♀ Female

ICD-10-PCS 2023   **613**

Ø Medical and Surgical
S Lower Joints
R Replacement Definition: Putting in or on biological or synthetic material that physically takes the place and/or function of all or a portion of a body part

Explanation: The body part may have been taken out or replaced, or may be taken out, physically eradicated, or rendered nonfunctional during the REPLACEMENT procedure. A REMOVAL procedure is coded for taking out the device used in a previous replacement procedure.

Body Part Character 4	Approach Character 5	Device Character 6	Qualifier Character 7
Ø Lumbar Vertebral Joint 　Lumbar facet joint 2 Lumbar Vertebral Disc `NC` 3 Lumbosacral Joint 　Lumbosacral facet joint 4 Lumbosacral Disc `NC` 5 Sacrococcygeal Joint 　Sacrococcygeal symphysis 6 Coccygeal Joint 7 Sacroiliac Joint, Right 8 Sacroiliac Joint, Left H Tarsal Joint, Right 　Calcaneocuboid joint 　Cuboideonavicular joint 　Cuneonavicular joint 　Intercuneiform joint 　Subtalar (talocalcaneal) joint 　Talocalcaneal (subtalar) joint 　Talocalcaneonavicular joint J Tarsal Joint, Left 　**See** H Tarsal Joint, Right K Tarsometatarsal Joint, Right L Tarsometatarsal Joint, Left M Metatarsal-Phalangeal Joint, Right 　Metatarsophalangeal (MTP) joint N Metatarsal-Phalangeal Joint, Left 　**See** M Metatarsal-Phalangeal Joint, Right P Toe Phalangeal Joint, Right 　Interphalangeal (IP) joint Q Toe Phalangeal Joint, Left 　**See** P Toe Phalangeal Joint, Right	Ø Open	7 Autologous Tissue Substitute J Synthetic Substitute K Nonautologous Tissue Substitute	Z No Qualifier
9 Hip Joint, Right ⊞ 　Acetabulofemoral joint B Hip Joint, Left ⊞ 　**See** 9 Hip Joint, Right	Ø Open	1 Synthetic Substitute, Metal 2 Synthetic Substitute, Metal on 　Polyethylene 3 Synthetic Substitute, Ceramic 4 Synthetic Substitute, Ceramic on 　Polyethylene 6 Synthetic Substitute, Oxidized 　Zirconium on Polyethylene J Synthetic Substitute	9 Cemented A Uncemented Z No Qualifier
9 Hip Joint, Right ⊞ 　Acetabulofemoral joint B Hip Joint, Left ⊞ 　**See** 9 Hip Joint, Right	Ø Open	7 Autologous Tissue Substitute E Articulating Spacer K Nonautologous Tissue Substitute	Z No Qualifier
A Hip Joint, Acetabular Surface, ⊞ 　Right E Hip Joint, Acetabular Surface, ⊞ 　Left	Ø Open	Ø Synthetic Substitute, Polyethylene 1 Synthetic Substitute, Metal 3 Synthetic Substitute, Ceramic J Synthetic Substitute	9 Cemented A Uncemented Z No Qualifier
A Hip Joint, Acetabular Surface, Right E Hip Joint, Acetabular Surface, Left	Ø Open	7 Autologous Tissue Substitute K Nonautologous Tissue Substitute	Z No Qualifier

`HAC` ØSR[9,B]Ø[1,2,3,4,6,J][9,A,Z] when reported with SDx of I26.Ø2-I26.Ø9, I26.92-I26.99, or I82.4Ø1-I82.4Z9

`HAC` ØSR[9,B]Ø[7,E,K]Z when reported with SDx of I26.Ø2-I26.Ø9, I26.92-I26.99, or I82.4Ø1-I82.4Z9

`HAC` ØSR[A,E]Ø[Ø,1,3,J][9,A,Z] when reported with SDx of I26.Ø2-I26.Ø9, I26.92-I26.99, or I82.4Ø1-I82.4Z9

`HAC` ØSR[A,E]Ø[7,K]Z when reported with SDx of I26.Ø2-I26.Ø9, I26.92-I26.99, or I82.4Ø1-I82.4Z9

`NC` ØSR[2,4]ØJZ when beneficiary age is over 6Ø

See Appendix L for Procedure Combinations
⊞ ØSR[9,B]Ø[1,2,3,4,6,J][9,A,Z]
⊞ ØSR[9,B]ØEZ
⊞ ØSR[A,E]Ø[Ø,1,3,J][9,A,Z]

ØSR Continued on next page

Non-OR Procedure   DRG Non-OR Procedure   Valid OR Procedure   HAC Associated Procedure   Combination Only   New/Revised April   New/Revised October

614   ICD-10-PCS 2023

ØSR–ØSR (side tab)

Ø   **Medical and Surgical**   *ØSR Continued*
S   **Lower Joints**
R   **Replacement**   Definition: Putting in or on biological or synthetic material that physically takes the place and/or function of all or a portion of a body part

Explanation: The body part may have been taken out or replaced, or may be taken out, physically eradicated, or rendered nonfunctional during the REPLACEMENT procedure. A REMOVAL procedure is coded for taking out the device used in a previous replacement procedure.

Body Part Character 4	Approach Character 5	Device Character 6	Qualifier Character 7

C   **Knee Joint, Right** ⊞
   Femoropatellar joint
   Femorotibial joint
   Lateral meniscus
   Medial meniscus
   Patellofemoral joint
   Tibiofemoral joint
D   **Knee Joint, Left** ⊞
   See C Knee Joint, Right
	Ø Open	6 Synthetic Substitute, Oxidized
		   Zirconium on Polyethylene
		J Synthetic Substitute
		L Synthetic Substitute, Unicondylar
		   Medial
		M Synthetic Substitute, Unicondylar
		   Lateral
		N Synthetic Substitute,
		   Patellofemoral
			9 Cemented
			A Uncemented
			Z No Qualifier

C   **Knee Joint, Right** ⊞
   Femoropatellar joint
   Femorotibial joint
   Lateral meniscus
   Medial meniscus
   Patellofemoral joint
   Tibiofemoral joint
D   **Knee Joint, Left** ⊞
   See C Knee Joint, Right
	Ø Open	7 Autologous Tissue Substitute
		E Articulating Spacer
		K Nonautologous Tissue Substitute
			Z No Qualifier

F   **Ankle Joint, Right**
   Inferior tibiofibular joint
   Talocrural joint
G   **Ankle Joint, Left**
   See F Ankle Joint, Right
T   **Knee Joint, Femoral Surface, Right**
   Femoropatellar joint
   Patellofemoral joint
U   **Knee Joint, Femoral Surface, Left**
   See T Knee Joint, Femoral Surface, Right
V   **Knee Joint, Tibial Surface, Right**
   Femorotibial joint
   Tibiofemoral joint
W   **Knee Joint, Tibial Surface, Left**
   See V Knee Joint, Tibial Surface, Right
	Ø Open	7 Autologous Tissue Substitute
		K Nonautologous Tissue Substitute
			Z No Qualifier

F   **Ankle Joint, Right**
   Inferior tibiofibular joint
   Talocrural joint
G   **Ankle Joint, Left**
   See F Ankle Joint, Right
T   **Knee Joint, Femoral Surface, Right** ⊞
   Femoropatellar joint
   Patellofemoral joint
U   **Knee Joint, Femoral Surface, Left** ⊞
   See T Knee Joint, Femoral Surface, Right
V   **Knee Joint, Tibial Surface, Right** ⊞
   Femorotibial joint
   Tibiofemoral joint
W   **Knee Joint, Tibial Surface, Left** ⊞
   See V Knee Joint, Tibial Surface, Right
	Ø Open	J Synthetic Substitute	9 Cemented
			A Uncemented
			Z No Qualifier

R **Hip Joint, Femoral Surface, Right** ⊞ S **Hip Joint, Femoral Surface, Left** ⊞	Ø Open	1 Synthetic Substitute, Metal 3 Synthetic Substitute, Ceramic J Synthetic Substitute	9 Cemented A Uncemented Z No Qualifier
R **Hip Joint, Femoral Surface, Right** S **Hip Joint, Femoral Surface, Left**	Ø Open	7 Autologous Tissue Substitute K Nonautologous Tissue Substitute	Z No Qualifier

HAC   ØSR[C,D]Ø[6,J,L,M,N][9,A,Z] when reported with SDx of I26.02-I26.09,
       I26.92-I26.99 or I82.401-I82.4Z9

HAC   ØSR[C,D]Ø[7,E,K]Z when reported with SDx of I26.02-I26.09, I26.92-I26.99
       or I82.401-I82.4Z9

HAC   ØSR[T,U,V,W]Ø[7,K]Z when reported with SDx of I26.02-I26.09,
       I26.92-I26.99 or I82.401-I82.4Z9

HAC   ØSR[T,U,V,W]ØJ[9,A,Z] when reported with SDx of I26.02-I26.09,
       I26.92-I26.99 or I82.401-I82.4Z9

HAC   ØSR[R,S]Ø[1,3,J][9,A,Z] when reported with SDx of I26.02-I26.09,
       I26.92-I26.99, or I82.401-I82.4Z9

HAC   ØSR[R,S]Ø[7,K]Z when reported with SDx of I26.02-I26.09, I26.92-I26.99,
       or I82.401-I82.4Z9

See Appendix L for Procedure Combinations
⊞   ØSR[C,D]Ø[6,J,L,M,N][9,A,Z]
⊞   ØSR[C,D]ØEZ
⊞   ØSR[T,U,V,W]ØJ[9,A,Z]
⊞   ØSR[R,S]Ø[1,3,J][9,A,Z]

NC Noncovered Procedure   **LC** Limited Coverage   **QA** Questionable OB Admit   **NT** New Tech Add-on   ⊞ Combination Member   ♂ Male   ♀ Female

ICD-10-PCS 2023   615

ØSR–ØSR

Ø Medical and Surgical
S Lower Joints
S Reposition Definition: Moving to its normal location, or other suitable location, all or a portion of a body part
Explanation: The body part is moved to a new location from an abnormal location, or from a normal location where it is not functioning correctly. The body part may or may not be cut out or off to be moved to the new location.

Body Part Character 4	Approach Character 5	Device Character 6	Qualifier Character 7
Ø Lumbar Vertebral Joint 　Lumbar facet joint **3 Lumbosacral Joint** 　Lumbosacral facet joint **5 Sacrococcygeal Joint** 　Sacrococcygeal symphysis **6 Coccygeal Joint** **7 Sacroiliac Joint, Right** **8 Sacroiliac Joint, Left**	**Ø Open** **3 Percutaneous** **4 Percutaneous Endoscopic** **X External**	**4 Internal Fixation Device** **Z No Device**	**Z No Qualifier**
9 Hip Joint, Right 　Acetabulofemoral joint **B Hip Joint, Left** 　See 9 Hip Joint, Right **C Knee Joint, Right** 　Femoropatellar joint 　Femorotibial joint 　Lateral meniscus 　Medial meniscus 　Patellofemoral joint 　Tibiofemoral joint **D Knee Joint, Left** 　See C Knee Joint, Right **F Ankle Joint, Right** 　Inferior tibiofibular joint 　Talocrural joint **G Ankle Joint, Left** 　See F Ankle Joint, Right **H Tarsal Joint, Right** 　Calcaneocuboid joint 　Cuboideonavicular joint 　Cuneonavicular joint 　Intercuneiform joint 　Subtalar (talocalcaneal) joint 　Talocalcaneal (subtalar) joint 　Talocalcaneonavicular joint **J Tarsal Joint, Left** 　See H Tarsal Joint, Right **K Tarsometatarsal Joint, Right** **L Tarsometatarsal Joint, Left** **M Metatarsal-Phalangeal Joint, Right** 　Metatarsophalangeal (MTP) joint **N Metatarsal-Phalangeal Joint, Left** 　See M Metatarsal-Phalangeal Joint, Right **P Toe Phalangeal Joint, Right** 　Interphalangeal (IP) joint **Q Toe Phalangeal Joint, Left** 　See P Toe Phalangeal Joint, Right	**Ø Open** **3 Percutaneous** **4 Percutaneous Endoscopic** **X External**	**4 Internal Fixation Device** **5 External Fixation Device** **Z No Device**	**Z No Qualifier**

Non-OR ØSS[Ø,3,5,6,][3,4,X][4,Z]Z
Non-OR ØSS[7,8]3ZZ
Non-OR ØSS[7,8][4,X][4,Z]Z
Non-OR ØSS[9,B]3ZZ
Non-OR ØSS[9,B][3,4,X]5Z
Non-OR ØSS[9,B][4,X][4,Z]Z
Non-OR ØSS[C,D,F,G,H,J,K,L,M,N,P,Q][3,4,X][4,5,Z]Z

Ø　Medical and Surgical
S　Lower Joints
T　Resection　　Definition: Cutting out or off, without replacement, all of a body part
　　　　　　　　　　Explanation: None

Body Part Character 4	Approach Character 5	Device Character 6	Qualifier Character 7
2 Lumbar Vertebral Disc	**Ø** Open	**Z** No Device	**Z** No Qualifier
4 Lumbosacral Disc			
5 Sacrococcygeal Joint 　Sacrococcygeal symphysis			
6 Coccygeal Joint			
7 Sacroiliac Joint, Right			
8 Sacroiliac Joint, Left			
9 Hip Joint, Right 　Acetabulofemoral joint			
B Hip Joint, Left 　See 9 Hip Joint, Right			
C Knee Joint, Right 　Femoropatellar joint 　Femorotibial joint 　Lateral meniscus 　Medial meniscus 　Patellofemoral joint 　Tibiofemoral joint			
D Knee Joint, Left 　See C Knee Joint, Right			
F Ankle Joint, Right 　Inferior tibiofibular joint 　Talocrural joint			
G Ankle Joint, Left 　See F Ankle Joint, Right			
H Tarsal Joint, Right 　Calcaneocuboid joint 　Cuboideonavicular joint 　Cuneonavicular joint 　Intercuneiform joint 　Subtalar (talocalcaneal) joint 　Talocalcaneal (subtalar) joint 　Talocalcaneonavicular joint			
J Tarsal Joint, Left 　See H Tarsal Joint, Right			
K Tarsometatarsal Joint, Right			
L Tarsometatarsal Joint, Left			
M Metatarsal-Phalangeal Joint, Right 　Metatarsophalangeal (MTP) joint			
N Metatarsal-Phalangeal Joint, Left 　See M Metatarsal-Phalangeal Joint, Right			
P Toe Phalangeal Joint, Right 　Interphalangeal (IP) joint			
Q Toe Phalangeal Joint, Left 　See P Toe Phalangeal Joint, Right			

Lower Joints

Ø   **Medical and Surgical**
S   **Lower Joints**
U   **Supplement**   Definition: Putting in or on biological or synthetic material that physically reinforces and/or augments the function of a portion of a body part
                     Explanation: The biological material is non-living, or is living and from the same individual. The body part may have been previously replaced, and the SUPPLEMENT procedure is performed to physically reinforce and/or augment the function of the replaced body part.

Body Part Character 4	Approach Character 5	Device Character 6	Qualifier Character 7

Ø   **Lumbar Vertebral Joint**
     Lumbar facet joint
2   **Lumbar Vertebral Disc**
3   **Lumbosacral Joint**
     Lumbosacral facet joint
4   **Lumbosacral Disc**
5   **Sacrococcygeal Joint**
     Sacrococcygeal symphysis
6   **Coccygeal Joint**
7   **Sacroiliac Joint, Right**
8   **Sacroiliac Joint, Left**
F   **Ankle Joint, Right**
     Inferior tibiofibular joint
     Talocrural joint
G   **Ankle Joint, Left**
     See F Ankle Joint, Right
H   **Tarsal Joint, Right**
     Calcaneocuboid joint
     Cuboideonavicular joint
     Cuneonavicular joint
     Intercuneiform joint
     Subtalar (talocalcaneal) joint
     Talocalcaneal (subtalar) joint
     Talocalcaneonavicular joint
J   **Tarsal Joint, Left**
     See H Tarsal Joint, Right
K   **Tarsometatarsal Joint, Right**
L   **Tarsometatarsal Joint, Left**
M   **Metatarsal-Phalangeal Joint, Right**
     Metatarsophalangeal (MTP) joint
N   **Metatarsal-Phalangeal Joint, Left**
     See M Metatarsal-Phalangeal Joint, Right
P   **Toe Phalangeal Joint, Right**
     Interphalangeal (IP) joint
Q   **Toe Phalangeal Joint, Left**
     See P Toe Phalangeal Joint, Right
	Ø Open
	3 Percutaneous
	4 Percutaneous Endoscopic
		7 Autologous Tissue Substitute
		J Synthetic Substitute
		K Nonautologous Tissue Substitute
			Z No Qualifier

9   **Hip Joint, Right** ⊞
     Acetabulofemoral joint
B   **Hip Joint, Left** ⊞
     See 9 Hip Joint, Right
	Ø Open	**7** Autologous Tissue Substitute
		9 Liner
		B Resurfacing Device
		J Synthetic Substitute
		K Nonautologous Tissue Substitute
			Z No Qualifier

9   **Hip Joint, Right**
     Acetabulofemoral joint
B   **Hip Joint, Left**
     See 9 Hip Joint, Right
	3 Percutaneous
	4 Percutaneous Endoscopic
		7 Autologous Tissue Substitute
		J Synthetic Substitute
		K Nonautologous Tissue Substitute
			Z No Qualifier

A **Hip Joint, Acetabular Surface, Right** ⊞ **E** **Hip Joint, Acetabular Surface, Left** ⊞ **R** **Hip Joint, Femoral Surface, Right** ⊞ **S** **Hip Joint, Femoral Surface, Left** ⊞	**Ø** Open	**9** Liner **B** Resurfacing Device	**Z** No Qualifier

C   **Knee Joint, Right**
     Femoropatellar joint
     Femorotibial joint
     Lateral meniscus
     Medial meniscus
     Patellofemoral joint
     Tibiofemoral joint
D   **Knee Joint, Left**
     See C Knee Joint, Right
	Ø Open	**7** Autologous Tissue Substitute
		J Synthetic Substitute
		K Nonautologous Tissue Substitute
			Z No Qualifier

C   **Knee Joint, Right**
     Femoropatellar joint
     Femorotibial joint
     Lateral meniscus
     Medial meniscus
     Patellofemoral joint
     Tibiofemoral joint
D   **Knee Joint, Left**
     See C Knee Joint, Right
	Ø Open	**9** Liner	**C** Patellar Surface
			Z No Qualifier

HAC   ØSU[9,B]ØBZ when reported with SDx of I26.Ø2-I26.Ø9, I26.92-I26.99, or I82.4Ø1-I82.4Z9
HAC   ØSU[A,E,R,S]ØBZ when reported with SDx of I26.Ø2-I26.Ø9, I26.92-I26.99, or I82.4Ø1-I82.4Z9

See Appendix L for Procedure Combinations
   ⊞   ØSU[9,B]Ø9Z
   ⊞   ØSU[A,E,R,S]Ø9Z

ØSU Continued on next page

Non-OR Procedure   DRG Non-OR Procedure   Valid OR Procedure   HAC Associated Procedure   Combination Only   New/Revised April   New/Revised October

Ø Medical and Surgical
S Lower Joints
U Supplement

ØSU Continued

Definition: Putting in or on biological or synthetic material that physically reinforces and/or augments the function of a portion of a body part

Explanation: The biological material is non-living, or is living and from the same individual. The body part may have been previously replaced, and the SUPPLEMENT procedure is performed to physically reinforce and/or augment the function of the replaced body part.

Body Part Character 4		Approach Character 5		Device Character 6		Qualifier Character 7	
C	Knee Joint, Right 　Femoropatellar joint 　Femorotibial joint 　Lateral meniscus 　Medial meniscus 　Patellofemoral joint 　Tibiofemoral joint D	Knee Joint, Left 　*See C Knee Joint, Right*	3 4	Percutaneous Percutaneous Endoscopic	7 J K	Autologous Tissue Substitute Synthetic Substitute Nonautologous Tissue Substitute	Z	No Qualifier
T	Knee Joint, Femoral Surface, Right 　Femoropatellar joint 　Patellofemoral joint U	Knee Joint, Femoral Surface, Left 　*See T Knee Joint, Femoral Surface, Right* V	Knee Joint, Tibial Surface, Right ⊞ 　Femorotibial joint 　Tibiofemoral joint W	Knee Joint, Tibial Surface, Left ⊞ 　*See V Knee Joint, Tibial Surface, Right*	Ø	Open	9	Liner	Z	No Qualifier

See Appendix L for Procedure Combinations
　⊞　ØSU[V,W]Ø9Z

NC Noncovered Procedure　　LC Limited Coverage　　QA Questionable OB Admit　　NT New Tech Add-on　　⊞ Combination Member　　♂ Male　　♀ Female

ICD-10-PCS 2023　　619

Lower Joints *(sidebar)*

Ø **Medical and Surgical**
S **Lower Joints**
W **Revision**

Definition: Correcting, to the extent possible, a portion of a malfunctioning device or the position of a displaced device
Explanation: Revision can include correcting a malfunctioning or displaced device by taking out or putting in components of the device such as a screw or pin

Body Part Character 4	Approach Character 5	Device Character 6	Qualifier Character 7
Ø Lumbar Vertebral Joint 　Lumbar facet joint 3 Lumbosacral Joint 　Lumbosacral facet joint	Ø Open 3 Percutaneous 4 Percutaneous Endoscopic X External	Ø Drainage Device 3 Infusion Device 4 Internal Fixation Device 7 Autologous Tissue Substitute 8 Spacer A Interbody Fusion Device J Synthetic Substitute K Nonautologous Tissue Substitute	Z No Qualifier
2 Lumbar Vertebral Disc 4 Lumbosacral Disc	Ø Open 3 Percutaneous 4 Percutaneous Endoscopic X External	Ø Drainage Device 3 Infusion Device 7 Autologous Tissue Substitute J Synthetic Substitute K Nonautologous Tissue Substitute	Z No Qualifier
5 Sacrococcygeal Joint 　Sacrococcygeal symphysis 6 Coccygeal Joint 7 Sacroiliac Joint, Right 8 Sacroiliac Joint, Left	Ø Open 3 Percutaneous 4 Percutaneous Endoscopic X External	Ø Drainage Device 3 Infusion Device 4 Internal Fixation Device 7 Autologous Tissue Substitute 8 Spacer J Synthetic Substitute K Nonautologous Tissue Substitute	Z No Qualifier
9 Hip Joint, Right 　Acetabulofemoral joint B Hip Joint, Left 　*See 9 Hip Joint, Right*	Ø Open	Ø Drainage Device 3 Infusion Device 4 Internal Fixation Device 5 External Fixation Device 7 Autologous Tissue Substitute 8 Spacer 9 Liner B Resurfacing Device J Synthetic Substitute K Nonautologous Tissue Substitute	Z No Qualifier
9 Hip Joint, Right 　Acetabulofemoral joint B Hip Joint, Left 　*See 9 Hip Joint, Right*	3 Percutaneous 4 Percutaneous Endoscopic X External	Ø Drainage Device 3 Infusion Device 4 Internal Fixation Device 5 External Fixation Device 7 Autologous Tissue Substitute 8 Spacer J Synthetic Substitute K Nonautologous Tissue Substitute	Z No Qualifier
A Hip Joint, Acetabular Surface, Right E Hip Joint, Acetabular Surface, Left R Hip Joint, Femoral Surface, Right S Hip Joint, Femoral Surface, Left T Knee Joint, Femoral Surface, Right 　Femoropatellar joint 　Patellofemoral joint U Knee Joint, Femoral Surface, Left 　*See T Knee Joint, Femoral Surface, Right* V Knee Joint, Tibial Surface, Right 　Femorotibial joint 　Tibiofemoral joint W Knee Joint, Tibial Surface, Left 　*See V Knee Joint, Tibial Surface, Right*	Ø Open 3 Percutaneous 4 Percutaneous Endoscopic X External	J Synthetic Substitute	Z No Qualifier
C Knee Joint, Right 　Femoropatellar joint 　Femorotibial joint 　Lateral meniscus 　Medial meniscus 　Patellofemoral joint 　Tibiofemoral joint D Knee Joint, Left 　*See C Knee Joint, Right*	Ø Open	Ø Drainage Device 3 Infusion Device 4 Internal Fixation Device 5 External Fixation Device 7 Autologous Tissue Substitute 8 Spacer 9 Liner K Nonautologous Tissue Substitute	Z No Qualifier

Non-OR　ØSW[Ø,3]X[Ø,3,4,7,8,A,J,K]Z
Non-OR　ØSW[2,4]X[Ø,3,7,J,K]Z
Non-OR　ØSW[5,6,7,8]X[Ø,3,4,7,8,J,K]Z
Non-OR　ØSW[9,B]X[Ø,3,4,5,7,8,J,K]Z
Non-OR　ØSW[A,E,R,S,T,U,V,W]XJZ

ØSW Continued on next page

Non-OR Procedure　　DRG Non-OR Procedure　　Valid OR Procedure　　HAC Associated Procedure　　Combination Only　　New/Revised April　　New/Revised October

Ø   Medical and Surgical
S   Lower Joints
W   Revision   *ØSW Continued*

Definition: Correcting, to the extent possible, a portion of a malfunctioning device or the position of a displaced device

Explanation: Revision can include correcting a malfunctioning or displaced device by taking out or putting in components of the device such as a screw or pin

Body Part Character 4	Approach Character 5	Device Character 6	Qualifier Character 7

C Knee Joint, Right
  Femoropatellar joint
  Femorotibial joint
  Lateral meniscus
  Medial meniscus
  Patellofemoral joint
  Tibiofemoral joint
D Knee Joint, Left
  See C Knee Joint, Right
	Ø Open	**J** Synthetic Substitute	**C** Patellar Surface
			Z No Qualifier

C Knee Joint, Right
  Femoropatellar joint
  Femorotibial joint
  Lateral meniscus
  Medial meniscus
  Patellofemoral joint
  Tibiofemoral joint
D Knee Joint, Left
  See C Knee Joint, Right
	3 Percutaneous
	4 Percutaneous Endoscopic
	X External
		Ø Drainage Device
		3 Infusion Device
		4 Internal Fixation Device
		5 External Fixation Device
		7 Autologous Tissue Substitute
		8 Spacer
		K Nonautologous Tissue Substitute
			Z No Qualifier

C Knee Joint, Right
  Femoropatellar joint
  Femorotibial joint
  Lateral meniscus
  Medial meniscus
  Patellofemoral joint
  Tibiofemoral joint
D Knee Joint, Left
  See C Knee Joint, Right
	3 Percutaneous
	4 Percutaneous Endoscopic
	X External
		J Synthetic Substitute	**C** Patellar Surface
			Z No Qualifier

F Ankle Joint, Right
  Inferior tibiofibular joint
  Talocrural joint
G Ankle Joint, Left
  See F Ankle Joint, Right
H Tarsal Joint, Right
  Calcaneocuboid joint
  Cuboideonavicular joint
  Cuneonavicular joint
  Intercuneiform joint
  Subtalar (talocalcaneal) joint
  Talocalcaneal (subtalar) joint
  Talocalcaneonavicular joint
J Tarsal Joint, Left
  See H Tarsal Joint, Right
K Tarsometatarsal Joint, Right
L Tarsometatarsal Joint, Left
M Metatarsal-Phalangeal Joint, Right
  Metatarsophalangeal (MTP) joint
N Metatarsal-Phalangeal Joint, Left
  See M Metatarsal-Phalangeal Joint, Right
P Toe Phalangeal Joint, Right
  Interphalangeal (IP) joint
Q Toe Phalangeal Joint, Left
  See P Toe Phalangeal Joint, Right
	Ø Open
	3 Percutaneous
	4 Percutaneous Endoscopic
	X External
		Ø Drainage Device
		3 Infusion Device
		4 Internal Fixation Device
		5 External Fixation Device
		7 Autologous Tissue Substitute
		8 Spacer
		J Synthetic Substitute
		K Nonautologous Tissue Substitute
			Z No Qualifier

Non-OR   ØSW[C,D]X[Ø,3,4,5,7,8,K]Z
Non-OR   ØSW[C,D]XJ[C,Z]
Non-OR   ØSW[F,G,H,J,K,L,M,N,P,Q]X[Ø,3,4,5,7,8,J,K]Z

NC Noncovered Procedure   LC Limited Coverage   QA Questionable OB Admit   NT New Tech Add-on   ⊞ Combination Member   ♂ Male   ♀ Female

ICD-10-PCS 2023   621

ØSW–ØSW

Urinary System ØT1–ØTY

Character Meanings

This Character Meaning table is provided as a guide to assist the user in the identification of character members that may be found in this section of code tables. It **SHOULD NOT** be used to build a PCS code.

Operation–Character 3	Body Part–Character 4	Approach–Character 5	Device–Character 6	Qualifier–Character 7
1 Bypass	Ø Kidney, Right	Ø Open	Ø Drainage Device	Ø Allogeneic
2 Change	1 Kidney, Left	3 Percutaneous	1 Radioactive Element	1 Syngeneic
5 Destruction	2 Kidneys, Bilateral	4 Percutaneous Endoscopic	2 Monitoring Device	2 Zooplastic
7 Dilation	3 Kidney Pelvis, Right	7 Via Natural or Artificial Opening	3 Infusion Device	3 Kidney Pelvis, Right
8 Division	4 Kidney Pelvis, Left	8 Via Natural or Artificial Opening Endoscopic	7 Autologous Tissue Substitute	4 Kidney Pelvis, Left
9 Drainage	5 Kidney	X External	C Extraluminal Device	6 Ureter, Right
B Excision	6 Ureter, Right		D Intraluminal Device	7 Ureter, Left
C Extirpation	7 Ureter, Left		J Synthetic Substitute	8 Colon
D Extraction	8 Ureters, Bilateral		K Nonautologous Tissue Substitute	9 Colocutaneous
F Fragmentation	9 Ureter		L Artificial Sphincter	A Ileum
H Insertion	B Bladder		M Stimulator Lead	B Bladder
J Inspection	C Bladder Neck		Y Other Device	C Ileocutaneous
L Occlusion	D Urethra		Z No Device	D Cutaneous
M Reattachment				X Diagnostic
N Release				Z No Qualifier
P Removal				
Q Repair				
R Replacement				
S Reposition				
T Resection				
U Supplement				
V Restriction				
W Revision				
Y Transplantation				

AHA Coding Clinic for table ØT1
2017, 3Q, 20   Creation of Indiana pouch
2017, 3Q, 21   Augmentation cystoplasty with Indiana pouch and continent urinary diversion
2017, 1Q, 37   Perineal urethrostomy
2015, 3Q, 34   Redo urinary diversion surgery via left ureteral reimplantation

AHA Coding Clinic for table ØT7
2019, 2Q, 16   Reimplantation of ureters with insertion of tubes
2017, 4Q, 111   Exchange of ureteral stent
2016, 2Q, 27   Exchange of ureteral stents
2015, 2Q, 8   Urinary calculi fragmentation and evacuation
2013, 4Q, 123   Urolift® procedure

AHA Coding Clinic for table ØT9
2017, 3Q, 19   Ureteral stent placement for urinary leakage
2017, 3Q, 20   Creation of Indiana pouch
2017, 3Q, 21   Augmentation cystoplasty with Indiana pouch and continent urinary diversion

AHA Coding Clinic for table ØTB
2016, 1Q, 19   Biopsy of neobladder malignancy
2015, 3Q, 34   Excision of Mitrofanoff polyp
2014, 2Q, 8   Ileoscopy with excision of polyp of Ileal loop urinary diversion

AHA Coding Clinic for table ØTC
2019, 3Q, 4   Evacuation of clots from bladder dome
2016, 3Q, 23   Ureteral stone migrating into bladder
2015, 2Q, 7   Urinary calculi fragmentation and evacuation
2015, 2Q, 8   Urinary calculi fragmentation and evacuation
2013, 4Q, 122   Laser lithotripsy with removal of fragments

AHA Coding Clinic for table ØTF
2015, 2Q, 7   Urinary calculi fragmentation and evacuation
2013, 4Q, 122   Extracorporeal shock wave lithotripsy
2013, 4Q, 122   Laser lithotripsy with removal of fragments

AHA Coding Clinic for table ØTH
2020, 4Q, 43-44 Insertion of radioactive element
2019, 2Q, 16   Reimplantation of ureters with insertion of tubes

AHA Coding Clinic for table ØTP
2017, 4Q, 111   Exchange of ureteral stent
2016, 2Q, 27   Exchange of ureteral stents

AHA Coding Clinic for table ØTQ
2018, 2Q, 27   Dismembered pyeloplasty
2017, 1Q, 37   Perineal urethrostomy

AHA Coding Clinic for table ØTR
2017, 3Q, 20   Creation of Indiana pouch

AHA Coding Clinic for table ØTS
2019, 1Q, 29   Young-Dees-Leadbetter bladder neck reconstruction
2018, 2Q, 27   Dismembered pyeloplasty
2017, 1Q, 36   Dismembered pyeloplasty
2016, 1Q, 15   Pubovaginal sling placement

AHA Coding Clinic for table ØTT
2014, 3Q, 16   Hand-assisted laparoscopy nephroureterectomy

AHA Coding Clinic for table ØTU
2019, 1Q, 29   Young-Dees-Leadbetter bladder neck reconstruction
2017, 3Q, 21   Augmentation cystoplasty with Indiana pouch and continent urinary diversion

AHA Coding Clinic for table ØTV
2015, 2Q, 11   Cystourethroscopic Deflux® injection

Urinary System

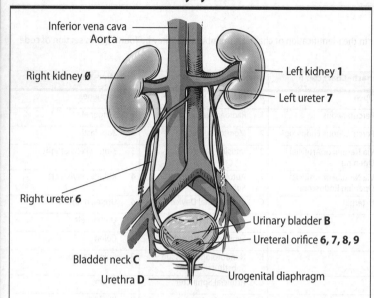

Urinary System

- Inferior vena cava
- Aorta
- Right kidney Ø
- Left kidney 1
- Left ureter 7
- Right ureter 6
- Urinary bladder B
- Ureteral orifice 6, 7, 8, 9
- Bladder neck C
- Urethra D
- Urogenital diaphragm

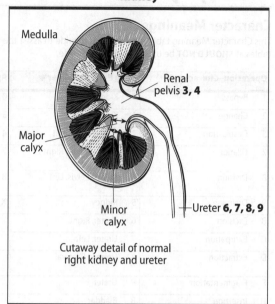

Kidney

- Medulla
- Renal pelvis 3, 4
- Major calyx
- Minor calyx
- Ureter 6, 7, 8, 9

Cutaway detail of normal right kidney and ureter

Bladder

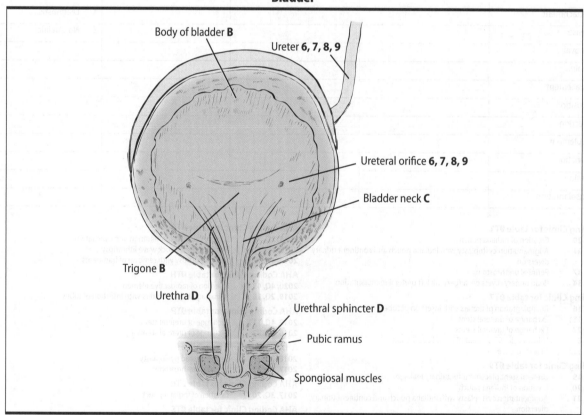

- Body of bladder B
- Ureter 6, 7, 8, 9
- Ureteral orifice 6, 7, 8, 9
- Bladder neck C
- Trigone B
- Urethra D
- Urethral sphincter D
- Pubic ramus
- Spongiosal muscles

Ø   Medical and Surgical
T   Urinary System
1   Bypass   Definition: Altering the route of passage of the contents of a tubular body part

Explanation: Rerouting contents of a body part to a downstream area of the normal route, to a similar route and body part, or to an abnormal route and dissimilar body part. Includes one or more anastomoses, with or without the use of a device.

Body Part Character 4	Approach Character 5	Device Character 6	Qualifier Character 7

3   **Kidney Pelvis, Right**
   Ureteropelvic junction (UPJ)
4   **Kidney Pelvis, Left**
   See 3 Kidney Pelvis, Right
	Ø Open
	4 Percutaneous Endoscopic
		7 Autologous Tissue Substitute
		J Synthetic Substitute
		K Nonautologous Tissue Substitute
		Z No Device
			3 Kidney Pelvis, Right
			4 Kidney Pelvis, Left
			6 Ureter, Right
			7 Ureter, Left
			8 Colon
			9 Colocutaneous
			A Ileum
			B Bladder
			C Ileocutaneous
			D Cutaneous

3   **Kidney Pelvis, Right**
   Ureteropelvic junction (UPJ)
4   **Kidney Pelvis, Left**
   See 3 Kidney Pelvis, Right
	3 Percutaneous	**J** Synthetic Substitute	**D** Cutaneous

6   **Ureter, Right**
   Ureteral orifice
   Ureterovesical orifice
7   **Ureter, Left**
   See 6 Ureter, Right
8   **Ureters, Bilateral**
   See 6 Ureter, Right
	Ø Open
	4 Percutaneous Endoscopic
		7 Autologous Tissue Substitute
		J Synthetic Substitute
		K Nonautologous Tissue Substitute
		Z No Device
			6 Ureter, Right
			7 Ureter, Left
			8 Colon
			9 Colocutaneous
			A Ileum
			B Bladder
			C Ileocutaneous
			D Cutaneous

6   **Ureter, Right**
   Ureteral orifice
   Ureterovesical orifice
7   **Ureter, Left**
   See 6 Ureter, Right
8   **Ureters, Bilateral**
   See 6 Ureter, Right
	3 Percutaneous	**J** Synthetic Substitute	**D** Cutaneous

B **Bladder** Trigone of bladder	**Ø** Open **4** Percutaneous Endoscopic	**7** Autologous Tissue Substitute **J** Synthetic Substitute **K** Nonautologous Tissue Substitute **Z** No Device	**9** Colocutaneous **C** Ileocutaneous **D** Cutaneous
B **Bladder** Trigone of bladder	**3** Percutaneous	**J** Synthetic Substitute	**D** Cutaneous

Ø   Medical and Surgical
T   Urinary System
2   Change   Definition: Taking out or off a device from a body part and putting back an identical or similar device in or on the same body part without cutting or puncturing the skin or a mucous membrane

Explanation: All CHANGE procedures are coded using the approach EXTERNAL

Body Part Character 4	Approach Character 5	Device Character 6	Qualifier Character 7

5   **Kidney**
   Renal calyx
   Renal capsule
   Renal cortex
   Renal segment
9   **Ureter**
   Ureteral orifice
   Ureterovesical orifice
B   **Bladder**
   Trigone of bladder
D   **Urethra**
   Bulbourethral (Cowper's) gland
   Cowper's (bulbourethral) gland
   External urethral sphincter
   Internal urethral sphincter
   Membranous urethra
   Penile urethra
   Prostatic urethra
	X External	**Ø** Drainage Device
		Y Other Device
			Z No Qualifier

Non-OR   All body part, approach, device, and qualifier values

NC Noncovered Procedure   **LC** Limited Coverage   **QA** Questionable OB Admit   **NT** New Tech Add-on   ⊞ Combination Member   ♂ Male   ♀ Female

ICD-10-PCS 2023   625

ØT1–ØT2

Urinary System (side margin)

Ø   **Medical and Surgical**
T   **Urinary System**
5   **Destruction**   Definition: Physical eradication of all or a portion of a body part by the direct use of energy, force, or a destructive agent

                 Explanation: None of the body part is physically taken out

Body Part Character 4	Approach Character 5	Device Character 6	Qualifier Character 7
Ø Kidney, Right Renal calyx Renal capsule Renal cortex Renal segment **1 Kidney, Left** *See Ø Kidney, Right* **3 Kidney Pelvis, Right** Ureteropelvic junction (UPJ) **4 Kidney Pelvis, Left** *See 3 Kidney Pelvis, Right* **6 Ureter, Right** Ureteral orifice Ureterovesical orifice **7 Ureter, Left** *See 6 Ureter, Right* **B Bladder** Trigone of bladder **C Bladder Neck**	**Ø Open** **3 Percutaneous** **4 Percutaneous Endoscopic** **7 Via Natural or Artificial Opening** **8 Via Natural or Artificial Opening Endoscopic**	**Z No Device**	**Z No Qualifier**
D Urethra Bulbourethral (Cowper's) gland Cowper's (bulbourethral) gland External urethral sphincter Internal urethral sphincter Membranous urethra Penile urethra Prostatic urethra	**Ø Open** **3 Percutaneous** **4 Percutaneous Endoscopic** **7 Via Natural or Artificial Opening** **8 Via Natural or Artificial Opening Endoscopic** **X External**	**Z No Device**	**Z No Qualifier**

Non-OR   ØT5D[Ø,3,4,7,8,X]ZZ

Ø   **Medical and Surgical**
T   **Urinary System**
7   **Dilation**   Definition: Expanding an orifice or the lumen of a tubular body part

                 Explanation: The orifice can be a natural orifice or an artificially created orifice. Accomplished by stretching a tubular body part using intraluminal pressure or by cutting part of the orifice or wall of the tubular body part.

Body Part Character 4	Approach Character 5	Device Character 6	Qualifier Character 7
3 Kidney Pelvis, Right Ureteropelvic junction (UPJ) **4 Kidney Pelvis, Left** *See 3 Kidney Pelvis, Right* **6 Ureter, Right** Ureteral orifice Ureterovesical orifice **7 Ureter, Left** *See 6 Ureter, Right* **8 Ureters, Bilateral** *See 6 Ureter, Right* **B Bladder** Trigone of bladder **C Bladder Neck** **D Urethra** Bulbourethral (Cowper's) gland Cowper's (bulbourethral) gland External urethral sphincter Internal urethral sphincter Membranous urethra Penile urethra Prostatic urethra	**Ø Open** **3 Percutaneous** **4 Percutaneous Endoscopic** **7 Via Natural or Artificial Opening** **8 Via Natural or Artificial Opening Endoscopic**	**D Intraluminal Device** **Z No Device**	**Z No Qualifier**

Non-OR   ØT7[6,7,8][Ø,3,4,7]DZ   Non-OR   ØT7B7[D,Z]Z   Non-OR   ØT7[C,D][7,8][D,Z]Z
Non-OR   ØT7[6,7,8]7ZZ   Non-OR   ØT7C[Ø,3,4]ZZ
Non-OR   ØT788ZZ   Non-OR   ØT7[C,D][Ø,3,4]DZ

Ø   **Medical and Surgical**
T   **Urinary System**
8   **Division**   Definition: Cutting into a body part, without draining fluids and/or gases from the body part, in order to separate or transect a body part

                 Explanation: All or a portion of the body part is separated into two or more portions

Body Part Character 4	Approach Character 5	Device Character 6	Qualifier Character 7
2 Kidneys, Bilateral Renal calyx Renal capsule Renal cortex Renal segment **C Bladder Neck**	**Ø Open** **3 Percutaneous** **4 Percutaneous Endoscopic**	**Z No Device**	**Z No Qualifier**

Non-OR Procedure   DRG Non-OR Procedure   Valid OR Procedure   HAC Associated Procedure   Combination Only   New/Revised April   New/Revised October

626   ICD-10-PCS 2023

ØT5–ØT8 (side margin)

0   Medical and Surgical
T   Urinary System
9   Drainage   Definition: Taking or letting out fluids and/or gases from a body part
                    Explanation: The qualifier DIAGNOSTIC is used to identify drainage procedures that are biopsies

Body Part Character 4	Approach Character 5	Device Character 6	Qualifier Character 7
0 Kidney, Right Renal calyx Renal capsule Renal cortex Renal segment **1 Kidney, Left** *See 0 Kidney, Right* **3 Kidney Pelvis, Right** Ureteropelvic junction (UPJ) **4 Kidney Pelvis, Left** *See 3 Kidney Pelvis, Right* **6 Ureter, Right** Ureteral orifice Ureterovesical orifice **7 Ureter, Left** *See 6 Ureter, Right* **8 Ureters, Bilateral** *See 6 Ureter, Right* **B Bladder** Trigone of bladder **C Bladder Neck**	**0** Open **3** Percutaneous **4** Percutaneous Endoscopic **7** Via Natural or Artificial Opening **8** Via Natural or Artificial Opening Endoscopic	**0** Drainage Device	**Z** No Qualifier
0 Kidney, Right Renal calyx Renal capsule Renal cortex Renal segment **1 Kidney, Left** *See 0 Kidney, Right* **3 Kidney Pelvis, Right** Ureteropelvic junction (UPJ) **4 Kidney Pelvis, Left** *See 3 Kidney Pelvis, Right* **6 Ureter, Right** Ureteral orifice Ureterovesical orifice **7 Ureter, Left** *See 6 Ureter, Right* **8 Ureters, Bilateral** *See 6 Ureter, Right* **B Bladder** Trigone of bladder **C Bladder Neck**	**0** Open **3** Percutaneous **4** Percutaneous Endoscopic **7** Via Natural or Artificial Opening **8** Via Natural or Artificial Opening Endoscopic	**Z** No Device	**X** Diagnostic **Z** No Qualifier
D Urethra Bulbourethral (Cowper's) gland Cowper's (bulbourethral) gland External urethral sphincter Internal urethral sphincter Membranous urethra Penile urethra Prostatic urethra	**0** Open **3** Percutaneous **4** Percutaneous Endoscopic **7** Via Natural or Artificial Opening **8** Via Natural or Artificial Opening Endoscopic **X** External	**0** Drainage Device	**Z** No Qualifier
D Urethra Bulbourethral (Cowper's) gland Cowper's (bulbourethral) gland External urethral sphincter Internal urethral sphincter Membranous urethra Penile urethra Prostatic urethra	**0** Open **3** Percutaneous **4** Percutaneous Endoscopic **7** Via Natural or Artificial Opening **8** Via Natural or Artificial Opening Endoscopic **X** External	**Z** No Device	**X** Diagnostic **Z** No Qualifier

Non-OR	0T9[0,1,3,4]30Z
Non-OR	0T9[6,7,8][0,3,4,7,8]0Z
Non-OR	0T9[B,C][3,4,7,8]0Z
Non-OR	0T9[0,1,3,4,6,7,8][3,4,7,8]ZX
Non-OR	0T9[0,1,3,4][3,4]ZZ
Non-OR	0T9[6,7,8]3ZZ
Non-OR	0T9[B,C][3,4,7,8]ZZ
Non-OR	0T9D30Z
Non-OR	0T9D[0,3,4,7,8,X]ZX
Non-OR	0T9D3ZZ

NC Noncovered Procedure   LC Limited Coverage   QA Questionable OB Admit   NT New Tech Add-on   ⊞ Combination Member   ♂Male   ♀Female

ICD-10-PCS 2023   627

Ø   **Medical and Surgical**
T   **Urinary System**
B   **Excision**   Definition: Cutting out or off, without replacement, a portion of a body part

            Explanation: The qualifier DIAGNOSTIC is used to identify excision procedures that are biopsies

Body Part Character 4	Approach Character 5	Device Character 6	Qualifier Character 7

Ø Kidney, Right
   Renal calyx
   Renal capsule
   Renal cortex
   Renal segment
1 Kidney, Left
   See Ø Kidney, Right
3 Kidney Pelvis, Right
   Ureteropelvic junction (UPJ)
4 Kidney Pelvis, Left
   See 3 Kidney Pelvis, Right
6 Ureter, Right
   Ureteral orifice
   Ureterovesical orifice
7 Ureter, Left
   See 6 Ureter, Right
B Bladder
   Trigone of bladder
C Bladder Neck
	Ø Open
	3 Percutaneous
	4 Percutaneous Endoscopic
	7 Via Natural or Artificial Opening
	8 Via Natural or Artificial Opening
	   Endoscopic
		Z No Device	**X** Diagnostic
			Z No Qualifier

D Urethra
   Bulbourethral (Cowper's) gland
   Cowper's (bulbourethral) gland
   External urethral sphincter
   Internal urethral sphincter
   Membranous urethra
   Penile urethra
   Prostatic urethra
	Ø Open
	3 Percutaneous
	4 Percutaneous Endoscopic
	7 Via Natural or Artificial Opening
	8 Via Natural or Artificial Opening
	   Endoscopic
	X External
		Z No Device	**X** Diagnostic
			Z No Qualifier

Non-OR   ØTB[Ø,1,3,4,6,7][3,4,7,8]ZX
Non-OR   ØTBD[Ø,3,4,7,8,X]ZX

Ø   **Medical and Surgical**
T   **Urinary System**
C   **Extirpation**   Definition: Taking or cutting out solid matter from a body part

            Explanation: The solid matter may be an abnormal byproduct of a biological function or a foreign body; it may be imbedded in a body part or in the lumen of a tubular body part. The solid matter may or may not have been previously broken into pieces.

Body Part Character 4	Approach Character 5	Device Character 6	Qualifier Character 7

Ø Kidney, Right
   Renal calyx
   Renal capsule
   Renal cortex
   Renal segment
1 Kidney, Left
   See Ø Kidney, Right
3 Kidney Pelvis, Right
   Ureteropelvic junction (UPJ)
4 Kidney Pelvis, Left
   See 3 Kidney Pelvis, Right
6 Ureter, Right
   Ureteral orifice
   Ureterovesical orifice
7 Ureter, Left
   See 6 Ureter, Right
B Bladder
   Trigone of bladder
C Bladder Neck
	Ø Open
	3 Percutaneous
	4 Percutaneous Endoscopic
	7 Via Natural or Artificial Opening
	8 Via Natural or Artificial Opening
	   Endoscopic
		Z No Device	**Z** No Qualifier

D Urethra
   Bulbourethral (Cowper's) gland
   Cowper's (bulbourethral) gland
   External urethral sphincter
   Internal urethral sphincter
   Membranous urethra
   Penile urethra
   Prostatic urethra
	Ø Open
	3 Percutaneous
	4 Percutaneous Endoscopic
	7 Via Natural or Artificial Opening
	8 Via Natural or Artificial Opening
	   Endoscopic
	X External
		Z No Device	**Z** No Qualifier

Non-OR   ØTC[Ø,1,3,4,6,7]8ZZ
Non-OR   ØTC[B,C][7,8]ZZ
Non-OR   ØTCD[7,8,X]ZZ

Non-OR Procedure   DRG Non-OR Procedure   Valid OR Procedure   HAC Associated Procedure   Combination Only   New/Revised April   New/Revised October

Ø   **Medical and Surgical**
T   **Urinary System**
D   **Extraction**   Definition: Pulling or stripping out or off all or a portion of a body part by the use of force

                        Explanation: The qualifier DIAGNOSTIC is used to identify extraction procedures that are biopsies

Body Part Character 4	Approach Character 5	Device Character 6	Qualifier Character 7

Ø Kidney, Right
   Renal calyx
   Renal capsule
   Renal cortex
   Renal segment
1 Kidney, Left
   See Ø Kidney, Right
	Ø Open
	3 Percutaneous
	4 Percutaneous Endoscopic
		Z No Device	**Z No Qualifier**

Ø   **Medical and Surgical**
T   **Urinary System**
F   **Fragmentation**   Definition: Breaking solid matter in a body part into pieces

                        Explanation: Physical force (e.g., manual, ultrasonic) applied directly or indirectly is used to break the solid matter into pieces. The solid matter may be an abnormal byproduct of a biological function or a foreign body. The pieces of solid matter are not taken out.

Body Part Character 4	Approach Character 5	Device Character 6	Qualifier Character 7

3 Kidney Pelvis, Right
   Ureteropelvic junction (UPJ)
4 Kidney Pelvis, Left
   See 3 Kidney Pelvis, Right
6 Ureter, Right
   Ureteral orifice
   Ureterovesical orifice
7 Ureter, Left
   See 6 Ureter, Right
B Bladder
   Trigone of bladder
C Bladder Neck
D Urethra NC
   Bulbourethral (Cowper's) gland
   Cowper's (bulbourethral) gland
   External urethral sphincter
   Internal urethral sphincter
   Membranous urethra
   Penile urethra
   Prostatic urethra
	Ø Open
	3 Percutaneous
	4 Percutaneous Endoscopic
	7 Via Natural or Artificial Opening
	8 Via Natural or Artificial Opening
	   Endoscopic
	X External
		Z No Device	**Z No Qualifier**

Non-OR	ØTF[3,4][Ø,7,8]ZZ
Non-OR	ØTF[6,7,B,C,D][Ø,3,4,7,8]ZZ
Non-OR	ØTF[3,4,6,7,B,C,D]XZZ
NC	ØTFDXZZ

Urinary System

Ø **Medical and Surgical**
T **Urinary System**
H **Insertion** Definition: Putting in a nonbiological appliance that monitors, assists, performs, or prevents a physiological function but does not physically take the place of a body part
Explanation: None

Body Part Character 4	Approach Character 5	Device Character 6	Qualifier Character 7
5 Kidney Renal calyx Renal capsule Renal cortex Renal segment	**Ø** Open **3** Percutaneous **4** Percutaneous Endoscopic **7** Via Natural or Artificial Opening **8** Via Natural or Artificial Opening Endoscopic	**1** Radioactive Element **2** Monitoring Device **3** Infusion Device **Y** Other Device	**Z** No Qualifier
9 Ureter Ureteral orifice Ureterovesical orifice	**Ø** Open **3** Percutaneous **4** Percutaneous Endoscopic **7** Via Natural or Artificial Opening **8** Via Natural or Artificial Opening Endoscopic	**1** Radioactive Element **2** Monitoring Device **3** Infusion Device **M** Stimulator Lead **Y** Other Device	**Z** No Qualifier
B Bladder NC Trigone of bladder	**Ø** Open **3** Percutaneous **4** Percutaneous Endoscopic **7** Via Natural or Artificial Opening **8** Via Natural or Artificial Opening Endoscopic	**1** Radioactive Element **2** Monitoring Device **3** Infusion Device **L** Artificial Sphincter **M** Stimulator Lead **Y** Other Device	**Z** No Qualifier
C Bladder Neck	**Ø** Open **3** Percutaneous **4** Percutaneous Endoscopic **7** Via Natural or Artificial Opening **8** Via Natural or Artificial Opening Endoscopic	**L** Artificial Sphincter	**Z** No Qualifier
D Urethra Bulbourethral (Cowper's) gland Cowper's (bulbourethral) gland External urethral sphincter Internal urethral sphincter Membranous urethra Penile urethra Prostatic urethra	**Ø** Open **3** Percutaneous **4** Percutaneous Endoscopic **7** Via Natural or Artificial Opening **8** Via Natural or Artificial Opening Endoscopic	**1** Radioactive Element **2** Monitoring Device **3** Infusion Device **L** Artificial Sphincter **Y** Other Device	**Z** No Qualifier
D Urethra Bulbourethral (Cowper's) gland Cowper's (bulbourethral) gland External urethral sphincter Internal urethral sphincter Membranous urethra Penile urethra Prostatic urethra	**X** External	**2** Monitoring Device **3** Infusion Device **L** Artificial Sphincter	**Z** No Qualifier

Non-OR ØTH5Ø3Z		**Non-OR** ØTHB3[1,3,Y]Z	
Non-OR ØTH53[1,3,Y]Z		**Non-OR** ØTHB4[3,Y]Z	
Non-OR ØTH54[3,Y]Z		**Non-OR** ØTHB7[1,2,3,Y]Z	
Non-OR ØTH57[1,2,3,Y]Z		**Non-OR** ØTHB8[2,3]Z	
Non-OR ØTH58[2,3]Z		**Non-OR** ØTHDØ3Z	
Non-OR ØTH9Ø3Z		**Non-OR** ØTHD3[1,3,Y]Z	
Non-OR ØTH93[1,3,Y]Z		**Non-OR** ØTHD4[3,Y]Z	
Non-OR ØTH94[3,Y]Z		**Non-OR** ØTHD7[1,2,3,Y]Z	
Non-OR ØTH97[1,2,3,Y]Z		**Non-OR** ØTHD8[2,3,Y]Z	
Non-OR ØTH98[2,3]Z		**Non-OR** ØTHDX3Z	
Non-OR ØTHBØ3Z		**NC** ØTHB[Ø,3,4,7,8]MZ	

Non-OR Procedure   DRG Non-OR Procedure   Valid OR Procedure   HAC Associated Procedure   Combination Only   New/Revised April   New/Revised October

630   ICD-10-PCS 2023

ØTH–ØTH

Ø   **Medical and Surgical**
T   **Urinary System**
J   **Inspection**   Definition: Visually and/or manually exploring a body part

Explanation: Visual exploration may be performed with or without optical instrumentation. Manual exploration may be performed directly or through intervening body layers.

Body Part Character 4	Approach Character 5	Device Character 6	Qualifier Character 7
5 Kidney Renal calyx Renal capsule Renal cortex Renal segment **9 Ureter** Ureteral orifice Ureterovesical orifice **B Bladder** Trigone of bladder **D Urethra** Bulbourethral (Cowper's) gland Cowper's (bulbourethral) gland External urethral sphincter Internal urethral sphincter Membranous urethra Penile urethra Prostatic urethra	**Ø** Open **3** Percutaneous **4** Percutaneous Endoscopic **7** Via Natural or Artificial Opening **8** Via Natural or Artificial Opening Endoscopic **X** External	**Z** No Device	**Z** No Qualifier

Non-OR	ØTJ[5,9,D][3,4,7,8,X]ZZ
Non-OR	ØTJB[3,7,8,X]ZZ

Ø   **Medical and Surgical**
T   **Urinary System**
L   **Occlusion**   Definition: Completely closing an orifice or the lumen of a tubular body part

Explanation: The orifice can be a natural orifice or an artificially created orifice

Body Part Character 4	Approach Character 5	Device Character 6	Qualifier Character 7
3 Kidney Pelvis, Right Ureteropelvic junction (UPJ) **4 Kidney Pelvis, Left** *See 3 Kidney Pelvis, Right* **6 Ureter, Right** Ureteral orifice Ureterovesical orifice **7 Ureter, Left** *See 6 Ureter, Right* **B Bladder** Trigone of bladder **C Bladder Neck**	**Ø** Open **3** Percutaneous **4** Percutaneous Endoscopic	**C** Extraluminal Device **D** Intraluminal Device **Z** No Device	**Z** No Qualifier
3 Kidney Pelvis, Right Ureteropelvic junction (UPJ) **4 Kidney Pelvis, Left** *See 3 Kidney Pelvis, Right* **6 Ureter, Right** Ureteral orifice Ureterovesical orifice **7 Ureter, Left** *See 6 Ureter, Right* **B Bladder** Trigone of bladder **C Bladder Neck**	**7** Via Natural or Artificial Opening **8** Via Natural or Artificial Opening Endoscopic	**D** Intraluminal Device **Z** No Device	**Z** No Qualifier
D Urethra Bulbourethral (Cowper's) gland Cowper's (bulbourethral) gland External urethral sphincter Internal urethral sphincter Membranous urethra Penile urethra Prostatic urethra	**Ø** Open **3** Percutaneous **4** Percutaneous Endoscopic **X** External	**C** Extraluminal Device **D** Intraluminal Device **Z** No Device	**Z** No Qualifier
D Urethra Bulbourethral (Cowper's) gland Cowper's (bulbourethral) gland External urethral sphincter Internal urethral sphincter Membranous urethra Penile urethra Prostatic urethra	**7** Via Natural or Artificial Opening **8** Via Natural or Artificial Opening Endoscopic	**D** Intraluminal Device **Z** No Device	**Z** No Qualifier

Ø   Medical and Surgical
T   Urinary System
M   Reattachment   Definition: Putting back in or on all or a portion of a separated body part to its normal location or other suitable location
                   Explanation: Vascular circulation and nervous pathways may or may not be reestablished

Body Part Character 4	Approach Character 5	Device Character 6	Qualifier Character 7

Ø   **Kidney, Right**
    Renal calyx
    Renal capsule
    Renal cortex
    Renal segment
1   **Kidney, Left**
    See Ø Kidney, Right
2   **Kidneys, Bilateral**
    See Ø Kidney, Right
3   **Kidney Pelvis, Right**
    Ureteropelvic junction (UPJ)
4   **Kidney Pelvis, Left**
    See 3 Kidney Pelvis, Right
6   **Ureter, Right**
    Ureteral orifice
    Ureterovesical orifice
7   **Ureter, Left**
    See 6 Ureter, Right
8   **Ureters, Bilateral**
    See 6 Ureter, Right
B   **Bladder**
    Trigone of bladder
C   **Bladder Neck**
D   **Urethra**
    Bulbourethral (Cowper's) gland
    Cowper's (bulbourethral) gland
    External urethral sphincter
    Internal urethral sphincter
    Membranous urethra
    Penile urethra
    Prostatic urethra
	Ø Open
	4 Percutaneous Endoscopic
		Z No Device	**Z** No Qualifier

Ø   Medical and Surgical
T   Urinary System
N   Release   Definition: Freeing a body part from an abnormal physical constraint by cutting or by the use of force
                 Explanation: Some of the restraining tissue may be taken out but none of the body part is taken out

Body Part Character 4	Approach Character 5	Device Character 6	Qualifier Character 7

Ø   **Kidney, Right**
    Renal calyx
    Renal capsule
    Renal cortex
    Renal segment
1   **Kidney, Left**
    See Ø Kidney, Right
3   **Kidney Pelvis, Right**
    Ureteropelvic junction (UPJ)
4   **Kidney Pelvis, Left**
    See 3 Kidney Pelvis, Right
6   **Ureter, Right**
    Ureteral orifice
    Ureterovesical orifice
7   **Ureter, Left**
    See 6 Ureter, Right
B   **Bladder**
    Trigone of bladder
C   **Bladder Neck**
	Ø Open
	3 Percutaneous
	4 Percutaneous Endoscopic
	7 Via Natural or Artificial Opening
	8 Via Natural or Artificial Opening
	    Endoscopic
		Z No Device	**Z** No Qualifier

D   **Urethra**
    Bulbourethral (Cowper's) gland
    Cowper's (bulbourethral) gland
    External urethral sphincter
    Internal urethral sphincter
    Membranous urethra
    Penile urethra
    Prostatic urethra
	Ø Open
	3 Percutaneous
	4 Percutaneous Endoscopic
	7 Via Natural or Artificial Opening
	8 Via Natural or Artificial Opening
	    Endoscopic
	X External
		Z No Device	**Z** No Qualifier

Non-OR Procedure   DRG Non-OR Procedure   Valid OR Procedure   HAC Associated Procedure   Combination Only   New/Revised April   New/Revised October

632   ICD-10-PCS 2023

Ø **Medical and Surgical**
T **Urinary System**
P **Removal**　　　Definition: Taking out or off a device from a body part

Explanation: If a device is taken out and a similar device put in without cutting or puncturing the skin or mucous membrane, the procedure is coded to the root operation CHANGE. Otherwise, the procedure for taking out the device is coded to the root operation REMOVAL.

Body Part Character 4	Approach Character 5	Device Character 6	Qualifier Character 7
5 Kidney Renal calyx Renal capsule Renal cortex Renal segment	**Ø** Open **3** Percutaneous **4** Percutaneous Endoscopic **7** Via Natural or Artificial Opening **8** Via Natural or Artificial Opening Endoscopic	**Ø** Drainage Device **2** Monitoring Device **3** Infusion Device **7** Autologous Tissue Substitute **C** Extraluminal Device **D** Intraluminal Device **J** Synthetic Substitute **K** Nonautologous Tissue Substitute **Y** Other Device	**Z** No Qualifier
5 Kidney Renal calyx Renal capsule Renal cortex Renal segment	**X** External	**Ø** Drainage Device **2** Monitoring Device **3** Infusion Device **D** Intraluminal Device	**Z** No Qualifier
9 Ureter Ureteral orifice Ureterovesical orifice	**Ø** Open **3** Percutaneous **4** Percutaneous Endoscopic **7** Via Natural or Artificial Opening **8** Via Natural or Artificial Opening Endoscopic	**Ø** Drainage Device **2** Monitoring Device **3** Infusion Device **7** Autologous Tissue Substitute **C** Extraluminal Device **D** Intraluminal Device **J** Synthetic Substitute **K** Nonautologous Tissue Substitute **M** Stimulator Lead **Y** Other Device	**Z** No Qualifier
9 Ureter Ureteral orifice Ureterovesical orifice	**X** External	**Ø** Drainage Device **2** Monitoring Device **3** Infusion Device **D** Intraluminal Device **M** Stimulator Lead	**Z** No Qualifier
B Bladder ▣NC Trigone of bladder	**Ø** Open **3** Percutaneous **4** Percutaneous Endoscopic **7** Via Natural or Artificial Opening **8** Via Natural or Artificial Opening Endoscopic	**Ø** Drainage Device **2** Monitoring Device **3** Infusion Device **7** Autologous Tissue Substitute **C** Extraluminal Device **D** Intraluminal Device **J** Synthetic Substitute **K** Nonautologous Tissue Substitute **L** Artificial Sphincter **M** Stimulator Lead **Y** Other Device	**Z** No Qualifier
B Bladder Trigone of bladder	**X** External	**Ø** Drainage Device **2** Monitoring Device **3** Infusion Device **D** Intraluminal Device **L** Artificial Sphincter **M** Stimulator Lead	**Z** No Qualifier
D Urethra Bulbourethral (Cowper's) gland Cowper's (bulbourethral) gland External urethral sphincter Internal urethral sphincter Membranous urethra Penile urethra Prostatic urethra	**Ø** Open **3** Percutaneous **4** Percutaneous Endoscopic **7** Via Natural or Artificial Opening **8** Via Natural or Artificial Opening Endoscopic	**Ø** Drainage Device **2** Monitoring Device **3** Infusion Device **7** Autologous Tissue Substitute **C** Extraluminal Device **D** Intraluminal Device **J** Synthetic Substitute **K** Nonautologous Tissue Substitute **L** Artificial Sphincter **Y** Other Device	**Z** No Qualifier
D Urethra Bulbourethral (Cowper's) gland Cowper's (bulbourethral) gland External urethral sphincter Internal urethral sphincter Membranous urethra Penile urethra Prostatic urethra	**X** External	**Ø** Drainage Device **2** Monitoring Device **3** Infusion Device **D** Intraluminal Device **L** Artificial Sphincter	**Z** No Qualifier

Non-OR ØTP5[3,4,7]YZ	**Non-OR** ØTP9[7,8][Ø,2,3,D]Z	**Non-OR** ØTPB[7,8][Ø,2,3,D]Z	**Non-OR** ØTPD[7,8][Ø,2,3,D,Y]Z
Non-OR ØTP5[7,8][Ø,2,3,D]Z	**Non-OR** ØTP9X[Ø,2,3,D]Z	**Non-OR** ØTPBX[Ø,2,3,D,L]Z	**Non-OR** ØTPDX[Ø,2,3,D]Z
Non-OR ØTP5X[Ø,2,3,D]Z	**Non-OR** ØTPB[3,4,7]YZ	**Non-OR** ØTPD[3,4]YZ	▣NC ØTPB[Ø,3,4,7,8]MZ
Non-OR ØTP9[3,4,7]YZ			

▣NC Noncovered Procedure　　▣LC Limited Coverage　　▣QA Questionable OB Admit　　▣NT New Tech Add-on　　✛ Combination Member　　♂ Male　　♀ Female

ICD-10-PCS 2023　　　　　　　　　　　　　　　　　　　　　　　　　　　　　　　　　　　　　　633

ØTP–ØTP

Ø   **Medical and Surgical**
T   **Urinary System**
Q   **Repair**   Definition: Restoring, to the extent possible, a body part to its normal anatomic structure and function

                 Explanation: Used only when the method to accomplish the repair is not one of the other root operations

Body Part Character 4	Approach Character 5	Device Character 6	Qualifier Character 7

Ø   **Kidney, Right**
    Renal calyx
    Renal capsule
    Renal cortex
    Renal segment
1   **Kidney, Left**
    See Ø Kidney, Right
3   **Kidney Pelvis, Right**
    Ureteropelvic junction (UPJ)
4   **Kidney Pelvis, Left**
    See 3 Kidney Pelvis, Right
6   **Ureter, Right**
    Ureteral orifice
    Ureterovesical orifice
7   **Ureter, Left**
    See 6 Ureter, Right
B   **Bladder**   ⊞
    Trigone of bladder
C   **Bladder Neck**
	Ø **Open**
	3 **Percutaneous**
	4 **Percutaneous Endoscopic**
	7 **Via Natural or Artificial Opening**
	8 **Via Natural or Artificial Opening**
	    Endoscopic
		Z **No Device**	Z **No Qualifier**

D   **Urethra**
    Bulbourethral (Cowper's) gland
    Cowper's (bulbourethral) gland
    External urethral sphincter
    Internal urethral sphincter
    Membranous urethra
    Penile urethra
    Prostatic urethra
	Ø **Open**
	3 **Percutaneous**
	4 **Percutaneous Endoscopic**
	7 **Via Natural or Artificial Opening**
	8 **Via Natural or Artificial Opening**
	    Endoscopic
	X **External**
		Z **No Device**	Z **No Qualifier**

See Appendix L for Procedure Combinations
   ⊞   ØTQB[Ø,3,4]ZZ

Ø   **Medical and Surgical**
T   **Urinary System**
R   **Replacement**   Definition: Putting in or on biological or synthetic material that physically takes the place and/or function of all or a portion of a body part

                      Explanation: The body part may have been taken out or replaced, or may be taken out, physically eradicated, or rendered nonfunctional during the REPLACEMENT procedure. A REMOVAL procedure is coded for taking out the device used in a previous replacement procedure.

Body Part Character 4	Approach Character 5	Device Character 6	Qualifier Character 7

3   **Kidney Pelvis, Right**
    Ureteropelvic junction (UPJ)
4   **Kidney Pelvis, Left**
    See 3 Kidney Pelvis, Right
6   **Ureter, Right**
    Ureteral orifice
    Ureterovesical orifice
7   **Ureter, Left**
    See 6 Ureter, Right
B   **Bladder**
    Trigone of bladder
C   **Bladder Neck**
	Ø **Open**
	4 **Percutaneous Endoscopic**
	7 **Via Natural or Artificial Opening**
	8 **Via Natural or Artificial Opening**
	    Endoscopic
		7 **Autologous Tissue Substitute**
		J **Synthetic Substitute**
		K **Nonautologous Tissue Substitute**
			Z **No Qualifier**

D   **Urethra**
    Bulbourethral (Cowper's) gland
    Cowper's (bulbourethral) gland
    External urethral sphincter
    Internal urethral sphincter
    Membranous urethra
    Penile urethra
    Prostatic urethra
	Ø **Open**
	4 **Percutaneous Endoscopic**
	7 **Via Natural or Artificial Opening**
	8 **Via Natural or Artificial Opening**
	    Endoscopic
	X **External**
		7 **Autologous Tissue Substitute**
		J **Synthetic Substitute**
		K **Nonautologous Tissue Substitute**
			Z **No Qualifier**

Non-OR Procedure   DRG Non-OR Procedure   Valid OR Procedure   HAC Associated Procedure   Combination Only   New/Revised April   New/Revised October

634   **ICD-10-PCS 2023**

ØTQ–ØTR

Ø   **Medical and Surgical**
T   **Urinary System**
S   **Reposition**   Definition: Moving to its normal location, or other suitable location, all or a portion of a body part

Explanation: The body part is moved to a new location from an abnormal location, or from a normal location where it is not functioning correctly. The body part may or may not be cut out or off to be moved to the new location.

Body Part Character 4	Approach Character 5	Device Character 6	Qualifier Character 7

Ø   **Kidney, Right**
    Renal calyx
    Renal capsule
    Renal cortex
    Renal segment
1   **Kidney, Left**
    See Ø Kidney, Right
2   **Kidneys, Bilateral**
    See Ø Kidney, Right
3   **Kidney Pelvis, Right**
    Ureteropelvic junction (UPJ)
4   **Kidney Pelvis, Left**
    See 3 Kidney Pelvis, Right
6   **Ureter, Right**
    Ureteral orifice
    Ureterovesical orifice
7   **Ureter, Left**
    See 6 Ureter, Right
8   **Ureters, Bilateral**
    See 6 Ureter, Right
B   **Bladder**
    Trigone of bladder
C   **Bladder Neck**
D   **Urethra**
    Bulbourethral (Cowper's) gland
    Cowper's (bulbourethral) gland
    External urethral sphincter
    Internal urethral sphincter
    Membranous urethra
    Penile urethra
    Prostatic urethra
	Ø Open
	4 Percutaneous Endoscopic
		Z No Device	**Z** No Qualifier

Ø   **Medical and Surgical**
T   **Urinary System**
T   **Resection**   Definition: Cutting out or off, without replacement, all of a body part

Explanation: None

Body Part Character 4	Approach Character 5	Device Character 6	Qualifier Character 7

Ø   **Kidney, Right**
    Renal calyx
    Renal capsule
    Renal cortex
    Renal segment
1   **Kidney, Left**
    See Ø Kidney, Right
2   **Kidneys, Bilateral**
    See Ø Kidney, Right
	Ø Open
	4 Percutaneous Endoscopic
		Z No Device	**Z** No Qualifier

3   **Kidney Pelvis, Right**
    Ureteropelvic junction (UPJ)
4   **Kidney Pelvis, Left**
    See 3 Kidney Pelvis, Right
6   **Ureter, Right**
    Ureteral orifice
    Ureterovesical orifice
7   **Ureter, Left**
    See 6 Ureter, Right
B   **Bladder**   ⊞
    Trigone of bladder
C   **Bladder Neck**
D   Urethra
    Bulbourethral (Cowper's) gland
    Cowper's (bulbourethral) gland
    External urethral sphincter
    Internal urethral sphincter
    Membranous urethra
    Penile urethra
    Prostatic urethra
	Ø Open
	4 Percutaneous Endoscopic
	7 Via Natural or Artificial Opening
	8 Via Natural or Artificial Opening
	    Endoscopic
		Z No Device	**Z** No Qualifier

Non-OR   ØTTD[4,7,8]ZZ

See Appendix L for Procedure Combinations
    Combo-only   ØTTDØZZ
    ⊞   ØTTBØZZ

NC Noncovered Procedure   **LC** Limited Coverage   **QA** Questionable OB Admit   **NT** New Tech Add-on   ⊞ Combination Member   ♂ Male   ♀ Female

ICD-10-PCS 2023   635

ØTS–ØTT

Urinary System

Ø   **Medical and Surgical**
T   **Urinary System**
U   **Supplement**   Definition: Putting in or on biological or synthetic material that physically reinforces and/or augments the function of a portion of a body part
Explanation: The biological material is non-living, or is living and from the same individual. The body part may have been previously replaced, and the SUPPLEMENT procedure is performed to physically reinforce and/or augment the function of the replaced body part.

Body Part Character 4	Approach Character 5	Device Character 6	Qualifier Character 7
3 **Kidney, Right** Ureteropelvic junction (UPJ) **4** **Kidney Pelvis, Left** *See 3 Kidney Pelvis, Right* **6** **Ureter, Right** Ureteral orifice Ureterovesical orifice **7** **Ureter, Left** *See 6 Ureter, Right* **B** **Bladder** Trigone of bladder **C** **Bladder Neck**	**Ø** Open **4** Percutaneous Endoscopic **7** Via Natural or Artificial Opening **8** Via Natural or Artificial Opening Endoscopic	**7** Autologous Tissue Substitute **J** Synthetic Substitute **K** Nonautologous Tissue Substitute	**Z** No Qualifier
D **Urethra** Bulbourethral (Cowper's) gland Cowper's (bulbourethral) gland External urethral sphincter Internal urethral sphincter Membranous urethra Penile urethra Prostatic urethra	**Ø** Open **4** Percutaneous Endoscopic **7** Via Natural or Artificial Opening **8** Via Natural or Artificial Opening Endoscopic **X** External	**7** Autologous Tissue Substitute **J** Synthetic Substitute **K** Nonautologous Tissue Substitute	**Z** No Qualifier

Ø   **Medical and Surgical**
T   **Urinary System**
V   **Restriction**   Definition: Partially closing an orifice or the lumen of a tubular body part
Explanation: The orifice can be a natural orifice or an artificially created orifice

Body Part Character 4	Approach Character 5	Device Character 6	Qualifier Character 7
3 **Kidney Pelvis, Right** Ureteropelvic junction (UPJ) **4** **Kidney Pelvis, Left** *See 3 Kidney Pelvis, Right* **6** **Ureter, Right** Ureteral orifice Ureterovesical orifice **7** **Ureter, Left** *See 6 Ureter, Right* **B** **Bladder** Trigone of bladder **C** **Bladder Neck**	**Ø** Open **3** Percutaneous **4** Percutaneous Endoscopic	**C** Extraluminal Device **D** Intraluminal Device **Z** No Device	**Z** No Qualifier
3 **Kidney Pelvis, Right** Ureteropelvic junction (UPJ) **4** **Kidney Pelvis, Left** *See 3 Kidney Pelvis, Right* **6** **Ureter, Right** Ureteral orifice Ureterovesical orifice **7** **Ureter, Left** *See 6 Ureter, Right* **B** **Bladder** Trigone of bladder **C** **Bladder Neck**	**7** Via Natural or Artificial Opening **8** Via Natural or Artificial Opening Endoscopic	**D** Intraluminal Device **Z** No Device	**Z** No Qualifier
D **Urethra** Bulbourethral (Cowper's) gland Cowper's (bulbourethral) gland External urethral sphincter Internal urethral sphincter Membranous urethra Penile urethra Prostatic urethra	**Ø** Open **3** Percutaneous **4** Percutaneous Endoscopic	**C** Extraluminal Device **D** Intraluminal Device **Z** No Device	**Z** No Qualifier
D **Urethra** Bulbourethral (Cowper's) gland Cowper's (bulbourethral) gland External urethral sphincter Internal urethral sphincter Membranous urethra Penile urethra Prostatic urethra	**7** Via Natural or Artificial Opening **8** Via Natural or Artificial Opening Endoscopic	**D** Intraluminal Device **Z** No Device	**Z** No Qualifier
D **Urethra** Bulbourethral (Cowper's) gland Cowper's (bulbourethral) gland External urethral sphincter Internal urethral sphincter Membranous urethra Penile urethra Prostatic urethra	**X** External	**Z** No Device	**Z** No Qualifier

Ø   **Medical and Surgical**
T   **Urinary System**
W   **Revision**   Definition: Correcting, to the extent possible, a portion of a malfunctioning device or the position of a displaced device
           Explanation: Revision can include correcting a malfunctioning or displaced device by taking out or putting in components of the device such as a screw or pin

Body Part Character 4	Approach Character 5	Device Character 6	Qualifier Character 7
5 Kidney Renal calyx Renal capsule Renal cortex Renal segment	**Ø** Open **3** Percutaneous **4** Percutaneous Endoscopic **7** Via Natural or Artificial Opening **8** Via Natural or Artificial Opening Endoscopic	**Ø** Drainage Device **2** Monitoring Device **3** Infusion Device **7** Autologous Tissue Substitute **C** Extraluminal Device **D** Intraluminal Device **J** Synthetic Substitute **K** Nonautologous Tissue Substitute **Y** Other Device	**Z** No Qualifier
5 Kidney Renal calyx Renal capsule Renal cortex Renal segment	**X** External	**Ø** Drainage Device **2** Monitoring Device **3** Infusion Device **7** Autologous Tissue Substitute **C** Extraluminal Device **D** Intraluminal Device **J** Synthetic Substitute **K** Nonautologous Tissue Substitute	**Z** No Qualifier
9 Ureter Ureteral orifice Ureterovesical orifice	**Ø** Open **3** Percutaneous **4** Percutaneous Endoscopic **7** Via Natural or Artificial Opening **8** Via Natural or Artificial Opening Endoscopic	**Ø** Drainage Device **2** Monitoring Device **3** Infusion Device **7** Autologous Tissue Substitute **C** Extraluminal Device **D** Intraluminal Device **J** Synthetic Substitute **K** Nonautologous Tissue Substitute **M** Stimulator Lead **Y** Other Device	**Z** No Qualifier
9 Ureter Ureteral orifice Ureterovesical orifice	**X** External	**Ø** Drainage Device **2** Monitoring Device **3** Infusion Device **7** Autologous Tissue Substitute **C** Extraluminal Device **D** Intraluminal Device **J** Synthetic Substitute **K** Nonautologous Tissue Substitute **M** Stimulator Lead	**Z** No Qualifier
B Bladder Trigone of bladder	**Ø** Open **3** Percutaneous **4** Percutaneous Endoscopic **7** Via Natural or Artificial Opening **8** Via Natural or Artificial Opening Endoscopic	**Ø** Drainage Device **2** Monitoring Device **3** Infusion Device **7** Autologous Tissue Substitute **C** Extraluminal Device **D** Intraluminal Device **J** Synthetic Substitute **K** Nonautologous Tissue Substitute **L** Artificial Sphincter **M** Stimulator Lead **Y** Other Device	**Z** No Qualifier
B Bladder Trigone of bladder	**X** External	**Ø** Drainage Device **2** Monitoring Device **3** Infusion Device **7** Autologous Tissue Substitute **C** Extraluminal Device **D** Intraluminal Device **J** Synthetic Substitute **K** Nonautologous Tissue Substitute **L** Artificial Sphincter **M** Stimulator Lead	**Z** No Qualifier

Non-OR	ØTW5[3,4,7]YZ		Non-OR	ØTW9X[Ø,2,3,7,C,D,J,K,M]Z
Non-OR	ØTW5X[Ø,2,3,7,C,D,J,K]Z		Non-OR	ØTWB[3,4,7]YZ
Non-OR	ØTW9[3,4,7]YZ		Non-OR	ØTWBX[Ø,2,3,7,C,D,J,K,L,M]Z

ØTW Continued on next page

NC Noncovered Procedure   LC Limited Coverage   QA Questionable OB Admit   NT New Tech Add-on   ⊞ Combination Member   ♂ Male   ♀ Female

ICD-10-PCS 2023   637

ØTW–ØTW

Urinary System (side tab)

Ø   **Medical and Surgical**   *ØTW Continued*
T   **Urinary System**
W   **Revision**   Definition: Correcting, to the extent possible, a portion of a malfunctioning device or the position of a displaced device

                      Explanation: Revision can include correcting a malfunctioning or displaced device by taking out or putting in components of the device such as a screw or pin

Body Part Character 4	Approach Character 5	Device Character 6	Qualifier Character 7
D Urethra Bulbourethral (Cowper's) gland Cowper's (bulbourethral) gland External urethral sphincter Internal urethral sphincter Membranous urethra Penile urethra Prostatic urethra	**Ø** Open **3** Percutaneous **4** Percutaneous Endoscopic **7** Via Natural or Artificial Opening **8** Via Natural or Artificial Opening Endoscopic	**Ø** Drainage Device **2** Monitoring Device **3** Infusion Device **7** Autologous Tissue Substitute **C** Extraluminal Device **D** Intraluminal Device **J** Synthetic Substitute **K** Nonautologous Tissue Substitute **L** Artificial Sphincter **Y** Other Device	**Z** No Qualifier
D Urethra Bulbourethral (Cowper's) gland Cowper's (bulbourethral) gland External urethral sphincter Internal urethral sphincter Membranous urethra Penile urethra Prostatic urethra	**X** External	**Ø** Drainage Device **2** Monitoring Device **3** Infusion Device **7** Autologous Tissue Substitute **C** Extraluminal Device **D** Intraluminal Device **J** Synthetic Substitute **K** Nonautologous Tissue Substitute **L** Artificial Sphincter	**Z** No Qualifier

Non-OR	ØTWD[3,4,7,8]YZ
Non-OR	ØTWDX[Ø,2,3,7,C,D,J,K,L]Z

Ø   **Medical and Surgical**
T   **Urinary System**
Y   **Transplantation**   Definition: Putting in or on all or a portion of a living body part taken from another individual or animal to physically take the place and/or function of all or a portion of a similar body part

                      Explanation: The native body part may or may not be taken out, and the transplanted body part may take over all or a portion of its function

Body Part Character 4	Approach Character 5	Device Character 6	Qualifier Character 7

Ø Kidney, Right LC ⊞
    Renal calyx
    Renal capsule
    Renal cortex
    Renal segment
1 Kidney, Left LC ⊞
    See Ø Kidney, Right
	Ø Open	**Z** No Device	**Ø** Allogeneic
			1 Syngeneic
			2 Zooplastic

LC	ØTY[Ø,1]ØZ[Ø,1,2]

See Appendix L for Procedure Combinations
⊞   ØTY[Ø,1]ØZ[Ø,1,2]

Non-OR Procedure   DRG Non-OR Procedure   Valid OR Procedure   HAC Associated Procedure   Combination Only   New/Revised April   New/Revised October

638   ICD-10-PCS 2023

Female Reproductive System ØU1–ØUY

Character Meanings

This Character Meaning table is provided as a guide to assist the user in the identification of character members that may be found in this section of code tables. It **SHOULD NOT** be used to build a PCS code.

Operation–Character 3	Body Part–Character 4	Approach–Character 5	Device–Character 6	Qualifier–Character 7
1 Bypass	Ø Ovary, Right	Ø Open	Ø Drainage Device	Ø Allogeneic
2 Change	1 Ovary, Left	3 Percutaneous	1 Radioactive Element	1 Syngeneic
5 Destruction	2 Ovaries, Bilateral	4 Percutaneous Endoscopic	3 Infusion Device	2 Zooplastic
7 Dilation	3 Ovary	7 Via Natural or Artificial Opening	7 Autologous Tissue Substitute	5 Fallopian Tube, Right
8 Division	4 Uterine Supporting Structure	8 Via Natural or Artificial Opening Endoscopic	C Extraluminal Device	6 Fallopian Tube, Left
9 Drainage	5 Fallopian Tube, Right	F Via Natural or Artificial Opening With Percutaneous Endoscopic Assistance	D Intraluminal Device	9 Uterus
B Excision	6 Fallopian Tube, Left	X External	G Intraluminal Device, Pessary	L Supracervical
C Extirpation	7 Fallopian Tubes, Bilateral		H Contraceptive Device	X Diagnostic
D Extraction	8 Fallopian Tube		J Synthetic Substitute	Z No Qualifier
F Fragmentation	9 Uterus		K Nonautologous Tissue Substitute	
H Insertion	B Endometrium		Y Other Device	
J Inspection	C Cervix		Z No Device	
L Occlusion	D Uterus and Cervix			
M Reattachment	F Cul-de-sac			
N Release	G Vagina			
P Removal	H Vagina and Cul-de-sac			
Q Repair	J Clitoris			
S Reposition	K Hymen			
T Resection	L Vestibular Gland			
U Supplement	M Vulva			
V Restriction	N Ova			
W Revision				
Y Transplantation				

AHA Coding Clinic for table ØU5
2015, 3Q, 31   Tubal ligation for sterilization

AHA Coding Clinic for table ØU7
2020, 2Q, 30   Duhrssen cervical incision

AHA Coding Clinic for table ØU9
2016, 4Q, 58   Longitudinal vaginal septum

AHA Coding Clinic for table ØUB
2018, 1Q, 23   Tubal ligation procedure
2015, 3Q, 31   Laparoscopic partial salpingectomy for ectopic pregnancy
2015, 3Q, 31   Tubal ligation for sterilization
2014, 4Q, 16   Excision of multiple uterine fibroids
2014, 3Q, 12   Excision of skin tag from labia majora

AHA Coding Clinic for table ØUC
2015, 3Q, 30   Removal of cervical cerclage
2013, 2Q, 38   Evacuation of clot post-partum

AHA Coding Clinic for table ØUH
2020, 4Q, 43-44   Insertion of radioactive element
2018, 1Q, 25   Intrauterine brachytherapy & placement of tandems & ovoids
2013, 2Q, 34   Placement of intrauterine device via open approach

AHA Coding Clinic for table ØUJ
2015, 1Q, 33   Robotic-assisted laparoscopic hysterectomy converted to open procedure

AHA Coding Clinic for table ØUL
2018, 1Q, 23   Tubal ligation procedure
2015, 3Q, 31   Tubal ligation for sterilization

AHA Coding Clinic for table ØUQ
2020, 4Q, 59-60   Extraction of ectopic products of conception
2014, 4Q, 18   Obstetrical periurethral laceration
2013, 4Q, 120   Repair of clitoral obstetric laceration

AHA Coding Clinic for table ØUS
2016, 1Q, 9   Anteversion of retroverted pregnant uterus

AHA Coding Clinic for table ØUT
2022, 1Q, 21   Gravid hysterectomy due to placenta increta
2017, 4Q, 68   New qualifier values - Supracervical hysterectomy
2015, 1Q, 33   Robotic-assisted laparoscopic hysterectomy converted to open procedure
2013, 3Q, 28   Total hysterectomy
2013, 1Q, 24   Excision versus Resection of remaining ovarian remnant following previous excision

AHA Coding Clinic for table ØUV
2015, 3Q, 30   Insertion of cervical cerclage

AHA Coding Clinic for table ØUY
2018, 4Q, 40   Uterus transplant

Female Reproductive System

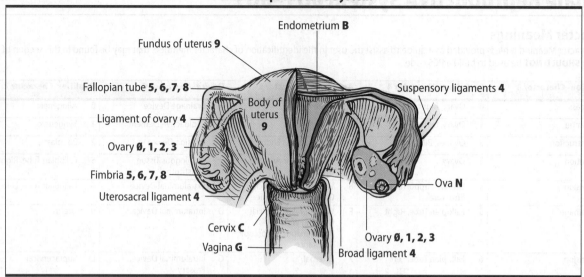

Female Internal/External Structures

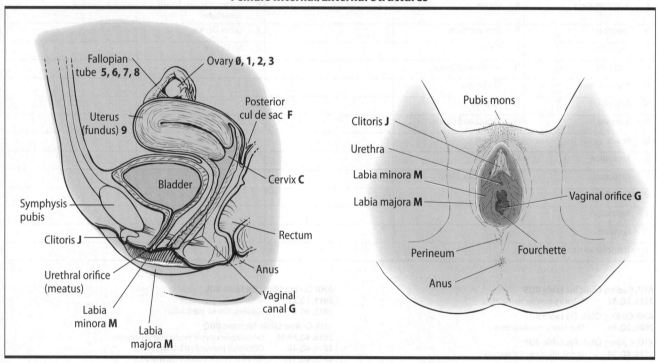

Ø   **Medical and Surgical**
U   **Female Reproductive System**
1   **Bypass**   Definition: Altering the route of passage of the contents of a tubular body part

                 Explanation: Rerouting contents of a body part to a downstream area of the normal route, to a similar route and body part, or to an abnormal route and dissimilar body part. Includes one or more anastomoses, with or without the use of a device.

Body Part Character 4		Approach Character 5	Device Character 6	Qualifier Character 7

5 Fallopian Tube, Right ♀
    Oviduct
    Salpinx
    Uterine tube
6 Fallopian Tube, Left ♀
    See 5 Fallopian Tube, Right
		Ø Open
		4 Percutaneous Endoscopic
			7 Autologous Tissue Substitute
			J Synthetic Substitute
			K Nonautologous Tissue Substitute
			Z No Device
				5 Fallopian Tube, Right
				6 Fallopian Tube, Left
				9 Uterus

      ♀   All body part, approach, device, and qualifier values

Ø   **Medical and Surgical**
U   **Female Reproductive System**
2   **Change**   Definition: Taking out or off a device from a body part and putting back an identical or similar device in or on the same body part without cutting or puncturing the skin or a mucous membrane

                 Explanation: All CHANGE procedures are coded using the approach EXTERNAL

Body Part Character 4		Approach Character 5	Device Character 6	Qualifier Character 7

3 Ovary ♀
8 Fallopian Tube ♀
M Vulva ♀
    Labia majora
    Labia minora
		X External	**Ø** Drainage Device
			Y Other Device
				Z No Qualifier

D Uterus and Cervix ♀		**X** External	**Ø** Drainage Device **H** Contraceptive Device **Y** Other Device	**Z** No Qualifier
H Vagina and Cul-de-sac ♀		**X** External	**Ø** Drainage Device **G** Intraluminal Device, Pessary **Y** Other Device	**Z** No Qualifier

     Non-OR   All body part, approach, device, and qualifier values   ♀   All body part, approach, device, and qualifier values

NC Noncovered Procedure   **LC** Limited Coverage   **QA** Questionable OB Admit   **NT** New Tech Add-on   ⊞ Combination Member   ♂ Male   ♀ Female

ICD-10-PCS 2023   **641**

Ø   **Medical and Surgical**
U   **Female Reproductive System**
5   **Destruction**   Definition: Physical eradication of all or a portion of a body part by the direct use of energy, force, or a destructive agent
                          Explanation: None of the body part is physically taken out

Body Part Character 4		Approach Character 5	Device Character 6	Qualifier Character 7
Ø Ovary, Right ♀ 1 Ovary, Left ♀ 2 Ovaries, Bilateral ♀ 4 Uterine Supporting Structure ♀ 　Broad ligament 　Infundibulopelvic ligament 　Ovarian ligament 　Round ligament of uterus		Ø Open 3 Percutaneous 4 Percutaneous Endoscopic 8 Via Natural or Artificial Opening 　Endoscopic	Z No Device	Z No Qualifier
5 Fallopian Tube, Right ♀ 　Oviduct 　Salpinx 　Uterine tube 6 Fallopian Tube, Left ♀ 　See 5 Fallopian Tube, Right 7 Fallopian Tubes, Bilateral NC♀ 9 Uterus ♀ 　Fundus uteri 　Myometrium 　Perimetrium 　Uterine cornu B Endometrium ♀ C Cervix ♀ F Cul-de-sac ♀		Ø Open 3 Percutaneous 4 Percutaneous Endoscopic 7 Via Natural or Artificial Opening 8 Via Natural or Artificial Opening 　Endoscopic	Z No Device	Z No Qualifier
G Vagina ♀ K Hymen ♀		Ø Open 3 Percutaneous 4 Percutaneous Endoscopic 7 Via Natural or Artificial Opening 8 Via Natural or Artificial Opening 　Endoscopic X External	Z No Device	Z No Qualifier
J Clitoris ♀ L Vestibular Gland ♀ 　Bartholin's (greater vestibular) gland 　Greater vestibular (Bartholin's) gland 　Paraurethral (Skene's) gland 　Skene's (paraurethral) gland M Vulva ♀ 　Labia majora 　Labia minora		Ø Open X External	Z No Device	Z No Qualifier

NC   ØU57[Ø,3,4,7,8]ZZ with principal or secondary diagnosis of Z3Ø.2   ♀   All body part, approach, device, and qualifier values

0	Medical and Surgical
U	Female Reproductive System
7	Dilation

Definition: Expanding an orifice or the lumen of a tubular body part

Explanation: The orifice can be a natural orifice or an artificially created orifice. Accomplished by stretching a tubular body part using intraluminal pressure or by cutting part of the orifice or wall of the tubular body part.

Body Part Character 4		Approach Character 5	Device Character 6	Qualifier Character 7
5 Fallopian Tube, Right Oviduct Salpinx Uterine tube	♀	**0** Open **3** Percutaneous **4** Percutaneous Endoscopic **7** Via Natural or Artificial Opening **8** Via Natural or Artificial Opening Endoscopic	**D** Intraluminal Device **Z** No Device	**Z** No Qualifier
6 Fallopian Tube, Left *See 5 Fallopian Tube, Right*	♀			
7 Fallopian Tubes, Bilateral	♀			
9 Uterus Fundus uteri Myometrium Perimetrium Uterine cornu	♀			
C Cervix	♀			
G Vagina	♀			
K Hymen	♀	**0** Open **3** Percutaneous **4** Percutaneous Endoscopic **7** Via Natural or Artificial Opening **8** Via Natural or Artificial Opening Endoscopic **X** External	**D** Intraluminal Device **Z** No Device	**Z** No Qualifier

Non-OR	0U7C[0,3,4,7,8][D,Z]Z	♀	All body part, approach, device, and qualifier values
Non-OR	0U7G[7,8][D,Z]Z		

0	Medical and Surgical
U	Female Reproductive System
8	Division

Definition: Cutting into a body part, without draining fluids and/or gases from the body part, in order to separate or transect a body part

Explanation: All or a portion of the body part is separated into two or more portions

Body Part Character 4		Approach Character 5	Device Character 6	Qualifier Character 7
0 Ovary, Right	♀	**0** Open **3** Percutaneous **4** Percutaneous Endoscopic	**Z** No Device	**Z** No Qualifier
1 Ovary, Left	♀			
2 Ovaries, Bilateral	♀			
4 Uterine Supporting Structure Broad ligament Infundibulopelvic ligament Ovarian ligament Round ligament of uterus	♀			
K Hymen	♀	**7** Via Natural or Artificial Opening **8** Via Natural or Artificial Opening Endoscopic **X** External	**Z** No Device	**Z** No Qualifier

Non-OR	0U8K[7,8,X]ZZ	♀	All body part, approach, device, and qualifier values

NC Noncovered Procedure   **LC** Limited Coverage   **QA** Questionable OB Admit   **NT** New Tech Add-on   ⊞ Combination Member   ♂ Male   ♀ Female

ICD-10-PCS 2023   **643**

Female Reproductive System

Ø   **Medical and Surgical**
U   **Female Reproductive System**
9   **Drainage**   Definition: Taking or letting out fluids and/or gases from a body part

                            Explanation: The qualifier DIAGNOSTIC is used to identify drainage procedures that are biopsies

Body Part Character 4	Approach Character 5	Device Character 6	Qualifier Character 7
Ø Ovary, Right ♀ 1 Ovary, Left ♀ 2 Ovaries, Bilateral ♀	Ø Open 3 Percutaneous 4 Percutaneous Endoscopic 8 Via Natural or Artificial Opening Endoscopic	Ø Drainage Device	Z No Qualifier
Ø Ovary, Right ♀ 1 Ovary, Left ♀ 2 Ovaries, Bilateral ♀	Ø Open 3 Percutaneous 4 Percutaneous Endoscopic 8 Via Natural or Artificial Opening Endoscopic	Z No Device	X Diagnostic Z No Qualifier
Ø Ovary, Right ♀ 1 Ovary, Left ♀ 2 Ovaries, Bilateral ♀	X External	Z No Device	Z No Qualifier

4 Uterine Supporting Structure ♀
  Broad ligament
  Infundibulopelvic ligament
  Ovarian ligament
  Round ligament of uterus
	Ø Open
	3 Percutaneous
	4 Percutaneous Endoscopic
	8 Via Natural or Artificial Opening Endoscopic
		Ø Drainage Device	Z No Qualifier

4 Uterine Supporting Structure ♀
  Broad ligament
  Infundibulopelvic ligament
  Ovarian ligament
  Round ligament of uterus
	Ø Open
	3 Percutaneous
	4 Percutaneous Endoscopic
	8 Via Natural or Artificial Opening Endoscopic
		Z No Device	X Diagnostic
			Z No Qualifier

5 Fallopian Tube, Right ♀
  Oviduct
  Salpinx
  Uterine tube
6 Fallopian Tube, Left ♀
  See 5 Fallopian Tube, Right
7 Fallopian Tubes, Bilateral ♀
9 Uterus ♀
  Fundus uteri
  Myometrium
  Perimetrium
  Uterine cornu
C Cervix ♀
F Cul-de-sac ♀
	Ø Open
	3 Percutaneous
	4 Percutaneous Endoscopic
	7 Via Natural or Artificial Opening
	8 Via Natural or Artificial Opening Endoscopic
		Ø Drainage Device	Z No Qualifier

5 Fallopian Tube, Right ♀
  Oviduct
  Salpinx
  Uterine tube
6 Fallopian Tube, Left ♀
  See 5 Fallopian Tube, Right
7 Fallopian Tubes, Bilateral ♀
9 Uterus ♀
  Fundus uteri
  Myometrium
  Perimetrium
  Uterine cornu
C Cervix ♀
F Cul-de-sac ♀
	Ø Open
	3 Percutaneous
	4 Percutaneous Endoscopic
	7 Via Natural or Artificial Opening
	8 Via Natural or Artificial Opening Endoscopic
		Z No Device	X Diagnostic
			Z No Qualifier

Non-OR ØU9[Ø,1,2][3,8]ØZ		Non-OR ØU9[5,6,7,9,C]3ØZ	
Non-OR ØU9[Ø,1,2][3,8]ZZ		Non-OR ØU9F[3,4]ØZ	
Non-OR ØU9[Ø,1,2]8ZX		Non-OR ØU9[5,6,7][3,4,7,8]ZZ	
Non-OR ØU94[3,8]ØZ		Non-OR ØU9[9,C]3ZZ	
Non-OR ØU94[3,8]ZZ		Non-OR ØU9F[3,4]ZZ	
Non-OR ØU948ZX		♀ All body part, approach, device, and qualifier values	

ØU9 Continued on next page

Non-OR Procedure   DRG Non-OR Procedure   Valid OR Procedure   HAC Associated Procedure   Combination Only   New/Revised April   New/Revised October

644   ICD-10-PCS 2023

Ø **Medical and Surgical**
U **Female Reproductive System**
9 **Drainage**   Definition: Taking or letting out fluids and/or gases from a body part

ØU9 Continued

                              Explanation: The qualifier DIAGNOSTIC is used to identify drainage procedures that are biopsies

Body Part Character 4	Approach Character 5	Device Character 6	Qualifier Character 7
G Vagina ♀ **K** Hymen ♀	**Ø** Open **3** Percutaneous **4** Percutaneous Endoscopic **7** Via Natural or Artificial Opening **8** Via Natural or Artificial Opening Endoscopic **X** External	**Ø** Drainage Device	**Z** No Qualifier
G Vagina ♀ **K** Hymen ♀	**Ø** Open **3** Percutaneous **4** Percutaneous Endoscopic **7** Via Natural or Artificial Opening **8** Via Natural or Artificial Opening Endoscopic **X** External	**Z** No Device	**X** Diagnostic **Z** No Qualifier

J Clitoris ♀
L Vestibular Gland ♀
    Bartholin's (greater vestibular) gland
    Greater vestibular (Bartholin's) gland
    Paraurethral (Skene's) gland
    Skene's (paraurethral) gland
M Vulva ♀
    Labia majora
    Labia minora
	Ø Open
	X External
		Ø Drainage Device	**Z** No Qualifier

J Clitoris ♀
L Vestibular Gland ♀
    Bartholin's (greater vestibular) gland
    Greater vestibular (Bartholin's) gland
    Paraurethral (Skene's) gland
    Skene's (paraurethral) gland
M Vulva ♀
    Labia majora
    Labia minora
	Ø Open
	X External
		Z No Device	**X** Diagnostic
			Z No Qualifier

Non-OR ØU9G3ØZ		**Non-OR** ØU9L[Ø,X]ØZ	
Non-OR ØU9K[Ø,3,4,7,8,X]ØZ		**Non-OR** ØU9L[Ø,X]Z[X,Z]	
Non-OR ØU9G3ZZ		♀ All body part, approach, device, and qualifier values	
Non-OR ØU9K[Ø,3,4,7,8,X]ZZ			

NC Noncovered Procedure   **LC** Limited Coverage   **QA** Questionable OB Admit   **NT** New Tech Add-on   ⊞ Combination Member   ♂ Male   ♀ Female

ICD-10-PCS 2023   645

Female Reproductive System

Ø   **Medical and Surgical**
U   **Female Reproductive System**
B   **Excision**   Definition: Cutting out or off, without replacement, a portion of a body part
                       Explanation: The qualifier DIAGNOSTIC is used to identify excision procedures that are biopsies

Body Part Character 4	Approach Character 5	Device Character 6	Qualifier Character 7

Ø Ovary, Right ♀
1 Ovary, Left ♀
2 Ovaries, Bilateral ♀
4 Uterine Supporting Structure ♀
   Broad ligament
   Infundibulopelvic ligament
   Ovarian ligament
   Round ligament of uterus
5 Fallopian Tube, Right ♀
   Oviduct
   Salpinx
   Uterine tube
6 Fallopian Tube, Left ♀
   See 5 Fallopian Tube, Right
7 Fallopian Tubes, Bilateral ♀
9 Uterus ♀
   Fundus uteri
   Myometrium
   Perimetrium
   Uterine cornu
C Cervix ♀
F Cul-de-sac ♀
	Ø Open
	3 Percutaneous
	4 Percutaneous Endoscopic
	7 Via Natural or Artificial Opening
	8 Via Natural or Artificial Opening
	   Endoscopic
		Z No Device	X Diagnostic
			Z No Qualifier

G Vagina ♀ K Hymen ♀	Ø Open 3 Percutaneous 4 Percutaneous Endoscopic 7 Via Natural or Artificial Opening 8 Via Natural or Artificial Opening Endoscopic X External	Z No Device	X Diagnostic Z No Qualifier

J Clitoris ♀
L Vestibular Gland ♀
   Bartholin's (greater vestibular) gland
   Greater vestibular (Bartholin's) gland
   Paraurethral (Skene's) gland
   Skene's (paraurethral) gland
M Vulva ♀
   Labia majora
   Labia minora
	Ø Open
	X External
		Z No Device	X Diagnostic
			Z No Qualifier

♀   All body part, approach, device, and qualifier values

Ø **Medical and Surgical**
U **Female Reproductive System**
C **Extirpation**　　　Definition: Taking or cutting out solid matter from a body part

Explanation: The solid matter may be an abnormal byproduct of a biological function or a foreign body; it may be imbedded in a body part or in the lumen of a tubular body part. The solid matter may or may not have been previously broken into pieces.

Body Part Character 4		Approach Character 5	Device Character 6	Qualifier Character 7
Ø Ovary, Right	♀	**Ø** Open	**Z** No Device	**Z** No Qualifier
1 Ovary, Left	♀	**3** Percutaneous		
2 Ovaries, Bilateral	♀	**4** Percutaneous Endoscopic		
4 Uterine Supporting Structure	♀	**8** Via Natural or Artificial Opening Endoscopic		
Broad ligament				
Infundibulopelvic ligament				
Ovarian ligament				
Round ligament of uterus				
5 Fallopian Tube, Right	♀	**Ø** Open	**Z** No Device	**Z** No Qualifier
Oviduct		**3** Percutaneous		
Salpinx		**4** Percutaneous Endoscopic		
Uterine tube		**7** Via Natural or Artificial Opening		
6 Fallopian Tube, Left	♀	**8** Via Natural or Artificial Opening Endoscopic		
See 5 Fallopian Tube, Right				
7 Fallopian Tubes, Bilateral	♀			
9 Uterus	♀			
Fundus uteri				
Myometrium				
Perimetrium				
Uterine cornu				
B Endometrium	♀			
C Cervix	♀			
F Cul-de-sac	♀			
G Vagina	♀	**Ø** Open	**Z** No Device	**Z** No Qualifier
K Hymen	♀	**3** Percutaneous		
		4 Percutaneous Endoscopic		
		7 Via Natural or Artificial Opening		
		8 Via Natural or Artificial Opening Endoscopic		
		X External		
J Clitoris	♀	**Ø** Open	**Z** No Device	**Z** No Qualifier
L Vestibular Gland	♀	**X** External		
Bartholin's (greater vestibular) gland				
Greater vestibular (Bartholin's) gland				
Paraurethral (Skene's) gland				
Skene's (paraurethral) gland				
M Vulva	♀			
Labia majora				
Labia minora				

Non-OR ØUC9[7,8]ZZ		**Non-OR** ØUCMXZZ	
Non-OR ØUCG[7,8,X]ZZ		♀	All body part, approach, device, and qualifier values
Non-OR ØUCK[Ø,3,4,7,8,X]ZZ			

Ø **Medical and Surgical**
U **Female Reproductive System**
D **Extraction**　　　Definition: Pulling or stripping out or off all or a portion of a body part by the use of force

Explanation: The qualifier DIAGNOSTIC is used to identify extraction procedures that are biopsies

Body Part Character 4		Approach Character 5	Device Character 6	Qualifier Character 7
B Endometrium	♀	**7** Via Natural or Artificial Opening	**Z** No Device	**X** Diagnostic
		8 Via Natural or Artificial Opening Endoscopic		**Z** No Qualifier
N Ova	♀	**Ø** Open	**Z** No Device	**Z** No Qualifier
		3 Percutaneous		
		4 Percutaneous Endoscopic		

♀	All body part, approach, device, and qualifier values

NC Noncovered Procedure　　**LC** Limited Coverage　　**QA** Questionable OB Admit　　**NT** New Tech Add-on　　✛ Combination Member　　♂ Male　　♀ Female

ICD-10-PCS 2023　　　　　　　　　　　　　　　　　　　　　　　　　　　　　　　　　　　　　647

ØUC–ØUD

Female Reproductive System

Ø   **Medical and Surgical**
U   **Female Reproductive System**
F   **Fragmentation**   Definition: Breaking solid matter in a body part into pieces

Explanation: Physical force (e.g., manual, ultrasonic) applied directly or indirectly is used to break the solid matter into pieces. The solid matter may be an abnormal byproduct of a biological function or a foreign body. The pieces of solid matter are not taken out.

Body Part Character 4	Approach Character 5	Device Character 6	Qualifier Character 7

5   Fallopian Tube, Right   NC ♀
   Oviduct
   Salpinx
   Uterine tube
6   Fallopian Tube, Left   NC ♀
   See 5 Fallopian Tube, Right
7   Fallopian Tubes, Bilateral   NC ♀
9   Uterus   NC ♀
   Fundus uteri
   Myometrium
   Perimetrium
   Uterine cornu
	Ø Open
	3 Percutaneous
	4 Percutaneous Endoscopic
	7 Via Natural or Artificial Opening
	8 Via Natural or Artificial Opening
	   Endoscopic
	X External
		Z No Device	Z No Qualifier

Non-OR	ØUF[5,6,7,9]XZZ
NC	ØUF[5,6,7,9]XZZ

♀   All body part, approach, device, and qualifier values

Ø   **Medical and Surgical**
U   **Female Reproductive System**
H   **Insertion**   Definition: Putting in a nonbiological appliance that monitors, assists, performs, or prevents a physiological function but does not physically take the place of a body part

Explanation: None

Body Part Character 4	Approach Character 5	Device Character 6	Qualifier Character 7
3 Ovary ♀	Ø Open 3 Percutaneous 4 Percutaneous Endoscopic	1 Radioactive Element 3 Infusion Device Y Other Device	Z No Qualifier
3 Ovary ♀	7 Via Natural or Artificial Opening 8 Via Natural or Artificial Opening Endoscopic	1 Radioactive Element Y Other Device	Z No Qualifier
8 Fallopian Tube ♀ D Uterus and Cervix ♀ H Vagina and Cul-de-sac ♀	Ø Open 3 Percutaneous 4 Percutaneous Endoscopic 7 Via Natural or Artificial Opening 8 Via Natural or Artificial Opening Endoscopic	3 Infusion Device Y Other Device	Z No Qualifier

9   Uterus   ♀
   Fundus uteri
   Myometrium
   Perimetrium
   Uterine cornu
	Ø Open
	7 Via Natural or Artificial Opening
	8 Via Natural or Artificial Opening
	   Endoscopic
		1 Radioactive Element
		H Contraceptive Device
			Z No Qualifier

C Cervix ♀	Ø Open 3 Percutaneous 4 Percutaneous Endoscopic	1 Radioactive Element	Z No Qualifier
C Cervix ♀	7 Via Natural or Artificial Opening 8 Via Natural or Artificial Opening Endoscopic	1 Radioactive Element H Contraceptive Device	Z No Qualifier
F Cul-de-sac ♀	7 Via Natural or Artificial Opening 8 Via Natural or Artificial Opening Endoscopic	G Intraluminal Device, Pessary	Z No Qualifier
G Vagina ♀	Ø Open 3 Percutaneous 4 Percutaneous Endoscopic X External	1 Radioactive Element	Z No Qualifier
G Vagina ♀	7 Via Natural or Artificial Opening 8 Via Natural or Artificial Opening Endoscopic	1 Radioactive Element G Intraluminal Device, Pessary	Z No Qualifier

Non-OR	ØUH3[Ø,4][3,Y]Z
Non-OR	ØUH33[1,3,Y]Z
Non-OR	ØUH3[7,8][1,Y]Z
Non-OR	ØUH[8,D][Ø,3,4,7,8][3,Y]Z
Non-OR	ØUHH[3,4]YZ
Non-OR	ØUHH[7,8][3,Y]Z

Non-OR	ØUH9[Ø,7,8][1,H]Z
Non-OR	ØUHC[7,8]HZ
Non-OR	ØUHF[7,8]HZ
Non-OR	ØUHG[7,8]HZ
♀	All body part, approach, device, and qualifier values

Ø   **Medical and Surgical**
U   **Female Reproductive System**
J   **Inspection**   Definition: Visually and/or manually exploring a body part

                    Explanation: Visual exploration may be performed with or without optical instrumentation. Manual exploration may be performed directly or through intervening body layers.

Body Part Character 4	Approach Character 5	Device Character 6	Qualifier Character 7
3 Ovary ♀	**Ø** Open **3** Percutaneous **4** Percutaneous Endoscopic **8** Via Natural or Artificial Opening Endoscopic **X** External	**Z** No Device	**Z** No Qualifier
8 Fallopian Tube ♀ **D** Uterus and Cervix ♀ **H** Vagina and Cul-de-sac ♀	**Ø** Open **3** Percutaneous **4** Percutaneous Endoscopic **7** Via Natural or Artificial Opening **8** Via Natural or Artificial Opening Endoscopic **X** External	**Z** No Device	**Z** No Qualifier

M Vulva   ♀
    Labia majora
    Labia minora
	Ø Open
	X External
		Z No Device	**Z** No Qualifier

Non-OR ØUJ3[3,8,X]ZZ		**Non-OR** ØUJMXZZ	
Non-OR ØUJ[8,D,H][3,7,8,X]ZZ		♀ All body part, approach, device, and qualifier values	

Ø   **Medical and Surgical**
U   **Female Reproductive System**
L   **Occlusion**   Definition: Completely closing an orifice or the lumen of a tubular body part

                    Explanation: The orifice can be a natural orifice or an artificially created orifice

Body Part Character 4	Approach Character 5	Device Character 6	Qualifier Character 7

5 Fallopian Tube, Right   ♀
    Oviduct
    Salpinx
    Uterine tube
6 Fallopian Tube, Left   ♀
    See 5 Fallopian Tube, Right
7 Fallopian Tubes, Bilateral **NC**♀
	Ø Open
	3 Percutaneous
	4 Percutaneous Endoscopic
		C Extraluminal Device
		D Intraluminal Device
		Z No Device
			Z No Qualifier

5 Fallopian Tube, Right   ♀
    Oviduct
    Salpinx
    Uterine tube
6 Fallopian Tube, Left   ♀
    See 5 Fallopian Tube, Right
7 Fallopian Tubes, Bilateral **NC**♀
	7 Via Natural or Artificial Opening
	8 Via Natural or Artificial Opening Endoscopic
		D Intraluminal Device
		Z No Device
			Z No Qualifier

F Cul-de-sac ♀ **G** Vagina ♀	**7** Via Natural or Artificial Opening **8** Via Natural or Artificial Opening Endoscopic	**D** Intraluminal Device **Z** No Device	**Z** No Qualifier

NC ØUL7[Ø,3,4][C,D,Z]Z with principal or secondary diagnosis of Z3Ø.2		♀ All body part, approach, device, and qualifier values	
NC ØUL7[7,8][D,Z]Z with principal or secondary diagnosis of Z3Ø.2			

Ø   Medical and Surgical
U   Female Reproductive System
M   Reattachment   Definition: Putting back in or on all or a portion of a separated body part to its normal location or other suitable location
                  Explanation: Vascular circulation and nervous pathways may or may not be reestablished

Body Part Character 4	Approach Character 5	Device Character 6	Qualifier Character 7

Ø **Ovary, Right** ♀
1 **Ovary, Left** ♀
2 **Ovaries, Bilateral** ♀
4 **Uterine Supporting Structure** ♀
    Broad ligament
    Infundibulopelvic ligament
    Ovarian ligament
    Round ligament of uterus
5 **Fallopian Tube, Right** ♀
    Oviduct
    Salpinx
    Uterine tube
6 **Fallopian Tube, Left** ♀
    See 5 Fallopian Tube, Right
7 **Fallopian Tubes, Bilateral** ♀
9 **Uterus** ♀
    Fundus uteri
    Myometrium
    Perimetrium
    Uterine cornu
C **Cervix** ♀
F **Cul-de-sac** ♀
G **Vagina** ♀
	Ø **Open**
	4 **Percutaneous Endoscopic**
		Z **No Device**	**Z** **No Qualifier**

J **Clitoris** ♀
M **Vulva** ♀
    Labia majora
    Labia minora
	X **External**	**Z** **No Device**	**Z** **No Qualifier**

K **Hymen** ♀	**Ø** **Open** **4** **Percutaneous Endoscopic** **X** **External**	**Z** **No Device**	**Z** **No Qualifier**

♀   All body part, approach, device, and qualifier values

Female Reproductive System

Ø   **Medical and Surgical**
U   **Female Reproductive System**
N   **Release**   Definition: Freeing a body part from an abnormal physical constraint by cutting or by the use of force
                          Explanation: Some of the restraining tissue may be taken out but none of the body part is taken out

Body Part Character 4	Approach Character 5	Device Character 6	Qualifier Character 7

Ø   Ovary, Right ♀
1   Ovary, Left ♀
2   Ovaries, Bilateral ♀
4   Uterine Supporting Structure ♀
     Broad ligament
     Infundibulopelvic ligament
     Ovarian ligament
     Round ligament of uterus
	Ø Open
	3 Percutaneous
	4 Percutaneous Endoscopic
	8 Via Natural or Artificial Opening
	     Endoscopic
		Z No Device	Z No Qualifier

5   Fallopian Tube, Right ♀
     Oviduct
     Salpinx
     Uterine tube
6   Fallopian Tube, Left ♀
     See 5 Fallopian Tube, Right
7   Fallopian Tubes, Bilateral ♀
9   Uterus ♀
     Fundus uteri
     Myometrium
     Perimetrium
     Uterine cornu
C   Cervix ♀
F   Cul-de-sac ♀
	Ø Open
	3 Percutaneous
	4 Percutaneous Endoscopic
	7 Via Natural or Artificial Opening
	8 Via Natural or Artificial Opening
	     Endoscopic
		Z No Device	Z No Qualifier

G Vagina ♀ K Hymen ♀	Ø Open 3 Percutaneous 4 Percutaneous Endoscopic 7 Via Natural or Artificial Opening 8 Via Natural or Artificial Opening Endoscopic X External	Z No Device	Z No Qualifier

J   Clitoris ♀
L   Vestibular Gland ♀
     Bartholin's (greater vestibular) gland
     Greater vestibular (Bartholin's) gland
     Paraurethral (Skene's) gland
     Skene's (paraurethral) gland
M   Vulva ♀
     Labia majora
     Labia minora
	Ø Open
	X External
		Z No Device	Z No Qualifier

♀   All body part, approach, device, and qualifier values

NC Noncovered Procedure   LC Limited Coverage   QA Questionable OB Admit   NT New Tech Add-on   ⊞ Combination Member   ♂ Male   ♀ Female

ICD-10-PCS 2023   651

Ø Medical and Surgical
U Female Reproductive System
P Removal   Definition: Taking out or off a device from a body part
Explanation: If a device is taken out and a similar device put in without cutting or puncturing the skin or mucous membrane, the procedure is coded to the root operation CHANGE. Otherwise, the procedure for taking out the device is coded to the root operation REMOVAL.

Body Part Character 4	Approach Character 5	Device Character 6	Qualifier Character 7
3 Ovary ♀	**Ø** Open **3** Percutaneous **4** Percutaneous Endoscopic	**Ø** Drainage Device **3** Infusion Device **Y** Other Device	**Z** No Qualifier
3 Ovary ♀	**7** Via Natural or Artificial Opening **8** Via Natural or Artificial Opening Endoscopic	**Y** Other Device	**Z** No Qualifier
3 Ovary ♀	**X** External	**Ø** Drainage Device **3** Infusion Device	**Z** No Qualifier
8 Fallopian Tube ♀	**Ø** Open **3** Percutaneous **4** Percutaneous Endoscopic **7** Via Natural or Artificial Opening **8** Via Natural or Artificial Opening Endoscopic	**Ø** Drainage Device **3** Infusion Device **7** Autologous Tissue Substitute **C** Extraluminal Device **D** Intraluminal Device **J** Synthetic Substitute **K** Nonautologous Tissue Substitute **Y** Other Device	**Z** No Qualifier
8 Fallopian Tube ♀	**X** External	**Ø** Drainage Device **3** Infusion Device **D** Intraluminal Device	**Z** No Qualifier
D Uterus and Cervix ♀	**Ø** Open **3** Percutaneous **4** Percutaneous Endoscopic **7** Via Natural or Artificial Opening **8** Via Natural or Artificial Opening Endoscopic	**Ø** Drainage Device **1** Radioactive Element **3** Infusion Device **7** Autologous Tissue Substitute **C** Extraluminal Device **D** Intraluminal Device **H** Contraceptive Device **J** Synthetic Substitute **K** Nonautologous Tissue Substitute **Y** Other Device	**Z** No Qualifier
D Uterus and Cervix ♀	**X** External	**Ø** Drainage Device **3** Infusion Device **D** Intraluminal Device **H** Contraceptive Device	**Z** No Qualifier
H Vagina and Cul-de-sac ♀	**Ø** Open **3** Percutaneous **4** Percutaneous Endoscopic **7** Via Natural or Artificial Opening **8** Via Natural or Artificial Opening Endoscopic	**Ø** Drainage Device **1** Radioactive Element **3** Infusion Device **7** Autologous Tissue Substitute **D** Intraluminal Device **J** Synthetic Substitute **K** Nonautologous Tissue Substitute **Y** Other Device	**Z** No Qualifier
H Vagina and Cul-de-sac ♀	**X** External	**Ø** Drainage Device **1** Radioactive Element **3** Infusion Device **D** Intraluminal Device	**Z** No Qualifier
M Vulva ♀ Labia majora Labia minora	**Ø** Open	**Ø** Drainage Device **7** Autologous Tissue Substitute **J** Synthetic Substitute **K** Nonautologous Tissue Substitute	**Z** No Qualifier
M Vulva ♀ Labia majora Labia minora	**X** External	**Ø** Drainage Device	**Z** No Qualifier

Non-OR ØUP3[3,4]YZ		**Non-OR** ØUPD[7,8][Ø,3,C,D,H,Y]Z	
Non-OR ØUP3[7,8]YZ		**Non-OR** ØUPDX[Ø,3,D,H]Z	
Non-OR ØUP3X[Ø,3]Z		**Non-OR** ØUPH[3,4]YZ	
Non-OR ØUP8[3,4]YZ		**Non-OR** ØUPH[7,8][Ø,3,D,Y]Z	
Non-OR ØUP8[7,8][Ø,3,D,Y]Z		**Non-OR** ØUPHX[Ø,1,3,D]Z	
Non-OR ØUP8X[Ø,3,D]Z		**Non-OR** ØUPMXØZ	
Non-OR ØUPD[3,4][C,Y]Z		♀ All body part, approach, device, and qualifier values	

Non-OR Procedure   DRG Non-OR Procedure   Valid OR Procedure   HAC Associated Procedure   Combination Only   New/Revised April   New/Revised October

652   ICD-10-PCS 2023

Ø **Medical and Surgical**
U **Female Reproductive System**
Q **Repair**　　Definition: Restoring, to the extent possible, a body part to its normal anatomic structure and function

Explanation: Used only when the method to accomplish the repair is not one of the other root operations

Body Part Character 4		Approach Character 5	Device Character 6	Qualifier Character 7
Ø Ovary, Right ♀ **1** Ovary, Left ♀ **2** Ovaries, Bilateral ♀ **4** Uterine Supporting Structure ♀ 　Broad ligament 　Infundibulopelvic ligament 　Ovarian ligament 　Round ligament of uterus		**Ø** Open **3** Percutaneous **4** Percutaneous Endoscopic **8** Via Natural or Artificial Opening 　　Endoscopic	**Z** No Device	**Z** No Qualifier
5 Fallopian Tube, Right ♀ 　Oviduct 　Salpinx 　Uterine tube **6** Fallopian Tube, Left ♀ 　*See* 5 Fallopian Tube, Right **7** Fallopian Tubes, Bilateral ♀ **9** Uterus ♀ 　Fundus uteri 　Myometrium 　Perimetrium 　Uterine cornu **C** Cervix ♀ **F** Cul-de-sac ♀		**Ø** Open **3** Percutaneous **4** Percutaneous Endoscopic **7** Via Natural or Artificial Opening **8** Via Natural or Artificial Opening 　　Endoscopic	**Z** No Device	**Z** No Qualifier
G Vagina ♀ **K** Hymen ♀		**Ø** Open **3** Percutaneous **4** Percutaneous Endoscopic **7** Via Natural or Artificial Opening **8** Via Natural or Artificial Opening 　　Endoscopic **X** External	**Z** No Device	**Z** No Qualifier
J Clitoris ♀ **L** Vestibular Gland ♀ 　Bartholin's (greater vestibular) gland 　Greater vestibular (Bartholin's) gland 　Paraurethral (Skene's) gland 　Skene's (paraurethral) gland **M** Vulva ♀ 　Labia majora 　Labia minora		**Ø** Open **X** External	**Z** No Device	**Z** No Qualifier

| Non-OR | ØUQG[7,X]ZZ |
| Non-OR | ØUQKXZZ |

| Non-OR | ØUQMXZZ |
| ♀ | All body part, approach, device, and qualifier values |

Ø **Medical and Surgical**
U **Female Reproductive System**
S **Reposition**　　Definition: Moving to its normal location, or other suitable location, all or a portion of a body part

Explanation: The body part is moved to a new location from an abnormal location, or from a normal location where it is not functioning correctly. The body part may or may not be cut out or off to be moved to the new location.

Body Part Character 4		Approach Character 5	Device Character 6	Qualifier Character 7
Ø Ovary, Right ♀ **1** Ovary, Left ♀ **2** Ovaries, Bilateral ♀ **4** Uterine Supporting Structure ♀ 　Broad ligament 　Infundibulopelvic ligament 　Ovarian ligament 　Round ligament of uterus **5** Fallopian Tube, Right ♀ 　Oviduct 　Salpinx 　Uterine tube **6** Fallopian Tube, Left ♀ 　*See* 5 Fallopian Tube, Right **7** Fallopian Tubes, Bilateral ♀ **C** Cervix ♀ **F** Cul-de-sac ♀		**Ø** Open **4** Percutaneous Endoscopic **8** Via Natural or Artificial Opening 　　Endoscopic	**Z** No Device	**Z** No Qualifier
9 Uterus ♀ 　Fundus uteri 　Myometrium 　Perimetrium 　Uterine cornu **G** Vagina ♀		**Ø** Open **4** Percutaneous Endoscopic **7** Via Natural or Artificial Opening **8** Via Natural or Artificial Opening 　　Endoscopic **X** External	**Z** No Device	**Z** No Qualifier

| Non-OR | ØUS9XZZ | | ♀ | All body part, approach, device, and qualifier values |

NC Noncovered Procedure　**LC** Limited Coverage　**QA** Questionable OB Admit　**NT** New Tech Add-on　⊞ Combination Member　♂ Male　♀ Female

Ø **Medical and Surgical**
U **Female Reproductive System**
T **Resection**   Definition: Cutting out or off, without replacement, all of a body part
                    Explanation: None

Body Part Character 4	Approach Character 5	Device Character 6	Qualifier Character 7

Ø Ovary, Right ♀
1 Ovary, Left ♀
2 Ovaries, Bilateral ⊞♀
5 Fallopian Tube, Right ♀
  Oviduct
  Salpinx
  Uterine tube
6 Fallopian Tube, Left ♀
  See 5 Fallopian Tube, Right
7 Fallopian Tubes, Bilateral ⊞♀
	Ø Open
	4 Percutaneous Endoscopic
	7 Via Natural or Artificial Opening
	8 Via Natural or Artificial Opening
	  Endoscopic
	F Via Natural or Artificial Opening
	  With Percutaneous Endoscopic
	  Assistance
		Z No Device	**Z** No Qualifier

4 Uterine Supporting Structure ⊞♀
  Broad ligament
  Infundibulopelvic ligament
  Ovarian ligament
  Round ligament of uterus
C Cervix ⊞♀
F Cul-de-sac ♀
G Vagina ⊞♀
	Ø Open
	4 Percutaneous Endoscopic
	7 Via Natural or Artificial Opening
	8 Via Natural or Artificial Opening
	  Endoscopic
		Z No Device	**Z** No Qualifier

9 Uterus ⊞♀
  Fundus uteri
  Myometrium
  Perimetrium
  Uterine cornu
	Ø Open
	4 Percutaneous Endoscopic
	7 Via Natural or Artificial Opening
	8 Via Natural or Artificial Opening
	  Endoscopic
	F Via Natural or Artificial Opening
	  With Percutaneous Endoscopic
	  Assistance
		Z No Device	**L** Supracervical
			Z No Qualifier

J Clitoris ♀
L Vestibular Gland ♀
  Bartholin's (greater vestibular)
    gland
  Greater vestibular (Bartholin's)
    gland
  Paraurethral (Skene's) gland
  Skene's (paraurethral) gland
M Vulva ⊞♀
  Labia majora
  Labia minora
	Ø Open
	X External
		Z No Device	**Z** No Qualifier

K Hymen ♀	**Ø** Open **4** Percutaneous Endoscopic **7** Via Natural or Artificial Opening **8** Via Natural or Artificial Opening Endoscopic **X** External	**Z** No Device	**Z** No Device

♀   All body part, approach, device, and qualifier values

See Appendix L for Procedure Combinations
⊞   ØUT[2,7]ØZZ
⊞   ØUT[4,C][Ø,4,7,8]ZZ
⊞   ØUTGØZZ
⊞   ØUT9[Ø,4,7,8,F]ZZ
⊞   ØUTM[Ø,X]ZZ

Ø   **Medical and Surgical**
U   **Female Reproductive System**
U   **Supplement**   Definition: Putting in or on biological or synthetic material that physically reinforces and/or augments the function of a portion of a body part

                       Explanation: The biological material is non-living, or is living and from the same individual. The body part may have been previously replaced, and the SUPPLEMENT procedure is performed to physically reinforce and/or augment the function of the replaced body part.

Body Part Character 4	Approach Character 5	Device Character 6	Qualifier Character 7

4 Uterine Supporting Structure ♀
    Broad ligament
    Infundibulopelvic ligament
    Ovarian ligament
    Round ligament of uterus
	Ø Open
	4 Percutaneous Endoscopic
		7 Autologous Tissue Substitute
		J Synthetic Substitute
		K Nonautologous Tissue Substitute
			Z No Qualifier

5 Fallopian Tube, Right ♀
    Oviduct
    Salpinx
    Uterine tube
6 Fallopian Tube, Left ♀
    See 5 Fallopian Tube, Right
7 Fallopian Tubes, Bilateral ♀
F Cul-de-sac ♀
	Ø Open
	4 Percutaneous Endoscopic
	7 Via Natural or Artificial Opening
	8 Via Natural or Artificial Opening Endoscopic
		7 Autologous Tissue Substitute
		J Synthetic Substitute
		K Nonautologous Tissue Substitute
			Z No Qualifier

G Vagina ♀ **K** Hymen ♀	**Ø** Open **4** Percutaneous Endoscopic **7** Via Natural or Artificial Opening **8** Via Natural or Artificial Opening Endoscopic **X** External	**7** Autologous Tissue Substitute **J** Synthetic Substitute **K** Nonautologous Tissue Substitute	**Z** No Qualifier

J Clitoris ♀
M Vulva ♀
    Labia majora
    Labia minora
	Ø Open
	X External
		7 Autologous Tissue Substitute
		J Synthetic Substitute
		K Nonautologous Tissue Substitute
			Z No Qualifier

♀   All body part, approach, device, and qualifier values

Ø   **Medical and Surgical**
U   **Female Reproductive System**
V   **Restriction**   Definition: Partially closing an orifice or the lumen of a tubular body part

                       Explanation: The orifice can be a natural orifice or an artificially created orifice

Body Part Character 4	Approach Character 5	Device Character 6	Qualifier Character 7
C Cervix ♀	**Ø** Open **3** Percutaneous **4** Percutaneous Endoscopic	**C** Extraluminal Device **D** Intraluminal Device **Z** No Device	**Z** No Qualifier
C Cervix ♀	**7** Via Natural or Artificial Opening **8** Via Natural or Artificial Opening Endoscopic	**D** Intraluminal Device **Z** No Device	**Z** No Qualifier

♀   All body part, approach, device, and qualifier values

NC Noncovered Procedure   **LC** Limited Coverage   **QA** Questionable OB Admit   **NT** New Tech Add-on   ⊞ Combination Member   ♂ Male   ♀ Female

ICD-10-PCS 2023   655

Female Reproductive System

Ø Medical and Surgical
U Female Reproductive System
W Revision   Definition: Correcting, to the extent possible, a portion of a malfunctioning device or the position of a displaced device
                      Explanation: Revision can include correcting a malfunctioning or displaced device by taking out or putting in components of the device such as a screw or pin

Body Part Character 4		Approach Character 5	Device Character 6	Qualifier Character 7
3 Ovary	♀	Ø Open 3 Percutaneous 4 Percutaneous Endoscopic	Ø Drainage Device 3 Infusion Device Y Other Device	Z No Qualifier
3 Ovary	♀	7 Via Natural or Artificial Opening 8 Via Natural or Artificial Opening Endoscopic	Y Other Device	Z No Qualifier
3 Ovary	♀	X External	Ø Drainage Device 3 Infusion Device	Z No Qualifier
8 Fallopian Tube	♀	Ø Open 3 Percutaneous 4 Percutaneous Endoscopic 7 Via Natural or Artificial Opening 8 Via Natural or Artificial Opening Endoscopic	Ø Drainage Device 3 Infusion Device 7 Autologous Tissue Substitute C Extraluminal Device D Intraluminal Device J Synthetic Substitute K Nonautologous Tissue Substitute Y Other Device	Z No Qualifier
8 Fallopian Tube	♀	X External	Ø Drainage Device 3 Infusion Device 7 Autologous Tissue Substitute C Extraluminal Device D Intraluminal Device J Synthetic Substitute K Nonautologous Tissue Substitute	Z No Qualifier
D Uterus and Cervix	♀	Ø Open 3 Percutaneous 4 Percutaneous Endoscopic 7 Via Natural or Artificial Opening 8 Via Natural or Artificial Opening Endoscopic	Ø Drainage Device 1 Radioactive Element 3 Infusion Device 7 Autologous Tissue Substitute C Extraluminal Device D Intraluminal Device H Contraceptive Device J Synthetic Substitute K Nonautologous Tissue Substitute Y Other Device	Z No Qualifier
D Uterus and Cervix	♀	X External	Ø Drainage Device 3 Infusion Device 7 Autologous Tissue Substitute C Extraluminal Device D Intraluminal Device H Contraceptive Device J Synthetic Substitute K Nonautologous Tissue Substitute	Z No Qualifier
H Vagina and Cul-de-sac	♀	Ø Open 3 Percutaneous 4 Percutaneous Endoscopic 7 Via Natural or Artificial Opening 8 Via Natural or Artificial Opening Endoscopic	Ø Drainage Device 1 Radioactive Element 3 Infusion Device 7 Autologous Tissue Substitute D Intraluminal Device J Synthetic Substitute K Nonautologous Tissue Substitute Y Other Device	Z No Qualifier
H Vagina and Cul-de-sac	♀	X External	Ø Drainage Device 3 Infusion Device 7 Autologous Tissue Substitute D Intraluminal Device J Synthetic Substitute K Nonautologous Tissue Substitute	Z No Qualifier

M Vulva
  Labia majora
  Labia minora
	♀	Ø Open
		X External
			Ø Drainage Device
			7 Autologous Tissue Substitute
			J Synthetic Substitute
			K Nonautologous Tissue Substitute
				Z No Qualifier

Non-OR	ØUW3[3,4]YZ		Non-OR	ØUWDX[Ø,3,7,C,D,H,J,K]Z
Non-OR	ØUW3[7,8]YZ		Non-OR	ØUWH[3,4,7,8]YZ
Non-OR	ØUW3X[Ø,3]Z		Non-OR	ØUWHX[Ø,3,7,D,J,K]Z
Non-OR	ØUW8[3,4,7,8]YZ		Non-OR	ØUWMX[Ø,7,J,K]Z
Non-OR	ØUW8X[Ø,3,7,C,D,J,K]Z		♀	All body part, approach, device, and qualifier values
Non-OR	ØUWD[3,4,7,8]YZ			

Non-OR Procedure   DRG Non-OR Procedure   Valid OR Procedure   HAC Associated Procedure   Combination Only   New/Revised April   New/Revised October

656   ICD-10-PCS 2023

Ø   Medical and Surgical
U   Female Reproductive System
Y   Transplantation   Definition: Putting in or on all or a portion of a living body part taken from another individual or animal to physically take the place and/or function of all or a portion of a similar body part

Explanation: The native body part may or may not be taken out, and the transplanted body part may take over all or a portion of its function

Body Part Character 4		Approach Character 5	Device Character 6	Qualifier Character 7
Ø Ovary, Right	♀	Ø Open	Z No Device	Ø Allogeneic
1 Ovary, Left	♀			1 Syngeneic
9 Uterus	♀			2 Zooplastic
♀ All body part, approach, device, and qualifier values				

NC Noncovered Procedure   **LC** Limited Coverage   **QA** Questionable OB Admit   **NT** New Tech Add-on   ⊞ Combination Member   ♂ Male   ♀ Female

ICD-10-PCS 2023   657

Male Reproductive System ØV1–ØVX

Character Meanings

This Character Meaning table is provided as a guide to assist the user in the identification of character members that may be found in this section of code tables. It **SHOULD NOT** be used to build a PCS code.

Operation–Character 3	Body Part–Character 4	Approach–Character 5	Device–Character 6	Qualifier–Character 7
1 Bypass	Ø Prostate	Ø Open	Ø Drainage Device	Ø Allogeneic
2 Change	1 Seminal Vesicle, Right	3 Percutaneous	1 Radioactive Element	1 Syngeneic
5 Destruction	2 Seminal Vesicle, Left	4 Percutaneous Endoscopic	3 Infusion Device	2 Zooplastic
7 Dilation	3 Seminal Vesicles, Bilateral	7 Via Natural or Artificial Opening	7 Autologous Tissue Substitute	3 Laser Interstitial Thermal Therapy
9 Drainage	4 Prostate and Seminal Vesicles	8 Via Natural or Artificial Opening Endoscopic	C Extraluminal Device	D Urethra
B Excision	5 Scrotum	X External	D Intraluminal Device	J Epididymis, Right
C Extirpation	6 Tunica Vaginalis, Right		J Synthetic Substitute	K Epididymis, Left
H Insertion	7 Tunica Vaginalis, Left		K Nonautologous Tissue Substitute	N Vas Deferens, Right
J Inspection	8 Scrotum and Tunica Vaginalis		Y Other Device	P Vas Deferens, Left
L Occlusion	9 Testis, Right		Z No Device	S Penis
M Reattachment	B Testis, Left			X Diagnostic
N Release	C Testes, Bilateral			Z No Qualifier
P Removal	D Testis			
Q Repair	F Spermatic Cord, Right			
R Replacement	G Spermatic Cord, Left			
S Reposition	H Spermatic Cords, Bilateral			
T Resection	J Epididymis, Right			
U Supplement	K Epididymis, Left			
W Revision	L Epididymis, Bilateral			
X Transfer	M Epididymis and Spermatic Cord			
Y Transplantation	N Vas Deferens, Right			
	P Vas Deferens, Left			
	Q Vas Deferens, Bilateral			
	R Vas Deferens			
	S Penis			
	T Prepuce			

AHA Coding Clinic for table ØV1
2018, 3Q, 12   Al-Ghorab distal penile shunt surgery

AHA Coding Clinic for table ØV9
2018, 3Q, 12   Al-Ghorab distal penile shunt surgery

AHA Coding Clinic for table ØVB
2020, 1Q, 31   Repair of buried penis
2019, 3Q, 18   Radical prostatectomy and lymph node dissection with biopsy of neurovascular bundle
2016, 1Q, 23   Transurethral resection of ejaculatory ducts
2014, 4Q, 33   Radical prostatectomy

AHA Coding Clinic for table ØVH
2020, 4Q, 43-44   Insertion of radioactive element

AHA Coding Clinic for table ØVP
2016, 2Q, 28   Removal of multi-component inflatable penile prosthesis with placement of new malleable device

AHA Coding Clinic for table ØVQ
2018, 3Q, 12   Al-Ghorab distal penile shunt surgery

AHA Coding Clinic for table ØVT
2020, 4Q, 99   Robotic-assisted prostatectomy with extension of incision for specimen removal
2019, 3Q, 18   Radical prostatectomy and lymph node dissection with biopsy of neurovascular bundle
2014, 4Q, 33   Radical prostatectomy

AHA Coding Clinic for table ØVU
2020, 1Q, 31   Repair of buried penis
2016, 2Q, 28   Removal of multi-component inflatable penile prosthesis with placement of new malleable device
2015, 3Q, 25   Placement of inflatable penile prosthesis

AHA Coding Clinic for table ØVX
2018, 4Q, 40   Transfer of prepuce

AHA Coding Clinic for table ØVY
2020, 4Q, 58   Male reproductive organ transplant

Male Reproductive System

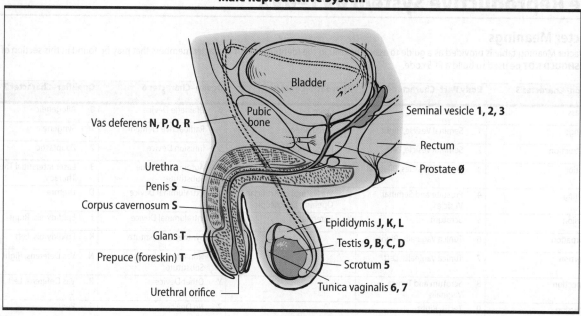

- Bladder
- Seminal vesicle **1, 2, 3**
- Pubic bone
- Vas deferens **N, P, Q, R**
- Rectum
- Prostate **Ø**
- Urethra
- Penis **S**
- Corpus cavernosum **S**
- Epididymis **J, K, L**
- Glans **T**
- Testis **9, B, C, D**
- Prepuce (foreskin) **T**
- Scrotum **5**
- Tunica vaginalis **6, 7**
- Urethral orifice

Penis

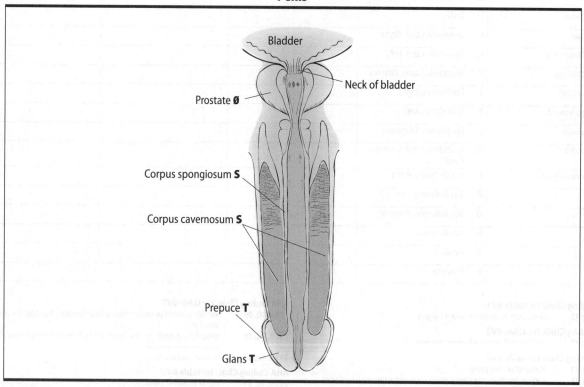

- Bladder
- Neck of bladder
- Prostate **Ø**
- Corpus spongiosum **S**
- Corpus cavernosum **S**
- Prepuce **T**
- Glans **T**

Ø   **Medical and Surgical**
V   **Male Reproductive System**
1   **Bypass**   Definition: Altering the route of passage of the contents of a tubular body part

Explanation: Rerouting contents of a body part to a downstream area of the normal route, to a similar route and body part, or to an abnormal route and dissimilar body part. Includes one or more anastomoses, with or without the use of a device.

Body Part Character 4	Approach Character 5	Device Character 6	Qualifier Character 7

N Vas Deferens, Right ♂
   Ductus deferens
   Ejaculatory duct
P Vas Deferens, Left ♂
   See N Vas Deferens, Right
Q Vas Deferens, Bilateral ♂
   See N Vas Deferens, Right
	Ø Open
	4 Percutaneous Endoscopic
		7 Autologous Tissue Substitute
		J Synthetic Substitute
		K Nonautologous Tissue Substitute
		Z No Device
			J Epididymis, Right
			K Epididymis, Left
			N Vas Deferens, Right
			P Vas Deferens, Left

♂   All body part, approach, device, and qualifier values

Ø   **Medical and Surgical**
V   **Male Reproductive System**
2   **Change**   Definition: Taking out or off a device from a body part and putting back an identical or similar device in or on the same body part without cutting or puncturing the skin or a mucous membrane

Explanation: All CHANGE procedures are coded using the approach EXTERNAL

Body Part Character 4	Approach Character 5	Device Character 6	Qualifier Character 7

4 Prostate and Seminal Vesicles ♂
8 Scrotum and Tunica Vaginalis ♂
D Testis ♂
M Epididymis and Spermatic Cord ♂
R Vas Deferens ♂
   Ductus deferens
   Ejaculatory duct
S Penis ♂
   Corpus cavernosum
   Corpus spongiosum
	X External	**Ø** Drainage Device
		Y Other Device
			Z No Qualifier

Non-OR   All body part, approach, device, and qualifier values   ♂   All body part, approach, device, and qualifier values

---

Ø   **Medical and Surgical**
V   **Male Reproductive System**
5   **Destruction**   Definition: Physical eradication of all or a portion of a body part by the direct use of energy, force, or a destructive agent

Explanation: None of the body part is physically taken out

Body Part Character 4	Approach Character 5	Device Character 6	Qualifier Character 7
Ø Prostate ♂	**Ø** Open **3** Percutaneous **4** Percutaneous Endoscopic	**Z** No Device	**3** Laser Interstitial Thermal Therapy **Z** No Qualifier
Ø Prostate ♂	**7** Via Natural or Artificial Opening **8** Via Natural or Artificial Opening Endoscopic	**Z** No Device	**Z** No Qualifier
1 Seminal Vesicle, Right ♂ **2** Seminal Vesicle, Left ♂ **3** Seminal Vesicles, Bilateral ♂ **6** Tunica Vaginalis, Right ♂ **7** Tunica Vaginalis, Left ♂ **9** Testis, Right ♂ **B** Testis, Left ♂ **C** Testes, Bilateral ♂	**Ø** Open **3** Percutaneous **4** Percutaneous Endoscopic	**Z** No Device	**Z** No Qualifier

5 Scrotum ♂
S Penis ♂
   Corpus cavernosum
   Corpus spongiosum
T Prepuce ♂
   Foreskin
   Glans penis
	Ø Open
	3 Percutaneous
	4 Percutaneous Endoscopic
	X External
		Z No Device	**Z** No Qualifier

F Spermatic Cord, Right ♂
G Spermatic Cord, Left ♂
H Spermatic Cords, Bilateral ♂
J Epididymis, Right ♂
K Epididymis, Left ♂
L Epididymis, Bilateral ♂
N Vas Deferens, Right NC ♂
   Ductus deferens
   Ejaculatory duct
P Vas Deferens, Left NC ♂
   See N Vas Deferens, Right
Q Vas Deferens, Bilateral NC ♂
   See N Vas Deferens, Right
	Ø Open
	3 Percutaneous
	4 Percutaneous Endoscopic
	8 Via Natural or Artificial Opening Endoscopic
		Z No Device	**Z** No Qualifier

Non-OR   ØV55[Ø,3,4,X]ZZ
Non-OR   ØV5[N,P,Q][Ø,3,4,8]ZZ

NC   ØV5[N,P,Q][Ø,3,4]ZZ with principal or secondary diagnosis of Z3Ø.2
♂   All body part, approach, device, and qualifier values

NC Noncovered Procedure   LC Limited Coverage   QA Questionable OB Admit   NT New Tech Add-on   ⊞ Combination Member   ♂ Male   ♀ Female

Ø   Medical and Surgical
V   Male Reproductive System
7   Dilation   Definition: Expanding an orifice or the lumen of a tubular body part

Explanation: The orifice can be a natural orifice or an artificially created orifice. Accomplished by stretching a tubular body part using intraluminal pressure or by cutting part of the orifice or wall of the tubular body part.

Body Part Character 4	Approach Character 5	Device Character 6	Qualifier Character 7

N Vas Deferens, Right ♂
   Ductus deferens
   Ejaculatory duct
P Vas Deferens, Left ♂
   See N Vas Deferens, Right
Q Vas Deferens, Bilateral ♂
   See N Vas Deferens, Right
	Ø Open
	3 Percutaneous
	4 Percutaneous Endoscopic
		D Intraluminal Device
		Z No Device
			Z No Qualifier

♂   All body part, approach, device, and qualifier values

Ø   Medical and Surgical
V   Male Reproductive System
9   Drainage   Definition: Taking or letting out fluids and/or gases from a body part

Explanation: The qualifier DIAGNOSTIC is used to identify drainage procedures that are biopsies

Body Part Character 4	Approach Character 5	Device Character 6	Qualifier Character 7
Ø Prostate ♂	Ø Open 3 Percutaneous 4 Percutaneous Endoscopic 7 Via Natural or Artificial Opening 8 Via Natural or Artificial Opening Endoscopic	Ø Drainage Device	Z No Qualifier
Ø Prostate ♂	Ø Open 3 Percutaneous 4 Percutaneous Endoscopic 7 Via Natural or Artificial Opening 8 Via Natural or Artificial Opening Endoscopic	Z No Device	X Diagnostic Z No Qualifier

1 Seminal Vesicle, Right ♂
2 Seminal Vesicle, Left ♂
3 Seminal Vesicles, Bilateral ♂
6 Tunica Vaginalis, Right ♂
7 Tunica Vaginalis, Left ♂
9 Testis, Right ♂
B Testis, Left ♂
C Testes, Bilateral ♂
F Spermatic Cord, Right ♂
G Spermatic Cord, Left ♂
H Spermatic Cords, Bilateral ♂
J Epididymis, Right ♂
K Epididymis, Left ♂
L Epididymis, Bilateral ♂
N Vas Deferens, Right ♂
   Ductus deferens
   Ejaculatory duct
P Vas Deferens, Left ♂
   See N Vas Deferens, Right
Q Vas Deferens, Bilateral ♂
   See N Vas Deferens, Right
	Ø Open
	3 Percutaneous
	4 Percutaneous Endoscopic
		Ø Drainage Device	Z No Qualifier

Non-OR ØV9Ø[3,4]ØZ	Non-OR ØV9[6,7,F,G,H,N,P,Q][Ø,3,4]ØZ
Non-OR ØV9Ø[3,4]Z[X,Z]	Non-OR ØV9[J,K,L]3ØZ
Non-OR ØV9Ø[7,8]ZX	♂ All body part, approach, device, and qualifier values
Non-OR ØV9[1,2,3,9,B,C][3,4]ØZ	

ØV9 Continued on next page

Ø   **Medical and Surgical**   *ØV9 Continued*
V   **Male Reproductive System**
9   **Drainage**   Definition: Taking or letting out fluids and/or gases from a body part

                           Explanation: The qualifier DIAGNOSTIC is used to identify drainage procedures that are biopsies

Body Part Character 4	Approach Character 5	Device Character 6	Qualifier Character 7
1 Seminal Vesicle, Right ♂	Ø Open	Z No Device	X Diagnostic
2 Seminal Vesicle, Left ♂	3 Percutaneous		Z No Qualifier
3 Seminal Vesicles, Bilateral ♂	4 Percutaneous Endoscopic		
6 Tunica Vaginalis, Right ♂			
7 Tunica Vaginalis, Left ♂			
9 Testis, Right ♂			
B Testis, Left ♂			
C Testes, Bilateral ♂			
F Spermatic Cord, Right ♂			
G Spermatic Cord, Left ♂			
H Spermatic Cords, Bilateral ♂			
J Epididymis, Right ♂			
K Epididymis, Left ♂			
L Epididymis, Bilateral ♂			
N Vas Deferens, Right ♂ Ductus deferens Ejaculatory duct			
P Vas Deferens, Left ♂ *See N Vas Deferens, Right*			
Q Vas Deferens, Bilateral ♂ *See N Vas Deferens, Right*			
5 Scrotum ♂	Ø Open	Ø Drainage Device	Z No Qualifier
S Penis ♂ Corpus cavernosum Corpus spongiosum	3 Percutaneous 4 Percutaneous Endoscopic X External		
T Prepuce ♂ Foreskin Glans penis			
5 Scrotum ♂	Ø Open	Z No Device	X Diagnostic
S Penis ♂ Corpus cavernosum Corpus spongiosum	3 Percutaneous 4 Percutaneous Endoscopic X External		Z No Qualifier
T Prepuce ♂ Foreskin Glans penis			

Non-OR ØV9[1,2,3,9,B,C][3,4]Z[X,Z]		**Non-OR** ØV9[S,T]3ØZ	
Non-OR ØV9[6,7,F,G,H,J,K,L,N,P,Q][Ø,3,4]ZX		**Non-OR** ØV95ØZX	
Non-OR ØV9[6,7,F,G,H,N,P,Q][Ø,3,4]ZZ		**Non-OR** ØV95[3,4,X]Z[X,Z]	
Non-OR ØV9[J,K,L]3ZZ		**Non-OR** ØV9[S,T]3ZZ	
Non-OR ØV95[Ø,3,4,X]ØZ		♂ All body part, approach, device, and qualifier values	

NC Noncovered Procedure   LC Limited Coverage   QA Questionable OB Admit   NT New Tech Add-on   ⊞ Combination Member   ♂ Male   ♀ Female

ICD-10-PCS 2023   663

Ø Medical and Surgical
V Male Reproductive System
B Excision   Definition: Cutting out or off, without replacement, a portion of a body part
                Explanation: The qualifier DIAGNOSTIC is used to identify excision procedures that are biopsies

Body Part Character 4	Approach Character 5	Device Character 6	Qualifier Character 7
Ø Prostate ♂	**Ø** Open **3** Percutaneous **4** Percutaneous Endoscopic **7** Via Natural or Artificial Opening **8** Via Natural or Artificial Opening Endoscopic	**Z** No Device	**X** Diagnostic **Z** No Qualifier
1 Seminal Vesicle, Right ♂ **2** Seminal Vesicle, Left ♂ **3** Seminal Vesicles, Bilateral ♂ **6** Tunica Vaginalis, Right ♂ **7** Tunica Vaginalis, Left ♂ **9** Testis, Right ♂ **B** Testis, Left ♂ **C** Testes, Bilateral ♂	**Ø** Open **3** Percutaneous **4** Percutaneous Endoscopic	**Z** No Device	**X** Diagnostic **Z** No Qualifier

5 Scrotum   ♂
S Penis   ♂
    Corpus cavernosum
    Corpus spongiosum
T Prepuce   ♂
    Foreskin
    Glans penis
	Ø Open
	3 Percutaneous
	4 Percutaneous Endoscopic
	X External
		Z No Device	**X** Diagnostic
			Z No Qualifier

F Spermatic Cord, Right   ♂
G Spermatic Cord, Left   ♂
H Spermatic Cords, Bilateral   ♂
J Epididymis, Right   ♂
K Epididymis, Left   ♂
L Epididymis, Bilateral   ♂
N Vas Deferens, Right   NC ♂
    Ductus deferens
    Ejaculatory duct
P Vas Deferens, Left   NC ♂
    See N Vas Deferens, Right
Q Vas Deferens, Bilateral   NC ♂
    See N Vas Deferens, Right
	Ø Open
	3 Percutaneous
	4 Percutaneous Endoscopic
	8 Via Natural or Artificial Opening Endoscopic
		Z No Device	**X** Diagnostic
			Z No Qualifier

Non-OR ØVBØ[3,4,7,8]ZX	**Non-OR** ØVB[F,G,H,J,K,L][Ø,3,4,8]ZX	
Non-OR ØVB[1,2,3,9,B,C][3,4]ZX	**Non-OR** ØVB[N,P,Q][Ø,3,4,8]Z[X,Z]	
Non-OR ØVB[6,7][Ø,3,4]ZX	**NC** ØVB[N,P,Q][Ø,3,4]ZZ with principal or secondary diagnosis of Z3Ø.2	
Non-OR ØVB5ØZX	♂ All body part, approach, device, and qualifier values	
Non-OR ØVB5[3,4,X]Z[X,Z]		

Non-OR Procedure   DRG Non-OR Procedure   Valid OR Procedure   HAC Associated Procedure   Combination Only   New/Revised April   New/Revised October

664   ICD-10-PCS 2023

Ø   Medical and Surgical
V   Male Reproductive System
C   Extirpation   Definition: Taking or cutting out solid matter from a body part

                Explanation: The solid matter may be an abnormal byproduct of a biological function or a foreign body; it may be imbedded in a body part or in the lumen of a tubular body part. The solid matter may or may not have been previously broken into pieces.

Body Part Character 4		Approach Character 5	Device Character 6	Qualifier Character 7
Ø Prostate	♂	Ø Open 3 Percutaneous 4 Percutaneous Endoscopic 7 Via Natural or Artificial Opening 8 Via Natural or Artificial Opening Endoscopic	Z No Device	Z No Qualifier

1   Seminal Vesicle, Right
2   Seminal Vesicle, Left
3   Seminal Vesicles, Bilateral
6   Tunica Vaginalis, Right
7   Tunica Vaginalis, Left
9   Testis, Right
B   Testis, Left
C   Testes, Bilateral
F   Spermatic Cord, Right
G   Spermatic Cord, Left
H   Spermatic Cords, Bilateral
J   Epididymis, Right
K   Epididymis, Left
L   Epididymis, Bilateral
N   Vas Deferens, Right
     Ductus deferens
     Ejaculatory duct
P   Vas Deferens, Left
     See N Vas Deferens, Right
Q   Vas Deferens, Bilateral
     See N Vas Deferens, Right
	♂
	♂
	♂
	♂
	♂
	♂
	♂
	♂
	♂
	♂
	♂
	♂
	♂
	♂
	♂
	
	♂
	
	♂
		Ø Open
		3 Percutaneous
		4 Percutaneous Endoscopic
			Z No Device	Z No Qualifier

5   Scrotum
S   Penis
     Corpus cavernosum
     Corpus spongiosum
T   Prepuce
     Foreskin
     Glans penis
	♂
	♂
	
	♂
		Ø Open
		3 Percutaneous
		4 Percutaneous Endoscopic
		X External
			Z No Device	Z No Qualifier

Non-OR	ØVC[6,7,N,P,Q][Ø,3,4]ZZ	**Non-OR**	ØVCSXZZ
Non-OR	ØVC5[3,4,X]ZZ	♂	All body part, approach, device, and qualifier values

NC Noncovered Procedure   LC Limited Coverage   OA Questionable OB Admit   NT New Tech Add-on   ⊞ Combination Member   ♂ Male   ♀ Female

ICD-10-PCS 2023   **665**

Ø Medical and Surgical
V Male Reproductive System
H Insertion   Definition: Putting in a nonbiological appliance that monitors, assists, performs, or prevents a physiological function but does not physically take the place of a body part
                        Explanation: None

Body Part Character 4	Approach Character 5	Device Character 6	Qualifier Character 7
Ø Prostate ♂	Ø Open 3 Percutaneous 4 Percutaneous Endoscopic 7 Via Natural or Artificial Opening 8 Via Natural or Artificial Opening Endoscopic	1 Radioactive Element	Z No Qualifier

4 Prostate and Seminal Vesicles ♂
8 Scrotum and Tunica Vaginalis ♂
M Epididymis and Spermatic Cord ♂
R Vas Deferens ♂
   Ductus deferens
   Ejaculatory duct
	Ø Open
	3 Percutaneous
	4 Percutaneous Endoscopic
	7 Via Natural or Artificial Opening
	8 Via Natural or Artificial Opening Endoscopic
		3 Infusion Device
		Y Other Device
			Z No Qualifier

D Testis ♂	Ø Open 3 Percutaneous 4 Percutaneous Endoscopic 7 Via Natural or Artificial Opening 8 Via Natural or Artificial Opening Endoscopic	1 Radioactive Element 3 Infusion Device Y Other Device	Z No Qualifier

S Penis ♂
   Corpus cavernosum
   Corpus spongiosum
	Ø Open
	3 Percutaneous
	4 Percutaneous Endoscopic
		3 Infusion Device
		Y Other Device
			Z No Qualifier

S Penis ♂
   Corpus cavernosum
   Corpus spongiosum
	7 Via Natural or Artificial Opening
	8 Via Natural or Artificial Opening Endoscopic
		Y Other Device	Z No Qualifier

S Penis ♂
   Corpus cavernosum
   Corpus spongiosum
	X External	3 Infusion Device	Z No Qualifier

Non-OR   ØVH[4,8,M,R][Ø,3,4,7,8][3,Y]Z
Non-OR   ØVHD[Ø,3,4,7,8][1,3,Y]Z
Non-OR   ØVHS[Ø,3,4][3,Y]Z
Non-OR   ØVHS[7,8]YZ

Non-OR   ØVHSX3Z
♂   All body part, approach, device, and qualifier values

Ø Medical and Surgical
V Male Reproductive System
J Inspection   Definition: Visually and/or manually exploring a body part
                         Explanation: Visual exploration may be performed with or without optical instrumentation. Manual exploration may be performed directly or through intervening body layers.

Body Part Character 4	Approach Character 5	Device Character 6	Qualifier Character 7

4 Prostate and Seminal Vesicles ♂
8 Scrotum and Tunica Vaginalis ♂
D Testis ♂
M Epididymis and Spermatic Cord ♂
R Vas Deferens ♂
   Ductus deferens
   Ejaculatory duct
S Penis ♂
   Corpus cavernosum
   Corpus spongiosum
	Ø Open
	3 Percutaneous
	4 Percutaneous Endoscopic
	X External
		Z No Device	Z No Qualifier

Non-OR   ØVJ[4,D,M,R][3,X]ZZ
Non-OR   ØVJ8[Ø,3,4,X]ZZ
Non-OR   ØVJS[3,4,X]ZZ

♂   All body part, approach, device, and qualifier values

Ø **Medical and Surgical**
V **Male Reproductive System**
L **Occlusion**   Definition: Completely closing an orifice or the lumen of a tubular body part
              Explanation: The orifice can be a natural orifice or an artificially created orifice

Body Part Character 4	Approach Character 5	Device Character 6	Qualifier Character 7

F Spermatic Cord, Right   NC ♂
G Spermatic Cord, Left   NC ♂
H Spermatic Cords, Bilateral   NC ♂
N Vas Deferens, Right   NC ♂
    Ductus deferens
    Ejaculatory duct
P Vas Deferens, Left   NC ♂
    See N Vas Deferens, Right
Q Vas Deferens, Bilateral   NC ♂
    See N Vas Deferens, Right
	Ø Open
	3 Percutaneous
	4 Percutaneous Endoscopic
	8 Via Natural or Artificial Opening
	    Endoscopic
		C Extraluminal Device
		D Intraluminal Device
		Z No Device
			Z No Qualifier

Non-OR ØVL[F,G,H][Ø,3,4,8][C,D,Z]Z	NC	ØVL[F,G,H][Ø,3,4][C,D,Z]Z with principal or secondary diagnosis of Z3Ø.2
Non-OR ØVL[N,P,Q][Ø,3,4,8][C,Z]Z	NC	ØVL[N,P,Q][Ø,3,4][C,Z]Z with principal or secondary diagnosis of Z3Ø.2
	♂	All body part, approach, device, and qualifier values

Ø **Medical and Surgical**
V **Male Reproductive System**
M **Reattachment**   Definition: Putting back in or on all or a portion of a separated body part to its normal location or other suitable location
              Explanation: Vascular circulation and nervous pathways may or may not be reestablished

Body Part Character 4	Approach Character 5	Device Character 6	Qualifier Character 7

5 Scrotum   ♂
S Penis   ♂
    Corpus cavernosum
    Corpus spongiosum
	X External	Z No Device	Z No Qualifier

6 Tunica Vaginalis, Right ♂ 7 Tunica Vaginalis, Left ♂ 9 Testis, Right ♂ B Testis, Left ♂ C Testes, Bilateral ♂ F Spermatic Cord, Right ♂ G Spermatic Cord, Left ♂ H Spermatic Cords, Bilateral ♂	Ø Open 4 Percutaneous Endoscopic	Z No Device	Z No Qualifier

♂	All body part, approach, device, and qualifier values

NC Noncovered Procedure   LC Limited Coverage   OA Questionable OB Admit   NT New Tech Add-on   ⊞ Combination Member   ♂ Male   ♀ Female

ICD-10-PCS 2023   **667**

Male Reproductive System

Ø   **Medical and Surgical**
V   **Male Reproductive System**
N   **Release**   Definition: Freeing a body part from an abnormal physical constraint by cutting or by the use of force
                     Explanation: Some of the restraining tissue may be taken out but none of the body part is taken out

Body Part Character 4		Approach Character 5	Device Character 6	Qualifier Character 7
Ø Prostate	♂	**Ø** Open **3** Percutaneous **4** Percutaneous Endoscopic **7** Via Natural or Artificial Opening **8** Via Natural or Artificial Opening Endoscopic	**Z** No Device	**Z** No Qualifier
1 Seminal Vesicle, Right **2** Seminal Vesicle, Left **3** Seminal Vesicles, Bilateral **6** Tunica Vaginalis, Right **7** Tunica Vaginalis, Left **9** Testis, Right **B** Testis, Left **C** Testes, Bilateral	♂ ♂ ♂ ♂ ♂ ♂ ♂ ♂	**Ø** Open **3** Percutaneous **4** Percutaneous Endoscopic	**Z** No Device	**Z** No Qualifier

5   Scrotum
S   Penis
     Corpus cavernosum
     Corpus spongiosum
T   Prepuce
     Foreskin
     Glans penis
	♂
	♂
	
	♂
		Ø Open
		3 Percutaneous
		4 Percutaneous Endoscopic
		X External
			Z No Device	**Z** No Qualifier

F   Spermatic Cord, Right
G   Spermatic Cord, Left
H   Spermatic Cords, Bilateral
J   Epididymis, Right
K   Epididymis, Left
L   Epididymis, Bilateral
N   Vas Deferens, Right
     Ductus deferens
     Ejaculatory duct
P   Vas Deferens, Left
     See N Vas Deferens, Right
Q   Vas Deferens, Bilateral
     See N Vas Deferens, Right
	♂
	♂
	♂
	♂
	♂
	♂
	♂
	
	♂
	
	♂
		Ø Open
		3 Percutaneous
		4 Percutaneous Endoscopic
		8 Via Natural or Artificial Opening Endoscopic
			Z No Device	**Z** No Qualifier

Non-OR	ØVN[9,B,C][Ø,3,4]ZZ	♂	All body part, approach, device, and qualifier values
Non-OR	ØVNT[Ø,3,4,X]ZZ		

Ø   Medical and Surgical
V   Male Reproductive System
P   Removal   Definition: Taking out or off a device from a body part

Explanation: If a device is taken out and a similar device put in without cutting or puncturing the skin or mucous membrane, the procedure is coded to the root operation CHANGE. Otherwise, the procedure for taking out the device is coded to the root operation REMOVAL.

Body Part Character 4		Approach Character 5	Device Character 6	Qualifier Character 7
4 Prostate and Seminal Vesicles	♂	Ø Open 3 Percutaneous 4 Percutaneous Endoscopic 7 Via Natural or Artificial Opening 8 Via Natural or Artificial Opening Endoscopic	Ø Drainage Device 1 Radioactive Element 3 Infusion Device 7 Autologous Tissue Substitute J Synthetic Substitute K Nonautologous Tissue Substitute Y Other Device	Z No Qualifier
4 Prostate and Seminal Vesicles	♂	X External	Ø Drainage Device 1 Radioactive Element 3 Infusion Device	Z No Qualifier

8   Scrotum and Tunica Vaginalis
D   Testis
S   Penis
     Corpus cavernosum
     Corpus spongiosum
	♂
	♂
	♂
		Ø Open
		3 Percutaneous
		4 Percutaneous Endoscopic
		7 Via Natural or Artificial Opening
		8 Via Natural or Artificial Opening
		     Endoscopic
			Ø Drainage Device
			3 Infusion Device
			7 Autologous Tissue Substitute
			J Synthetic Substitute
			K Nonautologous Tissue Substitute
			Y Other Device
				Z No Qualifier

8   Scrotum and Tunica Vaginalis
D   Testis
S   Penis
     Corpus cavernosum
     Corpus spongiosum
	♂
	♂
	♂
		X External	Ø Drainage Device
			3 Infusion Device
				Z No Qualifier

M Epididymis and Spermatic Cord	♂	Ø Open 3 Percutaneous 4 Percutaneous Endoscopic 7 Via Natural or Artificial Opening 8 Via Natural or Artificial Opening Endoscopic	Ø Drainage Device 3 Infusion Device 7 Autologous Tissue Substitute C Extraluminal Device J Synthetic Substitute K Nonautologous Tissue Substitute Y Other Device	Z No Qualifier
M Epididymis and Spermatic Cord	♂	X External	Ø Drainage Device 3 Infusion Device	Z No Qualifier

R   Vas Deferens
     Ductus deferens
     Ejaculatory duct
	♂	Ø Open
		3 Percutaneous
		4 Percutaneous Endoscopic
		7 Via Natural or Artificial Opening
		8 Via Natural or Artificial Opening
		     Endoscopic
			Ø Drainage Device
			3 Infusion Device
			7 Autologous Tissue Substitute
			C Extraluminal Device
			D Intraluminal Device
			J Synthetic Substitute
			K Nonautologous Tissue Substitute
			Y Other Device
				Z No Qualifier

R   Vas Deferens
     Ductus deferens
     Ejaculatory duct
	♂	X External	Ø Drainage Device
			3 Infusion Device
			D Intraluminal Device
				Z No Qualifier

Non-OR	ØVP4[3,4]YZ
Non-OR	ØVP4[7,8][Ø,3,Y]Z
Non-OR	ØVP4X[Ø,1,3]Z
Non-OR	ØVP8[Ø,3,4,7,8][Ø,3,7,J,K,Y]Z
Non-OR	ØVP[D,S][3,4]YZ
Non-OR	ØVP[D,S][7,8][Ø,3,Y]Z
Non-OR	ØVP[8,D,S]X[Ø,3]Z

Non-OR	ØVPM[3,4]YZ
Non-OR	ØVPM[7,8][Ø,3,Y]Z
Non-OR	ØVPMX[Ø,3]Z
Non-OR	ØVPR[Ø,3,4][Ø,3,7,C,J,K,Y]Z
Non-OR	ØVPR[7,8][Ø,3,7,C,D,J,K,Y]Z
Non-OR	ØVPRX[Ø,3,D]Z
♂	All body part, approach, device, and qualifier values

NC Noncovered Procedure   LC Limited Coverage   QA Questionable OB Admit   NT New Tech Add-on   ⊞ Combination Member   ♂ Male   ♀ Female

ICD-10-PCS 2023   **669**

Ø Medical and Surgical
V Male Reproductive System
Q Repair   Definition: Restoring, to the extent possible, a body part to its normal anatomic structure and function
                    Explanation: Used only when the method to accomplish the repair is not one of the other root operations

Body Part Character 4	Approach Character 5	Device Character 6	Qualifier Character 7
Ø Prostate ♂	Ø Open 3 Percutaneous 4 Percutaneous Endoscopic 7 Via Natural or Artificial Opening 8 Via Natural or Artificial Opening Endoscopic	Z No Device	Z No Qualifier
1 Seminal Vesicle, Right ♂ 2 Seminal Vesicle, Left ♂ 3 Seminal Vesicles, Bilateral ♂ 6 Tunica Vaginalis, Right ♂ 7 Tunica Vaginalis, Left ♂ 9 Testis, Right ♂ B Testis, Left ♂ C Testes, Bilateral ♂	Ø Open 3 Percutaneous 4 Percutaneous Endoscopic	Z No Device	Z No Qualifier

5 Scrotum ♂
S Penis ♂
   Corpus cavernosum
   Corpus spongiosum
T Prepuce ♂
   Foreskin
   Glans penis
	Ø Open
	3 Percutaneous
	4 Percutaneous Endoscopic
	X External
		Z No Device	Z No Qualifier

F Spermatic Cord, Right ♂
G Spermatic Cord, Left ♂
H Spermatic Cords, Bilateral ♂
J Epididymis, Right ♂
K Epididymis, Left ♂
L Epididymis, Bilateral ♂
N Vas Deferens, Right ♂
   Ductus deferens
   Ejaculatory duct
P Vas Deferens, Left ♂
   See N Vas Deferens, Right
Q Vas Deferens, Bilateral ♂
   See N Vas Deferens, Right
	Ø Open
	3 Percutaneous
	4 Percutaneous Endoscopic
	8 Via Natural or Artificial Opening Endoscopic
		Z No Device	Z No Qualifier

Non-OR	ØVQ[6,7][Ø,3,4]ZZ ♂	All body part, approach, device, and qualifier values
Non-OR	ØVQ5[Ø,3,4,X]ZZ	

Ø Medical and Surgical
V Male Reproductive System
R Replacement   Definition: Putting in or on biological or synthetic material that physically takes the place and/or function of all or a portion of a body part
                    Explanation: The body part may have been taken out or replaced, or may be taken out, physically eradicated, or rendered nonfunctional during the REPLACEMENT procedure. A REMOVAL procedure is coded for taking out the device used in a previous replacement procedure.

Body Part Character 4	Approach Character 5	Device Character 6	Qualifier Character 7
9 Testis, Right ♂ B Testis, Left ♂ C Testes, Bilateral ♂	Ø Open	J Synthetic Substitute	Z No Qualifier

♂	All body part, approach, device, and qualifier values

Ø Medical and Surgical
V Male Reproductive System
S Reposition   Definition: Moving to its normal location, or other suitable location, all or a portion of a body part
                    Explanation: The body part is moved to a new location from an abnormal location, or from a normal location where it is not functioning correctly. The body part may or may not be cut out or off to be moved to the new location.

Body Part Character 4	Approach Character 5	Device Character 6	Qualifier Character 7
9 Testis, Right ♂ B Testis, Left ♂ C Testes, Bilateral ♂ F Spermatic Cord, Right ♂ G Spermatic Cord, Left ♂ H Spermatic Cords, Bilateral ♂	Ø Open 3 Percutaneous 4 Percutaneous Endoscopic 8 Via Natural or Artificial Opening Endoscopic	Z No Device	Z No Qualifier

♂	All body part, approach, device, and qualifier values

Ø　**Medical and Surgical**
V　**Male Reproductive System**
T　**Resection**　　Definition: Cutting out or off, without replacement, all of a body part
　　　　　　　　　　　Explanation: None

Body Part Character 4	Approach Character 5	Device Character 6	Qualifier Character 7
Ø　Prostate　　　⊞♂	**Ø**　Open **4**　Percutaneous Endoscopic **7**　Via Natural or Artificial Opening **8**　Via Natural or Artificial Opening 　　Endoscopic	**Z**　No Device	**Z**　No Qualifier
1　Seminal Vesicle, Right　　♂ **2**　Seminal Vesicle, Left　　♂ **3**　Seminal Vesicles, Bilateral　⊞♂ **6**　Tunica Vaginalis, Right　　♂ **7**　Tunica Vaginalis, Left　　♂ **9**　Testis, Right　　♂ **B**　Testis, Left　　♂ **C**　Testes, Bilateral　　♂ **F**　Spermatic Cord, Right　　♂ **G**　Spermatic Cord, Left　　♂ **H**　Spermatic Cords, Bilateral　♂ **J**　Epididymis, Right　　♂ **K**　Epididymis, Left　　♂ **L**　Epididymis, Bilateral　　♂ **N**　Vas Deferens, Right　🆖♂ 　　Ductus deferens 　　Ejaculatory duct **P**　Vas Deferens, Left　🆖♂ 　　See N Vas Deferens, Right **Q**　Vas Deferens, Bilateral　🆖♂ 　　See N Vas Deferens, Right	**Ø**　Open **4**　Percutaneous Endoscopic	**Z**　No Device	**Z**　No Qualifier
5　Scrotum　　♂ **S**　Penis　　♂ 　　Corpus cavernosum 　　Corpus spongiosum **T**　Prepuce　　♂ 　　Foreskin 　　Glans penis	**Ø**　Open **4**　Percutaneous Endoscopic **X**　External	**Z**　No Device	**Z**　No Qualifier

Non-OR　ØVT[N,P,Q][Ø,4]ZZ	**See Appendix L for Procedure Combinations**
Non-OR　ØVT[5,T][Ø,4,X]ZZ	⊞　ØVTØ[Ø,4,7,8]ZZ
🆖　ØVT[N,P,Q][Ø,4]ZZ with principal or secondary diagnosis of Z3Ø.2	⊞　ØVT3[Ø,4]ZZ
♂　All body part, approach, device, and qualifier values	

🆖 Noncovered Procedure　　🆑 Limited Coverage　　🆀🅰 Questionable OB Admit　　🆕🆃 New Tech Add-on　　⊞ Combination Member　　♂ Male　　♀ Female

ICD-10-PCS 2023　　　**671**

ØVT–ØVT

Ø   **Medical and Surgical**
V   **Male Reproductive System**
U   **Supplement**   Definition: Putting in or on biological or synthetic material that physically reinforces and/or augments the function of a portion of a body part
                         Explanation: The biological material is non-living, or is living and from the same individual. The body part may have been previously replaced, and the SUPPLEMENT procedure is performed to physically reinforce and/or augment the function of the replaced body part.

Body Part Character 4		Approach Character 5	Device Character 6	Qualifier Character 7

1 Seminal Vesicle, Right ♂
2 Seminal Vesicle, Left ♂
3 Seminal Vesicles, Bilateral ♂
6 Tunica Vaginalis, Right ♂
7 Tunica Vaginalis, Left ♂
F Spermatic Cord, Right ♂
G Spermatic Cord, Left ♂
H Spermatic Cords, Bilateral ♂
J Epididymis, Right ♂
K Epididymis, Left ♂
L Epididymis, Bilateral ♂
N Vas Deferens, Right ♂
    Ductus deferens
    Ejaculatory duct
P Vas Deferens, Left ♂
    See N Vas Deferens, Right
Q Vas Deferens, Bilateral ♂
    See N Vas Deferens, Right
		Ø Open
		4 Percutaneous Endoscopic
		8 Via Natural or Artificial Opening Endoscopic
			7 Autologous Tissue Substitute
			J Synthetic Substitute
			K Nonautologous Tissue Substitute
				Z No Qualifier

5 Scrotum ♂
S Penis ♂
    Corpus cavernosum
    Corpus spongiosum
T Prepuce ♂
    Foreskin
    Glans penis
		Ø Open
		4 Percutaneous Endoscopic
		X External
			7 Autologous Tissue Substitute
			J Synthetic Substitute
			K Nonautologous Tissue Substitute
				Z No Qualifier

9 Testis, Right ♂ **B** Testis, Left ♂ **C** Testes, Bilateral ♂		**Ø** Open	**7** Autologous Tissue Substitute **J** Synthetic Substitute **K** Nonautologous Tissue Substitute	**Z** No Qualifier

Non-OR   ØVUSX[7,J,K]Z   ♂   All body part, approach, device, and qualifier values

Ø　**Medical and Surgical**
V　**Male Reproductive System**
W　**Revision**　　Definition: Correcting, to the extent possible, a portion of a malfunctioning device or the position of a displaced device
　　　　　　　　　　Explanation: Revision can include correcting a malfunctioning or displaced device by taking out or putting in components of the device such as a screw or pin

Body Part Character 4		Approach Character 5	Device Character 6	Qualifier Character 7
4　Prostate and Seminal Vesicles　♂ **8**　Scrotum and Tunica Vaginalis　♂ **D**　Testis　♂ **S**　Penis　♂ 　　　Corpus cavernosum 　　　Corpus spongiosum		**Ø**　Open **3**　Percutaneous **4**　Percutaneous Endoscopic **7**　Via Natural or Artificial Opening **8**　Via Natural or Artificial Opening 　　　Endoscopic	**Ø**　Drainage Device **3**　Infusion Device **7**　Autologous Tissue Substitute **J**　Synthetic Substitute **K**　Nonautologous Tissue Substitute **Y**　Other Device	**Z**　No Qualifier
4　Prostate and Seminal Vesicles　♂ **8**　Scrotum and Tunica Vaginalis　♂ **D**　Testis　♂ **S**　Penis　♂ 　　　Corpus cavernosum 　　　Corpus spongiosum		**X**　External	**Ø**　Drainage Device **3**　Infusion Device **7**　Autologous Tissue Substitute **J**　Synthetic Substitute **K**　Nonautologous Tissue Substitute	**Z**　No Qualifier
M　Epididymis and Spermatic Cord　♂		**Ø**　Open **3**　Percutaneous **4**　Percutaneous Endoscopic **7**　Via Natural or Artificial Opening **8**　Via Natural or Artificial Opening 　　　Endoscopic	**Ø**　Drainage Device **3**　Infusion Device **7**　Autologous Tissue Substitute **C**　Extraluminal Device **J**　Synthetic Substitute **K**　Nonautologous Tissue Substitute **Y**　Other Device	**Z**　No Qualifier
M　Epididymis and Spermatic Cord　♂		**X**　External	**Ø**　Drainage Device **3**　Infusion Device **7**　Autologous Tissue Substitute **C**　Extraluminal Device **J**　Synthetic Substitute **K**　Nonautologous Tissue Substitute	**Z**　No Qualifier
R　Vas Deferens　♂ 　　　Ductus deferens 　　　Ejaculatory duct		**Ø**　Open **3**　Percutaneous **4**　Percutaneous Endoscopic **7**　Via Natural or Artificial Opening **8**　Via Natural or Artificial Opening 　　　Endoscopic	**Ø**　Drainage Device **3**　Infusion Device **7**　Autologous Tissue Substitute **C**　Extraluminal Device **D**　Intraluminal Device **J**　Synthetic Substitute **K**　Nonautologous Tissue Substitute **Y**　Other Device	**Z**　No Qualifier
R　Vas Deferens　♂ 　　　Ductus deferens 　　　Ejaculatory duct		**X**　External	**Ø**　Drainage Device **3**　Infusion Device **7**　Autologous Tissue Substitute **C**　Extraluminal Device **D**　Intraluminal Device **J**　Synthetic Substitute **K**　Nonautologous Tissue Substitute	**Z**　No Qualifier

Non-OR　ØVW[4,D,S][3,4,7,8]YZ
Non-OR　ØVW8[Ø,3,4,7,8][Ø,3,7,J,K,Y]Z
Non-OR　ØVW[4,8,D,S]X[Ø,3,7,J,K]Z
Non-OR　ØVWM[3,4,7,8]YZ

Non-OR　ØVWMX[Ø,3,7,C,J,K]Z
Non-OR　ØVWR[Ø,3,4,7,8][Ø,3,7,C,D,J,K,Y]Z
Non-OR　ØVWRX[Ø,3,7,C,D,J,K]Z
♂　All body part, approach, device, and qualifier values

NC Noncovered Procedure　　LC Limited Coverage　　QA Questionable OB Admit　　NT New Tech Add-on　　⊞ Combination Member　　♂ Male　　♀ Female

ICD-10-PCS 2023　　　　　　　　　　　　　　　　　　　　　　　　　　　　　　　　　　673

Ø   Medical and Surgical
V   Male Reproductive System
X   Transfer   Definition: Moving, without taking out, all or a portion of a body part to another location to take over the function of all or a portion of a body part

Explanation: The body part transferred remains connected to its vascular and nervous supply

Body Part Character 4	Approach Character 5	Device Character 6	Qualifier Character 7

T   Prepuce
     Foreskin
     Glans penis
	Ø Open
	X External
		Z No Device	D Urethra
			S Penis

Ø   Medical and Surgical
V   Male Reproductive System
Y   Transplantation   Definition: Putting in or on all or a portion of a body part taken from another individual or animal to physically take the place and/or function of all or a portion of a similar body part

Explanation: The native body part may or may not be taken out, and the transplanted body part may take over all or a portion of its function

Body Part Character 4	Approach Character 5	Device Character 6	Qualifier Character 7

5   Scrotum   ♂
S   Penis   ♂
     Corpus cavernosum
     Corpus spongiosum
	Ø Open	Z No Device	Ø Allogeneic
			1 Syngeneic
			2 Zooplastic

♂ All body part, approach, device, and qualifier values			

Anatomical Regions, General ØWØ–ØWY

Character Meanings

This Character Meaning table is provided as a guide to assist the user in the identification of character members that may be found in this section of code tables. It **SHOULD NOT** be used to build a PCS code.

Operation–Character 3	Body Region–Character 4	Approach–Character 5	Device–Character 6	Qualifier–Character 7
Ø Alteration	Ø Head	Ø Open	Ø Drainage Device	Ø Vagina OR Allogeneic
1 Bypass	1 Cranial Cavity	3 Percutaneous	1 Radioactive Element	1 Penis OR Syngeneic
2 Change	2 Face	4 Percutaneous Endoscopic	3 Infusion Device	2 Stoma
3 Control	3 Oral Cavity and Throat	7 Via Natural or Artificial Opening	7 Autologous Tissue Substitute	4 Cutaneous
4 Creation	4 Upper Jaw	8 Via Natural or Artificial Opening Endoscopic	J Synthetic Substitute	6 Bladder
8 Division	5 Lower Jaw	X External	K Nonautologous Tissue Substitute	9 Pleural Cavity, Right
9 Drainage	6 Neck		Y Other Device	B Pleural Cavity, Left
B Excision	8 Chest Wall		Z No Device	G Peritoneal Cavity
C Extirpation	9 Pleural Cavity, Right			J Pelvic Cavity
F Fragmentation	B Pleural Cavity, Left			W Upper Vein
H Insertion	C Mediastinum			X Diagnostic
J Inspection	D Pericardial Cavity			Y Lower Vein
M Reattachment	F Abdominal Wall			Z No Qualifier
P Removal	G Peritoneal Cavity			
Q Repair	H Retroperitoneum			
U Supplement	J Pelvic Cavity			
W Revision	K Upper Back			
Y Transplantation	L Lower Back			
	M Perineum, Male			
	N Perineum, Female			
	P Gastrointestinal Tract			
	Q Respiratory Tract			
	R Genitourinary Tract			

AHA Coding Clinic for table ØWØ
2015, 1Q, 31   Bilateral browpexy

AHA Coding Clinic for table ØW1
2020, 4Q, 55   Insertion of subcutaneous pump system for ascites drainage
2018, 4Q, 41-42   Anatomical regions bypass qualifiers
2015, 2Q, 36   Insertion of infusion device into peritoneal cavity
2013, 4Q, 126-127 Creation of percutaneous cutaneoperitoneal fistula

AHA Coding Clinic for table ØW3
2021, 3Q, 26   Cavoatrial junction tear with repair and relief of cardiac tamponade
2019, 3Q, 4   Evacuation of subdural hematoma and control of bleeding artery
2018, 4Q, 38   Control of epistaxis
2018, 1Q, 19   Argon plasma coagulation of duodenal arteriovenous malformation
2018, 1Q, 19   Control of epistaxis via silver nitrate cauterization
2017, 4Q, 57-58   Added approach values - Transorifice esophageal vein banding
2017, 4Q, 105   Control of gastrointestinal bleeding
2017, 4Q, 106   Control of bleeding of external naris using suture
2017, 4Q, 106   Nasal packing for epistaxis
2016, 4Q, 99-100   Root operation Control
2014, 4Q, 44   Bakri balloon for control of postpartum hemorrhage
2013, 3Q, 23   Control of intraoperative bleeding

AHA Coding Clinic for table ØW4
2019, 4Q, 30   Transfer large intestine to vagina
2016, 4Q, 101   Root operation Creation

AHA Coding Clinic for table ØW9
2021, 3Q, 17   Incision and drainage of retropharyngeal space abscess
2021, 3Q, 21   Drainage of midline neck abscess
2021, 3Q, 26   Cavoatrial junction tear with repair and relief of cardiac tamponade
2020, 4Q, 52   Transvaginal drainage of pelvis
2017, 3Q, 12   Therapeutic and diagnostic paracentesis
2017, 2Q, 16   Incision and drainage of floor of mouth

AHA Coding Clinic for table ØWB
2021, 3Q, 21   Excision of thyroglossal duct cyst
2019, 1Q, 27   Excision of pelvic sidewall mass
2017, 2Q, 16   Excision of floor of mouth
2016, 1Q, 21   Excision of urachal mass
2013, 4Q, 119   Excision of inclusion cyst of perineum

AHA Coding Clinic for table ØWC
2022, 1Q, 42   Removal of fat necrosis from retroperitoneum and space of Retzius
2019, 4Q, 35   Extirpation of jaw
2017, 2Q, 16   Excision of floor of mouth

AHA Coding Clinic for table ØWH
2021, 2Q, 14   Peritoneal dialysis catheter placement
2019, 4Q, 43   Unidirectional source brachytherapy
2018, 1Q, 25   Intrauterine brachytherapy & placement of tandems & ovoids
2017, 4Q, 104   Intrauterine brachytherapy & placement of tandems & ovoids
2016, 2Q, 14   Insertion of peritoneal totally implantable venous access device
2015, 2Q, 36   Insertion of infusion device into peritoneal cavity

AHA Coding Clinic for table ØWJ
2021, 2Q, 19   Electromagnetic stealth guided ventriculoperitoneal shunt insertion with endoscopy
2019, 1Q, 3-8   Whipple procedure
2019, 1Q, 25   Laparoscopic appendectomy converted to open procedure
2018, 3Q, 29   Decommissioning of left ventricular assist device with exploration of mediastinum
2016, 4Q, 58   Longitudinal vaginal septum
2013, 2Q, 36   Insertion of ventriculoperitoneal shunt with laparoscopic assistance

AHA Coding Clinic for table ØWP
2021, 2Q, 14   Removal of peritoneal dialysis catheter

AHA Coding Clinic for table ØWQ
2017, 4Q, 106   Control of bleeding of external naris using suture
2017, 3Q, 8   Removal of silo and closure of gastroschisis
2016, 3Q, 3-7   Stoma creation & takedown procedures
2014, 4Q, 39   Abdominoplasty and abdominal wall plication for hernia repair
2014, 3Q, 28   Ileostomy takedown and parastomal hernia repair

AHA Coding Clinic for table ØWU
2017, 3Q, 8   First stage of gastroschisis repair with silo placement
2016, 3Q, 40   Omentoplasty
2015, 2Q, 29   Placement of Ioban™ antimicrobial drape over surgical wound
2014, 4Q, 39   Abdominal component release with placement of mesh for hernia repair
2012, 4Q, 101   Rib resection with reconstruction of anterior chest wall

AHA Coding Clinic for table ØWW
2015, 2Q, 9   Revision of ventriculoperitoneal (VP) shunt

AHA Coding Clinic for table ØWY
2016, 4Q, 112-113 Transplantation

Anatomical Regions, General

Ø   **Medical and Surgical**
W   **Anatomical Regions, General**
Ø   **Alteration**   Definition: Modifying the anatomic structure of a body part without affecting the function of the body part

                     Explanation: Principal purpose is to improve appearance

Body Part Character 4	Approach Character 5	Device Character 6	Qualifier Character 7
Ø Head	Ø Open	7 Autologous Tissue Substitute	Z No Qualifier
2 Face	3 Percutaneous	J Synthetic Substitute	
4 Upper Jaw	4 Percutaneous Endoscopic	K Nonautologous Tissue Substitute	
5 Lower Jaw		Z No Device	
6 Neck			
Parapharyngeal space			
Retropharyngeal space			
8 Chest Wall			
F Abdominal Wall			
K Upper Back			
L Lower Back			
M Perineum, Male ♂			
N Perineum, Female ♀			

♂   ØWØM[Ø,3,4][7,J,K,Z]Z
♀   ØWØN[Ø,3,4][7,J,K,Z]Z

Ø   **Medical and Surgical**
W   **Anatomical Regions, General**
1   **Bypass**   Definition: Altering the route of passage of the contents of a tubular body part

                     Explanation: Rerouting contents of a body part to a downstream area of the normal route, to a similar route and body part, or to an abnormal route and dissimilar body part. Includes one or more anastomoses, with or without the use of a device.

Body Part Character 4	Approach Character 5	Device Character 6	Qualifier Character 7
1 Cranial Cavity	Ø Open	J Synthetic Substitute	9 Pleural Cavity, Right
			B Pleural Cavity, Left
			G Peritoneal Cavity
			J Pelvic Cavity
9 Pleural Cavity, Right	Ø Open	J Synthetic Substitute	4 Cutaneous
B Pleural Cavity, Left	3 Percutaneous		9 Pleural Cavity, Right
J Pelvic Cavity	4 Percutaneous Endoscopic		B Pleural Cavity, Left
Retropubic space			G Peritoneal Cavity
			J Pelvic Cavity
			W Upper Vein
			Y Lower Vein
G Peritoneal Cavity	Ø Open	J Synthetic Substitute	4 Cutaneous
Abdominal cavity	3 Percutaneous		6 Bladder
	4 Percutaneous Endoscopic		9 Pleural Cavity, Right
			B Pleural Cavity, Left
			G Peritoneal Cavity
			J Pelvic Cavity
			W Upper Vein
			Y Lower Vein

Non-OR   ØW1[9,B][Ø,3,4]J[4,G,W,Y]
Non-OR   ØW1J[Ø,3,4]J[4,W,Y]
Non-OR   ØW1G[Ø,3,4]J[9,B,G,J]

Non-OR Procedure   DRG Non-OR Procedure   Valid OR Procedure   HAC Associated Procedure   Combination Only   New/Revised April   New/Revised October

676   ICD-10-PCS 2023

Ø   **Medical and Surgical**
W   **Anatomical Regions, General**
2   **Change**   Definition: Taking out or off a device from a body part and putting back an identical or similar device in or on the same body part without cutting or puncturing the skin or a mucous membrane
                           Explanation: All CHANGE procedures are coded using the approach EXTERNAL

Body Part Character 4	Approach Character 5	Device Character 6	Qualifier Character 7
Ø Head	**X** External	**Ø** Drainage Device	**Z** No Qualifier
1 Cranial Cavity		**Y** Other Device	
2 Face			
4 Upper Jaw			
5 Lower Jaw			
6 Neck			
Parapharyngeal space			
Retropharyngeal space			
8 Chest Wall			
9 Pleural Cavity, Right			
B Pleural Cavity, Left			
C Mediastinum			
Mediastinal cavity			
Mediastinal space			
D Pericardial Cavity			
F Abdominal Wall			
G Peritoneal Cavity			
Abdominal cavity			
H Retroperitoneum			
Retroperitoneal cavity			
Retroperitoneal space			
J Pelvic Cavity			
Retropubic space			
K Upper Back			
L Lower Back			
M Perineum, Male ♂			
N Perineum, Female ♀			

Non-OR	All body part, approach, device, and qualifier values	♂ ØW2MX[Ø,Y]Z
		♀ ØW2NX[Ø,Y]Z

Ø Medical and Surgical
W Anatomical Regions, General
3 Control   Definition: Stopping, or attempting to stop, postprocedural or other acute bleeding
               Explanation: None

Body Part Character 4	Approach Character 5	Device Character 6	Qualifier Character 7

Ø Head
1 Cranial Cavity
2 Face
4 Upper Jaw
5 Lower Jaw
6 Neck
  Parapharyngeal space
  Retropharyngeal space
8 Chest Wall
9 Pleural Cavity, Right
B Pleural Cavity, Left
C Mediastinum
  Mediastinal cavity
  Mediastinal space
D Pericardial Cavity
F Abdominal Wall
G Peritoneal Cavity
  Abdominal cavity
H Retroperitoneum
  Retroperitoneal cavity
  Retroperitoneal space
J Pelvic Cavity
  Retropubic space
K Upper Back
L Lower Back
M Perineum, Male ♂
N Perineum, Female ♀
	Ø Open
	3 Percutaneous
	4 Percutaneous Endoscopic
		Z No Device	Z No Qualifier

3 Oral Cavity and Throat	Ø Open 3 Percutaneous 4 Percutaneous Endoscopic 7 Via Natural or Artificial Opening 8 Via Natural or Artificial Opening Endoscopic X External	Z No Device	Z No Qualifier
P Gastrointestinal Tract Q Respiratory Tract R Genitourinary Tract	Ø Open 3 Percutaneous 4 Percutaneous Endoscopic 7 Via Natural or Artificial Opening 8 Via Natural or Artificial Opening Endoscopic	Z No Device	Z No Qualifier

Non-OR   ØW3P8ZZ
                                                ♂   ØW3M[Ø,3,4]ZZ
                                                ♀   ØW3N[Ø,3,4]ZZ

Ø Medical and Surgical
W Anatomical Regions, General
4 Creation   Definition: Putting in or on biological or synthetic material to form a new body part that to the extent possible replicates the anatomic structure or function of an absent body part
               Explanation: Used for gender reassignment surgery and corrective procedures in individuals with congenital anomalies

Body Part Character 4	Approach Character 5	Device Character 6	Qualifier Character 7
M Perineum, Male ♂	Ø Open	7 Autologous Tissue Substitute J Synthetic Substitute K Nonautologous Tissue Substitute	Ø Vagina
N Perineum, Female ♀	Ø Open	7 Autologous Tissue Substitute J Synthetic Substitute K Nonautologous Tissue Substitute	1 Penis

♂   ØW4MØ[7,J,K]Ø
♀   ØW4NØ[7,J,K]1

Ø Medical and Surgical
W Anatomical Regions, General
8 Division   Definition: Cutting into a body part, without draining fluids and/or gases from the body part, in order to separate or transect a body part
               Explanation: All or a portion of the body part is separated into two or more portions

Body Part Character 4	Approach Character 5	Device Character 6	Qualifier Character 7
N Perineum, Female ♀	X External	Z No Device	Z No Qualifier

Non-OR   ØW8NXZZ
                                                ♀   ØW8NXZZ

Ø   Medical and Surgical
W   Anatomical Regions, General
9   Drainage   Definition: Taking or letting out fluids and/or gases from a body part
                 Explanation: The qualifier DIAGNOSTIC is used to identify drainage procedures that are biopsies

Body Part Character 4	Approach Character 5	Device Character 6	Qualifier Character 7

Ø   Head
1   Cranial Cavity
2   Face
3   Oral Cavity and Throat
4   Upper Jaw
5   Lower Jaw
8   Chest Wall
9   Pleural Cavity, Right
B   Pleural Cavity, Left
C   Mediastinum
     Mediastinal cavity
     Mediastinal space
D   Pericardial Cavity
F   Abdominal Wall
G   Peritoneal Cavity
     Abdominal cavity
H   Retroperitoneum
     Retroperitoneal cavity
     Retroperitoneal space
K   Upper Back
L   Lower Back
M   Perineum, Male   ♂
N   Perineum, Female   ♀
	Ø Open
	3 Percutaneous
	4 Percutaneous Endoscopic
		Ø Drainage Device	Z No Qualifier

Ø   Head
1   Cranial Cavity
2   Face
3   Oral Cavity and Throat
4   Upper Jaw
5   Lower Jaw
8   Chest Wall
9   Pleural Cavity, Right
B   Pleural Cavity, Left
C   Mediastinum
     Mediastinal cavity
     Mediastinal space
D   Pericardial Cavity
F   Abdominal Wall
G   Peritoneal Cavity
     Abdominal cavity
H   Retroperitoneum
     Retroperitoneal cavity
     Retroperitoneal space
K   Upper Back
L   Lower Back
M   Perineum, Male   ♂
N   Perineum, Female   ♀
	Ø Open
	3 Percutaneous
	4 Percutaneous Endoscopic
		Z No Device	X Diagnostic
			Z No Qualifier

6   Neck
     Parapharyngeal space
     Retropharyngeal space
J   Pelvic Cavity
     Retropubic space
	Ø Open
	3 Percutaneous
	4 Percutaneous Endoscopic
	7 Via Natural or Artificial Opening
	8 Via Natural or Artificial Opening
	     Endoscopic
		Ø Drainage Device	Z No Qualifier

6   Neck
     Parapharyngeal space
     Retropharyngeal space
J   Pelvic Cavity
     Retropubic space
	Ø Open
	3 Percutaneous
	4 Percutaneous Endoscopic
	7 Via Natural or Artificial Opening
	8 Via Natural or Artificial Opening
	     Endoscopic
		Z No Device	X Diagnostic
			Z No Qualifier

Non-OR ØW9[Ø,8,9,B,K,L,M]ØØZ	**Non-OR** ØW9J[3,7,8]ØZ	
Non-OR ØW9[Ø,1,2,3,4,5,8,9,B,C,D,F,G,H,K,L,M,N]3ØZ	**Non-OR** ØW96[Ø,3,4]ZX	
Non-OR ØW9[Ø,1,8,F,K,L,M]4ØZ	**Non-OR** ØW9J[3,7,8]Z[X,Z]	
Non-OR ØW9[Ø,2,3,4,5,8,9,B,K,L,M,N]ØZX	**Non-OR** ØW963ZZ	
Non-OR ØW9[Ø,1,2,3,4,5,8,9,B,C,D,G,K,L,M,N]3ZX	♂ ØW9M[Ø,3,4]ØZ	
Non-OR ØW9[Ø,1,2,3,4,5,8,C,K,L,M,N]4ZX	♂ ØW9M[Ø,3,4]Z[X,Z]	
Non-OR ØW9[Ø,8,9,B,K,L,M]ØZZ	♀ ØW9N[Ø,3,4]ØZ	
Non-OR ØW9[Ø,1,2,3,4,5,8,9,B,C,D,F,G,H,K,L,M,N]3ZZ	♀ ØW9N[Ø,3]Z[X,Z]	
Non-OR ØW9[Ø,1,8,F,K,L,M]4ZZ	♀ ØW9N4ZZ	
Non-OR ØW963ØZ		

NC Noncovered Procedure   **LC** Limited Coverage   **QA** Questionable OB Admit   **NT** New Tech Add-on   ⊞ Combination Member   ♂ Male   ♀ Female

ICD-10-PCS 2023   679

Ø **Medical and Surgical**
W **Anatomical Regions, General**
B **Excision**   Definition: Cutting out or off, without replacement, a portion of a body part

Explanation: The qualifier DIAGNOSTIC is used to identify excision procedures that are biopsies

Body Part Character 4	Approach Character 5	Device Character 6	Qualifier Character 7
Ø Head 2 Face 3 Oral Cavity and Throat 4 Upper Jaw 5 Lower Jaw 8 Chest Wall K Upper Back L Lower Back M Perineum, Male ♂ N Perineum, Female ♀	Ø Open 3 Percutaneous 4 Percutaneous Endoscopic X External	Z No Device	X Diagnostic Z No Qualifier

6 Neck
   Parapharyngeal space
   Retropharyngeal space
F Abdominal Wall
	Ø Open
	3 Percutaneous
	4 Percutaneous Endoscopic
		Z No Device	X Diagnostic
			Z No Qualifier

6 Neck
   Parapharyngeal space
   Retropharyngeal space
F Abdominal Wall
	X External	Z No Device	2 Stoma
			X Diagnostic
			Z No Qualifier

C Mediastinum
   Mediastinal cavity
   Mediastinal space
H Retroperitoneum
   Retroperitoneal cavity
   Retroperitoneal space
	Ø Open
	3 Percutaneous
	4 Percutaneous Endoscopic
		Z No Device	X Diagnostic
			Z No Qualifier

Non-OR	ØWB[Ø,2,4,5,8,K,L,M][Ø,3,4,X]ZX	♂	ØWBM[Ø,3,4,X]Z[X,Z]
Non-OR	ØWB6[Ø,3,4]ZX	♀	ØWBN[Ø,3,4,X]Z[X,Z]
Non-OR	ØWB6XZX		
Non-OR	ØWBH[3,4]ZX		

Ø **Medical and Surgical**
W **Anatomical Regions, General**
C **Extirpation**   Definition: Taking or cutting out solid matter from a body part

Explanation: The solid matter may be an abnormal byproduct of a biological function or a foreign body; it may be imbedded in a body part or in the lumen of a tubular body part. The solid matter may or may not have been previously broken into pieces.

Body Part Character 4	Approach Character 5	Device Character 6	Qualifier Character 7

1 Cranial Cavity
3 Oral Cavity and Throat
9 Pleural Cavity, Right
B Pleural Cavity, Left
C Mediastinum
   Mediastinal cavity
   Mediastinal space
D Pericardial Cavity
G Peritoneal Cavity
   Abdominal cavity
H Retroperitoneum
   Retroperitoneal cavity
   Retroperitoneal space
J Pelvic Cavity
   Retropubic space
	Ø Open
	3 Percutaneous
	4 Percutaneous Endoscopic
	X External
		Z No Device	Z No Qualifier

4 Upper Jaw 5 Lower Jaw	Ø Open 3 Percutaneous 4 Percutaneous Endoscopic	Z No Device	Z No Qualifier
P Gastrointestinal Tract Q Respiratory Tract R Genitourinary Tract	Ø Open 3 Percutaneous 4 Percutaneous Endoscopic 7 Via Natural or Artificial Opening 8 Via Natural or Artificial Opening Endoscopic X External	Z No Device	Z No Qualifier

Non-OR	ØWC[1,3]XZZ
Non-OR	ØWC[9,B][Ø,3,4,X]ZZ
Non-OR	ØWC[C,D,G,H,J]XZZ
Non-OR	ØWC[4,5]3ZZ
Non-OR	ØWC[P,R][7,8,X]ZZ
Non-OR	ØWCQ[Ø,3,4,X]ZZ

Ø   **Medical and Surgical**
W   **Anatomical Regions, General**
F   **Fragmentation**   Definition: Breaking solid matter in a body part into pieces

Explanation: Physical force (e.g., manual, ultrasonic) applied directly or indirectly is used to break the solid matter into pieces. The solid matter may be an abnormal byproduct of a biological function or a foreign body. The pieces of solid matter are not taken out.

Body Part Character 4	Approach Character 5	Device Character 6	Qualifier Character 7

1 Cranial Cavity NC
3 Oral Cavity and Throat NC
9 Pleural Cavity, Right NC
B Pleural Cavity, Left NC
C Mediastinum NC
   Mediastinal cavity
   Mediastinal space
D Pericardial Cavity
G Peritoneal Cavity NC
   Abdominal cavity
J Pelvic Cavity NC
   Retropubic space
	Ø Open
	3 Percutaneous
	4 Percutaneous Endoscopic
	X External
		Z No Device	Z No Qualifier

P Gastrointestinal Tract NC Q Respiratory Tract NC R Genitourinary Tract	Ø Open 3 Percutaneous 4 Percutaneous Endoscopic 7 Via Natural or Artificial Opening 8 Via Natural or Artificial Opening Endoscopic X External	Z No Device	Z No Qualifier

Non-OR	ØWF[1,3,9,B,C,G]XZZ	NC	ØWF[1,3,9,B,C,G,J]XZZ
Non-OR	ØWFJ[Ø,3,4,X]ZZ	NC	ØWF[P,Q]XZZ
Non-OR	ØWFP[Ø,3,4,7,8,X]ZZ		
Non-OR	ØWFQXZZ		
Non-OR	ØWFR[Ø,3,4,7,8,X]ZZ		

Ø   **Medical and Surgical**
W   **Anatomical Regions, General**
H   **Insertion**   Definition: Putting in a nonbiological appliance that monitors, assists, performs, or prevents a physiological function but does not physically take the place of a body part

Explanation: None

Body Part Character 4	Approach Character 5	Device Character 6	Qualifier Character 7

Ø Head
1 Cranial Cavity
2 Face
3 Oral Cavity and Throat
4 Upper Jaw
5 Lower Jaw
6 Neck
   Parapharyngeal space
   Retropharyngeal space
8 Chest Wall
9 Pleural Cavity, Right
B Pleural Cavity, Left
C Mediastinum
   Mediastinal cavity
   Mediastinal space
D Pericardial Cavity
F Abdominal Wall
G Peritoneal Cavity
   Abdominal cavity
H Retroperitoneum
   Retroperitoneal cavity
   Retroperitoneal space
J Pelvic Cavity
   Retropubic space
K Upper Back
L Lower Back
M Perineum, Male
N Perineum, Female ♀
	Ø Open
	3 Percutaneous
	4 Percutaneous Endoscopic
		1 Radioactive Element
		3 Infusion Device
		Y Other Device
			Z No Qualifier

P Gastrointestinal Tract Q Respiratory Tract R Genitourinary Tract	Ø Open 3 Percutaneous 4 Percutaneous Endoscopic 7 Via Natural or Artificial Opening 8 Via Natural or Artificial Opening Endoscopic	1 Radioactive Element 3 Infusion Device Y Other Device	Z No Qualifier

DRG Non-OR	ØWH[Ø,2,4,5,6,K,L,M][Ø,3,4][3,Y]Z	Non-OR	ØWHP[3,4,7,8][3,Y]Z	
Non-OR	ØWH1[Ø,3,4]3Z	Non-OR	ØWHQ[Ø,7,8][3,Y]Z	
Non-OR	ØWH[8,9,B][Ø,3,4][3,Y]Z	Non-OR	ØWHR[Ø,3,4,7,8][3,Y]Z	
Non-OR	ØWHPØYZ	♀	ØWHN[Ø,3,4][3,Y]Z	

NC Noncovered Procedure   LC Limited Coverage   QA Questionable OB Admit   NT New Tech Add-on   ⊞ Combination Member   ♂ Male   ♀ Female

ICD-10-PCS 2023   681

Anatomical Regions, General

Ø   **Medical and Surgical**
W   **Anatomical Regions, General**
J   **Inspection**   Definition: Visually and/or manually exploring a body part

Explanation: Visual exploration may be performed with or without optical instrumentation. Manual exploration may be performed directly or through intervening body layers.

Body Part Character 4	Approach Character 5	Device Character 6	Qualifier Character 7

Ø Head
 2 Face
 3 Oral Cavity and Throat
 4 Upper Jaw
 5 Lower Jaw
 6 Neck
     Parapharyngeal space
     Retropharyngeal space
 8 Chest Wall
 F Abdominal Wall
 K Upper Back
 L Lower Back
 M Perineum, Male ♂
 N Perineum, Female ♀
	Ø Open
	 3 Percutaneous
	 4 Percutaneous Endoscopic
	 X External
		Z No Device	**Z** No Qualifier

1 Cranial Cavity
 9 Pleural Cavity, Right
 B Pleural Cavity, Left
 C Mediastinum
     Mediastinal cavity
     Mediastinal space
 D Pericardial Cavity
 G Peritoneal Cavity
     Abdominal cavity
 H Retroperitoneum
     Retroperitoneal cavity
     Retroperitoneal space
 J Pelvic Cavity
     Retropubic space
	Ø Open
	 3 Percutaneous
	 4 Percutaneous Endoscopic
		Z No Device	**Z** No Qualifier

P Gastrointestinal Tract **Q** Respiratory Tract **R** Genitourinary Tract	**Ø** Open **3** Percutaneous **4** Percutaneous Endoscopic **7** Via Natural or Artificial Opening **8** Via Natural or Artificial Opening Endoscopic	**Z** No Device	**Z** No Qualifier

DRG Non-OR	ØWJ[Ø,2,4,5,K,L]ØZZ	♂	ØWJM[Ø,3,4,X]ZZ
DRG Non-OR	ØWJM[Ø,4]ZZ	♀	ØWJN[Ø,3,4,X]ZZ
Non-OR	ØWJ3ØZZ		
Non-OR	ØWJ[Ø,2,3,4,5,6,8,F,K,L,M,N][3,X]ZZ		
Non-OR	ØWJ[Ø,2,3,4,5,K,L]4ZZ		
Non-OR	ØWJDØZZ		
Non-OR	ØWJ[1,9,B,C,D,G,H,J]3ZZ		
Non-OR	ØWJ[P,Q,R][3,7,8]ZZ		

Ø   **Medical and Surgical**
W   **Anatomical Regions, General**
M   **Reattachment**   Definition: Putting back in or on all or a portion of a separated body part to its normal location or other suitable location

Explanation: Vascular circulation and nervous pathways may or may not be reestablished

Body Part Character 4	Approach Character 5	Device Character 6	Qualifier Character 7

2 Face
 4 Upper Jaw
 5 Lower Jaw
 6 Neck
     Parapharyngeal space
     Retropharyngeal space
 8 Chest Wall
 F Abdominal Wall
 K Upper Back
 L Lower Back
 M Perineum, Male ♂
 N Perineum, Female ♀
	Ø Open	**Z** No Device	**Z** No Qualifier

♂	ØWMMØZZ
♀	ØWMNØZZ

Non-OR Procedure   DRG Non-OR Procedure   Valid OR Procedure   HAC Associated Procedure   Combination Only   New/Revised April   New/Revised October

Ø   **Medical and Surgical**
W   **Anatomical Regions, General**
P   **Removal**   Definition: Taking out or off a device from a body part

                Explanation: If a device is taken out and a similar device put in without cutting or puncturing the skin or mucous membrane, the procedure is coded to the root operation CHANGE. Otherwise, the procedure for taking out the device is coded to the root operation REMOVAL.

Body Part Character 4	Approach Character 5	Device Character 6	Qualifier Character 7

Ø   Head
2   Face
4   Upper Jaw
5   Lower Jaw
6   Neck
     Parapharyngeal space
     Retropharyngeal space
8   Chest Wall
C   Mediastinum
     Mediastinal cavity
     Mediastinal space
F   Abdominal Wall
K   Upper Back
L   Lower Back
M   Perineum, Male   ♂
N   Perineum, Female   ♀
	Ø Open
	3 Percutaneous
	4 Percutaneous Endoscopic
	X External
		Ø Drainage Device
		1 Radioactive Element
		3 Infusion Device
		7 Autologous Tissue Substitute
		J Synthetic Substitute
		K Nonautologous Tissue Substitute
		Y Other Device
			Z No Qualifier

1   Cranial Cavity
9   Pleural Cavity, Right
B   Pleural Cavity, Left
G   Peritoneal Cavity
     Abdominal cavity
J   Pelvic Cavity
     Retropubic space
	Ø Open
	3 Percutaneous
	4 Percutaneous Endoscopic
		Ø Drainage Device
		1 Radioactive Element
		3 Infusion Device
		J Synthetic Substitute
		Y Other Device
			Z No Qualifier

1   Cranial Cavity
9   Pleural Cavity, Right
B   Pleural Cavity, Left
G   Peritoneal Cavity
     Abdominal cavity
J   Pelvic Cavity
     Retropubic space
	X External	**Ø** Drainage Device
		1 Radioactive Element
		3 Infusion Device
			Z No Qualifier

D   Pericardial Cavity
H   Retroperitoneum
     Retroperitoneal cavity
     Retroperitoneal space
	Ø Open
	3 Percutaneous
	4 Percutaneous Endoscopic
		Ø Drainage Device
		1 Radioactive Element
		3 Infusion Device
		Y Other Device
			Z No Qualifier

D   Pericardial Cavity
H   Retroperitoneum
     Retroperitoneal cavity
     Retroperitoneal space
	X External	**Ø** Drainage Device
		1 Radioactive Element
		3 Infusion Device
			Z No Qualifier

P Gastrointestinal Tract **Q** Respiratory Tract **R** Genitourinary Tract	**Ø** Open **3** Percutaneous **4** Percutaneous Endoscopic **7** Via Natural or Artificial Opening **8** Via Natural or Artificial Opening Endoscopic **X** External	**1** Radioactive Element **3** Infusion Device **Y** Other Device	**Z** No Qualifier

Non-OR	ØWP[Ø,2,4,5,6,8][Ø,3,4,X][Ø,1,3,7,J,K,Y]Z	♂	ØWPM[Ø,3,4,X][Ø,1,3,7,J,K,Y]Z
Non-OR	ØWP[C,F]X[Ø,1,3,7,J,K,Y]Z	♀	ØWPN[Ø,3,4,X][Ø,1,3,7,J,K,Y]Z
Non-OR	ØWP[K,L][Ø,3,4,X][Ø,1,3,7,J,K,Y]Z		
Non-OR	ØWPM[Ø,3,4][Ø,1,3,J,Y]Z		
Non-OR	ØWPMX[Ø,1,3,Y]Z		
Non-OR	ØWPNX[Ø,1,3,7,J,K,Y]Z		
Non-OR	ØWP1[Ø,3,4]3Z		
Non-OR	ØWP[9,B,J][Ø,3,4][Ø,1,3,J,Y]Z		
Non-OR	ØWP[1,9,B,G,J]X[Ø,1,3]Z		
Non-OR	ØWP[D,H]X[Ø,1,3]Z		
Non-OR	ØWPP[3,4,7,8,X][1,3,Y]Z		
Non-OR	ØWPQ73Z		
Non-OR	ØWPQ8[3,Y]Z		
Non-OR	ØWPQ[Ø,X][1,3,Y]Z		
Non-OR	ØWPR[Ø,3,4,7,8,X][1,3,Y]Z		

NC Noncovered Procedure   **LC** Limited Coverage   **QA** Questionable OB Admit   **NT** New Tech Add-on   ⊞ Combination Member   ♂ Male   ♀ Female

ICD-10-PCS 2023   **683**

Ø   Medical and Surgical
W   Anatomical Regions, General
Q   Repair   Definition: Restoring, to the extent possible, a body part to its normal anatomic structure and function
                        Explanation: Used only when the method to accomplish the repair is not one of the other root operations

Body Part Character 4	Approach Character 5	Device Character 6	Qualifier Character 7
Ø Head 2 Face 3 Oral Cavity and Throat 4 Upper Jaw 5 Lower Jaw 8 Chest Wall K Upper Back L Lower Back M Perineum, Male ♂ N Perineum, Female ♀	Ø Open 3 Percutaneous 4 Percutaneous Endoscopic X External	Z No Device	Z No Qualifier

6 Neck
   Parapharyngeal space
   Retropharyngeal space
F Abdominal Wall
	Ø Open
	3 Percutaneous
	4 Percutaneous Endoscopic
		Z No Device	Z No Qualifier

6 Neck
   Parapharyngeal space
   Retropharyngeal space
F Abdominal Wall   ✚
	X External	Z No Device	2 Stoma
			Z No Qualifier

C Mediastinum
   Mediastinal cavity
   Mediastinal space
	Ø Open
	3 Percutaneous
	4 Percutaneous Endoscopic
		Z No Device	Z No Qualifier

Non-OR	ØWQNXZZ
♂	ØWQM[Ø,3,4,X]ZZ
♀	ØWQN[Ø,3,4,X]ZZ

See Appendix L for Procedure Combinations
✚   ØWQFXZ[2,Z]

Ø   Medical and Surgical
W   Anatomical Regions, General
U   Supplement   Definition: Putting in or on biological or synthetic material that physically reinforces and/or augments the function of a portion of a body part
                        Explanation: The biological material is non-living, or is living and from the same individual. The body part may have been previously replaced, and the SUPPLEMENT procedure is performed to physically reinforce and/or augment the function of the replaced body part.

Body Part Character 4	Approach Character 5	Device Character 6	Qualifier Character 7

Ø Head
2 Face
4 Upper Jaw
5 Lower Jaw
6 Neck
   Parapharyngeal space
   Retropharyngeal space
8 Chest Wall
C Mediastinum
   Mediastinal cavity
   Mediastinal space
F Abdominal Wall
K Upper Back
L Lower Back
M Perineum, Male   ♂
N Perineum, Female   ♀
	Ø Open
	4 Percutaneous Endoscopic
		7 Autologous Tissue Substitute
		J Synthetic Substitute
		K Nonautologous Tissue Substitute
			Z No Qualifier

♂	ØWUM[Ø,4][7,J,K]Z
♀	ØWUN[Ø,4][7,J,K]Z

Ø **Medical and Surgical**
W **Anatomical Regions, General**
W **Revision**   Definition: Correcting, to the extent possible, a portion of a malfunctioning device or the position of a displaced device

                Explanation: Revision can include correcting a malfunctioning or displaced device by taking out or putting in components of the device such as a screw or pin

Body Part Character 4	Approach Character 5	Device Character 6	Qualifier Character 7

Ø Head
2 Face
4 Upper Jaw
5 Lower Jaw
6 Neck
   Parapharyngeal space
   Retropharyngeal space
8 Chest Wall
C Mediastinum
   Mediastinal cavity
   Mediastinal space
F Abdominal Wall
K Upper Back
L Lower Back
M Perineum, Male   ♂
N Perineum, Female   ♀
	Ø Open
	3 Percutaneous
	4 Percutaneous Endoscopic
	X External
		Ø Drainage Device
		1 Radioactive Element
		3 Infusion Device
		7 Autologous Tissue Substitute
		J Synthetic Substitute
		K Nonautologous Tissue Substitute
		Y Other Device
			Z No Qualifier

1 Cranial Cavity
9 Pleural Cavity, Right
B Pleural Cavity, Left
G Peritoneal Cavity
   Abdominal cavity
J Pelvic Cavity
   Retropubic space
	Ø Open
	3 Percutaneous
	4 Percutaneous Endoscopic
	X External
		Ø Drainage Device
		1 Radioactive Element
		3 Infusion Device
		J Synthetic Substitute
		Y Other Device
			Z No Qualifier

D Pericardial Cavity
H Retroperitoneum
   Retroperitoneal cavity
   Retroperitoneal space
	Ø Open
	3 Percutaneous
	4 Percutaneous Endoscopic
	X External
		Ø Drainage Device
		1 Radioactive Element
		3 Infusion Device
		Y Other Device
			Z No Qualifier

P Gastrointestinal Tract Q Respiratory Tract R Genitourinary Tract	Ø Open 3 Percutaneous 4 Percutaneous Endoscopic 7 Via Natural or Artificial Opening 8 Via Natural or Artificial Opening Endoscopic X External	1 Radioactive Element 3 Infusion Device Y Other Device	Z No Qualifier

DRG Non-OR	ØWW[Ø,2,4,5,6,K,L][Ø,3,4][Ø,1,3,7,J,K,Y]Z	♂	ØWWM[Ø,3,4,X][Ø,1,3,7,K,Y]Z
DRG Non-OR	ØWWM[Ø,3,4][Ø,1,3,J,Y]Z	♀	ØWWN[Ø,3,4,X][Ø,1,3,7,K,Y]Z
Non-OR	ØWW[Ø,2,4,5,6,C,F,K,L,M,N]X[Ø,1,3,7,J,K,Y]Z		
Non-OR	ØWW8[Ø,3,4,X][Ø,1,3,7,J,K,Y]Z		
Non-OR	ØWW[1,G,J]X[Ø,1,3,J,Y]Z		
Non-OR	ØWW[9,B][Ø,3,4,X][Ø,1,3,J,Y]Z		
Non-OR	ØWW[D,H]X[Ø,1,3,Y]Z		
Non-OR	ØWWP[3,4,7,8,X][1,3,Y]Z		
Non-OR	ØWWQ[Ø,X][1,3,Y]Z		
Non-OR	ØWWR[Ø,3,4,7,8,X][1,3,Y]Z		

Ø **Medical and Surgical**
W **Anatomical Regions, General**
Y **Transplantation**   Definition: Putting in or on all or a portion of a living body part taken from another individual or animal to physically take the place and/or function of all or a portion of a similar body part

                Explanation: The native body part may or may not be taken out, and the transplanted body part may take over all or a portion of its function

Body Part Character 4	Approach Character 5	Device Character 6	Qualifier Character 7
2 Face	Ø Open	Z No Device	Ø Allogeneic 1 Syngeneic

NC Noncovered Procedure   **LC** Limited Coverage   **QA** Questionable OB Admit   **NT** New Tech Add-on   ⊞ Combination Member   ♂ Male   ♀ Female

ICD-10-PCS 2023   **685**

Anatomical Regions, Upper Extremities 0X0–0XY

Character Meanings

This Character Meaning table is provided as a guide to assist the user in the identification of character members that may be found in this section of code tables. It **SHOULD NOT** be used to build a PCS code.

Operation–Character 3		Body Part–Character 4		Approach–Character 5		Device–Character 6		Qualifier–Character 7	
0	Alteration	0	Forequarter, Right	0	Open	0	Drainage Device	0	Allogeneic OR Complete
2	Change	1	Forequarter, Left	3	Percutaneous	1	Radioactive Element	1	High OR Syngeneic
3	Control	2	Shoulder Region, Right	4	Percutaneous Endoscopic	3	Infusion Device	2	Mid
6	Detachment	3	Shoulder Region, Left	X	External	7	Autologous Tissue Substitute	3	Low
9	Drainage	4	Axilla, Right			J	Synthetic Substitute	4	Complete 1st Ray
B	Excision	5	Axilla, Left			K	Nonautologous Tissue Substitute	5	Complete 2nd Ray
H	Insertion	6	Upper Extremity, Right			Y	Other Device	6	Complete 3rd Ray
J	Inspection	7	Upper Extremity, Left			Z	No Device	7	Complete 4th Ray
M	Reattachment	8	Upper Arm, Right					8	Complete 5th Ray
P	Removal	9	Upper Arm, Left					9	Partial 1st Ray
Q	Repair	B	Elbow Region, Right					B	Partial 2nd Ray
R	Replacement	C	Elbow Region, Left					C	Partial 3rd Ray
U	Supplement	D	Lower Arm, Right					D	Partial 4th Ray
W	Revision	F	Lower Arm, Left					F	Partial 5th Ray
X	Transfer	G	Wrist Region, Right					L	Thumb, Right
Y	Transplantation	H	Wrist Region, Left					M	Thumb, Left
		J	Hand, Right					N	Toe, Right
		K	Hand, Left					P	Toe, Left
		L	Thumb, Right					X	Diagnostic
		M	Thumb, Left					Z	No Qualifier
		N	Index Finger, Right						
		P	Index Finger, Left						
		Q	Middle Finger, Right						
		R	Middle Finger, Left						
		S	Ring Finger, Right						
		T	Ring Finger, Left						
		V	Little Finger, Right						
		W	Little Finger, Left						

AHA Coding Clinic for table 0X3

2016, 4Q, 99	Root operation Control
2015, 1Q, 35	Evacuation of hematoma for control of postprocedural bleeding
2013, 3Q, 23	Control of intraoperative bleeding

AHA Coding Clinic for table 0X6

2017, 2Q, 3-4	Qualifiers for the root operation detachment
2017, 2Q, 18	Removal of polydactyl digits
2017, 1Q, 52	Further distal phalangeal amputation
2016, 3Q, 33	Traumatic amputation of fingers with further revision amputation

AHA Coding Clinic for table 0XH

2017, 2Q, 20	Exchange of intramedullary antibiotic impregnated spacer

AHA Coding Clinic for table 0XP

2017, 2Q, 20	Exchange of intramedullary antibiotic impregnated spacer

AHA Coding Clinic for table 0XY

2016, 4Q, 112-113	Transplantation

Detachment Qualifier Descriptions

Qualifier Definition	Upper Arm	Lower Arm
1 **High:** Amputation at the proximal portion of the shaft of the:	Humerus	Radius/Ulna
2 **Mid:** Amputation at the middle portion of the shaft of the:	Humerus	Radius/Ulna
3 **Low:** Amputation at the distal portion of the shaft of the:	Humerus	Radius/Ulna

Qualifier Definition	Hand
Ø Complete 1st through 5th Rays Ray: digit of hand or foot with corresponding metacarpus or metatarsus	Through carpo-metacarpal joint, **Wrist**
4 Complete 1st Ray	Through carpo-metacarpal joint, **Thumb**
5 Complete 2nd Ray	Through carpo-metacarpal joint, **Index Finger**
6 Complete 3rd Ray	Through carpo-metacarpal joint, **Middle Finger**
7 Complete 4th Ray	Through carpo-metacarpal joint, **Ring Finger**
8 Complete 5th Ray	Through carpo-metacarpal joint, **Little Finger**
9 Partial 1st Ray	Anywhere along shaft or head of metacarpal bone, **Thumb**
B Partial 2nd Ray	Anywhere along shaft or head of metacarpal bone, **Index Finger**
C Partial 3rd Ray	Anywhere along shaft or head of metacarpal bone, **Middle Finger**
D Partial 4th Ray	Anywhere along shaft or head of metacarpal bone, **Ring Finger**
F Partial 5th Ray	Anywhere along shaft or head of metacarpal bone, **Little Finger**

Qualifier Definition	Thumb/Finger
Ø Complete	At the metacarpophalangeal joint
1 High	Anywhere along the proximal phalanx
2 Mid	Through the proximal interphalangeal joint or anywhere along the middle phalanx
3 Low	Through the distal interphalangeal joint or anywhere along the distal phalanx

Ø   **Medical and Surgical**
X   **Anatomical Regions, Upper Extremities**
Ø   **Alteration**   Definition: Modifying the anatomic structure of a body part without affecting the function of the body part
                     Explanation: Principal purpose is to improve appearance

Body Part Character 4	Approach Character 5	Device Character 6	Qualifier Character 7
2 Shoulder Region, Right	Ø Open	7 Autologous Tissue Substitute	Z No Qualifier
3 Shoulder Region, Left	3 Percutaneous	J Synthetic Substitute	
4 Axilla, Right	4 Percutaneous Endoscopic	K Nonautologous Tissue Substitute	
5 Axilla, Left		Z No Device	
6 Upper Extremity, Right			
7 Upper Extremity, Left			
8 Upper Arm, Right			
9 Upper Arm, Left			
B Elbow Region, Right			
C Elbow Region, Left			
D Lower Arm, Right			
F Lower Arm, Left			
G Wrist Region, Right			
H Wrist Region, Left			

Ø   **Medical and Surgical**
X   **Anatomical Regions, Upper Extremities**
2   **Change**   Definition: Taking out or off a device from a body part and putting back an identical or similar device in or on the same body part without cutting or puncturing the skin or a mucous membrane
                     Explanation: All CHANGE procedures are coded using the approach EXTERNAL

Body Part Character 4	Approach Character 5	Device Character 6	Qualifier Character 7
6 Upper Extremity, Right	X External	Ø Drainage Device	Z No Qualifier
7 Upper Extremity, Left		Y Other Device	

Non-OR   All body part, approach, device, and qualifier values

Ø   **Medical and Surgical**
X   **Anatomical Regions, Upper Extremities**
3   **Control**   Definition: Stopping, or attempting to stop, postprocedural or other acute bleeding
                     Explanation: None

Body Part Character 4	Approach Character 5	Device Character 6	Qualifier Character 7
2 Shoulder Region, Right	Ø Open	Z No Device	Z No Qualifier
3 Shoulder Region, Left	3 Percutaneous		
4 Axilla, Right	4 Percutaneous Endoscopic		
5 Axilla, Left			
6 Upper Extremity, Right			
7 Upper Extremity, Left			
8 Upper Arm, Right			
9 Upper Arm, Left			
B Elbow Region, Right			
C Elbow Region, Left			
D Lower Arm, Right			
F Lower Arm, Left			
G Wrist Region, Right			
H Wrist Region, Left			
J Hand, Right			
K Hand, Left			

Ø   Medical and Surgical
X   Anatomical Regions, Upper Extremities
6   Detachment   Definition: Cutting off all or a portion of the upper or lower extremities

                     Explanation: The body part value is the site of the detachment, with a qualifier if applicable to further specify the level where the extremity was detached

Body Part Character 4	Approach Character 5	Device Character 6	Qualifier Character 7
Ø Forequarter, Right 1 Forequarter, Left 2 Shoulder Region, Right 3 Shoulder Region, Left B Elbow Region, Right C Elbow Region, Left	Ø Open	Z No Device	Z No Qualifier
8 Upper Arm, Right 9 Upper Arm, Left D Lower Arm, Right F Lower Arm, Left	Ø Open	Z No Device	1 High 2 Mid 3 Low
J Hand, Right K Hand, Left	Ø Open	Z No Device	Ø Complete 4 Complete 1st Ray 5 Complete 2nd Ray 6 Complete 3rd Ray 7 Complete 4th Ray 8 Complete 5th Ray 9 Partial 1st Ray B Partial 2nd Ray C Partial 3rd Ray D Partial 4th Ray F Partial 5th Ray
L Thumb, Right M Thumb, Left N Index Finger, Right P Index Finger, Left Q Middle Finger, Right R Middle Finger, Left S Ring Finger, Right T Ring Finger, Left V Little Finger, Right W Little Finger, Left	Ø Open	Z No Device	Ø Complete 1 High 2 Mid 3 Low

Ø   **Medical and Surgical**
X   **Anatomical Regions, Upper Extremities**
9   **Drainage**   Definition: Taking or letting out fluids and/or gases from a body part
                            Explanation: The qualifier DIAGNOSTIC is used to identify drainage procedures that are biopsies

Body Part Character 4	Approach Character 5	Device Character 6	Qualifier Character 7
2 Shoulder Region, Right **3** Shoulder Region, Left **4** Axilla, Right **5** Axilla, Left **6** Upper Extremity, Right **7** Upper Extremity, Left **8** Upper Arm, Right **9** Upper Arm, Left **B** Elbow Region, Right **C** Elbow Region, Left **D** Lower Arm, Right **F** Lower Arm, Left **G** Wrist Region, Right **H** Wrist Region, Left **J** Hand, Right **K** Hand, Left	**Ø** Open **3** Percutaneous **4** Percutaneous Endoscopic	**Ø** Drainage Device	**Z** No Qualifier
2 Shoulder Region, Right **3** Shoulder Region, Left **4** Axilla, Right **5** Axilla, Left **6** Upper Extremity, Right **7** Upper Extremity, Left **8** Upper Arm, Right **9** Upper Arm, Left **B** Elbow Region, Right **C** Elbow Region, Left **D** Lower Arm, Right **F** Lower Arm, Left **G** Wrist Region, Right **H** Wrist Region, Left **J** Hand, Right **K** Hand, Left	**Ø** Open **3** Percutaneous **4** Percutaneous Endoscopic	**Z** No Device	**X** Diagnostic **Z** No Qualifier

Non-OR   All body part, approach, device, and qualifier values

Ø   **Medical and Surgical**
X   **Anatomical Regions, Upper Extremities**
B   **Excision**   Definition: Cutting out or off, without replacement, a portion of a body part
                            Explanation: The qualifier DIAGNOSTIC is used to identify excision procedures that are biopsies

Body Part Character 4	Approach Character 5	Device Character 6	Qualifier Character 7
2 Shoulder Region, Right **3** Shoulder Region, Left **4** Axilla, Right **5** Axilla, Left **6** Upper Extremity, Right **7** Upper Extremity, Left **8** Upper Arm, Right **9** Upper Arm, Left **B** Elbow Region, Right **C** Elbow Region, Left **D** Lower Arm, Right **F** Lower Arm, Left **G** Wrist Region, Right **H** Wrist Region, Left **J** Hand, Right **K** Hand, Left	**Ø** Open **3** Percutaneous **4** Percutaneous Endoscopic	**Z** No Device	**X** Diagnostic **Z** No Qualifier

Non-OR   ØXB[2,3,4,5,6,7,8,9,B,C,D,F,G,H,J,K][Ø,3,4]ZX

NC Noncovered Procedure   **LC** Limited Coverage   **QA** Questionable OB Admit   **COM** New Tech Add-on   ⊞ Combination Member   ♂ Male   ♀ Female

ICD-10-PCS 2023   **691**

Ø   Medical and Surgical
X   Anatomical Regions, Upper Extremities
H   Insertion   Definition: Putting in a nonbiological appliance that monitors, assists, performs, or prevents a physiological function but does not physically take the place of a body part

                        Explanation: None

Body Part Character 4	Approach Character 5	Device Character 6	Qualifier Character 7
2 Shoulder Region, Right 3 Shoulder Region, Left 4 Axilla, Right 5 Axilla, Left 6 Upper Extremity, Right 7 Upper Extremity, Left 8 Upper Arm, Right 9 Upper Arm, Left B Elbow Region, Right C Elbow Region, Left D Lower Arm, Right F Lower Arm, Left G Wrist Region, Right H Wrist Region, Left J Hand, Right K Hand, Left	Ø Open 3 Percutaneous 4 Percutaneous Endoscopic	1 Radioactive Element 3 Infusion Device Y Other Device	Z No Qualifier

DRG Non-OR	ØXH[2,3,4,5,6,7,8,9,B,C,D,F,G,H,J,K][Ø,3,4][3,Y]Z

Ø   Medical and Surgical
X   Anatomical Regions, Upper Extremities
J   Inspection   Definition: Visually and/or manually exploring a body part

                        Explanation: Visual exploration may be performed with or without optical instrumentation. Manual exploration may be performed directly or through intervening body layers.

Body Part Character 4	Approach Character 5	Device Character 6	Qualifier Character 7
2 Shoulder Region, Right 3 Shoulder Region, Left 4 Axilla, Right 5 Axilla, Left 6 Upper Extremity, Right 7 Upper Extremity, Left 8 Upper Arm, Right 9 Upper Arm, Left B Elbow Region, Right C Elbow Region, Left D Lower Arm, Right F Lower Arm, Left G Wrist Region, Right H Wrist Region, Left J Hand, Right K Hand, Left	Ø Open 3 Percutaneous 4 Percutaneous Endoscopic X External	Z No Device	Z No Qualifier

DRG Non-OR	ØXJ[2,3,4,5,6,7,8,9,B,C,D,F,G,H,J,K]ØZZ
Non-OR	ØXJ[2,3,4,5,6,7,8,9,B,C,D,F,G,H][3,4,X]ZZ
Non-OR	ØXJ[J,K][3,X]ZZ

Ø　Medical and Surgical
X　Anatomical Regions, Upper Extremities
M　Reattachment　Definition: Putting back in or on all or a portion of a separated body part to its normal location or other suitable location
　　　　　　　　　Explanation: Vascular circulation and nervous pathways may or may not be reestablished

Body Part Character 4	Approach Character 5	Device Character 6	Qualifier Character 7
Ø　Forequarter, Right	Ø　Open	Z　No Device	Z　No Qualifier
1　Forequarter, Left			
2　Shoulder Region, Right			
3　Shoulder Region, Left			
4　Axilla, Right			
5　Axilla, Left			
6　Upper Extremity, Right			
7　Upper Extremity, Left			
8　Upper Arm, Right			
9　Upper Arm, Left			
B　Elbow Region, Right			
C　Elbow Region, Left			
D　Lower Arm, Right			
F　Lower Arm, Left			
G　Wrist Region, Right			
H　Wrist Region, Left			
J　Hand, Right			
K　Hand, Left			
L　Thumb, Right			
M　Thumb, Left			
N　Index Finger, Right			
P　Index Finger, Left			
Q　Middle Finger, Right			
R　Middle Finger, Left			
S　Ring Finger, Right			
T　Ring Finger, Left			
V　Little Finger, Right			
W　Little Finger, Left			

Ø　Medical and Surgical
X　Anatomical Regions, Upper Extremities
P　Removal　Definition: Taking out or off a device from a body part
　　　　　　Explanation: If a device is taken out and a similar device put in without cutting or puncturing the skin or mucous membrane, the procedure is coded to the root operation CHANGE. Otherwise, the procedure for taking out the device is coded to the root operation REMOVAL.

Body Part Character 4	Approach Character 5	Device Character 6	Qualifier Character 7
6　Upper Extremity, Right	Ø　Open	Ø　Drainage Device	Z　No Qualifier
7　Upper Extremity, Left	3　Percutaneous	1　Radioactive Element	
	4　Percutaneous Endoscopic	3　Infusion Device	
	X　External	7　Autologous Tissue Substitute	
		J　Synthetic Substitute	
		K　Nonautologous Tissue Substitute	
		Y　Other Device	

Non-OR	All body part, approach, device, and qualifier values

NC Noncovered Procedure　　LC Limited Coverage　　QA Questionable OB Admit　　COM New Tech Add-on　　⊞ Combination Member　　♂ Male　　♀ Female

ICD-10-PCS 2023　　　693

Ø   **Medical and Surgical**
X   **Anatomical Regions, Upper Extremities**
Q   **Repair**   Definition: Restoring, to the extent possible, a body part to its normal anatomic structure and function
                    Explanation: Used only when the method to accomplish the repair is not one of the other root operations

Body Part Character 4	Approach Character 5	Device Character 6	Qualifier Character 7
2 Shoulder Region, Right **3** Shoulder Region, Left **4** Axilla, Right **5** Axilla, Left **6** Upper Extremity, Right **7** Upper Extremity, Left **8** Upper Arm, Right **9** Upper Arm, Left **B** Elbow Region, Right **C** Elbow Region, Left **D** Lower Arm, Right **F** Lower Arm, Left **G** Wrist Region, Right **H** Wrist Region, Left **J** Hand, Right **K** Hand, Left **L** Thumb, Right **M** Thumb, Left **N** Index Finger, Right **P** Index Finger, Left **Q** Middle Finger, Right **R** Middle Finger, Left **S** Ring Finger, Right **T** Ring Finger, Left **V** Little Finger, Right **W** Little Finger, Left	**Ø** Open **3** Percutaneous **4** Percutaneous Endoscopic **X** External	**Z** No Device	**Z** No Qualifier

Ø   **Medical and Surgical**
X   **Anatomical Regions, Upper Extremities**
R   **Replacement**   Definition: Putting in or on biological or synthetic material that physically takes the place and/or function of all or a portion of a body part
                    Explanation: The body part may have been taken out or replaced, or may be taken out, physically eradicated, or rendered nonfunctional during the REPLACEMENT procedure. A REMOVAL procedure is coded for taking out the device used in a previous replacement procedure.

Body Part Character 4	Approach Character 5	Device Character 6	Qualifier Character 7
L Thumb, Right **M** Thumb, Left	**Ø** Open **4** Percutaneous Endoscopic	**7** Autologous Tissue Substitute	**N** Toe, Right **P** Toe, Left

Ø   Medical and Surgical
X   Anatomical Regions, Upper Extremities
U   Supplement   Definition: Putting in or on biological or synthetic material that physically reinforces and/or augments the function of a portion of a body part
                 Explanation: The biological material is non-living, or is living and from the same individual. The body part may have been previously replaced, and the SUPPLEMENT procedure is performed to physically reinforce and/or augment the function of the replaced body part.

Body Part Character 4	Approach Character 5	Device Character 6	Qualifier Character 7
2 Shoulder Region, Right	Ø Open	7 Autologous Tissue Substitute	Z No Qualifier
3 Shoulder Region, Left	4 Percutaneous Endoscopic	J Synthetic Substitute	
4 Axilla, Right		K Nonautologous Tissue Substitute	
5 Axilla, Left			
6 Upper Extremity, Right			
7 Upper Extremity, Left			
8 Upper Arm, Right			
9 Upper Arm, Left			
B Elbow Region, Right			
C Elbow Region, Left			
D Lower Arm, Right			
F Lower Arm, Left			
G Wrist Region, Right			
H Wrist Region, Left			
J Hand, Right			
K Hand, Left			
L Thumb, Right			
M Thumb, Left			
N Index Finger, Right			
P Index Finger, Left			
Q Middle Finger, Right			
R Middle Finger, Left			
S Ring Finger, Right			
T Ring Finger, Left			
V Little Finger, Right			
W Little Finger, Left			

Ø **Medical and Surgical**
X **Anatomical Regions, Upper Extremities**
W **Revision**   Definition: Correcting, to the extent possible, a portion of a malfunctioning device or the position of a displaced device

                Explanation: Revision can include correcting a malfunctioning or displaced device by taking out or putting in components of the device such as a screw or pin

Body Part Character 4	Approach Character 5	Device Character 6	Qualifier Character 7
6 Upper Extremity, Right	Ø Open	Ø Drainage Device	Z No Qualifier
7 Upper Extremity, Left	3 Percutaneous	3 Infusion Device	
	4 Percutaneous Endoscopic	7 Autologous Tissue Substitute	
	X External	J Synthetic Substitute	
		K Nonautologous Tissue Substitute	
		Y Other Device	

DRG Non-OR	ØXW[6,7][Ø,3,4][Ø,3,7,J,K,Y]Z
Non-OR	ØXW[6,7]X[Ø,3,7,J,K,Y]Z

Ø **Medical and Surgical**
X **Anatomical Regions, Upper Extremities**
X **Transfer**   Definition: Moving, without taking out, all or a portion of a body part to another location to take over the function of all or a portion of a body part

                Explanation: The body part transferred remains connected to its vascular and nervous supply

Body Part Character 4	Approach Character 5	Device Character 6	Qualifier Character 7
N Index Finger, Right	Ø Open	Z No Device	L Thumb, Right
P Index Finger, Left	Ø Open	Z No Device	M Thumb, Left

Ø **Medical and Surgical**
X **Anatomical Regions, Upper Extremities**
Y **Transplantation**   Definition: Putting in or on all or a portion of a living body part taken from another individual or animal to physically take the place and/or function of all or a portion of a similar body part

                Explanation: The native body part may or may not be taken out, and the transplanted body part may take over all or a portion of its function

Body Part Character 4	Approach Character 5	Device Character 6	Qualifier Character 7
J Hand, Right	Ø Open	Z No Device	Ø Allogeneic
K Hand, Left			1 Syngeneic

Anatomical Regions, Lower Extremities ØYØ–ØYW

Character Meanings

This Character Meaning table is provided as a guide to assist the user in the identification of character members that may be found in this section of code tables. It **SHOULD NOT** be used to build a PCS code.

Operation–Character 3		Body Part–Character 4		Approach–Character 5		Device–Character 6		Qualifier–Character 7	
Ø	Alteration	Ø	Buttock, Right	Ø	Open	Ø	Drainage Device	Ø	Complete
2	Change	1	Buttock, Left	3	Percutaneous	1	Radioactive Element	1	High
3	Control	2	Hindquarter, Right	4	Percutaneous Endoscopic	3	Infusion Device	2	Mid
6	Detachment	3	Hindquarter, Left	X	External	7	Autologous Tissue Substitute	3	Low
9	Drainage	4	Hindquarter, Bilateral			J	Synthetic Substitute	4	Complete 1st Ray
B	Excision	5	Inguinal Region, Right			K	Nonautologous Tissue Substitute	5	Complete 2nd Ray
H	Insertion	6	Inguinal Region, Left			Y	Other Device	6	Complete 3rd Ray
J	Inspection	7	Femoral Region, Right			Z	No Device	7	Complete 4th Ray
M	Reattachment	8	Femoral Region, Left					8	Complete 5th Ray
P	Removal	9	Lower Extremity, Right					9	Partial 1st Ray
Q	Repair	A	Inguinal Region, Bilateral					B	Partial 2nd Ray
U	Supplement	B	Lower Extremity, Left					C	Partial 3rd Ray
W	Revision	C	Upper Leg, Right					D	Partial 4th Ray
		D	Upper Leg, Left					F	Partial 5th Ray
		E	Femoral Region, Bilateral					X	Diagnostic
		F	Knee Region, Right					Z	No Qualifier
		G	Knee Region, Left						
		H	Lower Leg, Right						
		J	Lower Leg, Left						
		K	Ankle Region, Right						
		L	Ankle Region, Left						
		M	Foot, Right						
		N	Foot, Left						
		P	1st Toe, Right						
		Q	1st Toe, Left						
		R	2nd Toe, Right						
		S	2nd Toe, Left						
		T	3rd Toe, Right						
		U	3rd Toe, Left						
		V	4th Toe, Right						
		W	4th Toe, Left						
		X	5th Toe, Right						
		Y	5th Toe, Left						

AHA Coding Clinic for table ØY3

2016, 4Q, 99	Root operation Control
2013, 3Q, 23	Control of intraoperative bleeding

AHA Coding Clinic for table ØY6

2019, 2Q, 17	Cryoamputation of lower leg
2017, 2Q, 3-4	Qualifiers for the root operation detachment
2017, 1Q, 22	Chopart amputation of foot
2015, 2Q, 28	Partial amputation of hallux at interphalangeal Joint
2015, 1Q, 28	Mid-foot amputation

AHA Coding Clinic for table ØY9

2015, 1Q, 22	Incision and drainage of abscess of femoropopliteal bypass site
2015, 1Q, 22	Incision and drainage of groin abscess

Detachment Qualifier Descriptions

Qualifier Definition	Upper Leg	Lower Leg
1 **High:** Amputation at the proximal portion of the shaft of the:	Femur	Tibia/Fibula
2 **Mid:** Amputation at the middle portion of the shaft of the:	Femur	Tibia/Fibula
3 **Low:** Amputation at the distal portion of the shaft of the:	Femur	Tibia/Fibula

Qualifier Definition	Foot
Ø Complete 1st through 5th Rays Ray: digit of hand or foot with corresponding metacarpus or metatarsus	Through tarso-metatarsal Joint, **Ankle**
4 Complete 1st Ray	Through tarso-metatarsal joint, **Great Toe**
5 Complete 2nd Ray	Through tarso-metatarsal joint, **2nd Toe**
6 Complete 3rd Ray	Through tarso-metatarsal joint, **3rd Toe**
7 Complete 4th Ray	Through tarso-metatarsal joint, **4th Toe**
8 Complete 5th Ray	Through tarso-metatarsal joint, **Little Toe**
9 Partial 1st Ray	Anywhere along shaft or head of metatarsal bone, **Great Toe**
B Partial 2nd Ray	Anywhere along shaft or head of metatarsal bone, **2nd Toe**
C Partial 3rd Ray	Anywhere along shaft or head of metatarsal bone, **3rd Toe**
D Partial 4th Ray	Anywhere along shaft or head of metatarsal bone, **4th Toe**
F Partial 5th Ray	Anywhere along shaft or head of metatarsal bone, **Little Toe**

Qualifier Definition	Toe
Ø Complete	At the metatarsal-phalangeal joint
1 High	Anywhere along the proximal phalanx
2 Mid	Through the proximal interphalangeal joint or anywhere along the middle phalanx
3 Low	Through the distal interphalangeal joint or anywhere along the distal phalanx

Ø   Medical and Surgical
Y   Anatomical Regions, Lower Extremities
Ø   Alteration   Definition: Modifying the anatomic structure of a body part without affecting the function of the body part
          Explanation: Principal purpose is to improve appearance

Body Part Character 4	Approach Character 5	Device Character 6	Qualifier Character 7
Ø Buttock, Right	Ø Open	7 Autologous Tissue Substitute	Z No Qualifier
1 Buttock, Left	3 Percutaneous	J Synthetic Substitute	
9 Lower Extremity, Right	4 Percutaneous Endoscopic	K Nonautologous Tissue Substitute	
B Lower Extremity, Left		Z No Device	
C Upper Leg, Right			
D Upper Leg, Left			
F Knee Region, Right			
G Knee Region, Left			
H Lower Leg, Right			
J Lower Leg, Left			
K Ankle Region, Right			
L Ankle Region, Left			

Ø   Medical and Surgical
Y   Anatomical Regions, Lower Extremities
2   Change   Definition: Taking out or off a device from a body part and putting back an identical or similar device in or on the same body part without
          cutting or puncturing the skin or a mucous membrane
          Explanation: All CHANGE procedures are coded using the approach EXTERNAL

Body Part Character 4	Approach Character 5	Device Character 6	Qualifier Character 7
9 Lower Extremity, Right	X External	Ø Drainage Device	Z No Qualifier
B Lower Extremity, Left		Y Other Device	

    Non-OR   All body part, approach, device, and qualifier values

Ø   Medical and Surgical
Y   Anatomical Regions, Lower Extremities
3   Control   Definition: Stopping, or attempting to stop, postprocedural or other acute bleeding
          Explanation: None

Body Part Character 4	Approach Character 5	Device Character 6	Qualifier Character 7
Ø Buttock, Right	Ø Open	Z No Device	Z No Qualifier
1 Buttock, Left	3 Percutaneous		

5   Inguinal Region, Right
     Inguinal canal
     Inguinal triangle
	4 Percutaneous Endoscopic		

6 Inguinal Region, Left *See 5 Inguinal Region, Right*			
7 Femoral Region, Right			
8 Femoral Region, Left			
9 Lower Extremity, Right			
B Lower Extremity, Left			
C Upper Leg, Right			
D Upper Leg, Left			
F Knee Region, Right			
G Knee Region, Left			
H Lower Leg, Right			
J Lower Leg, Left			
K Ankle Region, Right			
L Ankle Region, Left			
M Foot, Right			
N Foot, Left			

NC Noncovered Procedure   **LC** Limited Coverage   **QA** Questionable OB Admit   **COM** New Tech Add-on   ⊞ Combination Member   ♂ Male   ♀ Female

ICD-10-PCS 2023   **699**

Ø   **Medical and Surgical**
Y   **Anatomical Regions, Lower Extremities**
6   **Detachment**   Definition: Cutting off all or a portion of the upper or lower extremities

                      Explanation: The body part value is the site of the detachment, with a qualifier if applicable to further specify the level where the extremity was detached

Body Part Character 4	Approach Character 5	Device Character 6	Qualifier Character 7
2 Hindquarter, Right 3 Hindquarter, Left 4 Hindquarter, Bilateral 7 Femoral Region, Right 8 Femoral Region, Left F Knee Region, Right G Knee Region, Left	Ø Open	Z No Device	Z No Qualifier
C Upper Leg, Right D Upper Leg, Left H Lower Leg, Right J Lower Leg, Left	Ø Open	Z No Device	1 High 2 Mid 3 Low
M Foot, Right N Foot, Left	Ø Open	Z No Device	Ø Complete 4 Complete 1st Ray 5 Complete 2nd Ray 6 Complete 3rd Ray 7 Complete 4th Ray 8 Complete 5th Ray 9 Partial 1st Ray B Partial 2nd Ray C Partial 3rd Ray D Partial 4th Ray F Partial 5th Ray

P 1st Toe, Right
    Hallux
Q 1st Toe, Left
    See 1st Toe, Right
R 2nd Toe, Right
S 2nd Toe, Left
T 3rd Toe, Right
U 3rd Toe, Left
V 4th Toe, Right
W 4th Toe, Left
X 5th Toe, Right
Y 5th Toe, Left
	Ø Open	Z No Device	Ø Complete
			1 High
			2 Mid
			3 Low

0   **Medical and Surgical**
Y   **Anatomical Regions, Lower Extremities**
9   **Drainage**   Definition: Taking or letting out fluids and/or gases from a body part
                        Explanation: The qualifier DIAGNOSTIC is used to identify drainage procedures that are biopsies

Body Part Character 4	Approach Character 5	Device Character 6	Qualifier Character 7

0 Buttock, Right
1 Buttock, Left
5 Inguinal Region, Right
   Inguinal canal
   Inguinal triangle
6 Inguinal Region, Left
   See 5 Inguinal Region, Right
7 Femoral Region, Right
8 Femoral Region, Left
9 Lower Extremity, Right
B Lower Extremity, Left
C Upper Leg, Right
D Upper Leg, Left
F Knee Region, Right
G Knee Region, Left
H Lower Leg, Right
J Lower Leg, Left
K Ankle Region, Right
L Ankle Region, Left
M Foot, Right
N Foot, Left
	0 Open
	3 Percutaneous
	4 Percutaneous Endoscopic
		0 Drainage Device	**Z** No Qualifier

0 Buttock, Right
1 Buttock, Left
5 Inguinal Region, Right
   Inguinal canal
   Inguinal triangle
6 Inguinal Region, Left
   See 5 Inguinal Region, Right
7 Femoral Region, Right
8 Femoral Region, Left
9 Lower Extremity, Right
B Lower Extremity, Left
C Upper Leg, Right
D Upper Leg, Left
F Knee Region, Right
G Knee Region, Left
H Lower Leg, Right
J Lower Leg, Left
K Ankle Region, Right
L Ankle Region, Left
M Foot, Right
N Foot, Left
	0 Open
	3 Percutaneous
	4 Percutaneous Endoscopic
		Z No Device	**X** Diagnostic
			Z No Qualifier

Non-OR   0Y9[0,1,7,8,9,B,C,D,F,G,H,J,K,L,M,N][0,3,4]0Z
Non-OR   0Y9[5,6]30Z
Non-OR   0Y9[0,1,7,8,9,B,C,D,F,G,H,J,K,L,M,N][0,3,4]Z[X,Z]
Non-OR   0Y9[5,6]3ZZ

NC Noncovered Procedure   **LC** Limited Coverage   **QA** Questionable OB Admit   **COM** New Tech Add-on   ⊞ Combination Member   ♂ Male   ♀ Female

ICD-10-PCS 2023   **701**

Anatomical Regions, Lower Extremities (side tab, left)

Ø   **Medical and Surgical**
Y   **Anatomical Regions, Lower Extremities**
B   **Excision**   Definition: Cutting out or off, without replacement, a portion of a body part
                          Explanation: The qualifier DIAGNOSTIC is used to identify excision procedures that are biopsies

Body Part Character 4	Approach Character 5	Device Character 6	Qualifier Character 7

Ø Buttock, Right
1 Buttock, Left
5 Inguinal Region, Right
  Inguinal canal
  Inguinal triangle
6 Inguinal Region, Left
  See 5 Inguinal Region, Right
7 Femoral Region, Right
8 Femoral Region, Left
9 Lower Extremity, Right
B Lower Extremity, Left
C Upper Leg, Right
D Upper Leg, Left
F Knee Region, Right
G Knee Region, Left
H Lower Leg, Right
J Lower Leg, Left
K Ankle Region, Right
L Ankle Region, Left
M Foot, Right
N Foot, Left
	Ø Open
	3 Percutaneous
	4 Percutaneous Endoscopic
		Z No Device	X Diagnostic
			Z No Qualifier

Non-OR   ØYB[Ø,1,9,B,C,D,F,G,H,J,K,L,M,N][Ø,3,4]ZX

Ø   **Medical and Surgical**
Y   **Anatomical Regions, Lower Extremities**
H   **Insertion**   Definition: Putting in a nonbiological appliance that monitors, assists, performs, or prevents a physiological function but does not physically
                          take the place of a body part
                          Explanation: None

Body Part Character 4	Approach Character 5	Device Character 6	Qualifier Character 7

Ø Buttock, Right
1 Buttock, Left
5 Inguinal Region, Right
  Inguinal canal
  Inguinal triangle
6 Inguinal Region, Left
  See 5 Inguinal Region, Right
7 Femoral Region, Right
8 Femoral Region, Left
9 Lower Extremity, Right
B Lower Extremity, Left
C Upper Leg, Right
D Upper Leg, Left
F Knee Region, Right
G Knee Region, Left
H Lower Leg, Right
J Lower Leg, Left
K Ankle Region, Right
L Ankle Region, Left
M Foot, Right
N Foot, Left
	Ø Open
	3 Percutaneous
	4 Percutaneous Endoscopic
		1 Radioactive Element
		3 Infusion Device
		Y Other Device
			Z No Qualifier

DRG Non-OR   ØYH[Ø,1,5,6,7,8,9,B,C,D,F,G,H,J,K,L,M,N][Ø,3,4][3,Y]Z

Non-OR Procedure   DRG Non-OR Procedure   Valid OR Procedure   HAC Associated Procedure   Combination Only   New/Revised GREEN

Ø   **Medical and Surgical**
Y   **Anatomical Regions, Lower Extremities**
J   **Inspection**   Definition: Visually and/or manually exploring a body part

                             Explanation: Visual exploration may be performed with or without optical instrumentation. Manual exploration may be performed directly or through intervening body layers.

Body Part Character 4	Approach Character 5	Device Character 6	Qualifier Character 7
Ø Buttock, Right	**Ø** Open	**Z** No Device	**Z** No Qualifier
1 Buttock, Left	**3** Percutaneous		
5 Inguinal Region, Right	**4** Percutaneous Endoscopic		
Inguinal canal	**X** External		
Inguinal triangle			
6 Inguinal Region, Left			
See 5 Inguinal Region, Right			
7 Femoral Region, Right			
8 Femoral Region, Left			
9 Lower Extremity, Right			
A Inguinal Region, Bilateral			
See 5 Inguinal Region, Right			
B Lower Extremity, Left			
C Upper Leg, Right			
D Upper Leg, Left			
E Femoral Region, Bilateral			
F Knee Region, Right			
G Knee Region, Left			
H Lower Leg, Right			
J Lower Leg, Left			
K Ankle Region, Right			
L Ankle Region, Left			
M Foot, Right			
N Foot, Left			

DRG Non-OR	ØYJ[Ø,1,8,9,B,C,D,E,F,G,H,J,K,L,M,N]ØZZ
Non-OR	ØYJ[Ø,1,9,B,C,D,F,G,H,J,K,L,M,N][3,4,X]ZZ
Non-OR	ØYJ[5,6,7,8,A,E][3,X]ZZ

Ø Medical and Surgical
Y Anatomical Regions, Lower Extremities
M Reattachment   Definition: Putting back in or on all or a portion of a separated body part to its normal location or other suitable location

                 Explanation: Vascular circulation and nervous pathways may or may not be reestablished

Body Part Character 4	Approach Character 5	Device Character 6	Qualifier Character 7
Ø Buttock, Right	Ø Open	Z No Device	Z No Qualifier
1 Buttock, Left			
2 Hindquarter, Right			
3 Hindquarter, Left			
4 Hindquarter, Bilateral			

5 Inguinal Region, Right
    Inguinal canal
    Inguinal triangle			

6 Inguinal Region, Left *See 5 Inguinal Region, Right*			
7 Femoral Region, Right			
8 Femoral Region, Left			
9 Lower Extremity, Right			
B Lower Extremity, Left			
C Upper Leg, Right			
D Upper Leg, Left			
F Knee Region, Right			
G Knee Region, Left			
H Lower Leg, Right			
J Lower Leg, Left			
K Ankle Region, Right			
L Ankle Region, Left			
M Foot, Right			
N Foot, Left			
P 1st Toe, Right Hallux			
Q 1st Toe, Left *See 1st Toe, Right*			
R 2nd Toe, Right			
S 2nd Toe, Left			
T 3rd Toe, Right			
U 3rd Toe, Left			
V 4th Toe, Right			
W 4th Toe, Left			
X 5th Toe, Right			
Y 5th Toe, Left			

Ø Medical and Surgical
Y Anatomical Regions, Lower Extremities
P Removal   Definition: Taking out or off a device from a body part

                Explanation: If a device is taken out and a similar device put in without cutting or puncturing the skin or mucous membrane, the procedure is coded to the root operation CHANGE. Otherwise, the procedure for taking out the device is coded to the root operation REMOVAL.

Body Part Character 4	Approach Character 5	Device Character 6	Qualifier Character 7
9 Lower Extremity, Right	Ø Open	Ø Drainage Device	Z No Qualifier
B Lower Extremity, Left	3 Percutaneous	1 Radioactive Element	
	4 Percutaneous Endoscopic	3 Infusion Device	
	X External	7 Autologous Tissue Substitute	
		J Synthetic Substitute	
		K Nonautologous Tissue Substitute	
		Y Other Device	

Non-OR   All body part, approach, device, and qualifier values

Ø   Medical and Surgical
Y   Anatomical Regions, Lower Extremities
Q   Repair   Definition: Restoring, to the extent possible, a body part to its normal anatomic structure and function
                       Explanation: Used only when the method to accomplish the repair is not one of the other root operations

Body Part Character 4	Approach Character 5	Device Character 6	Qualifier Character 7
Ø Buttock, Right	Ø Open	Z No Device	Z No Qualifier
1 Buttock, Left	3 Percutaneous		
5 Inguinal Region, Right	4 Percutaneous Endoscopic		
Inguinal canal	X External		
Inguinal triangle			
6 Inguinal Region, Left			
See 5 Inguinal Region, Right			
7 Femoral Region, Right			
8 Femoral Region, Left			
9 Lower Extremity, Right			
A Inguinal Region, Bilateral			
See 5 Inguinal Region, Right			
B Lower Extremity, Left			
C Upper Leg, Right			
D Upper Leg, Left			
E Femoral Region, Bilateral			
F Knee Region, Right			
G Knee Region, Left			
H Lower Leg, Right			
J Lower Leg, Left			
K Ankle Region, Right			
L Ankle Region, Left			
M Foot, Right			
N Foot, Left			
P 1st Toe, Right			
Hallux			
Q 1st Toe, Left			
See 1st Toe, Right			
R 2nd Toe, Right			
S 2nd Toe, Left			
T 3rd Toe, Right			
U 3rd Toe, Left			
V 4th Toe, Right			
W 4th Toe, Left			
X 5th Toe, Right			
Y 5th Toe, Left			

Non-OR   ØYQ[5,6,7,8,A,E]XZZ

NC Noncovered Procedure   **LC** Limited Coverage   **QA** Questionable OB Admit   **COM** New Tech Add-on   ⊞ Combination Member   ♂ Male   ♀ Female

ICD-10-PCS 2023   705

Ø   **Medical and Surgical**
Y   **Anatomical Regions, Lower Extremities**
U   **Supplement**   Definition: Putting in or on biological or synthetic material that physically reinforces and/or augments the function of a portion of a body part
                         Explanation: The biological material is non-living, or is living and from the same individual. The body part may have been previously replaced, and the SUPPLEMENT procedure is performed to physically reinforce and/or augment the function of the replaced body part.

Body Part Character 4	Approach Character 5	Device Character 6	Qualifier Character 7
Ø Buttock, Right	Ø Open	7 Autologous Tissue Substitute	Z No Qualifier
1 Buttock, Left	4 Percutaneous Endoscopic	J Synthetic Substitute	
5 Inguinal Region, Right		K Nonautologous Tissue Substitute	
Inguinal canal			
Inguinal triangle			
6 Inguinal Region, Left			
See 5 Inguinal Region, Right			
7 Femoral Region, Right			
8 Femoral Region, Left			
9 Lower Extremity, Right			
A Inguinal Region, Bilateral			
See 5 Inguinal Region, Right			
B Lower Extremity, Left			
C Upper Leg, Right			
D Upper Leg, Left			
E Femoral Region, Bilateral			
F Knee Region, Right			
G Knee Region, Left			
H Lower Leg, Right			
J Lower Leg, Left			
K Ankle Region, Right			
L Ankle Region, Left			
M Foot, Right			
N Foot, Left			
P 1st Toe, Right			
Hallux			
Q 1st Toe, Left			
See 1st Toe, Right			
R 2nd Toe, Right			
S 2nd Toe, Left			
T 3rd Toe, Right			
U 3rd Toe, Left			
V 4th Toe, Right			
W 4th Toe, Left			
X 5th Toe, Right			
Y 5th Toe, Left			

Ø   **Medical and Surgical**
Y   **Anatomical Regions, Lower Extremities**
W   **Revision**   Definition: Correcting, to the extent possible, a portion of a malfunctioning device or the position of a displaced device
                   Explanation: Revision can include correcting a malfunctioning or displaced device by taking out or putting in components of the device such as a screw or pin

Body Part Character 4	Approach Character 5	Device Character 6	Qualifier Character 7
9 Lower Extremity, Right	Ø Open	Ø Drainage Device	Z No Qualifier
B Lower Extremity, Left	3 Percutaneous	3 Infusion Device	
	4 Percutaneous Endoscopic	7 Autologous Tissue Substitute	
	X External	J Synthetic Substitute	
		K Nonautologous Tissue Substitute	
		Y Other Device	

DRG Non-OR   ØYW[9,B][Ø,3,4][Ø,3,7,J,K,Y]Z
Non-OR   ØYW[9,B]X[Ø,3,7,J,K,Y]Z

Obstetrics 1Ø2–1ØY

Character Meanings

This Character Meaning table is provided as a guide to assist the user in the identification of character members that may be found in this section of code tables. It **SHOULD NOT** be used to build a PCS code.

Ø: Pregnancy

Operation–Character 3		Body Part–Character 4		Approach–Character 5		Device–Character 6		Qualifier–Character 7	
2	Change	Ø	Products of Conception	Ø	Open	3	Monitoring Electrode	Ø	High
9	Drainage	1	Products of Conception, Retained	3	Percutaneous	Y	Other Device	1	Low
A	Abortion	2	Products of Conception, Ectopic	4	Percutaneous Endoscopic	Z	No Device	2	Extraperitoneal
D	Extraction			7	Via Natural or Artificial Opening			3	Low Forceps
E	Delivery			8	Via Natural or Artificial Opening Endoscopic			4	Mid Forceps
H	Insertion			X	External			5	High Forceps
J	Inspection							6	Vacuum
P	Removal							7	Internal Version
Q	Repair							8	Other
S	Reposition							9	Fetal Blood OR Manual
T	Resection							A	Fetal Cerebrospinal Fluid
Y	Transplantation							B	Fetal Fluid, Other
								C	Amniotic Fluid, Therapeutic
								D	Fluid, Other
								E	Nervous System
								F	Cardiovascular System
								G	Lymphatics & Hemic
								H	Eye
								J	Ear, Nose & Sinus
								K	Respiratory System
								L	Mouth & Throat
								M	Gastrointestinal System
								N	Hepatobiliary & Pancreas
								P	Endocrine System
								Q	Skin
								R	Musculoskeletal System
								S	Urinary System
								T	Female Reproductive System
								U	Amniotic Fluid, Diagnostic
								V	Male Reproductive System
								W	Laminaria
								X	Abortifacient
								Y	Other Body System
								Z	No Qualifier

AHA Coding Clinic for table 1Ø9

| 2014, 3Q, 12 | Fetoscopic laser photocoagulation and laser microseptostomy for twin-twin transfusion syndrome |
| 2014, 2Q, 9 | Pitocin administration to augment labor |

AHA Coding Clinic for table 1ØA

| 2022, 1Q, 21 | Gravid hysterectomy due to placenta increta |
| 2022, 1Q, 41 | Intrauterine Cook balloon placement for ectopic pregnancy |

AHA Coding Clinic for table 1ØD

2022, 1Q, 19	Spontaneous abortion with retained placenta of Twin B
2021, 1Q, 52	Removal of ectopic pregnancy via laparotomy
2020, 4Q, 59-60	Extraction of ectopic products of conception
2018, 4Q, 49-51	Revised qualifier values for root operation "extraction" (cesarean delivery)
2018, 2Q, 17	High transverse cesarean section
2016, 1Q, 9	Vaginal delivery assisted by vacuum and low forceps extraction
2014, 4Q, 43	Cesarean delivery assisted by vacuum extraction
2014, 4Q, 43	Vacuum dilation and curettage for blighted ovum

AHA Coding Clinic for table 1ØE

2017, 3Q, 5	Delivery of placenta
2016, 2Q, 34	Assisted vaginal delivery
2014, 4Q, 17	RH (D) alloimmunization (sensitization)
2014, 2Q, 9	Pitocin administration to augment labor

AHA Coding Clinic for table 1ØH

| 2013, 2Q, 36 | Intrauterine pressure monitor |

AHA Coding Clinic for table 1ØQ

| 2021, 2Q, 21 | Ex Utero intrapartum treatment procedure |
| 2014, 3Q, 12 | Fetoscopic laser photocoagulation and laser microseptostomy for twin-twin transfusion syndrome |

AHA Coding Clinic for table 1ØT

| 2020, 3Q, 47 | Removal of ectopic cornual pregnancy |
| 2015, 3Q, 31 | Laparoscopic partial salpingectomy for ectopic pregnancy |

1   Obstetrics
0   Pregnancy
2   Change

Definition: Taking out or off a device from a body part and putting back an identical or similar device in or on the same body part without cutting or puncturing the skin or a mucous membrane

Explanation: None

Body Part Character 4		Approach Character 5	Device Character 6	Qualifier Character 7
0 Products of Conception ♀	7	Via Natural or Artificial Opening	3 Monitoring Electrode Y Other Device	Z No Qualifier

Non-OR	All body part, approach, device, and qualifier values	♀	All body part, approach, device, and qualifier values

1   Obstetrics
0   Pregnancy
9   Drainage

Definition: Taking or letting out fluids and/or gases from a body part

Explanation: None

Body Part Character 4		Approach Character 5	Device Character 6	Qualifier Character 7
0 Products of Conception ♀	0 3 4 7 8	Open Percutaneous Percutaneous Endoscopic Via Natural or Artificial Opening Via Natural or Artificial Opening Endoscopic	Z No Device	9 Fetal Blood A Fetal Cerebrospinal Fluid B Fetal Fluid, Other C Amniotic Fluid, Therapeutic D Fluid, Other U Amniotic Fluid, Diagnostic

Non-OR	All body part, approach, device, and qualifier values	♀	All body part, approach, device, and qualifier values

1   Obstetrics
0   Pregnancy
A   Abortion

Definition: Artificially terminating a pregnancy

Explanation: None

Body Part Character 4		Approach Character 5	Device Character 6	Qualifier Character 7
0 Products of Conception ♀	0 3 4 8	Open Percutaneous Percutaneous Endoscopic Via Natural or Artificial Opening Endoscopic	Z No Device	Z No Qualifier
0 Products of Conception ♀	7	Via Natural or Artificial Opening	Z No Device	6 Vacuum W Laminaria X Abortifacient Z No Qualifier

Non-OR	10A07Z[6,W,X]	♀	All body part, approach, device, and qualifier values

1   Obstetrics
0   Pregnancy
D   Extraction

Definition: Pulling or stripping out or off all or a portion of a body part by the use of force

Explanation: None

Body Part Character 4		Approach Character 5	Device Character 6	Qualifier Character 7
0 Products of Conception QA ♀	0	Open	Z No Device	0 High 1 Low 2 Extraperitoneal
0 Products of Conception QA ♀	7	Via Natural or Artificial Opening	Z No Device	3 Low Forceps 4 Mid Forceps 5 High Forceps 6 Vacuum 7 Internal Version 8 Other
1 Products of Conception, Retained ♀	7 8	Via Natural or Artificial Opening Via Natural or Artificial Opening Endoscopic	Z No Device	9 Manual Z No Qualifier
2 Products of Conception, Ectopic ♀	0 4 7 8	Open Percutaneous Endoscopic Via Natural or Artificial Opening Via Natural or Artificial Opening Endoscopic	Z No Device	Z No Qualifier

DRG Non-OR QA QA	10D07Z[3,4,5,6,7,8] 10D00Z[0,1,2] except when a corresponding SDX of Z37.0-Z37.9 is also reported 10D07Z[3,4,5,7] except when a corresponding SDX of Z37.0-Z37.9 is also reported	♀	All body part, approach, device, and qualifier values

Non-OR Procedure   DRG Non-OR Procedure   Valid OR Procedure   HAC Associated Procedure   Combination Only   New/Revised April   New/Revised October

708   ICD-10-PCS 2023

1   Obstetrics
0   Pregnancy
E   Delivery   Definition: Assisting the passage of the products of conception from the genital canal

Explanation: None

Body Part Character 4	Approach Character 5	Device Character 6	Qualifier Character 7
0 Products of Conception QA ♀	X External	Z No Device	Z No Qualifier

DRG Non-OR	10E0XZZ		♀ All body part, approach, device, and qualifier values
QA	10E0XZZ except when a corresponding SDX of Z37.0-Z37.9 is also reported		

1   Obstetrics
0   Pregnancy
H   Insertion   Definition: Putting in a nonbiological appliance that monitors, assists, performs, or prevents a physiological function but does not physically take the place of a body part

Explanation: None

Body Part Character 4	Approach Character 5	Device Character 6	Qualifier Character 7
0 Products of Conception ♀	0 Open 7 Via Natural or Artificial Opening	3 Monitoring Electrode Y Other Device	Z No Qualifier

Non-OR	All body part, approach, device, and qualifier values	♀ All body part, approach, device, and qualifier values

1   Obstetrics
0   Pregnancy
J   Inspection   Definition: Visually and/or manually exploring a body part

Explanation: Visual exploration may be performed with or without optical instrumentation. Manual exploration may be performed directly or through intervening body layers.

Body Part Character 4	Approach Character 5	Device Character 6	Qualifier Character 7
0 Products of Conception ♀ 1 Products of Conception, Retained ♀ 2 Products of Conception, Ectopic ♀	0 Open 3 Percutaneous 4 Percutaneous Endoscopic 7 Via Natural or Artificial Opening 8 Via Natural or Artificial Opening Endoscopic X External	Z No Device	Z No Qualifier

Non-OR	All body part, approach, device, and qualifier values	♀ All body part, approach, device, and qualifier values

1   Obstetrics
0   Pregnancy
P   Removal   Definition: Taking out or off a device from a body part, region or orifice

Explanation: If a device is taken out and a similar device put in without cutting or puncturing the skin or mucous membrane, the procedure is coded to the root operation CHANGE. Otherwise, the procedure for taking out a device is coded to the root operation REMOVAL.

Body Part Character 4	Approach Character 5	Device Character 6	Qualifier Character 7
0 Products of Conception ♀	0 Open 7 Via Natural or Artificial Opening	3 Monitoring Electrode Y Other Device	Z No Qualifier

Non-OR	All body part, approach, device, and qualifier values	♀ All body part, approach, device, and qualifier values

1   Obstetrics
0   Pregnancy
Q   Repair   Definition: Restoring, to the extent possible, a body part to its normal anatomic structure and function

Explanation: Used only when the method to accomplish the repair is not one of the other root operations

Body Part Character 4	Approach Character 5	Device Character 6	Qualifier Character 7
0 Products of Conception ♀	0 Open 3 Percutaneous 4 Percutaneous Endoscopic 7 Via Natural or Artificial Opening 8 Via Natural or Artificial Opening Endoscopic	Y Other Device Z No Device	E Nervous System F Cardiovascular System G Lymphatics and Hemic H Eye J Ear, Nose and Sinus K Respiratory System L Mouth and Throat M Gastrointestinal System N Hepatobiliary and Pancreas P Endocrine System Q Skin R Musculoskeletal System S Urinary System T Female Reproductive System V Male Reproductive System Y Other Body System

Non-OR	All body part, approach, device, and qualifier values	♀ All body part, approach, device, and qualifier values

NC Noncovered Procedure   LC Limited Coverage   QA Questionable OB Admit   NT New Tech Add-on   ⊞ Combination Member   ♂ Male   ♀ Female

1   **Obstetrics**
Ø   **Pregnancy**
S   **Reposition**   Definition: Moving to its normal location, or other suitable location, all or a portion of a body part

Explanation: The body part is moved to a new location from an abnormal location, or from a normal location where it is not functioning correctly. The body part may or may not be cut out or off to be moved to the new location.

Body Part Character 4	Approach Character 5	Device Character 6	Qualifier Character 7
Ø Products of Conception ♀	**7** Via Natural or Artificial Opening **X** External	**Z** No Device	**Z** No Qualifier
2 Products of Conception, Ectopic ♀	**Ø** Open **3** Percutaneous **4** Percutaneous Endoscopic **7** Via Natural or Artificial Opening **8** Via Natural or Artificial Opening Endoscopic	**Z** No Device	**Z** No Qualifier

Non-OR	10SØ[7,X]ZZ	♀ All body part, approach, device, and qualifier values

1   **Obstetrics**
Ø   **Pregnancy**
T   **Resection**   Definition: Cutting out or off, without replacement, all of a body part

Explanation: None

Body Part Character 4	Approach Character 5	Device Character 6	Qualifier Character 7
2 Products of Conception, Ectopic ♀	**Ø** Open **3** Percutaneous **4** Percutaneous Endoscopic **7** Via Natural or Artificial Opening **8** Via Natural or Artificial Opening Endoscopic	**Z** No Device	**Z** No Qualifier

♀   All body part, approach, device, and qualifier values

1   **Obstetrics**
Ø   **Pregnancy**
Y   **Transplantation**   Definition: Putting in or on all or a portion of a living body part taken from another individual or animal to physically take the place and/or function of all or a portion of a similar body part

Explanation: The native body part may or may not be taken out, and the transplanted body part may take over all or a portion of its function

Body Part Character 4	Approach Character 5	Device Character 6	Qualifier Character 7
Ø Products of Conception ♀	**3** Percutaneous **4** Percutaneous Endoscopic **7** Via Natural or Artificial Opening	**Z** No Device	**E** Nervous System **F** Cardiovascular System **G** Lymphatics and Hemic **H** Eye **J** Ear, Nose and Sinus **K** Respiratory System **L** Mouth and Throat **M** Gastrointestinal System **N** Hepatobiliary and Pancreas **P** Endocrine System **Q** Skin **R** Musculoskeletal System **S** Urinary System **T** Female Reproductive System **V** Male Reproductive System **Y** Other Body System

Non-OR	All body part, approach, device, and qualifier values	♀ All body part, approach, device, and qualifier values

Non-OR Procedure   DRG Non-OR Procedure   Valid OR Procedure   HAC Associated Procedure   Combination Only   New/Revised April   New/Revised October

710   ICD-10-PCS 2023

10S–10Y

Placement 2W0–2Y5

AHA Coding Clinic for table 2W6
2015, 2Q, 35   Application of tongs to reduce and stabilize cervical fracture
2013, 2Q, 39   Application of cervical tongs for reduction of cervical fracture

AHA Coding Clinic for table 2Y4
2018, 4Q, 38   Control of epistaxis
2017, 4Q, 106   Nasal packing for epistaxis

2   Placement
W   Anatomical Regions
0   Change   Definition: Taking out or off a device from a body part and putting back an identical or similar device in or on the same body part without cutting or puncturing the skin or a mucous membrane

Body Region Character 4	Approach Character 5	Device Character 6	Qualifier Character 7
0 Head 2 Neck 3 Abdominal Wall 4 Chest Wall 5 Back 6 Inguinal Region, Right 7 Inguinal Region, Left 8 Upper Extremity, Right 9 Upper Extremity, Left A Upper Arm, Right B Upper Arm, Left C Lower Arm, Right D Lower Arm, Left E Hand, Right F Hand, Left G Thumb, Right H Thumb, Left J Finger, Right K Finger, Left L Lower Extremity, Right M Lower Extremity, Left N Upper Leg, Right P Upper Leg, Left Q Lower Leg, Right R Lower Leg, Left S Foot, Right T Foot, Left U Toe, Right V Toe, Left	X External	0 Traction Apparatus 1 Splint 2 Cast 3 Brace 4 Bandage 5 Packing Material 6 Pressure Dressing 7 Intermittent Pressure Device Y Other Device	Z No Qualifier
1 Face	X External	0 Traction Apparatus 1 Splint 2 Cast 3 Brace 4 Bandage 5 Packing Material 6 Pressure Dressing 7 Intermittent Pressure Device 9 Wire Y Other Device	Z No Qualifier

NC Noncovered Procedure   LC Limited Coverage   QA Questionable OB Admit   NT New Tech Add-on   ⊞ Combination Member   ♂ Male   ♀ Female

ICD-10-PCS 2023   711

Placement

Placement 2W0–2Y5

2 Placement
W Anatomical Regions
1 Compression Definition: Putting pressure on a body region

Body Region Character 4	Approach Character 5	Device Character 6	Qualifier Character 7
Ø Head	X External	6 Pressure Dressing	Z No Qualifier
1 Face		7 Intermittent Pressure Device	
2 Neck			
3 Abdominal Wall			
4 Chest Wall			
5 Back			
6 Inguinal Region, Right			
7 Inguinal Region, Left			
8 Upper Extremity, Right			
9 Upper Extremity, Left			
A Upper Arm, Right			
B Upper Arm, Left			
C Lower Arm, Right			
D Lower Arm, Left			
E Hand, Right			
F Hand, Left			
G Thumb, Right			
H Thumb, Left			
J Finger, Right			
K Finger, Left			
L Lower Extremity, Right			
M Lower Extremity, Left			
N Upper Leg, Right			
P Upper Leg, Left			
Q Lower Leg, Right			
R Lower Leg, Left			
S Foot, Right			
T Foot, Left			
U Toe, Right			
V Toe, Left			

2 Placement
W Anatomical Regions
2 Dressing Definition: Putting material on a body region for protection

Body Region Character 4	Approach Character 5	Device Character 6	Qualifier Character 7
Ø Head	X External	4 Bandage	Z No Qualifier
1 Face			
2 Neck			
3 Abdominal Wall			
4 Chest Wall			
5 Back			
6 Inguinal Region, Right			
7 Inguinal Region, Left			
8 Upper Extremity, Right			
9 Upper Extremity, Left			
A Upper Arm, Right			
B Upper Arm, Left			
C Lower Arm, Right			
D Lower Arm, Left			
E Hand, Right			
F Hand, Left			
G Thumb, Right			
H Thumb, Left			
J Finger, Right			
K Finger, Left			
L Lower Extremity, Right			
M Lower Extremity, Left			
N Upper Leg, Right			
P Upper Leg, Left			
Q Lower Leg, Right			
R Lower Leg, Left			
S Foot, Right			
T Foot, Left			
U Toe, Right			
V Toe, Left			

2　　Placement
W　　Anatomical Regions
3　　Immobilization　　Definition: Limiting or preventing motion of a body region

Body Region Character 4	Approach Character 5	Device Character 6	Qualifier Character 7
Ø Head 2 Neck 3 Abdominal Wall 4 Chest Wall 5 Back 6 Inguinal Region, Right 7 Inguinal Region, Left 8 Upper Extremity, Right 9 Upper Extremity, Left A Upper Arm, Right B Upper Arm, Left C Lower Arm, Right D Lower Arm, Left E Hand, Right F Hand, Left G Thumb, Right H Thumb, Left J Finger, Right K Finger, Left L Lower Extremity, Right M Lower Extremity, Left N Upper Leg, Right P Upper Leg, Left Q Lower Leg, Right R Lower Leg, Left S Foot, Right T Foot, Left U Toe, Right V Toe, Left	X External	1 Splint 2 Cast 3 Brace Y Other Device	Z No Qualifier
1 Face	X External	1 Splint 2 Cast 3 Brace 9 Wire Y Other Device	Z No Qualifier

2　　Placement
W　　Anatomical Regions
4　　Packing　　Definition: Putting material in a body region or orifice

Body Region Character 4	Approach Character 5	Device Character 6	Qualifier Character 7
Ø Head 1 Face 2 Neck 3 Abdominal Wall 4 Chest Wall 5 Back 6 Inguinal Region, Right 7 Inguinal Region, Left 8 Upper Extremity, Right 9 Upper Extremity, Left A Upper Arm, Right B Upper Arm, Left C Lower Arm, Right D Lower Arm, Left E Hand, Right F Hand, Left G Thumb, Right H Thumb, Left J Finger, Right K Finger, Left L Lower Extremity, Right M Lower Extremity, Left N Upper Leg, Right P Upper Leg, Left Q Lower Leg, Right R Lower Leg, Left S Foot, Right T Foot, Left U Toe, Right V Toe, Left	X External	5 Packing Material	Z No Qualifier

NC Noncovered Procedure　　LC Limited Coverage　　QA Questionable OB Admit　　NT New Tech Add-on　　⊞ Combination Member　　♂ Male　　♀ Female

ICD-10-PCS 2023　　　　　　　　　　　　　　　　　　　　　　　　　　　713

2W3–2W4

Placement

2　**Placement**
W　**Anatomical Regions**
5　**Removal**　　　Definition: Taking out or off a device from a body part

Body Region Character 4	Approach Character 5	Device Character 6	Qualifier Character 7
Ø Head	X External	Ø Traction Apparatus	Z No Qualifier
2 Neck		1 Splint	
3 Abdominal Wall		2 Cast	
4 Chest Wall		3 Brace	
5 Back		4 Bandage	
6 Inguinal Region, Right		5 Packing Material	
7 Inguinal Region, Left		6 Pressure Dressing	
8 Upper Extremity, Right		7 Intermittent Pressure Device	
9 Upper Extremity, Left		Y Other Device	
A Upper Arm, Right			
B Upper Arm, Left			
C Lower Arm, Right			
D Lower Arm, Left			
E Hand, Right			
F Hand, Left			
G Thumb, Right			
H Thumb, Left			
J Finger, Right			
K Finger, Left			
L Lower Extremity, Right			
M Lower Extremity, Left			
N Upper Leg, Right			
P Upper Leg, Left			
Q Lower Leg, Right			
R Lower Leg, Left			
S Foot, Right			
T Foot, Left			
U Toe, Right			
V Toe, Left			
1 Face	X External	Ø Traction Apparatus	Z No Qualifier
		1 Splint	
		2 Cast	
		3 Brace	
		4 Bandage	
		5 Packing Material	
		6 Pressure Dressing	
		7 Intermittent Pressure Device	
		9 Wire	
		Y Other Device	

2   **Placement**
W   **Anatomical Regions**
6   **Traction**   Definition: Exerting a pulling force on a body region in a distal direction

Body Region Character 4	Approach Character 5	Device Character 6	Qualifier Character 7
Ø Head 1 Face 2 Neck 3 Abdominal Wall 4 Chest Wall 5 Back 6 Inguinal Region, Right 7 Inguinal Region, Left 8 Upper Extremity, Right 9 Upper Extremity, Left A Upper Arm, Right B Upper Arm, Left C Lower Arm, Right D Lower Arm, Left E Hand, Right F Hand, Left G Thumb, Right H Thumb, Left J Finger, Right K Finger, Left L Lower Extremity, Right M Lower Extremity, Left N Upper Leg, Right P Upper Leg, Left Q Lower Leg, Right R Lower Leg, Left S Foot, Right T Foot, Left U Toe, Right V Toe, Left	X External	Ø Traction Apparatus Z No Device	Z No Qualifier

2   **Placement**
Y   **Anatomical Orifices**
Ø   **Change**   Definition: Taking out or off a device from a body part and putting back an identical or similar device in or on the same body part without cutting or puncturing the skin or a mucous membrane

Body Region Character 4	Approach Character 5	Device Character 6	Qualifier Character 7
Ø Mouth and Pharynx 1 Nasal 2 Ear 3 Anorectal 4 Female Genital Tract ♀ 5 Urethra	X External	5 Packing Material	Z No Qualifier

♀   2YØ4X5Z

2   Placement
Y   Anatomical Orifices
4   Packing   Definition: Putting material in a body region or orifice

Body Region Character 4	Approach Character 5	Device Character 6	Qualifier Character 7
0 Mouth and Pharynx 1 Nasal 2 Ear 3 Anorectal 4 Female Genital Tract ♀ 5 Urethra	X External	5 Packing Material	Z No Qualifier

♀   2Y44X5Z

2   Placement
Y   Anatomical Orifices
5   Removal   Definition: Taking out or off a device from a body part

Body Region Character 4	Approach Character 5	Device Character 6	Qualifier Character 7
0 Mouth and Pharynx 1 Nasal 2 Ear 3 Anorectal 4 Female Genital Tract ♀ 5 Urethra	X External	5 Packing Material	Z No Qualifier

♀   2Y54X5Z

Administration 3Ø2–3E1

AHA Coding Clinic for table 3Ø2

2021, 4Q, 54	Nonautologous pathogen reduced cryoprecipitated fibrinogen complex
2020, 4Q, 60-61	Transfusion stem cell progenitor cells
2019, 4Q, 35	Transfusion of blood products
2019, 4Q, 36	T-cell depleted hematopoietic stem cells for transplantation
2016, 4Q, 113	Bone marrow and stem cell transfusion (Transplantation)

AHA Coding Clinic for table 3EØ

2022, 1Q, 8	Other monoclonal antibody
2021, 4Q, 54-55	Antineoplastic monoclonal antibody
2021, 4Q, 110	New/revised frequently asked questions regarding ICD-10-CM/PCS coding for COVID-19
2021, 1Q, 49	Frequently asked questions regarding ICD-10-CM and ICD-10-PCS coding for COVID-19
2020, 4Q, 49-50	Intravascular ultrasound assisted thrombolysis
2020, 4Q, 95	Frequently asked questions regarding ICD-10-PCS coding for COVID-19
2020, 3Q, 17-21	New procedure codes for introduction or infusion of therapeutics
2019, 4Q, 36-37	Hyperthermic antineoplastic chemotherapy
2018, 3Q, 7	Coronary brachytherapy with angioplasty
2018, 1Q, 8	Placement of bone morphogenetic protein & spinal fusion surgery
2017, 2Q, 14	Infusion of tPA into pleural cavity
2017, 1Q, 37	Injection of glue into enteric fistula tract
2016, 4Q, 113-114	Substances applied to cranial cavity and brain
2016, 3Q, 29	Closure of bilateral alveolar clefts
2016, 1Q, 20	Metatarsophalangeal joint resection arthroplasty

AHA Coding Clinic for table 3EØ (Continued)

2015, 3Q, 24	Esophagogastroduodenoscopy with epinephrine injection for control of bleeding
2015, 3Q, 29	Placement of adhesion barrier
2015, 2Q, 29	Insertion of nasogastric tube for drainage and feeding
2015, 2Q, 31	Thoracoscopic talc pleurodesis
2015, 1Q, 31	Intrathecal chemotherapy
2015, 1Q, 38	Chemoembolization of the hepatic artery
2014, 4Q, 16	Administration of RH (D) immunoglobulin
2014, 4Q, 17	RH (D) alloimmunization (sensitization)
2014, 4Q, 19	Ultrasound accelerated thrombolysis
2014, 4Q, 34	Resection of brain malignancy with implantation of chemotherapeutic wafer
2014, 4Q, 38	Placement of saline and Seprafilm solution into abdominal cavity
2014, 3Q, 26	Coil embolization of gastroduodenal artery with chemoembolization of hepatic artery
2014, 2Q, 8	Medical induction of labor with Cervidil tampon insertion
2014, 2Q, 10	Prophylactic Neulasta injection for infection prevention
2013, 4Q, 124	Administration of tPA for stroke treatment prior to transfer
2013, 1Q, 27	Injection of sclerosing agent into an esophageal varix

AHA Coding Clinic for table 3E1

2021, 4Q, 55	Laparoscopic irrigation of peritoneal cavity
2019, 4Q, 38	Irrigation of joint using irrigating substance
2017, 3Q, 14	Bronchoscopy with suctioning and washings for removal of mucus plug

3   **Administration**
Ø   **Circulatory**
2   **Transfusion**   Definition: Putting in blood or blood products

Body System/Region Character 4	Approach Character 5	Substance Character 6	Qualifier Character 7
3 Peripheral Vein **NC** 4 Central Vein **NC**	3 Percutaneous	A Stem Cells, Embryonic	Z No Qualifier
3 Peripheral Vein 4 Central Vein	3 Percutaneous	C Hematopoietic Stem/Progenitor Cells, Genetically Modified	Ø Autologous
3 Peripheral Vein 4 Central Vein	3 Percutaneous	D Pathogen Reduced Cryoprecipitated Fibrinogen Complex **NT**	1 Nonautologous
3 Peripheral Vein **NC** 4 Central Vein **NC**	3 Percutaneous	G Bone Marrow X Stem Cells, Cord Blood Y Stem Cells, Hematopoietic	Ø Autologous 2 Allogeneic, Related 3 Allogeneic, Unrelated 4 Allogeneic, Unspecified
3 Peripheral Vein 4 Central Vein	3 Percutaneous	H Whole Blood J Serum Albumin K Frozen Plasma L Fresh Plasma M Plasma Cryoprecipitate N Red Blood Cells P Frozen Red Cells Q White Cells R Platelets S Globulin T Fibrinogen V Antihemophilic Factors W Factor IX	Ø Autologous 1 Nonautologous
3 Peripheral Vein 4 Central Vein	3 Percutaneous	U Stem Cells, T-cell Depleted Hematopoietic	2 Allogeneic, Related 3 Allogeneic, Unrelated 4 Allogeneic, Unspecified
7 Products of Conception,♀ Circulatory	3 Percutaneous 7 Via Natural or Artificial Opening	H Whole Blood J Serum Albumin K Frozen Plasma L Fresh Plasma M Plasma Cryoprecipitate N Red Blood Cells P Frozen Red Cells Q White Cells R Platelets S Globulin T Fibrinogen V Antihemophilic Factors W Factor IX	1 Nonautologous
8 Vein	3 Percutaneous	B 4-Factor Prothrombin Complex Concentrate	1 Nonautologous

DRG Non-OR	3Ø2[3,4]3AZ
DRG Non-OR	3Ø2[3,4]3CØ
DRG Non-OR	3Ø2[3,4]3[G,X,Y][Ø,2,3,4]
DRG Non-OR	3Ø2[3,4]3U[2,3,4]

NC   3Ø2[3,4]3AZ Only when reported with PDx or SDx of C91.ØØ, C92.ØØ, C92.1Ø, C92.11, C92.4Ø, C92.5Ø, C92.6Ø, C92.AØ, C93.ØØ, C94.ØØ, C95.ØØ

NC   3Ø2[3,4]3[G,Y]Ø Only when reported with PDx or SDx of C91.ØØ, C92.ØØ, C92.1Ø, C92.11, C92.4Ø, C92.5Ø, C92.6Ø, C92.AØ, C93.ØØ, C94.ØØ, C95.ØØ

NT   3Ø2[3,4]3D1 for Intercept® (PRCFC) in combination with dx code D62, D65, D68.2, D68.4, or D68.9

♀   3Ø27[3,7][H,J,K,L,M,N,P,Q,R,S,T,V,W]1

 NC Noncovered Procedure   **LC** Limited Coverage   **OA** Questionable OB Admit   **NT** New Tech Add-on   ⊞ Combination Member   ♂ Male   ♀ Female

3   **Administration**
C   **Indwelling Device**
1   **Irrigation**   Definition: Putting in or on a cleansing substance

Body System/Region Character 4	Approach Character 5	Substance Character 6	Qualifier Character 7
Z None	X External	8 Irrigating Substance	Z No Qualifier

3   **Administration**
E   **Physiological Systems and Anatomical Regions**
0   **Introduction**   Definition: Putting in or on a therapeutic, diagnostic, nutritional, physiological, or prophylactic substance except blood or blood products

Body System/Region Character 4	Approach Character 5	Substance Character 6	Qualifier Character 7
0 Skin and Mucous Membranes	X External	0 Antineoplastic	5 Other Antineoplastic M Monoclonal Antibody
0 Skin and Mucous Membranes	X External	2 Anti-infective	8 Oxazolidinones 9 Other Anti-infective
0 Skin and Mucous Membranes	X External	3 Anti-inflammatory 4 Serum, Toxoid and Vaccine B Anesthetic Agent K Other Diagnostic Substance M Pigment N Analgesics, Hypnotics, Sedatives T Destructive Agent	Z No Qualifier
0 Skin and Mucous Membranes	X External	G Other Therapeutic Substance	C Other Substance
1 Subcutaneous Tissue	0 Open	2 Anti-infective	A Anti-Infective Envelope
1 Subcutaneous Tissue	3 Percutaneous	0 Antineoplastic	5 Other Antineoplastic M Monoclonal Antibody
1 Subcutaneous Tissue	3 Percutaneous	2 Anti-infective	8 Oxazolidinones 9 Other Anti-infective A Anti-Infective Envelope
1 Subcutaneous Tissue	3 Percutaneous	3 Anti-inflammatory 6 Nutritional Substance 7 Electrolytic and Water Balance Substance B Anesthetic Agent H Radioactive Substance K Other Diagnostic Substance N Analgesics, Hypnotics, Sedatives T Destructive Agent	Z No Qualifier
1 Subcutaneous Tissue	3 Percutaneous	4 Serum, Toxoid and Vaccine	0 Influenza Vaccine Z No Qualifier
1 Subcutaneous Tissue	3 Percutaneous	G Other Therapeutic Substance	C Other Substance
1 Subcutaneous Tissue	3 Percutaneous	V Hormone	G Insulin J Other Hormone
2 Muscle	3 Percutaneous	0 Antineoplastic	5 Other Antineoplastic M Monoclonal Antibody
2 Muscle	3 Percutaneous	2 Anti-infective	8 Oxazolidinones 9 Other Anti-infective
2 Muscle	3 Percutaneous	3 Anti-inflammatory 6 Nutritional Substance 7 Electrolytic and Water Balance Substance B Anesthetic Agent H Radioactive Substance K Other Diagnostic Substance N Analgesics, Hypnotics, Sedatives T Destructive Agent	Z No Qualifier
2 Muscle	3 Percutaneous	4 Serum, Toxoid and Vaccine	0 Influenza Vaccine Z No Qualifier
2 Muscle	3 Percutaneous	G Other Therapeutic Substance	C Other Substance
3 Peripheral Vein	0 Open	0 Antineoplastic	2 High-dose Interleukin-2 3 Low-dose Interleukin-2 5 Other Antineoplastic M Monoclonal Antibody P Clofarabine
3 Peripheral Vein	0 Open	1 Thrombolytic	6 Recombinant Human- activated Protein C 7 Other Thrombolytic
3 Peripheral Vein	0 Open	2 Anti-infective	8 Oxazolidinones 9 Other Anti-infective

DRG Non-OR   3E03002
DRG Non-OR   3E03017

3E0 Continued on next page

3E0 Continued

3   Administration
E   Physiological Systems and Anatomical Regions
0   Introduction   Definition: Putting in or on a therapeutic, diagnostic, nutritional, physiological, or prophylactic substance except blood or blood products

Body System/Region Character 4	Approach Character 5	Substance Character 6	Qualifier Character 7
3 Peripheral Vein	0 Open	3 Anti-inflammatory 4 Serum, Toxoid and Vaccine 6 Nutritional Substance 7 Electrolytic and Water Balance Substance F Intracirculatory Anesthetic H Radioactive Substance K Other Diagnostic Substance N Analgesics, Hypnotics, Sedatives P Platelet Inhibitor R Antiarrhythmic T Destructive Agent X Vasopressor	Z No Qualifier
3 Peripheral Vein	0 Open	G Other Therapeutic Substance	C Other Substance N Blood Brain Barrier Disruption
3 Peripheral Vein	0 Open	U Pancreatic Islet Cells	0 Autologous 1 Nonautologous
3 Peripheral Vein	0 Open	V Hormone	G Insulin H Human B-type Natriuretic Peptide J Other Hormone
3 Peripheral Vein	0 Open	W Immunotherapeutic	K Immunostimulator L Immunosuppressive
3 Peripheral Vein	3 Percutaneous	0 Antineoplastic	2 High-dose Interleukin-2 3 Low-dose Interleukin-2 5 Other Antineoplastic M Monoclonal Antibody P Clofarabine
3 Peripheral Vein	3 Percutaneous	1 Thrombolytic	6 Recombinant Human- activated Protein C 7 Other Thrombolytic
3 Peripheral Vein	3 Percutaneous	2 Anti-infective	8 Oxazolidinones 9 Other Anti-infective
3 Peripheral Vein	3 Percutaneous	3 Anti-inflammatory 4 Serum, Toxoid and Vaccine 6 Nutritional Substance 7 Electrolytic and Water Balance Substance F Intracirculatory Anesthetic H Radioactive Substance K Other Diagnostic Substance N Analgesics, Hypnotics, Sedatives P Platelet Inhibitor R Antiarrhythmic T Destructive Agent X Vasopressor	Z No Qualifier
3 Peripheral Vein	3 Percutaneous	G Other Therapeutic Substance	C Other Substance N Blood Brain Barrier Disruption Q Glucarpidase R Other Therapeutic Monoclonal Antibody
3 Peripheral Vein	3 Percutaneous	U Pancreatic Islet Cells	0 Autologous 1 Nonautologous
3 Peripheral Vein	3 Percutaneous	V Hormone	G Insulin H Human B-type Natriuretic Peptide J Other Hormone
3 Peripheral Vein	3 Percutaneous	W Immunotherapeutic	K Immunostimulator L Immunosuppressive
4 Central Vein	0 Open	0 Antineoplastic	2 High-dose Interleukin-2 3 Low-dose Interleukin-2 5 Other Antineoplastic M Monoclonal Antibody P Clofarabine
4 Central Vein	0 Open	1 Thrombolytic	6 Recombinant Human- activated Protein C 7 Other Thrombolytic

Valid OR	3E030TZ	DRG Non-OR	3E033U[0,1]
DRG Non-OR	3E030U[0,1]	DRG Non-OR	3E04002
DRG Non-OR	3E03302	DRG Non-OR	3E04017
DRG Non-OR	3E03317		

3E0 Continued on next page

NC Noncovered Procedure   LC Limited Coverage   QA Questionable OB Admit   NT New Tech Add-on   ⊞ Combination Member   ♂ Male   ♀ Female

ICD-10-PCS 2023   719

3E0–3E0

Administration

3E0 Continued

3   **Administration**
E   **Physiological Systems and Anatomical Regions**
0   **Introduction**   Definition: Putting in or on a therapeutic, diagnostic, nutritional, physiological, or prophylactic substance except blood or blood products

Body System/Region Character 4	Approach Character 5	Substance Character 6	Qualifier Character 7
4 Central Vein	0 Open	2 Anti-infective	8 Oxazolidinones 9 Other Anti-infective
4 Central Vein	0 Open	3 Anti-inflammatory 4 Serum, Toxoid and Vaccine 6 Nutritional Substance 7 Electrolytic and Water Balance Substance F Intracirculatory Anesthetic H Radioactive Substance K Other Diagnostic Substance N Analgesics, Hypnotics, Sedatives P Platelet Inhibitor R Antiarrhythmic T Destructive Agent X Vasopressor	Z No Qualifier
4 Central Vein	0 Open	G Other Therapeutic Substance	C Other Substance N Blood Brain Barrier Disruption
4 Central Vein	0 Open	V Hormone	G Insulin H Human B-type Natriuretic Peptide J Other Hormone
4 Central Vein	0 Open	W Immunotherapeutic	K Immunostimulator L Immunosuppressive
4 Central Vein	3 Percutaneous	0 Antineoplastic	2 High-dose Interleukin-2 3 Low-dose Interleukin-2 5 Other Antineoplastic M Monoclonal Antibody P Clofarabine
4 Central Vein	3 Percutaneous	1 Thrombolytic	6 Recombinant Human- activated Protein C 7 Other Thrombolytic
4 Central Vein	3 Percutaneous	2 Anti-infective	8 Oxazolidinones 9 Other Anti-infective
4 Central Vein	3 Percutaneous	3 Anti-inflammatory 4 Serum, Toxoid and Vaccine 6 Nutritional Substance 7 Electrolytic and Water Balance Substance F Intracirculatory Anesthetic H Radioactive Substance K Other Diagnostic Substance N Analgesics, Hypnotics, Sedatives P Platelet Inhibitor R Antiarrhythmic T Destructive Agent X Vasopressor	Z No Qualifier
4 Central Vein	3 Percutaneous	G Other Therapeutic Substance	C Other Substance N Blood Brain Barrier Disruption Q Glucarpidase R Other Therapeutic Monoclonal Antibody
4 Central Vein	3 Percutaneous	V Hormone	G Insulin H Human B-type Natriuretic Peptide J Other Hormone
4 Central Vein	3 Percutaneous	W Immunotherapeutic	K Immunostimulator L Immunosuppressive
5 Peripheral Artery 6 Central Artery	0 Open 3 Percutaneous	0 Antineoplastic	2 High-dose Interleukin-2 3 Low-dose Interleukin-2 5 Other Antineoplastic M Monoclonal Antibody P Clofarabine
5 Peripheral Artery 6 Central Artery	0 Open 3 Percutaneous	1 Thrombolytic	6 Recombinant Human- activated Protein C 7 Other Thrombolytic
5 Peripheral Artery 6 Central Artery	0 Open 3 Percutaneous	2 Anti-infective	8 Oxazolidinones 9 Other Anti-infective

Valid OR	3E040TZ	**DRG Non-OR**	3E0[5,6][0,3]02
DRG Non-OR	3E04302	**DRG Non-OR**	3E0[5,6][0,3]17
DRG Non-OR	3E04317		

3E0 Continued on next page

Non-OR Procedure   DRG Non-OR Procedure   Valid OR Procedure   HAC Associated Procedure   Combination Only   New/Revised April   New/Revised October

720   ICD-10-PCS 2023

3   **Administration**
E   **Physiological Systems and Anatomical Regions**
Ø   **Introduction**   Definition: Putting in or on a therapeutic, diagnostic, nutritional, physiological, or prophylactic substance except blood or blood products

3EØ Continued

Body System/Region Character 4	Approach Character 5	Substance Character 6	Qualifier Character 7
5 Peripheral Artery 6 Central Artery	Ø Open 3 Percutaneous	3 Anti-inflammatory 4 Serum, Toxoid and Vaccine 6 Nutritional Substance 7 Electrolytic and Water Balance Substance F Intracirculatory Anesthetic H Radioactive Substance K Other Diagnostic Substance N Analgesics, Hypnotics, Sedatives P Platelet Inhibitor R Antiarrhythmic T Destructive Agent X Vasopressor	Z No Qualifier
5 Peripheral Artery 6 Central Artery	Ø Open 3 Percutaneous	G Other Therapeutic Substance	C Other Substance N Blood Brain Barrier Disruption
5 Peripheral Artery 6 Central Artery	Ø Open 3 Percutaneous	V Hormone	G Insulin H Human B-type Natriuretic Peptide J Other Hormone
5 Peripheral Artery 6 Central Artery	Ø Open 3 Percutaneous	W Immunotherapeutic	K Immunostimulator L Immunosuppressive
7 Coronary Artery 8 Heart	Ø Open 3 Percutaneous	1 Thrombolytic	6 Recombinant Human- activated Protein C 7 Other Thrombolytic
7 Coronary Artery 8 Heart	Ø Open 3 Percutaneous	G Other Therapeutic Substance	C Other Substance
7 Coronary Artery 8 Heart	Ø Open 3 Percutaneous	K Other Diagnostic Substance P Platelet Inhibitor	Z No Qualifier
7 Coronary Artery 8 Heart	4 Percutaneous Endoscopic	G Other Therapeutic Substance	C Other Substance
9 Nose	3 Percutaneous 7 Via Natural or Artificial Opening X External	Ø Antineoplastic	5 Other Antineoplastic M Monoclonal Antibody
9 Nose	3 Percutaneous 7 Via Natural or Artificial Opening X External	2 Anti-infective	8 Oxazolidinones 9 Other Anti-infective
9 Nose	3 Percutaneous 7 Via Natural or Artificial Opening X External	3 Anti-inflammatory 4 Serum, Toxoid and Vaccine B Anesthetic Agent H Radioactive Substance K Other Diagnostic Substance N Analgesics, Hypnotics, Sedatives T Destructive Agent	Z No Qualifier
9 Nose	3 Percutaneous 7 Via Natural or Artificial Opening X External	G Other Therapeutic Substance	C Other Substance
A Bone Marrow	3 Percutaneous	Ø Antineoplastic	5 Other Antineoplastic M Monoclonal Antibody
A Bone Marrow	3 Percutaneous	G Other Therapeutic Substance	C Other Substance
B Ear	3 Percutaneous 7 Via Natural or Artificial Opening X External	Ø Antineoplastic	4 Liquid Brachytherapy Radioisotope 5 Other Antineoplastic M Monoclonal Antibody
B Ear	3 Percutaneous 7 Via Natural or Artificial Opening X External	2 Anti-infective	8 Oxazolidinones 9 Other Anti-infective
B Ear	3 Percutaneous 7 Via Natural or Artificial Opening X External	3 Anti-inflammatory B Anesthetic Agent H Radioactive Substance K Other Diagnostic Substance N Analgesics, Hypnotics, Sedatives T Destructive Agent	Z No Qualifier
B Ear	3 Percutaneous 7 Via Natural or Artificial Opening X External	G Other Therapeutic Substance	C Other Substance

DRG Non-OR   3E08[Ø,3]17

3EØ Continued on next page

NC Noncovered Procedure   **LC** Limited Coverage   **QA** Questionable OB Admit   **NT** New Tech Add-on   ⊞ Combination Member   ♂ Male   ♀ Female

ICD-10-PCS 2023   721

3EØ-3EØ

Administration

3   **Administration**
E   **Physiological Systems and Anatomical Regions**
Ø   **Introduction**   Definition: Putting in or on a therapeutic, diagnostic, nutritional, physiological, or prophylactic substance except blood or blood products

3EØ Continued

Body System/Region Character 4	Approach Character 5	Substance Character 6	Qualifier Character 7
C Eye	3 Percutaneous 7 Via Natural or Artificial Opening X External	Ø Antineoplastic	4 Liquid Brachytherapy Radioisotope 5 Other Antineoplastic M Monoclonal Antibody
C Eye	3 Percutaneous 7 Via Natural or Artificial Opening X External	2 Anti-infective	8 Oxazolidinones 9 Other Anti-infective
C Eye	3 Percutaneous 7 Via Natural or Artificial Opening X External	3 Anti-inflammatory B Anesthetic Agent H Radioactive Substance K Other Diagnostic Substance M Pigment N Analgesics, Hypnotics, Sedatives T Destructive Agent	Z No Qualifier
C Eye	3 Percutaneous 7 Via Natural or Artificial Opening X External	G Other Therapeutic Substance	C Other Substance
C Eye	3 Percutaneous 7 Via Natural or Artificial Opening X External	S Gas	F Other Gas
D Mouth and Pharynx	3 Percutaneous 7 Via Natural or Artificial Opening X External	Ø Antineoplastic	4 Liquid Brachytherapy Radioisotope 5 Other Antineoplastic M Monoclonal Antibody
D Mouth and Pharynx	3 Percutaneous 7 Via Natural or Artificial Opening X External	2 Anti-infective	8 Oxazolidinones 9 Other Anti-infective
D Mouth and Pharynx	3 Percutaneous 7 Via Natural or Artificial Opening X External	3 Anti-inflammatory 4 Serum, Toxoid and Vaccine 6 Nutritional Substance 7 Electrolytic and Water Balance Substance B Anesthetic Agent H Radioactive Substance K Other Diagnostic Substance N Analgesics, Hypnotics, Sedatives R Antiarrhythmic T Destructive Agent	Z No Qualifier
D Mouth and Pharynx	3 Percutaneous 7 Via Natural or Artificial Opening X External	G Other Therapeutic Substance	C Other Substance
E Products of Conception ♀ G Upper GI H Lower GI K Genitourinary Tract N Male Reproductive ♂	3 Percutaneous 7 Via Natural or Artificial Opening 8 Via Natural or Artificial Opening Endoscopic	Ø Antineoplastic	4 Liquid Brachytherapy Radioisotope 5 Other Antineoplastic M Monoclonal Antibody
E Products of Conception ♀ G Upper GI H Lower GI K Genitourinary Tract N Male Reproductive ♂	3 Percutaneous 7 Via Natural or Artificial Opening 8 Via Natural or Artificial Opening Endoscopic	2 Anti-infective	8 Oxazolidinones 9 Other Anti-infective
E Products of Conception ♀ G Upper GI H Lower GI K Genitourinary Tract N Male Reproductive ♂	3 Percutaneous 7 Via Natural or Artificial Opening 8 Via Natural or Artificial Opening Endoscopic	3 Anti-inflammatory 6 Nutritional Substance 7 Electrolytic and Water Balance Substance B Anesthetic Agent H Radioactive Substance K Other Diagnostic Substance N Analgesics, Hypnotics, Sedatives T Destructive Agent	Z No Qualifier
E Products of Conception ♀ G Upper GI H Lower GI K Genitourinary Tract N Male Reproductive ♂	3 Percutaneous 7 Via Natural or Artificial Opening 8 Via Natural or Artificial Opening Endoscopic	G Other Therapeutic Substance	C Other Substance

♂   All approach, substance, and qualifier values for body system/region (character 4) with this icon
♀   All approach, substance, and qualifier values for body system/region (character 4) with this icon

3EØ Continued on next page

3 Administration
E Physiological Systems and Anatomical Regions
Ø Introduction Definition: Putting in or on a therapeutic, diagnostic, nutritional, physiological, or prophylactic substance except blood or blood products

3EØ Continued

Body System/Region Character 4	Approach Character 5	Substance Character 6	Qualifier Character 7
E Products of Conception ♀ G Upper GI H Lower GI K Genitourinary Tract N Male Reproductive ♂	3 Percutaneous 7 Via Natural or Artificial Opening 8 Via Natural or Artificial Opening Endoscopic	S Gas	F Other Gas
E Products of Conception ♀ G Upper GI H Lower GI K Genitourinary Tract N Male Reproductive ♂	4 Percutaneous Endoscopic	G Other Therapeutic Substance	C Other Substance
F Respiratory Tract	3 Percutaneous 7 Via Natural or Artificial Opening 8 Via Natural or Artificial Opening Endoscopic	Ø Antineoplastic	4 Liquid Brachytherapy Radioisotope 5 Other Antineoplastic M Monoclonal Antibody
F Respiratory Tract	3 Percutaneous 7 Via Natural or Artificial Opening 8 Via Natural or Artificial Opening Endoscopic	2 Anti-infective	8 Oxazolidinones 9 Other Anti-infective
F Respiratory Tract	3 Percutaneous 7 Via Natural or Artificial Opening 8 Via Natural or Artificial Opening Endoscopic	3 Anti-inflammatory 6 Nutritional Substance 7 Electrolytic and Water Balance Substance B Anesthetic Agent H Radioactive Substance K Other Diagnostic Substance N Analgesics, Hypnotics, Sedatives T Destructive Agent	Z No Qualifier
F Respiratory Tract	3 Percutaneous 7 Via Natural or Artificial Opening 8 Via Natural or Artificial Opening Endoscopic	G Other Therapeutic Substance	C Other Substance
F Respiratory Tract	3 Percutaneous 7 Via Natural or Artificial Opening 8 Via Natural or Artificial Opening Endoscopic	S Gas	D Nitric Oxide F Other Gas
F Respiratory Tract	4 Percutaneous Endoscopic	G Other Therapeutic Substance	C Other Substance
J Biliary and Pancreatic Tract	3 Percutaneous 7 Via Natural or Artificial Opening 8 Via Natural or Artificial Opening Endoscopic	Ø Antineoplastic	4 Liquid Brachytherapy Radioisotope 5 Other Antineoplastic M Monoclonal Antibody
J Biliary and Pancreatic Tract	3 Percutaneous 7 Via Natural or Artificial Opening 8 Via Natural or Artificial Opening Endoscopic	2 Anti-infective	8 Oxazolidinones 9 Other Anti-infective
J Biliary and Pancreatic Tract	3 Percutaneous 7 Via Natural or Artificial Opening 8 Via Natural or Artificial Opening Endoscopic	3 Anti-inflammatory 6 Nutritional Substance 7 Electrolytic and Water Balance Substance B Anesthetic Agent H Radioactive Substance K Other Diagnostic Substance N Analgesics, Hypnotics, Sedatives T Destructive Agent	Z No Qualifier
J Biliary and Pancreatic Tract	3 Percutaneous 7 Via Natural or Artificial Opening 8 Via Natural or Artificial Opening Endoscopic	G Other Therapeutic Substance	C Other Substance
J Biliary and Pancreatic Tract	3 Percutaneous 7 Via Natural or Artificial Opening 8 Via Natural or Artificial Opening Endoscopic	S Gas	F Other Gas

♂ All approach, substance, and qualifier values for body system/region (character 4) with this icon
♀ All approach, substance, and qualifier values for body system/region (character 4) with this icon

3EØ Continued on next page

3   Administration
E   Physiological Systems and Anatomical Regions
Ø   Introduction   Definition: Putting in or on a therapeutic, diagnostic, nutritional, physiological, or prophylactic substance except blood or blood products

3EØ Continued

Body System/Region Character 4	Approach Character 5	Substance Character 6	Qualifier Character 7
J Biliary and Pancreatic Tract	3 Percutaneous 7 Via Natural or Artificial Opening 8 Via Natural or Artificial Opening Endoscopic	U Pancreatic Islet Cells	Ø Autologous 1 Nonautologous
J Biliary and Pancreatic Tract	4 Percutaneous Endoscopic	G Other Therapeutic Substance	C Other Substance
L Pleural Cavity	Ø Open	5 Adhesion Barrier	Z No Qualifier
L Pleural Cavity	3 Percutaneous	Ø Antineoplastic	4 Liquid Brachytherapy Radioisotope 5 Other Antineoplastic M Monoclonal Antibody
L Pleural Cavity	3 Percutaneous	2 Anti-infective	8 Oxazolidinones 9 Other Anti-infective
L Pleural Cavity	3 Percutaneous	3 Anti-inflammatory 5 Adhesion Barrier 6 Nutritional Substance 7 Electrolytic and Water Balance Substance B Anesthetic Agent H Radioactive Substance K Other Diagnostic Substance N Analgesics, Hypnotics, Sedatives T Destructive Agent	Z No Qualifier
L Pleural Cavity	3 Percutaneous	G Other Therapeutic Substance	C Other Substance
L Pleural Cavity	3 Percutaneous	S Gas	F Other Gas
L Pleural Cavity	4 Percutaneous Endoscopic	5 Adhesion Barrier	Z No Qualifier
L Pleural Cavity	4 Percutaneous Endoscopic	G Other Therapeutic Substance	C Other Substance
L Pleural Cavity	7 Via Natural or Artificial Opening	Ø Antineoplastic	4 Liquid Brachytherapy Radioisotope 5 Other Antineoplastic M Monoclonal Antibody
L Pleural Cavity	7 Via Natural or Artificial Opening	S Gas	F Other Gas
M Peritoneal Cavity	Ø Open	5 Adhesion Barrier	Z No Qualifier
M Peritoneal Cavity	3 Percutaneous	Ø Antineoplastic	4 Liquid Brachytherapy Radioisotope 5 Other Antineoplastic M Monoclonal Antibody Y Hyperthermic
M Peritoneal Cavity	3 Percutaneous	2 Anti-infective	8 Oxazolidinones 9 Other Anti-infective
M Peritoneal Cavity	3 Percutaneous	3 Anti-inflammatory 5 Adhesion Barrier 6 Nutritional Substance 7 Electrolytic and Water Balance Substance B Anesthetic Agent H Radioactive Substance K Other Diagnostic Substance N Analgesics, Hypnotics, Sedatives T Destructive Agent	Z No Qualifier
M Peritoneal Cavity	3 Percutaneous	G Other Therapeutic Substance	C Other Substance
M Peritoneal Cavity	3 Percutaneous	S Gas	F Other Gas
M Peritoneal Cavity	4 Percutaneous Endoscopic	5 Adhesion Barrier	Z No Qualifier
M Peritoneal Cavity	4 Percutaneous Endoscopic	G Other Therapeutic Substance	C Other Substance
M Peritoneal Cavity	7 Via Natural or Artificial Opening	Ø Antineoplastic	4 Liquid Brachytherapy Radioisotope 5 Other Antineoplastic M Monoclonal Antibody
M Peritoneal Cavity	7 Via Natural or Artificial Opening	S Gas	F Other Gas
P Female Reproductive ♀	Ø Open	5 Adhesion Barrier	Z No Qualifier
P Female Reproductive ♀	3 Percutaneous	Ø Antineoplastic	4 Liquid Brachytherapy Radioisotope 5 Other Antineoplastic M Monoclonal Antibody
P Female Reproductive ♀	3 Percutaneous	2 Anti-infective	8 Oxazolidinones 9 Other Anti-infective

Valid OR	3EØL4GC
DRG Non-OR	3EØJ[3,7,8]U[Ø,1]
♀	All approach, substance, and qualifier values for body system/region (character 4) with this icon

3EØ Continued on next page

Non-OR Procedure   DRG Non-OR Procedure   Valid OR Procedure   HAC Associated Procedure   Combination Only   New/Revised April   New/Revised October

724   ICD-10-PCS 2023

3E0 Continued

3   **Administration**
E   **Physiological Systems and Anatomical Regions**
Ø   **Introduction**   Definition: Putting in or on a therapeutic, diagnostic, nutritional, physiological, or prophylactic substance except blood or blood products

Body System/Region Character 4		Approach Character 5	Substance Character 6	Qualifier Character 7
P	Female Reproductive ♀	3 Percutaneous	3 Anti-inflammatory 5 Adhesion Barrier 6 Nutritional Substance 7 Electrolytic and Water Balance Substance B Anesthetic Agent H Radioactive Substance K Other Diagnostic Substance L Sperm N Analgesics, Hypnotics, Sedatives T Destructive Agent V Hormone	Z No Qualifier
P	Female Reproductive ♀	3 Percutaneous	G Other Therapeutic Substance	C Other Substance
P	Female Reproductive ♀	3 Percutaneous	Q Fertilized Ovum	Ø Autologous 1 Nonautologous
P	Female Reproductive ♀	3 Percutaneous	S Gas	F Other Gas
P	Female Reproductive ♀	4 Percutaneous Endoscopic	5 Adhesion Barrier	Z No Qualifier
P	Female Reproductive ♀	4 Percutaneous Endoscopic	G Other Therapeutic Substance	C Other Substance
P	Female Reproductive ♀	7 Via Natural or Artificial Opening	Ø Antineoplastic	4 Liquid Brachytherapy Radioisotope 5 Other Antineoplastic M Monoclonal Antibody
P	Female Reproductive ♀	7 Via Natural or Artificial Opening	2 Anti-infective	8 Oxazolidinones 9 Other Anti-infective
P	Female Reproductive ♀	7 Via Natural or Artificial Opening	3 Anti-inflammatory 6 Nutritional Substance 7 Electrolytic and Water Balance Substance B Anesthetic Agent H Radioactive Substance K Other Diagnostic Substance L Sperm N Analgesics, Hypnotics, Sedatives T Destructive Agent V Hormone	Z No Qualifier
P	Female Reproductive ♀	7 Via Natural or Artificial Opening	G Other Therapeutic Substance	C Other Substance
P	Female Reproductive ♀	7 Via Natural or Artificial Opening	Q Fertilized Ovum	Ø Autologous 1 Nonautologous
P	Female Reproductive ♀	7 Via Natural or Artificial Opening	S Gas	F Other Gas
P	Female Reproductive ♀	8 Via Natural or Artificial Opening Endoscopic	Ø Antineoplastic	4 Liquid Brachytherapy Radioisotope 5 Other Antineoplastic M Monoclonal Antibody
P	Female Reproductive ♀	8 Via Natural or Artificial Opening Endoscopic	2 Anti-infective	8 Oxazolidinones 9 Other Anit-infective
P	Female Reproductive ♀	8 Via Natural or Artificial Opening Endoscopic	3 Anti-inflammatory 6 Nutritional Substance 7 Electrolytic and Water Balance Substance B Anesthetic Agent H Radioactive Substance K Other Diagnostic Substance N Analgesics, Hypnotics, Sedatives T Destructive Agent	Z No Qualifier
P	Female Reproductive ♀	8 Via Natural or Artificial Opening Endoscopic	G Other Therapeutic Substance	C Other Substance
P	Female Reproductive ♀	8 Via Natural or Artificial Opening Endoscopic	S Gas	F Other Gas
Q	Cranial Cavity and Brain	Ø Open 3 Percutaneous	Ø Antineoplastic	4 Liquid Brachytherapy Radioisotope 5 Other Antineoplastic M Monoclonal Antibody
Q	Cranial Cavity and Brain	Ø Open 3 Percutaneous	2 Anti-infective	8 Oxazolidinones 9 Other Anti-infective

Valid OR   3E0P3Q[Ø,1]
Valid OR   3E0P7Q[Ø,1]
DRG Non-OR   3E0Q[Ø,3]05
♀   All approach, substance, and qualifier values for body system/region (character 4) with this icon

3E0 Continued on next page

3   Administration
E   Physiological Systems and Anatomical Regions
Ø   Introduction   Definition: Putting in or on a therapeutic, diagnostic, nutritional, physiological, or prophylactic substance except blood or blood products

Body System/Region Character 4	Approach Character 5	Substance Character 6	Qualifier Character 7
Q Cranial Cavity and Brain	Ø Open 3 Percutaneous	3 Anti-inflammatory 6 Nutritional Substance 7 Electrolytic and Water Balance Substance A Stem Cells, Embryonic B Anesthetic Agent H Radioactive Substance K Other Diagnostic Substance N Analgesics, Hypnotics, Sedatives T Destructive Agent	Z No Qualifier
Q Cranial Cavity and Brain	Ø Open 3 Percutaneous	E Stem Cells, Somatic	Ø Autologous 1 Nonautologous
Q Cranial Cavity and Brain	Ø Open 3 Percutaneous	G Other Therapeutic Substance	C Other Substance
Q Cranial Cavity and Brain	Ø Open 3 Percutaneous	S Gas	F Other Gas
Q Cranial Cavity and Brain	7 Via Natural or Artificial Opening	Ø Antineoplastic	4 Liquid Brachytherapy Radioisotope 5 Other Antineoplastic M Monoclonal Antibody
Q Cranial Cavity and Brain	7 Via Natural or Artificial Opening	S Gas	F Other Gas
R Spinal Canal	Ø Open	A Stem Cells, Embryonic	Z No Qualifier
R Spinal Canal	Ø Open	E Stem Cells, Somatic	Ø Autologous 1 Nonautologous
R Spinal Canal	3 Percutaneous	Ø Antineoplastic	2 High-dose Interleukin-2 3 Low-dose Interleukin-2 4 Liquid Brachytherapy Radioisotope 5 Other Antineoplastic M Monoclonal Antibody
R Spinal Canal	3 Percutaneous	2 Anti-infective	8 Oxazolidinones 9 Other Anti-infective
R Spinal Canal	3 Percutaneous	3 Anti-inflammatory 6 Nutritional Substance 7 Electrolytic and Water Balance Substance A Stem Cells, Embryonic B Anesthetic Agent H Radioactive Substance K Other Diagnostic Substance N Analgesics, Hypnotics, Sedatives T Destructive Agent	Z No Qualifier
R Spinal Canal	3 Percutaneous	E Stem Cells, Somatic	Ø Autologous 1 Nonautologous
R Spinal Canal	3 Percutaneous	G Other Therapeutic Substance	C Other Substance
R Spinal Canal	3 Percutaneous	S Gas	F Other Gas
R Spinal Canal	7 Via Natural or Artificial Opening	S Gas	F Other Gas
S Epidural Space	3 Percutaneous	Ø Antineoplastic	2 High-dose Interleukin-2 3 Low-dose Interleukin-2 4 Liquid Brachytherapy Radioisotope 5 Other Antineoplastic M Monoclonal Antibody
S Epidural Space	3 Percutaneous	2 Anti-infective	8 Oxazolidinones 9 Other Anti-infective
S Epidural Space	3 Percutaneous	3 Anti-inflammatory 6 Nutritional Substance 7 Electrolytic and Water Balance Substance B Anesthetic Agent H Radioactive Substance K Other Diagnostic Substance N Analgesics, Hypnotics, Sedatives T Destructive Agent	Z No Qualifier

DRG Non-OR   3EØQ7Ø5
DRG Non-OR   3EØR3Ø2
DRG Non-OR   3EØS3Ø2

3EØ Continued on next page

Non-OR Procedure   DRG Non-OR Procedure   Valid OR Procedure   HAC Associated Procedure   Combination Only   New/Revised April   New/Revised October

3E0 Continued

3   **Administration**
E   **Physiological Systems and Anatomical Regions**
0   **Introduction**   Definition: Putting in or on a therapeutic, diagnostic, nutritional, physiological, or prophylactic substance except blood or blood products

Body System/Region Character 4	Approach Character 5	Substance Character 6	Qualifier Character 7
S Epidural Space	3 Percutaneous	G Other Therapeutic Substance	C Other Substance
S Epidural Space	3 Percutaneous	S Gas	F Other Gas
S Epidural Space	7 Via Natural or Artificial Opening	S Gas	F Other Gas
T Peripheral Nerves and Plexi X Cranial Nerves	3 Percutaneous	3 Anti-inflammatory B Anesthetic Agent T Destructive Agent	Z No Qualifier
T Peripheral Nerves and Plexi X Cranial Nerves	3 Percutaneous	G Other Therapeutic Substance	C Other Substance
U Joints	0 Open	2 Anti-infective	8 Oxazolidinones 9 Other Anti-infective
U Joints	0 Open	G Other Therapeutic Substance	B Recombinant Bone Morphogenetic Protein
U Joints	3 Percutaneous	0 Antineoplastic	4 Liquid Brachytherapy Radioisotope 5 Other Antineoplastic M Monoclonal Antibody
U Joints	3 Percutaneous	2 Anti-infective	8 Oxazolidinones 9 Other Anti-infective
U Joints	3 Percutaneous	3 Anti-inflammatory 6 Nutritional Substance 7 Electrolytic and Water Balance Substance B Anesthetic Agent H Radioactive Substance K Other Diagnostic Substance N Analgesics, Hypnotics, Sedatives T Destructive Agent	Z No Qualifier
U Joints	3 Percutaneous	G Other Therapeutic Substance	B Recombinant Bone Morphogenetic Protein C Other Substance
U Joints	3 Percutaneous	S Gas	F Other Gas
U Joints	4 Percutaneous Endoscopic	G Other Therapeutic Substance	C Other Substance
V Bones	0 Open	G Other Therapeutic Substance	B Recombinant Bone Morphogenetic Protein C Other Substance
V Bones	3 Percutaneous	0 Antineoplastic	5 Other Antineoplastic M Monoclonal Antibody
V Bones	3 Percutaneous	2 Anti-infective	8 Oxazolidinones 9 Other Anti-infective
V Bones	3 Percutaneous	3 Anti-inflammatory 6 Nutritional Substance 7 Electrolytic and Water Balance Substance B Anesthetic Agent H Radioactive Substance K Other Diagnostic Substance N Analgesics, Hypnotics, Sedatives T Destructive Agent	Z No Qualifier
V Bones	3 Percutaneous	G Other Therapeutic Substance	B Recombinant Bone Morphogenetic Protein C Other Substance
V Bones	4 Percutaneous Endoscopic	G Other Therapeutic Substance	C Other Substance
W Lymphatics	3 Percutaneous	0 Antineoplastic	5 Other Antineoplastic M Monoclonal Antibody
W Lymphatics	3 Percutaneous	2 Anti-infective	8 Oxazolidinones 9 Other Anti-infective
W Lymphatics	3 Percutaneous	3 Anti-inflammatory 6 Nutritional Substance 7 Electrolytic and Water Balance Substance B Anesthetic Agent H Radioactive Substance K Other Diagnostic Substance N Analgesics, Hypnotics, Sedatives T Destructive Agent	Z No Qualifier
W Lymphatics	3 Percutaneous	G Other Therapeutic Substance	C Other Substance

3E0 Continued on next page

3   Administration
E   Physiological Systems and Anatomical Regions
0   Introduction   Definition: Putting in or on a therapeutic, diagnostic, nutritional, physiological, or prophylactic substance except blood or blood products

3E0 Continued

Body System/Region Character 4	Approach Character 5	Substance Character 6	Qualifier Character 7
Y Pericardial Cavity	3 Percutaneous	0 Antineoplastic	4 Liquid Brachytherapy Radioisotope 5 Other Antineoplastic M Monoclonal Antibody
Y Pericardial Cavity	3 Percutaneous	2 Anti-infective	8 Oxazolidinones 9 Other Anti-infective
Y Pericardial Cavity	3 Percutaneous	3 Anti-inflammatory 6 Nutritional Substance 7 Electrolytic and Water Balance Substance B Anesthetic Agent H Radioactive Substance K Other Diagnostic Substance N Analgesics, Hypnotics, Sedatives T Destructive Agent	Z No Qualifier
Y Pericardial Cavity	3 Percutaneous	G Other Therapeutic Substance	C Other Substance
Y Pericardial Cavity	3 Percutaneous	S Gas	F Other Gas
Y Pericardial Cavity	4 Percutaneous Endoscopic	G Other Therapeutic Substance	C Other Substance
Y Pericardial Cavity	7 Via Natural or Artificial Opening	0 Antineoplastic	4 Liquid Brachytherapy Radioisotope 5 Other Antineoplastic M Monoclonal Antibody
Y Pericardial Cavity	7 Via Natural or Artificial Opening	S Gas	F Other Gas

3   Administration
E   Physiological Systems and Anatomical Regions
1   Irrigation   Definition: Putting in or on a cleansing substance

Body System/Region Character 4	Approach Character 5	Substance Character 6	Qualifier Character 7
0 Skin and Mucous Membranes C Eye	3 Percutaneous X External	8 Irrigating Substance	X Diagnostic Z No Qualifier
9 Nose B Ear F Respiratory Tract G Upper GI H Lower GI J Biliary and Pancreatic Tract K Genitourinary Tract N Male Reproductive ♂ P Female Reproductive ♀	3 Percutaneous 7 Via Natural or Artificial Opening 8 Via Natural or Artificial Opening Endoscopic	8 Irrigating Substance	X Diagnostic Z No Qualifier
L Pleural Cavity Q Cranial Cavity and Brain R Spinal Canal S Epidural Space Y Pericardial Cavity	3 Percutaneous	8 Irrigating Substance	X Diagnostic Z No Qualifier
M Peritoneal Cavity	3 Percutaneous	8 Irrigating Substance	X Diagnostic Z No Qualifier
M Peritoneal Cavity	3 Percutaneous	9 Dialysate	Z No Qualifier
M Peritoneal Cavity	4 Percutaneous Endoscopic	8 Irrigating Substance	X Diagnostic Z No Qualifier
U Joints	3 Percutaneous 4 Percutaneous Endoscopic	8 Irrigating Substance	X Diagnostic Z No Qualifier

♂   3E1N[3,7,8]8[X,Z]
♀   3E1P[3,7,8]8[X,Z]

Non-OR Procedure   DRG Non-OR Procedure   Valid OR Procedure   HAC Associated Procedure   Combination Only   New/Revised April   New/Revised October

728   ICD-10-PCS 2023

Measurement and Monitoring 4A0–4B0

AHA Coding Clinic for table 4A0

2022, 1Q, 46	Internal cardioversion
2020, 4Q, 62	Measurement of intracranial arterial flow
2020, 4Q, 62	Percutaneous endoscopic measurement of portal venous pressure
2020, 4Q, 63	Intercompartmental pressure measurement
2019, 3Q, 32	Endomyocardial biopsy and right heart catheterization
2018, 1Q, 12	Percutaneous balloon valvuloplasty & cardiac catheterization with ventriculogram
2016, 3Q, 37	Fractional flow reserve
2015, 3Q, 29	Approach value for esophageal electrophysiology study

AHA Coding Clinic for table 4B0

2021, 4Q, 55-56	Measurement of flow in a cerebral fluid shunt

AHA Coding Clinic for table 4A1

2019, 4Q, 38-39	Intraoperative fluorescence lymphatic mapping using Indocyanine green dye
2016, 4Q, 114	Fluorescence vascular angiography
2016, 2Q, 29	Decompressive craniectomy with cryopreservation and storage of bone flap
2016, 2Q, 33	Monitoring of arterial pressure & pulse
2015, 3Q, 35	Swan Ganz catheterization
2015, 2Q, 14	Intraoperative EMG monitoring via endotracheal tube
2015, 1Q, 26	Intraoperative monitoring using Sentio MMG®
2014, 4Q, 28	Removal and replacement of displaced growing rods

4   Measurement and Monitoring
A   Physiological Systems
0   Measurement   Definition: Determining the level of a physiological or physical function at a point in time

Body System Character 4	Approach Character 5	Function/Device Character 6	Qualifier Character 7
0 Central Nervous	0 Open	2 Conductivity 4 Electrical Activity B Pressure	Z No Qualifier
0 Central Nervous	3 Percutaneous 7 Via Natural or Artificial Opening 8 Via Natural or Artificial Opening Endoscopic	4 Electrical Activity	Z No Qualifier
0 Central Nervous	3 Percutaneous 7 Via Natural or Artificial Opening 8 Via Natural or Artificial Opening Endoscopic	B Pressure K Temperature R Saturation	D Intracranial
0 Central Nervous	X External	2 Conductivity 4 Electrical Activity	Z No Qualifier
1 Peripheral Nervous	0 Open 3 Percutaneous 7 Via Natural or Artificial Opening 8 Via Natural or Artificial Opening Endoscopic X External	2 Conductivity	9 Sensory B Motor
1 Peripheral Nervous	0 Open 3 Percutaneous 7 Via Natural or Artificial Opening 8 Via Natural or Artificial Opening Endoscopic X External	4 Electrical Activity	Z No Qualifier
2 Cardiac	0 Open 3 Percutaneous 7 Via Natural or Artificial Opening 8 Via Natural or Artificial Opening Endoscopic	4 Electrical Activity 9 Output C Rate F Rhythm H Sound P Action Currents	Z No Qualifier
2 Cardiac	0 Open 3 Percutaneous 7 Via Natural or Artificial Opening 8 Via Natural or Artificial Opening Endoscopic	N Sampling and Pressure	6 Right Heart 7 Left Heart 8 Bilateral
2 Cardiac	X External	4 Electrical Activity	A Guidance Z No Qualifier
2 Cardiac	X External	9 Output C Rate F Rhythm H Sound P Action Currents	Z No Qualifier
2 Cardiac	X External	M Total Activity	4 Stress
3 Arterial	0 Open 3 Percutaneous	5 Flow J Pulse	1 Peripheral 3 Pulmonary C Coronary
3 Arterial	0 Open 3 Percutaneous	B Pressure	1 Peripheral 3 Pulmonary C Coronary F Other Thoracic

DRG Non-OR	4A02[3,7,8]FZ
DRG Non-OR	4A02[0,3,7,8]N[6,7,8]

4A0 Continued on next page

NC Noncovered Procedure   LC Limited Coverage   QA Questionable OB Admit   NT New Tech Add-on   ⊞ Combination Member   ♂ Male   ♀ Female

ICD-10-PCS 2023   729

4 Measurement and Monitoring
A Physiological Systems
Ø Measurement   Definition: Determining the level of a physiological or physical function at a point in time

Body System Character 4	Approach Character 5	Function/Device Character 6	Qualifier Character 7
3 Arterial	Ø Open 3 Percutaneous	H Sound R Saturation	1 Peripheral
3 Arterial	X External	5 Flow	1 Peripheral D Intracranial
3 Arterial	X External	B Pressure H Sound J Pulse R Saturation	1 Peripheral
4 Venous	Ø Open 3 Percutaneous	5 Flow B Pressure J Pulse	Ø Central 1 Peripheral 2 Portal 3 Pulmonary
4 Venous	Ø Open 3 Percutaneous	R Saturation	1 Peripheral
4 Venous	4 Percutaneous Endoscopic	B Pressure	2 Portal
4 Venous	X External	5 Flow B Pressure J Pulse R Saturation	1 Peripheral
5 Circulatory	X External	L Volume	Z No Qualifier
6 Lymphatic	Ø Open 3 Percutaneous 7 Via Natural or Artificial Opening 8 Via Natural or Artificial Opening Endoscopic	5 Flow B Pressure	Z No Qualifier
7 Visual	X External	Ø Acuity 7 Mobility B Pressure	Z No Qualifier
8 Olfactory	X External	Ø Acuity	Z No Qualifier
9 Respiratory	7 Via Natural or Artificial Opening 8 Via Natural or Artificial Opening Endoscopic X External	1 Capacity 5 Flow C Rate D Resistance L Volume M Total Activity	Z No Qualifier
B Gastrointestinal	7 Via Natural or Artificial Opening 8 Via Natural or Artificial Opening Endoscopic	8 Motility B Pressure G Secretion	Z No Qualifier
C Biliary	3 Percutaneous 4 Percutaneous Endoscopic 7 Via Natural or Artificial Opening 8 Via Natural or Artificial Opening Endoscopic	5 Flow B Pressure	Z No Qualifier
D Urinary	7 Via Natural or Artificial Opening 8 Via Natural or Artificial Opening Endoscopic	3 Contractility 5 Flow B Pressure D Resistance L Volume	Z No Qualifier
F Musculoskeletal	3 Percutaneous	3 Contractility	Z No Qualifier
F Musculoskeletal	3 Percutaneous	B Pressure	E Compartment
F Musculoskeletal	X External	3 Contractility	Z No Qualifier
H Products of Conception, ♀ Cardiac	7 Via Natural or Artificial Opening 8 Via Natural or Artificial Opening Endoscopic X External	4 Electrical Activity C Rate F Rhythm H Sound	Z No Qualifier
J Products of Conception, ♀ Nervous	7 Via Natural or Artificial Opening 8 Via Natural or Artificial Opening Endoscopic X External	2 Conductivity 4 Electrical Activity B Pressure	Z No Qualifier
Z None	7 Via Natural or Artificial Opening	6 Metabolism K Temperature	Z No Qualifier
Z None	X External	6 Metabolism K Temperature Q Sleep	Z No Qualifier

Valid OR   4AØ6Ø[5,B]Z   ♀   4AØH[7,8,X][4,C,F,H]Z
Valid OR   4AØC4[5,B]Z   ♀   4AØJ[7,8,X][2,4,B]Z

Non-OR Procedure   DRG Non-OR Procedure   Valid OR Procedure   HAC Associated Procedure   Combination Only   New/Revised April   New/Revised October

4AØ Continued on next page

4   Measurement and Monitoring
A   Physiological Systems
1   Monitoring   Definition: Determining the level of a physiological or physical function repetitively over a period of time

Body System Character 4	Approach Character 5	Function/Device Character 6	Qualifier Character 7
Ø Central Nervous	Ø Open	2 Conductivity B Pressure	Z No Qualifier
Ø Central Nervous	Ø Open	4 Electrical Activity	G Intraoperative Z No Qualifier
Ø Central Nervous	3 Percutaneous 7 Via Natural or Artificial Opening 8 Via Natural or Artificial Opening Endoscopic	4 Electrical Activity	G Intraoperative Z No Qualifier
Ø Central Nervous	3 Percutaneous 7 Via Natural or Artificial Opening 8 Via Natural or Artificial Opening Endoscopic	B Pressure K Temperature R Saturation	D Intracranial
Ø Central Nervous	X External	2 Conductivity	Z No Qualifier
Ø Central Nervous	X External	4 Electrical Activity	G Intraoperative Z No Qualifier
1 Peripheral Nervous	Ø Open 3 Percutaneous 7 Via Natural or Artificial Opening 8 Via Natural or Artificial Opening Endoscopic X External	2 Conductivity	9 Sensory B Motor
1 Peripheral Nervous	Ø Open 3 Percutaneous 7 Via Natural or Artificial Opening 8 Via Natural or Artificial Opening Endoscopic X External	4 Electrical Activity	G Intraoperative Z No Qualifier
2 Cardiac	Ø Open 3 Percutaneous 7 Via Natural or Artificial Opening 8 Via Natural or Artificial Opening Endoscopic	4 Electrical Activity 9 Output C Rate F Rhythm H Sound	Z No Qualifier
2 Cardiac	X External	4 Electrical Activity	5 Ambulatory Z No Qualifier
2 Cardiac	X External	9 Output C Rate F Rhythm H Sound	Z No Qualifier
2 Cardiac	X External	M Total Activity	4 Stress
2 Cardiac	X External	S Vascular Perfusion	H Indocyanine Green Dye
3 Arterial	Ø Open 3 Percutaneous	5 Flow B Pressure J Pulse	1 Peripheral 3 Pulmonary C Coronary
3 Arterial	Ø Open 3 Percutaneous	H Sound R Saturation	1 Peripheral
3 Arterial	X External	5 Flow B Pressure H Sound J Pulse R Saturation	1 Peripheral
4 Venous	Ø Open 3 Percutaneous	5 Flow B Pressure J Pulse	Ø Central 1 Peripheral 2 Portal 3 Pulmonary
4 Venous	Ø Open 3 Percutaneous	R Saturation	Ø Central 2 Portal 3 Pulmonary
4 Venous	X External	5 Flow B Pressure J Pulse	1 Peripheral
6 Lymphatic	Ø Open 3 Percutaneous 7 Via Natural or Artificial Opening 8 Via Natural or Artificial Opening Endoscopic	5 Flow	H Indocyanine Green Dye Z No Qualifier

Valid OR   4A1605Z

4A1 Continued on next page

NC Noncovered Procedure   LC Limited Coverage   QA Questionable OB Admit   NT New Tech Add-on   ⊞ Combination Member   ♂ Male   ♀ Female

ICD-10-PCS 2023   731

4 Measurement and Monitoring
A Physiological Systems
1 Monitoring   Definition: Determining the level of a physiological or physical function repetitively over a period of time

Body System Character 4	Approach Character 5	Function/Device Character 6	Qualifier Character 7
6 Lymphatic	Ø Open 3 Percutaneous 7 Via Natural or Artificial Opening 8 Via Natural or Artificial Opening Endoscopic	B Pressure	Z No Qualifier
9 Respiratory	7 Via Natural or Artificial Opening X External	1 Capacity 5 Flow C Rate D Resistance L Volume	Z No Qualifier
B Gastrointestinal	7 Via Natural or Artificial Opening 8 Via Natural or Artificial Opening Endoscopic	8 Motility B Pressure G Secretion	Z No Qualifier
B Gastrointestinal	X External	S Vascular Perfusion	H Indocyanine Green Dye
D Urinary	7 Via Natural or Artificial Opening 8 Via Natural or Artificial Opening Endoscopic	3 Contractility 5 Flow B Pressure D Resistance L Volume	Z No Qualifier
G Skin and Breast	X External	S Vascular Perfusion	H Indocyanine Green Dye
H Products of Conception, ♀ Cardiac	7 Via Natural or Artificial Opening 8 Via Natural or Artificial Opening Endoscopic X External	4 Electrical Activity C Rate F Rhythm H Sound	Z No Qualifier
J Products of Conception, ♀ Nervous	7 Via Natural or Artificial Opening 8 Via Natural or Artificial Opening Endoscopic X External	2 Conductivity 4 Electrical Activity B Pressure	Z No Qualifier
Z None	7 Via Natural or Artificial Opening	K Temperature	Z No Qualifier
Z None	X External	K Temperature Q Sleep	Z No Qualifier

Valid OR 4A16ØBZ
♀   4A1H[7,8,X][4,C,F,H]Z
♀   4A1J[7,8,X][2,4,B]Z

4 Measurement and Monitoring
B Physiological Devices
Ø Measurement   Definition: Determining the level of a physiological or physical function at a point in time

Body System Character 4	Approach Character 5	Function/Device Character 6	Qualifier Character 7
Ø Central Nervous	X External	V Stimulator	Z No Qualifier
Ø Central Nervous	X External	W Cerebrospinal Fluid Shunt	Ø Wireless Sensor
1 Peripheral Nervous F Musculoskeletal	X External	V Stimulator	Z No Qualifier
2 Cardiac	X External	S Pacemaker T Defibrillator	Z No Qualifier
9 Respiratory	X External	S Pacemaker	Z No Qualifier

Non-OR Procedure   DRG Non-OR Procedure   Valid OR Procedure   HAC Associated Procedure   Combination Only   New/Revised April   New/Revised October

Extracorporeal or Systemic Assistance and Performance 5A0–5A2

AHA Coding Clinic for table 5A0

2021, 2Q, 12	Repositioning of displaced intra-aortic balloon pump
2020, 4Q, 64-65	Ventilatory assistance by high flow or high velocity nasal cannula devices
2020, 1Q, 10	Intermittent use of continuous positive airway pressure
2018, 2Q, 3-5	Intra-aortic balloon pump
2017, 4Q, 43-44	Insertion of external heart assist devices
2017, 3Q, 18	Intra-aortic balloon pump removal
2017, 1Q, 10-11	External heart assist device
2017, 1Q, 29	Newborn resuscitation using positive pressure ventilation
2017, 1Q, 29	Newborn noninvasive ventilation
2016, 4Q, 137-139	Heart assist device systems
2014, 4Q, 9	Mechanical ventilation
2014, 3Q, 19	Ablation of ventricular tachycardia with Impella® support
2013, 3Q, 18	Heart transplant surgery

AHA Coding Clinic for table 5A1

2022, 2Q, 25	Temporary-permanent pacemaker placement
2021, 4Q, 56	Automated chest compression
2019, 4Q, 39-41	Intraoperative extracorporeal membrane oxygenation
2019, 3Q, 19	Insertion of left ventricular catheter
2019, 3Q, 20	Removal and revision of ECMO component
2019, 3Q, 21	Exchange of extracorporeal membrane oxygenation component (oxygenator)

AHA Coding Clinic for table 5A1 (Continued)

2019, 2Q, 36	Veno-arterial extracorporeal membrane oxygenation via sternotomy
2019, 3Q, 22	Extracorporeal membrane oxygenation and Centrimag™ pump
2019, 3Q, 22	Extracorporeal membrane oxygenation transfers
2018, 4Q, 52-54	Percutaneous extracorporeal membrane oxygenation
2018, 1Q, 13	Mechanical ventilation using patient's equipment
2017, 4Q, 71-73	Hemodialysis and renal replacement therapy
2017, 3Q, 7	Senning procedure (arterial switch)
2017, 1Q, 19	Norwood Sano procedure
2016, 1Q, 27	Aortocoronary bypass graft utilizing Y-graft
2016, 1Q, 28	Extracorporeal liver assist device
2016, 1Q, 29	Duration of hemodialysis
2015, 4Q, 22-24	Congenital heart corrective procedures
2014, 4Q, 3-10	Mechanical ventilation
2014, 4Q, 11-15	Sequencing of mechanical ventilation with other procedures
2014, 3Q, 16	Repair of Tetralogy of Fallot
2014, 3Q, 20	MAZE procedure performed with coronary artery bypass graft
2014, 1Q, 10	Repair of thoracic aortic aneurysm & coronary artery bypass graft
2013, 3Q, 18	Heart transplant surgery

AHA Coding Clinic for table 5A2

2022, 1Q, 46	Internal cardioversion

5   **Extracorporeal or Systemic Assistance and Performance**
A   **Physiological Systems**
0   **Assistance**   Definition: Taking over a portion of a physiological function by extracorporeal means

Body System Character 4	Duration Character 5	Function Character 6	Qualifier Character 7
2 Cardiac	**1** Intermittent	**1** Output	**0** Balloon Pump **5** Pulsatile Compression **6** Other Pump **D** Impeller Pump
2 Cardiac	**2** Continuous	**1** Output	**0** Balloon Pump **5** Pulsatile Compression **6** Other Pump **D** Impeller Pump
2 Cardiac	**2** Continuous	**2** Oxygenation	**C** Supersaturated
5 Circulatory	**1** Intermittent **2** Continuous	**2** Oxygenation	**1** Hyperbaric
9 Respiratory	**2** Continuous	**0** Filtration	**Z** No Qualifier
9 Respiratory	**3** Less than 24 Consecutive Hours **4** 24-96 Consecutive Hours **5** Greater than 96 Consecutive Hours	**5** Ventilation	**7** Continuous Positive Airway Pressure **8** Intermittent Positive Airway Pressure **9** Continuous Negative Airway Pressure **A** High Nasal Flow/Velocity **B** Intermittent Negative Airway Pressure **Z** No Qualifier

Valid OR	5A0211[0,6,D]
Valid OR	5A0221[0,6,D]

NC Noncovered Procedure   **LC** Limited Coverage   **QA** Questionable OB Admit   **NT** New Tech Add-on   ⊞ Combination Member   ♂Male   ♀Female

ICD-10-PCS 2023   733

5 **Extracorporeal or Systemic Assistance and Performance**
A **Physiological Systems**
1 **Performance** Definition: Completely taking over a physiological function by extracorporeal means

Body System Character 4	Duration Character 5	Function Character 6	Qualifier Character 7
2 Cardiac	Ø Single	1 Output	2 Manual
2 Cardiac	1 Intermittent	3 Pacing	Z No Qualifier
2 Cardiac	2 Continuous	1 Output	J Automated Z No Qualifier
2 Cardiac	2 Continuous	3 Pacing	Z No Qualifier
5 Circulatory	2 Continuous A Intraoperative	2 Oxygenation	F Membrane, Central G Membrane, Peripheral Veno-arterial H Membrane, Peripheral Veno-venous
9 Respiratory	Ø Single	5 Ventilation	4 Nonmechanical
9 Respiratory	3 Less than 24 Consecutive Hours 4 24-96 Consecutive Hours 5 Greater than 96 Consecutive Hours	5 Ventilation	Z No Qualifier
C Biliary	Ø Single 6 Multiple	Ø Filtration	Z No Qualifier
D Urinary	7 Intermittent, Less than 6 Hours per day 8 Prolonged Intermittent, 6-18 Hours per day 9 Continuous, Greater than 18 Hours per day	Ø Filtration	Z No Qualifier

Valid OR	5A1522F
DRG Non-OR	5A1522[G,H]
DRG Non-OR	5A19[3,4]5Z
DRG Non-OR	5A1955Z Length of stay must be > 4 consecutive days.
DRG Non-OR	5A1D[7,8,9]ØZ

5 **Extracorporeal or Systemic Assistance and Performance**
A **Physiological Systems**
2 **Restoration** Definition: Returning, or attempting to return, a physiological function to its original state by extracorporeal means.

Body System Character 4	Duration Character 5	Function Character 6	Qualifier Character 7
2 Cardiac	Ø Single	4 Rhythm	Z No Qualifier

Extracorporeal or Systemic Therapies 6A0–6AB

AHA Coding Clinic for table 6A4
2019, 2Q, 17   Cryoamputation of lower leg

AHA Coding Clinic for table 6A5
2022, 1Q, 48   Umbilical cord blood sampling

AHA Coding Clinic for table 6A7
2014, 4Q, 19   Ultrasound accelerated thrombolysis

AHA Coding Clinic for table 6AB
2016, 4Q, 115   Donor organ perfusion

6   **Extracorporeal or Systemic Therapies**
A   **Physiological Systems**
0   **Atmospheric Control**   Definition: Extracorporeal control of atmospheric pressure and composition

Body System Character 4	Duration Character 5	Qualifier Character 6	Qualifier Character 7
Z None	0 Single 1 Multiple	Z No Qualifier	Z No Qualifier

6   **Extracorporeal or Systemic Therapies**
A   **Physiological Systems**
1   **Decompression**   Definition: Extracorporeal elimination of undissolved gas from body fluids

Body System Character 4	Duration Character 5	Qualifier Character 6	Qualifier Character 7
5 Circulatory	0 Single 1 Multiple	Z No Qualifier	Z No Qualifier

6   **Extracorporeal or Systemic Therapies**
A   **Physiological Systems**
2   **Electromagnetic Therapy**   Definition: Extracorporeal treatment by electromagnetic rays

Body System Character 4	Duration Character 5	Qualifier Character 6	Qualifier Character 7
1 Urinary 2 Central Nervous	0 Single 1 Multiple	Z No Qualifier	Z No Qualifier

6   **Extracorporeal or Systemic Therapies**
A   **Physiological Systems**
3   **Hyperthermia**   Definition: Extracorporeal raising of body temperature

Body System Character 4	Duration Character 5	Qualifier Character 6	Qualifier Character 7
Z None	0 Single 1 Multiple	Z No Qualifier	Z No Qualifier

6   **Extracorporeal or Systemic Therapies**
A   **Physiological Systems**
4   **Hypothermia**   Definition: Extracorporeal lowering of body temperature

Body System Character 4	Duration Character 5	Qualifier Character 6	Qualifier Character 7
Z None	0 Single 1 Multiple	Z No Qualifier	Z No Qualifier

6   **Extracorporeal or Systemic Therapies**
A   **Physiological Systems**
5   **Pheresis**   Definition: Extracorporeal separation of blood products

Body System Character 4	Duration Character 5	Qualifier Character 6	Qualifier Character 7
5 Circulatory	0 Single 1 Multiple	Z No Qualifier	0 Erythrocytes 1 Leukocytes 2 Platelets 3 Plasma T Stem Cells, Cord Blood V Stem Cells, Hematopoietic

---

NC Noncovered Procedure   LC Limited Coverage   QA Questionable OB Admit   NT New Tech Add-on   ⊞ Combination Member   ♂ Male   ♀ Female

6   Extracorporeal or Systemic Therapies
A   Physiological Systems
6   Phototherapy   Definition: Extracorporeal treatment by light rays

Body System Character 4	Duration Character 5	Qualifier Character 6	Qualifier Character 7
Ø Skin 5 Circulatory	Ø Single 1 Multiple	Z No Qualifier	Z No Qualifier

6   Extracorporeal or Systemic Therapies
A   Physiological Systems
7   Ultrasound Therapy   Definition: Extracorporeal treatment by ultrasound

Body System Character 4	Duration Character 5	Qualifier Character 6	Qualifier Character 7
5 Circulatory	Ø Single 1 Multiple	Z No Qualifier	4 Head and Neck Vessels 5 Heart 6 Peripheral Vessels 7 Other Vessels Z No Qualifier

6   Extracorporeal or Systemic Therapies
A   Physiological Systems
8   Ultraviolet Light Therapy   Definition: Extracorporeal treatment by ultraviolet light

Body System Character 4	Duration Character 5	Qualifier Character 6	Qualifier Character 7
Ø Skin	Ø Single 1 Multiple	Z No Qualifier	Z No Qualifier

6   Extracorporeal or Systemic Therapies
A   Physiological Systems
9   Shock Wave Therapy   Definition: Extracorporeal treatment by shock waves

Body System Character 4	Duration Character 5	Qualifier Character 6	Qualifier Character 7
3 Musculoskeletal	Ø Single 1 Multiple	Z No Qualifier	Z No Qualifier

6   Extracorporeal or Systemic Therapies
A   Physiological Systems
B   Perfusion   Definition: Extracorporeal treatment by diffusion of therapeutic fluid

Body System Character 4	Duration Character 5	Qualifier Character 6	Qualifier Character 7
5 Circulatory B Respiratory System F Hepatobiliary System and Pancreas T Urinary System	Ø Single	B Donor Organ	Z No Qualifier

Non-OR Procedure   DRG Non-OR Procedure   Valid OR Procedure   HAC Associated Procedure   Combination Only   New/Revised April   New/Revised October

736   ICD-10-PCS 2023

Osteopathic 7W0

7   **Osteopathic**
W   **Anatomical Regions**
0   **Treatment**   Definition: Manual treatment to eliminate or alleviate somatic dysfunction and related disorders

Body Region Character 4	Approach Character 5	Method Character 6	Qualifier Character 7
0 Head	X External	0 Articulatory-Raising	Z None
1 Cervical		1 Fascial Release	
2 Thoracic		2 General Mobilization	
3 Lumbar		3 High Velocity-Low Amplitude	
4 Sacrum		4 Indirect	
5 Pelvis		5 Low Velocity-High Amplitude	
6 Lower Extremities		6 Lymphatic Pump	
7 Upper Extremities		7 Muscle Energy-Isometric	
8 Rib Cage		8 Muscle Energy-Isotonic	
9 Abdomen		9 Other Method	

NC Noncovered Procedure   **LC** Limited Coverage   **QA** Questionable OB Admit   **NT** New Tech Add-on   ⊞ Combination Member   ♂ Male   ♀ Female

ICD-10-PCS 2023   **737**

Other Procedures 8C0–8E0

AHA Coding Clinic for table 8E0

2021, 4Q, 49	Division of liver for staged hepatectomy
2021, 2Q, 19	Electromagnetic stealth guided ventriculoperitoneal shunt insertion with endoscopy
2020, 4Q, 53	Bypass pancreatic duct to stomach
2020, 4Q, 65-66	Near infrared spectroscopy for tissue viability assessment
2020, 4Q, 99	Robotic-assisted prostatectomy with extension of incision for specimen removal
2020, 4Q, 100	Robotic-assisted sigmoid colectomy with extension of incision for specimen removal
2019, 4Q, 41-42	Intraoperative fluorescence guidance
2019, 1Q, 30	Laparoscopic-assisted rectopexy with manual reduction of prolapse
2015, 1Q, 33	Robotic-assisted laparoscopic hysterectomy converted to open procedure
2014, 4Q, 33	Radical prostatectomy

8   Other Procedures
C   Indwelling Device
0   Other Procedures   Definition: Methodologies which attempt to remediate or cure a disorder or disease

Body Region Character 4	Approach Character 5	Method Character 6	Qualifier Character 7
1 Nervous System	X External	6 Collection	J Cerebrospinal Fluid L Other Fluid
2 Circulatory System	X External	6 Collection	K Blood L Other Fluid

8   Other Procedures
E   Physiological Systems and Anatomical Regions
0   Other Procedures   Definition: Methodologies which attempt to remediate or cure a disorder or disease

Body Region Character 4	Approach Character 5	Method Character 6	Qualifier Character 7
1 Nervous System U Female Reproductive System ♀	X External	Y Other Method	7 Examination
2 Circulatory System	3 Percutaneous X External	D Near Infrared Spectroscopy	Z No Qualifier
9 Head and Neck Region	0 Open	C Robotic Assisted Procedure	Z No Qualifier
9 Head and Neck Region	0 Open	E Fluorescence Guided Procedure	M Aminolevulinic Acid Z No Qualifier
9 Head and Neck Region	3 Percutaneous 4 Percutaneous Endoscopic 7 Via Natural or Artificial Opening 8 Via Natural or Artificial Opening Endoscopic	C Robotic Assisted Procedure E Fluorescence Guided Procedure	Z No Qualifier
9 Head and Neck Region	X External	B Computer Assisted Procedure	F With Fluoroscopy G With Computerized Tomography H With Magnetic Resonance Imaging Z No Qualifier
9 Head and Neck Region	X External	C Robotic Assisted Procedure	Z No Qualifier
9 Head and Neck Region	X External	Y Other Method	8 Suture Removal
H Integumentary System and Breast	3 Percutaneous	0 Acupuncture	0 Anesthesia Z No Qualifier
H Integumentary System and Breast ♀	X External	6 Collection	2 Breast Milk
H Integumentary System and Breast	X External	Y Other Method	9 Piercing
K Musculoskeletal System	X External	1 Therapeutic Massage	Z No Qualifier
K Musculoskeletal System	X External	Y Other Method	7 Examination
V Male Reproductive System ♂	X External	1 Therapeutic Massage	C Prostate D Rectum
V Male Reproductive System ♂	X External	6 Collection	3 Sperm
W Trunk Region	0 Open 3 Percutaneous 4 Percutaneous Endoscopic 7 Via Natural or Artificial Opening 8 Via Natural or Artificial Opening Endoscopic	C Robotic Assisted Procedure E Fluorescence Guided Procedure	Z No Qualifier
W Trunk Region	X External	B Computer Assisted Procedure	F With Fluoroscopy G With Computerized Tomography H With Magnetic Resonance Imaging Z No Qualifier
W Trunk Region	X External	C Robotic Assisted Procedure	Z No Qualifier
W Trunk Region	X External	Y Other Method	8 Suture Removal
X Upper Extremity Y Lower Extremity	0 Open 3 Percutaneous 4 Percutaneous Endoscopic	C Robotic Assisted Procedure E Fluorescence Guided Procedure	Z No Qualifier

♂	8E0VX1C	♀	8E0UXY7
♂	8E0VX63	♀	8E0HX62

8E0 Continued on next page

NC Noncovered Procedure   LC Limited Coverage   QA Questionable OB Admit   NT New Tech Add-on   ⊞ Combination Member   ♂ Male   ♀ Female

ICD-10-PCS 2023   739

Other Procedures *(left margin)*

8E0 Continued

8   **Other Procedures**
E   **Physiological Systems and Anatomical Regions**
0   **Other Procedures**   Definition: Methodologies which attempt to remediate or cure a disorder or disease

Body Region Character 4	Approach Character 5	Method Character 6	Qualifier Character 7
X Upper Extremity **Y** Lower Extremity	**X** External	**B** Computer Assisted Procedure	**F** With Fluoroscopy **G** With Computerized Tomography **H** With Magnetic Resonance Imaging **Z** No Qualifier
X Upper Extremity **Y** Lower Extremity	**X** External	**C** Robotic Assisted Procedure	**Z** No Qualifier
X Upper Extremity **Y** Lower Extremity	**X** External	**Y** Other Method	**8** Suture Removal
Z None	**X** External	**Y** Other Method	**1** In Vitro Fertilization **4** Yoga Therapy **5** Meditation **6** Isolation

Chiropractic 9WB

9   **Chiropractic**
W   **Anatomical Regions**
B   **Manipulation**   Definition: Manual procedure that involves a directed thrust to move a joint past the physiological range of motion, without exceeding the anatomical limit

Body Region Character 4	Approach Character 5	Method Character 6	Qualifier Character 7
Ø Head	**X** External	**B** Non-Manual	**Z** None
1 Cervical		**C** Indirect Visceral	
2 Thoracic		**D** Extra-Articular	
3 Lumbar		**F** Direct Visceral	
4 Sacrum		**G** Long Lever Specific Contact	
5 Pelvis		**H** Short Lever Specific Contact	
6 Lower Extremities		**J** Long and Short Lever Specific Contact	
7 Upper Extremities		**K** Mechanically Assisted	
8 Rib Cage		**L** Other Method	
9 Abdomen			

NC Noncovered Procedure   **LC** Limited Coverage   **QA** Questionable OB Admit   **NT** New Tech Add-on   ⊞ Combination Member   ♂ Male   ♀ Female

ICD-10-PCS 2023   **741**

9WB–9WB

Imaging BØØ–BY4

AHA Coding Clinic for table B21

2018, 1Q, 12	Percutaneous balloon valvuloplasty & cardiac catheterization with ventriculogram
2016, 3Q, 36	Type of contrast medium for angiography (high osmolar, low osmolar, and other)

AHA Coding Clinic for table B41

2015, 3Q, 9	Aborted endovascular stenting of superficial femoral artery

AHA Coding Clinic for table B51

2015, 4Q, 30	Vascular access devices

AHA Coding Clinic for table BF1

2021, 4Q, 57	Fluoroscopic guidance of hepatobiliary sites

AHA Coding Clinic for table BF4

2014, 3Q, 15	Drainage of pancreatic pseudocyst
2020, 4Q, 66	Other imaging type

AHA Coding Clinic for table BF5

2020, 4Q, 66	Other imaging type
2020, 4Q, 66-67	Fluorescence imaging of hepatobiliary system

AHA Coding Clinic for table BW5

2020, 4Q, 66	Other imaging type
2020, 4Q, 68	Bacterial autofluorescence detection

Contrast Agents

High Osmolar (Ø)	Low Osmolar (1)	Other Contrast (Y)
cholografin meglumine	hexabrix	iodixanol
conray	iohexol	iotrolan
cysto-conray II	iomeprol	isovist
cystografin	iomeron	visipaque
cystografin-dilute	iopamidol	
diatrizoate	iopromide	
gastrografin	ioversol	
hypaque	ioxaglate	
iothalamate	ioxilan	
isopaque	isovue	
md-76r	omnipaque	
metrizoate	optiray	
reno-dip	oxilan	
sinografin	ultravist	

B   **Imaging**
Ø   **Central Nervous System**
Ø   **Plain Radiography**   Definition: Planar display of an image developed from the capture of external ionizing radiation on photographic or photoconductive plate

Body Part Character 4	Contrast Character 5	Qualifier Character 6	Qualifier Character 7
B Spinal Cord	**Ø** High Osmolar **1** Low Osmolar **Y** Other Contrast **Z** None	**Z** None	**Z** None

B   **Imaging**
Ø   **Central Nervous System**
1   **Fluoroscopy**   Definition: Single plane or bi-plane real time display of an image developed from the capture of external ionizing radiation on a fluorescent screen. The image may also be stored by either digital or analog means.

Body Part Character 4	Contrast Character 5	Qualifier Character 6	Qualifier Character 7
B Spinal Cord	**Ø** High Osmolar **1** Low Osmolar **Y** Other Contrast **Z** None	**Z** None	**Z** None

NC Noncovered Procedure   **LC** Limited Coverage   **OA** Questionable OB Admit   **NT** New Tech Add-on   ✚ Combination Member   ♂ Male   ♀ Female

ICD-10-PCS 2023   743

B   **Imaging**
0   **Central Nervous System**
2   **Computerized Tomography (CT Scan)**   Definition: Computer reformatted digital display of multiplanar images developed from the capture of multiple exposures of external ionizing radiation

Body Part Character 4	Contrast Character 5	Qualifier Character 6	Qualifier Character 7
0 Brain 7 Cisterna 8 Cerebral Ventricle(s) 9 Sella Turcica/Pituitary Gland B Spinal Cord	0 High Osmolar 1 Low Osmolar Y Other Contrast	0 Unenhanced and Enhanced Z None	Z None
0 Brain 7 Cisterna 8 Cerebral Ventricle(s) 9 Sella Turcica/Pituitary Gland B Spinal Cord	Z None	Z None	Z None

B   **Imaging**
0   **Central Nervous System**
3   **Magnetic Resonance Imaging (MRI)**   Definition: Computer reformatted digital display of multiplanar images developed from the capture of radio-frequency signals emitted by nuclei in a body site excited within a magnetic field

Body Part Character 4	Contrast Character 5	Qualifier Character 6	Qualifier Character 7
0 Brain 9 Sella Turcica/Pituitary Gland B Spinal Cord C Acoustic Nerves	Y Other Contrast	0 Unenhanced and Enhanced Z None	Z None
0 Brain 9 Sella Turcica/Pituitary Gland B Spinal Cord C Acoustic Nerves	Z None	Z None	Z None

B   **Imaging**
0   **Central Nervous System**
4   **Ultrasonography**   Definition: Real time display of images of anatomy or flow information developed from the capture of reflected and attenuated high frequency sound waves

Body Part Character 4	Contrast Character 5	Qualifier Character 6	Qualifier Character 7
0 Brain B Spinal Cord	Z None	Z None	Z None

B   **Imaging**
2   **Heart**
0   **Plain Radiography**   Definition: Planar display of an image developed from the capture of external ionizing radiation on photographic or photoconductive plate

Body Part Character 4	Contrast Character 5	Qualifier Character 6	Qualifier Character 7
0 Coronary Artery, Single 1 Coronary Arteries, Multiple 2 Coronary Artery Bypass Graft, Single 3 Coronary Artery Bypass Grafts, Multiple 4 Heart, Right 5 Heart, Left 6 Heart, Right and Left 7 Internal Mammary Bypass Graft, Right 8 Internal Mammary Bypass Graft, Left F Bypass Graft, Other	0 High Osmolar 1 Low Osmolar Y Other Contrast	Z None	Z None

DRG Non-OR   All body part, contrast, and qualifier values

Non-OR Procedure   DRG Non-OR Procedure   Valid OR Procedure   HAC Associated Procedure   Combination Only   New/Revised April   New/Revised October

B   Imaging
2   Heart
1   Fluoroscopy   Definition: Single plane or bi-plane real time display of an image developed from the capture of external ionizing radiation on a fluorescent screen. The image may also be stored by either digital or analog means.

Body Part Character 4	Contrast Character 5	Qualifier Character 6	Qualifier Character 7
Ø Coronary Artery, Single 1 Coronary Arteries, Multiple 2 Coronary Artery Bypass Graft, Single 3 Coronary Artery Bypass Grafts, Multiple	Ø High Osmolar 1 Low Osmolar Y Other Contrast	1 Laser	Ø Intraoperative
Ø Coronary Artery, Single 1 Coronary Arteries, Multiple 2 Coronary Artery Bypass Graft, Single 3 Coronary Artery Bypass Grafts, Multiple	Ø High Osmolar 1 Low Osmolar Y Other Contrast	Z None	Z None
4 Heart, Right 5 Heart, Left 6 Heart, Right and Left 7 Internal Mammary Bypass Graft, Right 8 Internal Mammary Bypass Graft, Left F Bypass Graft, Other	Ø High Osmolar 1 Low Osmolar Y Other Contrast	Z None	Z None

DRG Non-OR   B21[Ø,1,2,3][Ø,1,Y]ZZ
DRG Non-OR   B21[4,5,6,7,8,F][Ø,1,Y]ZZ

B   Imaging
2   Heart
2   Computerized Tomography (CT Scan)   Definition: Computer reformatted digital display of multiplanar images developed from the capture of multiple exposures of external ionizing radiation

Body Part Character 4	Contrast Character 5	Qualifier Character 6	Qualifier Character 7
1 Coronary Arteries, Multiple 3 Coronary Artery Bypass Grafts, Multiple 6 Heart, Right and Left	Ø High Osmolar 1 Low Osmolar Y Other Contrast	Ø Unenhanced and Enhanced Z None	Z None
1 Coronary Arteries, Multiple 3 Coronary Artery Bypass Grafts, Multiple 6 Heart, Right and Left	Z None	2 Intravascular Optical Coherence Z None	Z None

B   Imaging
2   Heart
3   Magnetic Resonance Imaging (MRI)   Definition: Computer reformatted digital display of multiplanar images developed from the capture of radio-frequency signals emitted by nuclei in a body site excited within a magnetic field

Body Part Character 4	Contrast Character 5	Qualifier Character 6	Qualifier Character 7
1 Coronary Arteries, Multiple 3 Coronary Artery Bypass Grafts, Multiple 6 Heart, Right and Left	Y Other Contrast	Ø Unenhanced and Enhanced Z None	Z None
1 Coronary Arteries, Multiple 3 Coronary Artery Bypass Grafts, Multiple 6 Heart, Right and Left	Z None	Z None	Z None

B   **Imaging**
2   **Heart**
4   **Ultrasonography**   Definition: Real time display of images of anatomy or flow information developed from the capture of reflected and attenuated high frequency sound waves

Body Part Character 4	Contrast Character 5	Qualifier Character 6	Qualifier Character 7
Ø Coronary Artery, Single 1 Coronary Arteries, Multiple 4 Heart, Right 5 Heart, Left 6 Heart, Right and Left B Heart with Aorta C Pericardium D Pediatric Heart	Y Other Contrast	Z None	Z None
Ø Coronary Artery, Single 1 Coronary Arteries, Multiple 4 Heart, Right 5 Heart, Left 6 Heart, Right and Left B Heart with Aorta C Pericardium D Pediatric Heart	Z None	Z None	3 Intravascular 4 Transesophageal Z None

B   **Imaging**
3   **Upper Arteries**
Ø   **Plain Radiography**   Definition: Planar display of an image developed from the capture of external ionizing radiation on photographic or photoconductive plate

Body Part Character 4	Contrast Character 5	Qualifier Character 6	Qualifier Character 7
Ø Thoracic Aorta 1 Brachiocephalic-Subclavian Artery, Right 2 Subclavian Artery, Left 3 Common Carotid Artery, Right 4 Common Carotid Artery, Left 5 Common Carotid Arteries, Bilateral 6 Internal Carotid Artery, Right 7 Internal Carotid Artery, Left 8 Internal Carotid Arteries, Bilateral 9 External Carotid Artery, Right B External Carotid Artery, Left C External Carotid Arteries, Bilateral D Vertebral Artery, Right F Vertebral Artery, Left G Vertebral Arteries, Bilateral H Upper Extremity Arteries, Right J Upper Extremity Arteries, Left K Upper Extremity Arteries, Bilateral L Intercostal and Bronchial Arteries M Spinal Arteries N Upper Arteries, Other P Thoraco-Abdominal Aorta Q Cervico-Cerebral Arch R Intracranial Arteries S Pulmonary Artery, Right T Pulmonary Artery, Left	Ø High Osmolar 1 Low Osmolar Y Other Contrast Z None	Z None	Z None

Non-OR Procedure   DRG Non-OR Procedure   Valid OR Procedure   HAC Associated Procedure   Combination Only   New/Revised April   New/Revised October

746   ICD-10-PCS 2023

B24–B3Ø

B   **Imaging**
3   **Upper Arteries**
1   **Fluoroscopy**   Definition: Single plane or bi-plane real time display of an image developed from the capture of external ionizing radiation on a fluorescent screen. The image may also be stored by either digital or analog means.

Body Part Character 4	Contrast Character 5	Qualifier Character 6	Qualifier Character 7
Ø Thoracic Aorta **1** Brachiocephalic-Subclavian Artery, Right **2** Subclavian Artery, Left **3** Common Carotid Artery, Right **4** Common Carotid Artery, Left **5** Common Carotid Arteries, Bilateral **6** Internal Carotid Artery, Right **7** Internal Carotid Artery, Left **8** Internal Carotid Arteries, Bilateral **9** External Carotid Artery, Right **B** External Carotid Artery, Left **C** External Carotid Arteries, Bilateral **D** Vertebral Artery, Right **F** Vertebral Artery, Left **G** Vertebral Arteries, Bilateral **H** Upper Extremity Arteries, Right **J** Upper Extremity Arteries, Left **K** Upper Extremity Arteries, Bilateral **L** Intercostal and Bronchial Arteries **M** Spinal Arteries **N** Upper Arteries, Other **P** Thoraco-Abdominal Aorta **Q** Cervico-Cerebral Arch **R** Intracranial Arteries **S** Pulmonary Artery, Right **T** Pulmonary Artery, Left **U** Pulmonary Trunk	**Ø** High Osmolar **1** Low Osmolar **Y** Other Contrast	**1** Laser	**Ø** Intraoperative
Ø Thoracic Aorta **1** Brachiocephalic-Subclavian Artery, Right **2** Subclavian Artery, Left **3** Common Carotid Artery, Right **4** Common Carotid Artery, Left **5** Common Carotid Arteries, Bilateral **6** Internal Carotid Artery, Right **7** Internal Carotid Artery, Left **8** Internal Carotid Arteries, Bilateral **9** External Carotid Artery, Right **B** External Carotid Artery, Left **C** External Carotid Arteries, Bilateral **D** Vertebral Artery, Right **F** Vertebral Artery, Left **G** Vertebral Arteries, Bilateral **H** Upper Extremity Arteries, Right **J** Upper Extremity Arteries, Left **K** Upper Extremity Arteries, Bilateral **L** Intercostal and Bronchial Arteries **M** Spinal Arteries **N** Upper Arteries, Other **P** Thoraco-Abdominal Aorta **Q** Cervico-Cerebral Arch **R** Intracranial Arteries **S** Pulmonary Artery, Right **T** Pulmonary Artery, Left **U** Pulmonary Trunk	**Ø** High Osmolar **1** Low Osmolar **Y** Other Contrast	**Z** None	**Z** None

B31 Continued on next page

NC Noncovered Procedure   **LC** Limited Coverage   **QA** Questionable OB Admit   **NT** New Tech Add-on   ⊞ Combination Member   ♂ Male   ♀ Female

ICD-10-PCS 2023   747

B31–B31

B	Imaging
3	**Upper Arteries**
1	**Fluoroscopy**

B31 Continued

Fluoroscopy Definition: Single plane or bi-plane real time display of an image developed from the capture of external ionizing radiation on a fluorescent screen. The image may also be stored by either digital or analog means.

Body Part Character 4	Contrast Character 5	Qualifier Character 6	Qualifier Character 7
0 Thoracic Aorta	Z None	Z None	Z None
1 Brachiocephalic-Subclavian Artery, Right			
2 Subclavian Artery, Left			
3 Common Carotid Artery, Right			
4 Common Carotid Artery, Left			
5 Common Carotid Arteries, Bilateral			
6 Internal Carotid Artery, Right			
7 Internal Carotid Artery, Left			
8 Internal Carotid Arteries, Bilateral			
9 External Carotid Artery, Right			
B External Carotid Artery, Left			
C External Carotid Arteries, Bilateral			
D Vertebral Artery, Right			
F Vertebral Artery, Left			
G Vertebral Arteries, Bilateral			
H Upper Extremity Arteries, Right			
J Upper Extremity Arteries, Left			
K Upper Extremity Arteries, Bilateral			
L Intercostal and Bronchial Arteries			
M Spinal Arteries			
N Upper Arteries, Other			
P Thoraco-Abdominal Aorta			
Q Cervico-Cerebral Arch			
R Intracranial Arteries			
S Pulmonary Artery, Right			
T Pulmonary Artery, Left			
U Pulmonary Trunk			

B	Imaging
3	**Upper Arteries**
2	**Computerized Tomography (CT Scan)**

Computerized Tomography (CT Scan) Definition: Computer reformatted digital display of multiplanar images developed from the capture of multiple exposures of external ionizing radiation

Body Part Character 4	Contrast Character 5	Qualifier Character 6	Qualifier Character 7
0 Thoracic Aorta	0 High Osmolar	Z None	Z None
5 Common Carotid Arteries, Bilateral	1 Low Osmolar		
8 Internal Carotid Arteries, Bilateral	Y Other Contrast		
G Vertebral Arteries, Bilateral			
R Intracranial Arteries			
S Pulmonary Artery, Right			
T Pulmonary Artery, Left			
0 Thoracic Aorta	Z None	2 Intravascular Optical Coherence	Z None
5 Common Carotid Arteries, Bilateral		Z None	
8 Internal Carotid Arteries, Bilateral			
G Vertebral Arteries, Bilateral			
R Intracranial Arteries			
S Pulmonary Artery, Right			
T Pulmonary Artery, Left			

Non-OR Procedure   DRG Non-OR Procedure   Valid OR Procedure   HAC Associated Procedure   Combination Only   New/Revised April   New/Revised October

748   ICD-10-PCS 2023

B   Imaging
3   Upper Arteries
3   Magnetic Resonance Imaging (MRI)   Definition: Computer reformatted digital display of multiplanar images developed from the capture of radio-frequency signals emitted by nuclei in a body site excited within a magnetic field

Body Part Character 4	Contrast Character 5	Qualifier Character 6	Qualifier Character 7
Ø Thoracic Aorta 5 Common Carotid Arteries, Bilateral 8 Internal Carotid Arteries, Bilateral G Vertebral Arteries, Bilateral H Upper Extremity Arteries, Right J Upper Extremity Arteries, Left K Upper Extremity Arteries, Bilateral M Spinal Arteries Q Cervico-Cerebral Arch R Intracranial Arteries	Y Other Contrast	Ø Unenhanced and Enhanced Z None	Z None
Ø Thoracic Aorta 5 Common Carotid Arteries, Bilateral 8 Internal Carotid Arteries, Bilateral G Vertebral Arteries, Bilateral H Upper Extremity Arteries, Right J Upper Extremity Arteries, Left K Upper Extremity Arteries, Bilateral M Spinal Arteries Q Cervico-Cerebral Arch R Intracranial Arteries	Z None	Z None	Z None

B   Imaging
3   Upper Arteries
4   Ultrasonography   Definition: Real time display of images of anatomy or flow information developed from the capture of reflected and attenuated high frequency sound waves

Body Part Character 4	Contrast Character 5	Qualifier Character 6	Qualifier Character 7
Ø Thoracic Aorta 1 Brachiocephalic-Subclavian Artery, Right 2 Subclavian Artery, Left 3 Common Carotid Artery, Right 4 Common Carotid Artery, Left 5 Common Carotid Arteries, Bilateral 6 Internal Carotid Artery, Right 7 Internal Carotid Artery, Left 8 Internal Carotid Arteries, Bilateral H Upper Extremity Arteries, Right J Upper Extremity Arteries, Left K Upper Extremity Arteries, Bilateral R Intracranial Arteries S Pulmonary Artery, Right T Pulmonary Artery, Left V Ophthalmic Arteries	Z None	Z None	3 Intravascular Z None

B   Imaging
4   Lower Arteries
Ø   Plain Radiography   Definition: Planar display of an image developed from the capture of external ionizing radiation on photographic or photoconductive plate

Body Part Character 4	Contrast Character 5	Qualifier Character 6	Qualifier Character 7
Ø Abdominal Aorta 2 Hepatic Artery 3 Splenic Arteries 4 Superior Mesenteric Artery 5 Inferior Mesenteric Artery 6 Renal Artery, Right 7 Renal Artery, Left 8 Renal Arteries, Bilateral 9 Lumbar Arteries B Intra-Abdominal Arteries, Other C Pelvic Arteries D Aorta and Bilateral Lower Extremity Arteries F Lower Extremity Arteries, Right G Lower Extremity Arteries, Left J Lower Arteries, Other M Renal Artery Transplant	Ø High Osmolar 1 Low Osmolar Y Other Contrast	Z None	Z None

NC Noncovered Procedure   **LC** Limited Coverage   **QA** Questionable OB Admit   **NT** New Tech Add-on   ⊞ Combination Member   ♂ Male   ♀ Female

ICD-10-PCS 2023   749

Imaging

B   Imaging
4   Lower Arteries
1   Fluoroscopy   Definition: Single plane or bi-plane real time display of an image developed from the capture of external ionizing radiation on a fluorescent screen. The image may also be stored by either digital or analog means.

Body Part Character 4	Contrast Character 5	Qualifier Character 6	Qualifier Character 7
0 Abdominal Aorta **2** Hepatic Artery **3** Splenic Arteries **4** Superior Mesenteric Artery **5** Inferior Mesenteric Artery **6** Renal Artery, Right **7** Renal Artery, Left **8** Renal Arteries, Bilateral **9** Lumbar Arteries **B** Intra-Abdominal Arteries, Other **C** Pelvic Arteries **D** Aorta and Bilateral Lower Extremity Arteries **F** Lower Extremity Arteries, Right **G** Lower Extremity Arteries, Left **J** Lower Arteries, Other	**0** High Osmolar **1** Low Osmolar **Y** Other Contrast	**1** Laser	**0** Intraoperative
0 Abdominal Aorta **2** Hepatic Artery **3** Splenic Arteries **4** Superior Mesenteric Artery **5** Inferior Mesenteric Artery **6** Renal Artery, Right **7** Renal Artery, Left **8** Renal Arteries, Bilateral **9** Lumbar Arteries **B** Intra-Abdominal Arteries, Other **C** Pelvic Arteries **D** Aorta and Bilateral Lower Extremity Arteries **F** Lower Extremity Arteries, Right **G** Lower Extremity Arteries, Left **J** Lower Arteries, Other	**0** High Osmolar **1** Low Osmolar **Y** Other Contrast	**Z** None	**Z** None
0 Abdominal Aorta **2** Hepatic Artery **3** Splenic Arteries **4** Superior Mesenteric Artery **5** Inferior Mesenteric Artery **6** Renal Artery, Right **7** Renal Artery, Left **8** Renal Arteries, Bilateral **9** Lumbar Arteries **B** Intra-Abdominal Arteries, Other **C** Pelvic Arteries **D** Aorta and Bilateral Lower Extremity Arteries **F** Lower Extremity Arteries, Right **G** Lower Extremity Arteries, Left **J** Lower Arteries, Other	**Z** None	**Z** None	**Z** None

Non-OR Procedure   DRG Non-OR Procedure   Valid OR Procedure   HAC Associated Procedure   Combination Only   New/Revised April   New/Revised October

750   ICD-10-PCS 2023

B   Imaging
4   Lower Arteries
2   Computerized Tomography (CT Scan) Definition: Computer reformatted digital display of multiplanar images developed from the capture of multiple exposures of external ionizing radiation

Body Part Character 4	Contrast Character 5	Qualifier Character 6	Qualifier Character 7
Ø Abdominal Aorta 1 Celiac Artery 4 Superior Mesenteric Artery 8 Renal Arteries, Bilateral C Pelvic Arteries F Lower Extremity Arteries, Right G Lower Extremity Arteries, Left H Lower Extremity Arteries, Bilateral M Renal Artery Transplant	Ø High Osmolar 1 Low Osmolar Y Other Contrast	Z None	Z None
Ø Abdominal Aorta 1 Celiac Artery 4 Superior Mesenteric Artery 8 Renal Arteries, Bilateral C Pelvic Arteries F Lower Extremity Arteries, Right G Lower Extremity Arteries, Left H Lower Extremity Arteries, Bilateral M Renal Artery Transplant	Z None	2 Intravascular Optical Coherence Z None	Z None

B   Imaging
4   Lower Arteries
3   Magnetic Resonance Imaging (MRI) Definition: Computer reformatted digital display of multiplanar images developed from the capture of radio-frequency signals emitted by nuclei in a body site excited within a magnetic field

Body Part Character 4	Contrast Character 5	Qualifier Character 6	Qualifier Character 7
Ø Abdominal Aorta 1 Celiac Artery 4 Superior Mesenteric Artery 8 Renal Arteries, Bilateral C Pelvic Arteries F Lower Extremity Arteries, Right G Lower Extremity Arteries, Left H Lower Extremity Arteries, Bilateral	Y Other Contrast	Ø Unenhanced and Enhanced Z None	Z None
Ø Abdominal Aorta 1 Celiac Artery 4 Superior Mesenteric Artery 8 Renal Arteries, Bilateral C Pelvic Arteries F Lower Extremity Arteries, Right G Lower Extremity Arteries, Left H Lower Extremity Arteries, Bilateral	Z None	Z None	Z None

B   Imaging
4   Lower Arteries
4   Ultrasonography Definition: Real time display of images of anatomy or flow information developed from the capture of reflected and attenuated high frequency sound waves

Body Part Character 4	Contrast Character 5	Qualifier Character 6	Qualifier Character 7
Ø Abdominal Aorta 4 Superior Mesenteric Artery 5 Inferior Mesenteric Artery 6 Renal Artery, Right 7 Renal Artery, Left 8 Renal Arteries, Bilateral B Intra-Abdominal Arteries, Other F Lower Extremity Arteries, Right G Lower Extremity Arteries, Left H Lower Extremity Arteries, Bilateral K Celiac and Mesenteric Arteries L Femoral Artery N Penile Arteries	Z None	Z None	3 Intravascular Z None

B   Imaging
5   Veins
Ø   Plain Radiography   Definition: Planar display of an image developed from the capture of external ionizing radiation on photographic or photoconductive plate

Body Part Character 4	Contrast Character 5	Qualifier Character 6	Qualifier Character 7
Ø Epidural Veins	Ø High Osmolar	Z None	Z None
1 Cerebral and Cerebellar Veins	1 Low Osmolar		
2 Intracranial Sinuses	Y Other Contrast		
3 Jugular Veins, Right			
4 Jugular Veins, Left			
5 Jugular Veins, Bilateral			
6 Subclavian Vein, Right			
7 Subclavian Vein, Left			
8 Superior Vena Cava			
9 Inferior Vena Cava			
B Lower Extremity Veins, Right			
C Lower Extremity Veins, Left			
D Lower Extremity Veins, Bilateral			
F Pelvic (Iliac) Veins, Right			
G Pelvic (Iliac) Veins, Left			
H Pelvic (Iliac) Veins, Bilateral			
J Renal Vein, Right			
K Renal Vein, Left			
L Renal Veins, Bilateral			
M Upper Extremity Veins, Right			
N Upper Extremity Veins, Left			
P Upper Extremity Veins, Bilateral			
Q Pulmonary Vein, Right			
R Pulmonary Vein, Left			
S Pulmonary Veins, Bilateral			
T Portal and Splanchnic Veins			
V Veins, Other			
W Dialysis Shunt/Fistula			

B   Imaging
5   Veins
1   Fluoroscopy   Definition: Single plane or bi-plane real time display of an image developed from the capture of external ionizing radiation on a fluorescent screen. The image may also be stored by either digital or analog means.

Body Part Character 4	Contrast Character 5	Qualifier Character 6	Qualifier Character 7
Ø Epidural Veins	Ø High Osmolar	Z None	A Guidance
1 Cerebral and Cerebellar Veins	1 Low Osmolar		Z None
2 Intracranial Sinuses	Y Other Contrast		
3 Jugular Veins, Right	Z None		
4 Jugular Veins, Left			
5 Jugular Veins, Bilateral			
6 Subclavian Vein, Right			
7 Subclavian Vein, Left			
8 Superior Vena Cava			
9 Inferior Vena Cava			
B Lower Extremity Veins, Right			
C Lower Extremity Veins, Left			
D Lower Extremity Veins, Bilateral			
F Pelvic (Iliac) Veins, Right			
G Pelvic (Iliac) Veins, Left			
H Pelvic (Iliac) Veins, Bilateral			
J Renal Vein, Right			
K Renal Vein, Left			
L Renal Veins, Bilateral			
M Upper Extremity Veins, Right			
N Upper Extremity Veins, Left			
P Upper Extremity Veins, Bilateral			
Q Pulmonary Vein, Right			
R Pulmonary Vein, Left			
S Pulmonary Veins, Bilateral			
T Portal and Splanchnic Veins			
V Veins, Other			
W Dialysis Shunt/Fistula			

B5Ø–B51

Non-OR Procedure   DRG Non-OR Procedure   Valid OR Procedure   HAC Associated Procedure   Combination Only   New/Revised April   New/Revised October

752   ICD-10-PCS 2023

B   **Imaging**
5   **Veins**
2   **Computerized Tomography (CT Scan)** Definition: Computer reformatted digital display of multiplanar images developed from the capture of multiple exposures of external ionizing radiation

Body Part Character 4	Contrast Character 5	Qualifier Character 6	Qualifier Character 7
2 Intracranial Sinuses **8** Superior Vena Cava **9** Inferior Vena Cava **F** Pelvic (Iliac) Veins, Right **G** Pelvic (Iliac) Veins, Left **H** Pelvic (Iliac) Veins, Bilateral **J** Renal Vein, Right **K** Renal Vein, Left **L** Renal Veins, Bilateral **Q** Pulmonary Vein, Right **R** Pulmonary Vein, Left **S** Pulmonary Veins, Bilateral **T** Portal and Splanchnic Veins	**Ø** High Osmolar **1** Low Osmolar **Y** Other Contrast	**Ø** Unenhanced and Enhanced **Z** None	**Z** None
2 Intracranial Sinuses **8** Superior Vena Cava **9** Inferior Vena Cava **F** Pelvic (Iliac) Veins, Right **G** Pelvic (Iliac) Veins, Left **H** Pelvic (Iliac) Veins, Bilateral **J** Renal Vein, Right **K** Renal Vein, Left **L** Renal Veins, Bilateral **Q** Pulmonary Vein, Right **R** Pulmonary Vein, Left **S** Pulmonary Veins, Bilateral **T** Portal and Splanchnic Veins	**Z** None	**2** Intravascular Optical Coherence **Z** None	**Z** None

B   **Imaging**
5   **Veins**
3   **Magnetic Resonance Imaging (MRI)**   Definition: Computer reformatted digital display of multiplanar images developed from the capture of radio-frequency signals emitted by nuclei in a body site excited within a magnetic field

Body Part Character 4	Contrast Character 5	Qualifier Character 6	Qualifier Character 7
1 Cerebral and Cerebellar Veins **2** Intracranial Sinuses **5** Jugular Veins, Bilateral **8** Superior Vena Cava **9** Inferior Vena Cava **B** Lower Extremity Veins, Right **C** Lower Extremity Veins, Left **D** Lower Extremity Veins, Bilateral **H** Pelvic (Iliac) Veins, Bilateral **L** Renal Veins, Bilateral **M** Upper Extremity Veins, Right **N** Upper Extremity Veins, Left **P** Upper Extremity Veins, Bilateral **S** Pulmonary Veins, Bilateral **T** Portal and Splanchnic Veins **V** Veins, Other	**Y** Other Contrast	**Ø** Unenhanced and Enhanced **Z** None	**Z** None
1 Cerebral and Cerebellar Veins **2** Intracranial Sinuses **5** Jugular Veins, Bilateral **8** Superior Vena Cava **9** Inferior Vena Cava **B** Lower Extremity Veins, Right **C** Lower Extremity Veins, Left **D** Lower Extremity Veins, Bilateral **H** Pelvic (Iliac) Veins, Bilateral **L** Renal Veins, Bilateral **M** Upper Extremity Veins, Right **N** Upper Extremity Veins, Left **P** Upper Extremity Veins, Bilateral **S** Pulmonary Veins, Bilateral **T** Portal and Splanchnic Veins **V** Veins, Other	**Z** None	**Z** None	**Z** None

B   Imaging
5   Veins
4   Ultrasonography   Definition: Real time display of images of anatomy or flow information developed from the capture of reflected and attenuated high frequency sound waves

Body Part Character 4	Contrast Character 5	Qualifier Character 6	Qualifier Character 7
3 Jugular Veins, Right 4 Jugular Veins, Left 6 Subclavian Vein, Right 7 Subclavian Vein, Left 8 Superior Vena Cava 9 Inferior Vena Cava B Lower Extremity Veins, Right C Lower Extremity Veins, Left D Lower Extremity Veins, Bilateral J Renal Vein, Right K Renal Vein, Left L Renal Veins, Bilateral M Upper Extremity Veins, Right N Upper Extremity Veins, Left P Upper Extremity Veins, Bilateral T Portal and Splanchnic Veins	Z None	Z None	3 Intravascular A Guidance Z None

B   Imaging
7   Lymphatic System
Ø   Plain Radiography   Definition: Planar display of an image developed from the capture of external ionizing radiation on photographic or photoconductive plate

Body Part Character 4	Contrast Character 5	Qualifier Character 6	Qualifier Character 7

Ø   Abdominal/Retroperitoneal
     Lymphatics, Unilateral
1   Abdominal/Retroperitoneal
     Lymphatics, Bilateral
4   Lymphatics, Head and Neck
5   Upper Extremity Lymphatics, Right
6   Upper Extremity Lymphatics, Left
7   Upper Extremity Lymphatics,
     Bilateral
8   Lower Extremity Lymphatics, Right
9   Lower Extremity Lymphatics, Left
B   Lower Extremity Lymphatics,
     Bilateral
C   Lymphatics, Pelvic
	Ø High Osmolar
	1 Low Osmolar
	Y Other Contrast
		Z None	Z None

B   Imaging
8   Eye
Ø   Plain Radiography   Definition: Planar display of an image developed from the capture of external ionizing radiation on photographic or photoconductive plate

Body Part Character 4	Contrast Character 5	Qualifier Character 6	Qualifier Character 7
Ø Lacrimal Duct, Right 1 Lacrimal Duct, Left 2 Lacrimal Ducts, Bilateral	Ø High Osmolar 1 Low Osmolar Y Other Contrast	Z None	Z None
3 Optic Foramina, Right 4 Optic Foramina, Left 5 Eye, Right 6 Eye, Left 7 Eyes, Bilateral	Z None	Z None	Z None

B   Imaging
8   Eye
2   Computerized Tomography (CT Scan)   Definition: Computer reformatted digital display of multiplanar images developed from the capture of multiple exposures of external ionizing radiation

Body Part Character 4	Contrast Character 5	Qualifier Character 6	Qualifier Character 7
5 Eye, Right 6 Eye, Left 7 Eyes, Bilateral	Ø High Osmolar 1 Low Osmolar Y Other Contrast	Ø Unenhanced and Enhanced Z None	Z None
5 Eye, Right 6 Eye, Left 7 Eyes, Bilateral	Z None	Z None	Z None

Non-OR Procedure   DRG Non-OR Procedure   Valid OR Procedure   HAC Associated Procedure   Combination Only   New/Revised April   New/Revised October

754   ICD-10-PCS 2023

B **Imaging**
8 **Eye**
3 **Magnetic Resonance Imaging (MRI)** Definition: Computer reformatted digital display of multiplanar images developed from the capture of radio-frequency signals emitted by nuclei in a body site excited within a magnetic field

Body Part Character 4	Contrast Character 5	Qualifier Character 6	Qualifier Character 7
5 Eye, Right 6 Eye, Left 7 Eyes, Bilateral	Y Other Contrast	Ø Unenhanced and Enhanced Z None	Z None
5 Eye, Right 6 Eye, Left 7 Eyes, Bilateral	Z None	Z None	Z None

B **Imaging**
8 **Eye**
4 **Ultrasonography** Definition: Real time display of images of anatomy or flow information developed from the capture of reflected and attenuated high frequency sound waves

Body Part Character 4	Contrast Character 5	Qualifier Character 6	Qualifier Character 7
5 Eye, Right 6 Eye, Left 7 Eyes, Bilateral	Z None	Z None	Z None

B **Imaging**
9 **Ear, Nose, Mouth and Throat**
Ø **Plain Radiography** Definition: Planar display of an image developed from the capture of external ionizing radiation on photographic or photoconductive plate

Body Part Character 4	Contrast Character 5	Qualifier Character 6	Qualifier Character 7
2 Paranasal Sinuses F Nasopharynx/Oropharynx H Mastoids	Z None	Z None	Z None
4 Parotid Gland, Right 5 Parotid Gland, Left 6 Parotid Glands, Bilateral 7 Submandibular Gland, Right 8 Submandibular Gland, Left 9 Submandibular Glands, Bilateral B Salivary Gland, Right C Salivary Gland, Left D Salivary Glands, Bilateral	Ø High Osmolar 1 Low Osmolar Y Other Contrast	Z None	Z None

B **Imaging**
9 **Ear, Nose, Mouth and Throat**
1 **Fluoroscopy** Definition: Single plane or bi-plane real time display of an image developed from the capture of external ionizing radiation on a fluorescent screen. The image may also be stored by either digital or analog means.

Body Part Character 4	Contrast Character 5	Qualifier Character 6	Qualifier Character 7
G Pharynx and Epiglottis J Larynx	Y Other Contrast Z None	Z None	Z None

B **Imaging**
9 **Ear, Nose, Mouth and Throat**
2 **Computerized Tomography (CT Scan)** Definition: Computer reformatted digital display of multiplanar images developed from the capture of multiple exposures of external ionizing radiation

Body Part Character 4	Contrast Character 5	Qualifier Character 6	Qualifier Character 7
Ø Ear 2 Paranasal Sinuses 6 Parotid Glands, Bilateral 9 Submandibular Glands, Bilateral D Salivary Glands, Bilateral F Nasopharynx/Oropharynx J Larynx	Ø High Osmolar 1 Low Osmolar Y Other Contrast	Ø Unenhanced and Enhanced Z None	Z None
Ø Ear 2 Paranasal Sinuses 6 Parotid Glands, Bilateral 9 Submandibular Glands, Bilateral D Salivary Glands, Bilateral F Nasopharynx/Oropharynx J Larynx	Z None	Z None	Z None

NC Noncovered Procedure **LC** Limited Coverage **QA** Questionable OB Admit **NT** New Tech Add-on ⊞ Combination Member ♂ Male ♀ Female

ICD-10-PCS 2023 755

B83–B92

B   **Imaging**
9   **Ear, Nose, Mouth and Throat**
3   **Magnetic Resonance Imaging (MRI)**   Definition: Computer reformatted digital display of multiplanar images developed from the capture of radio-frequency signals emitted by nuclei in a body site excited within a magnetic field

Body Part Character 4	Contrast Character 5	Qualifier Character 6	Qualifier Character 7
0 Ear 2 Paranasal Sinuses 6 Parotid Glands, Bilateral 9 Submandibular Glands, Bilateral D Salivary Glands, Bilateral F Nasopharynx/Oropharynx J Larynx	Y Other Contrast	0 Unenhanced and Enhanced Z None	Z None
0 Ear 2 Paranasal Sinuses 6 Parotid Glands, Bilateral 9 Submandibular Glands, Bilateral D Salivary Glands, Bilateral F Nasopharynx/Oropharynx J Larynx	Z None	Z None	Z None

B   **Imaging**
B   **Respiratory System**
0   **Plain Radiography**   Definition: Planar display of an image developed from the capture of external ionizing radiation on photographic or photoconductive plate

Body Part Character 4	Contrast Character 5	Qualifier Character 6	Qualifier Character 7
7 Tracheobronchial Tree, Right 8 Tracheobronchial Tree, Left 9 Tracheobronchial Trees, Bilateral	Y Other Contrast	Z None	Z None
D Upper Airways	Z None	Z None	Z None

B   **Imaging**
B   **Respiratory System**
1   **Fluoroscopy**   Definition: Single plane or bi-plane real time display of an image developed from the capture of external ionizing radiation on a fluorescent screen. The image may also be stored by either digital or analog means.

Body Part Character 4	Contrast Character 5	Qualifier Character 6	Qualifier Character 7
2 Lung, Right 3 Lung, Left 4 Lungs, Bilateral 6 Diaphragm C Mediastinum D Upper Airways	Z None	Z None	Z None
7 Tracheobronchial Tree, Right 8 Tracheobronchial Tree, Left 9 Tracheobronchial Trees, Bilateral	Y Other Contrast	Z None	Z None

B   **Imaging**
B   **Respiratory System**
2   **Computerized Tomography (CT Scan)**   Definition: Computer reformatted digital display of multiplanar images developed from the capture of multiple exposures of external ionizing radiation

Body Part Character 4	Contrast Character 5	Qualifier Character 6	Qualifier Character 7
4 Lungs, Bilateral 7 Tracheobronchial Tree, Right 8 Tracheobronchial Tree, Left 9 Tracheobronchial Trees, Bilateral F Trachea/Airways	0 High Osmolar 1 Low Osmolar Y Other Contrast	0 Unenhanced and Enhanced Z None	Z None
4 Lungs, Bilateral 7 Tracheobronchial Tree, Right 8 Tracheobronchial Tree, Left 9 Tracheobronchial Trees, Bilateral F Trachea/Airways	Z None	Z None	Z None

Non-OR Procedure   DRG Non-OR Procedure   Valid OR Procedure   HAC Associated Procedure   Combination Only   New/Revised April   New/Revised October

756

B93–BB2

ICD-10-PCS 2023

B   **Imaging**
B   **Respiratory System**
3   **Magnetic Resonance Imaging (MRI)**   Definition: Computer reformatted digital display of multiplanar images developed from the capture of radio-frequency signals emitted by nuclei in a body site excited within a magnetic field

Body Part Character 4	Contrast Character 5	Qualifier Character 6	Qualifier Character 7
4 Lungs, Bilateral	Z None	3 Hyperpolarized Xenon 129 (Xe-129)	Z None
G Lung Apices	Y Other Contrast	Ø Unenhanced and Enhanced Z None	Z None
G Lung Apices	Z None	Z None	Z None

B   **Imaging**
B   **Respiratory System**
4   **Ultrasonography**   Definition: Real time display of images of anatomy or flow information developed from the capture of reflected and attenuated high frequency sound waves

Body Part Character 4	Contrast Character 5	Qualifier Character 6	Qualifier Character 7
B Pleura C Mediastinum	Z None	Z None	Z None

B   **Imaging**
D   **Gastrointestinal System**
1   **Fluoroscopy**   Definition: Single plane or bi-plane real time display of an image developed from the capture of external ionizing radiation on a fluorescent screen. The image may also be stored by either digital or analog means.

Body Part Character 4	Contrast Character 5	Qualifier Character 6	Qualifier Character 7
1 Esophagus 2 Stomach 3 Small Bowel 4 Colon 5 Upper GI 6 Upper GI and Small Bowel 9 Duodenum B Mouth/Oropharynx	Y Other Contrast Z None	Z None	Z None

B   **Imaging**
D   **Gastrointestinal System**
2   **Computerized Tomography (CT Scan)**   Definition: Computer reformatted digital display of multiplanar images developed from the capture of multiple exposures of external ionizing radiation

Body Part Character 4	Contrast Character 5	Qualifier Character 6	Qualifier Character 7
4 Colon	Ø High Osmolar 1 Low Osmolar Y Other Contrast	Ø Unenhanced and Enhanced Z None	Z None
4 Colon	Z None	Z None	Z None

B   **Imaging**
D   **Gastrointestinal System**
4   **Ultrasonography**   Definition: Real time display of images of anatomy or flow information developed from the capture of reflected and attenuated high frequency sound waves

Body Part Character 4	Contrast Character 5	Qualifier Character 6	Qualifier Character 7
1 Esophagus 2 Stomach 7 Gastrointestinal Tract 8 Appendix 9 Duodenum C Rectum	Z None	Z None	Z None

B   **Imaging**
F   **Hepatobiliary System and Pancreas**
Ø   **Plain Radiography**   Definition: Planar display of an image developed from the capture of external ionizing radiation on photographic or photoconductive plate

Body Part Character 4	Contrast Character 5	Qualifier Character 6	Qualifier Character 7
Ø Bile Ducts 3 Gallbladder and Bile Ducts C Hepatobiliary System, All	Ø High Osmolar 1 Low Osmolar Y Other Contrast	Z None	Z None

NC Noncovered Procedure   LC Limited Coverage   QA Questionable OB Admit   NT New Tech Add-on   ⊞ Combination Member   ♂ Male   ♀ Female

ICD-10-PCS 2023   757

BB3–BFØ

B Imaging
F Hepatobiliary System and Pancreas
1 Fluoroscopy   Definition: Single plane or bi-plane real time display of an image developed from the capture of external ionizing radiation on a fluorescent screen. The image may also be stored by either digital or analog means.

Body Part Character 4	Contrast Character 5	Qualifier Character 6	Qualifier Character 7
0 Bile Ducts **1** Biliary and Pancreatic Ducts **2** Gallbladder **3** Gallbladder and Bile Ducts **4** Gallbladder, Bile Ducts and Pancreatic Ducts **8** Pancreatic Ducts	**0** High Osmolar **1** Low Osmolar **Y** Other Contrast	**Z** None	**Z** None
5 Liver	**0** High Osmolar **1** Low Osmolar **Y** Other Contrast	**Z** None	**Z** None
5 Liver	**Z** None	**Z** None	**A** Guidance

B Imaging
F Hepatobiliary System and Pancreas
2 Computerized Tomography (CT Scan)   Definition: Computer reformatted digital display of multiplanar images developed from the capture of multiple exposures of external ionizing radiation

Body Part Character 4	Contrast Character 5	Qualifier Character 6	Qualifier Character 7
5 Liver **6** Liver and Spleen **7** Pancreas **C** Hepatobiliary System, All	**0** High Osmolar **1** Low Osmolar **Y** Other Contrast	**0** Unenhanced and Enhanced **Z** None	**Z** None
5 Liver **6** Liver and Spleen **7** Pancreas **C** Hepatobiliary System, All	**Z** None	**Z** None	**Z** None

B Imaging
F Hepatobiliary System and Pancreas
3 Magnetic Resonance Imaging (MRI)   Definition: Computer reformatted digital display of multiplanar images developed from the capture of radio-frequency signals emitted by nuclei in a body site excited within a magnetic field

Body Part Character 4	Contrast Character 5	Qualifier Character 6	Qualifier Character 7
5 Liver **6** Liver and Spleen **7** Pancreas	**Y** Other Contrast	**0** Unenhanced and Enhanced **Z** None	**Z** None
5 Liver **6** Liver and Spleen **7** Pancreas	**Z** None	**Z** None	**Z** None

B Imaging
F Hepatobiliary System and Pancreas
4 Ultrasonography   Definition: Real time display of images of anatomy or flow information developed from the capture of reflected and attenuated high frequency sound waves

Body Part Character 4	Contrast Character 5	Qualifier Character 6	Qualifier Character 7
0 Bile Ducts **2** Gallbladder **3** Gallbladder and Bile Ducts **5** Liver **6** Liver and Spleen **7** Pancreas **C** Hepatobiliary System, All	**Z** None	**Z** None	**Z** None

B Imaging
F Hepatobiliary System and Pancreas
5 Other Imaging   Definition: Other specified modality for visualizing a body part

Body Part Character 4	Contrast Character 5	Qualifier Character 6	Qualifier Character 7
0 Bile Ducts **2** Gallbladder **3** Gallbladder and Bile Ducts **5** Liver **6** Liver and Spleen **7** Pancreas **C** Hepatobiliary System, All	**2** Fluorescing Agent	**0** Indocyanine Green Dye **Z** None	**0** Intraoperative **Z** None

Non-OR Procedure   DRG Non-OR Procedure   Valid OR Procedure   HAC Associated Procedure   Combination Only   New/Revised April   New/Revised October

758

ICD-10-PCS 2023

BF1–BF5

B   **Imaging**
G   **Endocrine System**
2   **Computerized Tomography (CT Scan)**   Definition: Computer reformatted digital display of multiplanar images developed from the capture of multiple exposures of external ionizing radiation

Body Part Character 4	Contrast Character 5	Qualifier Character 6	Qualifier Character 7
2 Adrenal Glands, Bilateral 3 Parathyroid Glands 4 Thyroid Gland	Ø High Osmolar 1 Low Osmolar Y Other Contrast	Ø Unenhanced and Enhanced Z None	Z None
2 Adrenal Glands, Bilateral 3 Parathyroid Glands 4 Thyroid Gland	Z None	Z None	Z None

B   **Imaging**
G   **Endocrine System**
3   **Magnetic Resonance Imaging (MRI)**   Definition: Computer reformatted digital display of multiplanar images developed from the capture of radio-frequency signals emitted by nuclei in a body site excited within a magnetic field

Body Part Character 4	Contrast Character 5	Qualifier Character 6	Qualifier Character 7
2 Adrenal Glands, Bilateral 3 Parathyroid Glands 4 Thyroid Gland	Y Other Contrast	Ø Unenhanced and Enhanced Z None	Z None
2 Adrenal Glands, Bilateral 3 Parathyroid Glands 4 Thyroid Gland	Z None	Z None	Z None

B   **Imaging**
G   **Endocrine System**
4   **Ultrasonography**   Definition: Real time display of images of anatomy or flow information developed from the capture of reflected and attenuated high frequency sound waves

Body Part Character 4	Contrast Character 5	Qualifier Character 6	Qualifier Character 7
Ø Adrenal Gland, Right 1 Adrenal Gland, Left 2 Adrenal Glands, Bilateral 3 Parathyroid Glands 4 Thyroid Gland	Z None	Z None	Z None

B   **Imaging**
H   **Skin, Subcutaneous Tissue and Breast**
Ø   **Plain Radiography**   Definition: Planar display of an image developed from the capture of external ionizing radiation on photographic or photoconductive plate

Body Part Character 4	Contrast Character 5	Qualifier Character 6	Qualifier Character 7
Ø Breast, Right 1 Breast, Left 2 Breasts, Bilateral	Z None	Z None	Z None
3 Single Mammary Duct, Right 4 Single Mammary Duct, Left 5 Multiple Mammary Ducts, Right 6 Multiple Mammary Ducts, Left	Ø High Osmolar 1 Low Osmolar Y Other Contrast Z None	Z None	Z None

B   **Imaging**
H   **Skin, Subcutaneous Tissue and Breast**
3   **Magnetic Resonance Imaging (MRI)**   Definition: Computer reformatted digital display of multiplanar images developed from the capture of radio-frequency signals emitted by nuclei in a body site excited within a magnetic field

Body Part Character 4	Contrast Character 5	Qualifier Character 6	Qualifier Character 7
Ø Breast, Right 1 Breast, Left 2 Breasts, Bilateral D Subcutaneous Tissue, Head/Neck F Subcutaneous Tissue, Upper Extremity G Subcutaneous Tissue, Thorax H Subcutaneous Tissue, Abdomen and Pelvis J Subcutaneous Tissue, Lower Extremity	Y Other Contrast	Ø Unenhanced and Enhanced Z None	Z None
Ø Breast, Right 1 Breast, Left 2 Breasts, Bilateral D Subcutaneous Tissue, Head/Neck F Subcutaneous Tissue, Upper Extremity G Subcutaneous Tissue, Thorax H Subcutaneous Tissue, Abdomen and Pelvis J Subcutaneous Tissue, Lower Extremity	Z None	Z None	Z None

B   **Imaging**
H   **Skin, Subcutaneous Tissue and Breast**
4   **Ultrasonography**   Definition: Real time display of images of anatomy or flow information developed from the capture of reflected and attenuated high frequency sound waves

Body Part Character 4	Contrast Character 5	Qualifier Character 6	Qualifier Character 7
Ø Breast, Right 1 Breast, Left 2 Breasts, Bilateral 7 Extremity, Upper 8 Extremity, Lower 9 Abdominal Wall B Chest Wall C Head and Neck	Z None	Z None	Z None

B   **Imaging**
L   **Connective Tissue**
3   **Magnetic Resonance Imaging (MRI)**   Definition: Computer reformatted digital display of multiplanar images developed from the capture of radio-frequency signals emitted by nuclei in a body site excited within a magnetic field

Body Part Character 4	Contrast Character 5	Qualifier Character 6	Qualifier Character 7
Ø Connective Tissue, Upper Extremity 1 Connective Tissue, Lower Extremity 2 Tendons, Upper Extremity 3 Tendons, Lower Extremity	Y Other Contrast	Ø Unenhanced and Enhanced Z None	Z None
Ø Connective Tissue, Upper Extremity 1 Connective Tissue, Lower Extremity 2 Tendons, Upper Extremity 3 Tendons, Lower Extremity	Z None	Z None	Z None

B   **Imaging**
L   **Connective Tissue**
4   **Ultrasonography**   Definition: Real time display of images of anatomy or flow information developed from the capture of reflected and attenuated high frequency sound waves

Body Part Character 4	Contrast Character 5	Qualifier Character 6	Qualifier Character 7
Ø Connective Tissue, Upper Extremity 1 Connective Tissue, Lower Extremity 2 Tendons, Upper Extremity 3 Tendons, Lower Extremity	Z None	Z None	Z None

Non-OR Procedure   DRG Non-OR Procedure   Valid OR Procedure   HAC Associated Procedure   Combination Only   New/Revised April   New/Revised October

760   ICD-10-PCS 2023

B   Imaging
N   Skull and Facial Bones
0   Plain Radiography   Definition: Planar display of an image developed from the capture of external ionizing radiation on photographic or photoconductive plate

Body Part Character 4	Contrast Character 5	Qualifier Character 6	Qualifier Character 7
0 Skull 1 Orbit, Right 2 Orbit, Left 3 Orbits, Bilateral 4 Nasal Bones 5 Facial Bones 6 Mandible B Zygomatic Arch, Right C Zygomatic Arch, Left D Zygomatic Arches, Bilateral G Tooth, Single H Teeth, Multiple J Teeth, All	Z None	Z None	Z None
7 Temporomandibular Joint, Right 8 Temporomandibular Joint, Left 9 Temporomandibular Joints, Bilateral	0 High Osmolar 1 Low Osmolar Y Other Contrast Z None	Z None	Z None

B   Imaging
N   Skull and Facial Bones
1   Fluoroscopy   Definition: Single plane or bi-plane real time display of an image developed from the capture of external ionizing radiation on a fluorescent screen. The image may also be stored by either digital or analog means.

Body Part Character 4	Contrast Character 5	Qualifier Character 6	Qualifier Character 7
7 Temporomandibular Joint, Right 8 Temporomandibular Joint, Left 9 Temporomandibular Joints, Bilateral	0 High Osmolar 1 Low Osmolar Y Other Contrast Z None	Z None	Z None

B   Imaging
N   Skull and Facial Bones
2   Computerized Tomography (CT Scan)   Definition: Computer reformatted digital display of multiplanar images developed from the capture of multiple exposures of external ionizing radiation

Body Part Character 4	Contrast Character 5	Qualifier Character 6	Qualifier Character 7
0 Skull 3 Orbits, Bilateral 5 Facial Bones 6 Mandible 9 Temporomandibular Joints, Bilateral F Temporal Bones	0 High Osmolar 1 Low Osmolar Y Other Contrast Z None	Z None	Z None

B   Imaging
N   Skull and Facial Bones
3   Magnetic Resonance Imaging (MRI)   Definition: Computer reformatted digital display of multiplanar images developed from the capture of radio-frequency signals emitted by nuclei in a body site excited within a magnetic field

Body Part Character 4	Contrast Character 5	Qualifier Character 6	Qualifier Character 7
9 Temporomandibular Joints, Bilateral	Y Other Contrast Z None	Z None	Z None

NC Noncovered Procedure   LC Limited Coverage   QA Questionable OB Admit   NT New Tech Add-on   ⊞ Combination Member   ♂Male   ♀Female

ICD-10-PCS 2023   761

B   **Imaging**
P   **Non-Axial Upper Bones**
0   **Plain Radiography**   Definition: Planar display of an image developed from the capture of external ionizing radiation on photographic or photoconductive plate

Body Part Character 4	Contrast Character 5	Qualifier Character 6	Qualifier Character 7
0 Sternoclavicular Joint, Right	Z None	Z None	Z None
1 Sternoclavicular Joint, Left			
2 Sternoclavicular Joints, Bilateral			
3 Acromioclavicular Joints, Bilateral			
4 Clavicle, Right			
5 Clavicle, Left			
6 Scapula, Right			
7 Scapula, Left			
A Humerus, Right			
B Humerus, Left			
E Upper Arm, Right			
F Upper Arm, Left			
J Forearm, Right			
K Forearm, Left			
N Hand, Right			
P Hand, Left			
R Finger(s), Right			
S Finger(s), Left			
X Ribs, Right			
Y Ribs, Left			
8 Shoulder, Right	0 High Osmolar	Z None	Z None
9 Shoulder, Left	1 Low Osmolar		
C Hand/Finger Joint, Right	Y Other Contrast		
D Hand/Finger Joint, Left	Z None		
G Elbow, Right			
H Elbow, Left			
L Wrist, Right			
M Wrist, Left			

B   **Imaging**
P   **Non-Axial Upper Bones**
1   **Fluoroscopy**   Definition: Single plane or bi-plane real time display of an image developed from the capture of external ionizing radiation on a fluorescent screen. The image may also be stored by either digital or analog means.

Body Part Character 4	Contrast Character 5	Qualifier Character 6	Qualifier Character 7
0 Sternoclavicular Joint, Right	Z None	Z None	Z None
1 Sternoclavicular Joint, Left			
2 Sternoclavicular Joints, Bilateral			
3 Acromioclavicular Joints, Bilateral			
4 Clavicle, Right			
5 Clavicle, Left			
6 Scapula, Right			
7 Scapula, Left			
A Humerus, Right			
B Humerus, Left			
E Upper Arm, Right			
F Upper Arm, Left			
J Forearm, Right			
K Forearm, Left			
N Hand, Right			
P Hand, Left			
R Finger(s), Right			
S Finger(s), Left			
X Ribs, Right			
Y Ribs, Left			
8 Shoulder, Right	0 High Osmolar	Z None	Z None
9 Shoulder, Left	1 Low Osmolar		
L Wrist, Right	Y Other Contrast		
M Wrist, Left	Z None		
C Hand/Finger Joint, Right	0 High Osmolar	Z None	Z None
D Hand/Finger Joint, Left	1 Low Osmolar		
G Elbow, Right	Y Other Contrast		
H Elbow, Left			

Non-OR Procedure   DRG Non-OR Procedure   Valid OR Procedure   HAC Associated Procedure   Combination Only   New/Revised April   New/Revised October

762   ICD-10-PCS 2023

B   **Imaging**
P   **Non-Axial Upper Bones**
2   **Computerized Tomography (CT Scan)** Definition: Computer reformatted digital display of multiplanar images developed from the capture of multiple exposures of external ionizing radiation

Body Part Character 4	Contrast Character 5	Qualifier Character 6	Qualifier Character 7
Ø Sternoclavicular Joint, Right 1 Sternoclavicular Joint, Left W Thorax	Ø High Osmolar 1 Low Osmolar Y Other Contrast	Z None	Z None
2 Sternoclavicular Joints, Bilateral 3 Acromioclavicular Joints, Bilateral 4 Clavicle, Right 5 Clavicle, Left 6 Scapula, Right 7 Scapula, Left 8 Shoulder, Right 9 Shoulder, Left A Humerus, Right B Humerus, Left E Upper Arm, Right F Upper Arm, Left G Elbow, Right H Elbow, Left J Forearm, Right K Forearm, Left L Wrist, Right M Wrist, Left N Hand, Right P Hand, Left Q Hands and Wrists, Bilateral R Finger(s), Right S Finger(s), Left T Upper Extremity, Right U Upper Extremity, Left V Upper Extremities, Bilateral X Ribs, Right Y Ribs, Left	Ø High Osmolar 1 Low Osmolar Y Other Contrast Z None	Z None	Z None
C Hand/Finger Joint, Right D Hand/Finger Joint, Left	Z None	Z None	Z None

B   **Imaging**
P   **Non-Axial Upper Bones**
3   **Magnetic Resonance Imaging (MRI)** Definition: Computer reformatted digital display of multiplanar images developed from the capture of radio-frequency signals emitted by nuclei in a body site excited within a magnetic field

Body Part Character 4	Contrast Character 5	Qualifier Character 6	Qualifier Character 7
8 Shoulder, Right 9 Shoulder, Left C Hand/Finger Joint, Right D Hand/Finger Joint, Left E Upper Arm, Right F Upper Arm, Left G Elbow, Right H Elbow, Left J Forearm, Right K Forearm, Left L Wrist, Right M Wrist, Left	Y Other Contrast	Ø Unenhanced and Enhanced Z None	Z None
8 Shoulder, Right 9 Shoulder, Left C Hand/Finger Joint, Right D Hand/Finger Joint, Left E Upper Arm, Right F Upper Arm, Left G Elbow, Right H Elbow, Left J Forearm, Right K Forearm, Left L Wrist, Right M Wrist, Left	Z None	Z None	Z None

NC Noncovered Procedure   LC Limited Coverage   QA Questionable OB Admit   NT New Tech Add-on   ⊞ Combination Member   ♂ Male   ♀ Female

ICD-10-PCS 2023   763

BP2–BP3

B   **Imaging**
P   **Non-Axial Upper Bones**
4   **Ultrasonography**   Definition: Real time display of images of anatomy or flow information developed from the capture of reflected and attenuated high frequency sound waves

Body Part Character 4	Contrast Character 5	Qualifier Character 6	Qualifier Character 7
8 Shoulder, Right 9 Shoulder, Left G Elbow, Right H Elbow, Left L Wrist, Right M Wrist, Left N Hand, Right P Hand, Left	Z None	Z None	1 Densitometry Z None

B   **Imaging**
Q   **Non-Axial Lower Bones**
0   **Plain Radiography**   Definition: Planar display of an image developed from the capture of external ionizing radiation on photographic or photoconductive plate

Body Part Character 4	Contrast Character 5	Qualifier Character 6	Qualifier Character 7
0 Hip, Right 1 Hip, Left	0 High Osmolar 1 Low Osmolar Y Other Contrast	Z None	Z None
0 Hip, Right 1 Hip, Left	Z None	Z None	1 Densitometry Z None
3 Femur, Right 4 Femur, Left	Z None	Z None	1 Densitometry Z None
7 Knee, Right 8 Knee, Left G Ankle, Right H Ankle, Left	0 High Osmolar 1 Low Osmolar Y Other Contrast Z None	Z None	Z None
D Lower Leg, Right F Lower Leg, Left J Calcaneus, Right K Calcaneus, Left L Foot, Right M Foot, Left P Toe(s), Right Q Toe(s), Left V Patella, Right W Patella, Left	Z None	Z None	Z None
X Foot/Toe Joint, Right Y Foot/Toe Joint, Left	0 High Osmolar 1 Low Osmolar Y Other Contrast	Z None	Z None

B   **Imaging**
Q   **Non-Axial Lower Bones**
1   **Fluoroscopy**   Definition: Single plane or bi-plane real time display of an image developed from the capture of external ionizing radiation on a fluorescent screen. The image may also be stored by either digital or analog means.

Body Part Character 4	Contrast Character 5	Qualifier Character 6	Qualifier Character 7
0 Hip, Right 1 Hip, Left 7 Knee, Right 8 Knee, Left G Ankle, Right H Ankle, Left X Foot/Toe Joint, Right Y Foot/Toe Joint, Left	0 High Osmolar 1 Low Osmolar Y Other Contrast Z None	Z None	Z None
3 Femur, Right 4 Femur, Left D Lower Leg, Right F Lower Leg, Left J Calcaneus, Right K Calcaneus, Left L Foot, Right M Foot, Left P Toe(s), Right Q Toe(s), Left V Patella, Right W Patella, Left	Z None	Z None	Z None

Non-OR Procedure   DRG Non-OR Procedure   Valid OR Procedure   HAC Associated Procedure   Combination Only   New/Revised April   New/Revised October

764

ICD-10-PCS 2023

BP4–BQ1

B   Imaging
Q   Non-Axial Lower Bones
2   Computerized Tomography (CT Scan) Definition: Computer reformatted digital display of multiplanar images developed from the capture of multiple exposures of external ionizing radiation

Body Part Character 4	Contrast Character 5	Qualifier Character 6	Qualifier Character 7
Ø Hip, Right 1 Hip, Left 3 Femur, Right 4 Femur, Left 7 Knee, Right 8 Knee, Left D Lower Leg, Right F Lower Leg, Left G Ankle, Right H Ankle, Left J Calcaneus, Right K Calcaneus, Left L Foot, Right M Foot, Left P Toe(s), Right Q Toe(s), Left R Lower Extremity, Right S Lower Extremity, Left V Patella, Right W Patella, Left X Foot/Toe Joint, Right Y Foot/Toe Joint, Left	Ø High Osmolar 1 Low Osmolar Y Other Contrast Z None	Z None	Z None
B Tibia/Fibula, Right C Tibia/Fibula, Left	Ø High Osmolar 1 Low Osmolar Y Other Contrast	Z None	Z None

B   Imaging
Q   Non-Axial Lower Bones
3   Magnetic Resonance Imaging (MRI) Definition: Computer reformatted digital display of multiplanar images developed from the capture of radio-frequency signals emitted by nuclei in a body site excited within a magnetic field

Body Part Character 4	Contrast Character 5	Qualifier Character 6	Qualifier Character 7
Ø Hip, Right 1 Hip, Left 3 Femur, Right 4 Femur, Left 7 Knee, Right 8 Knee, Left D Lower Leg, Right F Lower Leg, Left G Ankle, Right H Ankle, Left J Calcaneus, Right K Calcaneus, Left L Foot, Right M Foot, Left P Toe(s), Right Q Toe(s), Left V Patella, Right W Patella, Left	Y Other Contrast	Ø Unenhanced and Enhanced Z None	Z None
Ø Hip, Right 1 Hip, Left 3 Femur, Right 4 Femur, Left 7 Knee, Right 8 Knee, Left D Lower Leg, Right F Lower Leg, Left G Ankle, Right H Ankle, Left J Calcaneus, Right K Calcaneus, Left L Foot, Right M Foot, Left P Toe(s), Right Q Toe(s), Left V Patella, Right W Patella, Left	Z None	Z None	Z None

NC Noncovered Procedure   LC Limited Coverage   QA Questionable OB Admit   NT New Tech Add-on   ⊞ Combination Member   ♂ Male   ♀ Female

ICD-10-PCS 2023   765

BQ2–BQ3

B   **Imaging**
Q   **Non-Axial Lower Bones**
4   **Ultrasonography**   Definition: Real time display of images of anatomy or flow information developed from the capture of reflected and attenuated high frequency sound waves

Body Part Character 4	Contrast Character 5	Qualifier Character 6	Qualifier Character 7
0 Hip, Right 1 Hip, Left 2 Hips, Bilateral 7 Knee, Right 8 Knee, Left 9 Knees, Bilateral	Z None	Z None	Z None

B   **Imaging**
R   **Axial Skeleton, Except Skull and Facial Bones**
0   **Plain Radiography**   Definition: Planar display of an image developed from the capture of external ionizing radiation on photographic or photoconductive plate

Body Part Character 4	Contrast Character 5	Qualifier Character 6	Qualifier Character 7
0 Cervical Spine 7 Thoracic Spine 9 Lumbar Spine G Whole Spine	Z None	Z None	1 Densitometry Z None
1 Cervical Disc(s) 2 Thoracic Disc(s) 3 Lumbar Disc(s) 4 Cervical Facet Joint(s) 5 Thoracic Facet Joint(s) 6 Lumbar Facet Joint(s) D Sacroiliac Joints	0 High Osmolar 1 Low Osmolar Y Other Contrast Z None	Z None	Z None
8 Thoracolumbar Joint B Lumbosacral Joint C Pelvis F Sacrum and Coccyx H Sternum	Z None	Z None	Z None

B   **Imaging**
R   **Axial Skeleton, Except Skull and Facial Bones**
1   **Fluoroscopy**   Definition: Single plane or bi-plane real time display of an image developed from the capture of external ionizing radiation on a fluorescent screen. The image may also be stored by either digital or analog means.

Body Part Character 4	Contrast Character 5	Qualifier Character 6	Qualifier Character 7
0 Cervical Spine 1 Cervical Disc(s) 2 Thoracic Disc(s) 3 Lumbar Disc(s) 4 Cervical Facet Joint(s) 5 Thoracic Facet Joint(s) 6 Lumbar Facet Joint(s) 7 Thoracic Spine 8 Thoracolumbar Joint 9 Lumbar Spine B Lumbosacral Joint C Pelvis D Sacroiliac Joints F Sacrum and Coccyx G Whole Spine H Sternum	0 High Osmolar 1 Low Osmolar Y Other Contrast Z None	Z None	Z None

B   **Imaging**
R   **Axial Skeleton, Except Skull and Facial Bones**
2   **Computerized Tomography (CT Scan)**   Definition: Computer reformatted digital display of multiplanar images developed from the capture of multiple exposures of external ionizing radiation

Body Part Character 4	Contrast Character 5	Qualifier Character 6	Qualifier Character 7
0 Cervical Spine 7 Thoracic Spine 9 Lumbar Spine C Pelvis D Sacroiliac Joints F Sacrum and Coccyx	0 High Osmolar 1 Low Osmolar Y Other Contrast Z None	Z None	Z None

Non-OR Procedure   DRG Non-OR Procedure   Valid OR Procedure   HAC Associated Procedure   Combination Only   New/Revised April   New/Revised October

766   ICD-10-PCS 2023

B   **Imaging**
R   **Axial Skeleton, Except Skull and Facial Bones**
3   **Magnetic Resonance Imaging (MRI)**   Definition: Computer reformatted digital display of multiplanar images developed from the capture of radio-frequency signals emitted by nuclei in a body site excited within a magnetic field

Body Part Character 4	Contrast Character 5	Qualifier Character 6	Qualifier Character 7
Ø Cervical Spine 1 Cervical Disc(s) 2 Thoracic Disc(s) 3 Lumbar Disc(s) 7 Thoracic Spine 9 Lumbar Spine C Pelvis F Sacrum and Coccyx	Y Other Contrast	Ø Unenhanced and Enhanced Z None	Z None
Ø Cervical Spine 1 Cervical Disc(s) 2 Thoracic Disc(s) 3 Lumbar Disc(s) 7 Thoracic Spine 9 Lumbar Spine C Pelvis F Sacrum and Coccyx	Z None	Z None	Z None

B   **Imaging**
R   **Axial Skeleton, Except Skull and Facial Bones**
4   **Ultrasonography**   Definition: Real time display of images of anatomy or flow information developed from the capture of reflected and attenuated high frequency sound waves

Body Part Character 4	Contrast Character 5	Qualifier Character 6	Qualifier Character 7
Ø Cervical Spine 7 Thoracic Spine 9 Lumbar Spine F Sacrum and Coccyx	Z None	Z None	Z None

B   **Imaging**
T   **Urinary System**
Ø   **Plain Radiography**   Definition: Planar display of an image developed from the capture of external ionizing radiation on photographic or photoconductive plate

Body Part Character 4	Contrast Character 5	Qualifier Character 6	Qualifier Character 7
Ø Bladder 1 Kidney, Right 2 Kidney, Left 3 Kidneys, Bilateral 4 Kidneys, Ureters and Bladder 5 Urethra 6 Ureter, Right 7 Ureter, Left 8 Ureters, Bilateral B Bladder and Urethra C Ileal Diversion Loop	Ø High Osmolar 1 Low Osmolar Y Other Contrast Z None	Z None	Z None

B   **Imaging**
T   **Urinary System**
1   **Fluoroscopy**   Definition: Single plane or bi-plane real time display of an image developed from the capture of external ionizing radiation on a fluorescent screen. The image may also be stored by either digital or analog means.

Body Part Character 4	Contrast Character 5	Qualifier Character 6	Qualifier Character 7
Ø Bladder 1 Kidney, Right 2 Kidney, Left 3 Kidneys, Bilateral 4 Kidneys, Ureters and Bladder 5 Urethra 6 Ureter, Right 7 Ureter, Left B Bladder and Urethra C Ileal Diversion Loop D Kidney, Ureter and Bladder, Right F Kidney, Ureter and Bladder, Left G Ileal Loop, Ureters and Kidneys	Ø High Osmolar 1 Low Osmolar Y Other Contrast Z None	Z None	Z None

NC Noncovered Procedure   LC Limited Coverage   QA Questionable OB Admit   NT New Tech Add-on   ⊞ Combination Member   ♂ Male   ♀ Female

ICD-10-PCS 2023   767

BR3–BT1

B   Imaging
T   Urinary System
2   Computerized Tomography (CT Scan)   Definition: Computer reformatted digital display of multiplanar images developed from the capture of multiple exposures of external ionizing radiation

Body Part Character 4	Contrast Character 5	Qualifier Character 6	Qualifier Character 7
Ø Bladder 1 Kidney, Right 2 Kidney, Left 3 Kidneys, Bilateral 9 Kidney Transplant	Ø High Osmolar 1 Low Osmolar Y Other Contrast	Ø Unenhanced and Enhanced Z None	Z None
Ø Bladder 1 Kidney, Right 2 Kidney, Left 3 Kidneys, Bilateral 9 Kidney Transplant	Z None	Z None	Z None

B   Imaging
T   Urinary System
3   Magnetic Resonance Imaging (MRI)   Definition: Computer reformatted digital display of multiplanar images developed from the capture of radio-frequency signals emitted by nuclei in a body site excited within a magnetic field

Body Part Character 4	Contrast Character 5	Qualifier Character 6	Qualifier Character 7
Ø Bladder 1 Kidney, Right 2 Kidney, Left 3 Kidneys, Bilateral 9 Kidney Transplant	Y Other Contrast	Ø Unenhanced and Enhanced Z None	Z None
Ø Bladder 1 Kidney, Right 2 Kidney, Left 3 Kidneys, Bilateral 9 Kidney Transplant	Z None	Z None	Z None

B   Imaging
T   Urinary System
4   Ultrasonography   Definition: Real time display of images of anatomy or flow information developed from the capture of reflected and attenuated high frequency sound waves

Body Part Character 4	Contrast Character 5	Qualifier Character 6	Qualifier Character 7
Ø Bladder 1 Kidney, Right 2 Kidney, Left 3 Kidneys, Bilateral 5 Urethra 6 Ureter, Right 7 Ureter, Left 8 Ureters, Bilateral 9 Kidney Transplant J Kidneys and Bladder	Z None	Z None	Z None

B   Imaging
U   Female Reproductive System
Ø   Plain Radiography   Definition: Planar display of an image developed from the capture of external ionizing radiation on photographic or photoconductive plate

Body Part Character 4	Contrast Character 5	Qualifier Character 6	Qualifier Character 7
Ø Fallopian Tube, Right ♀ 1 Fallopian Tube, Left ♀ 2 Fallopian Tubes, Bilateral ♀ 6 Uterus ♀ 8 Uterus and Fallopian Tubes ♀ 9 Vagina ♀	Ø High Osmolar 1 Low Osmolar Y Other Contrast	Z None	Z None

♀   All body part, contrast, and qualifier values

Non-OR Procedure   DRG Non-OR Procedure   Valid OR Procedure   HAC Associated Procedure   Combination Only   New/Revised April   New/Revised October

768   ICD-10-PCS 2023

B Imaging
U Female Reproductive System
1 Fluoroscopy   Definition: Single plane or bi-plane real time display of an image developed from the capture of external ionizing radiation on a fluorescent screen. The image may also be stored by either digital or analog means.

Body Part Character 4		Contrast Character 5	Qualifier Character 6	Qualifier Character 7
Ø Fallopian Tube, Right ♀	Ø High Osmolar	Z None	Z None
1 Fallopian Tube, Left ♀	1 Low Osmolar		
2 Fallopian Tubes, Bilateral ♀	Y Other Contrast		
6 Uterus ♀	Z None		
8 Uterus and Fallopian Tubes ♀			
9 Vagina ♀			

♀   All body part, contrast, and qualifier values

B Imaging
U Female Reproductive System
3 Magnetic Resonance Imaging (MRI)   Definition: Computer reformatted digital display of multiplanar images developed from the capture of radio-frequency signals emitted by nuclei in a body site excited within a magnetic field

Body Part Character 4		Contrast Character 5	Qualifier Character 6	Qualifier Character 7
3 Ovary, Right ♀	Y Other Contrast	Ø Unenhanced and Enhanced	Z None
4 Ovary, Left ♀		Z None	
5 Ovaries, Bilateral ♀			
6 Uterus ♀			
9 Vagina ♀			
B Pregnant Uterus ♀			
C Uterus and Ovaries ♀			
3 Ovary, Right ♀	Z None	Z None	Z None
4 Ovary, Left ♀			
5 Ovaries, Bilateral ♀			
6 Uterus ♀			
9 Vagina ♀			
B Pregnant Uterus ♀			
C Uterus and Ovaries ♀			

♀   All body part, contrast, and qualifier values

B Imaging
U Female Reproductive System
4 Ultrasonography   Definition: Real time display of images of anatomy or flow information developed from the capture of reflected and attenuated high frequency sound waves

Body Part Character 4		Contrast Character 5	Qualifier Character 6	Qualifier Character 7
Ø Fallopian Tube, Right ♀	Y Other Contrast	Z None	Z None
1 Fallopian Tube, Left ♀	Z None		
2 Fallopian Tubes, Bilateral ♀			
3 Ovary, Right ♀			
4 Ovary, Left ♀			
5 Ovaries, Bilateral ♀			
6 Uterus ♀			
C Uterus and Ovaries ♀			

♀   All body part, contrast, and qualifier values

B Imaging
V Male Reproductive System
Ø Plain Radiography   Definition: Planar display of an image developed from the capture of external ionizing radiation on photographic or photoconductive plate

Body Part Character 4		Contrast Character 5	Qualifier Character 6	Qualifier Character 7
Ø Corpora Cavernosa ♂	Ø High Osmolar	Z None	Z None
1 Epididymis, Right ♂	1 Low Osmolar		
2 Epididymis, Left ♂	Y Other Contrast		
3 Prostate ♂			
5 Testicle, Right ♂			
6 Testicle, Left ♂			
8 Vasa Vasorum ♂			

♂   All body part, contrast, and qualifier values

NC Noncovered Procedure   LC Limited Coverage   QA Questionable OB Admit   NT New Tech Add-on   ⊞ Combination Member   ♂ Male   ♀ Female

B   **Imaging**
V   **Male Reproductive System**
1   **Fluoroscopy**   Definition: Single plane or bi-plane real time display of an image developed from the capture of external ionizing radiation on a fluorescent screen. The image may also be stored by either digital or analog means.

Body Part Character 4		Contrast Character 5	Qualifier Character 6	Qualifier Character 7
Ø Corpora Cavernosa	♂	Ø High Osmolar	Z None	Z None
8 Vasa Vasorum	♂	1 Low Osmolar		
		Y Other Contrast		
		Z None		

♂   All body part, contrast, and qualifier values

B   **Imaging**
V   **Male Reproductive System**
2   **Computerized Tomography (CT Scan)**   Definition: Computer reformatted digital display of multiplanar images developed from the capture of multiple exposures of external ionizing radiation

Body Part Character 4		Contrast Character 5	Qualifier Character 6	Qualifier Character 7
3 Prostate	♂	Ø High Osmolar	Ø Unenhanced and Enhanced	Z None
		1 Low Osmolar	Z None	
		Y Other Contrast		
3 Prostate	♂	Z None	Z None	Z None

♂   BV23[Ø,Y][Ø,Z]Z   ♂   BV23ZZZ
♂   BV231ØZ

B   **Imaging**
V   **Male Reproductive System**
3   **Magnetic Resonance Imaging (MRI)**   Definition: Computer reformatted digital display of multiplanar images developed from the capture of radio-frequency signals emitted by nuclei in a body site excited within a magnetic field

Body Part Character 4		Contrast Character 5	Qualifier Character 6	Qualifier Character 7
Ø Corpora Cavernosa	♂	Y Other Contrast	Ø Unenhanced and Enhanced	Z None
3 Prostate	♂		Z None	
4 Scrotum	♂			
5 Testicle, Right	♂			
6 Testicle, Left	♂			
7 Testicles, Bilateral	♂			
Ø Corpora Cavernosa	♂	Z None	Z None	Z None
3 Prostate	♂			
4 Scrotum	♂			
5 Testicle, Right	♂			
6 Testicle, Left	♂			
7 Testicles, Bilateral	♂			

♂   All body part, contrast, and qualifier values

B   **Imaging**
V   **Male Reproductive System**
4   **Ultrasonography**   Definition: Real time display of images of anatomy or flow information developed from the capture of reflected and attenuated high frequency sound waves

Body Part Character 4		Contrast Character 5	Qualifier Character 6	Qualifier Character 7
4 Scrotum	♂	Z None	Z None	Z None
9 Prostate and Seminal Vesicles	♂			
B Penis	♂			

♂   All body part, contrast, and qualifier values

B   **Imaging**
W   **Anatomical Regions**
Ø   **Plain Radiography**   Definition: Planar display of an image developed from the capture of external ionizing radiation on photographic or photoconductive plate

Body Part Character 4	Contrast Character 5	Qualifier Character 6	Qualifier Character 7
Ø Abdomen	Z None	Z None	Z None
1 Abdomen and Pelvis			
3 Chest			
B Long Bones, All			
C Lower Extremity			
J Upper Extremity			
K Whole Body			
L Whole Skeleton			
M Whole Body, Infant			

B   Imaging
W   Anatomical Regions
1   Fluoroscopy   Definition: Single plane or bi-plane real time display of an image developed from the capture of external ionizing radiation on a fluorescent screen. The image may also be stored by either digital or analog means.

Body Part Character 4	Contrast Character 5	Qualifier Character 6	Qualifier Character 7
1 Abdomen and Pelvis 9 Head and Neck C Lower Extremity J Upper Extremity	Ø High Osmolar 1 Low Osmolar Y Other Contrast Z None	Z None	Z None

B   Imaging
W   Anatomical Regions
2   Computerized Tomography (CT Scan)   Definition: Computer reformatted digital display of multiplanar images developed from the capture of multiple exposures of external ionizing radiation

Body Part Character 4	Contrast Character 5	Qualifier Character 6	Qualifier Character 7
Ø Abdomen 1 Abdomen and Pelvis 4 Chest and Abdomen 5 Chest, Abdomen and Pelvis 8 Head 9 Head and Neck F Neck G Pelvic Region	Ø High Osmolar 1 Low Osmolar Y Other Contrast	Ø Unenhanced and Enhanced Z None	Z None
Ø Abdomen 1 Abdomen and Pelvis 4 Chest and Abdomen 5 Chest, Abdomen and Pelvis 8 Head 9 Head and Neck F Neck G Pelvic Region	Z None	Z None	Z None

B   Imaging
W   Anatomical Regions
3   Magnetic Resonance Imaging (MRI)   Definition: Computer reformatted digital display of multiplanar images developed from the capture of radio-frequency signals emitted by nuclei in a body site excited within a magnetic field

Body Part Character 4	Contrast Character 5	Qualifier Character 6	Qualifier Character 7
Ø Abdomen 8 Head F Neck G Pelvic Region H Retroperitoneum P Brachial Plexus	Y Other Contrast	Ø Unenhanced and Enhanced Z None	Z None
Ø Abdomen 8 Head F Neck G Pelvic Region H Retroperitoneum P Brachial Plexus	Z None	Z None	Z None
3 Chest	Y Other Contrast	Ø Unenhanced and Enhanced Z None	Z None

B   Imaging
W   Anatomical Regions
4   Ultrasonography   Definition: Real time display of images of anatomy or flow information developed from the capture of reflected and attenuated high frequency sound waves

Body Part Character 4	Contrast Character 5	Qualifier Character 6	Qualifier Character 7
Ø Abdomen 1 Abdomen and Pelvis F Neck G Pelvic Region	Z None	Z None	Z None

NC Noncovered Procedure   LC Limited Coverage   QA Questionable OB Admit   NT New Tech Add-on   ⊞ Combination Member   ♂ Male   ♀ Female

ICD-10-PCS 2023   771

BW1–BW4

B **Imaging**
W **Anatomical Regions**
5 **Other Imaging**   Definition: Other specified modality for visualizing a body part

Body Part Character 4	Contrast Character 5	Qualifier Character 6	Qualifier Character 7
2 Trunk **9** Head and Neck **C** Lower Extremity **J** Upper Extremity	**Z** None	**1** Bacterial Autofluorescence	**Z** None

B **Imaging**
Y **Fetus and Obstetrical**
3 **Magnetic Resonance Imaging (MRI)**   Definition: Computer reformatted digital display of multiplanar images developed from the capture of radio-frequency signals emitted by nuclei in a body site excited within a magnetic field

Body Part Character 4	Contrast Character 5	Qualifier Character 6	Qualifier Character 7
0 Fetal Head ♀ **1** Fetal Heart ♀ **2** Fetal Thorax ♀ **3** Fetal Abdomen ♀ **4** Fetal Spine ♀ **5** Fetal Extremities ♀ **6** Whole Fetus ♀	**Y** Other Contrast	**0** Unenhanced and Enhanced **Z** None	**Z** None
0 Fetal Head ♀ **1** Fetal Heart ♀ **2** Fetal Thorax ♀ **3** Fetal Abdomen ♀ **4** Fetal Spine ♀ **5** Fetal Extremities ♀ **6** Whole Fetus ♀	**Z** None	**Z** None	**Z** None

♀   BY3[0,1,2,3,5,6]Y[0,Z]Z
♀   BY34YZZ
♀   BY3[0,1,2,3,4,5,6]ZZZ

B **Imaging**
Y **Fetus and Obstetrical**
4 **Ultrasonography**   Definition: Real time display of images of anatomy or flow information developed from the capture of reflected and attenuated high frequency sound waves

Body Part Character 4	Contrast Character 5	Qualifier Character 6	Qualifier Character 7
7 Fetal Umbilical Cord ♀ **8** Placenta ♀ **9** First Trimester, Single Fetus ♀ **B** First Trimester, Multiple Gestation ♀ **C** Second Trimester, Single Fetus ♀ **D** Second Trimester, Multiple Gestation ♀ **F** Third Trimester, Single Fetus ♀ **G** Third Trimester, Multiple Gestation ♀	**Z** None	**Z** None	**Z** None

♀   All body part, contrast, and qualifier values

Non-OR Procedure   DRG Non-OR Procedure   Valid OR Procedure   HAC Associated Procedure   Combination Only   New/Revised April   New/Revised October

772   ICD-10-PCS 2023

BW5–BY4

Nuclear Medicine C01–CW7

C   **Nuclear Medicine**
0   **Central Nervous System**
1   **Planar Nuclear Medicine Imaging**   Definition: Introduction of radioactive materials into the body for single plane display of images developed from the capture of radioactive emissions

Body Part Character 4	Radionuclide Character 5	Qualifier Character 6	Qualifier Character 7
0 Brain	**1** Technetium 99m (Tc-99m) **Y** Other Radionuclide	**Z** None	**Z** None
5 Cerebrospinal Fluid	**D** Indium 111 (In-111) **Y** Other Radionuclide	**Z** None	**Z** None
Y Central Nervous System	**Y** Other Radionuclide	**Z** None	**Z** None

C   **Nuclear Medicine**
0   **Central Nervous System**
2   **Tomographic (Tomo) Nuclear Medicine Imaging**   Definition: Introduction of radioactive materials into the body for three dimensional display of images developed from the capture of radioactive emissions

Body Part Character 4	Radionuclide Character 5	Qualifier Character 6	Qualifier Character 7
0 Brain	**1** Technetium 99m (Tc-99m) **F** Iodine 123 (I-123) **S** Thallium 201 (Tl-201) **Y** Other Radionuclide	**Z** None	**Z** None
5 Cerebrospinal Fluid	**D** Indium 111 (In-111) **Y** Other Radionuclide	**Z** None	**Z** None
Y Central Nervous System	**Y** Other Radionuclide	**Z** None	**Z** None

C   **Nuclear Medicine**
0   **Central Nervous System**
3   **Positron Emission Tomographic (PET) Imaging**   Definition: Introduction of radioactive materials into the body for three dimensional display of images developed from the simultaneous capture, 180 degrees apart, of radioactive emissions

Body Part Character 4	Radionuclide Character 5	Qualifier Character 6	Qualifier Character 7
0 Brain	**B** Carbon 11 (C-11) **K** Fluorine 18 (F-18) **M** Oxygen 15 (O-15) **Y** Other Radionuclide	**Z** None	**Z** None
Y Central Nervous System	**Y** Other Radionuclide	**Z** None	**Z** None

C   **Nuclear Medicine**
0   **Central Nervous System**
5   **Nonimaging Nuclear Medicine Probe**   Definition: Introduction of radioactive materials into the body for the study of distribution and fate of certain substances by the detection of radioactive emissions; or, alternatively, measurement of absorption of radioactive emissions from an external source

Body Part Character 4	Radionuclide Character 5	Qualifier Character 6	Qualifier Character 7
0 Brain	**V** Xenon 133 (Xe-133) **Y** Other Radionuclide	**Z** None	**Z** None
Y Central Nervous System	**Y** Other Radionuclide	**Z** None	**Z** None

C   **Nuclear Medicine**
2   **Heart**
1   **Planar Nuclear Medicine Imaging**   Definition: Introduction of radioactive materials into the body for single plane display of images developed from the capture of radioactive emissions

Body Part Character 4	Radionuclide Character 5	Qualifier Character 6	Qualifier Character 7
6 Heart, Right and Left	**1** Technetium 99m (Tc-99m) **Y** Other Radionuclide	**Z** None	**Z** None
G Myocardium	**1** Technetium 99m (Tc-99m) **D** Indium 111 (In-111) **S** Thallium 201 (Tl-201) **Y** Other Radionuclide **Z** None	**Z** None	**Z** None
Y Heart	**Y** Other Radionuclide	**Z** None	**Z** None

Nuclear Medicine

C   **Nuclear Medicine**
2   **Heart**
2   **Tomographic (Tomo) Nuclear Medicine Imaging**   Definition: Introduction of radioactive materials into the body for three dimensional display of images developed from the capture of radioactive emissions

Body Part Character 4	Radionuclide Character 5	Qualifier Character 6	Qualifier Character 7
6 Heart, Right and Left	**1** Technetium 99m (Tc-99m) **Y** Other Radionuclide	**Z** None	**Z** None
G Myocardium	**1** Technetium 99m (Tc-99m) **D** Indium 111 (In-111) **K** Fluorine 18 (F-18) **S** Thallium 201 (Tl-201) **Y** Other Radionuclide **Z** None	**Z** None	**Z** None
Y Heart	**Y** Other Radionuclide	**Z** None	**Z** None

C   **Nuclear Medicine**
2   **Heart**
3   **Positron Emission Tomographic (PET) Imaging**   Definition: Introduction of radioactive materials into the body for three dimensional display of images developed from the simultaneous capture, 180 degrees apart, of radioactive emissions

Body Part Character 4	Radionuclide Character 5	Qualifier Character 6	Qualifier Character 7
G Myocardium	**K** Fluorine 18 (F-18) **M** Oxygen 15 (O-15) **Q** Rubidium 82 (Rb-82) **R** Nitrogen 13 (N-13) **Y** Other Radionuclide	**Z** None	**Z** None
Y Heart	**Y** Other Radionuclide	**Z** None	**Z** None

C   **Nuclear Medicine**
2   **Heart**
5   **Nonimaging Nuclear Medicine Probe**   Definition: Introduction of radioactive materials into the body for the study of distribution and fate of certain substances by the detection of radioactive emissions; or, alternatively, measurement of absorption of radioactive emissions from an external source

Body Part Character 4	Radionuclide Character 5	Qualifier Character 6	Qualifier Character 7
6 Heart, Right and Left	**1** Technetium 99m (Tc-99m) **Y** Other Radionuclide	**Z** None	**Z** None
Y Heart	**Y** Other Radionuclide	**Z** None	**Z** None

C   **Nuclear Medicine**
5   **Veins**
1   **Planar Nuclear Medicine Imaging**   Definition: Introduction of radioactive materials into the body for single plane display of images developed from the capture of radioactive emissions

Body Part Character 4	Radionuclide Character 5	Qualifier Character 6	Qualifier Character 7
B Lower Extremity Veins, Right **C** Lower Extremity Veins, Left **D** Lower Extremity Veins, Bilateral **N** Upper Extremity Veins, Right **P** Upper Extremity Veins, Left **Q** Upper Extremity Veins, Bilateral **R** Central Veins	**1** Technetium 99m (Tc-99m) **Y** Other Radionuclide	**Z** None	**Z** None
Y Veins	**Y** Other Radionuclide	**Z** None	**Z** None

C   **Nuclear Medicine**
7   **Lymphatic and Hematologic System**
1   **Planar Nuclear Medicine Imaging**   Definition: Introduction of radioactive materials into the body for single plane display of images developed from the capture of radioactive emissions

Body Part Character 4	Radionuclide Character 5	Qualifier Character 6	Qualifier Character 7
Ø Bone Marrow	1 Technetium 99m (Tc-99m) D Indium 111 (In-111) Y Other Radionuclide	Z None	Z None
2 Spleen 5 Lymphatics, Head and Neck D Lymphatics, Pelvic J Lymphatics, Head K Lymphatics, Neck L Lymphatics, Upper Chest M Lymphatics, Trunk N Lymphatics, Upper Extremity P Lymphatics, Lower Extremity	1 Technetium 99m (Tc-99m) Y Other Radionuclide	Z None	Z None
3 Blood	D Indium 111 (In-111) Y Other Radionuclide	Z None	Z None
Y Lymphatic and Hematologic System	Y Other Radionuclide	Z None	Z None

C   **Nuclear Medicine**
7   **Lymphatic and Hematologic System**
2   **Tomographic (Tomo) Nuclear Medicine Imaging**   Definition: Introduction of radioactive materials into the body for three dimensional display of images developed from the capture of radioactive emissions

Body Part Character 4	Radionuclide Character 5	Qualifier Character 6	Qualifier Character 7
2 Spleen	1 Technetium 99m (Tc-99m) Y Other Radionuclide	Z None	Z None
Y Lymphatic and Hematologic System	Y Other Radionuclide	Z None	Z None

C   **Nuclear Medicine**
7   **Lymphatic and Hematologic System**
5   **Nonimaging Nuclear Medicine Probe**   Definition: Introduction of radioactive materials into the body for the study of distribution and fate of certain substances by the detection of radioactive emissions; or, alternatively, measurement of absorption of radioactive emissions from an external source

Body Part Character 4	Radionuclide Character 5	Qualifier Character 6	Qualifier Character 7
5 Lymphatics, Head and Neck D Lymphatics, Pelvic J Lymphatics, Head K Lymphatics, Neck L Lymphatics, Upper Chest M Lymphatics, Trunk N Lymphatics, Upper Extremity P Lymphatics, Lower Extremity	1 Technetium 99m (Tc-99m) Y Other Radionuclide	Z None	Z None
Y Lymphatic and Hematologic System	Y Other Radionuclide	Z None	Z None

C   **Nuclear Medicine**
7   **Lymphatic and Hematologic System**
6   **Nonimaging Nuclear Medicine Assay**   Definition: Introduction of radioactive materials into the body for the study of body fluids and blood elements, by the detection of radioactive emissions

Body Part Character 4	Radionuclide Character 5	Qualifier Character 6	Qualifier Character 7
3 Blood	1 Technetium 99m (Tc-99m) 7 Cobalt 58 (Co-58) C Cobalt 57 (Co-57) D Indium 111 (In-111) H Iodine 125 (I-125) W Chromium (Cr-51) Y Other Radionuclide	Z None	Z None
Y Lymphatic and Hematologic System	Y Other Radionuclide	Z None	Z None

NC Noncovered Procedure   **LC** Limited Coverage   **QA** Questionable OB Admit   **NT** New Tech Add-on   ⊞ Combination Member   ♂ Male   ♀ Female

ICD-10-PCS 2023   775

C71–C76

Nuclear Medicine

C Nuclear Medicine
8 Eye
1 Planar Nuclear Medicine Imaging   Definition: Introduction of radioactive materials into the body for single plane display of images developed from the capture of radioactive emissions

Body Part Character 4	Radionuclide Character 5	Qualifier Character 6	Qualifier Character 7
9 Lacrimal Ducts, Bilateral	1 Technetium 99m (Tc-99m) Y Other Radionuclide	Z None	Z None
Y Eye	Y Other Radionuclide	Z None	Z None

C Nuclear Medicine
9 Ear, Nose, Mouth and Throat
1 Planar Nuclear Medicine Imaging   Definition: Introduction of radioactive materials into the body for single plane display of images developed from the capture of radioactive emissions

Body Part Character 4	Radionuclide Character 5	Qualifier Character 6	Qualifier Character 7
B Salivary Glands, Bilateral	1 Technetium 99m (Tc-99m) Y Other Radionuclide	Z None	Z None
Y Ear, Nose, Mouth and Throat	Y Other Radionuclide	Z None	Z None

C Nuclear Medicine
B Respiratory System
1 Planar Nuclear Medicine Imaging   Definition: Introduction of radioactive materials into the body for single plane display of images developed from the capture of radioactive emissions

Body Part Character 4	Radionuclide Character 5	Qualifier Character 6	Qualifier Character 7
2 Lungs and Bronchi	1 Technetium 99m (Tc-99m) 9 Krypton (Kr-81m) T Xenon 127 (Xe-127) V Xenon 133 (Xe-133) Y Other Radionuclide	Z None	Z None
Y Respiratory System	Y Other Radionuclide	Z None	Z None

C Nuclear Medicine
B Respiratory System
2 Tomographic (Tomo) Nuclear Medicine Imaging   Definition: Introduction of radioactive materials into the body for three dimensional display of images developed from the capture of radioactive emissions

Body Part Character 4	Radionuclide Character 5	Qualifier Character 6	Qualifier Character 7
2 Lungs and Bronchi	1 Technetium 99m (Tc-99m) 9 Krypton (Kr-81m) Y Other Radionuclide	Z None	Z None
Y Respiratory System	Y Other Radionuclide	Z None	Z None

C Nuclear Medicine
B Respiratory System
3 Positron Emission Tomographic (PET) Imaging   Definition: Introduction of radioactive materials into the body for three dimensional display of images developed from the simultaneous capture, 180 degrees apart, of radioactive emissions

Body Part Character 4	Radionuclide Character 5	Qualifier Character 6	Qualifier Character 7
2 Lungs and Bronchi	K Fluorine 18 (F-18) Y Other Radionuclide	Z None	Z None
Y Respiratory System	Y Other Radionuclide	Z None	Z None

C Nuclear Medicine
D Gastrointestinal System
1 Planar Nuclear Medicine Imaging   Definition: Introduction of radioactive materials into the body for single plane display of images developed from the capture of radioactive emissions

Body Part Character 4	Radionuclide Character 5	Qualifier Character 6	Qualifier Character 7
5 Upper Gastrointestinal Tract 7 Gastrointestinal Tract	1 Technetium 99m (Tc-99m) D Indium 111 (In-111) Y Other Radionuclide	Z None	Z None
Y Digestive System	Y Other Radionuclide	Z None	Z None

C   **Nuclear Medicine**
D   **Gastrointestinal System**
2   **Tomographic (Tomo) Nuclear Medicine Imaging**   Definition: Introduction of radioactive materials into the body for three dimensional display of images developed from the capture of radioactive emissions

Body Part Character 4	Radionuclide Character 5	Qualifier Character 6	Qualifier Character 7
7 Gastrointestinal Tract	1 Technetium 99m (Tc-99m) D Indium 111 (In-111) Y Other Radionuclide	Z None	Z None
Y Digestive System	Y Other Radionuclide	Z None	Z None

C   **Nuclear Medicine**
F   **Hepatobiliary System and Pancreas**
1   **Planar Nuclear Medicine Imaging**   Definition: Introduction of radioactive materials into the body for single plane display of images developed from the capture of radioactive emissions

Body Part Character 4	Radionuclide Character 5	Qualifier Character 6	Qualifier Character 7
4 Gallbladder 5 Liver 6 Liver and Spleen C Hepatobiliary System, All	1 Technetium 99m (Tc-99m) Y Other Radionuclide	Z None	Z None
Y Hepatobiliary System and Pancreas	Y Other Radionuclide	Z None	Z None

C   **Nuclear Medicine**
F   **Hepatobiliary System and Pancreas**
2   **Tomographic (Tomo) Nuclear Medicine Imaging**   Definition: Introduction of radioactive materials into the body for three dimensional display of images developed from the capture of radioactive emissions

Body Part Character 4	Radionuclide Character 5	Qualifier Character 6	Qualifier Character 7
4 Gallbladder 5 Liver 6 Liver and Spleen	1 Technetium 99m (Tc-99m) Y Other Radionuclide	Z None	Z None
Y Hepatobiliary System and Pancreas	Y Other Radionuclide	Z None	Z None

C   **Nuclear Medicine**
G   **Endocrine System**
1   **Planar Nuclear Medicine Imaging**   Definition: Introduction of radioactive materials into the body for single plane display of images developed from the capture of radioactive emissions

Body Part Character 4	Radionuclide Character 5	Qualifier Character 6	Qualifier Character 7
1 Parathyroid Glands	1 Technetium 99m (Tc-99m) S Thallium 201 (Tl-201) Y Other Radionuclide	Z None	Z None
2 Thyroid Gland	1 Technetium 99m (Tc-99m) F Iodine 123 (I-123) G Iodine 131 (I-131) Y Other Radionuclide	Z None	Z None
4 Adrenal Glands, Bilateral	G Iodine 131 (I-131) Y Other Radionuclide	Z None	Z None
Y Endocrine System	Y Other Radionuclide	Z None	Z None

C   **Nuclear Medicine**
G   **Endocrine System**
2   **Tomographic (Tomo) Nuclear Medicine Imaging**   Definition: Introduction of radioactive materials into the body for three dimensional display of images developed from the capture of radioactive emissions

Body Part Character 4	Radionuclide Character 5	Qualifier Character 6	Qualifier Character 7
1 Parathyroid Glands	1 Technetium 99m (Tc-99m) S Thallium 201 (Tl-201) Y Other Radionuclide	Z None	Z None
Y Endocrine System	Y Other Radionuclide	Z None	Z None

C **Nuclear Medicine**
G **Endocrine System**
4 **Nonimaging Nuclear Medicine Uptake**   Definition: Introduction of radioactive materials into the body for measurements of organ function, from the detection of radioactive emissions

Body Part Character 4	Radionuclide Character 5	Qualifier Character 6	Qualifier Character 7
2 Thyroid Gland	1 Technetium 99m (Tc-99m) F Iodine 123 (I-123) G Iodine 131 (I-131) Y Other Radionuclide	Z None	Z None
Y Endocrine System	Y Other Radionuclide	Z None	Z None

C **Nuclear Medicine**
H **Skin, Subcutaneous Tissue and Breast**
1 **Planar Nuclear Medicine Imaging**   Definition: Introduction of radioactive materials into the body for single plane display of images developed from the capture of radioactive emissions

Body Part Character 4	Radionuclide Character 5	Qualifier Character 6	Qualifier Character 7
Ø Breast, Right 1 Breast, Left 2 Breasts, Bilateral	1 Technetium 99m (Tc-99m) S Thallium 201 (Tl-201) Y Other Radionuclide	Z None	Z None
Y Skin, Subcutaneous Tissue and Breast	Y Other Radionuclide	Z None	Z None

C **Nuclear Medicine**
H **Skin, Subcutaneous Tissue and Breast**
2 **Tomographic (Tomo) Nuclear Medicine Imaging** Definition: Introduction of radioactive materials into the body for three dimensional display of images developed from the capture of radioactive emissions

Body Part Character 4	Radionuclide Character 5	Qualifier Character 6	Qualifier Character 7
Ø Breast, Right 1 Breast, Left 2 Breasts, Bilateral	1 Technetium 99m (Tc-99m) S Thallium 201 (Tl-201) Y Other Radionuclide	Z None	Z None
Y Skin, Subcutaneous Tissue and Breast	Y Other Radionuclide	Z None	Z None

C **Nuclear Medicine**
P **Musculoskeletal System**
1 **Planar Nuclear Medicine Imaging**   Definition: Introduction of radioactive materials into the body for single plane display of images developed from the capture of radioactive emissions

Body Part Character 4	Radionuclide Character 5	Qualifier Character 6	Qualifier Character 7
1 Skull 4 Thorax 5 Spine 6 Pelvis 7 Spine and Pelvis 8 Upper Extremity, Right 9 Upper Extremity, Left B Upper Extremities, Bilateral C Lower Extremity, Right D Lower Extremity, Left F Lower Extremities, Bilateral Z Musculoskeletal System, All	1 Technetium 99m (Tc-99m) Y Other Radionuclide	Z None	Z None
Y Musculoskeletal System, Other	Y Other Radionuclide	Z None	Z None

C   **Nuclear Medicine**
P   **Musculoskeletal System**
2   **Tomographic (Tomo) Nuclear Medicine Imaging**   Definition: Introduction of radioactive materials into the body for three dimensional display of images developed from the capture of radioactive emissions

Body Part Character 4	Radionuclide Character 5	Qualifier Character 6	Qualifier Character 7
1 Skull 2 Cervical Spine 3 Skull and Cervical Spine 4 Thorax 6 Pelvis 7 Spine and Pelvis 8 Upper Extremity, Right 9 Upper Extremity, Left B Upper Extremities, Bilateral C Lower Extremity, Right D Lower Extremity, Left F Lower Extremities, Bilateral G Thoracic Spine H Lumbar Spine J Thoracolumbar Spine	1 Technetium 99m (Tc-99m) Y Other Radionuclide	Z None	Z None
Y Musculoskeletal System, Other	Y Other Radionuclide	Z None	Z None

C   **Nuclear Medicine**
P   **Musculoskeletal System**
5   **Nonimaging Nuclear Medicine Probe**   Definition: Introduction of radioactive materials into the body for the study of distribution and fate of certain substances by the detection of radioactive emissions; or, alternatively, measurement of absorption of radioactive emissions from an external source

Body Part Character 4	Radionuclide Character 5	Qualifier Character 6	Qualifier Character 7
5 Spine N Upper Extremities P Lower Extremities	Z None	Z None	Z None
Y Musculoskeletal System, Other	Y Other Radionuclide	Z None	Z None

C   **Nuclear Medicine**
T   **Urinary System**
1   **Planar Nuclear Medicine Imaging**   Definition: Introduction of radioactive materials into the body for single plane display of images developed from the capture of radioactive emissions

Body Part Character 4	Radionuclide Character 5	Qualifier Character 6	Qualifier Character 7
3 Kidneys, Ureters and Bladder	1 Technetium 99m (Tc-99m) F Iodine 123 (I-123) G Iodine 131 (I-131) Y Other Radionuclide	Z None	Z None
H Bladder and Ureters	1 Technetium 99m (Tc-99m) Y Other Radionuclide	Z None	Z None
Y Urinary System	Y Other Radionuclide	Z None	Z None

C   **Nuclear Medicine**
T   **Urinary System**
2   **Tomographic (Tomo) Nuclear Medicine Imaging**   Definition: Introduction of radioactive materials into the body for three dimensional display of images developed from the capture of radioactive emissions

Body Part Character 4	Radionuclide Character 5	Qualifier Character 6	Qualifier Character 7
3 Kidneys, Ureters and Bladder	1 Technetium 99m (Tc-99m) Y Other Radionuclide	Z None	Z None
Y Urinary System	Y Other Radionuclide	Z None	Z None

C   **Nuclear Medicine**
T   **Urinary System**
6   **Nonimaging Nuclear Medicine Assay**   Definition: Introduction of radioactive materials into the body for the study of body fluids and blood elements, by the detection of radioactive emissions

Body Part Character 4	Radionuclide Character 5	Qualifier Character 6	Qualifier Character 7
3 Kidneys, Ureters and Bladder	1 Technetium 99m (Tc-99m) F Iodine 123 (I-123) G Iodine 131 (I-131) H Iodine 125 (I-125) Y Other Radionuclide	Z None	Z None
Y Urinary System	Y Other Radionuclide	Z None	Z None

C   Nuclear Medicine
V   Male Reproductive System
1   Planar Nuclear Medicine Imaging   Definition: Introduction of radioactive materials into the body for single plane display of images developed from the capture of radioactive emissions

Body Part Character 4	Radionuclide Character 5	Qualifier Character 6	Qualifier Character 7
9 Testicles, Bilateral ♂	1 Technetium 99m (Tc-99m) Y Other Radionuclide	Z None	Z None
Y Male Reproductive System ♂	Y Other Radionuclide	Z None	Z None

♂   All body part, radionuclide, and qualifier values

C   Nuclear Medicine
W   Anatomical Regions
1   Planar Nuclear Medicine Imaging   Definition: Introduction of radioactive materials into the body for single plane display of images developed from the capture of radioactive emissions

Body Part Character 4	Radionuclide Character 5	Qualifier Character 6	Qualifier Character 7
Ø Abdomen 1 Abdomen and Pelvis 4 Chest and Abdomen 6 Chest and Neck B Head and Neck D Lower Extremity J Pelvic Region M Upper Extremity N Whole Body	1 Technetium 99m (Tc-99m) D Indium 111 (In-111) F Iodine 123 (I-123) G Iodine 131 (I-131) L Gallium 67 (Ga-67) S Thallium 201 (Tl-201) Y Other Radionuclide	Z None	Z None
3 Chest	1 Technetium 99m (Tc-99m) D Indium 111 (In-111) F Iodine 123 (I-123) G Iodine 131 (I-131) K Fluorine 18 (F-18) L Gallium 67 (Ga-67) S Thallium 201 (Tl-201) Y Other Radionuclide	Z None	Z None
Y Anatomical Regions, Multiple	Y Other Radionuclide	Z None	Z None
Z Anatomical Region, Other	Z None	Z None	Z None

C   Nuclear Medicine
W   Anatomical Regions
2   Tomographic (Tomo) Nuclear Medicine Imaging Definition: Introduction of radioactive materials into the body for three dimensional display of images developed from the capture of radioactive emissions

Body Part Character 4	Radionuclide Character 5	Qualifier Character 6	Qualifier Character 7
Ø Abdomen 1 Abdomen and Pelvis 3 Chest 4 Chest and Abdomen 6 Chest and Neck B Head and Neck D Lower Extremity J Pelvic Region M Upper Extremity	1 Technetium 99m (Tc-99m) D Indium 111 (In-111) F Iodine 123 (I-123) G Iodine 131 (I-131) K Fluorine 18 (F-18) L Gallium 67 (Ga-67) S Thallium 201 (Tl-201) Y Other Radionuclide	Z None	Z None
Y Anatomical Regions, Multiple	Y Other Radionuclide	Z None	Z None

C   Nuclear Medicine
W   Anatomical Regions
3   Positron Emission Tomographic (PET) Imaging   Definition: Introduction of radioactive materials into the body for three dimensional display of images developed from the simultaneous capture, 180 degrees apart, of radioactive emissions

Body Part Character 4	Radionuclide Character 5	Qualifier Character 6	Qualifier Character 7
N Whole Body	Y Other Radionuclide	Z None	Z None

Non-OR Procedure   DRG Non-OR Procedure   Valid OR Procedure   HAC Associated Procedure   Combination Only   New/Revised April   New/Revised October

780   ICD-10-PCS 2023

CV1–CW3

C Nuclear Medicine
W Anatomical Regions
5 Nonimaging Nuclear Medicine Probe   Definition: Introduction of radioactive materials into the body for the study of distribution and fate of certain substances by the detection of radioactive emissions; or, alternatively, measurement of absorption of radioactive emissions from an external source

Body Part Character 4	Radionuclide Character 5	Qualifier Character 6	Qualifier Character 7
Ø Abdomen **1** Abdomen and Pelvis **3** Chest **4** Chest and Abdomen **6** Chest and Neck **B** Head and Neck **D** Lower Extremity **J** Pelvic Region **M** Upper Extremity	**1** Technetium 99m (Tc-99m) **D** Indium 111 (In-111) **Y** Other Radionuclide	**Z** None	**Z** None

C Nuclear Medicine
W Anatomical Regions
7 Systemic Nuclear Medicine Therapy   Definition: Introduction of unsealed radioactive materials into the body for treatment

Body Part Character 4	Radionuclide Character 5	Qualifier Character 6	Qualifier Character 7
Ø Abdomen **3** Chest	**N** Phosphorus 32 (P-32) **Y** Other Radionuclide	**Z** None	**Z** None
G Thyroid	**G** Iodine 131 (I-131) **Y** Other Radionuclide	**Z** None	**Z** None
N Whole Body	**8** Samarium 153 (Sm-153) **G** Iodine 131 (I-131) **N** Phosphorus 32 (P-32) **P** Strontium 89 (Sr-89) **Y** Other Radionuclide	**Z** None	**Z** None
Y Anatomical Regions, Multiple	**Y** Other Radionuclide	**Z** None	**Z** None

NC Noncovered Procedure   **LC** Limited Coverage   **QA** Questionable OB Admit   **NT** New Tech Add-on   ⊞ Combination Member   ♂ Male   ♀ Female

ICD-10-PCS 2023   781

CW5–CW7

Radiation Therapy D00–DWY

AHA Coding Clinic for table D01
2020, 4Q, 43-44	Insertion of radioactive element
2020, 4Q, 69-70	Cesium 131 brachytherapy
2019, 4Q, 42-44	Unidirectional source brachytherapy

AHA Coding Clinic for table D0Y
2020, 4Q, 70	Intraoperative radiation therapy

AHA Coding Clinic for table D71
2020, 4Q, 43-44	Insertion of radioactive element
2020, 4Q, 69-70	Cesium 131 brachytherapy
2019, 4Q, 42-44	Unidirectional source brachytherapy

AHA Coding Clinic for table D81
2020, 4Q, 43-44	Insertion of radioactive element
2020, 4Q, 69-70	Cesium 131 brachytherapy
2019, 4Q, 42-44	Unidirectional source brachytherapy

AHA Coding Clinic for table D91
2020, 4Q, 43-44	Insertion of radioactive element
2020, 4Q, 69-70	Cesium 131 brachytherapy
2019, 4Q, 42-44	Unidirectional source brachytherapy

AHA Coding Clinic for table DB1
2020, 4Q, 43-44	Insertion of radioactive element
2020, 4Q, 69-70	Cesium 131 brachytherapy
2019, 4Q, 42-44	Unidirectional source brachytherapy

AHA Coding Clinic for table DD1
2020, 4Q, 43-44	Insertion of radioactive element
2020, 4Q, 69-70	Cesium 131 brachytherapy
2019, 4Q, 42-44	Unidirectional source brachytherapy

AHA Coding Clinic for table DF1
2022, 2Q, 26	Radioembolization of right hepatic lobe
2020, 4Q, 43-44	Insertion of radioactive element
2020, 4Q, 69-70	Cesium 131 brachytherapy
2019, 4Q, 42-44	Unidirectional source brachytherapy

AHA Coding Clinic for table DG1
2020, 4Q, 43-44	Insertion of radioactive element
2020, 4Q, 69-70	Cesium 131 brachytherapy
2019, 4Q, 42-44	Unidirectional source brachytherapy

AHA Coding Clinic for table DM1
2020, 4Q, 43-44	Insertion of radioactive element
2020, 4Q, 69-70	Cesium 131 brachytherapy
2019, 4Q, 42-44	Unidirectional source brachytherapy

AHA Coding Clinic for table DT1
2020, 4Q, 43-44	Insertion of radioactive element
2020, 4Q, 69-70	Cesium 131 brachytherapy
2019, 4Q, 42-44	Unidirectional source brachytherapy

AHA Coding Clinic for table DU1
2020, 4Q, 43-44	Insertion of radioactive element
2020, 4Q, 69-70	Cesium 131 brachytherapy
2019, 4Q, 42-44	Unidirectional source brachytherapy
2017, 4Q, 104	Intrauterine brachytherapy & placement of tandems & ovoids

AHA Coding Clinic for table DV1
2020, 4Q, 43-44	Insertion of radioactive element
2020, 4Q, 69-70	Cesium 131 brachytherapy
2019, 4Q, 42-44	Unidirectional source brachytherapy

AHA Coding Clinic for table DW1
2020, 4Q, 43-44	Insertion of radioactive element
2020, 4Q, 69-70	Cesium 131 brachytherapy
2019, 4Q, 42-44	Unidirectional source brachytherapy

AHA Coding Clinic for table DWY
2019, 4Q, 37	Hyperthermic antineoplastic chemotherapy

D　Radiation Therapy
0　Central and Peripheral Nervous System
0　Beam Radiation

Treatment Site Character 4	Modality Qualifier Character 5	Isotope Character 6	Qualifier Character 7
0　Brain 1　Brain Stem 6　Spinal Cord 7　Peripheral Nerve	0　Photons <1 MeV 1　Photons 1- 10 MeV 2　Photons >10 MeV 4　Heavy Particles (Protons, Ions) 5　Neutrons 6　Neutron Capture	Z　None	Z　None
0　Brain 1　Brain Stem 6　Spinal Cord 7　Peripheral Nerve	3　Electrons	Z　None	0　Intraoperative Z　None

D　Radiation Therapy
0　Central and Peripheral Nervous System
1　Brachytherapy

Treatment Site Character 4	Modality Qualifier Character 5	Isotope Character 6	Qualifier Character 7
0　Brain 1　Brain Stem 6　Spinal Cord 7　Peripheral Nerve	9　High Dose Rate (HDR)	7　Cesium 137 (Cs-137) 8　Iridium 192 (Ir-192) 9　Iodine 125 (I-125) B　Palladium 103 (Pd-103) C　Californium 252 (Cf-252) Y　Other Isotope	Z　None
0　Brain 1　Brain Stem 6　Spinal Cord 7　Peripheral Nerve	B　Low Dose Rate (LDR)	6　Cesium 131 (Cs-131) 7　Cesium 137 (Cs-137) 8　Iridium 192 (Ir-192) 9　Iodine 125 (I-125) C　Californium 252 (Cf-252) Y　Other Isotope	Z　None
0　Brain 1　Brain Stem 6　Spinal Cord 7　Peripheral Nerve	B　Low Dose Rate (LDR)	B　Palladium 103 (Pd-103)	1　Unidirectional Source Z　None

---

NC Noncovered Procedure　　**LC** Limited Coverage　　**QA** Questionable OB Admit　　**NT** New Tech Add-on　　⊞ Combination Member　　♂ Male　　♀ Female

Radiation Therapy

D   **Radiation Therapy**
Ø   **Central and Peripheral Nervous System**
2   **Stereotactic Radiosurgery**

Treatment Site Character 4	Modality Qualifier Character 5	Isotope Character 6	Qualifier Character 7

Ø   Brain
1   Brain Stem
6   Spinal Cord
7   Peripheral Nerve
	D Stereotactic Other Photon
	     Radiosurgery
	H Stereotactic Particulate
	     Radiosurgery
	J Stereotactic Gamma Beam
	     Radiosurgery
		Z None	Z None

DRG Non-OR   All treatment site, modality, isotope, and qualifier values

D   **Radiation Therapy**
Ø   **Central and Peripheral Nervous System**
Y   **Other Radiation**

Treatment Site Character 4	Modality Qualifier Character 5	Isotope Character 6	Qualifier Character 7
Ø Brain 1 Brain Stem 6 Spinal Cord 7 Peripheral Nerve	7 Contact Radiation 8 Hyperthermia C Intraoperative Radiation Therapy (IORT) F Plaque Radiation	Z None	Z None

D   **Radiation Therapy**
7   **Lymphatic and Hematologic System**
Ø   **Beam Radiation**

Treatment Site Character 4	Modality Qualifier Character 5	Isotope Character 6	Qualifier Character 7
Ø Bone Marrow 1 Thymus 2 Spleen 3 Lymphatics, Neck 4 Lymphatics, Axillary 5 Lymphatics, Thorax 6 Lymphatics, Abdomen 7 Lymphatics, Pelvis 8 Lymphatics, Inguinal	Ø Photons <1 MeV 1 Photons 1- 10 MeV 2 Photons >10 MeV 4 Heavy Particles (Protons, Ions) 5 Neutrons 6 Neutron Capture	Z None	Z None
Ø Bone Marrow 1 Thymus 2 Spleen 3 Lymphatics, Neck 4 Lymphatics, Axillary 5 Lymphatics, Thorax 6 Lymphatics, Abdomen 7 Lymphatics, Pelvis 8 Lymphatics, Inguinal	3 Electrons	Z None	Ø Intraoperative Z None

Radiation Therapy

D Radiation Therapy
7 Lymphatic and Hematologic System
1 Brachytherapy

Treatment Site Character 4	Modality Qualifier Character 5	Isotope Character 6	Qualifier Character 7
Ø Bone Marrow 1 Thymus 2 Spleen 3 Lymphatics, Neck 4 Lymphatics, Axillary 5 Lymphatics, Thorax 6 Lymphatics, Abdomen 7 Lymphatics, Pelvis 8 Lymphatics, Inguinal	9 High Dose Rate (HDR)	7 Cesium 137 (Cs-137) 8 Iridium 192 (Ir-192) 9 Iodine 125 (I-125) B Palladium 103 (Pd-103) C Californium 252 (Cf-252) Y Other Isotope	Z None
Ø Bone Marrow 1 Thymus 2 Spleen 3 Lymphatics, Neck 4 Lymphatics, Axillary 5 Lymphatics, Thorax 6 Lymphatics, Abdomen 7 Lymphatics, Pelvis 8 Lymphatics, Inguinal	B Low Dose Rate (LDR)	6 Cesium 131 (Cs-131) 7 Cesium 137 (Cs-137) 8 Iridium 192 (Ir-192) 9 Iodine 125 (I-125) C Californium 252 (Cf-252) Y Other Isotope	Z None
Ø Bone Marrow 1 Thymus 2 Spleen 3 Lymphatics, Neck 4 Lymphatics, Axillary 5 Lymphatics, Thorax 6 Lymphatics, Abdomen 7 Lymphatics, Pelvis 8 Lymphatics, Inguinal	B Low Dose Rate (LDR)	B Palladium 103 (Pd-103)	1 Unidirectional Source Z None

D Radiation Therapy
7 Lymphatic and Hematologic System
2 Stereotactic Radiosurgery

Treatment Site Character 4	Modality Qualifier Character 5	Isotope Character 6	Qualifier Character 7

Ø Bone Marrow
1 Thymus
2 Spleen
3 Lymphatics, Neck
4 Lymphatics, Axillary
5 Lymphatics, Thorax
6 Lymphatics, Abdomen
7 Lymphatics, Pelvis
8 Lymphatics, Inguinal
	D Stereotactic Other Photon
	    Radiosurgery
	H Stereotactic Particulate
	    Radiosurgery
	J Stereotactic Gamma Beam
	    Radiosurgery
		Z None	Z None

DRG Non-OR All treatment site, modality, isotope, and qualifier values

D Radiation Therapy
7 Lymphatic and Hematologic System
Y Other Radiation

Treatment Site Character 4	Modality Qualifier Character 5	Isotope Character 6	Qualifier Character 7
Ø Bone Marrow 1 Thymus 2 Spleen 3 Lymphatics, Neck 4 Lymphatics, Axillary 5 Lymphatics, Thorax 6 Lymphatics, Abdomen 7 Lymphatics, Pelvis 8 Lymphatics, Inguinal	8 Hyperthermia F Plaque Radiation	Z None	Z None

NC Noncovered Procedure   LC Limited Coverage   QA Questionable OB Admit   NT New Tech Add-on   ⊞ Combination Member   ♂ Male   ♀ Female

ICD-10-PCS 2023   785

D   Radiation Therapy
8   Eye
Ø   Beam Radiation

Treatment Site Character 4	Modality Qualifier Character 5	Isotope Character 6	Qualifier Character 7
Ø Eye	Ø Photons <1 MeV 1 Photons 1- 10 MeV 2 Photons >10 MeV 4 Heavy Particles (Protons, Ions) 5 Neutrons 6 Neutron Capture	Z None	Z None
Ø Eye	3 Electrons	Z None	Ø Intraoperative Z None

D   Radiation Therapy
8   Eye
1   Brachytherapy

Treatment Site Character 4	Modality Qualifier Character 5	Isotope Character 6	Qualifier Character 7
Ø Eye	9 High Dose Rate (HDR)	7 Cesium 137 (Cs-137) 8 Iridium 192 (Ir-192) 9 Iodine 125 (I-125) B Palladium 103 (Pd-103) C Californium 252 (Cf-252) Y Other Isotope	Z None
Ø Eye	B Low Dose Rate (LDR)	6 Cesium 131 (Cs-131) 7 Cesium 137 (Cs-137) 8 Iridium 192 (Ir-192) 9 Iodine 125 (I-125) C Californium 252 (Cf-252) Y Other Isotope	Z None
Ø Eye	B Low Dose Rate (LDR)	B Palladium 103 (Pd-103)	1 Unidirectional Source Z None

D   Radiation Therapy
8   Eye
2   Stereotactic Radiosurgery

Treatment Site Character 4	Modality Qualifier Character 5	Isotope Character 6	Qualifier Character 7
Ø Eye	D Stereotactic Other Photon Radiosurgery H Stereotactic Particulate Radiosurgery J Stereotactic Gamma Beam Radiosurgery	Z None	Z None

DRG Non-OR All treatment site, modality, isotope, and qualifier values

D   Radiation Therapy
8   Eye
Y   Other Radiation

Treatment Site Character 4	Modality Qualifier Character 5	Isotope Character 6	Qualifier Character 7
Ø Eye	7 Contact Radiation 8 Hyperthermia F Plaque Radiation	Z None	Z None

D   Radiation Therapy
9   Ear, Nose, Mouth and Throat
Ø   Beam Radiation

Treatment Site Character 4	Modality Qualifier Character 5	Isotope Character 6	Qualifier Character 7
Ø Ear 1 Nose 3 Hypopharynx 4 Mouth 5 Tongue 6 Salivary Glands 7 Sinuses 8 Hard Palate 9 Soft Palate B Larynx D Nasopharynx F Oropharynx	Ø Photons <1 MeV 1 Photons 1- 10 MeV 2 Photons >10 MeV 4 Heavy Particles (Protons, Ions) 5 Neutrons 6 Neutron Capture	Z None	Z None
Ø Ear 1 Nose 3 Hypopharynx 4 Mouth 5 Tongue 6 Salivary Glands 7 Sinuses 8 Hard Palate 9 Soft Palate B Larynx D Nasopharynx F Oropharynx	3 Electrons	Z None	Ø Intraoperative Z None

D   Radiation Therapy
9   Ear, Nose, Mouth and Throat
1   Brachytherapy

Treatment Site Character 4	Modality Qualifier Character 5	Isotope Character 6	Qualifier Character 7
Ø Ear 1 Nose 3 Hypopharynx 4 Mouth 5 Tongue 6 Salivary Glands 7 Sinuses 8 Hard Palate 9 Soft Palate B Larynx D Nasopharynx F Oropharynx	9 High Dose Rate (HDR)	7 Cesium 137 (Cs-137) 8 Iridium 192 (Ir-192) 9 Iodine 125 (I-125) B Palladium 103 (Pd-103) C Californium 252 (Cf-252) Y Other Isotope	Z None
Ø Ear 1 Nose 3 Hypopharynx 4 Mouth 5 Tongue 6 Salivary Glands 7 Sinuses 8 Hard Palate 9 Soft Palate B Larynx D Nasopharynx F Oropharynx	B Low Dose Rate (LDR)	6 Cesium 131 (Cs-131) 7 Cesium 137 (Cs-137) 8 Iridium 192 (Ir-192) 9 Iodine 125 (I-125) C Californium 252 (Cf-252) Y Other Isotope	Z None
Ø Ear 1 Nose 3 Hypopharynx 4 Mouth 5 Tongue 6 Salivary Glands 7 Sinuses 8 Hard Palate 9 Soft Palate B Larynx D Nasopharynx F Oropharynx	B Low Dose Rate (LDR)	B Palladium 103 (Pd-103)	1 Unidirectional Source Z None

NC Noncovered Procedure   LC Limited Coverage   QA Questionable OB Admit   NT New Tech Add-on   ⊞ Combination Member   ♂ Male   ♀ Female

ICD-10-PCS 2023   787

Radiation Therapy

D   Radiation Therapy
9   Ear, Nose, Mouth and Throat
2   Stereotactic Radiosurgery

Treatment Site Character 4	Modality Qualifier Character 5	Isotope Character 6	Qualifier Character 7

0   Ear
1   Nose
4   Mouth
5   Tongue
6   Salivary Glands
7   Sinuses
8   Hard Palate
9   Soft Palate
B   Larynx
C   Pharynx
D   Nasopharynx
	D Stereotactic Other Photon
	     Radiosurgery
	H Stereotactic Particulate
	     Radiosurgery
	J Stereotactic Gamma Beam
	     Radiosurgery
		Z None	Z None

DRG Non-OR   All treatment site, modality, isotope, and qualifier values

D   Radiation Therapy
9   Ear, Nose, Mouth and Throat
Y   Other Radiation

Treatment Site Character 4	Modality Qualifier Character 5	Isotope Character 6	Qualifier Character 7
0 Ear 1 Nose 5 Tongue 6 Salivary Glands 7 Sinuses 8 Hard Palate 9 Soft Palate	7 Contact Radiation 8 Hyperthermia F Plaque Radiation	Z None	Z None
3 Hypopharynx F Oropharynx	7 Contact Radiation 8 Hyperthermia	Z None	Z None
4 Mouth B Larynx D Nasopharynx	7 Contact Radiation 8 Hyperthermia C Intraoperative Radiation Therapy (IORT) F Plaque Radiation	Z None	Z None
C Pharynx	C Intraoperative Radiation Therapy (IORT) F Plaque Radiation	Z None	Z None

D   Radiation Therapy
B   Respiratory System
0   Beam Radiation

Treatment Site Character 4	Modality Qualifier Character 5	Isotope Character 6	Qualifier Character 7
0 Trachea 1 Bronchus 2 Lung 5 Pleura 6 Mediastinum 7 Chest Wall 8 Diaphragm	0 Photons <1 MeV 1 Photons 1- 10 MeV 2 Photons >10 MeV 4 Heavy Particles (Protons, Ions) 5 Neutrons 6 Neutron Capture	Z None	Z None
0 Trachea 1 Bronchus 2 Lung 5 Pleura 6 Mediastinum 7 Chest Wall 8 Diaphragm	3 Electrons	Z None	0 Intraoperative Z None

D Radiation Therapy
B Respiratory System
1 Brachytherapy

Treatment Site Character 4	Modality Qualifier Character 5	Isotope Character 6	Qualifier Character 7
0 Trachea 1 Bronchus 2 Lung 5 Pleura 6 Mediastinum 7 Chest Wall 8 Diaphragm	9 High Dose Rate (HDR)	7 Cesium 137 (Cs-137) 8 Iridium 192 (Ir-192) 9 Iodine 125 (I-125) B Palladium 103 (Pd-103) C Californium 252 (Cf-252) Y Other Isotope	Z None
0 Trachea 1 Bronchus 2 Lung 5 Pleura 6 Mediastinum 7 Chest Wall 8 Diaphragm	B Low Dose Rate (LDR)	6 Cesium 131 (Cs-131) 7 Cesium 137 (Cs-137) 8 Iridium 192 (Ir-192) 9 Iodine 125 (I-125) C Californium 252 (Cf-252) Y Other Isotope	Z None
0 Trachea 1 Bronchus 2 Lung 5 Pleura 6 Mediastinum 7 Chest Wall 8 Diaphragm	B Low Dose Rate (LDR)	B Palladium 103 (Pd-103)	1 Unidirectional Source Z None

D Radiation Therapy
B Respiratory System
2 Stereotactic Radiosurgery

Treatment Site Character 4	Modality Qualifier Character 5	Isotope Character 6	Qualifier Character 7

0 Trachea
1 Bronchus
2 Lung
5 Pleura
6 Mediastinum
7 Chest Wall
8 Diaphragm
	D Stereotactic Other Photon
	   Radiosurgery
	H Stereotactic Particulate
	   Radiosurgery
	J Stereotactic Gamma Beam
	   Radiosurgery
		Z None	Z None

DRG Non-OR All treatment site, modality, isotope, and qualifier values

D Radiation Therapy
B Respiratory System
Y Other Radiation

Treatment Site Character 4	Modality Qualifier Character 5	Isotope Character 6	Qualifier Character 7
0 Trachea 1 Bronchus 2 Lung 5 Pleura 6 Mediastinum 7 Chest Wall 8 Diaphragm	7 Contact Radiation 8 Hyperthermia F Plaque Radiation	Z None	Z None

NC Noncovered Procedure   **LC** Limited Coverage   **QA** Questionable OB Admit   **NT** New Tech Add-on   **⊞** Combination Member   ♂ Male   ♀ Female

ICD-10-PCS 2023   789

D   **Radiation Therapy**
D   **Gastrointestinal System**
0   **Beam Radiation**

Treatment Site Character 4	Modality Qualifier Character 5	Isotope Character 6	Qualifier Character 7
0 Esophagus 1 Stomach 2 Duodenum 3 Jejunum 4 Ileum 5 Colon 7 Rectum	0 Photons <1 MeV 1 Photons 1- 10 MeV 2 Photons >10 MeV 4 Heavy Particles (Protons, Ions) 5 Neutrons 6 Neutron Capture	Z None	Z None
0 Esophagus 1 Stomach 2 Duodenum 3 Jejunum 4 Ileum 5 Colon 7 Rectum	3 Electrons	Z None	0 Intraoperative Z None

D   **Radiation Therapy**
D   **Gastrointestinal System**
1   **Brachytherapy**

Treatment Site Character 4	Modality Qualifier Character 5	Isotope Character 6	Qualifier Character 7
0 Esophagus 1 Stomach 2 Duodenum 3 Jejunum 4 Ileum 5 Colon 7 Rectum	9 High Dose Rate (HDR)	7 Cesium 137 (Cs-137) 8 Iridium 192 (Ir-192) 9 Iodine 125 (I-125) B Palladium 103 (Pd-103) C Californium 252 (Cf-252) Y Other Isotope	Z None
0 Esophagus 1 Stomach 2 Duodenum 3 Jejunum 4 Ileum 5 Colon 7 Rectum	B Low Dose Rate (LDR)	6 Cesium 131 (Cs-131) 7 Cesium 137 (Cs-137) 8 Iridium 192 (Ir-192) 9 Iodine 125 (I-125) C Californium 252 (Cf-252) Y Other Isotope	Z None
0 Esophagus 1 Stomach 2 Duodenum 3 Jejunum 4 Ileum 5 Colon 7 Rectum	B Low Dose Rate (LDR)	B Palladium 103 (Pd-103)	1 Unidirectional Source Z None

D   **Radiation Therapy**
D   **Gastrointestinal System**
2   **Stereotactic Radiosurgery**

Treatment Site Character 4	Modality Qualifier Character 5	Isotope Character 6	Qualifier Character 7

0 Esophagus
1 Stomach
2 Duodenum
3 Jejunum
4 Ileum
5 Colon
7 Rectum
	D Stereotactic Other Photon
	   Radiosurgery
	H Stereotactic Particulate
	   Radiosurgery
	J Stereotactic Gamma Beam
	   Radiosurgery
		Z None	Z None

DRG Non-OR   All treatment site, modality, isotope, and qualifier values

Non-OR Procedure   DRG Non-OR Procedure   Valid OR Procedure   HAC Associated Procedure   Combination Only   New/Revised April   New/Revised October

790   ICD-10-PCS 2023

Radiation Therapy

D Radiation therapy
D Gastrointestinal System
Y Other Radiation

Treatment Site Character 4	Modality Qualifier Character 5	Isotope Character 6	Qualifier Character 7
0 Esophagus	7 Contact Radiation 8 Hyperthermia F Plaque Radiation	Z None	Z None
1 Stomach 2 Duodenum 3 Jejunum 4 Ileum 5 Colon 7 Rectum	7 Contact Radiation 8 Hyperthermia C Intraoperative Radiation Therapy (IORT) F Plaque Radiation	Z None	Z None
8 Anus	C Intraoperative Radiation Therapy (IORT) F Plaque Radiation	Z None	Z None

D Radiation Therapy
F Hepatobiliary System and Pancreas
0 Beam Radiation

Treatment Site Character 4	Modality Qualifier Character 5	Isotope Character 6	Qualifier Character 7
0 Liver 1 Gallbladder 2 Bile Ducts 3 Pancreas	0 Photons <1 MeV 1 Photons 1- 10 MeV 2 Photons >10 MeV 4 Heavy Particles (Protons, Ions) 5 Neutrons 6 Neutron Capture	Z None	Z None
0 Liver 1 Gallbladder 2 Bile Ducts 3 Pancreas	3 Electrons	Z None	0 Intraoperative Z None

D Radiation Therapy
F Hepatobiliary System and Pancreas
1 Brachytherapy

Treatment Site Character 4	Modality Qualifier Character 5	Isotope Character 6	Qualifier Character 7
0 Liver 1 Gallbladder 2 Bile Ducts 3 Pancreas	9 High Dose Rate (HDR)	7 Cesium 137 (Cs-137) 8 Iridium 192 (Ir-192) 9 Iodine 125 (I-125) B Palladium 103 (Pd-103) C Californium 252 (Cf-252) Y Other Isotope	Z None
0 Liver 1 Gallbladder 2 Bile Ducts 3 Pancreas	B Low Dose Rate (LDR)	6 Cesium 131 (Cs-131) 7 Cesium 137 (Cs-137) 8 Iridium 192 (Ir-192) 9 Iodine 125 (I-125) C Californium 252 (Cf-252) Y Other Isotope	Z None
0 Liver 1 Gallbladder 2 Bile Ducts 3 Pancreas	B Low Dose Rate (LDR)	B Palladium 103 (Pd-103)	1 Unidirectional Source Z None

D Radiation Therapy
F Hepatobiliary System and Pancreas
2 Stereotactic Radiosurgery

Treatment Site Character 4	Modality Qualifier Character 5	Isotope Character 6	Qualifier Character 7
0 Liver 1 Gallbladder 2 Bile Ducts 3 Pancreas	D Stereotactic Other Photon Radiosurgery H Stereotactic Particulate Radiosurgery J Stereotactic Gamma Beam Radiosurgery	Z None	Z None

DRG Non-OR All treatment site, modality, isotope, and qualifier values

D   Radiation Therapy
F   Hepatobiliary System and Pancreas
Y   Other Radiation

Treatment Site Character 4	Modality Qualifier Character 5	Isotope Character 6	Qualifier Character 7
Ø Liver 1 Gallbladder 2 Bile Ducts 3 Pancreas	7 Contact Radiation 8 Hyperthermia C Intraoperative Radiation Therapy (IORT) F Plaque Radiation	Z None	Z None

D   Radiation Therapy
G   Endocrine System
Ø   Beam Radiation

Treatment Site Character 4	Modality Qualifier Character 5	Isotope Character 6	Qualifier Character 7
Ø Pituitary Gland 1 Pineal Body 2 Adrenal Glands 4 Parathyroid Glands 5 Thyroid	Ø Photons <1 MeV 1 Photons 1- 10 MeV 2 Photons >10 MeV 5 Neutrons 6 Neutron Capture	Z None	Z None
Ø Pituitary Gland 1 Pineal Body 2 Adrenal Glands 4 Parathyroid Glands 5 Thyroid	3 Electrons	Z None	Ø Intraoperative Z None

D   Radiation Therapy
G   Endocrine System
1   Brachytherapy

Treatment Site Character 4	Modality Qualifier Character 5	Isotope Character 6	Qualifier Character 7
Ø Pituitary Gland 1 Pineal Body 2 Adrenal Glands 4 Parathyroid Glands 5 Thyroid	9 High Dose Rate (HDR)	7 Cesium 137 (Cs-137) 8 Iridium 192 (Ir-192) 9 Iodine 125 (I-125) B Palladium 103 (Pd-103) C Californium 252 (Cf-252) Y Other Isotope	Z None
Ø Pituitary Gland 1 Pineal Body 2 Adrenal Glands 4 Parathyroid Glands 5 Thyroid	B Low Dose Rate (LDR)	6 Cesium 131 (Cs-131) 7 Cesium 137 (Cs-137) 8 Iridium 192 (Ir-192) 9 Iodine 125 (I-125) C Californium 252 (Cf-252) Y Other Isotope	Z None
Ø Pituitary Gland 1 Pineal Body 2 Adrenal Glands 4 Parathyroid Glands 5 Thyroid	B Low Dose Rate (LDR)	B Palladium 103 (Pd-103)	1 Unidirectional Source Z None

D   Radiation Therapy
G   Endocrine System
2   Stereotactic Radiosurgery

Treatment Site Character 4	Modality Qualifier Character 5	Isotope Character 6	Qualifier Character 7

Ø Pituitary Gland
1 Pineal Body
2 Adrenal Glands
4 Parathyroid Glands
5 Thyroid
	D Stereotactic Other Photon
	  Radiosurgery
	H Stereotactic Particulate
	  Radiosurgery
	J Stereotactic Gamma Beam
	  Radiosurgery
		Z None	Z None

DRG Non-OR All treatment site, modality, isotope, and qualifier values

Non-OR Procedure   DRG Non-OR Procedure   Valid OR Procedure   HAC Associated Procedure   Combination Only   New/Revised April   New/Revised October

792
ICD-10-PCS 2023

D   **Radiation therapy**
G   **Endocrine System**
Y   **Other Radiation**

Treatment Site Character 4	Modality Qualifier Character 5	Isotope Character 6	Qualifier Character 7
Ø Pituitary Gland 1 Pineal Body 2 Adrenal Glands 4 Parathyroid Glands 5 Thyroid	7 Contact Radiation 8 Hyperthermia F Plaque Radiation	Z None	Z None

D   **Radiation Therapy**
H   **Skin**
Ø   **Beam Radiation**

Treatment Site Character 4	Modality Qualifier Character 5	Isotope Character 6	Qualifier Character 7
2 Skin, Face 3 Skin, Neck 4 Skin, Arm 6 Skin, Chest 7 Skin, Back 8 Skin, Abdomen 9 Skin, Buttock B Skin, Leg	Ø Photons <1 MeV 1 Photons 1- 10 MeV 2 Photons >10 MeV 4 Heavy Particles (Protons, Ions) 5 Neutrons 6 Neutron Capture	Z None	Z None
2 Skin, Face 3 Skin, Neck 4 Skin, Arm 6 Skin, Chest 7 Skin, Back 8 Skin, Abdomen 9 Skin, Buttock B Skin, Leg	3 Electrons	Z None	Ø Intraoperative Z None

D   **Radiation Therapy**
H   **Skin**
Y   **Other Radiation**

Treatment Site Character 4	Modality Qualifier Character 5	Isotope Character 6	Qualifier Character 7
2 Skin, Face 3 Skin, Neck 4 Skin, Arm 6 Skin, Chest 7 Skin, Back 8 Skin, Abdomen 9 Skin, Buttock B Skin, Leg	7 Contact Radiation 8 Hyperthermia F Plaque Radiation	Z None	Z None
5 Skin, Hand C Skin, Foot	F Plaque Radiation	Z None	Z None

D   **Radiation Therapy**
M   **Breast**
Ø   **Beam Radiation**

Treatment Site Character 4	Modality Qualifier Character 5	Isotope Character 6	Qualifier Character 7
Ø Breast, Left 1 Breast, Right	Ø Photons <1 MeV 1 Photons 1- 10 MeV 2 Photons >10 MeV 4 Heavy Particles (Protons, Ions) 5 Neutrons 6 Neutron Capture	Z None	Z None
Ø Breast, Left 1 Breast, Right	3 Electrons	Z None	Ø Intraoperative Z None

NC Noncovered Procedure   **LC** Limited Coverage   **QA** Questionable OB Admit   **NT** New Tech Add-on   ⊞ Combination Member   ♂ Male   ♀ Female

ICD-10-PCS 2023   **793**

Radiation Therapy

D   Radiation Therapy
M   Breast
1   Brachytherapy

Treatment Site Character 4	Modality Qualifier Character 5	Isotope Character 6	Qualifier Character 7
0 Breast, Left 1 Breast, Right	9 High Dose Rate (HDR)	7 Cesium 137 (Cs-137) 8 Iridium 192 (Ir-192) 9 Iodine 125 (I-125) B Palladium 103 (Pd-103) C Californium 252 (Cf-252) Y Other Isotope	Z None
0 Breast, Left 1 Breast, Right	B Low Dose Rate (LDR)	6 Cesium 131 (Cs-131) 7 Cesium 137 (Cs-137) 8 Iridium 192 (Ir-192) 9 Iodine 125 (I-125) C Californium 252 (Cf-252) Y Other Isotope	Z None
0 Breast, Left 1 Breast, Right	B Low Dose Rate (LDR)	B Palladium 103 (Pd-103)	1 Unidirectional Source Z None

D   Radiation Therapy
M   Breast
2   Stereotactic Radiosurgery

Treatment Site Character 4	Modality Qualifier Character 5	Isotope Character 6	Qualifier Character 7

0   Breast, Left
1   Breast, Right
	D Stereotactic Other Photon
	     Radiosurgery
	H Stereotactic Particulate
	     Radiosurgery
	J Stereotactic Gamma Beam
	     Radiosurgery
		Z None	Z None

DRG Non-OR   All treatment site, modality, isotope, and qualifier values

D   Radiation Therapy
M   Breast
Y   Other Radiation

Treatment Site Character 4	Modality Qualifier Character 5	Isotope Character 6	Qualifier Character 7
0 Breast, Left 1 Breast, Right	7 Contact Radiation 8 Hyperthermia F Plaque Radiation	Z None	Z None

D   Radiation Therapy
P   Musculoskeletal System
0   Beam Radiation

Treatment Site Character 4	Modality Qualifier Character 5	Isotope Character 6	Qualifier Character 7
0 Skull 2 Maxilla 3 Mandible 4 Sternum 5 Rib(s) 6 Humerus 7 Radius/Ulna 8 Pelvic Bones 9 Femur B Tibia/Fibula C Other Bone	0 Photons <1 MeV 1 Photons 1- 10 MeV 2 Photons >10 MeV 4 Heavy Particles (Protons, Ions) 5 Neutrons 6 Neutron Capture	Z None	Z None
0 Skull 2 Maxilla 3 Mandible 4 Sternum 5 Rib(s) 6 Humerus 7 Radius/Ulna 8 Pelvic Bones 9 Femur B Tibia/Fibula C Other Bone	3 Electrons	Z None	0 Intraoperative Z None

Non-OR Procedure   DRG Non-OR Procedure   Valid OR Procedure   HAC Associated Procedure   Combination Only   New/Revised April   New/Revised October

794   ICD-10-PCS 2023

D   **Radiation Therapy**
P   **Musculoskeletal System**
Y   **Other Radiation**

Treatment Site Character 4	Modality Qualifier Character 5	Isotope Character 6	Qualifier Character 7
Ø Skull	7 Contact Radiation	Z None	Z None
2 Maxilla	8 Hyperthermia		
3 Mandible	F Plaque Radiation		
4 Sternum			
5 Rib(s)			
6 Humerus			
7 Radius/Ulna			
8 Pelvic Bones			
9 Femur			
B Tibia/Fibula			
C Other Bone			

D   **Radiation Therapy**
T   **Urinary System**
Ø   **Beam Radiation**

Treatment Site Character 4	Modality Qualifier Character 5	Isotope Character 6	Qualifier Character 7
Ø Kidney	Ø Photons <1 MeV	Z None	Z None
1 Ureter	1 Photons 1- 10 MeV		
2 Bladder	2 Photons >10 MeV		
3 Urethra	4 Heavy Particles (Protons, Ions)		
	5 Neutrons		
	6 Neutron Capture		
Ø Kidney	3 Electrons	Z None	Ø Intraoperative
1 Ureter			Z None
2 Bladder			
3 Urethra			

D   **Radiation Therapy**
T   **Urinary System**
1   **Brachytherapy**

Treatment Site Character 4	Modality Qualifier Character 5	Isotope Character 6	Qualifier Character 7
Ø Kidney	9 High Dose Rate (HDR)	7 Cesium 137 (Cs-137)	Z None
1 Ureter		8 Iridium 192 (Ir-192)	
2 Bladder		9 Iodine 125 (I-125)	
3 Urethra		B Palladium 103 (Pd-103)	
		C Californium 252 (Cf-252)	
		Y Other Isotope	
Ø Kidney	B Low Dose Rate (LDR)	6 Cesium 131 (Cs-131)	Z None
1 Ureter		7 Cesium 137 (Cs-137)	
2 Bladder		8 Iridium 192 (Ir-192)	
3 Urethra		9 Iodine 125 (I-125)	
		C Californium 252 (Cf-252)	
		Y Other Isotope	
Ø Kidney	B Low Dose Rate (LDR)	B Palladium 103 (Pd-103)	1 Unidirectional Source
1 Ureter			Z None
2 Bladder			
3 Urethra			

D   **Radiation Therapy**
T   **Urinary System**
2   **Stereotactic Radiosurgery**

Treatment Site Character 4	Modality Qualifier Character 5	Isotope Character 6	Qualifier Character 7
Ø Kidney	D Stereotactic Other Photon Radiosurgery	Z None	Z None
1 Ureter	H Stereotactic Particulate Radiosurgery		
2 Bladder	J Stereotactic Gamma Beam Radiosurgery		
3 Urethra			

DRG Non-OR   All treatment site, modality, isotope, and qualifier values

---

NC Noncovered Procedure   **LC** Limited Coverage   **QA** Questionable OB Admit   **NT** New Tech Add-on   ✚ Combination Member   ♂ Male   ♀ Female

Radiation Therapy

D   Radiation Therapy
T   Urinary System
Y   Other Radiation

Treatment Site Character 4	Modality Qualifier Character 5	Isotope Character 6	Qualifier Character 7
Ø Kidney	7 Contact Radiation	Z None	Z None
1 Ureter	8 Hyperthermia		
2 Bladder	C Intraoperative Radiation Therapy (IORT)		
3 Urethra	F Plaque Radiation		

D   Radiation Therapy
U   Female Reproductive System
Ø   Beam Radiation

Treatment Site Character 4		Modality Qualifier Character 5	Isotope Character 6	Qualifier Character 7
Ø Ovary	♀	Ø Photons <1 MeV	Z None	Z None
1 Cervix	♀	1 Photons 1- 10 MeV		
2 Uterus	♀	2 Photons >10 MeV		
		4 Heavy Particles (Protons, Ions)		
		5 Neutrons		
		6 Neutron Capture		
Ø Ovary	♀	3 Electrons	Z None	Ø Intraoperative
1 Cervix	♀			Z None
2 Uterus	♀			

♀   All treatment site, modality, isotope, and qualifier values

D   Radiation Therapy
U   Female Reproductive System
1   Brachytherapy

Treatment Site Character 4		Modality Qualifier Character 5	Isotope Character 6	Qualifier Character 7
Ø Ovary	♀	9 High Dose Rate (HDR)	7 Cesium 137 (Cs-137)	Z None
1 Cervix	♀		8 Iridium 192 (Ir-192)	
2 Uterus	♀		9 Iodine 125 (I-125)	
			B Palladium 103 (Pd-103)	
			C Californium 252 (Cf-252)	
			Y Other Isotope	
Ø Ovary	♀	B Low Dose Rate (LDR)	6 Cesium 131 (Cs-131)	Z None
1 Cervix	♀		7 Cesium 137 (Cs-137)	
2 Uterus	♀		8 Iridium 192 (Ir-192)	
			9 Iodine 125 (I-125)	
			C Californium 252 (Cf-252)	
			Y Other Isotope	
Ø Ovary	♀	B Low Dose Rate (LDR)	B Palladium 103 (Pd-103)	1 Unidirectional Source
1 Cervix	♀			Z None
2 Uterus	♀			

♀   All treatment site, modality, isotope, and qualifier values

D   Radiation Therapy
U   Female Reproductive System
2   Stereotactic Radiosurgery

Treatment Site Character 4		Modality Qualifier Character 5	Isotope Character 6	Qualifier Character 7
Ø Ovary	♀	D Stereotactic Other Photon Radiosurgery	Z None	Z None
1 Cervix	♀	H Stereotactic Particulate Radiosurgery		
2 Uterus	♀	J Stereotactic Gamma Beam Radiosurgery		

DRG Non-OR   All treatment site, modality, isotope, and qualifier values
♀   All treatment site, modality, isotope, and qualifier values

Non-OR Procedure   DRG Non-OR Procedure   Valid OR Procedure   HAC Associated Procedure   Combination Only   New/Revised April   New/Revised October

D   Radiation Therapy
U   Female Reproductive System
Y   Other Radiation

Treatment Site Character 4		Modality Qualifier Character 5	Isotope Character 6	Qualifier Character 7
0 Ovary	♀	7 Contact Radiation	Z None	Z None
1 Cervix	♀	8 Hyperthermia		
2 Uterus	♀	C Intraoperative Radiation Therapy (IORT)		
		F Plaque Radiation		

   ♀   All treatment site, modality, isotope, and qualifier values

---

D   Radiation Therapy
V   Male Reproductive System
0   Beam Radiation

Treatment Site Character 4		Modality Qualifier Character 5	Isotope Character 6	Qualifier Character 7
0 Prostate	♂	0 Photons <1 MeV	Z None	Z None
1 Testis	♂	1 Photons 1- 10 MeV		
		2 Photons >10 MeV		
		4 Heavy Particles (Protons, Ions)		
		5 Neutrons		
		6 Neutron Capture		
0 Prostate	♂	3 Electrons	Z None	0 Intraoperative
1 Testis	♂			Z None

   ♂   All treatment site, modality, isotope, and qualifier values

---

D   Radiation Therapy
V   Male Reproductive System
1   Brachytherapy

Treatment Site Character 4		Modality Qualifier Character 5	Isotope Character 6	Qualifier Character 7
0 Prostate	♂	9 High Dose Rate (HDR)	7 Cesium 137 (Cs-137)	Z None
1 Testis	♂		8 Iridium 192 (Ir-192)	
			9 Iodine 125 (I-125)	
			B Palladium 103 (Pd-103)	
			C Californium 252 (Cf-252)	
			Y Other Isotope	
0 Prostate	♂	B Low Dose Rate (LDR)	6 Cesium 131 (Cs-131)	Z None
1 Testis	♂		7 Cesium 137 (Cs-137)	
			8 Iridium 192 (Ir-192)	
			9 Iodine 125 (I-125)	
			C Californium 252 (Cf-252)	
			Y Other Isotope	
0 Prostate	♂	B Low Dose Rate (LDR)	B Palladium 103 (Pd-103)	1 Unidirectional Source
1 Testis	♂			Z None

   ♂   All treatment site, modality, isotope, and qualifier values

---

D   Radiation Therapy
V   Male Reproductive System
2   Stereotactic Radiosurgery

Treatment Site Character 4		Modality Qualifier Character 5	Isotope Character 6	Qualifier Character 7
0 Prostate	♂	D Stereotactic Other Photon Radiosurgery	Z None	Z None
1 Testis	♂	H Stereotactic Particulate Radiosurgery		
		J Stereotactic Gamma Beam Radiosurgery		

   DRG Non-OR   All treatment site, modality, isotope, and qualifier values
   ♂   All treatment site, modality, isotope, and qualifier values

---

NC Noncovered Procedure   **LC** Limited Coverage   **QA** Questionable OB Admit   **NT** New Tech Add-on   ⊞ Combination Member   ♂ Male   ♀ Female

ICD-10-PCS 2023   **797**

D   Radiation Therapy
V   Male Reproductive System
Y   Other Radiation

Treatment Site Character 4	Modality Qualifier Character 5	Isotope Character 6	Qualifier Character 7
Ø Prostate ♂	7 Contact Radiation 8 Hyperthermia C Intraoperative Radiation Therapy (IORT) F Plaque Radiation	Z None	Z None
1 Testis ♂	7 Contact Radiation 8 Hyperthermia F Plaque Radiation	Z None	Z None

♂   All treatment site, modality, isotope, and qualifier values

D   Radiation Therapy
W   Anatomical Regions
Ø   Beam Radiation

Treatment Site Character 4	Modality Qualifier Character 5	Isotope Character 6	Qualifier Character 7
1 Head and Neck 2 Chest 3 Abdomen 4 Hemibody 5 Whole Body 6 Pelvic Region	Ø Photons <1 MeV 1 Photons 1- 10 MeV 2 Photons >10 MeV 4 Heavy Particles (Protons, Ions) 5 Neutrons 6 Neutron Capture	Z None	Z None
1 Head and Neck 2 Chest 3 Abdomen 4 Hemibody 5 Whole Body 6 Pelvic Region	3 Electrons	Z None	Ø Intraoperative Z None

D   Radiation Therapy
W   Anatomical Regions
1   Brachytherapy

Treatment Site Character 4	Modality Qualifier Character 5	Isotope Character 6	Qualifier Character 7
Ø Cranial Cavity K Upper Back L Lower Back P Gastrointestinal Tract Q Respiratory Tract R Genitourinary Tract X Upper Extremity Y Lower Extremity	B Low Dose Rate (LDR)	B Palladium 103 (Pd-103)	1 Unidirectional Source Z None
1 Head and Neck 2 Chest 3 Abdomen 6 Pelvic Region	9 High Dose Rate (HDR)	7 Cesium 137 (Cs-137) 8 Iridium 192 (Ir-192) 9 Iodine 125 (I-125) B Palladium 103 (Pd-103) C Californium 252 (Cf-252) Y Other Isotope	Z None
1 Head and Neck 2 Chest 3 Abdomen 6 Pelvic Region	B Low Dose Rate (LDR)	6 Cesium 131 (Cs-131) 7 Cesium 137 (Cs-137) 8 Iridium 192 (Ir-192) 9 Iodine 125 (I-125) C Californium 252 (Cf-252) Y Other Isotope	Z None
1 Head and Neck 2 Chest 3 Abdomen 6 Pelvic Region	B Low Dose Rate (LDR)	B Palladium 103 (Pd-103)	1 Unidirectional Source Z None

Non-OR Procedure   DRG Non-OR Procedure   Valid OR Procedure   HAC Associated Procedure   Combination Only   New/Revised April   New/Revised October

798   ICD-10-PCS 2023

Radiation Therapy

D   **Radiation Therapy**
W   **Anatomical Regions**
2   **Stereotactic Radiosurgery**

Treatment Site Character 4	Modality Qualifier Character 5	Isotope Character 6	Qualifier Character 7

1   Head and Neck
2   Chest
3   Abdomen
6   Pelvic Region
	D Stereotactic Other Photon
	     Radiosurgery
	H Stereotactic Particulate
	     Radiosurgery
	J Stereotactic Gamma Beam
	     Radiosurgery
		Z None	Z None

DRG Non-OR   All treatment site, modality, isotope, and qualifier values

D   **Radiation Therapy**
W   **Anatomical Regions**
Y   **Other Radiation**

Treatment Site Character 4	Modality Qualifier Character 5	Isotope Character 6	Qualifier Character 7
1 Head and Neck 2 Chest 3 Abdomen 4 Hemibody 6 Pelvic Region	7 Contact Radiation 8 Hyperthermia F Plaque Radiation	Z None	Z None
5 Whole Body	7 Contact Radiation 8 Hyperthermia F Plaque Radiation	Z None	Z None
5 Whole Body	G Isotope Administration	D Iodine 131 (I-131) F Phosphorus 32 (P-32) G Strontium 89 (Sr-89) H Strontium 90 (Sr-90) Y Other Isotope	Z None

NC Noncovered Procedure   **LC** Limited Coverage   **QA** Questionable OB Admit   **NT** New Tech Add-on   ⊞ Combination Member   ♂ Male   ♀ Female

ICD-10-PCS 2023   **799**

Physical Rehabilitation and Diagnostic Audiology F00–F15

F   **Physical Rehabilitation and Diagnostic Audiology**
0   **Rehabilitation**
0   **Speech Assessment**   Definition: Measurement of speech and related functions

Body System/Region Character 4	Type Qualifier Character 5	Equipment Character 6	Qualifier Character 7

3 Neurological System - Whole Body	G Communicative/Cognitive
	    Integration Skills
		K Audiovisual
		M Augmentative / Alternative
		    Communication
		P Computer
		Y Other Equipment
		Z None
			Z None

Z None	0 Filtered Speech 3 Staggered Spondaic Word Q Performance Intensity Phonetically Balanced Speech Discrimination R Brief Tone Stimuli S Distorted Speech T Dichotic Stimuli V Temporal Ordering of Stimuli W Masking Patterns	1 Audiometer 2 Sound Field / Booth K Audiovisual Z None	Z None
Z None	1 Speech Threshold 2 Speech/Word Recognition	1 Audiometer 2 Sound Field / Booth 9 Cochlear Implant K Audiovisual Z None	Z None
Z None	4 Sensorineural Acuity Level	1 Audiometer 2 Sound Field / Booth Z None	Z None
Z None	5 Synthetic Sentence Identification	1 Audiometer 2 Sound Field / Booth 9 Cochlear Implant K Audiovisual	Z None

Z None	6 Speech and/or Language Screening
	7 Nonspoken Language
	8 Receptive/Expressive Language
	C Aphasia
	G Communicative/Cognitive
	    Integration Skills
	L Augmentative/Alternative
	    Communication System
		K Audiovisual
		M Augmentative / Alternative
		    Communication
		P Computer
		Y Other Equipment
		Z None
			Z None

Z None	9 Articulation/Phonology	K Audiovisual P Computer Q Speech Analysis Y Other Equipment Z None	Z None
Z None	B Motor Speech	K Audiovisual N Biosensory Feedback P Computer Q Speech Analysis T Aerodynamic Function Y Other Equipment Z None	Z None
Z None	D Fluency	K Audiovisual N Biosensory Feedback P Computer Q Speech Analysis S Voice Analysis T Aerodynamic Function Y Other Equipment Z None	Z None
Z None	F Voice	K Audiovisual N Biosensory Feedback P Computer S Voice Analysis T Aerodynamic Function Y Other Equipment Z None	Z None

DRG Non-OR   All body system/region, type qualifier, equipment, and qualifier values

F00 Continued on next page

NC Noncovered Procedure   LC Limited Coverage   QA Questionable OB Admit   NT New Tech Add-on   ⊞ Combination Member   ♂ Male   ♀ Female

ICD-10-PCS 2023   801

F Physical Rehabilitation and Diagnostic Audiology
Ø Rehabilitation
Ø Speech Assessment   Definition: Measurement of speech and related functions

Body System/Region Character 4	Type Qualifier Character 5	Equipment Character 6	Qualifier Character 7
Z None	H Bedside Swallowing and Oral Function P Oral Peripheral Mechanism	Y Other Equipment Z None	Z None
Z None	J Instrumental Swallowing and Oral Function	T Aerodynamic Function W Swallowing Y Other Equipment	Z None
Z None	K Orofacial Myofunctional	K Audiovisual P Computer Y Other Equipment Z None	Z None
Z None	M Voice Prosthetic	K Audiovisual P Computer S Voice Analysis V Speech Prosthesis Y Other Equipment Z None	Z None
Z None	N Non-invasive Instrumental Status	N Biosensory Feedback P Computer Q Speech Analysis S Voice Analysis T Aerodynamic Function Y Other Equipment	Z None
Z None	X Other Specified Central Auditory Processing	Z None	Z None

DRG Non-OR   All body system/region, type qualifier, equipment, and qualifier values

F Physical Rehabilitation and Diagnostic Audiology
Ø Rehabilitation
1 Motor and/or Nerve Function Assessment   Definition: Measurement of motor, nerve, and related functions

Body System/Region Character 4	Type Qualifier Character 5	Equipment Character 6	Qualifier Character 7
Ø Neurological System - Head and Neck 1 Neurological System - Upper Back/ Upper Extremity 2 Neurological System - Lower Back/ Lower Extremity 3 Neurological System - Whole Body	Ø Muscle Performance	E Orthosis F Assistive, Adaptive, Supportive or Protective U Prosthesis Y Other Equipment Z None	Z None
Ø Neurological System - Head and Neck 1 Neurological System - Upper Back/ Upper Extremity 2 Neurological System - Lower Back/ Lower Extremity 3 Neurological System - Whole Body	1 Integumentary Integrity 3 Coordination/Dexterity 4 Motor Function G Reflex Integrity	Z None	Z None
Ø Neurological System - Head and Neck 1 Neurological System - Upper Back/ Upper Extremity 2 Neurological System - Lower Back/ Lower Extremity 3 Neurological System - Whole Body	5 Range of Motion and Joint Integrity 6 Sensory Awareness/Processing/ Integrity	Y Other Equipment Z None	Z None
D Integumentary System - Head and Neck F Integumentary System - Upper Back/ Upper Extremity G Integumentary System - Lower Back/ Lower Extremity H Integumentary System - Whole Body J Musculoskeletal System - Head and Neck K Musculoskeletal System - Upper Back/ Upper Extremity L Musculoskeletal System - Lower Back/ Lower Extremity M Musculoskeletal System - Whole Body	Ø Muscle Performance	E Orthosis F Assistive, Adaptive, Supportive or Protective U Prosthesis Y Other Equipment Z None	Z None

DRG Non-OR   All body system/region, type qualifier, equipment, and qualifier values

F01 Continued on next page

F **Physical Rehabilitation and Diagnostic Audiology**
Ø **Rehabilitation**
1 **Motor and/or Nerve Function Assessment**　Definition: Measurement of motor, nerve, and related functions

Body System/Region Character 4	Type Qualifier Character 5	Equipment Character 6	Qualifier Character 7
D Integumentary System - Head and Neck **F** Integumentary System - Upper Back/ Upper Extremity **G** Integumentary System - Lower Back/ Lower Extremity **H** Integumentary System - Whole Body **J** Musculoskeletal System - Head and Neck **K** Musculoskeletal System - Upper Back/ Upper Extremity **L** Musculoskeletal System - Lower Back/ Lower Extremity **M** Musculoskeletal System - Whole Body	**1** Integumentary Integrity	**Z** None	**Z** None
D Integumentary System - Head and Neck **F** Integumentary System - Upper Back/ Upper Extremity **G** Integumentary System - Lower Back/ Lower Extremity **H** Integumentary System - Whole Body **J** Musculoskeletal System - Head and Neck **K** Musculoskeletal System - Upper Back/ Upper Extremity **L** Musculoskeletal System - Lower Back/ Lower Extremity **M** Musculoskeletal System - Whole Body	**5** Range of Motion and Joint Integrity **6** Sensory Awareness/Processing/ Integrity	**Y** Other Equipment **Z** None	**Z** None
N Genitourinary System	**Ø** Muscle Performance	**E** Orthosis **F** Assistive, Adaptive, Supportive or Protective **U** Prosthesis **Y** Other Equipment **Z** None	**Z** None
Z None	**2** Visual Motor Integration	**K** Audiovisual **M** Augmentative / Alternative Communication **N** Biosensory Feedback **P** Computer **Q** Speech Analysis **S** Voice Analysis **Y** Other Equipment **Z** None	**Z** None
Z None	**7** Facial Nerve Function	**7** Electrophysiologic	**Z** None
Z None	**9** Somatosensory Evoked Potentials	**J** Somatosensory	**Z** None
Z None	**B** Bed Mobility **C** Transfer **F** Wheelchair Mobility	**E** Orthosis **F** Assistive, Adaptive, Supportive or Protective **U** Prosthesis **Z** None	**Z** None
Z None	**D** Gait and/or Balance	**E** Orthosis **F** Assistive, Adaptive, Supportive or Protective **U** Prosthesis **Y** Other Equipment **Z** None	**Z** None

DRG Non-OR All body system/region, type qualifier, equipment, and qualifier values

NC Noncovered Procedure　　**LC** Limited Coverage　　**QA** Questionable OB Admit　　**NT** New Tech Add-on　　⊞ Combination Member　　♂Male　♀Female

ICD-10-PCS 2023

803

F   **Physical Rehabilitation and Diagnostic Audiology**
Ø   **Rehabilitation**
2   **Activities of Daily Living Assessment**   Definition: Measurement of functional level for activities of daily living

Body System/Region Character 4	Type Qualifier Character 5	Equipment Character 6	Qualifier Character 7
Ø Neurological System - Head and Neck	**9** Cranial Nerve Integrity **D** Neuromotor Development	**Y** Other Equipment **Z** None	**Z** None
1 Neurological System - Upper Back/Upper Extremity **2** Neurological System - Lower Back/Lower Extremity **3** Neurological System - Whole Body	**D** Neuromotor Development	**Y** Other Equipment **Z** None	**Z** None
4 Circulatory System - Head and Neck **5** Circulatory System - Upper Back/Upper Extremity **6** Circulatory System - Lower Back/Lower Extremity **8** Respiratory System - Head and Neck **9** Respiratory System - Upper Back/Upper Extremity **B** Respiratory System - Lower Back/Lower Extremity	**G** Ventilation, Respiration and Circulation	**C** Mechanical **G** Aerobic Endurance and Conditioning **Y** Other Equipment **Z** None	**Z** None
7 Circulatory System - Whole Body **C** Respiratory System - Whole Body	**7** Aerobic Capacity and Endurance	**E** Orthosis **G** Aerobic Endurance and Conditioning **U** Prosthesis **Y** Other Equipment **Z** None	**Z** None
7 Circulatory System - Whole Body **C** Respiratory System - Whole Body	**G** Ventilation, Respiration and Circulation	**C** Mechanical **G** Aerobic Endurance and Conditioning **Y** Other Equipment **Z** None	**Z** None
Z None	**Ø** Bathing/Showering **1** Dressing **3** Grooming/Personal Hygiene **4** Home Management	**E** Orthosis **F** Assistive, Adaptive, Supportive or Protective **U** Prosthesis **Z** None	**Z** None
Z None	**2** Feeding/Eating **8** Anthropometric Characteristics **F** Pain	**Y** Other Equipment **Z** None	**Z** None
Z None	**5** Perceptual Processing	**K** Audiovisual **M** Augmentative / Alternative Communication **N** Biosensory Feedback **P** Computer **Q** Speech Analysis **S** Voice Analysis **Y** Other Equipment **Z** None	**Z** None
Z None	**6** Psychosocial Skills	**Z** None	**Z** None
Z None	**B** Environmental, Home and Work Barriers **C** Ergonomics and Body Mechanics	**E** Orthosis **F** Assistive, Adaptive, Supportive or Protective **U** Prosthesis **Y** Other Equipment **Z** None	**Z** None
Z None	**H** Vocational Activities and Functional Community or Work Reintegration Skills	**E** Orthosis **F** Assistive, Adaptive, Supportive or Protective **G** Aerobic Endurance and Conditioning **U** Prosthesis **Y** Other Equipment **Z** None	**Z** None

DRG Non-OR   All body system/region, type qualifier, equipment, and qualifier values

---

Non-OR Procedure   DRG Non-OR Procedure   Valid OR Procedure   HAC Associated Procedure   Combination Only   New/Revised April   New/Revised October

F   **Physical Rehabilitation and Diagnostic Audiology**
Ø   **Rehabilitation**
6   **Speech Treatment**   Definition: Application of techniques to improve, augment, or compensate for speech and related functional impairment

Body System/Region Character 4	Type Qualifier Character 5	Equipment Character 6	Qualifier Character 7
3 Neurological System - Whole Body	**6** Communicative/Cognitive Integration Skills	**K** Audiovisual **M** Augmentative / Alternative Communication **P** Computer **Y** Other Equipment **Z** None	**Z** None
Z None	**Ø** Nonspoken Language **3** Aphasia **6** Communicative/Cognitive Integration Skills	**K** Audiovisual **M** Augmentative / Alternative Communication **P** Computer **Y** Other Equipment **Z** None	**Z** None
Z None	**1** Speech-Language Pathology and Related Disorders Counseling **2** Speech-Language Pathology and Related Disorders Prevention	**K** Audiovisual **Z** None	**Z** None
Z None	**4** Articulation/Phonology	**K** Audiovisual **P** Computer **Q** Speech Analysis **T** Aerodynamic Function **Y** Other Equipment **Z** None	**Z** None
Z None	**5** Aural Rehabilitation	**K** Audiovisual **L** Assistive Listening **M** Augmentative / Alternative Communication **N** Biosensory Feedback **P** Computer **Q** Speech Analysis **S** Voice Analysis **Y** Other Equipment **Z** None	**Z** None
Z None	**7** Fluency	**4** Electroacoustic Immitance / Acoustic Reflex **K** Audiovisual **N** Biosensory Feedback **Q** Speech Analysis **S** Voice Analysis **T** Aerodynamic Function **Y** Other Equipment **Z** None	**Z** None
Z None	**8** Motor Speech	**K** Audiovisual **N** Biosensory Feedback **P** Computer **Q** Speech Analysis **S** Voice Analysis **T** Aerodynamic Function **Y** Other Equipment **Z** None	**Z** None
Z None	**9** Orofacial Myofunctional	**K** Audiovisual **P** Computer **Y** Other Equipment **Z** None	**Z** None
Z None	**B** Receptive/Expressive Language	**K** Audiovisual **L** Assistive Listening **M** Augmentative / Alternative Communication **P** Computer **Y** Other Equipment **Z** None	**Z** None

DRG Non-OR   All body system/region, type qualifier, equipment, and qualifier values

F06 Continued on next page

NC Noncovered Procedure   **LC** Limited Coverage   **QA** Questionable OB Admit   **NT** New Tech Add-on   ⊞ Combination Member   ♂ Male   ♀ Female

Physical Rehabilitation and Diagnostic Audiology

F06 Continued

F   Physical Rehabilitation and Diagnostic Audiology
Ø   Rehabilitation
6   Speech Treatment   Definition: Application of techniques to improve, augment, or compensate for speech and related functional impairment

Body System/Region Character 4	Type Qualifier Character 5	Equipment Character 6	Qualifier Character 7
Z None	C Voice	K Audiovisual N Biosensory Feedback P Computer S Voice Analysis T Aerodynamic Function V Speech Prosthesis Y Other Equipment Z None	Z None
Z None	D Swallowing Dysfunction	M Augmentative / Alternative Communication T Aerodynamic Function V Speech Prosthesis Y Other Equipment Z None	Z None

DRG Non-OR   All body system/region, type qualifier, equipment, and qualifier values

F   Physical Rehabilitation and Diagnostic Audiology
Ø   Rehabilitation
7   Motor Treatment   Definition: Exercise or activities to increase or facilitate motor function

Body System/Region Character 4	Type Qualifier Character 5	Equipment Character 6	Qualifier Character 7
Ø Neurological System - Head and Neck 1 Neurological System - Upper Back/Upper Extremity 2 Neurological System - Lower Back/Lower Extremity 3 Neurological System - Whole Body D Integumentary System - Head and Neck F Integumentary System - Upper Back/Upper Extremity G Integumentary System - Lower Back/Lower Extremity H Integumentary System - Whole Body J Musculoskeletal System - Head and Neck K Musculoskeletal System - Upper Back/Upper Extremity L Musculoskeletal System - Lower Back/Lower Extremity M Musculoskeletal System - Whole Body	Ø Range of Motion and Joint Mobility 1 Muscle Performance 2 Coordination/Dexterity 3 Motor Function	E Orthosis F Assistive, Adaptive, Supportive or Protective U Prosthesis Y Other Equipment Z None	Z None
Ø Neurological System - Head and Neck 1 Neurological System - Upper Back/Upper Extremity 2 Neurological System - Lower Back/Lower Extremity 3 Neurological System - Whole Body D Integumentary System - Head and Neck F Integumentary System - Upper Back/Upper Extremity G Integumentary System - Lower Back/Lower Extremity H Integumentary System - Whole Body J Musculoskeletal System - Head and Neck K Musculoskeletal System - Upper Back/Upper Extremity L Musculoskeletal System - Lower Back/Lower Extremity M Musculoskeletal System - Whole Body	6 Therapeutic Exercise	B Physical Agents C Mechanical D Electrotherapeutic E Orthosis F Assistive, Adaptive, Supportive or Protective G Aerobic Endurance and Conditioning H Mechanical or Electromechanical U Prosthesis Y Other Equipment Z None	Z None

DRG Non-OR   All body system/region, type qualifier, equipment, and qualifier values

F07 Continued on next page

Non-OR Procedure   DRG Non-OR Procedure   Valid OR Procedure   HAC Associated Procedure   Combination Only   New/Revised April   New/Revised October

806   ICD-10-PCS 2023

F   **Physical Rehabilitation and Diagnostic Audiology**
0   **Rehabilitation**
7   **Motor Treatment**   Definition: Exercise or activities to increase or facilitate motor function

F07 Continued

Body System/Region Character 4	Type Qualifier Character 5	Equipment Character 6	Qualifier Character 7
0 Neurological System - Head and Neck **1** Neurological System - Upper Back/Upper Extremity **2** Neurological System - Lower Back/Lower Extremity **3** Neurological System - Whole Body **D** Integumentary System - Head and Neck **F** Integumentary System - Upper Back/Upper Extremity **G** Integumentary System - Lower Back/Lower Extremity **H** Integumentary System - Whole Body **J** Musculoskeletal System - Head and Neck **K** Musculoskeletal System - Upper Back/Upper Extremity **L** Musculoskeletal System - Lower Back/Lower Extremity **M** Musculoskeletal System - Whole Body	**7** Manual Therapy Techniques	**Z** None	**Z** None
4 Circulatory System - Head and Neck **5** Circulatory System - Upper Back / Upper Extremity **6** Circulatory System - Lower Back/Lower Extremity **7** Circulatory System - Whole Body **8** Respiratory System - Head and Neck **9** Respiratory System - Upper Back / Upper Extremity **B** Respiratory System - Lower Back / Lower Extremity **C** Respiratory System - Whole Body	**6** Therapeutic Exercise	**B** Physical Agents **C** Mechanical **D** Electrotherapeutic **E** Orthosis **F** Assistive, Adaptive, Supportive or Protective **G** Aerobic Endurance and Conditioning **H** Mechanical or Electromechanical **U** Prosthesis **Y** Other Equipment **Z** None	**Z** None
N Genitourinary System	**1** Muscle Performance	**E** Orthosis **F** Assistive, Adaptive, Supportive or Protective **U** Prosthesis **Y** Other Equipment **Z** None	**Z** None
N Genitourinary System	**6** Therapeutic Exercise	**B** Physical Agents **C** Mechanical **D** Electrotherapeutic **E** Orthosis **F** Assistive, Adaptive, Supportive or Protective **G** Aerobic Endurance and Conditioning **H** Mechanical or Electromechanical **U** Prosthesis **Y** Other Equipment **Z** None	**Z** None
Z None	**4** Wheelchair Mobility	**D** Electrotherapeutic **E** Orthosis **F** Assistive, Adaptive, Supportive or Protective **U** Prosthesis **Y** Other Equipment **Z** None	**Z** None
Z None	**5** Bed Mobility	**C** Mechanical **E** Orthosis **F** Assistive, Adaptive, Supportive or Protective **U** Prosthesis **Y** Other Equipment **Z** None	**Z** None
Z None	**8** Transfer Training	**C** Mechanical **D** Electrotherapeutic **E** Orthosis **F** Assistive, Adaptive, Supportive or Protective **U** Prosthesis **Y** Other Equipment **Z** None	**Z** None

DRG Non-OR   All body system/region, type qualifier, equipment, and qualifier values

F07 Continued on next page

NC Noncovered Procedure   **LC** Limited Coverage   **QA** Questionable OB Admit   **NT** New Tech Add-on   ⊞ Combination Member   ♂ Male   ♀ Female

ICD-10-PCS 2023   807

Physical Rehabilitation and Diagnostic Audiology *(side tab)*

F07 Continued

F   **Physical Rehabilitation and Diagnostic Audiology**
Ø   **Rehabilitation**
7   **Motor Treatment**   Definition: Exercise or activities to increase or facilitate motor function

Body System/Region Character 4	Type Qualifier Character 5	Equipment Character 6	Qualifier Character 7
Z None	9 Gait Training/Functional Ambulation	C Mechanical D Electrotherapeutic E Orthosis F Assistive, Adaptive, Supportive or Protective G Aerobic Endurance and Conditioning U Prosthesis Y Other Equipment Z None	Z None

DRG Non-OR   All body system/region, type qualifier, equipment, and qualifier values

F   **Physical Rehabilitation and Diagnostic Audiology**
Ø   **Rehabilitation**
8   **Activities of Daily Living Treatment**   Definition: Exercise or activities to facilitate functional competence for activities of daily living

Body System/Region Character 4	Type Qualifier Character 5	Equipment Character 6	Qualifier Character 7
D Integumentary System - Head and Neck F Integumentary System - Upper Back/Upper Extremity G Integumentary System - Lower Back/Lower Extremity H Integumentary System - Whole Body J Musculoskeletal System - Head and Neck K Musculoskeletal System - Upper Back/Upper Extremity L Musculoskeletal System - Lower Back/Lower Extremity M Musculoskeletal System - Whole Body	5 Wound Management	B Physical Agents C Mechanical D Electrotherapeutic E Orthosis F Assistive, Adaptive, Supportive or Protective U Prosthesis Y Other Equipment Z None	Z None
Z None	Ø Bathing/Showering Techniques 1 Dressing Techniques 2 Grooming/Personal Hygiene	E Orthosis F Assistive, Adaptive, Supportive or Protective U Prosthesis Y Other Equipment Z None	Z None
Z None	3 Feeding/Eating	C Mechanical D Electrotherapeutic E Orthosis F Assistive, Adaptive, Supportive or Protective U Prosthesis Y Other Equipment Z None	Z None
Z None	4 Home Management	D Electrotherapeutic E Orthosis F Assistive, Adaptive, Supportive or Protective U Prosthesis Y Other Equipment Z None	Z None
Z None	6 Psychosocial Skills	Z None	Z None
Z None	7 Vocational Activities and Functional Community or Work Reintegration Skills	B Physical Agents C Mechanical D Electrotherapeutic E Orthosis F Assistive, Adaptive, Supportive or Protective G Aerobic Endurance and Conditioning U Prosthesis Y Other Equipment Z None	Z None

DRG Non-OR   All body system/region, type qualifier, equipment, and qualifier values

Non-OR Procedure   DRG Non-OR Procedure   Valid OR Procedure   HAC Associated Procedure   Combination Only   New/Revised April   New/Revised October

808

ICD-10-PCS 2023

F   **Physical Rehabilitation and Diagnostic Audiology**
Ø   **Rehabilitation**
9   **Hearing Treatment**   Definition: Application of techniques to improve, augment, or compensate for hearing and related functional impairment

Body System/Region Character 4	Type Qualifier Character 5	Equipment Character 6	Qualifier Character 7
Z None	Ø Hearing and Related Disorders Counseling 1 Hearing and Related Disorders Prevention	K Audiovisual Z None	Z None
Z None	2 Auditory Processing	K Audiovisual L Assistive Listening P Computer Y Other Equipment Z None	Z None
Z None	3 Cerumen Management	X Cerumen Management Z None	Z None

DRG Non-OR   All body system/region, type qualifier, equipment, and qualifier values

F   **Physical Rehabilitation and Diagnostic Audiology**
Ø   **Rehabilitation**
B   **Cochlear Implant Treatment**   Definition: Application of techniques to improve the communication abilities of individuals with cochlear implant

Body System/Region Character 4	Type Qualifier Character 5	Equipment Character 6	Qualifier Character 7
Z None	Ø Cochlear Implant Rehabilitation	1 Audiometer 2 Sound Field / Booth 9 Cochlear Implant K Audiovisual P Computer Y Other Equipment	Z None

DRG Non-OR   All body system/region, type qualifier, equipment, and qualifier values

F   **Physical Rehabilitation and Diagnostic Audiology**
Ø   **Rehabilitation**
C   **Vestibular Treatment**   Definition: Application of techniques to improve, augment, or compensate for vestibular and related functional impairment

Body System/Region Character 4	Type Qualifier Character 5	Equipment Character 6	Qualifier Character 7
3 Neurological System - Whole Body H Integumentary System - Whole Body M Musculoskeletal System - Whole Body	3 Postural Control	E Orthosis F Assistive, Adaptive, Supportive or Protective U Prosthesis Y Other Equipment Z None	Z None
Z None	Ø Vestibular	8 Vestibular / Balance Z None	Z None
Z None	1 Perceptual Processing 2 Visual Motor Integration	K Audiovisual L Assistive Listening N Biosensory Feedback P Computer Q Speech Analysis S Voice Analysis T Aerodynamic Function Y Other Equipment Z None	Z None

DRG Non-OR   All body system/region, type qualifier, equipment, and qualifier values

NC Noncovered Procedure   **LC** Limited Coverage   **QA** Questionable OB Admit   **NT** New Tech Add-on   ⊞ Combination Member   ♂ Male   ♀ Female

ICD-10-PCS 2023   **809**

F   **Physical Rehabilitation and Diagnostic Audiology**
0   **Rehabilitation**
D   **Device Fitting**   Definition: Fitting of a device designed to facilitate or support achievement of a higher level of function

Body System/Region Character 4	Type Qualifier Character 5	Equipment Character 6	Qualifier Character 7
Z None	**0** Tinnitus Masker	**5** Hearing Aid Selection / Fitting / Test **Z** None	**Z** None
Z None	**1** Monaural Hearing Aid **2** Binaural Hearing Aid **5** Assistive Listening Device	**1** Audiometer **2** Sound Field / Booth **5** Hearing Aid Selection / Fitting / Test **K** Audiovisual **L** Assistive Listening **Z** None	**Z** None
Z None	**3** Augmentative/Alternative Communication System	**M** Augmentative / Alternative Communication	**Z** None
Z None	**4** Voice Prosthetic	**S** Voice Analysis **V** Speech Prosthesis	**Z** None
Z None	**6** Dynamic Orthosis **7** Static Orthosis **8** Prosthesis **9** Assistive, Adaptive, Supportive or Protective Devices	**E** Orthosis **F** Assistive, Adaptive, Supportive or Protective **U** Prosthesis **Z** None	**Z** None

DRG Non-OR	F0DZ0[5,Z]Z
DRG Non-OR	F0DZ[1, 2,5][1,2,5, K,L,Z]Z
DRG Non-OR	F0DZ3MZ
DRG Non-OR	F0DZ4[S,V]Z
DRG Non-OR	F0DZ[6,7][E,F,U,Z]Z
DRG Non-OR	F0DZ8[E,F,U]Z

F   **Physical Rehabilitation and Diagnostic Audiology**
0   **Rehabilitation**
F   **Caregiver Training**   Definition: Training in activities to support patient's optimal level of function

Body System/Region Character 4	Type Qualifier Character 5	Equipment Character 6	Qualifier Character 7
Z None	**0** Bathing/Showering Technique **1** Dressing **2** Feeding and Eating **3** Grooming/Personal Hygiene **4** Bed Mobility **5** Transfer **6** Wheelchair Mobility **7** Therapeutic Exercise **8** Airway Clearance Techniques **9** Wound Management **B** Vocational Activities and Functional Community or Work Reintegration Skills **C** Gait Training/Functional Ambulation **D** Application, Proper Use and Care of Devices **F** Application, Proper Use and Care of Orthoses **G** Application, Proper Use and Care of Prosthesis **H** Home Management	**E** Orthosis **F** Assistive, Adaptive, Supportive or Protective **U** Prosthesis **Z** None	**Z** None
Z None	**J** Communication Skills	**K** Audiovisual **L** Assistive Listening **M** Augmentative / Alternative Communication **P** Computer **Z** None	**Z** None

DRG Non-OR	All body system/region, type qualifier, equipment, and qualifier values

Non-OR Procedure   DRG Non-OR Procedure   Valid OR Procedure   HAC Associated Procedure   Combination Only   New/Revised April   New/Revised October

810   ICD-10-PCS 2023

F Physical Rehabilitation and Diagnostic Audiology
1 Diagnostic Audiology
3 Hearing Assessment   Definition: Measurement of hearing and related functions

Body System/Region Character 4	Type Qualifier Character 5	Equipment Character 6	Qualifier Character 7
Z None	0 Hearing Screening	0 Occupational Hearing 1 Audiometer 2 Sound Field / Booth 3 Tympanometer 8 Vestibular / Balance 9 Cochlear Implant Z None	Z None
Z None	1 Pure Tone Audiometry, Air 2 Pure Tone Audiometry, Air and Bone	0 Occupational Hearing 1 Audiometer 2 Sound Field / Booth Z None	Z None
Z None	3 Bekesy Audiometry 6 Visual Reinforcement Audiometry 9 Short Increment Sensitivity Index B Stenger C Pure Tone Stenger	1 Audiometer 2 Sound Field / Booth Z None	Z None
Z None	4 Conditioned Play Audiometry 5 Select Picture Audiometry	1 Audiometer 2 Sound Field / Booth K Audiovisual Z None	Z None
Z None	7 Alternate Binaural or Monaural Loudness Balance	1 Audiometer K Audiovisual Z None	Z None
Z None	8 Tone Decay D Tympanometry F Eustachian Tube Function G Acoustic Reflex Patterns H Acoustic Reflex Threshold J Acoustic Reflex Decay	3 Tympanometer 4 Electroacoustic Immitance / Acoustic Reflex Z None	Z None
Z None	K Electrocochleography L Auditory Evoked Potentials	7 Electrophysiologic Z None	Z None

Z None	M Evoked Otoacoustic Emissions,
	   Screening
	N Evoked Otoacoustic Emissions,
	   Diagnostic
		6 Otoacoustic Emission (OAE)
		Z None
			Z None

Z None	P Aural Rehabilitation Status	1 Audiometer 2 Sound Field / Booth 4 Electroacoustic Immitance / Acoustic Reflex 9 Cochlear Implant K Audiovisual L Assistive Listening P Computer Z None	Z None
Z None	Q Auditory Processing	K Audiovisual P Computer Y Other Equipment Z None	Z None

NC Noncovered Procedure   **LC** Limited Coverage   **QA** Questionable OB Admit   **NT** New Tech Add-on   ⊞ Combination Member   ♂ Male   ♀ Female

ICD-10-PCS 2023   811

F Physical Rehabilitation and Diagnostic Audiology
1 Diagnostic Audiology
4 Hearing Aid Assessment   Definition: Measurement of the appropriateness and/or effectiveness of a hearing device

Body System/Region Character 4	Type Qualifier Character 5	Equipment Character 6	Qualifier Character 7
Z None	Ø Cochlear Implant	1 Audiometer 2 Sound Field / Booth 3 Tympanometer 4 Electroacoustic Immitance / Acoustic Reflex 5 Hearing Aid Selection / Fitting / Test 7 Electrophysiologic 9 Cochlear Implant K Audiovisual L Assistive Listening P Computer Y Other Equipment Z None	Z None

Z None	1 Ear Canal Probe Microphone
	6 Binaural Electroacoustic Hearing
	   Aid Check
	8 Monaural Electroacoustic Hearing
	   Aid Check
		5 Hearing Aid Selection / Fitting / Test
		Z None
			Z None

Z None	2 Monaural Hearing Aid 3 Binaural Hearing Aid	1 Audiometer 2 Sound Field / Booth 3 Tympanometer 4 Electroacoustic Immitance / Acoustic Reflex 5 Hearing Aid Selection / Fitting / Test K Audiovisual L Assistive Listening P Computer Z None	Z None

Z None	4 Assistive Listening System/Device
	   Selection
		1 Audiometer
		2 Sound Field / Booth
		3 Tympanometer
		4 Electroacoustic Immitance /
		   Acoustic Reflex
		K Audiovisual
		L Assistive Listening
		Z None
			Z None

Z None	5 Sensory Aids	1 Audiometer 2 Sound Field / Booth 3 Tympanometer 4 Electroacoustic Immitance / Acoustic Reflex 5 Hearing Aid Selection / Fitting / Test K Audiovisual L Assistive Listening Z None	Z None
Z None	7 Ear Protector Attentuation	Ø Occupational Hearing Z None	Z None

F Physical Rehabilitation and Diagnostic Audiology
1 Diagnostic Audiology
5 Vestibular Assessment   Definition: Measurement of the vestibular system and related functions

Body System/Region Character 4	Type Qualifier Character 5	Equipment Character 6	Qualifier Character 7

Z None	Ø Bithermal, Binaural Caloric
	   Irrigation
	1 Bithermal, Monaural Caloric
	   Irrigation
	2 Unithermal Binaural Screen
	3 Oscillating Tracking
	4 Sinusoidal Vertical Axis Rotational
	5 Dix-Hallpike Dynamic
	6 Computerized Dynamic
	   Posturography
		8 Vestibular / Balance
		Z None
			Z None

Z None	7 Tinnitus Masker	5 Hearing Aid Selection / Fitting / Test Z None	Z None

Mental Health GZ1–GZJ

G   **Mental Health**
Z   **None**
1   **Psychological Tests**   Definition: The administration and interpretation of standardized psychological tests and measurement instruments for the assessment of psychological function

Qualifier Character 4	Qualifier Character 5	Qualifier Character 6	Qualifier Character 7
Ø Developmental 1 Personality and Behavioral 2 Intellectual and Psychoeducational 3 Neuropsychological 4 Neurobehavioral and Cognitive Status	Z None	Z None	Z None

G   **Mental Health**
Z   **None**
2   **Crisis Intervention**   Definition: Treatment of a traumatized, acutely disturbed or distressed individual for the purpose of short-term stabilization

Qualifier Character 4	Qualifier Character 5	Qualifier Character 6	Qualifier Character 7
Z None	Z None	Z None	Z None

G   **Mental Health**
Z   **None**
3   **Medication Management**   Definition: Monitoring and adjusting the use of medications for the treatment of a mental health disorder

Qualifier Character 4	Qualifier Character 5	Qualifier Character 6	Qualifier Character 7
Z None	Z None	Z None	Z None

G   **Mental Health**
Z   **None**
5   **Individual Psychotherapy**   Definition: Treatment of an individual with a mental health disorder by behavioral, cognitive, psychoanalytic, psychodynamic or psychophysiological means to improve functioning or well-being

Qualifier Character 4	Qualifier Character 5	Qualifier Character 6	Qualifier Character 7
Ø Interactive 1 Behavioral 2 Cognitive 3 Interpersonal 4 Psychoanalysis 5 Psychodynamic 6 Supportive 8 Cognitive-Behavioral 9 Psychophysiological	Z None	Z None	Z None

G   **Mental Health**
Z   **None**
6   **Counseling**   Definition: The application of psychological methods to treat an individual with normal developmental issues and psychological problems in order to increase function, improve well-being, alleviate distress, maladjustment or resolve crises

Qualifier Character 4	Qualifier Character 5	Qualifier Character 6	Qualifier Character 7
Ø Educational 1 Vocational 3 Other Counseling	Z None	Z None	Z None

G   **Mental Health**
Z   **None**
7   **Family Psychotherapy**   Definition: Treatment that includes one or more family members of an individual with a mental health disorder by behavioral, cognitive, psychoanalytic, psychodynamic or psychophysiological means to improve functioning or well-being

Explanation: Remediation of emotional or behavioral problems presented by one or more family members in cases where psychotherapy with more than one family member is indicated

Qualifier Character 4	Qualifier Character 5	Qualifier Character 6	Qualifier Character 7
2 Other Family Psychotherapy	Z None	Z None	Z None

NC Noncovered Procedure   **LC** Limited Coverage   **QA** Questionable OB Admit   **NT** New Tech Add-on   ⊞ Combination Member   ♂ Male   ♀ Female

ICD-10-PCS 2023   **813**

GZ1–GZ7

G   **Mental Health**
Z   **None**
B   **Electroconvulsive Therapy**   Definition: The application of controlled electrical voltages to treat a mental health disorder

Qualifier Character 4	Qualifier Character 5	Qualifier Character 6	Qualifier Character 7
Ø Unilateral-Single Seizure 1 Unilateral-Multiple Seizure 2 Bilateral-Single Seizure 3 Bilateral-Multiple Seizure 4 Other Electroconvulsive Therapy	Z None	Z None	Z None

G   **Mental Health**
Z   **None**
C   **Biofeedback**   Definition: Provision of information from the monitoring and regulating of physiological processes in conjunction with cognitive-behavioral techniques to improve patient functioning or well-being

Qualifier Character 4	Qualifier Character 5	Qualifier Character 6	Qualifier Character 7
9 Other Biofeedback	Z None	Z None	Z None

G   **Mental Health**
Z   **None**
F   **Hypnosis**   Definition: Induction of a state of heightened suggestibility by auditory, visual and tactile techniques to elicit an emotional or behavioral response

Qualifier Character 4	Qualifier Character 5	Qualifier Character 6	Qualifier Character 7
Z None	Z None	Z None	Z None

G   **Mental Health**
Z   **None**
G   **Narcosynthesis**   Definition: Administration of intravenous barbiturates in order to release suppressed or repressed thoughts

Qualifier Character 4	Qualifier Character 5	Qualifier Character 6	Qualifier Character 7
Z None	Z None	Z None	Z None

G   **Mental Health**
Z   **None**
H   **Group Psychotherapy**   Definition: Treatment of two or more individuals with a mental health disorder by behavioral, cognitive, psychoanalytic, psychodynamic or psychophysiological means to improve functioning or well-being

Qualifier Character 4	Qualifier Character 5	Qualifier Character 6	Qualifier Character 7
Z None	Z None	Z None	Z None

G   **Mental Health**
Z   **None**
J   **Light Therapy**   Definition: Application of specialized light treatments to improve functioning or well-being

Qualifier Character 4	Qualifier Character 5	Qualifier Character 6	Qualifier Character 7
Z None	Z None	Z None	Z None

Substance Abuse Treatment HZ2–HZ9

AHA Coding Clinic for table HZ2
2020, 1Q, 21   Inpatient detoxification services

AHA Coding Clinic for table HZ9
2020, 1Q, 21   Inpatient detoxification services

H   **Substance Abuse Treatment**
Z   **None**
2   **Detoxification Services**   Definition: Detoxification from alcohol and/or drugs

Explanation: Not a treatment modality, but helps the patient stabilize physically and psychologically until the body becomes free of drugs and the effects of alcohol

Qualifier Character 4	Qualifier Character 5	Qualifier Character 6	Qualifier Character 7
Z None	**Z** None	**Z** None	**Z** None

H   **Substance Abuse Treatment**
Z   **None**
3   **Individual Counseling**   Definition: The application of psychological methods to treat an individual with addictive behavior

Explanation: Comprised of several different techniques, which apply various strategies to address drug addiction

Qualifier Character 4	Qualifier Character 5	Qualifier Character 6	Qualifier Character 7
0 Cognitive **1** Behavioral **2** Cognitive-Behavioral **3** 12-Step **4** Interpersonal **5** Vocational **6** Psychoeducation **7** Motivational Enhancement **8** Confrontational **9** Continuing Care **B** Spiritual **C** Pre/Post-Test Infectious Disease	**Z** None	**Z** None	**Z** None

DRG Non-OR   HZ3[0,1,2,3,4,5,6,7,8,9,B]ZZZ

H   **Substance Abuse Treatment**
Z   **None**
4   **Group Counseling**   Definition: The application of psychological methods to treat two or more individuals with addictive behavior

Explanation: Provides structured group counseling sessions and healing power through the connection with others

Qualifier Character 4	Qualifier Character 5	Qualifier Character 6	Qualifier Character 7
0 Cognitive **1** Behavioral **2** Cognitive-Behavioral **3** 12-Step **4** Interpersonal **5** Vocational **6** Psychoeducation **7** Motivational Enhancement **8** Confrontational **9** Continuing Care **B** Spiritual **C** Pre/Post-Test Infectious Disease	**Z** None	**Z** None	**Z** None

DRG Non-OR   HZ4[0,1,2,3,4,5,6,7,8,9,B]ZZZ

NC Noncovered Procedure   **LC** Limited Coverage   **QA** Questionable OB Admit   **NT** New Tech Add-on   ⊞ Combination Member   ♂ Male   ♀ Female

ICD-10-PCS 2023   **815**

H Substance Abuse Treatment
Z None
5 Individual Psychotherapy Definition: Treatment of an individual with addictive behavior by behavioral, cognitive, psychoanalytic, psychodynamic or psychophysiological means

Qualifier Character 4	Qualifier Character 5	Qualifier Character 6	Qualifier Character 7
0 Cognitive	Z None	Z None	Z None
1 Behavioral			
2 Cognitive-Behavioral			
3 12-Step			
4 Interpersonal			
5 Interactive			
6 Psychoeducation			
7 Motivational Enhancement			
8 Confrontational			
9 Supportive			
B Psychoanalysis			
C Psychodynamic			
D Psychophysiological			

DRG Non-OR For all qualifier values

H Substance Abuse Treatment
Z None
6 Family Counseling Definition: The application of psychological methods that includes one or more family members to treat an individual with addictive behavior

Explanation: Provides support and education for family members of addicted individuals. Family member participation is seen as a critical area of substance abuse treatment

Qualifier Character 4	Qualifier Character 5	Qualifier Character 6	Qualifier Character 7
3 Other Family Counseling	Z None	Z None	Z None

H Substance Abuse Treatment
Z None
8 Medication Management Definition: Monitoring or adjusting the use of replacement medications for the treatment of addiction

Qualifier Character 4	Qualifier Character 5	Qualifier Character 6	Qualifier Character 7
0 Nicotine Replacement	Z None	Z None	Z None
1 Methadone Maintenance			
2 Levo-alpha-acetyl-methadol (LAAM)			
3 Antabuse			
4 Naltrexone			
5 Naloxone			
6 Clonidine			
7 Bupropion			
8 Psychiatric Medication			
9 Other Replacement Medication			

H Substance Abuse Treatment
Z None
9 Pharmacotherapy Definition: The use of replacement medications for the treatment of addiction

Qualifier Character 4	Qualifier Character 5	Qualifier Character 6	Qualifier Character 7
0 Nicotine Replacement	Z None	Z None	Z None
1 Methadone Maintenance			
2 Levo-alpha-acetyl-methadol (LAAM)			
3 Antabuse			
4 Naltrexone			
5 Naloxone			
6 Clonidine			
7 Bupropion			
8 Psychiatric Medication			
9 Other Replacement Medication			

Non-OR Procedure   DRG Non-OR Procedure   Valid OR Procedure   HAC Associated Procedure   Combination Only   New/Revised April   New/Revised October

816

ICD-10-PCS 2023

New Technology X27–XY0

AHA Coding Clinic for all tables in the New Technology Section
2015, 4Q, 8-11   New Section X codes - New Technology procedures

AHA Coding Clinic for table X27
2019, 4Q, 45-46   Sustained released drug-eluting stent

AHA Coding Clinic for table X2A
2021, 1Q, 16   Placement of Sentinel™ embolic protection device with deployment of single filter
2020, 4Q, 70-71   Cerebral embolic filtration extracorporeal flow reversal circuit
2019, 4Q, 46   Cerebral embolic filtration
2016, 4Q, 115-116   Cerebral embolic filtration

AHA Coding Clinic for table X2C
2021, 4Q, 58-59   Computer-aided mechanical aspiration thrombectomy
2016, 4Q, 82-83   Coronary artery, number of arteries
2015, 4Q, 8-14   New Section X codes—New Technology procedures

AHA Coding Clinic for table X2J
2021, 4Q, 59   Transthoracic echocardiography with computer-aided image acquisition

AHA Coding Clinic for table X2K
2021, 4Q, 60   Percutaneous creation of arteriovenous fistula using thermal resistance energy

AHA Coding Clinic for table X2R
2021, 4Q, 61-62   Replacement combined with restriction of descending thoracic aorta
2016, 4Q, 116   Aortic valve rapid deployment
2015, 4Q, 8-12   New Section X codes—New Technology procedures

AHA Coding Clinic for table X2V
2021, 4Q, 61-62   Replacement combined with restriction of descending thoracic aorta
2021, 4Q, 63   Restriction of coronary sinus

AHA Coding Clinic for table XD2
2021, 4Q, 63-64   Monitoring of tissue oxygen saturation in gastrointestinal tract

AHA Coding Clinic for table XDP
2021, 4Q, 64-65   Colonic irrigation for colonoscopy

AHA Coding Clinic for table XFJ
2021, 4Q, 65-66   Single-use duodenoscope during endoscopic retrograde cholangiopancreatography

AHA Coding Clinic for table XHR
2021, 4Q, 66   Application of bioengineered allogeneic construct
2016, 4Q, 116   Application of wound matrix

AHA Coding Clinic for table XK0
2017, 4Q, 74   Intramuscular autologous bone marrow cell therapy

AHA Coding Clinic for table XNS
2021, 4Q, 67   Posterior dynamic distraction
2017, 4Q, 74-75   Magnetic growth rods
2016, 4Q, 117   Placement of magnetic growth rods

AHA Coding Clinic for table XNU
2020, 4Q, 72   Implantation of vertebral mechanically expandable device

AHA Coding Clinic for table XRG
2021, 4Q, 68   Customizable interbody fusion
2017, 4Q, 76   Radiolucent porous interbody fusion device

AHA Coding Clinic for table XT2
2019, 4Q, 46-47   Renal function monitoring

AHA Coding Clinic for table XV5
2018, 4Q, 55   Robotic waterjet ablation

AHA Coding Clinic for table XW0
2022, 1Q, 5-6   COVID-19 vaccine administration
2022, 1Q, 7   Fostamatinib
2022, 1Q, 7-8   Tixagevimab and cilgavimab
2022, 1Q, 8   Other monoclonal antibody
2021, 4Q, 69-71   Introduction of new therapeutic substances
2021, 4Q, 71-74   Chimeric antigen receptor T-cell immunotherapy
2021, 4Q, 74-75   Antibiotic-eluting bone void filler
2021, 4Q, 110   New/revised frequently asked questions regarding ICD-10-CM/PCS coding for COVID-19
2021, 1Q, 49   Frequently asked questions regarding ICD-10-CM and ICD-10-PCS coding for COVID-19
2020, 4Q, 72-76   Introduction of new therapeutic substances
2020, 4Q, 95   Frequently asked questions regarding ICD-10-PCS coding for COVID-19
2020, 3Q, 17-21   New procedure codes for introduction or infusion of therapeutics
2019, 4Q, 47-50   New therapeutic substances
2018, 4Q, 56   New therapeutic substances
2015, 4Q, 8-15   New Section X codes—New Technology procedures

AHA Coding Clinic for table XW1
2021, 4Q, 76   Transfusion of hyperimmune globulin and high-dose immune globulin
2020, 3Q, 17-21   New procedure codes for introduction or infusion of therapeutics

AHA Coding Clinic for table XWH
2021, 4Q, 76-77   Pharyngeal electrical stimulation

AHA Coding Clinic for table XXE
2021, 4Q, 77   Computer-aided assessment of intracranial vascular activity
2021, 4Q, 77-78   Computer-aided triage and notification of pulmonary artery flow
2021, 4Q, 78-79   Mechanical initial specimen diversion of whole blood using active negative pressure
2021, 4Q, 79-80   Concurrent measurement of mRNA, PCR test and detection of antibodies
2020, 4Q, 78-79   Measurement of infection
2020, 4Q, 78-79   Positive blood culture fluorescence hybridization
2020, 4Q, 79   Nucleic acid-base microbial detection
2019, 4Q, 50-51   Whole blood nucleic acid-base microbial detection

AHA Coding Clinic for table XY0
2021, 4Q, 80   Regional anticoagulation for renal replacement therapy
2017, 4Q, 78   Intraoperative treatment of vascular grafts

X   **New Technology**
0   **Nervous System**
H   **Insertion**   Definition: Putting in a nonbiological appliance that monitors, assists, performs, or prevents a physiological function but does not physically take the place of a body part
       Explanation: None

Body Part Character 4	Approach Character 5	Device/Substance/Technology Character 6	Qualifier Character 7
K Sphenopalatine Ganglion	3 Percutaneous	Q Neurostimulator Lead	8 New Technology Group 8
Q Vagus Nerve	3 Percutaneous	R Neurostimulator Lead with Paired Stimulation System	8 New Technology Group 8

X   **New Technology**
0   **Nervous System**
Z   **Other Procedures**   Definition: Methodologies which attempt to remediate or cure a disorder or disease
                Explanation: None

Body Part Character 4	Approach Character 5	Device/Substance/Technology Character 6	Qualifier Character 7
0 Prefrontal Cortex	X External	1 Computer-assisted Transcranial Magnetic Stimulation	8 New Technology Group 8

NC Noncovered Procedure   **LC** Limited Coverage   **QA** Questionable OB Admit   **NT** New Tech Add-on   ⊞ Combination Member   ♂ Male   ♀ Female

ICD-10-PCS 2023   817

X New Technology
2 Cardiovascular System
7 Dilation   Definition: Expanding an orifice or the lumen of a tubular body part

Explanation: The orifice can be a natural orifice or an artificially created orifice. Accomplished by stretching a tubular body part using intraluminal pressure or by cutting part of the orifice or wall of the tubular body part.

Body Part Character 4	Approach Character 5	Device/Substance/Technology Character 6	Qualifier Character 7
H Femoral Artery, Right **J** Femoral Artery, Left **K** Popliteal Artery, Proximal Right **L** Popliteal Artery, Proximal Left **M** Popliteal Artery, Distal Right **N** Popliteal Artery, Distal Left **P** Anterior Tibial Artery, Right **Q** Anterior Tibial Artery, Left **R** Posterior Tibial Artery, Right **S** Posterior Tibial Artery, Left **T** Peroneal Artery, Right **U** Peroneal Artery, Left	**3** Percutaneous	**8** Intraluminal Device, Sustained Release Drug-eluting **9** Intraluminal Device, Sustained Release Drug-eluting, Two **B** Intraluminal Device, Sustained Release Drug-eluting, Three **C** Intraluminal Device, Sustained Release Drug-eluting, Four or More	**5** New Technology Group 5

Valid OR All body part, approach, device/substance/technology, and qualifier values

X New Technology
2 Cardiovascular System
A Assistance   Definition: Taking over a portion of a physiological function by extracorporeal means

Explanation: None

Body Part Character 4	Approach Character 5	Device/Substance/Technology Character 6	Qualifier Character 7
5 Innominate Artery and Left Common Carotid Artery	**3** Percutaneous	**1** Cerebral Embolic Filtration, Dual Filter	**2** New Technology Group 2
6 Aortic Arch	**3** Percutaneous	**2** Cerebral Embolic Filtration, Single Deflection Filter	**5** New Technology Group 5
7 Coronary Sinus	**3** Percutaneous	**5** Intermittent Coronary Sinus Occlusion	**8** New Technology Group 8
H Common Carotid Artery, Right **J** Common Carotid Artery, Left	**3** Percutaneous	**3** Cerebral Embolic Filtration, Extracorporeal Flow Reversal Circuit	**6** New Technology Group 6

DRG Non-OR X2A7358

X New Technology
2 Cardiovascular System
C Extirpation   Definition: Taking or cutting out solid matter from a body part

Explanation: The solid matter may be an abnormal byproduct of a biological function or a foreign body; it may be imbedded in a body part or in the lumen of a tubular body part. The solid matter may or may not have been previously broken into pieces.

Body Part Character 4	Approach Character 5	Device/Substance/Technology Character 6	Qualifier Character 7
P Abdominal Aorta **Q** Upper Extremity Vein, Right **R** Upper Extremity Vein, Left **S** Lower Extremity Artery, Right **T** Lower Extremity Artery, Left **U** Lower Extremity Vein, Right **V** Lower Extremity Vein, Left **Y** Great Vessel	**3** Percutaneous	**T** Computer-aided Mechanical Aspiration	**7** New Technology Group 7

Valid OR All body part, approach, device/substance/technology, and qualifier values

X New Technology
2 Cardiovascular System
J Inspection   Definition: Visually and/or manually exploring a body part

Explanation: None

Body Part Character 4	Approach Character 5	Device/Substance/Technology Character 6	Qualifier Character 7
A Heart	**X** External	**4** Transthoracic Echocardiography, Computer-aided Guidance 〖NT〗	**7** New Technology Group 7

〖NT〗 X2JAX47 for Caption Guidance™

X New Technology
2 Cardiovascular System
K Bypass   Definition: Altering the route of passage of the contents of a tubular body part

Explanation: None

Body Part Character 4	Approach Character 5	Device/Substance/Technology Character 6	Qualifier Character 7
B Radial Artery, Right **C** Radial Artery, Left	**3** Percutaneous	**1** Thermal Resistance Energy	**7** New Technology Group 7

Valid OR All body part, approach, device/substance/technology, and qualifier values

Non-OR Procedure   DRG Non-OR Procedure   Valid OR Procedure   HAC Associated Procedure   Combination Only   New/Revised April   New/Revised October

X New Technology
2 Cardiovascular System
R Replacement   Definition: Putting in or on biological or synthetic material that physically takes the place and/or function of all or a portion of a body part
     Explanation: None

Body Part Character 4	Approach Character 5	Device/Substance/Technology Character 6	Qualifier Character 7
X Thoracic Aorta, Arch	Ø Open	N Branched Synthetic Substitute with Intraluminal Device	7 New Technology Group 7

Valid OR   All body part, approach, device/substance/technology, and qualifier values

X New Technology
2 Cardiovascular System
V Restriction   Definition: Partially closing an orifice or the lumen of a tubular body part
     Explanation: None

Body Part Character 4	Approach Character 5	Device/Substance/Technology Character 6	Qualifier Character 7
7 Coronary Sinus	3 Percutaneous	Q Reduction Device	7 New Technology Group 7
W Thoracic Aorta, Descending	Ø Open	N Branched Synthetic Substitute with Intraluminal Device	7 New Technology Group 7

Valid OR   All body part, approach, device/substance/technology, and qualifier values

X New Technology
D Gastrointestinal System
2 Monitoring   Definition: Determining the level of a physiological or physical function repetitively over a period of time
     Explanation: None

Body Part Character 4	Approach Character 5	Device/Substance/Technology Character 6	Qualifier Character 7
G Upper GI H Lower GI	4 Percutaneous Endoscopic 8 Via Natural or Artificial Opening Endoscopic	V Oxygen Saturation	7 New Technology Group 7

X New Technology
D Gastrointestinal System
P Irrigation   Definition: Putting in or on a cleansing substance
     Explanation: None

Body Part Character 4	Approach Character 5	Device/Substance/Technology Character 6	Qualifier Character 7
H Lower GI	8 Via Natural or Artificial Opening Endoscopic	K Intraoperative Single-use Oversleeve	7 New Technology Group 7

X New Technology
F Hepatobiliary System and Pancreas
5 Destruction   Definition: Physical eradication of all or a portion of a body part by the direct use of energy, force, or a destructive agent
     Explanation: None of the body part is physically taken out

Body Part Character 4	Approach Character 5	Device/Substance/Technology Character 6	Qualifier Character 7
Ø Liver 1 Liver, Right Lobe 2 Liver, Left Lobe	X External	Ø Ultrasound-guided Cavitation	8 New Technology Group 8

DRG Non-OR   All body part, approach, device/substance/technology, and qualifier values

X New Technology
F Hepatobiliary System and Pancreas
J Inspection   Definition: Visually and/or manually exploring a body part
     Explanation: None

Body Part Character 4	Approach Character 5	Device/Substance/Technology Character 6	Qualifier Character 7
B Hepatobiliary Duct D Pancreatic Duct	8 Via Natural or Artificial Opening Endoscopic	A Single-use Duodenoscope **NT**	7 New Technology Group 7

NT   XFJ[B,D]8A7 for aScope® Duodeno

NC Noncovered Procedure   **LC** Limited Coverage   **QA** Questionable OB Admit   **NT** New Tech Add-on   ⊞ Combination Member   ♂ Male   ♀ Female

ICD-10-PCS 2023   819

X2R–XFJ

New Technology

X	New Technology
H	Skin, Subcutaneous Tissue, Fascia and Breast
R	Replacement

Definition: Putting in or on biological or synthetic material that physically takes the place and/or function of all or a portion of a body part

Explanation: None

Body Part Character 4	Approach Character 5	Device/Substance/Technology Character 6	Qualifier Character 7
P Skin	X External	F Bioengineered Allogeneic [NT] Construct	7 New Technology Group 7

Valid OR XHRPXF7
[NT] XHRPXF7 for StrataGraft®

X	New Technology
K	Muscles, Tendons, Bursae and Ligaments
U	Supplement

Definition: Putting in or on biological or synthetic material that physically reinforces and/or augments the function of a portion of a body part

Explanation: None

Body Part Character 4	Approach Character 5	Device/Substance/Technology Character 6	Qualifier Character 7
C Upper Spine Bursa and Ligament D Lower Spine Bursa and Ligament	Ø Open	6 Posterior Vertebral Tether	8 New Technology Group 8

X	New Technology
N	Bones
H	Insertion

Definition: Putting in a nonbiological appliance that monitors, assists, performs, or prevents a physiological function but does not physically take the place of a body part

Explanation: None

Body Part Character 4	Approach Character 5	Device/Substance/Technology Character 6	Qualifier Character 7
6 Pelvic Bone, Right 7 Pelvic Bone, Left	Ø Open 3 Percutaneous	5 Internal Fixation Device with Tulip Connector	8 New Technology Group 8

X	New Technology
N	Bones
S	Reposition

Definition: Moving to its normal location, or other suitable location, all or a portion of a body part

Explanation: The body part is moved to a new location from an abnormal location, or from a normal location where it is not functioning correctly. The body part may or may not be cut out or off to be moved to the new location.

Body Part Character 4	Approach Character 5	Device/Substance/Technology Character 6	Qualifier Character 7
Ø Lumbar Vertebra	Ø Open	3 Magnetically Controlled Growth Rod(s)	2 New Technology Group 2
Ø Lumbar Vertebra	Ø Open	C Posterior (Dynamic) Distraction Device	7 New Technology Group 7
Ø Lumbar Vertebra	3 Percutaneous	3 Magnetically Controlled Growth Rod(s)	2 New Technology Group 2
Ø Lumbar Vertebra	3 Percutaneous	C Posterior (Dynamic) Distraction Device	7 New Technology Group 7
3 Cervical Vertebra	Ø Open 3 Percutaneous	3 Magnetically Controlled Growth Rod(s)	2 New Technology Group 2
4 Thoracic Vertebra	Ø Open	3 Magnetically Controlled Growth Rod(s)	2 New Technology Group 2
4 Thoracic Vertebra	Ø Open	C Posterior (Dynamic) Distraction Device	7 New Technology Group 7
4 Thoracic Vertebra	3 Percutaneous	3 Magnetically Controlled Growth Rod(s)	2 New Technology Group 2
4 Thoracic Vertebra	3 Percutaneous	C Posterior (Dynamic) Distraction Device	7 New Technology Group 7

Valid OR All body part, approach, device/substance/technology, and qualifier values

X	New Technology
N	Bones
U	Supplement

Definition: Putting in or on biological or synthetic material that physically reinforces and/or augments the function of a portion of a body part

Explanation: None

Body Part Character 4	Approach Character 5	Device/Substance/Technology Character 6	Qualifier Character 7
Ø Lumbar Vertebra 4 Thoracic Vertebra	3 Percutaneous	5 Synthetic Substitute, Mechanically Expandable (Paired)	6 New Technology Group 6

Valid OR XNU[Ø,4]356

X   **New Technology**
R   **Joints**
G   **Fusion**   Definition: Joining together portions of an articular body part rendering the articular body part immobile
                    Explanation: None

Body Part Character 4	Approach Character 5	Device/Substance/Technology Character 6	Qualifier Character 7
A Thoracolumbar Vertebral Joint B Lumbar Vertebral Joint C Lumbar Vertebral Joints, 2 or more ⊞ D Lumbosacral Joint	Ø Open 3 Percutaneous 4 Percutaneous Endoscopic	R Interbody Fusion Device, **NT** Customizable	7 New Technology Group 7
E Sacroiliac Joint, Right F Sacroiliac Joint, Left	Ø Open 3 Percutaneous	5 Internal Fixation Device with Tulip Connector	8 New Technology Group 8

Valid OR   XRG[A,B,C,D][Ø,3,4]R7
HAC   XRG[A,B,C,D][Ø,3,4]R7 when reported with SDx K68.11 or T81.40-T81.49,
              T84.60-T84.619, T84.63-T84.7 with 7th character A
NT   XRG[A,B,C,D][Ø,3,4]R7 for aprevo® Intervertebral Body Fusion Device

See Appendix L for Procedure Combinations
    ⊞   XRGC[Ø,3,4]R7

X   **New Technology**
R   **Joints**
H   **Insertion**   Definition: Putting in a nonbiological appliance that monitors, assists, performs, or prevents a physiological function but does not physically
                     take the place of a body part
                     Explanation: None

Body Part Character 4	Approach Character 5	Device/Substance/Technology Character 6	Qualifier Character 7
B Lumbar Vertebral Joint D Lumbosacral Joint	Ø Open	1 Posterior Spinal Motion Preservation Device	8 New Technology Group 8

X   **New Technology**
R   **Joints**
R   **Replacement**   Definition: Putting in or on biological or synthetic material that physically takes the place and/or function of all or a portion of a body part
                         Explanation: None

Body Part Character 4	Approach Character 5	Device/Substance/Technology Character 6	Qualifier Character 7

G   Knee Joint, Right   ⊞
H   Knee Joint, Left   ⊞
	Ø Open	L Synthetic Substitute, Lateral
		      Meniscus
		M Synthetic Substitute, Medial
		       Meniscus
			8 New Technology Group 8

Valid OR   All body part, approach, device/substance/technology, and qualifier values
HAC   XRR[G,H]Ø[L,M]8 when reported with SDx of I26.02-I26.09, I26.92-I26.99, or I82.401-I82.4Z9

See Appendix L for Procedure Combinations
    ⊞   XRR[G,H]Ø[L,M]8

X   **New Technology**
T   **Urinary System**
2   **Monitoring**   Definition: Determining the level of a physiological or physical function repetitively over a period of time
                     Explanation: None

Body Part Character 4	Approach Character 5	Device/Substance/Technology Character 6	Qualifier Character 7
5 Kidney	X External	E Fluorescent Pyrazine	5 New Technology Group 5

X   **New Technology**
V   **Male Reproductive System**
5   **Destruction**   Definition: Physical eradication of all or a portion of a body part by the direct use of energy, force, or a destructive agent
                     Explanation: None of the body part is physically taken out

Body Part Character 4	Approach Character 5	Device/Substance/Technology Character 6	Qualifier Character 7
Ø Prostate	8 Via Natural or Artificial Opening Endoscopic	A Robotic Waterjet Ablation	4 New Technology Group 4

Valid OR   All body part, approach, device/substance/technology, and qualifier values

NC Noncovered Procedure   **LC** Limited Coverage   **QA** Questionable OB Admit   **NT** New Tech Add-on   ⊞ Combination Member   ♂ Male   ♀ Female

ICD-10-PCS 2023   821

New Technology

X **New Technology**
W **Anatomical Regions**
Ø **Introduction**   Definition: Putting in or on a therapeutic, diagnostic, nutritional, physiological, or prophylactic substance except blood or blood products
Explanation: None

Body Part Character 4	Approach Character 5	Device/Substance/Technology Character 6	Qualifier Character 7
Ø Skin	X External	2 Bromelain-enriched Proteolytic Enzyme	7 New Technology Group 7
1 Subcutaneous Tissue	3 Percutaneous	1 Daratumumab and Hyaluronidase-fihj 4 Teclistamab Antineoplastic	8 New Technology Group 8
1 Subcutaneous Tissue	3 Percutaneous	9 Satralizumab-mwge	7 New Technology Group 7
1 Subcutaneous Tissue	3 Percutaneous	F Other New Technology Therapeutic Substance	5 New Technology Group 5
1 Subcutaneous Tissue	3 Percutaneous	H Other New Technology Monoclonal Antibody K Leronlimab Monoclonal Antibody S COVID-19 Vaccine Dose 1 T COVID-19 Vaccine Dose 2 U COVID-19 Vaccine	6 New Technology Group 6
1 Subcutaneous Tissue	3 Percutaneous	V COVID-19 Vaccine Dose 3	7 New Technology Group 7
1 Subcutaneous Tissue	3 Percutaneous	W Caplacizumab	5 New Technology Group 5
1 Subcutaneous Tissue	3 Percutaneous	W COVID-19 Vaccine Booster	7 New Technology Group 7
1 Subcutaneous Tissue	X External	2 Bromelain-enriched Proteolytic Enzyme	7 New Technology Group 7
2 Muscle	Ø Open	D Engineered Allogeneic Thymus Tissue	8 New Technology Group 8
2 Muscle	3 Percutaneous	S COVID-19 Vaccine Dose 1 T COVID-19 Vaccine Dose 2 U COVID-19 Vaccine	6 New Technology Group 6
2 Muscle	3 Percutaneous	V COVID-19 Vaccine Dose 3 W COVID-19 Vaccine Booster X Tixagevimab and Cilgavimab Monoclonal Antibody Y Other New Technology Monoclonal Antibody	7 New Technology Group 7
3 Peripheral Vein	3 Percutaneous	Ø Brexanolone	6 New Technology Group 6
3 Peripheral Vein	3 Percutaneous	Ø Spesolimab Monoclonal Antibody	8 New Technology Group 8
3 Peripheral Vein	3 Percutaneous	2 Nerinitide 3 Durvalumab Antineoplastic	6 New Technology Group 6
3 Peripheral Vein	3 Percutaneous	5 Narsoplimab Monoclonal Antibody	7 New Technology Group 7
3 Peripheral Vein	3 Percutaneous	5 Mosunetuzumab Antineoplastic	8 New Technology Group 8
3 Peripheral Vein	3 Percutaneous	6 Lefamulin Anti-infective	6 New Technology Group 6
3 Peripheral Vein	3 Percutaneous	6 Terlipressin	7 New Technology Group 7
3 Peripheral Vein	3 Percutaneous	6 Afamitresgene Autoleucel Immunotherapy	8 New Technology Group 8
3 Peripheral Vein	3 Percutaneous	7 Coagulation Factor Xa, Inactivated	2 New Technology Group 2
3 Peripheral Vein	3 Percutaneous	7 Trilaciclib [NT]	7 New Technology Group 7
3 Peripheral Vein	3 Percutaneous	7 Tabelecleucel Immunotherapy	8 New Technology Group 8
3 Peripheral Vein	3 Percutaneous	8 Lurbinectedin [NT]	7 New Technology Group 7
3 Peripheral Vein	3 Percutaneous	8 Treosulfan	8 New Technology Group 8
3 Peripheral Vein	3 Percutaneous	9 Ceftolozane/Tazobactam Anti-infective	6 New Technology Group 6
3 Peripheral Vein	3 Percutaneous	9 Inebilizumab-cdon	8 New Technology Group 8
3 Peripheral Vein	3 Percutaneous	A Cefiderocol Anti-infective [NT]	6 New Technology Group 6
3 Peripheral Vein	3 Percutaneous	A Ciltacabtagene Autoleucel	7 New Technology Group 7
3 Peripheral Vein	3 Percutaneous	B Cytarabine and Daunorubicin Liposome Antineoplastic	3 New Technology Group 3
3 Peripheral Vein	3 Percutaneous	B Omadacycline Anti-infective	6 New Technology Group 6
3 Peripheral Vein	3 Percutaneous	B Amivantamab Monoclonal Antibody [NT]	7 New Technology Group 7
3 Peripheral Vein	3 Percutaneous	C Eculizumab	6 New Technology Group 6
3 Peripheral Vein	3 Percutaneous	C Engineered Chimeric Antigen Receptor T-cell Immunotherapy, Autologous	7 New Technology Group 7
3 Peripheral Vein	3 Percutaneous	D Atezolizumab Antineoplastic	6 New Technology Group 6
3 Peripheral Vein	3 Percutaneous	E Remdesivir Anti-infective [NT]	5 New Technology Group 5
3 Peripheral Vein	3 Percutaneous	E Etesevimab Monoclonal Antibody	6 New Technology Group 6
3 Peripheral Vein	3 Percutaneous	F Other New Technology Therapeutic Substance	3 New Technology Group 3
3 Peripheral Vein	3 Percutaneous	F Other New Technology Therapeutic Substance	5 New Technology Group 5

DRG Non-OR   XWØ33A7
DRG Non-OR   XWØ33C7
[NT]   XWØ3377
[NT]   XWØ3387
[NT]   XWØ33A6 in combination with dx code Y95 and one of the following: J14, J15.Ø, J15.1, J15.5, J15.6, J15.8, OR dx code J95.851 and one of the following: B96.1, B96.2Ø, B96.21, B96.22, B96.23, B96.29, B96.3, B96.5, or B96.89
[NT]   XWØ33B7
[NT]   XWØ33E5

* For all codes with NT icon *see* Appendix I for registered or trade name of substance

XWØ Continued on next page

Non-OR Procedure   DRG Non-OR Procedure   Valid OR Procedure   HAC Associated Procedure   Combination Only   New/Revised April   New/Revised October

X   New Technology
W   Anatomical Regions
Ø   Introduction   Definition: Putting in or on a therapeutic, diagnostic, nutritional, physiological, or prophylactic substance except blood or blood products
                   Explanation: None

XWØ Continued

Body Part Character 4		Approach Character 5		Device/Substance/Technology Character 6		Qualifier Character 7	
3	Peripheral Vein	3	Percutaneous	F	Bamlanivimab Monoclonal Antibody	6	New Technology Group 6
3	Peripheral Vein	3	Percutaneous	G	Plazomicin Anti-infective	4	New Technology Group 4
3	Peripheral Vein	3	Percutaneous	G	Sarilumab	5	New Technology Group 5
3	Peripheral Vein	3	Percutaneous	G	REGN-COV2 Monoclonal Antibody	6	New Technology Group 6
3	Peripheral Vein	3	Percutaneous	G	Engineered Chimeric Antigen Receptor T-cell Immunotherapy, Allogeneic	7	New Technology Group 7
3	Peripheral Vein	3	Percutaneous	H	Synthetic Human Angiotensin II	4	New Technology Group 4
3	Peripheral Vein	3	Percutaneous	H	Tocilizumab	5	New Technology Group 5
3	Peripheral Vein	3	Percutaneous	H	Other New Technology Monoclonal Antibody	6	New Technology Group 6
3	Peripheral Vein	3	Percutaneous	H J	Axicabtagene Ciloleucel Immunotherapy Tisagenlecleucel Immunotherapy	7	New Technology Group 7
3	Peripheral Vein	3	Percutaneous	K	Fosfomycin Anti-infective	5	New Technology Group 5
3	Peripheral Vein	3	Percutaneous	K	Idecabtagene Vicleucel **NT** Immunotherapy	7	New Technology Group 7
3	Peripheral Vein	3	Percutaneous	L	CD24Fc Immunomodulator	6	New Technology Group 6
3	Peripheral Vein	3	Percutaneous	L M	Lifileucel Immunotherapy Brexucabtagene Autoleucel **NT** Immunotherapy	7	New Technology Group 7
3	Peripheral Vein	3	Percutaneous	N	Meropenem-vaborbactam Anti-infective	5	New Technology Group 5
3	Peripheral Vein	3	Percutaneous	N	Lisocabtagene Maraleucel Immunotherapy	7	New Technology Group 7
3	Peripheral Vein	3	Percutaneous	Q S U W	Tagraxofusp-erzs Antineoplastic Iobenguane I-131 Antineoplastic Imipenem-cilastatin-relebactam **NT** Anti-infective Caplacizumab	5	New Technology Group 5
4	Central Vein	3	Percutaneous	Ø	Brexanolone	6	New Technology Group 6
4	Central Vein	3	Percutaneous	Ø	Spesolimab Monoclonal Antibody	8	New Technology Group 8
4	Central Vein	3	Percutaneous	2 3	Nerinitide Durvalumab Antineoplastic	6	New Technology Group 6
4	Central Vein	3	Percutaneous	5	Narsoplimab Monoclonal Antibody	7	New Technology Group 7
4	Central Vein	3	Percutaneous	5	Mosunetuzumab Antineoplastic	8	New Technology Group 8
4	Central Vein	3	Percutaneous	6	Lefamulin Anti-infective	6	New Technology Group 6
4	Central Vein	3	Percutaneous	6	Terlipressin	7	New Technology Group 7
4	Central Vein	3	Percutaneous	6	Afamitresgene Autoleucel Immunotherapy	8	New Technology Group 8
4	Central Vein	3	Percutaneous	7	Coagulation Factor Xa, Inactivated	2	New Technology Group 2
4	Central Vein	3	Percutaneous	7	Trilaciclib **NT**	7	New Technology Group 7
4	Central Vein	3	Percutaneous	7	Tabelecleucel Immunotherapy	8	New Technology Group 8
4	Central Vein	3	Percutaneous	8	Lurbinectedin **NT**	7	New Technology Group 7
4	Central Vein	3	Percutaneous	8	Treosulfan	8	New Technology Group 8
4	Central Vein	3	Percutaneous	9	Ceftolozane/Tazobactam Anti-infective	6	New Technology Group 6
4	Central Vein	3	Percutaneous	9	Inebilizumab-cdon	8	New Technology Group 8
4	Central Vein	3	Percutaneous	A	Cefiderocol Anti-infective **NT**	6	New Technology Group 6
4	Central Vein	3	Percutaneous	A	Ciltacabtagene Autoleucel	7	New Technology Group 7
4	Central Vein	3	Percutaneous	B	Cytarabine and Daunorubicin Liposome Antineoplastic	3	New Technology Group 3
4	Central Vein	3	Percutaneous	B	Omadacycline Anti-infective	6	New Technology Group 6
4	Central Vein	3	Percutaneous	B	Amivantamab Monoclonal Antibody **NT**	7	New Technology Group 7
4	Central Vein	3	Percutaneous	C	Eculizumab	6	New Technology Group 6
4	Central Vein	3	Percutaneous	C	Engineered Chimeric Antigen Receptor T-cell Immunotherapy, Autologous	7	New Technology Group 7
4	Central Vein	3	Percutaneous	D	Atezolizumab Antineoplastic	6	New Technology Group 6
4	Central Vein	3	Percutaneous	E	Remdesivir Anti-infective **NT**	5	New Technology Group 5
4	Central Vein	3	Percutaneous	E	Etesevimab Monoclonal Antibody	6	New Technology Group 6

DRG Non-OR	XW033G7	**NT**	XW033K7	
DRG Non-OR	XW033[H,J]7	**NT**	XW033M7	
DRG Non-OR	XW033K7	**NT**	XW033U5 in combination with dx code Y95 and one of the following: J14, J15.Ø, J15.1, J15.5, J15.6, J15.8, OR dx code J95.851 and one of the following: B96.1, B96.2Ø, B96.21, B96.22, B96.23, B96.29, B96.3, B96.5, or B96.89	
DRG Non-OR	XW033[L,M]7			
DRG Non-OR	XW033N7	**NT**	XW04377	
DRG Non-OR	XW043A7	**NT**	XW04387	
DRG Non-OR	XW043C7	**NT**	XW043A6 in combination with dx code Y95 and one of the following: J14, J15.Ø, J15.1, J15.5, J15.6, J15.8 OR dx code J95.851 and one of the following: B96.1, B96.2Ø, B96.21, B96.22, B96.23, B96.29, B96.3, B96.5, or B96.89	
		NT	XW043B7	
		NT	XW043E5	

* For all codes with NT icon *see* Appendix I for registered or trade name of substance

XWØ Continued on next page

NC Noncovered Procedure   **LC** Limited Coverage   **QA** Questionable OB Admit   **NT** New Tech Add-on   ⊞ Combination Member   ♂ Male   ♀ Female

ICD-10-PCS 2023   823

XWØ–XWØ

X　**New Technology**
W　**Anatomical Regions**
Ø　**Introduction**　　Definition: Putting in or on a therapeutic, diagnostic, nutritional, physiological, or prophylactic substance except blood or blood products
　　　　　　　　　　Explanation: None

XWØ Continued

Body Part Character 4	Approach Character 5	Device/Substance/Technology Character 6	Qualifier Character 7
4　Central Vein	3　Percutaneous	F　Other New Technology Therapeutic Substance	3　New Technology Group 3
4　Central Vein	3　Percutaneous	F　Other New Technology Therapeutic Substance	5　New Technology Group 5
4　Central Vein	3　Percutaneous	F　Bamlanivimab Monoclonal Antibody	6　New Technology Group 6
4　Central Vein	3　Percutaneous	G　Plazomicin Anti-infective	4　New Technology Group 4
4　Central Vein	3　Percutaneous	G　Sarilumab	5　New Technology Group 5
4　Central Vein	3　Percutaneous	G　REGN-COV2 Monoclonal Antibody	6　New Technology Group 6
4　Central Vein	3　Percutaneous	G　Engineered Chimeric Antigen Receptor T-cell Immunotherapy, Allogeneic	7　New Technology Group 7
4　Central Vein	3　Percutaneous	H　Synthetic Human Angiotensin II	4　New Technology Group 4
4　Central Vein	3　Percutaneous	H　Tocilizumab	5　New Technology Group 5
4　Central Vein	3　Percutaneous	H　Other New Technology Monoclonal Antibody	6　New Technology Group 6
4　Central Vein	3　Percutaneous	H　Axicabtagene Ciloleucel Immunotherapy J　Tisagenlecleucel Immunotherapy	7　New Technology Group 7
4　Central Vein	3　Percutaneous	K　Fosfomycin Anti-infective	5　New Technology Group 5
4　Central Vein	3　Percutaneous	K　Idecabtagene Vicleucel Immunotherapy　NT	7　New Technology Group 7
4　Central Vein	3　Percutaneous	L　CD24Fc Immunomodulator	6　New Technology Group 6
4　Central Vein	3　Percutaneous	L　Lifileucel Immunotherapy M　Brexucabtagene Autoleucel Immunotherapy　NT	7　New Technology Group 7
4　Central Vein	3　Percutaneous	N　Meropenem-vaborbactam Anti-infective	5　New Technology Group 5
4　Central Vein	3　Percutaneous	N　Lisocabtagene Maraleucel Immunotherapy	7　New Technology Group 7
4　Central Vein	3　Percutaneous	Q　Tagraxofusp-erzs Antineoplastic S　Iobenguane I-131 Antineoplastic U　Imipenem-cilastatin-relebactam Anti-infective　NT W　Caplacizumab	5　New Technology Group 5
9　Nose	7　Via Natural or Artificial Opening	M　Esketamine Hydrochloride	5　New Technology Group 5
D　Mouth and Pharynx	X　External	3　Maribavir Anti-infective	8　New Technology Group 8
D　Mouth and Pharynx	X　External	6　Lefamulin Anti-infective	6　New Technology Group 6
D　Mouth and Pharynx	X　External	8　Uridine Triacetate	2　New Technology Group 2
D　Mouth and Pharynx	X　External	F　Other New Technology Therapeutic Substance J　Apalutamide Antineoplastic L　Erdafitinib Antineoplastic	5　New Technology Group 5
D　Mouth and Pharynx	X　External	M　Baricitinib　NT	6　New Technology Group 6
D　Mouth and Pharynx	X　External	R　Venetoclax Antineoplastic	5　New Technology Group 5
D　Mouth and Pharynx	X　External	R　Fostamatinib	7　New Technology Group 7
D　Mouth and Pharynx	X　External	T　Ruxolitinib V　Gilteritinib Antineoplastic	5　New Technology Group 5
G　Upper GI	7　Via Natural or Artificial Opening	3　Maribavir Anti-infective	8　New Technology Group 8
G　Upper GI	7　Via Natural or Artificial Opening	M　Baricitinib　NT	6　New Technology Group 6
G　Upper GI	7　Via Natural or Artificial Opening	R　Fostamatinib	7　New Technology Group 7
G　Upper GI	8　Via Natural or Artificial Opening Endoscopic	8　Mineral-based Topical Hemostatic Agent	6　New Technology Group 6
H　Lower GI	7　Via Natural or Artificial Opening	3　Maribavir Anti-infective	8　New Technology Group 8
H　Lower GI	7　Via Natural or Artificial Opening	M　Baricitinib　NT	6　New Technology Group 6
H　Lower GI	7　Via Natural or Artificial Opening	R　Fostamatinib	7　New Technology Group 7
H　Lower GI	7　Via Natural or Artificial Opening	X　Broad Consortium Microbiota-based Live Biotherapeutic Suspension	8　New Technology Group 8
H　Lower GI	8　Via Natural or Artificial Opening Endoscopic	8　Mineral-based Topical HemostaticAgent	6　New Technology Group 6
Q　Cranial Cavity and Brain	3　Percutaneous	1　Eladocagene exuparvovec	6　New Technology Group 6
V　Bones	Ø　Open	P　Antibiotic-eluting Bone Void Filler	7　New Technology Group 7

Valid OR	XWØQ316	NT	XWØ43K7
DRG Non-OR	XWØ43G7	NT	XWØ43M7
DRG Non-OR	XWØ43[H,J]7	NT	XWØ43U5 in combination with dx code Y95 and one of the following: J14, J15.Ø, J15.1, J15.5, J15.6, J15.8, OR dx code
DRG Non-OR	XWØ43K7		J95.851 and one of the following: B96.1, B96.2Ø, B96.21, B96.22, B96.23, B96.29, B96.3, B96.5, or B96.89
DRG Non-OR	XWØ43[L,M]7	NT	XWØDXM6
DRG Non-OR	XWØ43N7	NT	XWØG7M6
		NT	XWØH7M6

* For all codes with NT icon see Appendix I for registered or trade name of substance

Non-OR Procedure　　DRG Non-OR Procedure　　Valid OR Procedure　　HAC Associated Procedure　　Combination Only　　New/Revised April　　New/Revised October

X   New Technology
W   Anatomical Regions
1   Transfusion   Definition: Putting in blood or blood products
                  Explanation: None

Body Part Character 4	Approach Character 5	Device/Substance/Technology Character 6	Qualifier Character 7
3 Peripheral Vein	**3** Percutaneous	**2** Plasma, Convalescent NT (Nonautologous)	**5** New Technology Group 5
3 Peripheral Vein	**3** Percutaneous	**B** Betibeglogene Autotemcel **C** Omidubicel	**8** New Technology Group 8
3 Peripheral Vein	**3** Percutaneous	**D** High-Dose Intravenous Immune Globulin **E** Hyperimmune Globulin	**7** New Technology Group 7
3 Peripheral Vein	**3** Percutaneous	**F** OTL-103 **G** OTL-200	**8** New Technology Group 8
4 Central Vein	**3** Percutaneous	**2** Plasma, Convalescent NT (Nonautologous)	**5** New Technology Group 5
4 Central Vein	**3** Percutaneous	**B** Betibeglogene Autotemcel **C** Omidubicel	**8** New Technology Group 8
4 Central Vein	**3** Percutaneous	**D** High-Dose Intravenous Immune Globulin **E** Hyperimmune Globulin	**7** New Technology Group 7
4 Central Vein	**3** Percutaneous	**F** OTL-103 **G** OTL-200	**8** New Technology Group 8

NT   XW13325
NT   XW14325

X   New Technology
W   Anatomical Regions
H   Insertion   Definition: Putting in a nonbiological appliance that monitors, assists, performs, or prevents a physiological function but does not physically
                  take the place of a body part
                  Explanation: None

Body Part Character 4	Approach Character 5	Device/Substance/Technology Character 6	Qualifier Character 7
D Mouth and Pharynx	**7** Via Natural or Artificial Opening	**Q** Neurostimulator Lead	**7** New Technology Group 7

X New Technology
X Physiological Systems
E Measurement Definition: Determining the level of a physiological or physical function at a point in time
Explanation: None

Body Part Character 4	Approach Character 5	Device/Substance/Technology Character 6	Qualifier Character 7
Ø Central Nervous	X External	Ø Intracranial Vascular Activity, Computer-aided Assessment	7 New Technology Group 7
Ø Central Nervous	X External	4 Brain Electrical Activity, Computer-aided Semiologic Analysis	8 New Technology Group 8
3 Arterial	X External	2 Pulmonary Artery Flow, Computer-aided Triage and Notification	7 New Technology Group 7
3 Arterial	X External	5 Coronary Artery Flow, Quantitative Flow Ratio Analysis	8 New Technology Group 8
		6 Coronary Artery Flow, Computer-aided Valve Modeling and Notification	
5 Circulatory	X External	3 Infection, Whole Blood Reverse Transcription and Quantitative Real-time Polymerase Chain Reaction	8 New Technology Group 8
5 Circulatory	X External	M Infection, Whole Blood Nucleic Acid-base Microbial Detection	5 New Technology Group 5
5 Circulatory	X External	N Infection, Positive Blood Culture Fluorescence Hybridization for Organism Identification, Concentration and Susceptibility	6 New Technology Group 6
5 Circulatory	X External	R Infection, Mechanical Initial Specimen Diversion Technique Using Active Negative Pressure	7 New Technology Group 7
		T Intracranial Arterial Flow, Whole Blood mRNA	
		V Infection, Serum/Plasma Nanoparticle Fluorescence SARS-CoV-2 Antibody Detection	
9 Nose	7 Via Natural or Artificial Opening	U Infection, Nasopharyngeal Fluid SARS-CoV-2 Polymerase Chain Reaction	7 New Technology Group 7
B Respiratory	X External	Q Infection, Lower Respiratory Fluid Nucleic Acid-base Microbial Detection	6 New Technology Group 6

X New Technology
Y Extracorporeal
Ø Introduction Definition: Putting in or on a therapeutic, diagnostic, nutritional, physiological, or prophylactic substance except blood or blood products
Explanation: None

Body Part Character 4	Approach Character 5	Device/Substance/Technology Character 6	Qualifier Character 7
V Vein Graft	X External	8 Endothelial Damage Inhibitor	3 New Technology Group 3
Y Extracorporeal	X External	2 Taurolidine Anti-infective and Heparin Anticoagulant	8 New Technology Group 8
Y Extracorporeal	X External	3 Nafamostat Anticoagulant	7 New Technology Group 7

Non-OR Procedure   DRG Non-OR Procedure   Valid OR Procedure   HAC Associated Procedure   Combination Only   New/Revised April   New/Revised October

826

ICD-10-PCS 2023

Appendixes

Appendix A: Components of the Medical and Surgical Approach Definitions

ICD-10-PCS Value	Definition	Access Location	Method	Type of Instrumentation	Example
Open (Ø)	Cutting through the skin or mucous membrane and any other body layers necessary to expose the site of the procedure	Skin or mucous membrane, any other body layers	Cutting	None	Abdominal hysterectomy
Percutaneous (3)	Entry, by puncture or minor incision, of instrumentation through the skin or mucous membrane and any other body layers necessary to reach the site of the procedure	Skin or mucous membrane, any other body layers	Puncture or minor incision	Without visualization	Needle biopsy of liver, Liposuction
Percutaneous endoscopic (4)	Entry, by puncture or minor incision, of instrumentation through the skin or mucous membrane and any other body layers necessary to reach and visualize the site of the procedure	Skin or mucous membrane, any other body layers	Puncture or minor incision	With visualization	Arthroscopy, Laparoscopic cholecystectomy
Via natural or artificial opening (7)	Entry of instrumentation through a natural or artificial external opening to reach the site of the procedure	Natural or artificial external opening	Direct entry	Without visualization	Endotracheal tube insertion, Foley catheter placement
Via natural or artificial opening endoscopic (8)	Entry of instrumentation through a natural or artificial external opening to reach and visualize the site of the procedure	Natural or artificial external opening	Direct entry	With visualization	Sigmoidoscopy, EGD, ERCP
Via natural or artificial opening with percutaneous endoscopic assistance (F)	Entry of instrumentation through a natural or artificial external opening and entry, by puncture or minor incision, of instrumentation through the skin or mucous membrane and any other body layers necessary to aid in the performance of the procedure	Skin or mucous membrane, any other body layers	Direct entry with puncture or minor incision for instrumentation only	With visualization	Laparoscopic-assisted vaginal hysterectomy
External (X)	Procedures performed directly on the skin or mucous membrane and procedures performed indirectly by the application of external force through the skin or mucous membrane	Skin or mucous membrane	Direct or indirect application	None	Closed fracture reduction, Resection of tonsils

The approach comprises three components: the access location, method, and type of instrumentation.

Access location: For procedures performed on an internal body part, the access location specifies the external site through which the site of the procedure is reached. There are two general types of access locations: skin or mucous membranes, and external orifices. Every approach value except external includes one of these two access locations. The skin or mucous membrane can be cut or punctured to reach the procedure site. All open and percutaneous approach values use this access location. The site of a procedure can also be reached through an external opening. External openings can be natural (e.g., mouth) or artificial (e.g., colostomy stoma).

Method: For procedures performed on an internal body part, the method specifies how the external access location is entered. An open method specifies cutting through the skin or mucous membrane and any other intervening body layers necessary to expose the site of the procedure. An instrumentation method specifies the entry of instrumentation through the access location to the internal procedure site. Instrumentation can be introduced by puncture or minor incision, or through an external opening. The puncture or minor incision does not constitute an open approach because it does not expose the site of the procedure. An approach can define multiple methods. For example, Via Natural or Artificial Opening with Percutaneous Endoscopic Assistance includes both the initial entry of instrumentation to reach the site of the procedure, and the placement of additional percutaneous instrumentation into the body part to visualize and assist in the performance of the procedure.

Type of instrumentation: For procedures performed on an internal body part, instrumentation means that specialized equipment is used to perform the procedure. Instrumentation is used in all internal approaches other than the basic open approach. Instrumentation may or may not include the capacity to visualize the procedure site. For example, the instrumentation used to perform a sigmoidoscopy permits the internal site of the procedure to be visualized, while the instrumentation used to perform a needle biopsy of the liver does not. The term "endoscopic" as used in approach values refers to instrumentation that permits a site to be visualized.

Procedures performed directly on the skin or mucous membrane are identified by the external approach (e.g., skin excision). Procedures performed indirectly by the application of external force are also identified by the external approach (e.g., closed reduction of fracture).

Appendices

Appendix A: Components of the Medical and Surgical Approach Definitions

Open (Ø)

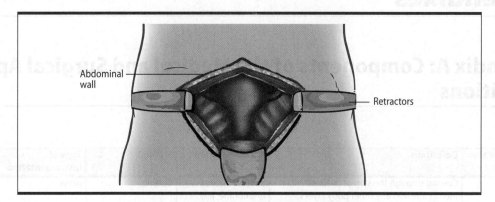

Percutaneous (3)

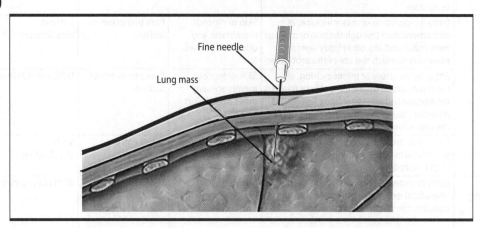

Percutaneous Endoscopic (4)

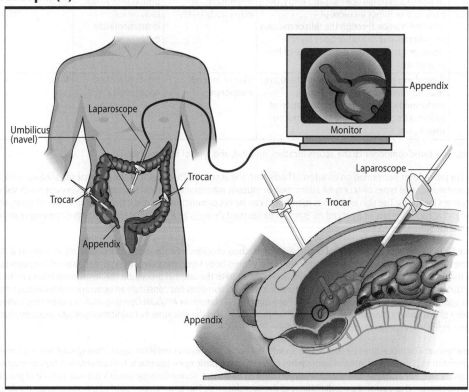

Via Natural or Artificial Opening (7)

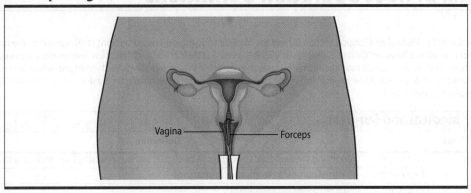

Via Natural or Artificial Opening, Endoscopic (8)

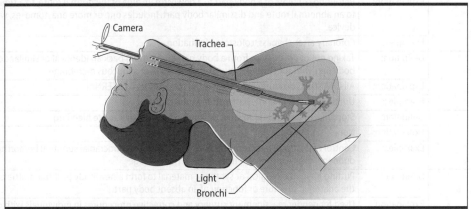

Via Natural or Artificial Opening with Percutaneous Endoscopic Assistance (F)

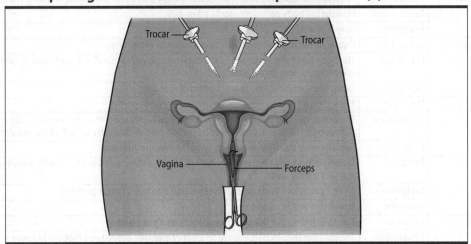

External (X)

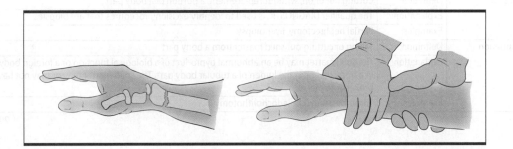

Appendix B: Root Operation Definitions

The character 3 value in the Medical and Surgical section (Ø) and the Medical and Surgical-related sections (1-9) represents the root operation. This resource provides each root operation (character 3) value, found in sections Ø-9, as well as their associated definition, explanation, and examples, where applicable. The Ancillary sections (B-H) do not include root operations; instead, the character 3 value represents the type of procedure performed with additional detail provided by the character 4 or 5 value, when applicable. For the character 3, character 4, and character 5 values used in the Ancillary sections of B-H, along with their definitions, see appendix J.

Ø	Medical and Surgical		
ICD-1Ø-PCS Value			**Definition**
Ø	Alteration	Definition:	Modifying the anatomic structure of a body part without affecting the function of the body part
		Explanation:	Principal purpose is to improve appearance
		Examples:	Face lift, breast augmentation
1	Bypass	Definition:	Altering the route of passage of the contents of a tubular body part
		Explanation:	Rerouting contents of a body part to a downstream area of the normal route, to a similar route and body part, or to an abnormal route and dissimilar body part. Includes one or more anastomoses, with or without the use of a device.
		Examples:	Coronary artery bypass, colostomy formation
2	Change	Definition:	Taking out or off a device from a body part and putting back an identical or similar device in or on the same body part without cutting or puncturing the skin or a mucous membrane
		Explanation:	All CHANGE procedures are coded using the approach EXTERNAL
		Examples:	Urinary catheter change, gastrostomy tube change
3	Control	Definition:	Stopping, or attempting to stop, postprocedural or other acute bleeding
		Explanation:	None
		Examples:	Control of post-prostatectomy hemorrhage, control of intracranial subdural hemorrhage, control of bleeding duodenal ulcer, control of retroperitoneal hemorrhage
4	Creation	Definition:	Putting in or on biological or synthetic material to form a new body part that to the extent possible replicates the anatomic structure or function of an absent body part
		Explanation:	Used for gender reassignment surgery and corrective procedures in individuals with congenital anomalies
		Examples:	Creation of vagina in a male, creation of right and left atrioventricular valve from common atrioventricular valve
5	Destruction	Definition:	Physical eradication of all or a portion of a body part by the direct use of energy, force, or a destructive agent
		Explanation:	None of the body part is physically taken out
		Examples:	Fulguration of rectal polyp, cautery of skin lesion
6	Detachment	Definition:	Cutting off all or a portion of the upper or lower extremities
		Explanation:	The body part value is the site of the detachment, with a qualifier if applicable to further specify the level where the extremity was detached
		Examples:	Below knee amputation, disarticulation of shoulder
7	Dilation	Definition:	Expanding an orifice or the lumen of a tubular body part
		Explanation:	The orifice can be a natural orifice or an artificially created orifice. Accomplished by stretching a tubular body part using intraluminal pressure or by cutting part of the orifice or wall of the tubular body part.
		Examples:	Percutaneous transluminal angioplasty, internal urethrotomy
8	Division	Definition:	Cutting into a body part, without draining fluids and/or gases from the body part, in order to separate or transect a body part
		Explanation:	All or a portion of the body part is separated into two or more portions
		Examples:	Spinal cordotomy, osteotomy
9	Drainage	Definition:	Taking or letting out fluids and/or gases from a body part
		Explanation:	The qualifier DIAGNOSTIC is used to identify drainage procedures that are biopsies
		Examples:	Thoracentesis, incision and drainage
B	Excision	Definition:	Cutting out or off, without replacement, a portion of a body part
		Explanation:	The qualifier DIAGNOSTIC is used to identify excision procedures that are biopsies
		Examples:	Partial nephrectomy, liver biopsy
C	Extirpation	Definition:	Taking or cutting out solid matter from a body part
		Explanation:	The solid matter may be an abnormal byproduct of a biological function or a foreign body; it may be imbedded in a body part or in the lumen of a tubular body part. The solid matter may or may not have been previously broken into pieces.
		Examples:	Thrombectomy, choledocholithotomy

Continued on next page

Ø	**Medical and Surgical**			*Continued from previous page*
	ICD-1Ø-PCS Value			**Definition**
D	Extraction	Definition:		Pulling or stripping out or off all or a portion of a body part by the use of force
		Explanation:		The qualifier DIAGNOSTIC is used to identify extractions that are biopsies
		Examples:		Dilation and curettage, vein stripping
F	Fragmentation	Definition:		Breaking solid matter in a body part into pieces
		Explanation:		Physical force (e.g., manual, ultrasonic) applied directly or indirectly is used to break the solid matter into pieces. The solid matter may be an abnormal byproduct of a biological function or a foreign body. The pieces of solid matter are not taken out.
		Examples:		Extracorporeal shockwave lithotripsy, transurethral lithotripsy
G	Fusion	Definition:		Joining together portions of an articular body part rendering the articular body part immobile
		Explanation:		The body part is joined together by fixation device, bone graft, or other means
		Examples:		Spinal fusion, ankle arthrodesis
H	Insertion	Definition:		Putting in a nonbiological appliance that monitors, assists, performs, or prevents a physiological function but does not physically take the place of a body part
		Explanation:		None
		Examples:		Insertion of radioactive implant, insertion of central venous catheter
J	Inspection	Definition:		Visually and/or manually exploring a body part
		Explanation:		Visual exploration may be performed with or without optical instrumentation. Manual exploration may be performed directly or through intervening body layers.
		Examples:		Diagnostic arthroscopy, exploratory laparotomy
K	Map	Definition:		Locating the route of passage of electrical impulses and/or locating functional areas in a body part
		Explanation:		Applicable only to the cardiac conduction mechanism and the central nervous system
		Examples:		Cardiac mapping, cortical mapping
L	Occlusion	Definition:		Completely closing an orifice or lumen of a tubular body part
		Explanation:		The orifice can be a natural orifice or an artificially created orifice
		Examples:		Fallopian tube ligation, ligation of inferior vena cava
M	Reattachment	Definition:		Putting back in or on all or a portion of a separated body part to its normal location or other suitable location
		Explanation:		Vascular circulation and nervous pathways may or may not be reestablished
		Examples:		Reattachment of hand, reattachment of avulsed kidney
N	Release	Definition:		Freeing a body part from an abnormal physical constraint by cutting or by use of force
		Explanation:		Some of the restraining tissue may be taken out but none of the body part is taken out
		Examples:		Adhesiolysis, carpal tunnel release
P	Removal	Definition:		Taking out or off a device from a body part
		Explanation:		If a device is taken out and a similar device put in without cutting or puncturing the skin or mucous membrane, the procedure is coded to the root operation CHANGE. Otherwise, the procedure for taking out a device is coded to the root operation REMOVAL.
		Examples:		Drainage tube removal, cardiac pacemaker removal
Q	Repair	Definition:		Restoring, to the extent possible, a body part to its normal anatomic structure and function
		Explanation:		Used only when the method to accomplish the repair is not one of the other root operations
		Examples:		Colostomy takedown, suture of laceration
R	Replacement	Definition:		Putting in or on biological or synthetic material that physically takes the place and/or function of all or a portion of a body part
		Explanation:		The body part may have been taken out or replaced, or may be taken out, physically eradicated, or rendered nonfunctional during the REPLACEMENT procedure. A REMOVAL procedure is coded for taking out the device used in a previous replacement procedure.
		Examples:		Total hip replacement, bone graft, free skin graft
S	Reposition	Definition:		Moving to its normal location, or other suitable location, all or a portion of a body part
		Explanation:		The body part is moved to a new location from an abnormal location, or from a normal location where it is not functioning correctly. The body part may or may not be cut out or off to be moved to the new location.
		Examples:		Reposition of undescended testicle, fracture reduction
T	Resection	Definition:		Cutting out or off, without replacement, all of a body part
		Explanation:		None
		Examples:		Total nephrectomy, total lobectomy of lung
V	Restriction	Definition:		Partially closing an orifice or the lumen of a tubular body part
		Explanation:		The orifice can be a natural orifice or an artificially created orifice
		Examples:		Esophagogastric fundoplication, cervical cerclage

Continued on next page

Ø   Medical and Surgical

Continued from previous page

ICD-10-PCS Value			Definition
W	Revision	Definition:	Correcting, to the extent possible, a portion of a malfunctioning device or the position of a displaced device
		Explanation:	Revision can include correcting a malfunctioning or displaced device by taking out or putting in components of the device such as a screw or pin
		Examples:	Adjustment of position of pacemaker lead, recementing of hip prosthesis
U	Supplement	Definition:	Putting in or on biological or synthetic material that physically reinforces and/or augments the function of a portion of a body part
		Explanation:	The biological material is non-living, or is living and from the same individual. The body part may have been previously replaced, and the SUPPLEMENT procedure is performed to physically reinforce and/or augment the function of the replaced body part.
		Examples:	Herniorrhaphy using mesh, mitral valve ring annuloplasty, put a new acetabular liner in a previous hip replacement
X	Transfer	Definition:	Moving, without taking out, all or a portion of a body part to another location to take over the function of all or a portion of a body part
		Explanation:	The body part transferred remains connected to its vascular and nervous supply
		Examples:	Tendon transfer, skin pedicle flap transfer
Y	Transplantation	Definition:	Putting in or on all or a portion of a living body part taken from another individual or animal to physically take the place and/or function of all or a portion of a similar body part
		Explanation:	The native body part may or may not be taken out, and the transplanted body part may take over all or a portion of its function
		Examples:	Kidney transplant, heart transplant

Root Operation Definitions for Other Sections

1   Obstetrics

ICD-10-PCS Value			Definition
2	Change	Definition:	Taking out or off a device from a body part and putting back an identical or similar device in or on the same body part without cutting or puncturing the skin or a mucous membrane
		Explanation:	None
		Example:	Replacement of fetal scalp electrode
9	Drainage	Definition:	Taking or letting out fluids and/or gases from a body part
		Explanation:	None
		Example:	Biopsy of amniotic fluid
A	Abortion	Definition:	Artificially terminating a pregnancy
		Explanation:	None
		Example:	Transvaginal abortion using vacuum aspiration technique
D	Extraction	Definition:	Pulling or stripping out or off all or a portion of a body part by the use of force
		Explanation:	None
		Example:	Low-transverse C-section
E	Delivery	Definition:	Assisting the passage of the products of conception from the genital canal
		Explanation:	None
		Example:	Manually-assisted delivery
H	Insertion	Definition:	Putting in a nonbiological appliance that monitors, assists, performs, or prevents a physiological function but does not physically take the place of a body part
		Explanation:	None
		Example:	Placement of fetal scalp electrode
J	Inspection	Definition:	Visually and/or manually exploring a body part
		Explanation:	Visual exploration may be performed with or without optical instrumentation. Manual exploration may be performed directly or through intervening body layers.
		Example:	Bimanual pregnancy exam
P	Removal	Definition:	Taking out or off a device from a body part, region or orifice
		Explanation:	If a device is taken out and a similar device put in without cutting or puncturing the skin or mucous membrane, the procedure is coded to the root operation CHANGE. Otherwise, the procedure for taking out a device is coded to the root operation REMOVAL.
		Example:	Removal of fetal monitoring electrode

Continued on next page

1   Obstetrics

Continued from previous page

ICD-10-PCS Value			Definition
Q	Repair	Definition:	Restoring, to the extent possible, a body part to its normal anatomic structure and function
		Explanation:	Used only when the method to accomplish the repair is not one of the other root operations
		Example:	In utero repair of congenital diaphragmatic hernia
S	Reposition	Definition:	Moving to its normal location, or other suitable location, all or a portion of a body part
		Explanation:	The body part is moved to a new location from an abnormal location, or from a normal location where it is not functioning correctly. The body part may or may not be cut out or off to be moved to the new location.
		Example:	External version of fetus
T	Resection	Definition:	Cutting out or off, without replacement, all of a body part
		Explanation:	None
		Example:	Total excision of tubal pregnancy
Y	Transplantation	Definition:	Putting in or on all or a portion of a living body part taken from another individual or animal to physically take the place and/or function of all or a portion of a similar body part
		Explanation:	The native body part may or may not be taken out, and the transplanted body part may take over all or a portion of its function
		Example:	In utero fetal kidney transplant

2   Placement

ICD-10-PCS Value			Definition
Ø	Change	Definition:	Taking out or off a device from a body part and putting back an identical or similar device in or on the same body part without cutting or puncturing the skin or a mucous membrane
		Example:	Change of vaginal packing
1	Compression	Definition:	Putting pressure on a body region
		Example:	Placement of pressure dressing on abdominal wall
2	Dressing	Definition:	Putting material on a body region for protection
		Example:	Application of sterile dressing to head wound
3	Immobilization	Definition:	Limiting or preventing motion of a body region
		Example:	Placement of splint on left finger
4	Packing	Definition:	Putting material in a body region or orifice
		Example:	Placement of nasal packing
5	Removal	Definition:	Taking out or off a device from a body part
		Example:	Removal of stereotactic head frame
6	Traction	Definition:	Exerting a pulling force on a body region in a distal direction
		Example:	Lumbar traction using motorized split-traction table

3   Administration

ICD-10-PCS Value			Definition
Ø	Introduction	Definition:	Putting in or on a therapeutic, diagnostic, nutritional, physiological, or prophylactic substance except blood or blood products
		Example:	Nerve block injection to median nerve
1	Irrigation	Definition:	Putting in or on a cleansing substance
		Example:	Flushing of eye
2	Transfusion	Definition:	Putting in blood or blood products
		Example:	Transfusion of cell saver red cells into central venous line

4   Measurement and Monitoring

ICD-10-PCS Value			Definition
Ø	Measurement	Definition:	Determining the level of a physiological or physical function at a point in time
		Example:	External electrocardiogram(EKG), single reading
1	Monitoring	Definition:	Determining the level of a physiological or physical function repetitively over a period of time
		Example:	Urinary pressure monitoring

5   Extracorporeal or Systemic Assistance and Performance

ICD-10-PCS Value			Definition
Ø	Assistance	Definition:	Taking over a portion of a physiological function by extracorporeal means
		Example:	Hyperbaric oxygenation of wound
1	Performance	Definition:	Completely taking over a physiological function by extracorporeal means
		Example:	Cardiopulmonary bypass in conjunction with CABG
2	Restoration	Definition:	Returning, or attempting to return, a physiological function to its original state by extracorporeal means
		Example:	Attempted cardiac defibrillation, unsuccessful

6   Extracorporeal or Systemic Therapies

ICD-10-PCS Value			Definition
Ø	Atmospheric Control	Definition:	Extracorporeal control of atmospheric pressure and composition
		Example:	Antigen-free air conditioning, series treatment
1	Decompression	Definition:	Extracorporeal elimination of undissolved gas from body fluids
		Example:	Hyperbaric decompression treatment, single
2	Electromagnetic Therapy	Definition:	Extracorporeal treatment by electromagnetic rays
		Example:	TMS (transcranial magnetic stimulation), series treatment
3	Hyperthermia	Definition:	Extracorporeal raising of body temperature
		Example:	None
4	Hypothermia	Definition:	Extracorporeal lowering of body temperature
		Example:	Whole body hypothermia treatment for temperature imbalances, series
5	Pheresis	Definition:	Extracorporeal separation of blood products
		Example:	Therapeutic leukopheresis, single treatment
6	Phototherapy	Definition:	Extracorporeal treatment by light rays
		Example:	Phototherapy of circulatory system, series treatment
7	Ultrasound Therapy	Definition:	Extracorporeal treatment by ultrasound
		Example:	Therapeutic ultrasound of peripheral vessels, single treatment
8	Ultraviolet Light Therapy	Definition:	Extracorporeal treatment by ultraviolet light
		Example:	Ultraviolet light phototherapy, series treatment
9	Shock Wave Therapy	Definition:	Extracorporeal treatment by shock waves
		Example:	Shockwave therapy of plantar fascia, single treatment
B	Perfusion	Definition:	Extracorporeal treatment by diffusion of therapeutic fluid
		Example:	Perfusion of donor liver while preparing transplant patient

7   Osteopathic

ICD-10-PCS Value			Definition
Ø	Treatment	Definition:	Manual treatment to eliminate or alleviate somatic dysfunction and related disorders
		Examples:	Fascial release of abdomen, osteopathic treatment

8   Other Procedures

ICD-10-PCS Value			Definition
Ø	Other Procedures	Definition:	Methodologies which attempt to remediate or cure a disorder or disease
		Examples:	Acupuncture, yoga therapy

9   Chiropractic

ICD-10-PCS Value			Definition
B	Manipulation	Definition:	Manual procedure that involves a directed thrust to move a joint past the physiological range of motion, without exceeding the anatomical limit
		Example:	Chiropractic treatment of cervical spine, short lever specific contact

Appendix C: Comparison of Medical and Surgical Root Operations

Note: The character associated with each operation appears in parentheses after its title.

Procedures That Take Out Some or All of a Body Part

Root Operation	Objective of Procedure	Site of Procedure	Example
Destruction (5)	Eradicating without taking out or replacement	Some/all of a body part	Fulguration of endometrium
Detachment (6)	Cutting out/off without replacement	Extremity only, any level	Amputation above elbow
Excision (B)	Cutting out/off without replacement	Some of a body part	Breast lumpectomy
Extraction (D)	Pulling out/off without replacement	Some/all of a body part	Suction D&C
Resection (T)	Cutting out/off without replacement	All of a body part	Total mastectomy

Procedures That Put In/Put Back or Move Some/All of a Body Part

Root Operation	Objective of Procedure	Site of Procedure	Example
Reattachment (M)	Putting back a detached body part	Some/all of a body part	Reattach finger
Reposition (S)	Moving a body part to normal or other suitable location	Some/all of a body part	Move undescended testicle
Transfer (X)	Moving a body part to function for a similar body part	Some/all of a body part	Skin pedicle transfer flap
Transplantation (Y)	Putting in a living body part from a person/animal	Some/all of a body part	Kidney transplant

Procedures That Take Out or Eliminate Solid Matter, Fluids, or Gases From a Body Part

Root Operation	Objective of Procedure	Site of Procedure	Example
Drainage (9)	Taking or letting out	Fluids and/or gases from a body part	Incision and drainage
Extirpation (C)	Taking or cutting out	Solid matter in a body part	Thrombectomy
Fragmentation (F)	Breaking into pieces	Solid matter within a body part	Lithotripsy

Procedures That Involve Only Examination of Body Parts and Regions

Root Operation	Objective of Procedure	Site of Procedure	Example
Inspection (J)	Visual/manual exploration	Some/all of a body part	Diagnostic cystoscopy Exploratory laparoscopy
Map (K)	Locating electrical impulse route/functional areas	Brain/cardiac conduction mechanism	Cardiac mapping

Procedures That Alter the Diameter/Route of a Tubular Body Part

Root Operation	Objective of Procedure	Site of Procedure	Example
Bypass (1)	Altering route of passage of contents	Tubular body part	Coronary artery bypass graft (CABG)
Dilation (7)	Expanding natural or artificially created orifice/lumen	Tubular body part	Percutaneous transluminal coronary angioplasty (PTCA)
Occlusion (L)	Completely closing natural or artificially created orifice/lumen	Tubular body part	Fallopian tube ligation
Restriction (V)	Partially closing natural or artificially created orifice/lumen	Tubular body part	Gastroesophageal fundoplication

Procedures That Always Involve Devices

Root Operation	Objective of Procedure	Site of Procedure	Example
Change (2) **DVC**	Exchanging device w/out cutting/puncturing	In/on a body part	Gastrostomy tube change
Insertion (H) **DVC**	Putting in nonbiological device	In/on a body part	Central line insertion
Removal (P) **DVC**	Taking out device	In/on a body part	Central line removal
Replacement (R) **DVC**	Putting in device that replaces a body part	Some/all of a body part	Total hip replacement
Revision (W) **DVC**	Correcting a malfunctioning/displaced device	In/on a body part	Revision of pacemaker
Supplement (U) **DVC**	Putting in device that reinforces or augments a body part	In/on a body part	Abdominal wall herniorrhaphy using mesh

DVC = Device involved in root operation

Procedures Involving Cutting or Separation Only

Root Operation	Objective of Procedure	Site of Procedure	Example
Division (8)	Cutting into/separating	A body part	Neurotomy
Release (N)	Freeing a body part from constraint	Around a body part	Adhesiolysis

Procedures That Define Other Repairs

Root Operation	Objective of Procedure	Site of Procedure	Example
Control (3)	Stopping/attempting to stop postprocedural or other acute bleeding	Anatomical region or nasal mucosa/soft tissue	Post-prostatectomy bleeding control, control subdural hemorrhage, bleeding ulcer, retroperitoneal hemorrhage
Repair (Q)	Restoring body part to its normal structure/function	Some/all of a body part	Suture laceration

Procedures That Define Other Objectives

Root Operation	Objective of Procedure	Site of Procedure	Example
Alteration (Ø)	Modifying body part for cosmetic purposes without affecting function	Some/all of a body part	Face lift
Creation (4)	Using biological or synthetic material to form a new body part that replicates the anatomic structure or function of a missing body part	Perineum, valve	Sex change/artificial vagina/penis, atrioventricular valve creation
Fusion (G)	Unification or immobilization	Joint or articular body part	Spinal fusion

Appendix D: Body Part Key

Term	ICD-10-PCS Value
Abdominal aortic plexus	Abdominal Sympathetic Nerve
Abdominal cavity	Peritoneal Cavity
Abdominal esophagus	Esophagus, Lower
Abductor hallucis muscle	Foot Muscle, Right
	Foot Muscle, Left
Accessory cephalic vein	Cephalic Vein, Right
	Cephalic Vein, Left
Accessory obturator nerve	Lumbar Plexus
Accessory phrenic nerve	Phrenic nerve
Accessory spleen	Spleen
Acetabulofemoral joint	Hip Joint, Right
	Hip Joint, Left
Achilles tendon	Lower Leg Tendon, Right
	Lower Leg Tendon, Left
Acromioclavicular ligament	Shoulder Bursa and Ligament, Right
	Shoulder Bursa and Ligament, Left
Acromion (process)	Scapula, Right
	Scapula, Left
Adductor brevis muscle	Upper Leg Muscle, Right
	Upper Leg Muscle, Left
Adductor hallucis muscle	Foot Muscle, Right
	Foot Muscle, Left
Adductor longus muscle	Upper Leg Muscle, Right
	Upper Leg Muscle, Left
Adductor magnus muscle	Upper Leg Muscle, Right
	Upper Leg Muscle, Left
Adenohypophysis	Pituitary Gland
Alar ligament of axis	Head and Neck Bursa and Ligament
Alveolar process of mandible	Mandible, Right
	Mandible, Left
Alveolar process of maxilla	Maxilla
Anal orifice	Anus
Anatomical snuffbox	Lower Arm and Wrist Muscle, Right
	Lower Arm and Wrist Muscle, Left
Angular artery	Face Artery
Angular vein	Face Vein, Right
	Face Vein, Left
Annular ligament	Elbow Bursa and Ligament, Right
	Elbow Bursa and Ligament, Left
Anorectal junction	Rectum
Ansa cervicalis	Cervical Plexus
Antebrachial fascia	Subcutaneous Tissue and Fascia, Right Lower Arm
	Subcutaneous Tissue and Fascia, Left Lower Arm
Anterior (pectoral) lymph node	Lymphatic, Right Axillary
	Lymphatic, Left Axillary
Anterior cerebral artery	Intracranial Artery
Anterior cerebral vein	Intracranial Vein
Anterior choroidal artery	Intracranial Artery
Anterior circumflex humeral artery	Axillary Artery, Right
	Axillary Artery, Left
Anterior communicating artery	Intracranial Artery

Term	ICD-10-PCS Value
Anterior cruciate ligament (ACL)	Knee Bursa and Ligament, Right
	Knee Bursa and Ligament, Left
Anterior crural nerve	Femoral Nerve
Anterior facial vein	Face Vein, Right
	Face Vein, Left
Anterior intercostal artery	Internal Mammary Artery, Right
	Internal Mammary Artery, Left
Anterior interosseous nerve	Median Nerve
Anterior lateral malleolar artery	Anterior Tibial Artery, Right
	Anterior Tibial Artery, Left
Anterior lingual gland	Minor Salivary Gland
Anterior medial malleolar artery	Anterior Tibial Artery, Right
	Anterior Tibial Artery, Left
Anterior spinal artery	Vertebral Artery, Right
	Vertebral Artery, Left
Anterior tibial recurrent artery	Anterior Tibial Artery, Right
	Anterior Tibial Artery, Left
Anterior ulnar recurrent artery	Ulnar Artery, Right
	Ulnar Artery, Left
Anterior vagal trunk	Vagus Nerve
Anterior vertebral muscle	Neck Muscle, Right
	Neck Muscle, Left
Antihelix	External Ear, Right
	External Ear, Left
	External Ear, Bilateral
Antitragus	External Ear, Right
	External Ear, Left
	External Ear, Bilateral
Antrum of Highmore	Maxillary Sinus, Right
	Maxillary Sinus, Left
Aortic annulus	Aortic Valve
Aortic arch	Thoracic Aorta, Ascending/Arch
Aortic intercostal artery	Upper Artery
Apical (subclavicular) lymph node	Lymphatic, Right Axillary
	Lymphatic, Left Axillary
Apneustic center	Pons
Aqueduct of Sylvius	Cerebral Ventricle
Aqueous humour	Anterior Chamber, Right
	Anterior Chamber, Left
Arachnoid mater, intracranial	Cerebral Meninges
Arachnoid mater, spinal	Spinal Meninges
Arcuate artery	Foot Artery, Right
	Foot Artery, Left
Areola	Nipple, Right
	Nipple, Left
Arterial canal (duct)	Pulmonary Artery, Left
Aryepiglottic fold	Larynx
Arytenoid cartilage	Larynx
Arytenoid muscle	Neck Muscle, Right
	Neck Muscle, Left
Ascending aorta	Thoracic Aorta, Ascending/Arch
Ascending palatine artery	Face Artery
Ascending pharyngeal artery	External Carotid Artery, Right
	External Carotid Artery, Left

Term	ICD-10-PCS Value
Atlantoaxial joint	Cervical Vertebral Joint
Atrioventricular node	Conduction Mechanism
Atrium dextrum cordis	Atrium, Right
Atrium pulmonale	Atrium, Left
Auditory tube	Eustachian Tube, Right
	Eustachian Tube, Left
Auerbach's (myenteric) plexus	Abdominal Sympathetic Nerve
Auricle	External Ear, Right
	External Ear, Left
	External Ear, Bilateral
Auricularis muscle	Head Muscle
Axillary fascia	Subcutaneous Tissue and Fascia, Right Upper Arm
	Subcutaneous Tissue and Fascia, Left Upper Arm
Axillary nerve	Brachial Plexus
Bartholin's (greater vestibular) gland	Vestibular Gland
Basal (internal) cerebral vein	Intracranial Vein
Basal nuclei	Basal Ganglia
Base of tongue	Pharynx
Basilar artery	Intracranial Artery
Basis pontis	Pons
Biceps brachii muscle	Upper Arm Muscle, Right
	Upper Arm Muscle, Left
Biceps femoris muscle	Upper Leg Muscle, Right
	Upper Leg Muscle, Left
Bicipital aponeurosis	Subcutaneous Tissue and Fascia, Right Lower Arm
	Subcutaneous Tissue and Fascia, Left Lower Arm
Bicuspid valve	Mitral Valve
Body of femur	Femoral Shaft, Right
	Femoral Shaft, Left
Body of fibula	Fibula, Right
	Fibula, Left
Bony labyrinth	Inner Ear, Right
	Inner Ear, Left
Bony orbit	Orbit, Right
	Orbit, Left
Bony vestibule	Inner Ear, Right
	Inner Ear, Left
Botallo's duct	Pulmonary Artery, Left
Brachial (lateral) lymph node	Lymphatic, Right Axillary
	Lymphatic, Left Axillary
Brachialis muscle	Upper Arm Muscle, Right
	Upper Arm Muscle, Left
Brachiocephalic artery	Innominate Artery
Brachiocephalic trunk	Innominate Artery
Brachiocephalic vein	Innominate Vein, Right
	Innominate Vein, Left
Brachioradialis muscle	Lower Arm and Wrist Muscle, Right
	Lower Arm and Wrist Muscle, Left
Breast procedures, skin only	Skin, Chest
Broad ligament	Uterine Supporting Structure
Bronchial artery	Upper Artery
Bronchus intermedius	Main Bronchus, Right

Term	ICD-10-PCS Value
Buccal gland	Buccal Mucosa
Buccinator lymph node	Lymphatic, Head
Buccinator muscle	Facial Muscle
Bulbospongiosus muscle	Perineum Muscle
Bulbourethral (Cowper's) gland	Urethra
Bundle of His	Conduction Mechanism
Bundle of Kent	Conduction Mechanism
Calcaneocuboid joint	Tarsal Joint, Right
	Tarsal Joint, Left
Calcaneocuboid ligament	Foot Bursa and Ligament, Right
	Foot Bursa and Ligament, Left
Calcaneofibular ligament	Ankle Bursa and Ligament, Right
	Ankle Bursa and Ligament, Left
Calcaneus	Tarsal, Right
	Tarsal, Left
Capitate bone	Carpal, Right
	Carpal, Left
Cardia	Esophagogastric Junction
Cardiac plexus	Thoracic Sympathetic Nerve
Cardioesophageal junction	Esophagogastric Junction
Caroticotympanic artery	Internal Carotid Artery, Right
	Internal Carotid Artery, Left
Carotid glomus	Carotid Body, Right
	Carotid Body, Left
	Carotid Bodies, Bilateral
Carotid sinus	Internal Carotid Artery, Right
	Internal Carotid Artery, Left
Carotid sinus nerve	Glossopharyngeal Nerve
Carpometacarpal ligament	Hand Bursa and Ligament, Right
	Hand Bursa and Ligament, Left
Cauda equina	Lumbar Spinal Cord
Cavernous plexus	Head and Neck Sympathetic Nerve
Cavoatrial junction	Superior Vena Cava
Celiac ganglion	Abdominal Sympathetic Nerve
Celiac (solar) plexus	Abdominal Sympathetic Nerve
Celiac lymph node	Lymphatic, Aortic
Celiac trunk	Celiac Artery
Central axillary lymph node	Lymphatic, Right Axillary
	Lymphatic, Left Axillary
Cerebral aqueduct (Sylvius)	Cerebral Ventricle
Cerebrum	Brain
Cervical esophagus	Esophagus, Upper
Cervical facet joint	Cervical Vertebral Joint
	Cervical Vertebral Joints, 2 or more
Cervical ganglion	Head and Neck Sympathetic Nerve
Cervical interspinous ligament	Head and Neck Bursa and Ligament
Cervical intertransverse ligament	Head and Neck Bursa and Ligament
Cervical ligamentum flavum	Head and Neck Bursa and Ligament
Cervical lymph node	Lymphatic, Right Neck
	Lymphatic, Left Neck
Cervicothoracic facet joint	Cervicothoracic Vertebral Joint
Choana	Nasopharynx
Chondroglossus muscle	Tongue, Palate, Pharynx Muscle
Chorda tympani	Facial Nerve
Choroid plexus	Cerebral Ventricle

Term	ICD-10-PCS Value
Ciliary body	Eye, Right
	Eye, Left
Ciliary ganglion	Head and Neck Sympathetic Nerve
Circle of Willis	Intracranial Artery
Circumflex iliac artery	Femoral Artery, Right
	Femoral Artery, Left
Claustrum	Basal Ganglia
Coccygeal body	Coccygeal Glomus
Coccygeus muscle	Trunk Muscle, Right
	Trunk Muscle, Left
Cochlea	Inner Ear, Right
	Inner Ear, Left
Cochlear nerve	Acoustic Nerve
Columella	Nasal Mucosa and Soft Tissue
Common digital vein	Foot Vein, Right
	Foot Vein, Left
Common facial vein	Face Vein, Right
	Face Vein, Left
Common fibular nerve	Peroneal Nerve
Common hepatic artery	Hepatic Artery
Common iliac (subaortic) lymph node	Lymphatic, Pelvis
Common interosseous artery	Ulnar Artery, Right
	Ulnar Artery, Left
Common peroneal nerve	Peroneal Nerve
Condyloid process	Mandible, Right
	Mandible, Left
Conus arteriosus	Ventricle, Right
Conus medullaris	Lumbar Spinal Cord
Coracoacromial ligament	Shoulder Bursa and Ligament, Right
	Shoulder Bursa and Ligament, Left
Coracobrachialis muscle	Upper Arm Muscle, Right
	Upper Arm Muscle, Left
Coracoclavicular ligament	Shoulder Bursa and Ligament, Right
	Shoulder Bursa and Ligament, Left
Coracohumeral ligament	Shoulder Bursa and Ligament, Right
	Shoulder Bursa and Ligament, Left
Coracoid process	Scapula, Right
	Scapula, Left
Corniculate cartilage	Larynx
Corpus callosum	Brain
Corpus cavernosum	Penis
Corpus spongiosum	Penis
Corpus striatum	Basal Ganglia
Corrugator supercilii muscle	Facial Muscle
Costocervical trunk	Subclavian Artery, Right
	Subclavian Artery, Left
Costoclavicular ligament	Shoulder Bursa and Ligament, Right
	Shoulder Bursa and Ligament, Left
Costotransverse joint	Thoracic Vertebral Joint
Costotransverse ligament	Rib(s) Bursa and Ligament
Costovertebral joint	Thoracic Vertebral Joint
Costoxiphoid ligament	Sternum Bursa and Ligament
Cowper's (bulbourethral) gland	Urethra
Cremaster muscle	Perineum Muscle
Cribriform plate	Ethmoid Bone, Right
	Ethmoid Bone, Left

Term	ICD-10-PCS Value
Cricoid cartilage	Trachea
Cricothyroid artery	Thyroid Artery, Right
	Thyroid Artery, Left
Cricothyroid muscle	Neck Muscle, Right
	Neck Muscle, Left
Crural fascia	Subcutaneous Tissue and Fascia, Right Upper Leg
	Subcutaneous Tissue and Fascia, Left Upper Leg
Cubital lymph node	Lymphatic, Right Upper Extremity
	Lymphatic, Left Upper Extremity
Cubital nerve	Ulnar Nerve
Cuboid bone	Tarsal, Right
	Tarsal, Left
Cuboideonavicular joint	Tarsal Joint, Right
	Tarsal Joint, Left
Culmen	Cerebellum
Cuneiform cartilage	Larynx
Cuneonavicular joint	Tarsal Joint, Right
	Tarsal Joint, Left
Cuneonavicular ligament	Foot Bursa and Ligament, Right
	Foot Bursa and Ligament, Left
Cutaneous (transverse) cervical nerve	Cervical Plexus
Deep cervical fascia	Subcutaneous Tissue and Fascia, Right Neck
	Subcutaneous Tissue and Fascia, Left Neck
Deep cervical vein	Vertebral Vein, Right
	Vertebral Vein, Left
Deep circumflex iliac artery	External Iliac Artery, Right
	External Iliac Artery, Left
Deep facial vein	Face Vein, Right
	Face Vein, Left
Deep femoral artery	Femoral Artery, Right
	Femoral Artery, Left
Deep femoral (profunda femoris) vein	Femoral Vein, Right
	Femoral Vein, Left
Deep palmar arch	Hand Artery, Right
	Hand Artery, Left
Deep transverse perineal muscle	Perineum Muscle
Deferential artery	Internal Iliac Artery, Right
	Internal Iliac Artery, Left
Deltoid fascia	Subcutaneous Tissue and Fascia, Right Upper Arm
	Subcutaneous Tissue and Fascia, Left Upper Arm
Deltoid ligament	Ankle Bursa and Ligament, Right
	Ankle Bursa and Ligament, Left
Deltoid muscle	Shoulder Muscle, Right
	Shoulder Muscle, Left
Deltopectoral (infraclavicular) lymph node	Lymphatic, Right Upper Extremity
	Lymphatic, Left Upper Extremity
Dens	Cervical Vertebra
Denticulate (dentate) ligament	Spinal Meninges
Depressor anguli oris muscle	Facial Muscle
Depressor labii inferioris muscle	Facial Muscle

Term	ICD-10-PCS Value
Depressor septi nasi muscle	Facial Muscle
Depressor supercilii muscle	Facial Muscle
Dermis	Skin
Descending genicular artery	Femoral Artery, Right
	Femoral Artery, Left
Diaphragma sellae	Dura Mater
Distal humerus	Humeral Shaft, Right
	Humeral Shaft, Left
Distal humerus, involving joint	Elbow Joint, Right
	Elbow Joint, Left
Distal radioulnar joint	Wrist Joint, Right
	Wrist Joint, Left
Dorsal digital nerve	Radial Nerve
Dorsal metacarpal vein	Hand Vein, Right
	Hand Vein, Left
Dorsal metatarsal artery	Foot Artery, Right
	Foot Artery, Left
Dorsal metatarsal vein	Foot Vein, Right
	Foot Vein, Left
Dorsal root ganglion	Cervical Spinal Cord
	Lumbar Spinal Cord
	Spinal Cord
	Thoracic Spinal Cord
Dorsal scapular artery	Subclavian Artery, Right
	Subclavian Artery, Left
Dorsal scapular nerve	Brachial Plexus
Dorsal venous arch	Foot Vein, Right
	Foot Vein, Left
Dorsalis pedis artery	Anterior Tibial Artery, Right
	Anterior Tibial Artery, Left
Duct of Santorini	Pancreatic Duct, Accessory
Duct of Wirsung	Pancreatic Duct
Ductus deferens	Vas Deferens, Right
	Vas Deferens, Left
	Vas Deferens, Bilateral
	Vas Deferens
Duodenal ampulla	Ampulla of Vater
Duodenojejunal flexure	Jejunum
Dura mater, intracranial	Dura Mater
Dura mater, spinal	Spinal Meninges
Dural venous sinus	Intracranial Vein
Earlobe	External Ear, Right
	External Ear, Left
	External Ear, Bilateral
Eighth cranial nerve	Acoustic Nerve
Ejaculatory duct	Vas Deferens, Right
	Vas Deferens, Left
	Vas Deferens, Bilateral
	Vas Deferens
Eleventh cranial nerve	Accessory Nerve
Encephalon	Brain
Ependyma	Cerebral Ventricle
Epidermis	Skin
Epidural space, spinal	Spinal Canal
Epiploic foramen	Peritoneum
Epithalamus	Thalamus
Epitrochlear lymph node	Lymphatic, Right Upper Extremity
	Lymphatic, Left Upper Extremity

Term	ICD-10-PCS Value
Erector spinae muscle	Trunk Muscle, Right
	Trunk Muscle, Left
Esophageal artery	Upper Artery
Esophageal plexus	Thoracic Sympathetic Nerve
Ethmoidal air cell	Ethmoid Sinus, Right
	Ethmoid Sinus, Left
Extensor carpi radialis muscle	Lower Arm and Wrist Muscle, Right
	Lower Arm and Wrist Muscle, Left
Extensor carpi ulnaris muscle	Lower Arm and Wrist Muscle, Right
	Lower Arm and Wrist Muscle, Left
Extensor digitorum brevis muscle	Foot Muscle, Right
	Foot Muscle, Left
Extensor digitorum longus muscle	Lower Leg Muscle, Right
	Lower Leg Muscle, Left
Extensor hallucis brevis muscle	Foot Muscle, Right
	Foot Muscle, Left
Extensor hallucis longus muscle	Lower Leg Muscle, Right
	Lower Leg Muscle, Left
External anal sphincter	Anal Sphincter
External auditory meatus	External Auditory Canal, Right
	External Auditory Canal, Left
External maxillary artery	Face Artery
External naris	Nasal Mucosa and Soft Tissue
External oblique aponeurosis	Subcutaneous Tissue and Fascia, Trunk
External oblique muscle	Abdomen Muscle, Right
	Abdomen Muscle, Left
External popliteal nerve	Peroneal Nerve
External pudendal artery	Femoral Artery, Right
	Femoral Artery, Left
External pudendal vein	Saphenous Vein, Right
	Saphenous Vein, Left
External urethral sphincter	Urethra
Extradural space, intracranial	Epidural Space, Intracranial
Extradural space, spinal	Spinal Canal
Facial artery	Face Artery
False vocal cord	Larynx
Falx cerebri	Dura Mater
Fascia lata	Subcutaneous Tissue and Fascia, Right Upper Leg
	Subcutaneous Tissue and Fascia, Left Upper Leg
Femoral head	Upper Femur, Right
	Upper Femur, Left
Femoral lymph node	Lymphatic, Right Lower Extremity
	Lymphatic, Left Lower Extremity
Femoropatellar joint	Knee Joint, Right
	Knee Joint, Left
	Knee Joint, Femoral Surface, Right
	Knee Joint, Femoral Surface, Left
Femorotibial joint	Knee Joint, Right
	Knee Joint, Left
	Knee Joint, Tibial Surface, Right
	Knee Joint, Tibial Surface, Left
Fibular artery	Peroneal Artery, Right
	Peroneal Artery, Left
Fibular sesamoid	Metatarsal, Right
	Metatarsal, Left

Term	ICD-10-PCS Value
Fibularis brevis muscle	Lower Leg Muscle, Right
	Lower Leg Muscle, Left
Fibularis longus muscle	Lower Leg Muscle, Right
	Lower Leg Muscle, Left
Fifth cranial nerve	Trigeminal Nerve
Filum terminale	Spinal Meninges
First cranial nerve	Olfactory Nerve
First intercostal nerve	Brachial Plexus
Flexor carpi radialis muscle	Lower Arm and Wrist Muscle, Right
	Lower Arm and Wrist Muscle, Left
Flexor carpi ulnaris muscle	Lower Arm and Wrist Muscle, Right
	Lower Arm and Wrist Muscle, Left
Flexor digitorum brevis muscle	Foot Muscle, Right
	Foot Muscle, Left
Flexor digitorum longus muscle	Lower Leg Muscle, Right
	Lower Leg Muscle, Left
Flexor hallucis brevis muscle	Foot Muscle, Right
	Foot Muscle, Left
Flexor hallucis longus muscle	Lower Leg Muscle, Right
	Lower Leg Muscle, Left
Flexor pollicis longus muscle	Lower Arm and Wrist Muscle, Right
	Lower Arm and Wrist Muscle, Left
Foramen magnum	Occipital Bone
Foramen of Monro (intraventricular)	Cerebral Ventricle
Foreskin	Prepuce
Fossa of Rosenmuller	Nasopharynx
Fourth cranial nerve	Trochlear Nerve
Fourth ventricle	Cerebral Ventricle
Fovea	Retina, Right
	Retina, Left
Frenulum labii inferioris	Lower Lip
Frenulum labii superioris	Upper Lip
Frenulum linguae	Tongue
Frontal lobe	Cerebral Hemisphere
Frontal vein	Face Vein, Right
	Face Vein, Left
Fundus uteri	Uterus
Galea aponeurotica	Subcutaneous Tissue and Fascia, Scalp
Ganglion impar (ganglion of Walther)	Sacral Sympathetic Nerve
Gasserian ganglion	Trigeminal Nerve
Gastric lymph node	Lymphatic, Aortic
Gastric plexus	Abdominal Sympathetic Nerve
Gastrocnemius muscle	Lower Leg Muscle, Right
	Lower Leg Muscle, Left
Gastrocolic ligament	Omentum
Gastrocolic omentum	Omentum
Gastroduodenal artery	Hepatic Artery
Gastroesophageal (GE) junction	Esophagogastric Junction
Gastrohepatic omentum	Omentum
Gastrophrenic ligament	Omentum
Gastrosplenic ligament	Omentum
Gemellus muscle	Hip Muscle, Right
	Hip Muscle, Left
Geniculate ganglion	Facial Nerve
Geniculate nucleus	Thalamus
Genioglossus muscle	Tongue, Palate, Pharynx Muscle

Term	ICD-10-PCS Value
Genitofemoral nerve	Lumbar Plexus
Glans penis	Prepuce
Glenohumeral joint	Shoulder Joint, Right
	Shoulder Joint, Left
Glenohumeral ligament	Shoulder Bursa and Ligament, Right
	Shoulder Bursa and Ligament, Left
Glenoid fossa (of scapula)	Glenoid Cavity, Right
	Glenoid Cavity, Left
Glenoid ligament (labrum)	Shoulder Joint, Right
	Shoulder Joint, Left
Globus pallidus	Basal Ganglia
Glossoepiglottic fold	Epiglottis
Glottis	Larynx
Gluteal lymph node	Lymphatic, Pelvis
Gluteal vein	Hypogastric Vein, Right
	Hypogastric Vein, Left
Gluteus maximus muscle	Hip Muscle, Right
	Hip Muscle, Left
Gluteus medius muscle	Hip Muscle, Right
	Hip Muscle, Left
Gluteus minimus muscle	Hip Muscle, Right
	Hip Muscle, Left
Gracilis muscle	Upper Leg Muscle, Right
	Upper Leg Muscle, Left
Great auricular nerve	Cervical Plexus
Great cerebral vein	Intracranial Vein
Great(er) saphenous vein	Saphenous Vein, Right
	Saphenous Vein, Left
Greater alar cartilage	Nasal Mucosa and Soft Tissue
Greater occipital nerve	Cervical Nerve
Greater omentum	Omentum
Greater splanchnic nerve	Thoracic Sympathetic Nerve
Greater superficial petrosal nerve	Facial Nerve
Greater trochanter	Upper Femur, Right
	Upper Femur, Left
Greater tuberosity	Humeral Head, Right
	Humeral Head, Left
Greater vestibular (Bartholin's) gland	Vestibular Gland
Greater wing	Sphenoid Bone
Hallux	1st Toe, Right
	1st Toe, Left
Hamate bone	Carpal, Right
	Carpal, Left
Head of fibula	Fibula, Right
	Fibula, Left
Helix	External Ear, Right
	External Ear, Left
	External Ear, Bilateral
Hepatic artery proper	Hepatic Artery
Hepatic flexure	Transverse Colon
Hepatic lymph node	Lymphatic, Aortic
Hepatic plexus	Abdominal Sympathetic Nerve
Hepatic portal vein	Portal Vein
Hepatogastric ligament	Omentum
Hepatopancreatic ampulla	Ampulla of Vater

Term	ICD-10-PCS Value
Humeroradial joint	Elbow Joint, Right
	Elbow Joint, Left
Humeroulnar joint	Elbow Joint, Right
	Elbow Joint, Left
Humerus, distal	Humeral Shaft, Right
	Humeral Shaft, Left
Hyoglossus muscle	Tongue, Palate, Pharynx Muscle
Hyoid artery	Thyroid Artery, Right
	Thyroid Artery, Left
Hypogastric artery	Internal Iliac Artery, Right
	Internal Iliac Artery, Left
Hypopharynx	Pharynx
Hypophysis	Pituitary Gland
Hypothenar muscle	Hand Muscle, Right
	Hand Muscle, Left
Ileal artery	Superior Mesenteric Artery
Ileocolic artery	Superior Mesenteric Artery
Ileocolic vein	Colic Vein
Iliac crest	Pelvic Bone, Right
	Pelvic Bone, Left
Iliac fascia	Subcutaneous Tissue and Fascia, Right Upper Leg
	Subcutaneous Tissue and Fascia, Left Upper Leg
Iliac lymph node	Lymphatic, Pelvis
Iliacus muscle	Hip Muscle, Right
	Hip Muscle, Left
Iliofemoral ligament	Hip Bursa and Ligament, Right
	Hip Bursa and Ligament, Left
Iliohypogastric nerve	Lumbar Plexus
Ilioinguinal nerve	Lumbar Plexus
Iliolumbar artery	Internal Iliac Artery, Right
	Internal Iliac Artery, Left
Iliolumbar ligament	Lower Spine Bursa and Ligament
Iliotibial tract (band)	Subcutaneous Tissue and Fascia, Right Upper Leg
	Subcutaneous Tissue and Fascia, Left Upper Leg
Ilium	Pelvic Bone, Right
	Pelvic Bone, Left
Incus	Auditory Ossicle, Right
	Auditory Ossicle, Left
Inferior cardiac nerve	Thoracic Sympathetic Nerve
Inferior cerebellar vein	Intracranial Vein
Inferior cerebral vein	Intracranial Vein
Inferior epigastric artery	External Iliac Artery, Right
	External Iliac Artery, Left
Inferior epigastric lymph node	Lymphatic, Pelvis
Inferior genicular artery	Popliteal Artery, Right
	Popliteal Artery, Left
Inferior gluteal artery	Internal Iliac Artery, Right
	Internal Iliac Artery, Left
Inferior gluteal nerve	Sacral Plexus
Inferior hypogastric plexus	Abdominal Sympathetic Nerve
Inferior labial artery	Face Artery
Inferior longitudinal muscle	Tongue, Palate, Pharynx Muscle
Inferior mesenteric ganglion	Abdominal Sympathetic Nerve

Term	ICD-10-PCS Value
Inferior mesenteric lymph node	Lymphatic, Mesenteric
Inferior mesenteric plexus	Abdominal Sympathetic Nerve
Inferior oblique muscle	Extraocular Muscle, Right
	Extraocular Muscle, Left
Inferior pancreaticoduo-denal artery	Superior Mesenteric Artery
Inferior phrenic artery	Abdominal Aorta
Inferior rectus muscle	Extraocular Muscle, Right
	Extraocular Muscle, Left
Inferior suprarenal artery	Renal Artery, Right
	Renal Artery, Left
Inferior tarsal plate	Lower Eyelid, Right
	Lower Eyelid, Left
Inferior thyroid vein	Innominate Vein, Right
	Innominate Vein, Left
Inferior tibiofibular joint	Ankle Joint, Right
	Ankle Joint, Left
Inferior turbinate	Nasal Turbinate
Inferior ulnar collateral artery	Brachial Artery, Right
	Brachial Artery, Left
Inferior vesical artery	Internal Iliac Artery, Right
	Internal Iliac Artery, Left
Infraauricular lymph node	Lymphatic, Head
Infraclavicular (deltopectoral) lymph node	Lymphatic, Right Upper Extremity
	Lymphatic, Left Upper Extremity
Infrahyoid muscle	Neck Muscle, Right
	Neck Muscle, Left
Infraparotid lymph node	Lymphatic, Head
Infraspinatus fascia	Subcutaneous Tissue and Fascia, Right Upper Arm
	Subcutaneous Tissue and Fascia, Left Upper Arm
Infraspinatus muscle	Shoulder Muscle, Right
	Shoulder Muscle, Left
Infundibulopelvic ligament	Uterine Supporting Structure
Inguinal canal	Inguinal Region, Right
	Inguinal Region, Left
	Inguinal Region, Bilateral
Inguinal triangle	Inguinal Region, Right
	Inguinal Region, Left
	Inguinal Region, Bilateral
Interatrial septum	Atrial Septum
Intercarpal joint	Carpal Joint, Right
	Carpal Joint, Left
Intercarpal ligament	Hand Bursa and Ligament, Right
	Hand Bursa and Ligament, Left
Interclavicular ligament	Shoulder Bursa and Ligament, Right
	Shoulder Bursa and Ligament, Left
Intercostal lymph node	Lymphatic, Thorax
Intercostal muscle	Thorax Muscle, Right
	Thorax Muscle, Left
Intercostal nerve	Thoracic Nerve
Intercostobrachial nerve	Thoracic Nerve
Intercuneiform joint	Tarsal Joint, Right
	Tarsal Joint, Left
Intercuneiform ligament	Foot Bursa and Ligament, Right
	Foot Bursa and Ligament, Left
Intermediate bronchus	Main Bronchus, Right

Term	ICD-10-PCS Value
Intermediate cuneiform bone	Tarsal, Right
	Tarsal, Left
Internal anal sphincter	Anal Sphincter
Internal (basal) cerebral vein	Intracranial Vein
Internal carotid artery, intracranial portion	Intracranial Artery
Internal carotid plexus	Head and Neck Sympathetic Nerve
Internal iliac vein	Hypogastric Vein, Right
	Hypogastric Vein, Left
Internal maxillary artery	External Carotid Artery, Right
	External Carotid Artery, Left
Internal naris	Nasal Mucosa and Soft Tissue
Internal oblique muscle	Abdomen Muscle, Right
	Abdomen Muscle, Left
Internal pudendal artery	Internal Iliac Artery, Right
	Internal Iliac Artery, Left
Internal pudendal vein	Hypogastric Vein, Right
	Hypogastric Vein, Left
Internal thoracic artery	Internal Mammary Artery, Right
	Internal Mammary Artery, Left
	Subclavian Artery, Right
	Subclavian Artery, Left
Internal urethral sphincter	Urethra
Interphalangeal (IP) joint	Finger Phalangeal Joint, Right
	Finger Phalangeal Joint, Left
	Toe Phalangeal Joint, Right
	Toe Phalangeal Joint, Left
Interphalangeal ligament	Foot Bursa and Ligament, Right
	Foot Bursa and Ligament, Left
	Hand Bursa and Ligament, Right
	Hand Bursa and Ligament, Left
Interspinalis muscle	Trunk Muscle, Right
	Trunk Muscle, Left
Interspinous ligament, cervical	Head and Neck Bursa and Ligament
Interspinous ligament, lumbar	Lower Spine Bursa and Ligament
Interspinous ligament, thoracic	Upper Spine Bursa and Ligament
Intertransversarius muscle	Trunk Muscle, Right
	Trunk Muscle, Left
Intertransverse ligament, cervical	Head and Neck Bursa and Ligament
Intertransverse ligament, lumbar	Lower Spine Bursa and Ligament
Intertransverse ligament, thoracic	Upper Spine Bursa and Ligament
Interventricular foramen (Monro)	Cerebral Ventricle
Interventricular septum	Ventricular Septum
Intestinal lymphatic trunk	Cisterna Chyli
Ischiatic nerve	Sciatic Nerve
Ischiocavernosus muscle	Perineum Muscle
Ischiofemoral ligament	Hip Bursa and Ligament, Right
	Hip Bursa and Ligament, Left
Ischium	Pelvic Bone, Right
	Pelvic Bone, Left
Jejunal artery	Superior Mesenteric Artery
Jugular body	Glomus Jugulare

Term	ICD-10-PCS Value
Jugular lymph node	Lymphatic, Right Neck
	Lymphatic, Left Neck
Labia majora	Vulva
Labia minora	Vulva
Labial gland	Upper Lip
	Lower Lip
Lacrimal canaliculus	Lacrimal Duct, Right
	Lacrimal Duct, Left
Lacrimal punctum	Lacrimal Duct, Right
	Lacrimal Duct, Left
Lacrimal sac	Lacrimal Duct, Right
	Lacrimal Duct, Left
Laryngopharynx	Pharynx
Lateral (brachial) lymph node	Lymphatic, Right Axillary
	Lymphatic, Left Axillary
Lateral canthus	Upper Eyelid, Right
	Upper Eyelid, Left
Lateral collateral ligament (LCL)	Knee Bursa and Ligament, Right
	Knee Bursa and Ligament, Left
Lateral condyle of femur	Lower Femur, Right
	Lower Femur, Left
Lateral condyle of tibia	Tibia, Right
	Tibia, Left
Lateral cuneiform bone	Tarsal, Right
	Tarsal, Left
Lateral epicondyle of femur	Lower Femur, Right
	Lower Femur, Left
Lateral epicondyle of humerus	Humeral Shaft, Right
	Humeral Shaft, Left
Lateral femoral cutaneous nerve	Lumbar Plexus
Lateral malleolus	Fibula, Right
	Fibula, Left
Lateral meniscus	Knee Joint, Right
	Knee Joint, Left
Lateral nasal cartilage	Nasal Mucosa and Soft Tissue
Lateral plantar artery	Foot Artery, Right
	Foot Artery, Left
Lateral plantar nerve	Tibial Nerve
Lateral rectus muscle	Extraocular Muscle, Right
	Extraocular Muscle, Left
Lateral sacral artery	Internal Iliac Artery, Right
	Internal Iliac Artery, Left
Lateral sacral vein	Hypogastric Vein, Right
	Hypogastric Vein, Left
Lateral sural cutaneous nerve	Peroneal Nerve
Lateral tarsal artery	Foot Artery, Right
	Foot Artery, Left
Lateral temporo-mandibular ligament	Head and Neck Bursa and Ligament
Lateral thoracic artery	Axillary Artery, Right
	Axillary Artery, Left
Latissimus dorsi muscle	Trunk Muscle, Right
	Trunk Muscle, Left
Least splanchnic nerve	Thoracic Sympathetic Nerve
Left ascending lumbar vein	Hemiazygos Vein
Left atrioventricular valve	Mitral Valve
Left auricular appendix	Atrium, Left

Term	ICD-10-PCS Value
Left colic vein	Colic Vein
Left coronary sulcus	Heart, Left
Left gastric artery	Gastric Artery
Left gastroepiploic artery	Splenic Artery
Left gastroepiploic vein	Splenic Vein
Left inferior phrenic vein	Renal Vein, Left
Left inferior pulmonary vein	Pulmonary Vein, Left
Left jugular trunk	Thoracic Duct
Left lateral ventricle	Cerebral Ventricle
Left ovarian vein	Renal Vein, Left
Left second lumbar vein	Renal Vein, Left
Left subclavian trunk	Thoracic Duct
Left subcostal vein	Hemiazygos Vein
Left superior pulmonary vein	Pulmonary Vein, Left
Left suprarenal vein	Renal Vein, Left
Left testicular vein	Renal Vein, Left
Leptomeninges, intracranial	Cerebral Meninges
Leptomeninges, spinal	Spinal Meninges
Lesser alar cartilage	Nasal Mucosa and Soft Tissue
Lesser occipital nerve	Cervical Plexus
Lesser omentum	Omentum
Lesser saphenous vein	Saphenous Vein, Right
	Saphenous Vein, Left
Lesser splanchnic nerve	Thoracic Sympathetic Nerve
Lesser trochanter	Upper Femur, Right
	Upper Femur, Left
Lesser tuberosity	Humeral Head, Right
	Humeral Head, Left
Lesser wing	Sphenoid Bone
Levator anguli oris muscle	Facial Muscle
Levator ani muscle	Perineum Muscle
Levator labii superioris alaeque nasi muscle	Facial Muscle
Levator labii superioris muscle	Facial Muscle
Levator palpebrae superioris muscle	Upper Eyelid, Right
	Upper Eyelid, Left
Levator scapulae muscle	Neck Muscle, Right
	Neck Muscle, Left
Levator veli palatini muscle	Tongue, Palate, Pharynx Muscle
Levatores costarum muscle	Thorax Muscle, Right
	Thorax Muscle, Left
Ligament of head of fibula	Knee Bursa and Ligament, Right
	Knee Bursa and Ligament, Left
Ligament of the lateral malleolus	Ankle Bursa and Ligament, Right
	Ankle Bursa and Ligament, Left
Ligamentum flavum, cervical	Head and Neck Bursa and Ligament
Ligamentum flavum, lumbar	Lower Spine Bursa and Ligament
Ligamentum flavum, thoracic	Upper Spine Bursa and Ligament
Lingual artery	External Carotid Artery, Right
	External Carotid Artery, Left
Lingual tonsil	Pharynx
Locus ceruleus	Pons
Long thoracic nerve	Brachial Plexus

Term	ICD-10-PCS Value
Lumbar artery	Abdominal Aorta
Lumbar facet joint	Lumbar Vertebral Joint
Lumbar ganglion	Lumbar Sympathetic Nerve
Lumbar lymph node	Lymphatic, Aortic
Lumbar lymphatic trunk	Cisterna Chyli
Lumbar splanchnic nerve	Lumbar Sympathetic Nerve
Lumbosacral facet joint	Lumbosacral Joint
Lumbosacral trunk	Lumbar Nerve
Lunate bone	Carpal, Right
	Carpal, Left
Lunotriquetral ligament	Hand Bursa and Ligament, Right
	Hand Bursa and Ligament, Left
Macula	Retina, Right
	Retina, Left
Malleus	Auditory Ossicle, Right
	Auditory Ossicle, Left
Mammary duct	Breast, Right
	Breast, Left
	Breast, Bilateral
Mammary gland	Breast, Right
	Breast, Left
	Breast, Bilateral
Mammillary body	Hypothalamus
Mandibular nerve	Trigeminal Nerve
Mandibular notch	Mandible, Right
	Mandible, Left
Manubrium	Sternum
Masseter muscle	Head Muscle
Masseteric fascia	Subcutaneous Tissue and Fascia, Face
Mastoid (postauricular) lymph node	Lymphatic, Right Neck
	Lymphatic, Left Neck
Mastoid air cells	Mastoid Sinus, Right
	Mastoid Sinus, Left
Mastoid process	Temporal Bone, Right
	Temporal Bone, Left
Maxillary artery	External Carotid Artery, Right
	External Carotid Artery, Left
Maxillary nerve	Trigeminal Nerve
Medial canthus	Lower Eyelid, Right
	Lower Eyelid, Left
Medial collateral ligament (MCL)	Knee Bursa and Ligament, Right
	Knee Bursa and Ligament, Left
Medial condyle of femur	Lower Femur, Right
	Lower Femur, Left
Medial condyle of tibia	Tibia, Right
	Tibia, Left
Medial cuneiform bone	Tarsal, Right
	Tarsal, Left
Medial epicondyle of femur	Lower Femur, Right
	Lower Femur, Left
Medial epicondyle of humerus	Humeral Shaft, Right
	Humeral Shaft, Left
Medial malleolus	Tibia, Right
	Tibia, Left
Medial meniscus	Knee Joint, Right
	Knee Joint, Left
Medial plantar artery	Foot Artery, Right
	Foot Artery, Left

Term	ICD-10-PCS Value
Medial plantar nerve	Tibial Nerve
Medial popliteal nerve	Tibial Nerve
Medial rectus muscle	Extraocular Muscle, Right
	Extraocular Muscle, Left
Medial sural cutaneous nerve	Tibial Nerve
Median antebrachial vein	Basilic Vein, Right
	Basilic Vein, Left
Median cubital vein	Basilic Vein, Right
	Basilic Vein, Left
Median sacral artery	Abdominal Aorta
Mediastinal cavity	Mediastinum
Mediastinal lymph node	Lymphatic, Thorax
Mediastinal space	Mediastinum
Meissner's (submucous) plexus	Abdominal Sympathetic Nerve
Membranous urethra	Urethra
Mental foramen	Mandible, Right
	Mandible, Left
Mentalis muscle	Facial Muscle
Mesoappendix	Mesentery
Mesocolon	Mesentery
Metacarpal ligament	Hand Bursa and Ligament, Right
	Hand Bursa and Ligament, Left
Metacarpophalangeal ligament	Hand Bursa and Ligament, Right
	Hand Bursa and Ligament, Left
Metatarsal ligament	Foot Bursa and Ligament, Right
	Foot Bursa and Ligament, Left
Metatarsophalangeal ligament	Foot Bursa and Ligament, Right
	Foot Bursa and Ligament, Left
Metatarsophalangeal (MTP) joint	Metatarsal-Phalangeal Joint, Right
	Metatarsal-Phalangeal Joint, Left
Metathalamus	Thalamus
Midcarpal joint	Carpal Joint, Right
	Carpal Joint, Left
Middle cardiac nerve	Thoracic Sympathetic Nerve
Middle cerebral artery	Intracranial Artery
Middle cerebral vein	Intracranial Vein
Middle colic vein	Colic Vein
Middle genicular artery	Popliteal Artery, Right
	Popliteal Artery, Left
Middle hemorrhoidal vein	Hypogastric Vein, Right
	Hypogastric Vein, Left
Middle rectal artery	Internal Iliac Artery, Right
	Internal Iliac Artery, Left
Middle suprarenal artery	Abdominal Aorta
Middle temporal artery	Temporal Artery, Right
	Temporal Artery, Left
Middle turbinate	Nasal Turbinate
Mitral annulus	Mitral Valve
Molar gland	Buccal Mucosa
Musculocutaneous nerve	Brachial Plexus
Musculophrenic artery	Internal Mammary Artery, Right
	Internal Mammary Artery, Left
Musculospiral nerve	Radial Nerve
Myelencephalon	Medulla Oblongata
Myenteric (Auerbach's) plexus	Abdominal Sympathetic Nerve
Myometrium	Uterus

Term	ICD-10-PCS Value
Nail bed	Finger Nail
	Toe Nail
Nail plate	Finger Nail
	Toe Nail
Nasal cavity	Nasal Mucosa and Soft Tissue
Nasal concha	Nasal Turbinate
Nasalis muscle	Facial Muscle
Nasolacrimal duct	Lacrimal Duct, Right
	Lacrimal Duct, Left
Navicular bone	Tarsal, Right
	Tarsal, Left
Neck of femur	Upper Femur, Right
	Upper Femur, Left
Neck of humerus (anatomical) (surgical)	Humeral Head, Right
	Humeral Head, Left
Nerve to the stapedius	Facial Nerve
Neurohypophysis	Pituitary Gland
Ninth cranial nerve	Glossopharyngeal Nerve
Nostril	Nasal Mucosa and Soft Tissue
Obturator artery	Internal Iliac Artery, Right
	Internal Iliac Artery, Left
Obturator lymph node	Lymphatic, Pelvis
Obturator muscle	Hip Muscle, Right
	Hip Muscle, Left
Obturator nerve	Lumbar Plexus
Obturator vein	Hypogastric Vein, Right
	Hypogastric Vein, Left
Obtuse margin	Heart, Left
Occipital artery	External Carotid Artery, Right
	External Carotid Artery, Left
Occipital lobe	Cerebral Hemisphere
Occipital lymph node	Lymphatic, Right Neck
	Lymphatic, Left Neck
Occipitofrontalis muscle	Facial Muscle
Odontoid process	Cervical Vertebra
Olecranon bursa	Elbow Bursa and Ligament, Right
	Elbow Bursa and Ligament, Left
Olecranon process	Ulna, Right
	Ulna, Left
Olfactory bulb	Olfactory Nerve
Ophthalmic artery	Intracranial Artery
Ophthalmic nerve	Trigeminal Nerve
Ophthalmic vein	Intracranial Vein
Optic chiasma	Optic Nerve
Optic disc	Retina, Right
	Retina, Left
Optic foramen	Sphenoid Bone
Orbicularis oculi muscle	Upper Eyelid, Right
	Upper Eyelid, Left
Orbicularis oris muscle	Facial Muscle
Orbital fascia	Subcutaneous Tissue and Fascia, Face
Orbital portion of ethmoid bone	Orbit, Right
	Orbit, Left
Orbital portion of frontal bone	Orbit, Right
	Orbit, Left
Orbital portion of lacrimal bone	Orbit, Right
	Orbit, Left

Appendix D: Body Part Key

Term	ICD-10-PCS Value
Orbital portion of maxilla	Orbit, Right
	Orbit, Left
Orbital portion of palatine bone	Orbit, Right
	Orbit, Left
Orbital portion of sphenoid bone	Orbit, Right
	Orbit, Left
Orbital portion of zygomatic bone	Orbit, Right
	Orbit, Left
Oropharynx	Pharynx
Otic ganglion	Head and Neck Sympathetic Nerve
Oval window	Middle Ear, Right
	Middle Ear, Left
Ovarian artery	Abdominal Aorta
Ovarian ligament	Uterine Supporting Structure
Oviduct	Fallopian Tube, Right
	Fallopian Tube, Left
Palatine gland	Buccal Mucosa
Palatine tonsil	Tonsils
Palatine uvula	Uvula
Palatoglossal muscle	Tongue, Palate, Pharynx Muscle
Palatopharyngeal muscle	Tongue, Palate, Pharynx Muscle
Palmar (volar) digital vein	Hand Vein, Right
	Hand Vein, Left
Palmar (volar) metacarpal vein	Hand Vein, Right
	Hand Vein, Left
Palmar cutaneous nerve	Median Nerve
	Radial Nerve
Palmar fascia (aponeurosis)	Subcutaneous Tissue and Fascia, Right Hand
	Subcutaneous Tissue and Fascia, Left Hand
Palmar interosseous muscle	Hand Muscle, Right
	Hand Muscle, Left
Palmar ulnocarpal ligament	Wrist Bursa and Ligament, Right
	Wrist Bursa and Ligament, Left
Palmaris longus muscle	Lower Arm and Wrist Muscle, Right
	Lower Arm and Wrist Muscle, Left
Pancreatic artery	Splenic Artery
Pancreatic plexus	Abdominal Sympathetic Nerve
Pancreatic vein	Splenic Vein
Pancreaticosplenic lymph node	Lymphatic, Aortic
Paraaortic lymph node	Lymphatic, Aortic
Parapharyngeal space	Neck
Pararectal lymph node	Lymphatic, Mesenteric
Parasternal lymph node	Lymphatic, Thorax
Paratracheal lymph node	Lymphatic, Thorax
Paraurethral (Skene's) gland	Vestibular Gland
Parietal lobe	Cerebral Hemisphere
Parotid lymph node	Lymphatic, Head
Parotid plexus	Facial Nerve
Pars flaccida	Tympanic Membrane, Right
	Tympanic Membrane, Left
Patellar ligament	Knee Bursa and Ligament, Right
	Knee Bursa and Ligament, Left
Patellar tendon	Knee Tendon, Right
	Knee Tendon, Left

Term	ICD-10-PCS Value
Patellofemoral joint	Knee Joint, Right
	Knee Joint, Left
	Knee Joint, Femoral Surface, Right
	Knee Joint, Femoral Surface, Left
Pectineus muscle	Upper Leg Muscle, Right
	Upper Leg Muscle, Left
Pectoral (anterior) lymph node	Lymphatic, Right Axillary
	Lymphatic, Left Axillary
Pectoral fascia	Subcutaneous Tissue and Fascia, Chest
Pectoralis major muscle	Thorax Muscle, Right
	Thorax Muscle, Left
Pectoralis minor muscle	Thorax Muscle, Right
	Thorax Muscle, Left
Pelvic splanchnic nerve	Abdominal Sympathetic Nerve
	Sacral Sympathetic Nerve
Penile urethra	Urethra
Perianal skin	Skin, Perineum
Pericardiophrenic artery	Internal Mammary Artery, Right
	Internal Mammary Artery, Left
Perimetrium	Uterus
Peroneus brevis muscle	Lower Leg Muscle, Right
	Lower Leg Muscle, Left
Peroneus longus muscle	Lower Leg Muscle, Right
	Lower Leg Muscle, Left
Petrous part of temoporal bone	Temporal Bone, Right
	Temporal Bone, Left
Pharyngeal constrictor muscle	Tongue, Palate, Pharynx Muscle
Pharyngeal plexus	Vagus Nerve
Pharyngeal recess	Nasopharynx
Pharyngeal tonsil	Adenoids
Pharyngotympanic tube	Eustachian Tube, Right
	Eustachian Tube, Left
Pia mater, intracranial	Cerebral Meninges
Pia mater, spinal	Spinal Meninges
Pinna	External Ear, Right
	External Ear, Left
	External Ear, Bilateral
Piriform recess (sinus)	Pharynx
Piriformis muscle	Hip Muscle, Right
	Hip Muscle, Left
Pisiform bone	Carpal, Right
	Carpal, Left
Pisohamate ligament	Hand Bursa and Ligament, Right
	Hand Bursa and Ligament, Left
Pisometacarpal ligament	Hand Bursa and Ligament, Right
	Hand Bursa and Ligament, Left
Plantar digital vein	Foot Vein, Right
	Foot Vein, Left
Plantar fascia (aponeurosis)	Subcutaneous Tissue and Fascia, Right Foot
	Subcutaneous Tissue and Fascia, Left Foot
Plantar metatarsal vein	Foot Vein, Right
	Foot Vein, Left
Plantar venous arch	Foot Vein, Right
	Foot Vein, Left
Platysma muscle	Neck Muscle, Right
	Neck Muscle, Left

Term	ICD-10-PCS Value
Plica semilunaris	Conjunctiva, Right
	Conjunctiva, Left
Pneumogastric nerve	Vagus Nerve
Pneumotaxic center	Pons
Pontine tegmentum	Pons
Popliteal ligament	Knee Bursa and Ligament, Right
	Knee Bursa and Ligament, Left
Popliteal lymph node	Lymphatic, Left Lower Extremity
	Lymphatic, Right Lower Extremity
Popliteal vein	Femoral Vein, Right
	Femoral Vein, Left
Popliteus muscle	Lower Leg Muscle, Right
	Lower Leg Muscle, Left
Postauricular (mastoid) lymph node	Lymphatic, Right Neck
	Lymphatic, Left Neck
Postcava	Inferior Vena Cava
Posterior (subscapular) lymph node	Lymphatic, Right Axillary
	Lymphatic, Left Axillary
Posterior auricular artery	External Carotid Artery, Right
	External Carotid Artery, Left
Posterior auricular nerve	Facial Nerve
Posterior auricular vein	External Jugular Vein, Right
	External Jugular Vein, Left
Posterior cerebral artery	Intracranial Artery
Posterior chamber	Eye, Right
	Eye, Left
Posterior circumflex humeral artery	Axillary Artery, Right
	Axillary Artery, Left
Posterior communicating artery	Intracranial Artery
Posterior cruciate ligament (PCL)	Knee Bursa and Ligament, Right
	Knee Bursa and Ligament, Left
Posterior facial (retromandibular) vein	Face Vein, Right
	Face Vein, Left
Posterior femoral cutaneous nerve	Sacral Plexus
Posterior inferior cerebellar artery (PICA)	Intracranial Artery
Posterior interosseous nerve	Radial Nerve
Posterior labial nerve	Pudendal Nerve
Posterior scrotal nerve	Pudendal Nerve
Posterior spinal artery	Vertebral Artery, Right
	Vertebral Artery, Left
Posterior tibial recurrent artery	Anterior Tibial Artery, Right
	Anterior Tibial Artery, Left
Posterior ulnar recurrent artery	Ulnar Artery, Right
	Ulnar Artery, Left
Posterior vagal trunk	Vagus Nerve
Preauricular lymph node	Lymphatic, Head
Precava	Superior Vena Cava
Prepatellar bursa	Knee Bursa and Ligament, Right
	Knee Bursa and Ligament, Left
Pretracheal fascia	Subcutaneous Tissue and Fascia, Right Neck
	Subcutaneous Tissue and Fascia, Left Neck
Prevertebral fascia	Subcutaneous Tissue and Fascia, Right Neck
	Subcutaneous Tissue and Fascia, Left Neck

Term	ICD-10-PCS Value
Princeps pollicis artery	Hand Artery, Right
	Hand Artery, Left
Procerus muscle	Facial Muscle
Profunda brachii	Brachial Artery, Right
	Brachial Artery, Left
Profunda femoris (deep femoral) vein	Femoral Vein, Right
	Femoral Vein, Left
Pronator quadratus muscle	Lower Arm and Wrist Muscle, Right
	Lower Arm and Wrist Muscle, Left
Pronator teres muscle	Lower Arm and Wrist Muscle, Right
	Lower Arm and Wrist Muscle, Left
Prostatic artery	Internal Iliac Artery, Right
	Internal Iliac Artery, Left
Prostatic urethra	Urethra
Proximal radioulnar joint	Elbow Joint, Right
	Elbow Joint, Left
Psoas muscle	Hip Muscle, Right
	Hip Muscle, Left
Pterygoid muscle	Head Muscle
Pterygoid process	Sphenoid Bone
Pterygopalatine (sphenopalatine) ganglion	Head and Neck Sympathetic Nerve
Pubis	Pelvic Bone, Right
	Pelvic Bone, Left
Pubofemoral ligament	Hip Bursa and Ligament, Right
	Hip Bursa and Ligament, Left
Pudendal nerve	Sacral Plexus
Pulmoaortic canal	Pulmonary Artery, Left
Pulmonary annulus	Pulmonary Valve
Pulmonary plexus	Thoracic Sympathetic Nerve
	Vagus Nerve
Pulmonic valve	Pulmonary Valve
Pulvinar	Thalamus
Pyloric antrum	Stomach, Pylorus
Pyloric canal	Stomach, Pylorus
Pyloric sphincter	Stomach, Pylorus
Pyramidalis muscle	Abdomen Muscle, Right
	Abdomen Muscle, Left
Quadrangular cartilage	Nasal Septum
Quadrate lobe	Liver
Quadratus femoris muscle	Hip Muscle, Right
	Hip Muscle, Left
Quadratus lumborum muscle	Trunk Muscle, Right
	Trunk Muscle, Left
Quadratus plantae muscle	Foot Muscle, Right
	Foot Muscle, Left
Quadriceps (femoris)	Upper Leg Muscle, Right
	Upper Leg Muscle, Left
Radial collateral carpal ligament	Wrist Bursa and Ligament, Right
	Wrist Bursa and Ligament, Left
Radial collateral ligament	Elbow Bursa and Ligament, Right
	Elbow Bursa and Ligament, Left
Radial notch	Ulna, Right
	Ulna, Left
Radial recurrent artery	Radial Artery, Right
	Radial Artery, Left
Radial vein	Brachial Vein, Right
	Brachial Vein, Left

Term	ICD-10-PCS Value
Radialis indicis	Hand Artery, Right
	Hand Artery, Left
Radiocarpal joint	Wrist Joint, Right
	Wrist Joint, Left
Radiocarpal ligament	Wrist Bursa and Ligament, Right
	Wrist Bursa and Ligament, Left
Radioulnar ligament	Wrist Bursa and Ligament, Right
	Wrist Bursa and Ligament, Left
Rectosigmoid junction	Sigmoid Colon
Rectus abdominis muscle	Abdomen Muscle, Right
	Abdomen Muscle, Left
Rectus femoris muscle	Upper Leg Muscle, Right
	Upper Leg Muscle, Left
Recurrent laryngeal nerve	Vagus Nerve
Renal calyx	Kidney, Right
	Kidney, Left
	Kidneys, Bilateral
	Kidney
Renal capsule	Kidney, Right
	Kidney, Left
	Kidneys, Bilateral
	Kidney
Renal cortex	Kidney, Right
	Kidney, Left
	Kidneys, Bilateral
	Kidney
Renal nerve	Abdominal sympathetic Nerve
Renal plexus	Abdominal Sympathetic Nerve
Renal segment	Kidney, Right
	Kidney, Left
	Kidneys, Bilateral
	Kidney
Renal segmental artery	Renal Artery, Right
	Renal Artery, Left
Retroperitoneal cavity	Retroperitoneum
Retroperitoneal lymph node	Lymphatic, Aortic
Retroperitoneal space	Retroperitoneum
Retropharyngeal lymph node	Lymphatic, Right Neck
	Lymphatic, Left Neck
Retropharyngeal space	Neck
Retropubic space	Pelvic Cavity
Rhinopharynx	Nasopharynx
Rhomboid major muscle	Trunk Muscle, Right
	Trunk Muscle, Left
Rhomboid minor muscle	Trunk Muscle, Right
	Trunk Muscle, Left
Right ascending lumbar vein	Azygos Vein
Right atrioventricular valve	Tricuspid Valve
Right auricular appendix	Atrium, Right
Right colic vein	Colic Vein
Right coronary sulcus	Heart, Right
Right gastric artery	Gastric Artery
Right gastroepiploic vein	Superior Mesenteric Vein
Right inferior phrenic vein	Inferior Vena Cava
Right inferior pulmonary vein	Pulmonary Vein, Right
Right jugular trunk	Lymphatic, Right Neck

Term	ICD-10-PCS Value
Right lateral ventricle	Cerebral Ventricle
Right lymphatic duct	Lymphatic, Right Neck
Right ovarian vein	Inferior Vena Cava
Right second lumbar vein	Inferior Vena Cava
Right subclavian trunk	Lymphatic, Right Neck
Right subcostal vein	Azygos Vein
Right superior pulmonary vein	Pulmonary Vein, Right
Right suprarenal vein	Inferior Vena Cava
Right testicular vein	Inferior Vena Cava
Rima glottidis	Larynx
Risorius muscle	Facial Muscle
Round ligament of uterus	Uterine Supporting Structure
Round window	Inner Ear, Right
	Inner Ear, Left
Sacral ganglion	Sacral Sympathetic Nerve
Sacral lymph node	Lymphatic, Pelvis
Sacral splanchnic nerve	Sacral Sympathetic Nerve
Sacrococcygeal ligament	Lower Spine Bursa and Ligament
Sacrococcygeal symphysis	Sacrococcygeal Joint
Sacroiliac ligament	Lower Spine Bursa and Ligament
Sacrospinous ligament	Lower Spine Bursa and Ligament
Sacrotuberous ligament	Lower Spine Bursa and Ligament
Salpingopharyngeus muscle	Tongue, Palate, Pharynx Muscle
Salpinx	Fallopian Tube, Right
	Fallopian Tube, Left
Saphenous nerve	Femoral Nerve
Sartorius muscle	Upper Leg Muscle, Right
	Upper Leg Muscle, Left
Scalene muscle	Neck Muscle, Right
	Neck Muscle, Left
Scaphoid bone	Carpal, Right
	Carpal, Left
Scapholunate ligament	Wrist Bursa and Ligament, Right
	Wrist Bursa and Ligament, Left
Scaphotrapezium ligament	Hand Bursa and Ligament, Right
	Hand Bursa and Ligament, Left
Scarpa's (vestibular) ganglion	Acoustic Nerve
Sebaceous gland	Skin
Second cranial nerve	Optic Nerve
Sella turcica	Sphenoid Bone
Semicircular canal	Inner Ear, Right
	Inner Ear, Left
Semimembranosus muscle	Upper Leg Muscle, Right
	Upper Leg Muscle, Left
Semitendinosus muscle	Upper Leg Muscle, Right
	Upper Leg Muscle, Left
Septal cartilage	Nasal Septum
Serratus anterior muscle	Thorax Muscle, Right
	Thorax Muscle, Left
Serratus posterior muscle	Trunk Muscle, Right
	Trunk Muscle, Left
Seventh cranial nerve	Facial Nerve
Short gastric artery	Splenic Artery
Sigmoid artery	Inferior Mesenteric Artery
Sigmoid flexure	Sigmoid Colon
Sigmoid vein	Inferior Mesenteric Vein

Term	ICD-10-PCS Value
Sinoatrial node	Conduction Mechanism
Sinus venosus	Atrium, Right
Sixth cranial nerve	Abducens Nerve
Skene's (paraurethral) gland	Vestibular Gland
Small saphenous vein	Saphenous Vein, Right
	Saphenous Vein, Left
Solar (celiac) plexus	Abdominal Sympathetic Nerve
Soleus muscle	Lower Leg Muscle, Right
	Lower Leg Muscle, Left
Sphenomandibular ligament	Head and Neck Bursa and Ligament
Sphenopalatine (pterygopalatine) ganglion	Head and Neck Sympathetic Nerve
Spinal nerve, cervical	Cervical Nerve
Spinal nerve, lumbar	Lumbar Nerve
Spinal nerve, sacral	Sacral Nerve
Spinal nerve, thoracic	Thoracic Nerve
Spinous process	Cervical Vertebra
	Lumbar Vertebra
	Thoracic Vertebra
Spiral ganglion	Acoustic Nerve
Splenic flexure	Transverse Colon
Splenic plexus	Abdominal Sympathetic Nerve
Splenius capitis muscle	Head Muscle
Splenius cervicis muscle	Neck Muscle, Right
	Neck Muscle, Left
Stapes	Auditory Ossicle, Right
	Auditory Ossicle, Left
Stellate ganglion	Head and Neck Sympathetic Nerve
Stensen's duct	Parotid Duct, Right
	Parotid Duct, Left
Sternoclavicular ligament	Shoulder Bursa and Ligament, Right
	Shoulder Bursa and Ligament, Left
Sternocleidomastoid artery	Thyroid Artery, Right
	Thyroid Artery, Left
Sternocleidomastoid muscle	Neck Muscle, Right
	Neck Muscle, Left
Sternocostal ligament	Sternum Bursa and Ligament
Styloglossus muscle	Tongue, Palate, Pharynx Muscle
Stylomandibular ligament	Head and Neck Bursa and Ligament
Stylopharyngeus muscle	Tongue, Palate, Pharynx Muscle
Subacromial bursa	Shoulder Bursa and Ligament, Right
	Shoulder Bursa and Ligament, Left
Subaortic (common iliac) lymph node	Lymphatic, Pelvis
Subarachnoid space, spinal	Spinal Canal
Subclavicular (apical) lymph node	Lymphatic, Right Axillary
	Lymphatic, Left Axillary
Subclavius muscle	Thorax Muscle, Right
	Thorax Muscle, Left
Subclavius nerve	Brachial Plexus
Subcostal artery	Upper Artery
Subcostal muscle	Thorax Muscle, Right
	Thorax Muscle, Left
Subcostal nerve	Thoracic Nerve
Subdural space, spinal	Spinal Canal
Submandibular ganglion	Facial Nerve
	Head and Neck Sympathetic Nerve

Term	ICD-10-PCS Value
Submandibular gland	Submaxillary Gland, Right
	Submaxillary Gland, Left
Submandibular lymph node	Lymphatic, Head
Submandibular space	Subcutaneous Tissue and Fascia, Face
Submaxillary ganglion	Head and Neck Sympathetic Nerve
Submaxillary lymph node	Lymphatic, Head
Submental artery	Face Artery
Submental lymph node	Lymphatic, Head
Submucous (Meissner's) plexus	Abdominal Sympathetic Nerve
Suboccipital nerve	Cervical Nerve
Suboccipital venous plexus	Vertebral Vein, Right
	Vertebral Vein, Left
Subparotid lymph node	Lymphatic, Head
Subscapular aponeurosis	Subcutaneous Tissue and Fascia, Right Upper Arm
	Subcutaneous Tissue and Fascia, Left Upper Arm
Subscapular artery	Axillary Artery, Right
	Axillary Artery, Left
Subscapular (posterior) lymph node	Lymphatic, Right Axillary
	Lymphatic, Left Axillary
Subscapularis muscle	Shoulder Muscle, Right
	Shoulder Muscle, Left
Substantia nigra	Basal Ganglia
Subtalar (talocalcaneal) joint	Tarsal Joint, Right
	Tarsal Joint, Left
Subtalar ligament	Foot Bursa and Ligament, Right
	Foot Bursa and Ligament, Left
Subthalamic nucleus	Basal Ganglia
Superficial circumflex iliac vein	Saphenous Vein, Right
	Saphenous Vein, Left
Superficial epigastric artery	Femoral Artery, Right
	Femoral Artery, Left
Superficial epigastric vein	Saphenous Vein, Right
	Saphenous Vein, Left
Superficial palmar arch	Hand Artery, Right
	Hand Artery, Left
Superficial palmar venous arch	Hand Vein, Right
	Hand Vein, Left
Superficial temporal artery	Temporal Artery, Right
	Temporal Artery, Left
Superficial transverse perineal muscle	Perineum Muscle
Superior cardiac nerve	Thoracic Sympathetic Nerve
Superior cerebellar vein	Intracranial Vein
Superior cerebral vein	Intracranial Vein
Superior clunic (cluneal) nerve	Lumbar Nerve
Superior epigastric artery	Internal Mammary Artery, Right
	Internal Mammary Artery, Left
Superior genicular artery	Popliteal Artery, Right
	Popliteal Artery, Left
Superior gluteal artery	Internal Iliac Artery, Right
	Internal Iliac Artery, Left
Superior gluteal nerve	Lumbar Plexus
Superior hypogastric plexus	Abdominal Sympathetic Nerve
Superior labial artery	Face Artery

Appendix D: Body Part Key

Term	ICD-10-PCS Value
Superior laryngeal artery	Thyroid Artery, Right
	Thyroid Artery, Left
Superior laryngeal nerve	Vagus Nerve
Superior longitudinal muscle	Tongue, Palate, Pharynx Muscle
Superior mesenteric ganglion	Abdominal Sympathetic Nerve
Superior mesenteric lymph node	Lymphatic, Mesenteric
Superior mesenteric plexus	Abdominal Sympathetic Nerve
Superior oblique muscle	Extraocular Muscle, Right
	Extraocular Muscle, Left
Superior olivary nucleus	Pons
Superior rectal artery	Inferior Mesenteric Artery
Superior rectal vein	Inferior Mesenteric Vein
Superior rectus muscle	Extraocular Muscle, Right
	Extraocular Muscle, Left
Superior tarsal plate	Upper Eyelid, Right
	Upper Eyelid, Left
Superior thoracic artery	Axillary Artery, Right
	Axillary Artery, Left
Superior thyroid artery	External Carotid Artery, Right
	External Carotid Artery, Left
	Thyroid Artery, Right
	Thyroid Artery, Left
Superior turbinate	Nasal Turbinate
Superior ulnar collateral artery	Brachial Artery, Right
	Brachial Artery, Left
Superior vesical artery	Internal Iliac Artery, Right
	Internal Iliac Artery, Left
Supraclavicular nerve	Cervical Plexus
Supraclavicular (Virchow's) lymph node	Lymphatic, Right Neck
	Lymphatic, Left Neck
Suprahyoid lymph node	Lymphatic, Head
Suprahyoid muscle	Neck Muscle, Right
	Neck Muscle, Left
Suprainguinal lymph node	Lymphatic, Pelvis
Supraorbital vein	Face Vein, Right
	Face Vein, Left
Suprarenal gland	Adrenal Gland, Right
	Adrenal Gland, Left
	Adrenal Glands, Bilateral
	Adrenal Gland
Suprarenal plexus	Abdominal Sympathetic Nerve
Suprascapular nerve	Brachial Plexus
Supraspinatus fascia	Subcutaneous Tissue and Fascia, Right Upper Arm
	Subcutaneous Tissue and Fascia, Left Upper Arm
Supraspinatus muscle	Shoulder Muscle, Right
	Shoulder Muscle, Left
Supraspinous ligament	Upper Spine Bursa and Ligament
	Lower Spine Bursa and Ligament
Suprasternal notch	Sternum
Supratrochlear lymph node	Lymphatic, Right Upper Extremity
	Lymphatic, Left Upper Extremity
Sural artery	Popliteal Artery, Right
	Popliteal Artery, Left
Sweat gland	Skin

Term	ICD-10-PCS Value
Talocalcaneal ligament	Foot Bursa and Ligament, Right
	Foot Bursa and Ligament, Left
Talocalcaneal (subtalar) joint	Tarsal Joint, Right
	Tarsal Joint, Left
Talocalcaneonavicular joint	Tarsal Joint, Right
	Tarsal Joint, Left
Talocalcaneonavicular ligament	Foot Bursa and Ligament, Right
	Foot Bursa and Ligament, Left
Talocrural joint	Ankle Joint, Right
	Ankle Joint, Left
Talofibular ligament	Ankle Bursa and Ligament, Right
	Ankle Bursa and Ligament, Left
Talus bone	Tarsal, Right
	Tarsal, Left
Tarsometatarsal ligament	Foot Bursa and Ligament, Right
	Foot Bursa and Ligament, Left
Temporal lobe	Cerebral Hemisphere
Temporalis muscle	Head Muscle
Temporoparietalis muscle	Head Muscle
Tensor fasciae latae muscle	Hip Muscle, Right
	Hip Muscle, Left
Tensor veli palatini muscle	Tongue, Palate, Pharynx Muscle
Tenth cranial nerve	Vagus Nerve
Tentorium cerebelli	Dura Mater
Teres major muscle	Shoulder Muscle, Right
	Shoulder Muscle, Left
Teres minor muscle	Shoulder Muscle, Right
	Shoulder Muscle, Left
Testicular artery	Abdominal Aorta
Thenar muscle	Hand Muscle, Right
	Hand Muscle, Left
Third cranial nerve	Oculomotor Nerve
Third occipital nerve	Cervical Nerve
Third ventricle	Cerebral Ventricle
Thoracic aortic plexus	Thoracic Sympathetic Nerve
Thoracic esophagus	Esophagus, Middle
Thoracic facet joint	Thoracic Vertebral Joint
Thoracic ganglion	Thoracic Sympathetic Nerve
Thoracoacromial artery	Axillary Artery, Right
	Axillary Artery, Left
Thoracolumbar facet joint	Thoracolumbar Vertebral Joint
Thymus gland	Thymus
Thyroarytenoid muscle	Neck Muscle, Right
	Neck Muscle, Left
Thyrocervical trunk	Thyroid Artery, Right
	Thyroid Artery, Left
Thyroid cartilage	Larynx
Tibial sesamoid	Metatarsal, Right
	Metatarsal, Left
Tibialis anterior muscle	Lower Leg Muscle, Right
	Lower Leg Muscle, Left
Tibialis posterior muscle	Lower Leg Muscle, Right
	Lower Leg Muscle, Left
Tibiofemoral joint	Knee Joint, Right
	Knee Joint, Left
	Knee Joint, Tibial Surface, Right
	Knee Joint, Tibial Surface, Left

Term	ICD-10-PCS Value
Tibioperoneal trunk	Popliteal Artery, Right
	Popliteal Artery, Left
Tongue, base of	Pharynx
Tracheobronchial lymph node	Lymphatic, Thorax
Tragus	External Ear, Right
	External Ear, Left
	External Ear, Bilateral
Transversalis fascia	Subcutaneous Tissue and Fascia, Trunk
Transverse acetabular ligament	Hip Bursa and Ligament, Right
	Hip Bursa and Ligament, Left
Transverse (cutaneous) cervical nerve	Cervical Plexus
Transverse facial artery	Temporal Artery, Right
	Temporal Artery, Left
Transverse foramen	Cervical Vertebra
Transverse humeral ligament	Shoulder Bursa and Ligament, Right
	Shoulder Bursa and Ligament, Left
Transverse ligament of atlas	Head and Neck Bursa and Ligament
Transverse process	Cervical Vertebra
	Thoracic Vertebra
	Lumbar Vertebra
Transverse scapular ligament	Shoulder Bursa and Ligament, Right
	Shoulder Bursa and Ligament, Left
Transverse thoracis muscle	Thorax Muscle, Right
	Thorax Muscle, Left
Transversospinalis muscle	Trunk Muscle, Right
	Trunk Muscle, Left
Transversus abdominis muscle	Abdomen Muscle, Right
	Abdomen Muscle, Left
Trapezium bone	Carpal, Right
	Carpal, Left
Trapezius muscle	Trunk Muscle, Right
	Trunk Muscle, Left
Trapezoid bone	Carpal, Right
	Carpal, Left
Triceps brachii muscle	Upper Arm Muscle, Right
	Upper Arm Muscle, Left
Tricuspid annulus	Tricuspid Valve
Trifacial nerve	Trigeminal Nerve
Trigone of bladder	Bladder
Triquetral bone	Carpal, Right
	Carpal, Left
Trochanteric bursa	Hip Bursa and Ligament, Right
	Hip Bursa and Ligament, Left
Twelfth cranial nerve	Hypoglossal Nerve
Tympanic cavity	Middle Ear, Right
	Middle Ear, Left
Tympanic nerve	Glossopharyngeal Nerve
Tympanic part of temoporal bone	Temporal Bone, Right
	Temporal Bone, Left
Ulnar collateral carpal ligament	Wrist Bursa and Ligament, Right
	Wrist Bursa and Ligament, Left
Ulnar collateral ligament	Elbow Bursa and Ligament, Right
	Elbow Bursa and Ligament, Left
Ulnar notch	Radius, Right
	Radius, Left

Term	ICD-10-PCS Value
Ulnar vein	Brachial Vein, Right
	Brachial Vein, Left
Umbilical artery	Internal Iliac Artery, Right
	Internal Iliac Artery, Left
	Lower Artery
Ureteral orifice	Ureter, Right
	Ureter, Left
	Ureters, Bilateral
	Ureter
Ureteropelvic junction (UPJ)	Kidney Pelvis, Right
	Kidney Pelvis, Left
Ureterovesical orifice	Ureter, Right
	Ureter, Left
	Ureters, Bilateral
	Ureter
Uterine artery	Internal Iliac Artery, Right
	Internal Iliac Artery, Left
Uterine cornu	Uterus
Uterine tube	Fallopian Tube, Right
	Fallopian Tube, Left
Uterine vein	Hypogastric Vein, Right
	Hypogastric Vein, Left
Vaginal artery	Internal Iliac Artery, Right
	Internal Iliac Artery, Left
Vaginal vein	Hypogastric Vein, Right
	Hypogastric Vein, Left
Vastus intermedius muscle	Upper Leg Muscle, Right
	Upper Leg Muscle, Left
Vastus lateralis muscle	Upper Leg Muscle, Right
	Upper Leg Muscle, Left
Vastus medialis muscle	Upper Leg Muscle, Right
	Upper Leg Muscle, Left
Ventricular fold	Larynx
Vermiform appendix	Appendix
Vermilion border	Upper Lip
	Lower Lip
Vertebral arch	Cervical Vertebra
	Lumbar Vertebra
	Thoracic Vertebra
Vertebral body	Cervical Vertebra
	Lumbar Vertebra
	Thoracic Vertebra
Vertebral canal	Spinal Canal
Vertebral foramen	Cervical Vertebra
	Lumbar Vertebra
	Thoracic Vertebra
Vertebral lamina	Cervical Vertebra
	Lumbar Vertebra
	Thoracic Vertebra
Vertebral pedicle	Cervical Vertebra
	Lumbar Vertebra
	Thoracic Vertebra
Vesical vein	Hypogastric Vein, Right
	Hypogastric Vein, Left
Vestibular (Scarpa's) ganglion	Acoustic Nerve
Vestibular nerve	Acoustic Nerve
Vestibulocochlear nerve	Acoustic Nerve

Term	ICD-10-PCS Value
Virchow's (supraclavicular) lymph node	Lymphatic, Right Neck
	Lymphatic, Left Neck
Vitreous body	Vitreous, Right
	Vitreous, Left
Vocal fold	Vocal Cord, Right
	Vocal Cord, Left
Volar (palmar) digital vein	Hand Vein, Right
	Hand Vein, Left
Volar (palmar) metacarpal vein	Hand Vein, Right
	Hand Vein, Left
Vomer bone	Nasal Septum
Vomer of nasal septum	Nasal Bone
Xiphoid process	Sternum
Zonule of Zinn	Lens, Right
	Lens, Left
Zygomatic process of frontal bone	Frontal Bone
Zygomatic process of temporal bone	Temporal Bone, Right
	Temporal Bone, Left
Zygomaticus muscle	Facial Muscle

Appendix E: Body Part Definitions

ICD-10-PCS Value	Definition
1st Toe, Left 1st Toe, Right	**Includes:** Hallux
Abdomen Muscle, Left Abdomen Muscle, Right	**Includes:** External oblique muscle Internal oblique muscle Pyramidalis muscle Rectus abdominis muscle Transversus abdominis muscle
Abdominal Aorta	**Includes:** Inferior phrenic artery Lumbar artery Median sacral artery Middle suprarenal artery Ovarian artery Testicular artery
Abdominal Sympathetic Nerve	**Includes:** Abdominal aortic plexus Auerbach's (myenteric) plexus Celiac (solar) plexus Celiac ganglion Gastric plexus Hepatic plexus Inferior hypogastric plexus Inferior mesenteric ganglion Inferior mesenteric plexus Meissner's (submucous) plexus Myenteric (Auerbach's) plexus Pancreatic plexus Pelvic splanchnic nerve Renal nerve Renal plexus Solar (celiac) plexus Splenic plexus Submucous (Meissner's) plexus Superior hypogastric plexus Superior mesenteric ganglion Superior mesenteric plexus Suprarenal plexus
Abducens Nerve	**Includes:** Sixth cranial nerve
Accessory Nerve	**Includes:** Eleventh cranial nerve
Acoustic Nerve	**Includes:** Cochlear nerve Eighth cranial nerve Scarpa's (vestibular) ganglion Spiral ganglion Vestibular (Scarpa's) ganglion Vestibular nerve Vestibulocochlear nerve
Adenoids	**Includes:** Pharyngeal tonsil
Adrenal Gland Adrenal Gland, Left Adrenal Gland, Right Adrenal Glands, Bilateral	**Includes:** Suprarenal gland
Ampulla of Vater	**Includes:** Duodenal ampulla Hepatopancreatic ampulla
Anal Sphincter	**Includes:** External anal sphincter Internal anal sphincter

ICD-10-PCS Value	Definition
Ankle Bursa and Ligament, Left Ankle Bursa and Ligament, Right	**Includes:** Calcaneofibular ligament Deltoid ligament Ligament of the lateral malleolus Talofibular ligament
Ankle Joint, Left Ankle Joint, Right	**Includes:** Inferior tibiofibular joint Talocrural joint
Anterior Chamber, Left Anterior Chamber, Right	**Includes:** Aqueous humour
Anterior Tibial Artery, Left Anterior Tibial Artery, Right	**Includes:** Anterior lateral malleolar artery Anterior medial malleolar artery Anterior tibial recurrent artery Dorsalis pedis artery Posterior tibial recurrent artery
Anus	**Includes:** Anal orifice
Aortic Valve	**Includes:** Aortic annulus
Appendix	**Includes:** Vermiform appendix
Atrial Septum	**Includes:** Interatrial septum
Atrium, Left	**Includes:** Atrium pulmonale Left auricular appendix
Atrium, Right	**Includes:** Atrium dextrum cordis Right auricular appendix Sinus venosus
Auditory Ossicle, Left Auditory Ossicle, Right	**Includes:** Incus Malleus Stapes
Axillary Artery, Left Axillary Artery, Right	**Includes:** Anterior circumflex humeral artery Lateral thoracic artery Posterior circumflex humeral artery Subscapular artery Superior thoracic artery Thoracoacromial artery
Azygos Vein	**Includes:** Right ascending lumbar vein Right subcostal vein
Basal Ganglia	**Includes:** Basal nuclei Claustrum Corpus striatum Globus pallidus Substantia nigra Subthalamic nucleus
Basilic Vein, Left Basilic Vein, Right	**Includes:** Median antebrachial vein Median cubital vein
Bladder	**Includes:** Trigone of bladder
Brachial Artery, Left Brachial Artery, Right	**Includes:** Inferior ulnar collateral artery Profunda brachii Superior ulnar collateral artery

Appendix E: Body Part Definitions

ICD-10-PCS Value	Definition
Brachial Plexus	**Includes:** Axillary nerve Dorsal scapular nerve First intercostal nerve Long thoracic nerve Musculocutaneous nerve Subclavius nerve Suprascapular nerve
Brachial Vein, Left Brachial Vein, Right	**Includes:** Radial vein Ulnar vein
Brain	**Includes:** Cerebrum Corpus callosum Encephalon
Breast, Bilateral Breast, Left Breast, Right	**Includes:** Mammary duct Mammary gland
Buccal Mucosa	**Includes:** Buccal gland Molar gland Palatine gland
Carotid Bodies, Bilateral Carotid Body, Left Carotid Body, Right	**Includes:** Carotid glomus
Carpal Joint, Left Carpal Joint, Right	**Includes:** Intercarpal joint Midcarpal joint
Carpal, Left Carpal, Right	**Includes:** Capitate bone Hamate bone Lunate bone Pisiform bone Scaphoid bone Trapezium bone Trapezoid bone Triquetral bone
Celiac Artery	**Includes:** Celiac trunk
Cephalic Vein, Left Cephalic Vein, Right	**Includes:** Accessory cephalic vein
Cerebellum	**Includes:** Culmen
Cerebral Hemisphere	**Includes:** Frontal lobe Occipital lobe Parietal lobe Temporal lobe
Cerebral Meninges	**Includes:** Arachnoid mater, intracranial Leptomeninges, intracranial Pia mater, intracranial
Cerebral Ventricle	**Includes:** Aqueduct of Sylvius Cerebral aqueduct (Sylvius) Choroid plexus Ependyma Foramen of Monro (intraventricular) Fourth ventricle Interventricular foramen (Monro) Left lateral ventricle Right lateral ventricle Third ventricle
Cervical Nerve	**Includes:** Greater occipital nerve Spinal nerve, cervical Suboccipital nerve Third occipital nerve

ICD-10-PCS Value	Definition
Cervical Plexus	**Includes:** Ansa cervicalis Cutaneous (transverse) cervical nerve Great auricular nerve Lesser occipital nerve Supraclavicular nerve Transverse (cutaneous) cervical nerve
Cervical Spinal Cord	**Includes:** Dorsal root ganglion
Cervical Vertebra	**Includes:** Dens Odontoid process Spinous process Transverse foramen Transverse process Vertebral arch Vertebral body Vertebral foramen Vertebral lamina Vertebral pedicle
Cervical Vertebral Joint	**Includes:** Atlantoaxial joint Cervical facet joint
Cervical Vertebral Joints, 2 or more	**Includes:** Cervical facet joint
Cervicothoracic Vertebral Joint	**Includes:** Cervicothoracic facet joint
Cisterna Chyli	**Includes:** Intestinal lymphatic trunk Lumbar lymphatic trunk
Coccygeal Glomus	**Includes:** Coccygeal body
Colic Vein	**Includes:** Ileocolic vein Left colic vein Middle colic vein Right colic vein
Conduction Mechanism	**Includes:** Atrioventricular node Bundle of His Bundle of Kent Sinoatrial node
Conjunctiva, Left Conjunctiva, Right	**Includes:** Plica semilunaris
Dura Mater	**Includes:** Diaphragma sellae Dura mater, intracranial Falx cerebri Tentorium cerebelli
Elbow Bursa and Ligament, Left Elbow Bursa and Ligament, Right	**Includes:** Annular ligament Olecranon bursa Radial collateral ligament Ulnar collateral ligament
Elbow Joint, Left Elbow Joint, Right	**Includes:** Distal humerus, involving joint Humeroradial joint Humeroulnar joint Proximal radioulnar joint
Epidural Space, Intracranial	**Includes:** Extradural space, intracranial
Epiglottis	**Includes:** Glossoepiglottic fold
Esophagogastric Junction	**Includes:** Cardia Cardioesophageal junction Gastroesophageal (GE) junction

ICD-10-PCS Value	Definition
Esophagus, Lower	**Includes:** Abdominal esophagus
Esophagus, Middle	**Includes:** Thoracic esophagus
Esophagus, Upper	**Includes:** Cervical esophagus
Ethmoid Bone, Left Ethmoid Bone, Right	**Includes:** Cribriform plate
Ethmoid Sinus, Left Ethmoid Sinus, Right	**Includes:** Ethmoidal air cell
Eustachian Tube, Left Eustachian Tube, Right	**Includes:** Auditory tube Pharyngotympanic tube
External Auditory Canal, Left External Auditory Canal, Right	**Includes:** External auditory meatus
External Carotid Artery, Left External Carotid Artery, Right	**Includes:** Ascending pharyngeal artery Internal maxillary artery Lingual artery Maxillary artery Occipital artery Posterior auricular artery Superior thyroid artery
External Ear, Bilateral External Ear, Left External Ear, Right	**Includes:** Antihelix Antitragus Auricle Earlobe Helix Pinna Tragus
External Iliac Artery, Left External Iliac Artery, Right	**Includes:** Deep circumflex iliac artery Inferior epigastric artery
External Jugular Vein, Left External Jugular Vein, Right	**Includes:** Posterior auricular vein
Extraocular Muscle, Left Extraocular Muscle, Right	**Includes:** Inferior oblique muscle Inferior rectus muscle Lateral rectus muscle Medial rectus muscle Superior oblique muscle Superior rectus muscle
Eye, Left Eye, Right	**Includes:** Ciliary body Posterior chamber
Face Artery	**Includes:** Angular artery Ascending palatine artery External maxillary artery Facial artery Inferior labial artery Submental artery Superior labial artery
Face Vein, Left Face Vein, Right	**Includes:** Angular vein Anterior facial vein Common facial vein Deep facial vein Frontal vein Posterior facial (retromandibular) vein Supraorbital vein

ICD-10-PCS Value	Definition
Facial Muscle	**Includes:** Buccinator muscle Corrugator supercilii muscle Depressor anguli oris muscle Depressor labii inferioris muscle Depressor septi nasi muscle Depressor supercilii muscle Levator anguli oris muscle Levator labii superioris alaeque nasi muscle Levator labii superioris muscle Mentalis muscle Nasalis muscle Occipitofrontalis muscle Orbicularis oris muscle Procerus muscle Risorius muscle Zygomaticus muscle
Facial Nerve	**Includes:** Chorda tympani Geniculate ganglion Greater superficial petrosal nerve Nerve to the stapedius Parotid plexus Posterior auricular nerve Seventh cranial nerve Submandibular ganglion
Fallopian Tube, Left Fallopian Tube, Right	**Includes:** Oviduct Salpinx Uterine tube
Femoral Artery, Left Femoral Artery, Right	**Includes:** Circumflex iliac artery Deep femoral artery Descending genicular artery External pudendal artery Superficial epigastric artery
Femoral Nerve	**Includes:** Anterior crural nerve Saphenous nerve
Femoral Shaft, Left Femoral Shaft, Right	**Includes:** Body of femur
Femoral Vein, Left Femoral Vein, Right	**Includes:** Deep femoral (profunda femoris) vein Popliteal vein Profunda femoris (deep femoral) vein
Fibula, Left Fibula, Right	**Includes:** Body of fibula Head of fibula Lateral malleolus
Finger Nail	**Includes:** Nail bed Nail plate
Finger Phalangeal Joint, Left Finger Phalangeal Joint, Right	**Includes:** Interphalangeal (IP) joint
Foot Artery, Left Foot Artery, Right	**Includes:** Arcuate artery Dorsal metatarsal artery Lateral plantar artery Lateral tarsal artery Medial plantar artery

ICD-10-PCS Value	Definition
Foot Bursa and Ligament, Left **Foot Bursa and Ligament, Right**	**Includes:** Calcaneocuboid ligament Cuneonavicular ligament Intercuneiform ligament Interphalangeal ligament Metatarsal ligament Metatarsophalangeal ligament Subtalar ligament Talocalcaneal ligament Talocalcaneonavicular ligament Tarsometatarsal ligament
Foot Muscle, Left **Foot Muscle, Right**	**Includes:** Abductor hallucis muscle Adductor hallucis muscle Extensor digitorum brevis muscle Extensor hallucis brevis muscle Flexor digitorum brevis muscle Flexor hallucis brevis muscle Quadratus plantae muscle
Foot Vein, Left **Foot Vein, Right**	**Includes:** Common digital vein Dorsal metatarsal vein Dorsal venous arch Plantar digital vein Plantar metatarsal vein Plantar venous arch
Frontal Bone	**Includes:** Zygomatic process of frontal bone
Gastric Artery	**Includes:** Left gastric artery Right gastric artery
Glenoid Cavity, Left **Glenoid Cavity, Right**	**Includes:** Glenoid fossa (of scapula)
Glomus Jugulare	**Includes:** Jugular body
Glossopharyngeal Nerve	**Includes:** Carotid sinus nerve Ninth cranial nerve Tympanic nerve
Hand Artery, Left **Hand Artery, Right**	**Includes:** Deep palmar arch Princeps pollicis artery Radialis indicis Superficial palmar arch
Hand Bursa and Ligament, Left **Hand Bursa and Ligament, Right**	**Includes:** Carpometacarpal ligament Intercarpal ligament Interphalangeal ligament Lunotriquetral ligament Metacarpal ligament Metacarpophalangeal ligament Pisohamate ligament Pisometacarpal ligament Scaphotrapezium ligament
Hand Muscle, Left **Hand Muscle, Right**	**Includes:** Hypothenar muscle Palmar interosseous muscle Thenar muscle
Hand Vein, Left **Hand Vein, Right**	**Includes:** Dorsal metacarpal vein Palmar (volar) digital vein Palmar (volar) metacarpal vein Superficial palmar venous arch Volar (palmar) digital vein Volar (palmar) metacarpal vein

ICD-10-PCS Value	Definition
Head and Neck Bursa and Ligament	**Includes:** Alar ligament of axis Cervical interspinous ligament Cervical intertransverse ligament Cervical ligamentum flavum Interspinous ligament, cervical Intertransverse ligament, cervical Lateral temporomandibular ligament Ligamentum flavum, cervical Sphenomandibular ligament Stylomandibular ligament Transverse ligament of atlas
Head and Neck Sympathetic Nerve	**Includes:** Cavernous plexus Cervical ganglion Ciliary ganglion Internal carotid plexus Otic ganglion Pterygopalatine (sphenopalatine) ganglion Sphenopalatine (pterygopalatine) ganglion Stellate ganglion Submandibular ganglion Submaxillary ganglion
Head Muscle	**Includes:** Auricularis muscle Masseter muscle Pterygoid muscle Splenius capitis muscle Temporalis muscle Temporoparietalis muscle
Heart, Left	**Includes:** Left coronary sulcus Obtuse margin
Heart, Right	**Includes:** Right coronary sulcus
Hemiazygos Vein	**Includes:** Left ascending lumbar vein Left subcostal vein
Hepatic Artery	**Includes:** Common hepatic artery Gastroduodenal artery Hepatic artery proper
Hip Bursa and Ligament, Left **Hip Bursa and Ligament, Right**	**Includes:** Iliofemoral ligament Ischiofemoral ligament Pubofemoral ligament Transverse acetabular ligament Trochanteric bursa
Hip Joint, Left **Hip Joint, Right**	**Includes:** Acetabulofemoral joint
Hip Muscle, Left **Hip Muscle, Right**	**Includes:** Gemellus muscle Gluteus maximus muscle Gluteus medius muscle Gluteus minimus muscle Iliacus muscle Obturator muscle Piriformis muscle Psoas muscle Quadratus femoris muscle Tensor fasciae latae muscle
Humeral Head, Left **Humeral Head, Right**	**Includes:** Greater tuberosity Lesser tuberosity Neck of humerus (anatomical)(surgical)

ICD-10-PCS Value	Definition
Humeral Shaft, Left Humeral Shaft, Right	**Includes:** Distal humerus Humerus, distal Lateral epicondyle of humerus Medial epicondyle of humerus
Hypogastric Vein, Left Hypogastric Vein, Right	**Includes:** Gluteal vein Internal iliac vein Internal pudendal vein Lateral sacral vein Middle hemorrhoidal vein Obturator vein Uterine vein Vaginal vein Vesical vein
Hypoglossal Nerve	**Includes:** Twelfth cranial nerve
Hypothalamus	**Includes:** Mammillary body
Inferior Mesenteric Artery	**Includes:** Sigmoid artery Superior rectal artery
Inferior Mesenteric Vein	**Includes:** Sigmoid vein Superior rectal vein
Inferior Vena Cava	**Includes:** Postcava Right inferior phrenic vein Right ovarian vein Right second lumbar vein Right suprarenal vein Right testicular vein
Inguinal Region, Bilateral Inguinal Region, Left Inguinal Region, Right	**Includes:** Inguinal canal Inguinal triangle
Inner Ear, Left Inner Ear, Right	**Includes:** Bony labyrinth Bony vestibule Cochlea Round window Semicircular canal
Innominate Artery	**Includes:** Brachiocephalic artery Brachiocephalic trunk
Innominate Vein, Left Innominate Vein, Right	**Includes:** Brachiocephalic vein Inferior thyroid vein
Internal Carotid Artery, Left Internal Carotid Artery, Right	**Includes:** Caroticotympanic artery Carotid sinus
Internal Iliac Artery, Left Internal Iliac Artery, Right	**Includes:** Deferential artery Hypogastric artery Iliolumbar artery Inferior gluteal artery Inferior vesical artery Internal pudendal artery Lateral sacral artery Middle rectal artery Obturator artery Prostatic artery Superior gluteal artery Superior vesical artery Umbilical artery Uterine artery Vaginal artery

ICD-10-PCS Value	Definition
Internal Mammary Artery, Left Internal Mammary Artery, Right	**Includes:** Anterior intercostal artery Internal thoracic artery Musculophrenic artery Pericardiophrenic artery Superior epigastric artery
Intracranial Artery	**Includes:** Anterior cerebral artery Anterior choroidal artery Anterior communicating artery Basilar artery Circle of Willis Internal carotid artery, intracranial portion Middle cerebral artery Ophthalmic artery Posterior cerebral artery Posterior communicating artery Posterior inferior cerebellar artery (PICA)
Intracranial Vein	**Includes:** Anterior cerebral vein Basal (internal) cerebral vein Dural venous sinus Great cerebral vein Inferior cerebellar vein Inferior cerebral vein Internal (basal) cerebral vein Middle cerebral vein Ophthalmic vein Superior cerebellar vein Superior cerebral vein
Jejunum	**Includes:** Duodenojejunal flexure
Kidney	**Includes:** Renal calyx Renal capsule Renal cortex Renal segment
Kidney Pelvis, Left Kidney Pelvis, Right	**Includes:** Ureteropelvic junction (UPJ)
Kidney, Left Kidney, Right Kidneys, Bilateral	**Includes:** Renal calyx Renal capsule Renal cortex Renal segment
Knee Bursa and Ligament, Left Knee Bursa and Ligament, Right	**Includes:** Anterior cruciate ligament (ACL) Lateral collateral ligament (LCL) Ligament of head of fibula Medial collateral ligament (MCL) Patellar ligament Popliteal ligament Posterior cruciate ligament (PCL) Prepatellar bursa
Knee Joint, Femoral Surface, Left Knee Joint, Femoral Surface, Right	**Includes:** Femoropatellar joint Patellofemoral joint
Knee Joint, Left Knee Joint, Right	**Includes:** Femoropatellar joint Femorotibial joint Lateral meniscus Medial meniscus Patellofemoral joint Tibiofemoral joint
Knee Joint, Tibial Surface, Left Knee Joint, Tibial Surface, Right	**Includes:** Femorotibial joint Tibiofemoral joint
Knee Tendon, Left Knee Tendon, Right	**Includes:** Patellar tendon

ICD-10-PCS Value	Definition
Lacrimal Duct, Left **Lacrimal Duct, Right**	**Includes:** Lacrimal canaliculus Lacrimal punctum Lacrimal sac Nasolacrimal duct
Larynx	**Includes:** Aryepiglottic fold Arytenoid cartilage Corniculate cartilage Cuneiform cartilage False vocal cord Glottis Rima glottidis Thyroid cartilage Ventricular fold
Lens, Left **Lens, Right**	**Includes:** Zonule of Zinn
Liver	**Includes:** Quadrate lobe
Lower Arm and Wrist Muscle, Left **Lower Arm and Wrist Muscle, Right**	**Includes:** Anatomical snuffbox Brachioradialis muscle Extensor carpi radialis muscle Extensor carpi ulnaris muscle Flexor carpi radialis muscle Flexor carpi ulnaris muscle Flexor pollicis longus muscle Palmaris longus muscle Pronator quadratus muscle Pronator teres muscle
Lower Artery	**Includes:** Umbilical artery
Lower Eyelid, Left **Lower Eyelid, Right**	**Includes:** Inferior tarsal plate Medial canthus
Lower Femur, Left **Lower Femur, Right**	**Includes:** Lateral condyle of femur Lateral epicondyle of femur Medial condyle of femur Medial epicondyle of femur
Lower Leg Muscle, Left **Lower Leg Muscle, Right**	**Includes:** Extensor digitorum longus muscle Extensor hallucis longus muscle Fibularis brevis muscle Fibularis longus muscle Flexor digitorum longus muscle Flexor hallucis longus muscle Gastrocnemius muscle Peroneus brevis muscle Peroneus longus muscle Popliteus muscle Soleus muscle Tibialis anterior muscle Tibialis posterior muscle
Lower Leg Tendon, Left **Lower Leg Tendon, Right**	**Includes:** Achilles tendon
Lower Lip	**Includes:** Frenulum labii inferioris Labial gland Vermilion border

ICD-10-PCS Value	Definition
Lower Spine Bursa and Ligament	**Includes:** Iliolumbar ligament Interspinous ligament, lumbar Intertransverse ligament, lumbar Ligamentum flavum, lumbar Sacrococcygeal ligament Sacroiliac ligament Sacrospinous ligament Sacrotuberous ligament Supraspinous ligament
Lumbar Nerve	**Includes:** Lumbosacral trunk Spinal nerve, lumbar Superior clunic (cluneal) nerve
Lumbar Plexus	**Includes:** Accessory obturator nerve Genitofemoral nerve Iliohypogastric nerve Ilioinguinal nerve Lateral femoral cutaneous nerve Obturator nerve Superior gluteal nerve
Lumbar Spinal Cord	**Includes:** Cauda equina Conus medullaris Dorsal root ganglion
Lumbar Sympathetic Nerve	**Includes:** Lumbar ganglion Lumbar splanchnic nerve
Lumbar Vertebra	**Includes:** Spinous process Transverse process Vertebral arch Vertebral body Vertebral foramen Vertebral lamina Vertebral pedicle
Lumbar Vertebral Joint	**Includes:** Lumbar facet joint
Lumbosacral Joint	**Includes:** Lumbosacral facet joint
Lymphatic, Aortic	**Includes:** Celiac lymph node Gastric lymph node Hepatic lymph node Lumbar lymph node Pancreaticosplenic lymph node Paraaortic lymph node Retroperitoneal lymph node
Lymphatic, Head	**Includes:** Buccinator lymph node Infraauricular lymph node Infraparotid lymph node Parotid lymph node Preauricular lymph node Submandibular lymph node Submaxillary lymph node Submental lymph node Subparotid lymph node Suprahyoid lymph node
Lymphatic, Left Axillary	**Includes:** Anterior (pectoral) lymph node Apical (subclavicular) lymph node Brachial (lateral) lymph node Central axillary lymph node Lateral (brachial) lymph node Pectoral (anterior) lymph node Posterior (subscapular) lymph node Subclavicular (apical) lymph node Subscapular (posterior) lymph node

ICD-10-PCS Value	Definition
Lymphatic, Left Lower Extremity	**Includes:** Femoral lymph node Popliteal lymph node
Lymphatic, Left Neck	**Includes:** Cervical lymph node Jugular lymph node Mastoid (postauricular) lymph node Occipital lymph node Postauricular (mastoid) lymph node Retropharyngeal lymph node Supraclavicular (Virchow's) lymph node Virchow's (supraclavicular) lymph node
Lymphatic, Left Upper Extremity	**Includes:** Cubital lymph node Deltopectoral (infraclavicular) lymph node Epitrochlear lymph node Infraclavicular (deltopectoral) lymph node Supratrochlear lymph node
Lymphatic, Mesenteric	**Includes:** Inferior mesenteric lymph node Pararectal lymph node Superior mesenteric lymph node
Lymphatic, Pelvis	**Includes:** Common iliac (subaortic) lymph node Gluteal lymph node Iliac lymph node Inferior epigastric lymph node Obturator lymph node Sacral lymph node Subaortic (common iliac) lymph node Suprainguinal lymph node
Lymphatic, Right Axillary	**Includes:** Anterior (pectoral) lymph node Apical (subclavicular) lymph node Brachial (lateral) lymph node Central axillary lymph node Lateral (brachial) lymph node Pectoral (anterior) lymph node Posterior (subscapular) lymph node Subclavicular (apical) lymph node Subscapular (posterior) lymph node
Lymphatic, Right Lower Extremity	**Includes:** Femoral lymph node Popliteal lymph node
Lymphatic, Right Neck	**Includes:** Cervical lymph node Jugular lymph node Mastoid (postauricular) lymph node Occipital lymph node Postauricular (mastoid) lymph node Retropharyngeal lymph node Right jugular trunk Right lymphatic duct Right subclavian trunk Supraclavicular (Virchow's) lymph node Virchow's (supraclavicular) lymph node
Lymphatic, Right Upper Extremity	**Includes:** Cubital lymph node Deltopectoral (infraclavicular) lymph node Epitrochlear lymph node Infraclavicular (deltopectoral) lymph node Supratrochlear lymph node
Lymphatic, Thorax	**Includes:** Intercostal lymph node Mediastinal lymph node Parasternal lymph node Paratracheal lymph node Tracheobronchial lymph node

ICD-10-PCS Value	Definition
Main Bronchus, Right	**Includes:** Bronchus intermedius Intermediate bronchus
Mandible, Left Mandible, Right	**Includes:** Alveolar process of mandible Condyloid process Mandibular notch Mental foramen
Mastoid Sinus, Left Mastoid Sinus, Right	**Includes:** Mastoid air cells
Metatarsal, Left Metatarsal, Right	**Includes:** Fibular sesamoid Tibial sesamoid
Maxilla	**Includes:** Alveolar process of maxilla
Maxillary Sinus, Left Maxillary Sinus, Right	**Includes:** Antrum of Highmore
Median Nerve	**Includes:** Anterior interosseous nerve Palmar cutaneous nerve
Mediastinum	**Includes:** Mediastinal cavity Mediastinal space
Medulla Oblongata	**Includes:** Myelencephalon
Mesentery	**Includes:** Mesoappendix Mesocolon
Metatarsal, Right Metatarsal, Left	**Includes:** Fibular sesamoid Tibial sesamoid
Metatarsal-Phalangeal Joint, Left Metatarsal-Phalangeal Joint, Right	**Includes:** Metatarsophalangeal (MTP) joint
Middle Ear, Left Middle Ear, Right	**Includes:** Oval window Tympanic cavity
Minor Salivary Gland	**Includes:** Anterior lingual gland
Mitral Valve	**Includes:** Bicuspid valve Left atrioventricular valve Mitral annulus
Nasal Bone	**Includes:** Vomer of nasal septum
Nasal Mucosa and Soft Tissue	**Includes:** Columella External naris Greater alar cartilage Internal naris Lateral nasal cartilage Lesser alar cartilage Nasal cavity Nostril
Nasal Septum	**Includes:** Quadrangular cartilage Septal cartilage Vomer bone
Nasal Turbinate	**Includes:** Inferior turbinate Middle turbinate Nasal concha Superior turbinate

Appendix E: Body Part Definitions

ICD-10-PCS Value	Definition
Nasopharynx	**Includes:** Choana Fossa of Rosenmuller Pharyngeal recess Rhinopharynx
Neck	**Includes:** Parapharyngeal space Retropharyngeal space
Neck Muscle, Left Neck Muscle, Right	**Includes:** Anterior vertebral muscle Arytenoid muscle Cricothyroid muscle Infrahyoid muscle Levator scapulae muscle Platysma muscle Scalene muscle Splenius cervicis muscle Sternocleidomastoid muscle Suprahyoid muscle Thyroarytenoid muscle
Nipple, Left Nipple, Right	**Includes:** Areola
Occipital Bone	**Includes:** Foramen magnum
Oculomotor Nerve	**Includes:** Third cranial nerve
Olfactory Nerve	**Includes:** First cranial nerve Olfactory bulb
Omentum	**Includes:** Gastrocolic ligament Gastrocolic omentum Gastrohepatic omentum Gastrophrenic ligament Gastrosplenic ligament Greater Omentum Hepatogastric ligament Lesser Omentum
Optic Nerve	**Includes:** Optic chiasma Second cranial nerve
Orbit, Left Orbit, Right	**Includes:** Bony orbit Orbital portion of ethmoid bone Orbital portion of frontal bone Orbital portion of lacrimal bone Orbital portion of maxilla Orbital portion of palatine bone Orbital portion of sphenoid bone Orbital portion of zygomatic bone
Pancreatic Duct	**Includes:** Duct of Wirsung
Pancreatic Duct, Accessory	**Includes:** Duct of Santorini
Parotid Duct, Left Parotid Duct, Right	**Includes:** Stensen's duct
Pelvic Bone, Left Pelvic Bone, Right	**Includes:** Iliac crest Ilium Ischium Pubis
Pelvic Cavity	**Includes:** Retropubic space
Penis	**Includes:** Corpus cavernosum Corpus spongiosum

ICD-10-PCS Value	Definition
Perineum Muscle	**Includes:** Bulbospongiosus muscle Cremaster muscle Deep transverse perineal muscle Ischiocavernosus muscle Levator ani muscle Superficial transverse perineal muscle
Peritoneal Cavity	**Includes:** Abdominal cavity
Peritoneum	**Includes:** Epiploic foramen
Peroneal Artery, Left Peroneal Artery, Right	**Includes:** Fibular artery
Peroneal Nerve	**Includes:** Common fibular nerve Common peroneal nerve External popliteal nerve Lateral sural cutaneous nerve
Pharynx	**Includes:** Base of Tongue Hypopharynx Laryngopharynx Lingual tonsil Oropharynx Piriform recess (sinus) Tongue, base of
Phrenic Nerve	**Includes:** Accessory phrenic nerve
Pituitary Gland	**Includes:** Adenohypophysis Hypophysis Neurohypophysis
Pons	**Includes:** Apneustic center Basis pontis Locus ceruleus Pneumotaxic center Pontine tegmentum Superior olivary nucleus
Popliteal Artery, Left Popliteal Artery, Right	**Includes:** Inferior genicular artery Middle genicular artery Superior genicular artery Sural artery Tibioperoneal trunk
Portal Vein	**Includes:** Hepatic portal vein
Prepuce	**Includes:** Foreskin Glans penis
Pudendal Nerve	**Includes:** Posterior labial nerve Posterior scrotal nerve
Pulmonary Artery, Left	**Includes:** Arterial canal (duct) Botallo's duct Pulmoaortic canal
Pulmonary Valve	**Includes:** Pulmonary annulus Pulmonic valve
Pulmonary Vein, Left	**Includes:** Left inferior pulmonary vein Left superior pulmonary vein
Pulmonary Vein, Right	**Includes:** Right inferior pulmonary vein Right superior pulmonary vein
Radial Artery, Left Radial Artery, Right	**Includes:** Radial recurrent artery

ICD-10-PCS Value	Definition
Radial Nerve	**Includes:** Dorsal digital nerve Musculospiral nerve Palmar cutaneous nerve Posterior interosseous nerve
Radius, Left Radius, Right	**Includes:** Ulnar notch
Rectum	**Includes:** Anorectal junction
Renal Artery, Left Renal Artery, Right	**Includes:** Inferior suprarenal artery Renal segmental artery
Renal Vein, Left	**Includes:** Left inferior phrenic vein Left ovarian vein Left second lumbar vein Left suprarenal vein Left testicular vein
Retina, Left Retina, Right	**Includes:** Fovea Macula Optic disc
Retroperitoneum	**Includes:** Retroperitoneal cavity Retroperitoneal space
Rib(s) Bursa and Ligament	**Includes:** Costotransverse ligament
Sacral Nerve	**Includes:** Spinal nerve, sacral
Sacral Plexus	**Includes:** Inferior gluteal nerve Posterior femoral cutaneous nerve Pudendal nerve
Sacral Sympathetic Nerve	**Includes:** Ganglion impar (ganglion of Walther) Pelvic splanchnic nerve Sacral ganglion Sacral splanchnic nerve
Sacrococcygeal Joint	**Includes:** Sacrococcygeal symphysis
Saphenous Vein, Left Saphenous Vein, Right	**Includes:** External pudendal vein Great(er) saphenous vein Lesser saphenous vein Small saphenous vein Superficial circumflex iliac vein Superficial epigastric vein
Scapula, Left Scapula, Right	**Includes:** Acromion (process) Coracoid process
Sciatic Nerve	**Includes:** Ischiatic nerve
Shoulder Bursa and Ligament, Left Shoulder Bursa and Ligament, Right	**Includes:** Acromioclavicular ligament Coracoacromial ligament Coracoclavicular ligament Coracohumeral ligament Costoclavicular ligament Glenohumeral ligament Interclavicular ligament Sternoclavicular ligament Subacromial bursa Transverse humeral ligament Transverse scapular ligament
Shoulder Joint, Left Shoulder Joint, Right	**Includes:** Glenohumeral joint Glenoid ligament (labrum)

ICD-10-PCS Value	Definition
Shoulder Muscle, Left Shoulder Muscle, Right	**Includes:** Deltoid muscle Infraspinatus muscle Subscapularis muscle Supraspinatus muscle Teres major muscle Teres minor muscle
Sigmoid Colon	**Includes:** Rectosigmoid junction Sigmoid flexure
Skin	**Includes:** Dermis Epidermis Sebaceous gland Sweat gland
Skin, Chest	**Includes:** Breast procedures, skin only
Skin, Perineum	**Includes:** Perianal skin
Sphenoid Bone	**Includes:** Greater wing Lesser wing Optic foramen Pterygoid process Sella turcica
Spinal Canal	**Includes:** Epidural space, spinal Extradural space, spinal Subarachnoid space, spinal Subdural space, spinal Vertebral canal
Spinal Cord	**Includes:** Dorsal root ganglion
Spinal Meninges	**Includes:** Arachnoid mater, spinal Denticulate (dentate) ligament Dura mater, spinal Filum terminale Leptomeninges, spinal Pia mater, spinal
Spleen	**Includes:** Accessory spleen
Splenic Artery	**Includes:** Left gastroepiploic artery Pancreatic artery Short gastric artery
Splenic Vein	**Includes:** Left gastroepiploic vein Pancreatic vein
Sternum	**Includes:** Manubrium Suprasternal notch Xiphoid process
Sternum Bursa and Ligament	**Includes:** Costoxiphoid ligament Sternocostal ligament
Stomach, Pylorus	**Includes:** Pyloric antrum Pyloric canal Pyloric sphincter
Subclavian Artery, Left Subclavian Artery, Right	**Includes:** Costocervical trunk Dorsal scapular artery Internal thoracic artery
Subcutaneous Tissue and Fascia, Chest	**Includes:** Pectoral fascia

ICD-10-PCS Value	Definition
Subcutaneous Tissue and Fascia, Face	**Includes:** Masseteric fascia Orbital fascia Submandibular space
Subcutaneous Tissue and Fascia, Left Foot	**Includes:** Plantar fascia (aponeurosis)
Subcutaneous Tissue and Fascia, Left Hand	**Includes:** Palmar fascia (aponeurosis)
Subcutaneous Tissue and Fascia, Left Lower Arm	**Includes:** Antebrachial fascia Bicipital aponeurosis
Subcutaneous Tissue and Fascia, Left Neck	**Includes:** Deep cervical fascia Pretracheal fascia Prevertebral fascia
Subcutaneous Tissue and Fascia, Left Upper Arm	**Includes:** Axillary fascia Deltoid fascia Infraspinatus fascia Subscapular aponeurosis Supraspinatus fascia
Subcutaneous Tissue and Fascia, Left Upper Leg	**Includes:** Crural fascia Fascia lata Iliac fascia Iliotibial tract (band)
Subcutaneous Tissue and Fascia, Right Foot	**Includes:** Plantar fascia (aponeurosis)
Subcutaneous Tissue and Fascia, Right Hand	**Includes:** Palmar fascia (aponeurosis)
Subcutaneous Tissue and Fascia, Right Lower Arm	**Includes:** Antebrachial fascia Bicipital aponeurosis
Subcutaneous Tissue and Fascia, Right Neck	**Includes:** Deep cervical fascia Pretracheal fascia Prevertebral fascia
Subcutaneous Tissue and Fascia, Right Upper Arm	**Includes:** Axillary fascia Deltoid fascia Infraspinatus fascia Subscapular aponeurosis Supraspinatus fascia
Subcutaneous Tissue and Fascia, Right Upper Leg	**Includes:** Crural fascia Fascia lata Iliac fascia Iliotibial tract (band)
Subcutaneous Tissue and Fascia, Scalp	**Includes:** Galea aponeurotica
Subcutaneous Tissue and Fascia, Trunk	**Includes:** External oblique aponeurosis Transversalis fascia
Submaxillary Gland, Left Submaxillary Gland, Right	**Includes:** Submandibular gland
Superior Mesenteric Artery	**Includes:** Ileal artery Ileocolic artery Inferior pancreaticoduodenal artery Jejunal artery
Superior Mesenteric Vein	**Includes:** Right gastroepiploic vein
Superior Vena Cava	**Includes:** Cavoatrial junction Precava

ICD-10-PCS Value	Definition
Tarsal Joint, Left Tarsal Joint, Right	**Includes:** Calcaneocuboid joint Cuboideonavicular joint Cuneonavicular joint Intercuneiform joint Subtalar (talocalcaneal) joint Talocalcaneal (subtalar) joint Talocalcaneonavicular joint
Tarsal, Left Tarsal, Right	**Includes:** Calcaneus Cuboid bone Intermediate cuneiform bone Lateral cuneiform bone Medial cuneiform bone Navicular bone Talus bone
Temporal Artery, Left Temporal Artery, Right	**Includes:** Middle temporal artery Superficial temporal artery Transverse facial artery
Temporal Bone, Left Temporal Bone, Right	**Includes:** Mastoid process Petrous part of temporal bone Tympanic part of temporal bone Zygomatic process of temporal bone
Thalamus	**Includes:** Epithalamus Geniculate nucleus Metathalamus Pulvinar
Thoracic Aorta, Ascending/Arch	**Includes:** Aortic arch Ascending aorta
Thoracic Duct	**Includes:** Left jugular trunk Left subclavian trunk
Thoracic Nerve	**Includes:** Intercostal nerve Intercostobrachial nerve Spinal nerve, thoracic Subcostal nerve
Thoracic Spinal Cord	**Includes:** Dorsal root ganglion
Thoracic Sympathetic Nerve	**Includes:** Cardiac plexus Esophageal plexus Greater splanchnic nerve Inferior cardiac nerve Least splanchnic nerve Lesser splanchnic nerve Middle cardiac nerve Pulmonary plexus Superior cardiac nerve Thoracic aortic plexus Thoracic ganglion
Thoracic Vertebra	**Includes:** Spinous process Transverse process Vertebral arch Vertebral body Vertebral foramen Vertebral lamina Vertebral pedicle
Thoracic Vertebral Joint	**Includes:** Costotransverse joint Costovertebral joint Thoracic facet joint
Thoracolumbar Vertebral Joint	**Includes:** Thoracolumbar facet joint

Appendix E: Body Part Definitions

ICD-10-PCS Value	Definition
Thorax Muscle, Left Thorax Muscle, Right	**Includes:** Intercostal muscle Levatores costarum muscle Pectoralis major muscle Pectoralis minor muscle Serratus anterior muscle Subclavius muscle Subcostal muscle Transverse thoracis muscle
Thymus	**Includes:** Thymus gland
Thyroid Artery, Left Thyroid Artery, Right	**Includes:** Cricothyroid artery Hyoid artery Sternocleidomastoid artery Superior laryngeal artery Superior thyroid artery Thyrocervical trunk
Tibia, Left Tibia, Right	**Includes:** Lateral condyle of tibia Medial condyle of tibia Medial malleolus
Tibial Nerve	**Includes:** Lateral plantar nerve Medial plantar nerve Medial popliteal nerve Medial sural cutaneous nerve
Toe Nail	**Includes:** Nail bed Nail plate
Toe Phalangeal Joint, Left Toe Phalangeal Joint, Right	**Includes:** Interphalangeal (IP) joint
Tongue	**Includes:** Frenulum linguae
Tongue, Palate, Pharynx Muscle	**Includes:** Chondroglossus muscle Genioglossus muscle Hyoglossus muscle Inferior longitudinal muscle Levator veli palatini muscle Palatoglossal muscle Palatopharyngeal muscle Pharyngeal constrictor muscle Salpingopharyngeus muscle Styloglossus muscle Stylopharyngeus muscle Superior longitudinal muscle Tensor veli palatini muscle
Tonsils	**Includes:** Palatine tonsil
Trachea	**Includes:** Cricoid cartilage
Transverse Colon	**Includes:** Hepatic flexure Splenic flexure
Tricuspid Valve	**Includes:** Right atrioventricular valve Tricuspid annulus
Trigeminal Nerve	**Includes:** Fifth cranial nerve Gasserian ganglion Mandibular nerve Maxillary nerve Ophthalmic nerve Trifacial nerve
Trochlear Nerve	**Includes:** Fourth cranial nerve

ICD-10-PCS Value	Definition
Trunk Muscle, Left Trunk Muscle, Right	**Includes:** Coccygeus muscle Erector spinae muscle Interspinalis muscle Intertransversarius muscle Latissimus dorsi muscle Quadratus lumborum muscle Rhomboid major muscle Rhomboid minor muscle Serratus posterior muscle Transversospinalis muscle Trapezius muscle
Tympanic Membrane, Left Tympanic Membrane, Right	**Includes:** Pars flaccida
Ulna, Left Ulna, Right	**Includes:** Olecranon process Radial notch
Ulnar Artery, Left Ulnar Artery, Right	**Includes:** Anterior ulnar recurrent artery Common interosseous artery Posterior ulnar recurrent artery
Ulnar Nerve	**Includes:** Cubital nerve
Upper Arm Muscle, Left Upper Arm Muscle, Right	**Includes:** Biceps brachii muscle Brachialis muscle Coracobrachialis muscle Triceps brachii muscle
Upper Artery	**Includes:** Aortic intercostal artery Bronchial artery Esophageal artery Subcostal artery
Upper Eyelid, Left Upper Eyelid, Right	**Includes:** Lateral canthus Levator palpebrae superioris muscle Orbicularis oculi muscle Superior tarsal plate
Upper Femur, Left Upper Femur, Right	**Includes:** Femoral head Greater trochanter Lesser trochanter Neck of femur
Upper Leg Muscle, Left Upper Leg Muscle, Right	**Includes:** Adductor brevis muscle Adductor longus muscle Adductor magnus muscle Biceps femoris muscle Gracilis muscle Pectineus muscle Quadriceps (femoris) Rectus femoris muscle Sartorius muscle Semimembranosus muscle Semitendinosus muscle Vastus intermedius muscle Vastus lateralis muscle Vastus medialis muscle
Upper Lip	**Includes:** Frenulum labii superioris Labial gland Vermilion border
Upper Spine Bursa and Ligament	**Includes:** Interspinous ligament, thoracic Intertransverse ligament, thoracic Ligamentum flavum, thoracic Supraspinous ligament

ICD-10-PCS Value	Definition
Ureter Ureter, Left Ureter, Right Ureters, Bilateral	Includes: Ureteral orifice Ureterovesical orifice
Urethra	Includes: Bulbourethral (Cowper's) gland Cowper's (bulbourethral) gland External urethral sphincter Internal urethral sphincter Membranous urethra Penile urethra Prostatic urethra
Uterine Supporting Structure	Includes: Broad ligament Infundibulopelvic ligament Ovarian ligament Round ligament of uterus
Uterus	Includes: Fundus uteri Myometrium Perimetrium Uterine cornu
Uvula	Includes: Palatine uvula
Vagus Nerve	Includes: Anterior vagal trunk Pharyngeal plexus Pneumogastric nerve Posterior vagal trunk Pulmonary plexus Recurrent laryngeal nerve Superior laryngeal nerve Tenth cranial nerve
Vas Deferens Vas Deferens, Bilateral Vas Deferens, Left Vas Deferens, Right	Includes: Ductus deferens Ejaculatory duct
Ventricle, Right	Includes: Conus arteriosus
Ventricular Septum	Includes: Interventricular septum
Vertebral Artery, Left Vertebral Artery, Right	Includes: Anterior spinal artery Posterior spinal artery
Vertebral Vein, Left Vertebral Vein, Right	Includes: Deep cervical vein Suboccipital venous plexus
Vestibular Gland	Includes: Bartholin's (greater vestibular) gland Greater vestibular (Bartholin's) gland Paraurethral (Skene's) gland Skene's (paraurethral) gland
Vitreous, Left Vitreous, Right	Includes: Vitreous body
Vocal Cord, Left Vocal Cord, Right	Includes: Vocal fold
Vulva	Includes: Labia majora Labia minora
Wrist Bursa and Ligament, Left Wrist Bursa and Ligament, Right	Includes: Palmar ulnocarpal ligament Radial collateral carpal ligament Radiocarpal ligament Radioulnar ligament Scapholunate ligament Ulnar collateral carpal ligament
Wrist Joint, Left Wrist Joint, Right	Includes: Distal radioulnar joint Radiocarpal joint

Appendix F: Device Classification

In most PCS codes, the sixth character of the code classifies the device. The sixth character device value "defines the material or appliance used to accomplish the objective of the procedure that remains in or on the procedure site at the end of the procedure." If the device is the means by which the procedural objective is accomplished, then a specific device value is coded in the sixth character. If no device is used to accomplish the objective of the procedure, the device value *No Device* is coded in the sixth character. In limited root operations, the classification provides the qualifier values *Temporary* and *Intraoperative*, for specific procedures involving clinically significant devices whose purpose is brief use during the procedure or current inpatient stay.

Material that is classified as a PCS device is distinguished from material classified as a PCS substance by its having a specific location. A device is intended to maintain a fixed location at the procedure site where it was put, whereas a substance is intended to disperse or be absorbed in the body. There are circumstances in which a device does not stay where it was put and may need to be "revised" in a subsequent procedure to move the device back to its intended location.

Material classified as a PCS device is also distinguishable by the fact that it is removable. Although it may not be practical to remove some types of devices, once they become established at the site, it is physically possible to remove a device for some time after the procedure. A skin graft, for example, once it "takes," may be nearly indistinguishable from the surrounding skin and so is no longer clearly identifiable as a device. Nevertheless, procedures that involve material coded as a device can for the most part be "reversed" by removing the device from the procedure site.

General Device Types

Device Type	Definition	Examples
Grafts	Biological or synthetic material that **takes the place of all or a portion of a body part.**	Full- or partial-thickness skin grafts: • Autologous • Nonautologous • Synthetic • Zooplastic Other tissue grafts: • Bone • Tendon • Vascular
Prosthesis	Biological or synthetic material that **takes the place of all or a portion of a body part.**	Joint prosthesis: • Autologous • Nonautologous • Synthetic
Implants	**Therapeutic** material that is not absorbed by, eliminated by, or incorporated into a body part.	External fixation device Internal fixation device: • Orthopaedic pins • Intramedullary rods Radioactive element implant Mesh
Simple or mechanical appliances	Biological or synthetic material that **assists or prevents a physiological function.**	Drainage device Extraluminal device Endobrachial device Fusion device Intraluminal device (can be temporary) Tracheostomy device IUD
Electronic appliances	Electronic appliances used to **assist, monitor, take the pace of, or prevent a physiological function.**	Cardiac leads Diaphragmatic pacemaker External heart assist system Short-term external heart assist system (Intraoperative) Fetal monitoring Hearing device Monitoring device Neurostimulator
External appliances	Performed without making an incision or a puncture, external appliances are used for the purpose of **protection, immobilization, stretching, compression, or packing.**	Bandage Cast Packing material Pressure dressing Traction apparatus

Transplant/Grafting Tissue Type Terminology

Tissue Type	Terminology
Tissue or organ transferred into a new position in **the body of the same individual**	Autograft Autologous Autoplastic
Having to do with individuals or tissues that have **identical genes**, such as identical twins	Isograft Isologous Syngeneic Syngraft
Tissue or organ taken from **different individuals** of the same species	Allogeneic Allograft Homologous Homograft
Tissue or organ from a **cadaver**	Nonautologous
Tissue or organ from individuals of **different species**	Heterogeneic Heterologous Xenogeneic Xenograft Zooplastic

Appendix G: Device Key and Aggregation Table

This **NT** symbol next to a device in the Term column identifies that the device has been approved for NTAP (new technology add-on payment). CMS provides incremental payment, in addition to the DRG payment, for technologies that have received an NTAP designation.

Device Key

Term	ICD-10-PCS Value
3f (Aortic) Bioprosthesis valve	Zooplastic Tissue in Heart and Great Vessels
AbioCor® Total Replacement Heart	Synthetic Substitute
Absolute Pro Vascular (OTW) Self-Expanding Stent System	Intraluminal Device
Acculink (RX) Carotid Stent System	Intraluminal Device
Acellular Hydrated Dermis	Nonautologous Tissue Substitute
Acetabular cup	Liner in Lower Joints
Activa PC neurostimulator	Stimulator Generator, Multiple Array for Insertion in Subcutaneous Tissue and Fascia
Activa RC neurostimulator	Stimulator Generator, Multiple Array Rechargeable for Insertion in Subcutaneous Tissue and Fascia
Activa SC neurostimulator	Stimulator Generator, Single Array for Insertion in Subcutaneous Tissue and Fascia
ACUITY™ Steerable Lead	Cardiac Lead, Pacemaker for Insertion in Heart and Great Vessels Cardiac Lead, Defibrillator for Insertion in Heart and Great Vessels
Advisa (MRI)	Pacemaker, Dual Chamber for Insertion in Subcutaneous Tissue and Fascia
AFX® Endovascular AAA System	Intraluminal Device
Alfapump® system	Other Device
AMPLATZER® Muscular VSD Occluder	Synthetic Substitute
AMS 800® Urinary Control System	Artificial Sphincter in Urinary System
AneuRx® AAA Advantage®	Intraluminal Device
Annuloplasty ring	Synthetic Substitute
ApiFix® Minimally Invasive Deformity Correction (MID-C) System (C)	Posterior (Dynamic) Distraction Device in New Technology
aprevo™	Interbody Fusion Device, Customizable in New Technology
Articulating Spacer (Antibiotic)	Articulating Spacer in Lower Joints
Artificial anal sphincter (AAS)	Artificial Sphincter in Gastrointestinal System
Artificial bowel sphincter (neosphincter)	Artificial Sphincter in Gastrointestinal System
Artificial urinary sphincter (AUS)	Artificial Sphincter in Urinary System
Ascenda Intrathecal Catheter	Infusion Device
Assurant (Cobalt) stent	Intraluminal Device
AtriClip LAA Exclusion System	Extraluminal Device
Attain Ability® Lead	Cardiac Lead, Pacemaker for Insertion in Heart and Great Vessels Cardiac Lead, Defibrillator for Insertion in Heart and Great Vessels

Term	ICD-10-PCS Value
Attain StarFix® (OTW) Lead	Cardiac Lead, Pacemaker for Insertion in Heart and Great Vessels Cardiac Lead, Defibrillator for Insertion in Heart and Great Vessels
Autograft	Autologous Tissue Substitute
Autologous artery graft	Autologous Arterial Tissue in Heart and Great Vessels Autologous Arterial Tissue in Upper Arteries Autologous Arterial Tissue in Lower Arteries Autologous Arterial Tissue in Upper Veins Autologous Arterial Tissue in Lower Veins
Autologous vein graft	Autologous Venous Tissue in Heart and Great Vessels Autologous Venous Tissue in Upper Arteries Autologous Venous Tissue in Lower Arteries Autologous Venous Tissue in Upper Veins Autologous Venous Tissue in Lower Veins
Axial Lumbar Interbody Fusion System	Interbody Fusion Device in Lower Joints
AxiaLIF® System	Interbody Fusion Device in Lower Joints
BAK/C® Interbody Cervical Fusion System	Interbody Fusion Device in Upper Joints
Bard® Composix® (E/X)(LP) mesh	Synthetic Substitute
Bard® Composix® Kugel® patch	Synthetic Substitute
Bard® Dulex™ mesh	Synthetic Substitute
Bard® Ventralex™ hernia patch	Synthetic Substitute
Baroreflex Activation Therapy® (BAT®)	Stimulator Lead in Upper Arteries Stimulator Generator in Subcutaneous Tissue and Fascia
Barricaid® Annular Closure Device (ACD)	Synthetic Substitute
Berlin Heart Ventricular Assist Device	Implantable Heart Assist System in Heart and Great Vessels
Bioactive embolization coil(s)	Intraluminal Device, Bioactive in Upper Arteries
Biventricular external heart assist system	Short-term External Heart Assist System in Heart and Great Vessels
Blood glucose monitoring system	Monitoring Device
Bone anchored hearing device	Hearing Device, Bone Conduction for Insertion in Ear, Nose, Sinus Hearing Device, in Head and Facial Bones
Bone bank bone graft	Nonautologous Tissue Substitute
Bone screw (interlocking)(lag)(pedicle)(recessed)	Internal Fixation Device in Head and Facial Bones Internal Fixation Device in Upper Bones Internal Fixation Device in Lower Bones
Bovine pericardial valve	Zooplastic Tissue in Heart and Great Vessels
Bovine pericardium graft	Zooplastic Tissue in Heart and Great Vessels
Brachytherapy seeds	Radioactive Element
BRYAN® Cervical Disc System	Synthetic Substitute
BVS 5000 Ventricular Assist Device	Short-term External Heart Assist System in Heart and Great Vessels

Term	ICD-10-PCS Value
Cardiac contractility modulation lead	Cardiac Lead in Heart and Great Vessels
Cardiac event recorder	Monitoring Device
Cardiac resynchronization therapy (CRT) lead	Cardiac Lead, Pacemaker for Insertion in Heart and Great Vessels Cardiac Lead, Defibrillator for Insertion in Heart and Great Vessels
CardioMEMS® pressure sensor	Monitoring Device, Pressure Sensor for Insertion in Heart and Great Vessels
Carmat total artificial heart (TAH)	Biologic with Synthetic Substitute, Autoregulated Electrohydraulic for Replacement in Heart and Great Vessels
Carotid (artery) sinus (baroreceptor) lead	Stimulator Lead in Upper Arteries
Carotid WALLSTENT® Monorail® Endoprosthesis	Intraluminal Device
Centrimag® Blood Pump	Short-term External Heart Assist System in Heart and Great Vessels
Ceramic on ceramic bearing surface	Synthetic Substitute, Ceramic for Replacement in Lower Joints
Cesium-131 Collagen Implant	Radioactive Element, Cesium-131 Collagen Implant for Insertion in Central Nervous System and Cranial Nerves
CivaSheet®	Radioactive Element
Clamp and rod internal fixation system (CRIF)	Internal Fixation Device in Upper Bones Internal Fixation Device in Lower Bones
COALESCE® radiolucent interbody fusion device	Interbody Fusion Device in Upper Joints Interbody Fusion Device in Lower Joints
CoAxia NeuroFlo catheter	Intraluminal Device
Cobalt/chromium head and polyethylene socket	Synthetic Substitute, Metal on Polyethylene for Replacement in Lower Joints
Cobalt/chromium head and socket	Synthetic Substitute, Metal for Replacement in Lower Joints
Cochlear implant (CI), multiple channel (electrode)	Hearing Device, Multiple Channel Cochlear Prosthesis for Insertion in Ear, Nose, Sinus
Cochlear implant (CI), single channel (electrode)	Hearing Device, Single Channel Cochlear Prosthesis for Insertion in Ear, Nose, Sinus
COGNIS® CRT-D	Cardiac Resynchronization Defibrillator Pulse Generator for Insertion in Subcutaneous Tissue and Fascia
COHERE® radiolucent interbody fusion device	Interbody Fusion Device in Upper Joints Interbody Fusion Device in Lower Joints
Colonic Z-Stent®	Intraluminal Device
Complete (SE) stent	Intraluminal Device
Concerto II CRT-D	Cardiac Resynchronization Defibrillator Pulse Generator for Insertion in Subcutaneous Tissue and Fascia
CONSERVE® PLUS Total Resurfacing Hip System	Resurfacing Device in Lower Joints
Consulta CRT-D	Cardiac Resynchronization Defibrillator Pulse Generator for Insertion in Subcutaneous Tissue and Fascia
Consulta CRT-P	Cardiac Resynchronization Pacemaker Pulse Generator for Insertion in Subcutaneous Tissue and Fascia
CONTAK RENEWAL® 3 RF (HE) CRT-D	Cardiac Resynchronization Defibrillator Pulse Generator for Insertion in Subcutaneous Tissue and Fascia
Contegra Pulmonary Valved Conduit	Zooplastic Tissue in Heart and Great Vessels

Term	ICD-10-PCS Value
Continuous Glucose Monitoring (CGM) device	Monitoring Device
Cook Biodesign® Fistula Plug(s)	Nonautologous Tissue Substitute
Cook Biodesign® Hernia Graft(s)	Nonautologous Tissue Substitute
Cook Biodesign® Layered Graft(s)	Nonautologous Tissue Substitute
Cook Zenapro™ Layered Graft(s)	Nonautologous Tissue Substitute
Cook Zenith AAA Endovascular Graft	Intraluminal Device
Cook Zenith® Fenestrated AAA Endovascular Graft	Intraluminal Device, Branched or Fenestrated, One or Two Arteries for Restriction in Lower Arteries Intraluminal Device, Branched or Fenestrated, Three or More Arteries for Restriction in Lower Arteries
CoreValve transcatheter aortic valve	Zooplastic Tissue in Heart and Great Vessels
Cormet Hip Resurfacing System	Resurfacing Device in Lower Joints
CoRoent® XL	Interbody Fusion Device in Lower Joints
Corox (OTW) Bipolar Lead	Cardiac Lead, Pacemaker for Insertion in Heart and Great Vessels Cardiac Lead, Defibrillator for Insertion in Heart and Great Vessels
Cortical strip neurostimulator lead	Neurostimulator Lead in Central Nervous System and Cranial Nerves
Corvia IASD®	Synthetic Substitute
Cultured epidermal cell autograft	Autologous Tissue Substitute
CYPHER® Stent	Intraluminal Device, Drug-eluting in Heart and Great Vessels
Cystostomy tube	Drainage Device
DBS lead	Neurostimulator Lead in Central Nervous System and Cranial Nerves
DeBakey Left Ventricular Assist Device	Implantable Heart Assist System in Heart and Great Vessels
Deep brain neurostimulator lead	Neurostimulator Lead in Central Nervous System and Cranial Nerves
Delta frame external fixator	External Fixation Device, Hybrid for Insertion in Upper Bones External Fixation Device, Hybrid for Reposition in Upper Bones External Fixation Device, Hybrid for Insertion in Lower Bones External Fixation Device, Hybrid for Reposition in Lower Bones
Delta III Reverse shoulder prosthesis	Synthetic Substitute, Reverse Ball and Socket for Replacement in Upper Joints
Diaphragmatic pacemaker generator	Stimulator Generator in Subcutaneous Tissue and Fascia
Direct Lateral Interbody Fusion (DLIF) device	Interbody Fusion Device in Lower Joints
Driver stent (RX) (OTW)	Intraluminal Device
DuraHeart Left Ventricular Assist System	Implantable Heart Assist System in Heart and Great Vessels
Durata® Defibrillation Lead	Cardiac Lead, Defibrillator for Insertion in Heart and Great Vessels
DynaClip® (Forte)	Internal Fixation Device, Sustained Compression for Fusion in Upper Joints Internal Fixation Device, Sustained Compression for Fusion in Lower Joints

Term	ICD-10-PCS Value
DynaNail® (Hybrid) (Mini)	Internal Fixation Device, Sustained Compression for Fusion in Upper Joints Internal Fixation Device, Sustained Compression for Fusion in Lower Joints
Dynesys® Dynamic Stabilization System	Spinal Stabilization Device, Pedicle-Based for Insertion in Upper Joints Spinal Stabilization Device, Pedicle-Based for Insertion in Lower Joints
E-Luminexx™ (Biliary)(Vascular) Stent	Intraluminal Device
Electrical bone growth stimulator (EBGS)	Bone Growth Stimulator in Head and Facial Bones Bone Growth Stimulator in Upper Bones Bone Growth Stimulator in Lower Bones
Electrical muscle stimulation (EMS) lead	Stimulator Lead in Muscles
Electronic muscle stimulator lead	Stimulator Lead in Muscles
Eluvia™ Drug-eluting Vascular Stent System	Intraluminal Device, Sustained Release Drug-eluting in New Technology Intraluminal Device, Sustained Release Drug-eluting, Two in New Technology Intraluminal Device, Sustained Release Drug-eluting, Three in New Technology Intraluminal Device, Sustained Release Drug-eluting, Four or More in New Technology
Embolization coil(s)	Intraluminal Device
Endeavor® (III)(IV) (Sprint) Zotarolimus-eluting Coronary Stent System	Intraluminal Device, Drug-eluting in Heart and Great Vessels
Endologix AFX® Endovascular AAA System	Intraluminal Device
EndoSure® sensor	Monitoring Device, Pressure Sensor for Insertion in Heart and Great Vessels
ENDOTAK RELIANCE® (G) Defibrillation Lead	Cardiac Lead, Defibrillator for Insertion in Heart and Great Vessels
Endotracheal tube (cuffed)(double-lumen)	Intraluminal Device, Endotracheal Airway in Respiratory System
Endurant® Endovascular Stent Graft	Intraluminal Device
Endurant® II AAA stent graft system	Intraluminal Device
EnRhythm	Pacemaker, Dual Chamber for Insertion in Subcutaneous Tissue and Fascia
Enterra gastric neurostimulator	Stimulator Generator, Multiple Array for Insertion in Subcutaneous Tissue and Fascia
Epic™ Stented Tissue Valve (aortic)	Zooplastic Tissue in Heart and Great Vessels
Epicel® cultured epidermal autograft	Autologous Tissue Substitute
Esophageal obturator airway (EOA)	Intraluminal Device, Airway in Gastrointestinal System
Esteem® implantable hearing system	Hearing Device in Ear, Nose, Sinus
Evera (XT)(S)(DR/VR)	Defibrillator Generator for Insertion in Subcutaneous Tissue and Fascia
Everolimus-eluting coronary stent	Intraluminal Device, Drug-eluting in Heart and Great Vessels
Ex-PRESS™ mini glaucoma shunt	Synthetic Substitute

Term	ICD-10-PCS Value
EXCLUDER® AAA Endoprosthesis	Intraluminal Device Intraluminal Device, Branched or Fenestrated, One or Two Arteries for Restriction in Lower Arteries Intraluminal Device, Branched or Fenestrated, Three or More Arteries for Restriction in Lower Arteries
EXCLUDER® IBE Endoprosthesis	Intraluminal Device, Branched or Fenestrated, One or Two Arteries for Restriction in Lower Arteries
Express® (LD) Premounted Stent System	Intraluminal Device
Express® Biliary SD Monorail® Premounted Stent System	Intraluminal Device
Express® SD Renal Monorail® Premounted Stent System	Intraluminal Device
External fixator	External Fixation Device in Head and Facial Bones External Fixation Device in Upper Bones External Fixation Device in Lower Bones External Fixation Device in Upper Joints External Fixation Device in Lower Joints
EXtreme Lateral Interbody Fusion (XLIF) device	Interbody Fusion Device in Lower Joints
Facet replacement spinal stabilization device	Spinal Stabilization Device, Facet Replacement for Insertion in Upper Joints Spinal Stabilization Device, Facet Replacement for Insertion in Lower Joints
FLAIR® Endovascular Stent Graft	Intraluminal Device
Flexible Composite Mesh	Synthetic Substitute
Flow Diverter embolization device	Intraluminal Device, Flow Diverter for Restriction in Upper Arteries
Foley catheter	Drainage Device
Formula™ Balloon-Expandable Renal Stent System	Intraluminal Device
Freestyle (Stentless) Aortic Root Bioprosthesis	Zooplastic Tissue in Heart and Great Vessels
Fusion screw (compression)(lag)(locking)	Internal Fixation Device in Upper Joints Internal Fixation Device in Lower Joints
GammaTile™	Radioactive Element, Cesium-131 Collagen Implant for Insertion in Central Nervous System and Cranial Nerves
Gastric electrical stimulation (GES) lead	Stimulator Lead in Gastrointestinal System
Gastric pacemaker lead	Stimulator Lead in Gastrointestinal System
GORE EXCLUDER® AAA Endoprosthesis	Intraluminal Device Intraluminal Device, Branched or Fenestrated, One or Two Arteries for Restriction in Lower Arteries Intraluminal Device, Branched or Fenestrated, Three or More Arteries for Restriction in Lower Arteries
GORE EXCLUDER® IBE Endoprosthesis	Intraluminal Device, Branched or Fenestrated, One or Two Arteries for Restriction in Lower Arteries
GORE TAG® Thoracic Endoprosthesis	Intraluminal Device
GORE® DUALMESH®	Synthetic Substitute
Guedel airway	Intraluminal Device, Airway in Mouth and Throat

Term	ICD-10-PCS Value
Hancock Bioprosthesis (aortic)(mitral) valve	Zooplastic Tissue in Heart and Great Vessels
Hancock Bioprosthetic Valved Conduit	Zooplastic Tissue in Heart and Great Vessels
HeartMate 3™ LVAS	Implantable Heart Assist System in Heart and Great Vessels
HeartMate II® Left Ventricular Assist Device (LVAD)	Implantable Heart Assist System in Heart and Great Vessels
HeartMate XVE® Left Ventricular Assist Device (LVAD)	Implantable Heart Assist System in Heart and Great Vessels
Herculink (RX) Elite Renal Stent System	Intraluminal Device
Hip (joint) liner	Liner in Lower Joints
Holter valve ventricular shunt	Synthetic Substitute
IASD® (InterAtrial Shunt Device), Corvia	Synthetic Substitute
iFuse Bedrock™ Granite Implant System	Internal Fixation Device with Tulip Connector in New Technology
Ilizarov external fixator	External Fixation Device, Ring for Insertion in Upper Bones External Fixation Device, Ring for Reposition in Upper Bones External Fixation Device, Ring for Insertion in Lower Bones External Fixation Device, Ring for Reposition in Lower Bones
Ilizarov-Vecklich device	External Fixation Device, Limb Lengthening for Insertion in Upper Bones External Fixation Device, Limb Lengthening for Insertion in Lower Bones
Impella® heart pump	Short-term External Heart Assist System in Heart and Great Vessels
Implantable cardioverter-defibrillator (ICD)	Defibrillator Generator for Insertion in Subcutaneous Tissue and Fascia
Implantable drug infusion pump (anti-spasmodic) (chemotherapy)(pain)	Infusion Device, Pump in Subcutaneous Tissue and Fascia
Implantable glucose monitoring device	Monitoring Device
Implantable hemodynamic monitor (IHM)	Monitoring Device, Hemodynamic for Insertion in Subcutaneous Tissue and Fascia
Implantable hemodynamic monitoring system (IHMS)	Monitoring Device, Hemodynamic for Insertion in Subcutaneous Tissue and Fascia
Implantable Miniature Telescope™ (IMT)	Synthetic Substitute, Intraocular Telescope for Replacement in Eye
Implanted (venous)(access) port	Vascular Access Device, Totally Implantable in Subcutaneous Tissue and Fascia
InDura, intrathecal catheter (1P) (spinal)	Infusion Device
Injection reservoir, port	Vascular Access Device, Totally Implantable in Subcutaneous Tissue and Fascia
Injection reservoir, pump	Infusion Device, Pump in Subcutaneous Tissue and Fascia
InterAtrial Shunt Device IASD®, Corvia	Synthetic Substitute
Interbody fusion (spine) cage	Interbody Fusion Device in Upper Joints Interbody Fusion Device in Lower Joints

Term	ICD-10-PCS Value
Interspinous process spinal stabilization device	Spinal Stabilization Device, Interspinous Process for Insertion in Upper Joints Spinal Stabilization Device, Interspinous Process for Insertion in Lower Joints
InterStim™ Micro Therapy neurostimulator	Stimulator Generator, Single Array Rechargeable for Insertion in Subcutaneous Tissue and Fascia
InterStim® Therapy lead	Neurostimulator Lead in Peripheral Nervous System
InterStim™ II Therapy neurostimulator	Stimulator Generator, Single Array for Insertion in Subcutaneous Tissue and Fascia
Intramedullary (IM) rod (nail)	Internal Fixation Device, Intramedullary in Upper Bones Internal Fixation Device, Intramedullary in Lower Bones
Intramedullary skeletal kinetic distractor (ISKD)	Internal Fixation Device, Intramedullary in Upper Bones Internal Fixation Device, Intramedullary in Lower Bones
Intrauterine Device (IUD)	Contraceptive Device in Female Reproductive System
Ischemic Stroke System (ISS500)	Neurostimulator Lead in New Technology
ISS500 (Ischemic Stroke System)	Neurostimulator Lead in New Technology
Itrel (3)(4) neurostimulator	Stimulator Generator, Single Array for Insertion in Subcutaneous Tissue and Fascia
Joint fixation plate	Internal Fixation Device in Upper Joints Internal Fixation Device in Lower Joints
Joint liner (insert)	Liner in Lower Joints
Joint spacer (antibiotic)	Spacer in Upper Joints Spacer in Lower Joints
Kappa	Pacemaker, Dual Chamber for Insertion in Subcutaneous Tissue and Fascia
Kirschner wire (K-wire)	Internal Fixation Device in Head and Facial Bones Internal Fixation Device in Upper Bones Internal Fixation Device in Lower Bones Internal Fixation Device in Upper Joints Internal Fixation Device in Lower Joints
Knee (implant) insert	Liner in Lower Joints
Kuntscher nail	Internal Fixation Device, Intramedullary in Upper Bones Internal Fixation Device, Intramedullary in Lower Bones
LAP-BAND® adjustable gastric banding system	Extraluminal Device
LifeStent® (Flexstar)(XL) Vascular Stent System	Intraluminal Device
LigaPASS 2.0™ PJK Prevention System	Posterior Vertebral Tether in New Technology
LIVIAN™ CRT-D	Cardiac Resynchronization Defibrillator Pulse Generator for Insertion in Subcutaneous Tissue and Fascia
Loop recorder, implantable	Monitoring Device
MAGEC® Spinal Bracing and Distraction System	Magnetically Controlled Growth Rod(s) in New Technology
Mark IV Breathing Pacemaker System	Stimulator Generator in Subcutaneous Tissue and Fascia
Maximo II DR (VR)	Defibrillator Generator for Insertion in Subcutaneous Tissue and Fascia

Term	ICD-10-PCS Value
Maximo II DR CRT-D	Cardiac Resynchronization Defibrillator Pulse Generator for Insertion in Subcutaneous Tissue and Fascia
Medtronic Endurant® II AAA stent graft system	Intraluminal Device
Melody® transcatheter pulmonary valve	Zooplastic Tissue in Heart and Great Vessels
Metal on metal bearing surface	Synthetic Substitute, Metal for Replacement in Lower Joints
Micro-Driver stent (RX) (OTW)	Intraluminal Device
MicroMed HeartAssist	Implantable Heart Assist System in Heart and Great Vessels
Micrus CERECYTE microcoil	Intraluminal Device, Bioactive in Upper Arteries
MIRODERM™ Biologic Wound Matrix	Nonautologous Tissue Substitute
MitraClip valve repair system	Synthetic Substitute
Mitroflow® Aortic Pericardial Heart Valve	Zooplastic Tissue in Heart and Great Vessels
Mosaic Bioprosthesis (aortic) (mitral) valve	Zooplastic Tissue in Heart and Great Vessels
MULTI-LINK (VISION)(MINI-VISION)(ULTRA) Coronary Stent System	Intraluminal Device
nanoLOCK™ interbody fusion device	Interbody Fusion Device in Upper Joints Interbody Fusion Device in Lower Joints
Nasopharyngeal airway (NPA)	Intraluminal Device, Airway in Ear, Nose, Sinus
Neovasc Reducer™	Reduction Device in New Technology
Neuromuscular electrical stimulation (NEMS) lead	Stimulator Lead in Muscles
Neurostimulator generator, multiple channel	Stimulator Generator, Multiple Array for Insertion in Subcutaneous Tissue and Fascia
Neurostimulator generator, multiple channel rechargeable	Stimulator Generator, Multiple Array Rechargeable for Insertion in Subcutaneous Tissue and Fascia
Neurostimulator generator, single channel	Stimulator Generator, Single Array for Insertion in Subcutaneous Tissue and Fascia
Neurostimulator generator, single channel rechargeable	Stimulator Generator, Single Array Rechargeable for Insertion in Subcutaneous Tissue and Fascia
Neutralization plate	Internal Fixation Device in Head and Facial Bones Internal Fixation Device in Upper Bones Internal Fixation Device in Lower Bones
Nitinol framed polymer mesh	Synthetic Substitute
Non-tunneled central venous catheter	Infusion Device
Novacor Left Ventricular Assist Device	Implantable Heart Assist System in Heart and Great Vessels
Novation® Ceramic AHS® (Articulation Hip System)	Synthetic Substitute, Ceramic for Replacement in Lower Joints
NUsurface® Meniscus Implant	Synthetic Substitute, Lateral Meniscus in New Technology Synthetic Substitute, Medial Meniscus in New Technology
Omnilink Elite Vascular Balloon Expandable Stent System	Intraluminal Device

Term	ICD-10-PCS Value
Open Pivot Aortic Valve Graft (AVG)	Synthetic Substitute
Open Pivot (mechanical) Valve	Synthetic Substitute
Optimizer™ III implantable pulse generator	Contractility Modulation Device for Insertion in Subcutaneous Tissue and Fascia
Oropharyngeal airway (OPA)	Intraluminal Device, Airway in Mouth and Throat
Ovatio™ CRT-D	Cardiac Resynchronization Defibrillator Pulse Generator for Insertion in Subcutaneous Tissue and Fascia
OXINIUM	Synthetic Substitute, Oxidized Zirconium on Polyethylene for Replacement in Lower Joints
Paclitaxel-eluting coronary stent	Intraluminal Device, Drug-eluting in Heart and Great Vessels
Paclitaxel-eluting peripheral stent	Intraluminal Device, Drug-eluting in Upper Arteries Intraluminal Device, Drug-eluting in Lower Arteries
Partially absorbable mesh	Synthetic Substitute
Pedicle-based dynamic stabilization device	Spinal Stabilization Device, Pedicle-Based for Insertion in Upper Joints Spinal Stabilization Device, Pedicle-Based for Insertion in Lower Joints
PERCEPT™ PC neurostimulator	Stimulator Generator, Multiple Array for Insertion in Subcutaneous Tissue and Fascia
Percutaneous endoscopic gastrojejunostomy (PEG/J) tube	Feeding Device in Gastrointestinal System
Percutaneous endoscopic gastrostomy (PEG) tube	Feeding Device in Gastrointestinal System
Percutaneous nephrostomy catheter	Drainage Device
Peripherally inserted central catheter (PICC)	Infusion Device
Pessary ring	Intraluminal Device, Pessary in Female Reproductive System
Phrenic nerve stimulator generator	Stimulator Generator in Subcutaneous Tissue and Fascia
Phrenic nerve stimulator lead	Diaphragmatic Pacemaker Lead in Respiratory System
PHYSIOMESH™ Flexible Composite Mesh	Synthetic Substitute
Pipeline™ (Flex) embolization device	Intraluminal Device, Flow Diverter for Restriction in Upper Arteries
Polyethylene socket	Synthetic Substitute, Polyethylene for Replacement in Lower Joints
Polymethylmethacrylate (PMMA)	Synthetic Substitute
Polypropylene mesh	Synthetic Substitute
Porcine (bioprosthetic) valve	Zooplastic Tissue in Heart and Great Vessels
PRECICE intramedullary limb lengthening system	Internal Fixation Device, Intramedullary Limb Lengthening for Insertion in Upper Bones Internal Fixation Device, Intramedullary Limb Lengthening for Insertion in Lower Bones
PRESTIGE® Cervical Disc	Synthetic Substitute
PrimeAdvanced neurostimulator (SureScan)(MRI Safe)	Stimulator Generator, Multiple Array for Insertion in Subcutaneous Tissue and Fascia

Term	ICD-10-PCS Value
PROCEED™ Ventral Patch	Synthetic Substitute
Prodisc-C	Synthetic Substitute
Prodisc-L	Synthetic Substitute
PROLENE Polypropylene Hernia System (PHS)	Synthetic Substitute
Protecta XT CRT-D	Cardiac Resynchronization Defibrillator Pulse Generator for Insertion in Subcutaneous Tissue and Fascia
Protecta XT DR (XT VR)	Defibrillator Generator for Insertion in Subcutaneous Tissue and Fascia
Protégé® RX Carotid Stent System	Intraluminal Device
Pump reservoir	Infusion Device, Pump in Subcutaneous Tissue and Fascia
REALIZE® Adjustable Gastric Band	Extraluminal Device
Rebound HRD® (Hernia Repair Device)	Synthetic Substitute
Reducer™ System	Reduction Device in New Technology
RestoreAdvanced neurostimulator (SureScan)(MRI Safe)	Stimulator Generator, Multiple Array Rechargeable for Insertion in Subcutaneous Tissue and Fascia
RestoreSensor neurostimulator (SureScan)(MRI Safe)	Stimulator Generator, Multiple Array Rechargeable for Insertion in Subcutaneous Tissue and Fascia
RestoreUltra neurostimulator (SureScan)(MRI Safe)	Stimulator Generator, Multiple Array Rechargeable for Insertion in Subcutaneous Tissue and Fascia
Reveal (LINQ)(DX)(XT)	Monitoring Device
Reverse® Shoulder Prosthesis	Synthetic Substitute, Reverse Ball and Socket for Replacement in Upper Joints
Revo MRI™ SureScan® pacemaker	Pacemaker, Dual Chamber for Insertion in Subcutaneous Tissue and Fascia
Rheos® System device	Stimulator Generator in Subcutaneous Tissue and Fascia
Rheos® System lead	Stimulator Lead in Upper Arteries
RNS System lead	Neurostimulator Lead in Central Nervous System and Cranial Nerves
RNS system neurostimulator generator	Neurostimulator Generator in Head and Facial Bones
S-ICD™ lead	Subcutaneous Defibrillator Lead in Subcutaneous Tissue and Fascia
Sacral nerve modulation (SNM) lead	Stimulator Lead in Urinary System
Sacral neuromodulation lead	Stimulator Lead in Urinary System
SAPIEN transcatheter aortic valve	Zooplastic Tissue in Heart and Great Vessels
SAVAL below-the-knee (BTK) drug-eluting stent system	Intraluminal Device, Sustained Release Drug-eluting in New Technology Intraluminal Device, Sustained Release Drug-eluting, Two in New Technology Intraluminal Device, Sustained Release Drug-eluting, Three in New Technology Intraluminal Device, Sustained Release Drug-eluting, Four or More in New Technology
Secura (DR) (VR)	Defibrillator Generator for Insertion in Subcutaneous Tissue and Fascia

Term	ICD-10-PCS Value
Sheffield hybrid external fixator	External Fixation Device, Hybrid for Insertion in Upper Bones External Fixation Device, Hybrid for Reposition in Upper Bones External Fixation Device, Hybrid for Insertion in Lower Bones External Fixation Device, Hybrid for Reposition in Lower Bones
Sheffield ring external fixator	External Fixation Device, Ring for Insertion in Upper Bones External Fixation Device, Ring for Reposition in Upper Bones External Fixation Device, Ring for Insertion in Lower Bones External Fixation Device, Ring for Reposition in Lower Bones
Single lead pacemaker (atrium)(ventricle)	Pacemaker, Single Chamber for Insertion in Subcutaneous Tissue and Fascia
Single lead rate responsive pacemaker (atrium)(ventricle)	Pacemaker, Single Chamber Rate Responsive for Insertion in Subcutaneous Tissue and Fascia
Sirolimus-eluting coronary stent	Intraluminal Device, Drug-eluting in Heart and Great Vessels
SJM Biocor® Stented Valve System	Zooplastic Tissue in Heart and Great Vessels
Spacer, Articulating (Antibiotic)	Articulating Spacer in Lower Joints
Spacer, Static (Antibiotic)	Spacer in Lower Joints
Spinal cord neurostimulator lead	Neurostimulator Lead in Central Nervous System and Cranial Nerves
Spinal growth rods, magnetically controlled	Magnetically Controlled Growth Rod(s) in New Technology
SpineJack® system	Synthetic Substitute, Mechanically Expandable (Paired) in New Technology
Spiration IBV™ Valve System	Intraluminal Device, Endobronchial Valve in Respiratory System
Static Spacer (Antibiotic)	Spacer in Lower Joints
Stent, intraluminal (cardiovascular) (gastrointestinal) (hepatobiliary)(urinary)	Intraluminal Device
Stented tissue valve	Zooplastic Tissue in Heart and Great Vessels
Stratos LV	Cardiac Resynchronization Pacemaker Pulse Generator for Insertion in Subcutaneous Tissue and Fascia
Subcutaneous injection reservoir, port	Vascular Access Device, Totally Implantable in Subcutaneous Tissue and Fascia
Subcutaneous injection reservoir, pump	Infusion Device, Pump in Subcutaneous Tissue and Fascia
Subdermal progesterone implant	Contraceptive Device in Subcutaneous Tissue and Fascia
Surpass Streamline™ Flow Diverter	Intraluminal Device, Flow Diverter for Restriction in Upper Arteries
SynCardia (temporary) Total Artificial Heart (TAH)	Synthetic Substitute, Pneumatic for Replacement in Heart and Great Vessels
SynCardia Total Artificial Heart	Synthetic Substitute
Synchra CRT-P	Cardiac Resynchronization Pacemaker Pulse Generator for Insertion in Subcutaneous Tissue and Fascia
SynchroMed Pump	Infusion Device, Pump in Subcutaneous Tissue and Fascia
Talent® Converter	Intraluminal Device

Term	ICD-10-PCS Value
Talent® Occluder	Intraluminal Device
Talent® Stent Graft (abdominal)(thoracic)	Intraluminal Device
TandemHeart® System	Short-term External Heart Assist System in Heart and Great Vessels
TAXUS® Liberté® Paclitaxel-eluting Coronary Stent System	Intraluminal Device, Drug-eluting in Heart and Great Vessels
Therapeutic occlusion coil(s)	Intraluminal Device
Thoracostomy tube	Drainage Device
Thoraflex™ Hybrid device	Branched Synthetic Substitute with Intraluminal Device in New Technology
Thoratec IVAD (Implantable Ventricular Assist Device)	Implantable Heart Assist System in Heart and Great Vessels
Thoratec Paracorporeal Ventricular Assist Device	Short-term External Heart Assist System in Heart and Great Vessels
Tibial insert	Liner in Lower Joints
Tissue bank graft	Nonautologous Tissue Substitute
Tissue expander (inflatable)(injectable)	Tissue Expander in Skin and Breast Tissue Expander in Subcutaneous Tissue and Fascia
Titan Endoskeleton™	Interbody Fusion Device in Upper Joints Interbody Fusion Device in Lower Joints
Titanium Sternal Fixation System (TSFS)	Internal Fixation Device, Rigid Plate for Insertion in Upper Bones Internal Fixation Device, Rigid Plate for Reposition in Upper Bones
TOPS™ System	Posterior Spinal Motion Preservation Device in New Technology
Total artificial (replacement) heart	Synthetic Substitute
Tracheostomy tube	Tracheostomy Device in Respiratory System
Trifecta™ Valve (aortic)	Zooplastic Tissue in Heart and Great Vessels
Tunneled central venous catheter	Vascular Access Device, Tunneled in Subcutaneous Tissue and Fascia
Tunneled spinal (intrathecal) catheter	Infusion Device
Two lead pacemaker	Pacemaker, Dual Chamber for Insertion in Subcutaneous Tissue and Fascia
Ultraflex™ Precision Colonic Stent System	Intraluminal Device
ULTRAPRO Hernia System (UHS)	Synthetic Substitute
ULTRAPRO Partially Absorbable Lightweight Mesh	Synthetic Substitute
ULTRAPRO Plug	Synthetic Substitute
Ultrasonic osteogenic stimulator	Bone Growth Stimulator in Head and Facial Bones Bone Growth Stimulator in Upper Bones Bone Growth Stimulator in Lower Bones
Ultrasound bone healing system	Bone Growth Stimulator in Head and Facial Bones Bone Growth Stimulator in Upper Bones Bone Growth Stimulator in Lower Bones
Uniplanar external fixator	External Fixation Device, Monoplanar for Insertion in Upper Bones External Fixation Device, Monoplanar for Reposition in Upper Bones External Fixation Device, Monoplanar for Insertion in Lower Bones External Fixation Device, Monoplanar for Reposition in Lower Bones

Term	ICD-10-PCS Value
Urinary incontinence stimulator lead	Stimulator Lead in Urinary System
V-Wave Interatrial Shunt System	Synthetic Substitute
Vaginal pessary	Intraluminal Device, Pessary in Female Reproductive System
Valiant Thoracic Stent Graft	Intraluminal Device
Vectra® Vascular Access Graft	Vascular Access Device, Tunneled in Subcutaneous Tissue and Fascia
Ventrio™ Hernia Patch	Synthetic Substitute
Versa	Pacemaker, Dual Chamber for Insertion in Subcutaneous Tissue and Fascia
Virtuoso (II) (DR) (VR)	Defibrillator Generator for Insertion in Subcutaneous Tissue and Fascia
Viva(XT)(S)	Cardiac Resynchronization Defibrillator Pulse Generator for Insertion in Subcutaneous Tissue and Fascia
Vivistim® Paired VNS System Lead	Neurostimulator Lead with Paired Stimulation System in New Technology
WALLSTENT® Endoprosthesis	Intraluminal Device
X-Spine Axle Cage	Spinal Stabilization Device, Interspinous Process for Insertion in Upper Joints Spinal Stabilization Device, Interspinous Process for Insertion in Lower Joints
X-STOP® Spacer	Spinal Stabilization Device, Interspinous Process for Insertion in Upper Joints Spinal Stabilization Device, Interspinous Process for Insertion in Lower Joints
Xact Carotid Stent System	Intraluminal Device
Xenograft	Zooplastic Tissue in Heart and Great Vessels
XIENCE Everolimus Eluting Coronary Stent System	Intraluminal Device, Drug-eluting in Heart and Great Vessels
XLIF® System	Interbody Fusion Device in Lower Joints
Zenith AAA Endovascular Graft	Intraluminal Device
Zenith® Fenestrated AAA Endovascular Graft	Intraluminal Device, Branched or Fenestrated, One or Two Arteries for Restriction in Lower Arteries Intraluminal Device, Branched or Fenestrated, Three or More Arteries for Restriction in Lower Arteries
Zenith Flex® AAA Endovascular Graft	Intraluminal Device
Zenith® Renu™ AAA Ancillary Graft	Intraluminal Device
Zenith TX2® TAA Endovascular Graft	Intraluminal Device
Zilver® PTX® (paclitaxel) Drug-Eluting Peripheral Stent	Intraluminal Device, Drug-eluting in Upper Arteries Intraluminal Device, Drug-eluting in Lower Arteries
Zimmer® NexGen® LPS Mobile Bearing Knee	Synthetic Substitute
Zimmer® NexGen® LPS-Flex Mobile Knee	Synthetic Substitute
Zotarolimus-eluting coronary stent	Intraluminal Device, Drug-eluting in Heart and Great Vessels

Device Aggregation Table

This table crosswalks specific device character value definitions for specific root operations in a specific body system to the more general device character value to be used when the root operation covers a wide range of body parts and the device character represents an entire family of devices.

Specific Device	for Operation	in Body System	General Device	
Autologous Arterial Tissue (A)	All applicable	Heart and Great Vessels Lower Arteries Lower Veins Upper Arteries Upper Veins	7	Autologous Tissue Substitute
Autologous Venous Tissue (9)	All applicable	Heart and Great Vessels Lower Arteries Lower Veins Upper Arteries Upper Veins	7	Autologous Tissue Substitute
Cardiac Lead, Defibrillator (K)	Insertion	Heart and Great Vessels	M	Cardiac Lead
Cardiac Lead, Pacemaker (J)	Insertion	Heart and Great Vessels	M	Cardiac Lead
Cardiac Resynchronization Defibrillator Pulse Generator (9)	Insertion	Subcutaneous Tissue and Fascia	P	Cardiac Rhythm Related Device
Cardiac Resynchronization Pacemaker Pulse Generator (7)	Insertion	Subcutaneous Tissue and Fascia	P	Cardiac Rhythm Related Device
Contractility Modulation Device (A)	Insertion	Subcutaneous Tissue and Fascia	P	Cardiac Rhythm Related Device
Defibrillator Generator (8)	Insertion	Subcutaneous Tissue and Fascia	P	Cardiac Rhythm Related Device
Epiretinal Visual Prosthesis (5)	All applicable	Eye	J	Synthetic Substitute
External Fixation Device, Hybrid (D)	Insertion	Lower Bones Upper Bones	5	External Fixation Device
External Fixation Device, Hybrid (D)	Reposition	Lower Bones Upper Bones	5	External Fixation Device
External Fixation Device, Limb Lengthening (8)	Insertion	Lower Bones Upper Bones	5	External Fixation Device
External Fixation Device, Monoplanar (B)	Insertion	Lower Bones Upper Bones	5	External Fixation Device
External Fixation Device, Monoplanar (B)	Reposition	Lower Bones Upper Bones	5	External Fixation Device
External Fixation Device, Ring (C)	Insertion	Lower Bones Upper Bones	5	External Fixation Device
External Fixation Device, Ring (C)	Reposition	Lower Bones Upper Bones	5	External Fixation Device
Hearing Device, Bone Conduction (4)	Insertion	Ear, Nose, Sinus	S	Hearing Device
Hearing Device, Multiple Channel Cochlear Prosthesis (6)	Insertion	Ear, Nose, Sinus	S	Hearing Device
Hearing Device, Single Channel Cochlear Prosthesis (5)	Insertion	Ear, Nose, Sinus	S	Hearing Device
Internal Fixation Device, Intramedullary (6)	All applicable	Lower Bones Upper Bones	4	Internal Fixation Device
Internal Fixation Device, Intramedullary Limb Lengthening (7)	Insertion	Lower Bones Upper Bones	6	Internal Fixation Device, Intramedullary
Internal Fixation Device, Rigid Plate (Ø)	Insertion	Upper Bones	4	Internal Fixation Device
Internal Fixation Device, Rigid Plate (Ø)	Reposition	Upper Bones	4	Internal Fixation Device
Intraluminal Device, Airway (B)	All applicable	Ear, Nose, Sinus Gastrointestinal System Mouth and Throat	D	Intraluminal Device
Intraluminal Device, Bioactive (B)	All applicable	Upper Arteries	D	Intraluminal Device
Intraluminal Device, Branched or Fenestrated, One or Two Arteries (E)	Restriction	Heart and Great Vessels Lower Arteries	D	Intraluminal Device
Intraluminal Device, Branched or Fenestrated, Three or More Arteries (F)	Restriction	Heart and Great Vessels Lower Arteries	D	Intraluminal Device
Intraluminal Device, Drug-eluting (4)	All applicable	Heart and Great Vessels Lower Arteries Upper Arteries	D	Intraluminal Device
Intraluminal Device, Drug-eluting, Four or More (7)	All applicable	Heart and Great Vessels Lower Arteries Upper Arteries	D	Intraluminal Device

Specific Device	for Operation	in Body System	General Device	
Intraluminal Device, Drug-eluting, Three (6)	All applicable	Heart and Great Vessels Lower Arteries Upper Arteries	D	Intraluminal Device
Intraluminal Device, Drug-eluting, Two (5)	All applicable	Heart and Great Vessels Lower Arteries Upper Arteries	D	Intraluminal Device
Intraluminal Device, Endobronchial Valve (G)	All applicable	Respiratory System	D	Intraluminal Device
Intraluminal Device, Endotracheal Airway (E)	All applicable	Respiratory System	D	Intraluminal Device
Intraluminal Device, Flow Diverter (H)	Restriction	Upper Arteries	D	Intraluminal Device
Intraluminal Device, Four or More (G)	All applicable	Heart and Great Vessels Lower Arteries Upper Arteries	D	Intraluminal Device
Intraluminal Device, Pessary (G)	All applicable	Female Reproductive System	D	Intraluminal Device
Intraluminal Device, Radioactive (T)	All applicable	Heart and Great Vessels	D	Intraluminal Device
Intraluminal Device, Three (F)	All applicable	Heart and Great Vessels Lower Arteries Upper Arteries	D	Intraluminal Device
Intraluminal Device, Two (E)	All applicable	Heart and Great Vessels Lower Arteries Upper Arteries	D	Intraluminal Device
Monitoring Device, Hemodynamic (Ø)	Insertion	Subcutaneous Tissue and Fascia	2	Monitoring Device
Monitoring Device, Pressure Sensor (Ø)	Insertion	Heart and Great Vessels	2	Monitoring Device
Pacemaker, Dual Chamber (6)	Insertion	Subcutaneous Tissue and Fascia	P	Cardiac Rhythm Related Device
Pacemaker, Single Chamber (4)	Insertion	Subcutaneous Tissue and Fascia	P	Cardiac Rhythm Related Device
Pacemaker, Single Chamber Rate Responsive (5)	Insertion	Subcutaneous Tissue and Fascia	P	Cardiac Rhythm Related Device
Spinal Stabilization Device, Facet Replacement (D)	Insertion	Lower Joints Upper Joints	4	Internal Fixation Device
Spinal Stabilization Device, Interspinous Process (B)	Insertion	Lower Joints Upper Joints	4	Internal Fixation Device
Spinal Stabilization Device, Pedicle-Based (C)	Insertion	Lower Joints Upper Joints	4	Internal Fixation Device
Spinal Stabilization Device, Vertebral Body Tether (3)	Reposition	Lower Bones Upper Bones	4	Internal Fixation Device
Stimulator Generator, Multiple Array (D)	Insertion	Subcutaneous Tissue and Fascia	M	Stimulator Generator
Stimulator Generator, Multiple Array Rechargeable (E)	Insertion	Subcutaneous Tissue and Fascia	M	Stimulator Generator
Stimulator Generator, Single Array (B)	Insertion	Subcutaneous Tissue and Fascia	M	Stimulator Generator
Stimulator Generator, Single Array Rechargeable (C)	Insertion	Subcutaneous Tissue and Fascia	M	Stimulator Generator
Synthetic Substitute, Ceramic (3)	Replacement	Lower Joints	J	Synthetic Substitute
Synthetic Substitute, Ceramic on Polyethylene (4)	Replacement	Lower Joints	J	Synthetic Substitute
Synthetic Substitute, Intraocular Telescope (Ø)	Replacement	Eye	J	Synthetic Substitute
Synthetic Substitute, Metal (1)	Replacement	Lower Joints	J	Synthetic Substitute
Synthetic Substitute, Metal on Polyethylene (2)	Replacement	Lower Joints	J	Synthetic Substitute
Synthetic Substitute, Oxidized Zirconium on Polyethylene (6)	Replacement	Lower Joints	J	Synthetic Substitute
Synthetic Substitute, Polyethylene (Ø)	Replacement	Lower Joints	J	Synthetic Substitute
Synthetic Substitute, Reverse Ball and Socket (Ø)	Replacement	Upper Joints	J	Synthetic Substitute

Appendix H: Device Definitions

This **NT** symbol next to a device in the Definition column identifies that the device has been approved for NTAP (new technology add-on payment). CMS provides incremental payment, in addition to the DRG payment, for technologies that have received an NTAP designation.

ICD-10-PCS Value	Definition
Articulating Spacer in Lower Joints	**Includes:** Articulating Spacer (Antibiotic) Spacer, Articulating (Antibiotic)
Artificial Sphincter in Gastrointestinal System	**Includes:** Artificial anal sphincter (AAS) Artificial bowel sphincter (neosphincter)
Artificial Sphincter in Urinary System	**Includes:** AMS 800® Urinary Control System Artificial urinary sphincter (AUS)
Autologous Arterial Tissue in Heart and Great Vessels	**Includes:** Autologous artery graft
Autologous Arterial Tissue in Lower Arteries	**Includes:** Autologous artery graft
Autologous Arterial Tissue in Lower Veins	**Includes:** Autologous artery graft
Autologous Arterial Tissue in Upper Arteries	**Includes:** Autologous artery graft
Autologous Arterial Tissue in Upper Veins	**Includes:** Autologous artery graft
Autologous Tissue Substitute	**Includes:** Autograft Cultured epidermal cell autograft Epicel® cultured epidermal autograft
Autologous Venous Tissue in Heart and Great Vessels	**Includes:** Autologous vein graft
Autologous Venous Tissue in Lower Arteries	**Includes:** Autologous vein graft
Autologous Venous Tissue in Lower Veins	**Includes:** Autologous vein graft
Autologous Venous Tissue in Upper Arteries	**Includes:** Autologous vein graft
Autologous Venous Tissue in Upper Veins	**Includes:** Autologous vein graft
Biologic with Synthetic Substitute, Autoregulated Electrohydraulic for Replacement in Heart and Great Vessels	**Includes:** Carmat total artificial heart (TAH)
Bone Growth Stimulator in Head and Facial Bones	**Includes:** Electrical bone growth stimulator (EBGS) Ultrasonic osteogenic stimulator Ultrasound bone healing system
Bone Growth Stimulator in Lower Bones	**Includes:** Electrical bone growth stimulator (EBGS) Ultrasonic osteogenic stimulator Ultrasound bone healing system
Bone Growth Stimulator in Upper Bones	**Includes:** Electrical bone growth stimulator (EBGS) Ultrasonic osteogenic stimulator Ultrasound bone healing system
Branched Synthetic Substitute with Intraluminal Device in New Technology	**Includes:** Thoraflex™ Hybrid device
Cardiac Lead in Heart and Great Vessels	**Includes:** Cardiac contractility modulation lead

ICD-10-PCS Value	Definition
Cardiac Lead, Defibrillator for Insertion in Heart and Great Vessels	**Includes:** ACUITY™ Steerable Lead Attain Ability® lead Attain StarFix® (OTW) lead Cardiac resynchronization therapy (CRT) lead Corox (OTW) Bipolar Lead Durata® Defibrillation Lead ENDOTAK RELIANCE® (G) Defibrillation Lead
Cardiac Lead, Pacemaker for Insertion in Heart and Great Vessels	**Includes:** ACUITY™ Steerable Lead Attain Ability® lead Attain StarFix® (OTW) lead Cardiac resynchronization therapy (CRT) lead Corox (OTW) Bipolar Lead
Cardiac Resynchronization Defibrillator Pulse Generator for Insertion in Subcutaneous Tissue and Fascia	**Includes:** COGNIS® CRT-D Concerto II CRT-D Consulta CRT-D CONTAK RENEWA® 3 RF (HE) CRT-D LIVIAN™ CRT-D Maximo II DR CRT-D Ovatio™ CRT-D Protecta XT CRT-D Viva (XT)(S)
Cardiac Resynchronization Pacemaker Pulse Generator for Insertion in Subcutaneous Tissue and Fascia	**Includes:** Consulta CRT-P Stratos LV Synchra CRT-P
Contraceptive Device in Female Reproductive System	**Includes:** Intrauterine device (IUD)
Contraceptive Device in Subcutaneous Tissue and Fascia	**Includes:** Subdermal progesterone implant
Contractility Modulation Device for Insertion in Subcutaneous Tissue and Fascia	**Includes:** Optimizer™ III implantable pulse generator
Defibrillator Generator for Insertion in Subcutaneous Tissue and Fascia	**Includes:** Evera (XT)(S)(DR/VR) Implantable cardioverter-defibrillator (ICD) Maximo II DR (VR) Protecta XT DR (XT VR) Secura (DR) (VR) Virtuoso (II) (DR) (VR)
Diaphragmatic Pacemaker Lead in Respiratory System	**Includes:** Phrenic nerve stimulator lead
Drainage Device	**Includes:** Cystostomy tube Foley catheter Percutaneous nephrostomy catheter Thoracostomy tube
External Fixation Device in Head and Facial Bones	**Includes:** External fixator

ICD-10-PCS Value	Definition
External Fixation Device in Lower Bones	**Includes:** External fixator
External Fixation Device in Lower Joints	**Includes:** External fixator
External Fixation Device in Upper Bones	**Includes:** External fixator
External Fixation Device in Upper Joints	**Includes:** External fixator
External Fixation Device, Hybrid for Insertion in Lower Bones	**Includes:** Delta frame external fixator Sheffield hybrid external fixator
External Fixation Device, Hybrid for Insertion in Upper Bones	**Includes:** Delta frame external fixator Sheffield hybrid external fixator
External Fixation Device, Hybrid for Reposition in Lower Bones	**Includes:** Delta frame external fixator Sheffield hybrid external fixator
External Fixation Device, Hybrid for Reposition in Upper Bones	**Includes:** Delta frame external fixator Sheffield hybrid external fixator
External Fixation Device, Limb Lengthening for Insertion in Lower Bones	**Includes:** Ilizarov-Vecklich device
External Fixation Device, Limb Lengthening for Insertion in Upper Bones	**Includes:** Ilizarov-Vecklich device
External Fixation Device, Monoplanar for Insertion in Lower Bones	**Includes:** Uniplanar external fixator
External Fixation Device, Monoplanar for Insertion in Upper Bones	**Includes:** Uniplanar external fixator
External Fixation Device, Monoplanar for Reposition in Lower Bones	**Includes:** Uniplanar external fixator
External Fixation Device, Monoplanar for Reposition in Upper Bones	**Includes:** Uniplanar external fixator
External Fixation Device, Ring for Insertion in Lower Bones	**Includes:** Ilizarov external fixator Sheffield ring external fixator
External Fixation Device, Ring for Insertion in Upper Bones	**Includes:** Ilizarov external fixator Sheffield ring external fixator
External Fixation Device, Ring for Reposition in Lower Bones	**Includes:** Ilizarov external fixator Sheffield ring external fixator
External Fixation Device, Ring for Reposition in Upper Bones	**Includes:** Ilizarov external fixator Sheffield ring external fixator
Extraluminal Device	**Includes:** AtriClip LAA Exclusion System LAP-BAND® adjustable gastric banding system REALIZE® Adjustable Gastric Band
Feeding Device in Gastrointestinal System	**Includes:** Percutaneous endoscopic gastrojejunostomy (PEG/J) tube Percutaneous endoscopic gastrostomy (PEG) tube
Hearing Device in Ear, Nose, Sinus	**Includes:** Esteem® implantable hearing system
Hearing Device in Head and Facial Bones	**Includes:** Bone anchored hearing device

ICD-10-PCS Value	Definition
Hearing Device, Bone Conduction for Insertion in Ear, Nose, Sinus	**Includes:** Bone anchored hearing device
Hearing Device, Multiple Channel Cochlear Prosthesis for Insertion in Ear, Nose, Sinus	**Includes:** Cochlear implant (CI), multiple channel (electrode)
Hearing Device, Single Channel Cochlear Prosthesis for Insertion in Ear, Nose, Sinus	**Includes:** Cochlear implant (CI), single channel (electrode)
Implantable Heart Assist System in Heart and Great Vessels	**Includes:** Berlin Heart Ventricular Assist Device DeBakey Left Ventricular Assist Device DuraHeart Left Ventricular Assist System HeartMate 3™ LVAS HeartMate II® Left Ventricular Assist Device (LVAD) HeartMate XVE® Left Ventricular Assist Device (LVAD) MicroMed HeartAssist Novacor Left Ventricular Assist Device Thoratec IVAD (Implantable Ventricular Assist Device)
Infusion Device	**Includes:** Ascenda Intrathecal Catheter InDura, intrathecal catheter (1P) (spinal) Non-tunneled central venous catheter Peripherally inserted central catheter (PICC) Tunneled spinal (intrathecal) catheter
Infusion Device, Pump in Subcutaneous Tissue and Fascia	**Includes:** Implantable drug infusion pump (anti-spasmodic)(chemotherapy) (pain) Injection reservoir, pump Pump reservoir Subcutaneous injection reservoir, pump SynchroMed pump
Interbody Fusion Device, Customizable in New Technology	**Includes:** aprevo™
Interbody Fusion Device in Lower Joints	**Includes:** Axial Lumbar Interbody Fusion System AxiaLIF® System COALESCE® radiolucent interbody fusion device COHERE® radiolucent interbody fusion device CoRoent® XL Direct Lateral Interbody Fusion (DLIF) device EXtreme Lateral Interbody Fusion (XLIF) device Interbody fusion (spine) cage nanoLOCK™ interbody fusion device Titan Endoskeleton™ XLIF® System
Interbody Fusion Device in Upper Joints	**Includes:** BAK/C® Interbody Cervical Fusion System COALESCE® radiolucent interbody fusion device COHERE® radiolucent interbody fusion device Interbody fusion (spine) cage nanoLOCK™ interbody fusion device Titan Endoskeleton™

Appendix H: Device Definitions

ICD-10-PCS Value	Definition
Internal Fixation Device in Head and Facial Bones	**Includes:** Bone screw (interlocking)(lag)(pedicle) (recessed) Kirschner wire (K-wire) Neutralization plate
Internal Fixation Device in Lower Bones	**Includes:** Bone screw (interlocking)(lag)(pedicle) (recessed) Clamp and rod internal fixation system (CRIF) Kirschner wire (K-wire) Neutralization plate
Internal Fixation Device in Lower Joints	**Includes:** Fusion screw (compression)(lag)(locking) Joint fixation plate Kirschner wire (K-wire)
Internal Fixation Device in Upper Bones	**Includes:** Bone screw (interlocking)(lag)(pedicle) (recessed) Clamp and rod internal fixation system (CRIF) Kirschner wire (K-wire) Neutralization plate
Internal Fixation Device in Upper Joints	**Includes:** Fusion screw (compression)(lag)(locking) Joint fixation plate Kirschner wire (K-wire)
Internal Fixation Device, Intramedullary in Lower Bones	**Includes:** Intramedullary (IM) rod (nail) Intramedullary skeletal kinetic distractor (ISKD) Kuntscher nail
Internal Fixation Device, Intramedullary in Upper Bones	**Includes:** Intramedullary (IM) rod (nail) Intramedullary skeletal kinetic distractor (ISKD) Kuntscher nail
Internal Fixation Device Intramedullary Limb Lengthening for Insertion in Lower Bones	**Includes:** PRECICE intramedullary limb lengthening system
Internal Fixation Device Intramedullary Limb Lengthening for Insertion in Upper Bones	**Includes:** PRECICE intramedullary limb lengthening system
Internal Fixation Device, Rigid Plate for Insertion in Upper Bones	**Includes:** Titanium Sternal Fixation System (TSFS)
Internal Fixation Device, Rigid Plate for Reposition in Upper Bones	**Includes:** Titanium Sternal Fixation System (TSFS)
Internal Fixation Device, Sustained Compression for Fusion in Lower Joints	**Includes:** DynaClip® (Forte) DynaNail® (Hybrid) (Mini)
Internal Fixation Device, Sustained Compression for Fusion in Upper Joints	**Includes:** DynaClip® (Forte) DynaNail® (Hybrid) (Mini)
Internal Fixation Device with Tulip Connector in New Technology	**Includes:** iFuse Bedrock™ Granite Implant System

ICD-10-PCS Value	Definition
Intraluminal Device	**Includes:** Absolute Pro Vascular (OTW) Self-Expanding Stent System Acculink (RX) Carotid Stent System AFX® Endovascular AAA System AneuRx® AAA Advantage® Assurant (Cobalt) stent Carotid WALLSTENT® Monorail® Endoprosthesis CoAxia NeuroFlo catheter Colonic Z-Stent® Complete (SE) stent Cook Zenith AAA Endovascular Graft Driver stent (RX) (OTW) E-Luminexx™ (Biliary)(Vascular) Stent Embolization coil(s) Endologix AFX® Endovascular AAA System Endurant® Endovascular Stent Graft Endurant® II AAA stent graft system EXCLUDER® AAA Endoprosthesis Express® (LD) Premounted Stent System Express® Biliary SD Monorail® Premounted Stent System Express® SD Renal Monorail® Premounted Stent System FLAIR® Endovascular Stent Graft Formula™ Balloon-Expandable Renal Stent System GORE EXCLUDER® AAA Endoprosthesis GORE TAG® Thoracic Endoprosthesis Herculink (RX) Elite Renal Stent System LifeStent® (Flexstar)(XL) Vascular Stent System Medtronic Endurant® II AAA stent graft system Micro-Driver stent (RX) (OTW) MULTI-LINK (VISION)(MINI-VISION)(ULTRA) Coronary Stent System Omnilink Elite Vascular Balloon Expandable Stent System Protege® RX Carotid Stent System Stent, intraluminal (cardiovascular) (gastrointestinal)(hepatobiliary) (urinary) Talent® Converter Talent® Occluder Talent® Stent Graft (abdominal)(thoracic) Therapeutic occlusion coil(s) Ultraflex™ Precision Colonic Stent System Valiant Thoracic Stent Graft WALLSTENT® Endoprosthesis Xact Carotid Stent System Zenith AAA Endovascular Graft Zenith Flex® AAA Endovascular Graft Zenith TX2® TAA Endovascular Graft Zenith® Renu™ AAA Ancillary Graft
Intraluminal Device, Airway in Ear, Nose, Sinus	**Includes:** Nasopharyngeal airway (NPA)
Intraluminal Device, Airway in Gastrointestinal System	**Includes:** Esophageal obturator airway (EOA)
Intraluminal Device, Airway in Mouth and Throat	**Includes:** Guedel airway Oropharyngeal airway (OPA)
Intraluminal Device, Bioactive in Upper Arteries	**Includes:** Bioactive embolization coil(s) Micrus CERECYTE microcoil

ICD-10-PCS Value	Definition
Intraluminal Device, Branched or Fenestrated, One or Two Arteries for Restriction in Lower Arteries	**Includes:** Cook Zenith® Fenestrated AAA Endovascular Graft EXCLUDER® AAA Endoprosthesis EXCLUDER® IBE Endoprosthesis GORE EXCLUDER® AAA Endoprosthesis GORE EXCLUDER®IBE Endoprosthesis Zenith® Fenestrated AAA Endovascular Graft
Intraluminal Device, Branched or Fenestrated, Three or More Arteries for Restriction in Lower Arteries	**Includes:** Cook Zenith® Fenestrated AAA Endovascular Graft EXCLUDER® AAA Endoprosthesis GORE EXCLUDER® AAA Endoprosthesis Zenith® Fenestrated AAA Endovascular Graft
Intraluminal Device, Drug-eluting in Heart and Great Vessels	**Includes:** CYPHER® Stent Endeavor® (III)(IV) (Sprint) Zotarolimus-eluting Coronary Stent System Everolimus-eluting coronary stent Paclitaxel-eluting coronary stent Sirolimus-eluting coronary stent TAXUS® Liberte® Paclitaxel-eluting Coronary Stent System XIENCE Everolimus Eluting Coronary Stent System Zotarolimus-eluting coronary stent
Intraluminal Device, Drug-eluting in Lower Arteries	**Includes:** Paclitaxel-eluting peripheral stent Zilver® PTX® (paclitaxel) Drug-Eluting Peripheral Stent
Intraluminal Device, Drug-eluting in Upper Arteries	**Includes:** Paclitaxel-eluting peripheral stent Zilver® PTX® (paclitaxel) Drug-Eluting Peripheral Stent
Intraluminal Device, Endobronchial Valve in Respiratory System	**Includes:** Spiration IBV™ Valve System
Intraluminal Device, Endotracheal Airway in Respiratory System	**Includes:** Endotracheal tube (cuffed)(double-lumen)
Intraluminal Device, Flow Diverter for Restriction in Upper Arteries	**Includes:** Flow Diverter embolization device Pipeline™ (Flex) embolization device Surpass Streamline™ Flow Diverter
Intraluminal Device, Pessary in Female Reproductive System	**Includes:** Pessary ring Vaginal pessary
Intraluminal Device, Sustained Release Drug-eluting in New Technology	**Includes:** Eluvia™ Drug-eluting Vascular Stent System SAVAL below-the-knee (BTK) drug-eluting stent system
Intraluminal Device, Sustained Release Drug-eluting, Four or More in New Technology	**Includes:** Eluvia™ Drug-eluting Vascular Stent System SAVAL below-the-knee (BTK) drug-eluting stent system
Intraluminal Device, Sustained Release Drug-eluting, Three in New Technology	**Includes:** Eluvia™ Drug-eluting Vascular Stent System SAVAL below-the-knee (BTK) drug-eluting stent system

ICD-10-PCS Value	Definition
Intraluminal Device, Sustained Release Drug-eluting, Two in New Technology	**Includes:** Eluvia™ Drug-eluting Vascular Stent System SAVAL below-the-knee (BTK) drug-eluting stent system
Liner in Lower Joints	**Includes:** Acetabular cup Hip (joint) liner Joint liner (insert) Knee (implant) insert Tibial insert
Magnetically Controlled Growth Rod(s) in New Technology	**Includes:** MAGEC® Spinal Bracing and Distraction System Spinal growth rods, magnetically controlled
Monitoring Device	**Includes:** Blood glucose monitoring system Cardiac event recorder Continuous Glucose Monitoring (CGM) device Implantable glucose monitoring device Loop recorder, implantable Reveal (LINQ)(DX)(XT)
Monitoring Device, Hemodynamic for Insertion in Subcutaneous Tissue and Fascia	**Includes:** Implantable hemodynamic monitor (IHM) Implantable hemodynamic monitoring system (IHMS)
Monitoring Device, Pressure Sensor for Insertion in Heart and Great Vessels	**Includes:** CardioMEMS® pressure sensor EndoSure® sensor
Neurostimulator Generator in Head and Facial Bones	**Includes:** RNS system neurostimulator generator
Neurostimulator Lead in Central Nervous System and Cranial Nerves	**Includes:** Cortical strip neurostimulator lead DBS lead Deep brain neurostimulator lead RNS System lead Spinal cord neurostimulator lead
Neurostimulator Lead in Peripheral Nervous System	**Includes:** InterStim® Therapy lead
Neurostimulator Lead in New Technology	**Includes:** Ischemic Stroke System (ISS500) ISS500 (Ischemic Stroke System)
Neurostimulator Lead with Paired Stimulation System in New Technology	**Includes:** Vivistim® Paired VNS System Lead
Nonautologous Tissue Substitute	**Includes:** Acellular Hydrated Dermis Bone bank bone graft Cook Biodesign® Fistula Plug(s) Cook Biodesign® Hernia Graft(s) Cook Biodesign® Layered Graft(s) Cook Zenapro™ Layered Graft(s) MIRODERM™ Biologic Wound Matrix Tissue bank graft
Other Device	**Includes:** Alfapump® system
Pacemaker, Dual Chamber for Insertion in Subcutaneous Tissue and Fascia	**Includes:** Advisa (MRI) EnRhythm Kappa Revo MRI™ SureScan® pacemaker Two lead pacemaker Versa

Appendix H: Device Definitions

ICD-10-PCS Value	Definition
Pacemaker, Single Chamber for Insertion in Subcutaneous Tissue and Fascia	**Includes:** Single lead pacemaker (atrium)(ventricle)
Pacemaker, Single Chamber Rate Responsive for Insertion in Subcutaneous Tissue and Fascia	**Includes:** Single lead rate responsive pacemaker (atrium)(ventricle)
Posterior (Dynamic) Distraction Device in New Technology	**Includes:** ApiFix® Minimally Invasive Deformity Correction (MID-C) System
Posterior Spinal Motion Preservation Device in New Technology	**Includes:** TOPS™ System
Posterior Vertebral Tether in New Technology	**Includes:** LigaPASS 2.0™ PJK Prevention System
Radioactive Element	**Includes:** Brachytherapy seeds CivaSheet®
Radioactive Element, Cesium-131 Collagen Implant for Insertion in Central Nervous System and Cranial Nerves	**Includes:** Cesium-131 Collagen Implant GammaTile™
Reduction Device in New Technology	**Includes:** Neovasc Reducer™ Reducer™ System
Resurfacing Device in Lower Joints	**Includes:** CONSERVE® PLUS Total Resurfacing Hip System Cormet Hip Resurfacing System
Short-term External Heart Assist System in Heart and Great Vessels	**Includes:** Biventricular external heart assist system BVS 5000 Ventricular Assist Device Centrimag® Blood Pump Impella® heart pump TandemHeart® System Thoratec Paracorporeal Ventricular Assist Device
Spacer in Lower Joints	**Includes:** Joint spacer (antibiotic) Spacer, Static (Antibiotic) Static Spacer (Antibiotic)
Spacer in Upper Joints	**Includes:** Joint spacer (antibiotic)
Spinal Stabilization Device, Facet Replacement for Insertion in Lower Joints	**Includes:** Facet replacement spinal stabilization device
Spinal Stabilization Device, Facet Replacement for Insertion in Upper Joints	**Includes:** Facet replacement spinal stabilization device
Spinal Stabilization Device, Interspinous Process for Insertion in Lower Joints	**Includes:** Interspinous process spinal stabilization device X-Spine Axle Cage X-STOP® Spacer
Spinal Stabilization Device, Interspinous Process for Insertion in Upper Joints	**Includes:** Interspinous process spinal stabilization device X-Spine Axle Cage X-STOP® Spacer

ICD-10-PCS Value	Definition
Spinal Stabilization Device, Pedicle- Based for Insertion in Lower Joints	**Includes:** Dynesys® Dynamic Stabilization System Pedicle-based dynamic stabilization device
Spinal Stabilization Device, Pedicle-Based for Insertion in Upper Joints	**Includes:** Dynesys® Dynamic Stabilization System Pedicle-based dynamic stabilization device
Stimulator Generator in Subcutaneous Tissue and Fascia	**Includes:** Baroreflex Activation Therapy® (BAT®) Diaphragmatic pacemaker generator Mark IV Breathing Pacemaker System Phrenic nerve stimulator generator Rheos® System device
Stimulator Generator, Multiple Array for Insertion in Subcutaneous Tissue and Fascia	**Includes:** Activa PC neurostimulator Enterra gastric neurostimulator Neurostimulator generator, multiple channel PERCEPT™ PC neurostimulator PrimeAdvanced neurostimulator (SureScan)(MRI Safe)
Stimulator Generator, Multiple Array Rechargeable for Insertion in Subcutaneous Tissue and Fascia	**Includes:** Activa RC neurostimulator Neurostimulator generator, multiple channel rechargeable RestoreAdvanced neurostimulator (SureScan)(MRI Safe) RestoreSensor neurostimulator (SureScan)(MRI Safe) RestoreUltra neurostimulator (SureScan)(MRI Safe)
Stimulator Generator, Single Array for Insertion in Subcutaneous Tissue and Fascia	**Includes:** Activa SC neurostimulator InterStim™ II Therapy neurostimulator Itrel (3)(4) neurostimulator Neurostimulator generator, single channel
Stimulator Generator, Single Array Rechargeable for Insertion in Subcutaneous Tissue and Fascia	**Includes:** InterStim™ Micro Therapy neurostimulator Neurostimulator generator, single channel rechargeable
Stimulator Lead in Gastrointestinal System	**Includes:** Gastric electrical stimulation (GES) lead Gastric pacemaker lead
Stimulator Lead in Muscles	**Includes:** Electrical muscle stimulation (EMS) lead Electronic muscle stimulator lead Neuromuscular electrical stimulation (NEMS) lead
Stimulator Lead in Upper Arteries	**Includes:** Baroreflex Activation Therapy® (BAT®) Carotid (artery) sinus (baroreceptor) lead Rheos® System lead
Stimulator Lead in Urinary System	**Includes:** Sacral nerve modulation (SNM) lead Sacral neuromodulation lead Urinary incontinence stimulator lead
Subcutaneous Defibrillator Lead in Subcutaneous Tissue and Fascia	**Includes:** S-ICD™ lead

ICD-10-PCS Value	Definition	ICD-10-PCS Value	Definition

Synthetic Substitute	**Includes:**
	AbioCor® Total Replacement Heart
	AMPLATZER® Muscular VSD Occluder
	Annuloplasty ring
	Bard® Composix® (E/X) (LP) mesh
	Bard® Composix® Kugel® patch
	Bard® Dulex™ mesh
	Bard® Ventralex® hernia patch
	Barricaid® Annular Closure Device (ACD)
	BRYAN® Cervical Disc System
	Corvia IASD®
	Ex-PRESS™ mini glaucoma shunt
	Flexible Composite Mesh
	GORE® DUALMESH®
	Holter valve ventricular shunt
	IASD® (InterAtrial Shunt Device), Corvia
	InterAtrial Shunt Device IASD®, Corvia
	MitraClip valve repair system
	Nitinol framed polymer mesh
	Open Pivot (mechanical) valve
	Open Pivot Aortic Valve Graft (AVG)
	Partially absorbable mesh
	PHYSIOMESH™ Flexible Composite Mesh
	Polymethylmethacrylate (PMMA)
	Polypropylene mesh
	PRESTIGE® Cervical Disc
	PROCEED™ Ventral Patch
	Prodisc-C
	Prodisc-L
	PROLENE Polypropylene Hernia System
	  (PHS)
	Rebound HRD® (Hernia Repair Device)
	SynCardia Total Artificial Heart
	Total artificial (replacement) heart
	ULTRAPRO Hernia System (UHS)
	ULTRAPRO Partially Absorbable
	  Lightweight Mesh
	ULTRAPRO Plug
	V-Wave Interatrial Shunt System
	Ventrio™ Hernia Patch
	Zimmer® NexGen® LPS Mobile Bearing
	  Knee
	Zimmer® NexGen® LPS-Flex Mobile Knee
		Synthetic Substitute, Oxidized Zirconium on Polyethylene for Replacement in Lower Joints	**Includes:**
			OXINIUM

		Synthetic Substitute, Pneumatic for Replacement in Heart and Great Vessels	**Includes:** SynCardia (temporary) total artificial heart (TAH)
		Synthetic Substitute, Polyethylene for Replacement in Lower Joints	**Includes:** Polyethylene socket
		Synthetic Substitute, Reverse Ball and Socket for Replacement in Upper Joints	**Includes:** Delta III Reverse shoulder prosthesis Reverse® Shoulder Prosthesis
		Tissue Expander in Skin and Breast	**Includes:** Tissue expander (inflatable) (injectable)
		Tissue Expander in Subcutaneous Tissue and Fascia	**Includes:** Tissue expander (inflatable) (injectable)
		Tracheostomy Device in Respiratory System	**Includes:** Tracheostomy tube
		Vascular Access Device, Totally Implantable in Subcutaneous Tissue and Fascia	**Includes:** Implanted (venous)(access) port Injection reservoir, port Subcutaneous injection reservoir, port
		Vascular Access Device, Tunneled in Subcutaneous Tissue and Fascia	**Includes:** Tunneled central venous catheter Vectra® Vascular Access Graft

		Zooplastic Tissue in Heart and Great Vessels	**Includes:**
			3f (Aortic) Bioprosthesis valve
			Bovine pericardial valve
			Bovine pericardium graft
			Contegra Pulmonary Valved Conduit
			CoreValve transcatheter aortic valve
			Epic™ Stented Tissue Valve (aortic)
			Freestyle (Stentless) Aortic Root
			  Bioprosthesis
			Hancock Bioprosthesis (aortic) (mitral)
			  valve
			Hancock Bioprosthetic Valved Conduit
			Melody® transcatheter pulmonary valve
			Mitroflow® Aortic Pericardial Heart Valve
			Mosaic Bioprosthesis (aortic) (mitral) valve
			Porcine (bioprosthetic) valve
			SAPIEN transcatheter aortic valve
			SJM Biocor® Stented Valve System
			Stented tissue valve
			Trifecta™ Valve (aortic)
			Xenograft

Synthetic Substitute, Ceramic for Replacement in Lower Joints	**Includes:** Ceramic on ceramic bearing surface Novation® Ceramic AHS® (Articulation Hip System)		
Synthetic Substitute, Intraocular Telescope for Replacement in Eye	**Includes:** Implantable Miniature Telescope™ (IMT)		
Synthetic Substitute, Lateral Meniscus in New Technology	**Includes:** NUsurface® Meniscus Implant		
Synthetic Substitute, Mechanically Expandable (Paired) in New Technology	**Includes:** SpineJack® system		
Synthetic Substitute, Medial Meniscus in New Technology	**Includes:** NUsurface® Meniscus Implant		
Synthetic Substitute, Metal for Replacement in Lower Joints	**Includes:** Cobalt/chromium head and socket Metal on metal bearing surface		
Synthetic Substitute, Metal on Polyethylene for Replacement in Lower Joints	**Includes:** Cobalt/chromium head and polyethylene socket		

Appendix I: Substance Key/Substance Definitions

Substance Key

This table crosswalks a specific substance, listed by trade name or synonym, to the PCS value that would be used to represent that substance in either the Administration or New Technology section. The ICD-10-PCS value may be located in either the 6th-character Substance column or the 7th-character Qualifier column depending on the section/table to which it is classified. The most specific character is listed in the table.

This **NT** symbol next to a substance/technology in the Trade Name or Synonym column identifies that the substance/technology has been approved for NTAP (new technology add-on payment). CMS provides incremental payment, in addition to the DRG payment, for technologies that have received an NTAP designation.

Substances denoted by an asterisk (*) in the Trade Name or Synonym column, although not included in the official ICD-10-PCS classification, were added based on information provided in the FY 2023 IPPS proposed rule.

Trade Name or Synonym	ICD-10-PCS Value	PCS Section
ABECMA® **NT**	Idecabtagene Vicleucel Immunotherapy (K)	New Technology (X)
ACTEMRA®	Tocilizumab (H)	New Technology (X)
afami-cel	Afamitresgene Autoleucel Immunotherapy (6)	New Technology (X)
AIGISRx Antibacterial Envelope	Anti-Infective Envelope (A)	Administration (3)
Andexanet Alfa, Factor Xa Inhibitor Reversal Agent	Coagulation Factor Xa, Inactivated (7)	New Technology (X)
Andexxa	Coagulation Factor Xa, Inactivated (7)	New Technology (X)
Angiotensin II	Synthetic Human Angiotensin II (H)	New Technology (X)
Antibacterial Envelope (TYRX) (AIGISRx)	Anti-Infective Envelope (A)	Administration (3)
Antimicrobial envelope	Anti-Infective Envelope (A)	Administration (3)
Anti-SARS-CoV-2 hyperimmune globulin	Hyperimmune Globulin (E)	New Technology (X)
AVYCAZ® (ceftazidime-avibactam)	Other Anti-infective (9)	Administration (3)
Axicabtagene Ciloleucel	Axicabtagene Ciloleucel Immunotherapy (H)	New Technology (X)
AZEDRA®	Iobenguane I-131 Antineoplastic (S)	New Technology (X)
*Balversa™	Erdafitinib Antineoplastic (L)	New Technology (X)
beti-cel	Betibeglogene Autotemcel (B)	New Technology (X)
Blinatumomab	Other Antineoplastic (5)	Administration (3)
BLINCYTO® (blinatumomab)	Other Antineoplastic (5)	Administration (3)
Bone morphogenetic protein 2 (BMP 2)	Recombinant Bone Morphogenetic Protein (B)	Administration (3)
Brexucabtagene Autoleucel	Brexucabtagene Autoleucel Immunotherapy (4)	New Technology (X)
Breyanzi®	Lisocabtagene Maraleucel Immunotherapy (N)	New Technology (X)
*CABLIVI®	Caplacizumab (W)	New Technology (X)
CARVYKTI™	Ciltacabtagene Autoleucel (A)	New Technology (X)
Casirivimab (REGN10933) and Imdevimab (REGN10987)	REGN-COV2 Monoclonal Antibody (G)	New Technology (X)
CBMA (Concentrated Bone Marrow Aspirate)	Other Substance (C)	Administration (3)
Ceftazidime-avibactam	Other Anti-infective (9)	Administration (3)
CERAMENT® G	Antibiotic-eluting Bone Void Filler (P)	New Technology (X)
cilta-cel	Ciltacabtagene Autoleucel (A)	New Technology (X)
Clolar	Clofarabine (P)	Administration (3)
Coagulation Factor Xa, (Recombinant) Inactivated	Coagulation Factor Xa, Inactivated (7)	New Technology (X)
CONTEPO™	Fosfomycin Anti-infective (K)	New Technology (X)
COSELA™ **NT**	Trilaciclib (7)	New Technology (X)
CRESEMBA® (isavuconazonium sulfate)	Other Anti-infective (9)	Administration (3)
Darzalex Faspro®	Daratumumab and Hyaluronidase-fihj (1)	New Technology (X)
DefenCath™	Taurolidine Anti-infective and Heparin Anticoagulant (2)	New Technology (X)
Defitelio	Other Substance (C)	Administration (3)
DuraGraft® Endothelial Damage Inhibitor	Endothelial Damage Inhibitor (8)	New Technology (X)
ELZONRIS™	Tagraxofusp-erzs Antineoplastic (Q)	New Technology (X)
ENSPRYNG™	Satralizumab-mwge (9)	New Technology (X)
ERLEADA™	Apalutamide Antineoplastic (J)	New Technology (X)
EVUSHELD™	Tixagevimab and Cilgavimab Monoclonal Antibody (X)	New Technology (X)
Factor Xa Inhibitor Reversal Agent, Andexanet Alfa	Coagulation Factor Xa, Inactivated (7)	New Technology (X)
FETROJA® **NT**	Cefiderocol Anti-infective (A)	New Technology (X)
Fosfomycin injection	Fosfomycin Anti-infective (K)	New Technology (X)
Gammaglobulin	Globulin (S)	Administration (3)

Trade Name or Synonym	ICD-10-PCS Value	PCS Section
GAMUNEX-C, for COVID-19 treatment	High-Dose Intravenous Immune Globulin (D)	New Technology (X)
GIAPREZA™	Synthetic Human Angiotensin II (H)	New Technology (X)
GS-5734	Remdesivir Anti-infective (E)	New Technology (X)
hdIVIG (high-dose intravenous immunoglobulin), for COVID-19 treatment	High-Dose Intravenous Immune Globulin (D)	New Technology (X)
Hemospray® Endoscopic Hemostat	Mineral-based Topical Hemostatic Agent (8)	New Technology (X)
HIG (hyperimmune globulin), for COVID-19 treatment	Hyperimmune Globulin (E)	New Technology (X)
High-dose intravenous immunoglobulin (hdIVIG), for COVID-19 treatment	High-Dose Intravenous Immune Globulin (D)	New Technology (X)
hIVIG (hyperimmune intravenous immunoglobulin), for COVID-19 treatment	Hyperimmune Globulin (E)	New Technology (X)
Human angiotensin II, synthetic	Synthetic Human Angiotensin II (H)	New Technology (X)
Hyperimmune globulin	Globulin (S)	Administration (3)
Hyperimmune intravenous immunoglobulin (hIVIG), for COVID-19 treatment	Hyperimmune Globulin (E)	New Technology (X)
Idarucizumab, Pradaxa® (dabigatran) reversal agent	Other Therapeutic Substance (G)	Administration (3)
Idecabtagene Vicleucel	Idecabtagene Vicleucel Immunotherapy (K)	New Technology (X)
Ide-cel	Idecabtagene Vicleucel Immunotherapy (K)	New Technology (X)
IGIV-C, for COVID-19 treatment	Hyperimmune Globulin (E)	New Technology (X)
Imdevimab (REGN10987) and Casirivimab (REGN10933)	REGN-COV2 Monoclonal Antibody (G)	New Technology (X)
IMFINZI®	Durvalumab Antineoplastic (3)	New Technology (X)
IMI/REL	Imipenem-cilastatin-relebactam Anti-infective (U)	New Technology (X)
Immunoglobulin	Globulin (S)	Administration (3)
INTERCEPT Blood System for Plasma Pathogen Reduced Cryoprecipitated Fibrinogen Complex `NT`	Pathogen Reduced Cryoprecipitated Fibrinogen Complex (D)	Administration (3)
INTERCEPT Fibrinogen Complex `NT`	Pathogen Reduced Cryoprecipitated Fibrinogen Complex (D)	Administration (3)
Iobenguane I-131, High Specific Activity (HSA)	Iobenguane I-131 Antineoplastic (S)	New Technology (X)
Isavuconazole (isavuconazonium sulfate)	Other Anti-infective (9)	Administration (3)
Jakafi®	Ruxolitinib (T)	New Technology (X)
Kcentra	4-Factor Prothrombin Complex Concentrate (B)	Administration (3)
KEVZARA®	Sarilumab (G)	New Technology (X)
KYMRIAH ®	Tisagenlecleucel Immunotherapy (J)	New Technology (X)
Lifileucel	Lifileucel Immunotherapy (L)	New Technology (X)
Lisocabtagene Maraleucel	Lisocabtagene Maraleucel Immunotherapy (7)	New Technology (X)
LIVTENCITY™	Maribavir Anti-infective (3)	New Technology (X)
LTX Regional Anticoagulant	Nafamostat Anticoagulant (3)	New Technology (X)
MarrowStim™ PAD Kit for CBMA (Concentrated Bone Marrow Aspirate)	Other Substance (C)	Administration (3)
NA-1 (Nerinitide)	Nerinitide (2)	New Technology (X)
Nesiritide	Human B-type Natriuretic Peptide (H)	Administration (3)
NexoBrid™	Bromelain-enriched Proteolytic Enzyme (2)	New Technology (X)
Niyad™	Nafamostat Anticoagulant (3)	New Technology (X)
NUZYRA™	Omadacycline Anti-infective (B)	New Technology (X)
Octagam 10%, for COVID-19 treatment	High-Dose Intravenous Immune Globulin (D)	New Technology (X)
Olumiant® `NT`	Baricitinib (M)	New Technology (X)
OTL-101	Hematopoietic Stem/Progenitor Cells, Genetically Modified (C)	Administration (3)
Polyclonal hyperimmune globulin	Globulin (S)	Administration (3)
Praxbind® (idarucizumab), Pradaxa® (dabigatran) reversal agent	Other Therapeutic Substance (G)	Administration (3)
REBYOTA®	Broad Consortium Microbiota-based Live Biotherapeutic Suspension (X)	New Technology (X)
*RECARBRIO™ `NT`	Imipenem-cilastatin-relebactam Anti-infective (U)	New Technology (X)
RETHYMIC®	Engineered Allogeneic Thymus Tissue (D)	New Technology (X)
rhBMP-2	Recombinant Bone Morphogenetic Protein (B)	Administration (3)
RYBREVANT™ `NT`	Amivantamab Monoclonal Antibody (B)	New Technology (X)
Seprafilm	Adhesion Barrier (5)	Administration (3)
Soliris®	Eculizumab (C)	New Technology (X)
SPRAVATO™	Esketamine Hydrochloride (M)	New Technology (X)
STELARA®	Other New Technology Therapeutic Substance (F)	New Technology (X)

Trade Name or Synonym		ICD-10-PCS Value	PCS Section
StrataGraft®	NT	Bioengineered Allogeneic Construct (F)	New Technology (X)
tab-cel®		Tabelecleucel Immunotherapy (7)	New Technology (X)
TECARTUS™	NT	Brexucabtagene Autoleucel Immunotherapy (M)	New Technology (X)
TECENTRIQ®		Atezolizumab Antineoplastic (D)	New Technology (X)
TERLIVAZ®		Terlipressin (6)	New Technology (X)
Tisagenlecleucel		Tisagenlecleucel Immunotherapy (J)	New Technology (X)
Tissue Plasminogen Activator (tPA)(r-tPA)		Other Thrombolytic (7)	Administration (3)
TYRX Antibacterial Envelope		Anti-Infective Envelope (A)	Administration (3)
UPLIZNA®		Inebilizumab-cdon (9)	New Technology (X)
Ustekinumab		Other New Technology Therapeutic Substance (F)	New Technology (X)
Vabomere™		Meropenem-vaborbactam Anti-infective (N)	New Technology (X)
Veklury	NT	Remdesivir Anti-infective (E)	New Technology (X)
Venclexta®		Venetoclax Antineoplastic (R)	New Technology (X)
Vistogard®		Uridine Triacetate (8)	New Technology (X)
Voraxaze		Glucarpidase (Q)	Administration (3)
VYXEOS™		Cytarabine and Daunorubicin Liposome Antineoplastic (B)	New Technology (X)
XENLETA™		Lefamulin Anti-infective (6)	New Technology (X)
XOSPATA®		Gilteritinib Antineoplastic (V)	New Technology (X)
Yescarta®		Axicabtagene Ciloleucel Immunotherapy (H)	New Technology (X)
*ZEMDRI®		Plazomicin Anti-infective (6)	New Technology (X)
ZEPZELCA™	NT	Lurbinectedin (8)	New Technology (X)
ZERBAXA®		Ceftolozane/Tazobactam Anti-infective (9)	New Technology (X)
ZULRESSO™		Brexanolone (Ø)	New Technology (X)
Zyvox		Oxazolidinones (8)	Administration (3)

Substance Definitions

This table crosswalks a PCS value, used in the Administration or New Technology section, to a specific substance. The specific substances are listed by trade name or synonym. The ICD-10-PCS value may be located in either the 6th-character Substance column or the 7th-character Qualifier column depending on the section/table to which it is classified.

This **NT** symbol next to a substance/technology in the Trade Name or Synonym column identifies that the substance/technology has been approved for NTAP (new technology add-on payment). CMS provides incremental payment, in addition to the DRG payment, for technologies that have received an NTAP designation.

Substances denoted by an asterisk (*) in the Trade Name or Synonym column, although not included in the official ICD-10-PCS classification, were added based on information provided in the FY 2023 IPPS proposed rule.

ICD-10-PCS Value	Trade Name or Synonym			PCS Section
4-Factor Prothrombin Complex Concentrate (B)	Includes:	Kcentra		Administration (3)
Afamitresgene Autoleucel Immunotherapy (6)	Includes:	afami-cel		New Technology (X)
Adhesion Barrier (5)	Includes:	Seprafilm		Administration (3)
Amivantamab Monoclonal Antibody (B)	Includes:	RYBREVANT™	NT	New Technology (X)
Antibiotic-eluting Bone Void Filler (P)	Includes:	CERAMENT® G		New Technology (X)
Anti-Infective Envelope (A)	Includes:	AIGISRx Antibacterial Envelope Antibacterial Envelope (TYRX) (AIGISRx) Antimicrobial envelope TYRX Antibacterial Envelope		Administration (3)
Apalutamide Antineoplastic (J)	Includes:	ERLEADA™		New Technology (X)
Atezolizumab Antineoplastic (D)	Includes:	TECENTRIQ®		New Technology (X)
Axicabtagene Ciloleucel Immunotherapy (H)	Includes:	Axicabtagene Ciloleucel Yescarta®		New Technology (X)
Baricitinib (M)	Includes:	Olumiant®	NT	New Technology (X)
Betibeglogene Autotemcel (B)	Includes:	beti-cel		New Technology (X)
Bioengineered Allogeneic Construct (F)	Includes:	StrataGraft®	NT	New Technology (X)
Brexanolone (Ø)	Includes:	ZULRESSO™		New Technology (X)
Brexucabtagene Autoleucel Immunotherapy (M)	Includes:	TECARTUS™	NT	New Technology (X)
Broad Consortium Microbiota-based Live Biotherapeutic Suspension (X)	Includes:	REBYOTA®		New Technology (X)
Bromelain-enriched Proteolytic Enzyme (2)	Includes:	NexoBrid™		New Technology (X)
Caplacizumab (W)	Includes:	*CABLIVI®		New Technology (X)

ICD-10-PCS Value	Trade Name or Synonym		PCS Section
Cefiderocol Anti-infective (A)	Includes:	FETROJA® [NT]	New Technology (X)
Ceftolozane/Tazobactam Anti- infective (9)	Includes:	ZERBAXA®	New Technology (X)
Ciltacabtagene Autoleucel (A)	Includes:	CARVYKTI™ cilta-cel	New Technology (X)
Clofarabine (P)	Includes:	Clolar	Administration (3)
Coagulation Factor Xa, Inactivated (7)	Includes:	Andexanet Alfa, Factor Xa Inhibitor Reversal Agent Andexxa Coagulation Factor Xa, (Recombinant) Inactivated Factor Xa Inhibitor Reversal Agent, Andexanet Alfa	New Technology (X)
Cytarabine and Daunorubicin Liposome Antineoplastic (B)	Includes:	VYXEOS™	New Technology (X)
Daratumumab and Hyaluronidase-fihj (1)	Includes:	Darzalex Faspro®	New Technology (X)
Durvalumab Antineoplastic (3)	Includes:	IMFINZI®	New Technology (X)
Eculizumab (C)	Includes:	Soliris®	New Technology (X)
Endothelial Damage Inhibitor (8)	Includes:	DuraGraft® Endothelial Damage Inhibitor	New Technology (X)
Erdafitinib Antineoplastic (L)	Includes:	*Balversa™	New Technology (X)
Engineered Allogeneic Thymus Tissue (D)	Includes:	RETHYMIC®	New Technology (X)
Esketamine Hydrochloride (M)	Includes:	SPRAVATO™	New Technology (X)
Fosfomycin Anti-infective (K)	Includes:	CONTEPO™ Fosfomycin injection	New Technology (X)
Gilteritinib Antineoplastic (V)	Includes:	XOSPATA®	New Technology (X)
Globulin (S)	Includes:	Gammaglobulin Hyperimmune globulin Immunoglobulin Polyclonal hyperimmune globulin	Administration (3)
Glucarpidase (Q)	Includes:	Voraxaze	Administration (3)
Hematopoietic Stem/Progenitor Cells, Genetically Modified (C)	Includes:	OTL-101	Administration (3)
High-Dose Intravenous Immune Globulin (D)	Includes:	GAMUNEX-C, for COVID-19 treatment hdIVIG (high-dose intravenous immunoglobulin), for COVID-19 treatment High-dose intravenous immunoglobulin (hdIVIG), for COVID-19 treatment Octagam 10%, for COVID-19 treatment	New Technology (X)
Human B-type Natriuretic Peptide (H)	Includes:	Nesiritide	Administration (3)
Hyperimmune Globulin (E)	Includes:	Anti-SARS-CoV-2 hyperimmune globulin HIG (hyperimmune globulin), for COVID-19 treatment hIVIG (hyperimmune intravenous immunoglobulin), for COVID-19 treatment Hyperimmune intravenous immunoglobulin (hIVIG), for COVID-19 treatment IGIV-C, for COVID-19 treatment	New Technology (X)
Idecabtagene Vicleucel Immunotherapy (K)	Includes:	ABECMA® [NT] Idecabtagene Vicleucel Ide-cel	New Technology (X)
Imipenem-cilastatin-relebactam Anti-infective (U)	Includes:	IMI/REL *RECARBRIO™ [NT]	New Technology (X)
Inebilizumab-cdon (9)	Includes:	UPLIZNA®	New Technology (X)
Iobenguane I-131 Antineoplastic (S)	Includes:	AZEDRA® Iobenguane I-131, High Specific Activity (HSA)	New Technology (X)
Lefamulin Anti-infective (6)	Includes:	XENLETA™	New Technology (X)
Lifileucel Immunotherapy (L)	Includes:	Lifileucel	New Technology (X)
Lisocabtagene Maraleucel Immunotherapy (7)	Includes:	Breyanzi® Lisocabtagene Maraleucel	New Technology (X)
Lurbinectedin (8)	Includes:	ZEPZELCA™ [NT]	New Technology (X)
Maribavir Anti-infective (3)	Includes:	LIVTENCITY™	New Technology (X)
Meropenem-vaborbactam Anti-infective (N)	Includes:	Vabomere™	New Technology (X)
Mineral-based Topical Hemostatic Agent (8)	Includes:	Hemospray® Endoscopic Hemostat	New Technology (X)
Nafamostat Anticoagulant (3)	Includes:	LTX Regional Anticoagulant Niyad™	New Technology (X)
Nerinitide (2)	Includes:	NA-1 (Nerinitide)	New Technology (X)
Omadacycline Anti-infective (B)	Includes:	NUZYRA™	New Technology (X)

ICD-10-PCS Value	Trade Name or Synonym		PCS Section
Other Anti-infective (9)	Includes:	AVYCAZ® (ceftazidime-avibactam) Ceftazidime-avibactam CRESEMBA® (isavuconazonium sulfate) Isavuconazole (isavuconazonium sulfate)	Administration (3)
Other Antineoplastic (5)	Includes:	Blinatumomab BLINCYTO® (blinatumomab)	Administration (3)
Other New Technology Therapeutic Substance (F)	Includes:	STELARA® Ustekinumab	New Technology (X)
Other Substance (C)	Includes:	CBMA (Concentrated Bone Marrow Aspirate) Defitelio MarrowStim™ PAD Kit for CBMA (Concentrated Bone Marrow Aspirate)	Administration (3)
Other Therapeutic Substance (G)	Includes:	Idarucizumab, Pradaxa® (dabigatran) reversal agent Praxbind® (idarucizumab), Pradaxa® (dabigatran) reversal agent	Administration (3)
Other Thrombolytic (7)	Includes:	Tissue Plasminogen Activator (tPA)(r-tPA)	Administration (3)
Oxazolidinones (8)	Includes:	Zyvox	Administration (3)
Pathogen Reduced Cryoprecipitated Fibrinogen Complex (D)	Includes:	INTERCEPT Blood System for Plasma Pathogen Reduced Cryoprecipitated Fibrinogen Complex `NT` INTERCEPT Fibrinogen Complex `NT`	Administration (3)
Plazomicin Anti-infective (G)	Includes:	*ZEMDRI®	New Technology (X)
Recombinant Bone Morphogenetic Protein (B)	Includes:	Bone morphogenetic protein 2 (BMP 2) rhBMP-2	Administration (3)
REGN-COV2 Monoclonal Antibody (G)	Includes:	Casirivimab (REGN10933) and Imdevimab (REGN10987) Imdevimab (REGN10987) and Casirivimab (REGN10933)	New Technology (X)
Remdesivir Anti-infective (E)	Includes:	GS-5734 Veklury `NT`	New Technology (X)
Ruxolitinib (T)	Includes:	Jakafi®	New Technology (X)
Sarilumab (G)	Includes:	KEVZARA®	New Technology (X)
Satralizumab-mwge (9)	Includes:	ENSPRYNG™	New Technology (X)
Synthetic Human Angiotensin II (H)	Includes:	Angiotensin II GIAPREZA™ Human angiotensin II, synthetic	New Technology (X)
Tabelecleucel Immunotherapy (7)	Includes:	tab-cel®	New Technology (X)
Tagraxofusp-erzs Antineoplastic (Q)	Includes:	ELZONRIS™	New Technology (X)
Taurolidine Anti-infective and Heparin Anticoagulant (2)	Includes:	DefenCath™	New Technology (X)
Terlipressin (6)	Includes:	TERLIVAZ®	New Technology (X)
Tisagenlecleucel Immunotherapy (J)	Includes:	KYMRIAH® Tisagenlecleucel	New Technology (X)
Tixagevimab and Cilgavimab Monoclonal Antibody (X)	Includes:	EVUSHELD™	New Technology (X)
Tocilizumab (H)	Includes:	ACTEMRA®	New Technology (X)
Trilaciclib (7)	Includes:	COSELA™ `NT`	New Technology (X)
Uridine Triacetate (8)	Includes:	Vistogard®	New Technology (X)
Venetoclax Antineoplastic (R)	Includes:	Venclexta®	New Technology (X)

Appendix J: Sections B–H Character Definitions

Sections B-H (Imaging through Substance Abuse Treatment) do not include root operations. Instead, the character 3 value represents the type of procedure performed with additional details about that procedure provided by the character 4 or 5 value, when appropriate. This resource provides the specific ICD-10-PCS value and its associated definition for the character 3, character 4, and character 5 values in the ancillary sections of B-H.

Section B–Imaging

ICD-10-PCS Value (Character 3)	Definition
Computerized Tomography (CT Scan) (2)	Computer reformatted digital display of multiplanar images developed from the capture of multiple exposures of external ionizing radiation
Fluoroscopy (1)	Single plane or bi-plane real time display of an image developed from the capture of external ionizing radiation on a fluorescent screen. The image may also be stored by either digital or analog means.
Magnetic Resonance Imaging (MRI) (3)	Computer reformatted digital display of multiplanar images developed from the capture of radiofrequency signals emitted by nuclei in a body site excited within a magnetic field
Other Imaging (5)	Other specified modality for visualizing a body part
Plain Radiography (Ø)	Planar display of an image developed from the capture of external ionizing radiation on photographic or photoconductive plate
Ultrasonography (4)	Real time display of images of anatomy or flow information developed from the capture of reflected and attenuated high frequency sound waves

Section C–Nuclear Medicine

ICD-10-PCS Value (Character 3)	Definition
Nonimaging Nuclear Medicine Assay (6)	Introduction of radioactive materials into the body for the study of body fluids and blood elements, by the detection of radioactive emissions
Nonimaging Nuclear Medicine Probe (5)	Introduction of radioactive materials into the body for the study of distribution and fate of certain substances by the detection of radioactive emissions; or, alternatively, measurement of absorption of radioactive emissions from an external source
Nonimaging Nuclear Medicine Uptake (4)	Introduction of radioactive materials into the body for measurements of organ function, from the detection of radioactive emissions
Planar Nuclear Medicine Imaging (1)	Introduction of radioactive materials into the body for single plane display of images developed from the capture of radioactive emissions
Positron Emission Tomographic (PET) Imaging (3)	Introduction of radioactive materials into the body for three dimensional display of images developed from the simultaneous capture, 18Ø degrees apart, of radioactive emissions
Systemic Nuclear Medicine Therapy (7)	Introduction of unsealed radioactive materials into the body for treatment
Tomographic (Tomo) Nuclear Medicine Imaging (2)	Introduction of radioactive materials into the body for three dimensional display of images developed from the capture of radioactive emissions

Section F–Physical Rehabilitation and Diagnostic Audiology

ICD-10-PCS Value (Character 3)	Definition
Activities of Daily Living Assessment (2)	Measurement of functional level for activities of daily living
Activities of Daily Living Treatment (8)	Exercise or activities to facilitate functional competence for activities of daily living
Caregiver Training (F)	Training in activities to support patient's optimal level of function
Cochlear Implant Treatment (B)	Application of techniques to improve the communication abilities of individuals with cochlear implant
Device Fitting (D)	Fitting of a device designed to facilitate or support achievement of a higher level of function
Hearing Aid Assessment (4)	Measurement of the appropriateness and/or effectiveness of a hearing device
Hearing Assessment (3)	Measurement of hearing and related functions
Hearing Treatment (9)	Application of techniques to improve, augment, or compensate for hearing and related functional impairment
Motor and/or Nerve Function Assessment (1)	Measurement of motor, nerve, and related functions

Continued on next page

Section F–Physical Rehabilitation and Diagnostic Audiology

Continued from previous page

ICD-10-PCS Value (Character 3)	Definition
Motor Treatment (7)	Exercise or activities to increase or facilitate motor function
Speech Assessment (0)	Measurement of speech and related functions
Speech Treatment (6)	Application of techniques to improve, augment, or compensate for speech and related functional impairment
Vestibular Assessment (5)	Measurement of the vestibular system and related functions
Vestibular Treatment (C)	Application of techniques to improve, augment, or compensate for vestibular and related functional impairment

Section F–Physical Rehabilitation and Diagnostic Audiology

ICD-10-PCS Value Qualifier (Character 5)	Definition
Acoustic Reflex Decay (J)	Measures reduction in size/strength of acoustic reflex over time Includes/Examples: Includes site of lesion test
Acoustic Reflex Patterns (G)	Defines site of lesion based upon presence/absence of acoustic reflexes with ipsilateral vs. contralateral stimulation
Acoustic Reflex Threshold (H)	Determines minimal intensity that acoustic reflex occurs with ipsilateral and/or contralateral stimulation
Aerobic Capacity and Endurance (7)	Measures autonomic responses to positional changes; perceived exertion, dyspnea or angina during activity; performance during exercise protocols; standard vital signs; and blood gas analysis or oxygen consumption
Alternate Binaural or Monaural Loudness Balance (7)	Determines auditory stimulus parameter that yields the same objective sensation Includes/Examples: Sound intensities that yield same loudness perception
Anthropometric Characteristics (B)	Measures edema, body fat composition, height, weight, length and girth
Aphasia (Assessment) (C)	Measures expressive and receptive speech and language function including reading and writing
Aphasia (Treatment) (3)	Applying techniques to improve, augment, or compensate for receptive/ expressive language impairments
Articulation/Phonology (Assessment) (9)	Measures speech production
Articulation/Phonology (Treatment) (4)	Applying techniques to correct, improve, or compensate for speech productive impairment
Assistive Listening Device (5)	Assists in use of effective and appropriate assistive listening device/system
Assistive Listening System/Device Selection (4)	Measures the effectiveness and appropriateness of assistive listening systems/devices
Assistive, Adaptive, Supportive or Protective Devices (9)	Explanation: Devices to facilitate or support achievement of a higher level of function in wheelchair mobility; bed mobility; transfer or ambulation ability; bath and showering ability; dressing; grooming; personal hygiene; play or leisure
Auditory Evoked Potentials (L)	Measures electric responses produced by the VIIIth cranial nerve and brainstem following auditory stimulation
Auditory Processing (Assessment) (Q)	Evaluates ability to receive and process auditory information and comprehension of spoken language
Auditory Processing (Treatment) (2)	Applying techniques to improve the receiving and processing of auditory information and comprehension of spoken language
Augmentative/Alternative Communication System (Assessment) (L)	Determines the appropriateness of aids, techniques, symbols, and/or strategies to augment or replace speech and enhance communication Includes/Examples: Includes the use of telephones, writing equipment, emergency equipment, and TDD
Augmentative/Alternative Communication System (Treatment) (3)	Includes/Examples: Includes augmentative communication devices and aids
Aural Rehabilitation (5)	Applying techniques to improve the communication abilities associated with hearing loss
Aural Rehabilitation Status (P)	Measures impact of a hearing loss including evaluation of receptive and expressive communication skills
Bathing/Showering (0)	Includes/Examples: Includes obtaining and using supplies; soaping, rinsing, and drying body parts; maintaining bathing position; and transferring to and from bathing positions

Continued on next page

Section F–Physical Rehabilitation and Diagnostic Audiology

Continued from previous page

ICD-10-PCS Value Qualifier (Character 5)	Definition
Bathing/Showering Techniques (Ø)	Activities to facilitate obtaining and using supplies, soaping, rinsing and drying body parts, maintaining bathing position, and transferring to and from bathing positions
Bed Mobility (Assessment) (B)	Transitional movement within bed
Bed Mobility (Treatment) (5)	Exercise or activities to facilitate transitional movements within bed
Bedside Swallowing and Oral Function (H)	Includes/Examples: Bedside swallowing includes assessment of sucking, masticating, coughing, and swallowing. Oral function includes assessment of musculature for controlled movements, structures, and functions to determine coordination and phonation.
Bekesy Audiometry (3)	Uses an instrument that provides a choice of discrete or continuously varying pure tones; choice of pulsed or continuous signal
Binaural Electroacoustic Hearing Aid Check (6)	Determines mechanical and electroacoustic function of bilateral hearing aids using hearing aid test box
Binaural Hearing Aid (Assessment) (3)	Measures the candidacy, effectiveness, and appropriateness of a hearing aid Explanation: Measures bilateral fit
Binaural Hearing Aid (Treatment) (2)	Explanation: Assists in achieving maximum understanding and performance
Bithermal, Binaural Caloric Irrigation (Ø)	Measures the rhythmic eye movements stimulated by changing the temperature of the vestibular system
Bithermal, Monaural Caloric Irrigation (1)	Measures the rhythmic eye movements stimulated by changing the temperature of the vestibular system in one ear
Brief Tone Stimuli (R)	Measures specific central auditory process
Cerumen Management (3)	Includes examination of external auditory canal and tympanic membrane and removal of cerumen from external ear canal
Cochlear Implant (Ø)	Measures candidacy for cochlear implant
Cochlear Implant Rehabilitation (Ø)	Applying techniques to improve the communication abilities of individuals with cochlear implant; includes programming the device, providing patients/families with information
Communicative/Cognitive Integration Skills (Assessment) (G)	Measures ability to use higher cortical functions Includes/Examples: Includes orientation, recognition, attention span, initiation and termination of activity, memory, sequencing, categorizing, concept formation, spatial operations, judgment, problem solving, generalization and pragmatic communication
Communicative/Cognitive Integration Skills (Treatment) (6)	Activities to facilitate the use of higher cortical functions Includes/Examples: Includes level of arousal, orientation, recognition, attention span, initiation and termination of activity, memory sequencing, judgment and problem solving, learning and generalization, and pragmatic communication
Computerized Dynamic Posturography (6)	Measures the status of the peripheral and central vestibular system and the sensory/motor component of balance; evaluates the efficacy of vestibular rehabilitation
Conditioned Play Audiometry (4)	Behavioral measures using nonspeech and speech stimuli to obtain frequency-specific and ear-specific information on auditory status from the patient Explanation: Obtains speech reception threshold by having patient point to pictures of spondaic words
Coordination/Dexterity (Assessment) (3)	Measures large and small muscle groups for controlled goal-directed movements Explanation: Dexterity includes object manipulation
Coordination/Dexterity (Treatment) (2)	Exercise or activities to facilitate gross coordination and fine coordination
Cranial Nerve Integrity (9)	Measures cranial nerve sensory and motor functions, including tastes, smell and facial expression
Dichotic Stimuli (T)	Measures specific central auditory process
Distorted Speech (S)	Measures specific central auditory process
Dix-Hallpike Dynamic (5)	Measures nystagmus following Dix-Hallpike maneuver
Dressing (1)	Includes/Examples: Includes selecting clothing and accessories, obtaining clothing from storage, dressing, fastening and adjusting clothing and shoes, and applying and removing personal devices, prosthesis or orthosis
Dressing Techniques (1)	Activities to facilitate selecting clothing and accessories, dressing and undressing, adjusting clothing and shoes, applying and removing devices, prostheses or orthoses
Dynamic Orthosis (6)	Includes/Examples: Includes customized and prefabricated splints, inhibitory casts, spinal and other braces, and protective devices; allows motion through transfer of movement from other body parts or by use of outside forces

Continued on next page

Section F–Physical Rehabilitation and Diagnostic Audiology

Continued from previous page

ICD-10-PCS Value Qualifier (Character 5)	Definition
Ear Canal Probe Microphone (1)	Real ear measures
Ear Protector Attentuation (7)	Measures ear protector fit and effectiveness
Electrocochleography (K)	Measures the VIIIth cranial nerve action potential
Environmental, Home, Work Barriers (B)	Measures current and potential barriers to optimal function, including safety hazards, access problems and home or office design
Ergonomics and Body Mechanics (C)	Ergonomic measurement of job tasks, work hardening or work conditioning needs; functional capacity; and body mechanics
Eustachian Tube Function (F)	Measures eustachian tube function and patency of eustachian tube
Evoked Otoacoustic Emissions, Diagnostic (N)	Measures auditory evoked potentials in a diagnostic format
Evoked Otoacoustic Emissions, Screening (M)	Measures auditory evoked potentials in a screening format
Facial Nerve Function (7)	Measures electrical activity of the VIIth cranial nerve (facial nerve)
Feeding/Eating (Assessment) (2)	Includes/Examples: Includes setting up food, selecting and using utensils and tableware, bringing food or drink to mouth, cleaning face, hands, and clothing, and management of alternative methods of nourishment
Feeding/Eating (Treatment) (3)	Exercise or activities to facilitate setting up food, selecting and using utensils and tableware, bringing food or drink to mouth, cleaning face, hands, and clothing, and management of alternative methods of nourishment
Filtered Speech (0)	Uses high or low pass filtered speech stimuli to assess central auditory processing disorders, site of lesion testing
Fluency (Assessment) (D)	Measures speech fluency or stuttering
Fluency (Treatment) (7)	Applying techniques to improve and augment fluent speech
Gait and/or Balance (D)	Measures biomechanical, arthrokinematic and other spatial and temporal characteristics of gait and balance
Gait Training/Functional Ambulation (9)	Exercise or activities to facilitate ambulation on a variety of surfaces and in a variety of environments
Grooming/Personal Hygiene (Assessment) (3)	Includes/Examples: Includes ability to obtain and use supplies in a sequential fashion, general grooming, oral hygiene, toilet hygiene, personal care devices, including care for artificial airways
Grooming/Personal Hygiene (Treatment) (2)	Activities to facilitate obtaining and using supplies in a sequential fashion: general grooming, oral hygiene, toilet hygiene, cleaning body, and personal care devices, including artificial airways
Hearing and Related Disorders Counseling (0)	Provides patients/families/caregivers with information, support, referrals to facilitate recovery from a communication disorder Includes/Examples: Includes strategies for psychosocial adjustment to hearing loss for clients and families/caregivers
Hearing and Related Disorders Prevention (1)	Provides patients/families/caregivers with information and support to prevent communication disorders
Hearing Screening (0)	Pass/refer measures designed to identify need for further audiologic assessment
Home Management (Assessment) (4)	Obtaining and maintaining personal and household possessions and environment Includes/Examples: Includes clothing care, cleaning, meal preparation and cleanup, shopping, money management, household maintenance, safety procedures, and childcare/parenting
Home Management (Treatment) (4)	Activities to facilitate obtaining and maintaining personal household possessions and environment Includes/Examples: Includes clothing care, cleaning, meal preparation and clean-up, shopping, money management, household maintenance, safety procedures, childcare/parenting
Instrumental Swallowing and Oral Function (J)	Measures swallowing function using instrumental diagnostic procedures Explanation: Methods include videofluoroscopy, ultrasound, manometry, endoscopy
Integumentary Integrity (1)	Includes/Examples: Includes burns, skin conditions, ecchymosis, bleeding, blisters, scar tissue, wounds and other traumas, tissue mobility, turgor and texture
Manual Therapy Techniques (7)	Techniques in which the therapist uses his/her hands to administer skilled movements Includes/Examples: Includes connective tissue massage, joint mobilization and manipulation, manual lymph drainage, manual traction, soft tissue mobilization and manipulation
Masking Patterns (W)	Measures central auditory processing status

Continued on next page

Section F–Physical Rehabilitation and Diagnostic Audiology

Continued from previous page

ICD-10-PCS Value Qualifier (Character 5)	Definition
Monaural Electroacoustic Hearing Aid Check (8)	Determines mechanical and electroacoustic function of one hearing aid using hearing aid test box
Monaural Hearing Aid (Assessment) (2)	Measures the candidacy, effectiveness, and appropriateness of a hearing aid Explanation: Measures unilateral fit
Monaural Hearing Aid (Treatment) (1)	Explanation: Assists in achieving maximum understanding and performance
Motor Function (Assessment) (4)	Measures the body's functional and versatile movement patterns Includes/Examples: Includes motor assessment scales, analysis of head, trunk and limb movement, and assessment of motor learning
Motor Function (Treatment) (3)	Exercise or activities to facilitate crossing midline, laterality, bilateral integration, praxis, neuromuscular relaxation, inhibition, facilitation, motor function and motor learning
Motor Speech (Assessment) (B)	Measures neurological motor aspects of speech production
Motor Speech (Treatment) (8)	Applying techniques to improve and augment the impaired neurological motor aspects of speech production
Muscle Performance (Assessment) (Ø)	Measures muscle strength, power and endurance using manual testing, dynamometry or computer-assisted electromechanical muscle test; functional muscle strength, power and endurance; muscle pain, tone, or soreness; or pelvic-floor musculature Explanation: Muscle endurance refers to the ability to contract a muscle repeatedly over time
Muscle Performance (Treatment) (1)	Exercise or activities to increase the capacity of a muscle to do work in terms of strength, power, and/or endurance Explanation: Muscle strength is the force exerted to overcome resistance in one maximal effort. Muscle power is work produced per unit of time, or the product of strength and speed. Muscle endurance is the ability to contract a muscle repeatedly over time.
Neuromotor Development (D)	Measures motor development, righting and equilibrium reactions, and reflex and equilibrium reactions
Non-invasive Instrumental Status (N)	Instrumental measures of oral, nasal, vocal, and velopharyngeal functions as they pertain to speech production
Nonspoken Language (Assessment) (7)	Measures nonspoken language (print, sign, symbols) for communication
Nonspoken Language (Treatment) (Ø)	Applying techniques that improve, augment, or compensate spoken communication
Oral Peripheral Mechanism (P)	Structural measures of face, jaw, lips, tongue, teeth, hard and soft palate, pharynx as related to speech production
Orofacial Myofunctional (Assessment) (K)	Measures orofacial myofunctional patterns for speech and related functions
Orofacial Myofunctional (Treatment) (9)	Applying techniques to improve, alter, or augment impaired orofacial myofunctional patterns and related speech production errors
Oscillating Tracking (3)	Measures ability to visually track
Pain (F)	Measures muscle soreness, pain and soreness with joint movement, and pain perception Includes/Examples: Includes questionnaires, graphs, symptom magnification scales or visual analog scales
Perceptual Processing (Assessment) (5)	Measures stereognosis, kinesthesia, body schema, right-left discrimination, form constancy, position in space, visual closure, figure-ground, depth perception, spatial relations and topographical orientation
Perceptual Processing (Treatment) (1)	Exercise and activities to facilitate perceptual processing Explanation: Includes stereognosis, kinesthesia, body schema, right-left discrimination, form constancy, position in space, visual closure, figure-ground, depth perception, spatial relations, and topographical orientation Includes/Examples: Includes stereognosis, kinesthesia, body schema, right-left discrimination, form constancy, position in space, visual closure, figure-ground, depth perception, spatial relations, and topographical orientation
Performance Intensity Phonetically Balanced Speech Discrimination (Q)	Measures word recognition over varying intensity levels
Postural Control (3)	Exercise or activities to increase postural alignment and control
Prosthesis (8)	Explanation: Artificial substitutes for missing body parts that augment performance or function Includes/Examples: Limb prosthesis, ocular prosthesis

Continued on next page

Section F–Physical Rehabilitation and Diagnostic Audiology

Continued from previous page

ICD-10-PCS Value Qualifier (Character 5)	Definition
Psychosocial Skills (Assessment) (6)	The ability to interact in society and to process emotions Includes/Examples: Includes psychological (values, interests, self-concept); social (role performance, social conduct, interpersonal skills, self expression); self-management (coping skills, time management, self-control)
Psychosocial Skills (Treatment) (6)	The ability to interact in society and to process emotions Includes/Examples: Includes psychological (values, interests, self-concept); social (role performance, social conduct, interpersonal skills, self expression); self-management (coping skills, time management, self-control)
Pure Tone Audiometry, Air (1)	Air-conduction pure tone threshold measures with appropriate masking
Pure Tone Audiometry, Air and Bone (2)	Air-conduction and bone-conduction pure tone threshold measures with appropriate masking
Pure Tone Stenger (C)	Measures unilateral nonorganic hearing loss based on simultaneous presentation of pure tones of differing volume
Range of Motion and Joint Integrity (5)	Measures quantity, quality, grade, and classification of joint movement and/or mobility Explanation: Range of Motion is the space, distance or angle through which movement occurs at a joint or series of joints. Joint integrity is the conformance of joints to expected anatomic, biomechanical and kinematic norms.
Range of Motion and Joint Mobility (Ø)	Exercise or activities to increase muscle length and joint mobility
Receptive/Expressive Language (Assessment) (8)	Measures receptive and expressive language
Receptive/Expressive Language (Treatment) (B)	Applying techniques to improve and augment receptive/expressive language
Reflex Integrity (G)	Measures the presence, absence, or exaggeration of developmentally appropriate, pathologic or normal reflexes
Select Picture Audiometry (5)	Establishes hearing threshold levels for speech using pictures
Sensorineural Acuity Level (4)	Measures sensorineural acuity masking presented via bone conduction
Sensory Aids (5)	Determines the appropriateness of a sensory prosthetic device, other than a hearing aid or assistive listening system/device
Sensory Awareness/ Processing/ Integrity (6)	Includes/Examples: Includes light touch, pressure, temperature, pain, sharp/dull, proprioception, vestibular, visual, auditory, gustatory, and olfactory
Short Increment Sensitivity Index (9)	Measures the ear's ability to detect small intensity changes; site of lesion test requiring a behavioral response
Sinusoidal Vertical Axis Rotational (4)	Measures nystagmus following rotation
Somatosensory Evoked Potentials (9)	Measures neural activity from sites throughout the body
Speech/Language Screening (6)	Identifies need for further speech and/or language evaluation
Speech Threshold (1)	Measures minimal intensity needed to repeat spondaic words
Speech-Language Pathology and Related Disorders Counseling (1)	Provides patients/families with information, support, referrals to facilitate recovery from a communication disorder
Speech-Language Pathology and Related Disorders Prevention (2)	Applying techniques to avoid or minimize onset and/or development of a communication disorder
Speech/Word Recognition (2)	Measures ability to repeat/identify single syllable words; scores given as a percentage; includes word recognition/speech discrimination
Staggered Spondaic Word (3)	Measures central auditory processing site of lesion based upon dichotic presentation of spondaic words
Static Orthosis (7)	Includes/Examples: Includes customized and prefabricated splints, inhibitory casts, spinal and other braces, and protective devices; has no moving parts, maintains joint(s) in desired position
Stenger (B)	Measures unilateral nonorganic hearing loss based on simultaneous presentation of signals of differing volume
Swallowing Dysfunction (D)	Activities to improve swallowing function in coordination with respiratory function Includes/Examples: Includes function and coordination of sucking, mastication, coughing, swallowing
Synthetic Sentence Identification (5)	Measures central auditory dysfunction using identification of third order approximations of sentences and competing messages

Continued on next page

Section F–Physical Rehabilitation and Diagnostic Audiology   *Continued from previous page*

ICD-10-PCS Value Qualifier (Character 5)	Definition
Temporal Ordering of Stimuli (V)	Measures specific central auditory process
Therapeutic Exercise (6)	Exercise or activities to facilitate sensory awareness, sensory processing, sensory integration, balance training, conditioning, reconditioning Includes/Examples: Includes developmental activities, breathing exercises, aerobic endurance activities, aquatic exercises, stretching and ventilatory muscle training
Tinnitus Masker (Assessment) (7)	Determines candidacy for tinnitus masker
Tinnitus Masker (Treatment) (Ø)	Explanation: Used to verify physical fit, acoustic appropriateness, and benefit; assists in achieving maximum benefit
Tone Decay (8)	Measures decrease in hearing sensitivity to a tone; site of lesion test requiring a behavioral response
Transfer (C)	Transitional movement from one surface to another
Transfer Training (8)	Exercise or activities to facilitate movement from one surface to another
Tympanometry (D)	Measures the integrity of the middle ear; measures ease at which sound flows through the tympanic membrane while air pressure against the membrane is varied
Unithermal Binaural Screen (2)	Measures the rhythmic eye movements stimulated by changing the temperature of the vestibular system in both ears using warm water, screening format
Ventilation/Respiration/Circulation (G)	Measures ventilatory muscle strength, power and endurance, pulmonary function and ventilatory mechanics Includes/Examples: Includes ability to clear airway, activities that aggravate or relieve edema, pain, dyspnea or other symptoms, chest wall mobility, cardiopulmonary response to performance of ADL and IAD, cough and sputum, standard vital signs
Vestibular (Ø)	Applying techniques to compensate for balance disorders; includes habituation, exercise therapy, and balance retraining
Visual Motor Integration (Assessment) (2)	Coordinating the interaction of information from the eyes with body movement during activity
Visual Motor Integration (Treatment) (2)	Exercise or activities to facilitate coordinating the interaction of information from eyes with body movement during activity
Visual Reinforcement Audiometry (6)	Behavioral measures using nonspeech and speech stimuli to obtain frequency/ear-specific information on auditory status Includes/Examples: Includes a conditioned response of looking toward a visual reinforcer (e.g., lights, animated toy) every time auditory stimuli are heard
Vocational Activities and Functional Community or Work Reintegration Skills (Assessment) (H)	Measures environmental, home, work (job/school/play) barriers that keep patients from functioning optimally in their environment Includes/Examples: Includes assessment of vocational skills and interests, environment of work (job/school/play), injury potential and injury prevention or reduction, ergonomic stressors, transportation skills, and ability to access and use community resources
Vocational Activities and Functional Community or Work Reintegration Skills (Treatment) (7)	Activities to facilitate vocational exploration, body mechanics training, job acquisition, and environmental or work (job/school/play) task adaptation Includes/Examples: Includes injury prevention and reduction, ergonomic stressor reduction, job coaching and simulation, work hardening and conditioning, driving training, transportation skills, and use of community resources
Voice (Assessment) (F)	Measures vocal structure, function and production
Voice (Treatment) (C)	Applying techniques to improve voice and vocal function
Voice Prosthetic (Assessment) (M)	Determines the appropriateness of voice prosthetic/adaptive device to enhance or facilitate communication
Voice Prosthetic (Treatment) (4)	Includes/Examples: Includes electrolarynx, and other assistive, adaptive, supportive devices
Wheelchair Mobility (Assessment) (F)	Measures fit and functional abilities within wheelchair in a variety of environments
Wheelchair Mobility (Treatment) (4)	Management, maintenance and controlled operation of a wheelchair, scooter or other device, in and on a variety of surfaces and environments
Wound Management (5)	Includes/Examples: Includes non-selective and selective debridement (enzymes, autolysis, sharp debridement), dressings (wound coverings, hydrogel, vacuum-assisted closure), topical agents, etc.

Section G–Mental Health

ICD-10-PCS Value (Character 3)	Definition
Biofeedback (C)	Provision of information from the monitoring and regulating of physiological processes in conjunction with cognitive-behavioral techniques to improve patient functioning or well-being Includes/Examples: Includes EEG, blood pressure, skin temperature or peripheral blood flow, ECG, electrooculogram, EMG, respirometry or capnometry, GSR/EDR, perineometry to monitor/regulate bowel/bladder activity, electrogastrogram to monitor/regulate gastric motility
Counseling (6)	The application of psychological methods to treat an individual with normal developmental issues and psychological problems in order to increase function, improve well-being, alleviate distress, maladjustment or resolve crises
Crisis Intervention (2)	Treatment of a traumatized, acutely disturbed or distressed individual for the purpose of short-term stabilization Includes/Examples: Includes defusing, debriefing, counseling, psychotherapy and/or coordination of care with other providers or agencies
Electroconvulsive Therapy (B)	The application of controlled electrical voltages to treat a mental health disorder Includes/Examples: Includes appropriate sedation and other preparation of the individual
Family Psychotherapy (7)	Treatment that includes one or more family members of an individual with a mental health disorder by behavioral, cognitive, psychoanalytic, psychodynamic or psychophysiological means to improve functioning or well-being Explanation: Remediation of emotional or behavioral problems presented by one or more family members in cases where psychotherapy with more than one family member is indicated
Group Psychotherapy (H)	Treatment of two or more individuals with a mental health disorder by behavioral, cognitive, psychoanalytic, psychodynamic or psychophysiological means to improve functioning or well-being
Hypnosis (F)	Induction of a state of heightened suggestibility by auditory, visual and tactile techniques to elicit an emotional or behavioral response
Individual Psychotherapy (5)	Treatment of an individual with a mental health disorder by behavioral, cognitive, psychoanalytic, psychodynamic or psychophysiological means to improve functioning or well-being
Light Therapy (J)	Application of specialized light treatments to improve functioning or well-being
Medication Management (3)	Monitoring and adjusting the use of medications for the treatment of a mental health disorder
Narcosynthesis (G)	Administration of intravenous barbiturates in order to release suppressed or repressed thoughts
Psychological Tests (1)	The administration and interpretation of standardized psychological tests and measurement instruments for the assessment of psychological function
Behavioral (1)	Primarily to modify behavior Includes/Examples: Includes modeling and role playing, positive reinforcement of target behaviors, response cost, and training of self-management skills
Cognitive (2)	Primarily to correct cognitive distortions and errors
Cognitive-Behavioral (8)	Combining cognitive and behavioral treatment strategies to improve functioning Explanation: Maladaptive responses are examined to determine how cognitions relate to behavior patterns in response to an event. Uses learning principles and information-processing models.
Developmental (Ø)	Age-normed developmental status of cognitive, social and adaptive behavior skills
Intellectual and Psychoeducational (2)	Intellectual abilities, academic achievement and learning capabilities (including behaviors and emotional factors affecting learning)
Interactive (Ø)	Uses primarily physical aids and other forms of non-oral interaction with a patient who is physically, psychologically or developmentally unable to use ordinary language for communication Includes/Examples: Includes the use of toys in symbolic play
Interpersonal (3)	Helps an individual make changes in interpersonal behaviors to reduce psychological dysfunction Includes/Examples: Includes exploratory techniques, encouragement of affective expression, clarification of patient statements, analysis of communication patterns, use of therapy relationship and behavior change techniques
Neurobehavioral and Cognitive Status (4)	Includes neurobehavioral status exam, interview(s), and observation for the clinical assessment of thinking, reasoning and judgment, acquired knowledge, attention, memory, visual spatial abilities, language functions, and planning
Neuropsychological (3)	Thinking, reasoning and judgment, acquired knowledge, attention, memory, visual spatial abilities, language functions, planning
Personality and Behavioral (1)	Mood, emotion, behavior, social functioning, psychopathological conditions, personality traits and characteristics

Continued on next page

Section G–Mental Health

Continued from previous page

ICD-10-PCS Value (Character 3)	Definition
Psychoanalysis (4)	Methods of obtaining a detailed account of past and present mental and emotional experiences to determine the source and eliminate or diminish the undesirable effects of unconscious conflicts Explanation: Accomplished by making the individual aware of their existence, origin, and inappropriate expression in emotions and behavior
Psychodynamic (5)	Exploration of past and present emotional experiences to understand motives and drives using insight-oriented techniques to reduce the undesirable effects of internal conflicts on emotions and behavior Explanation: Techniques include empathetic listening, clarifying self-defeating behavior patterns, and exploring adaptive alternatives
Psychophysiological (9)	Monitoring and alteration of physiological processes to help the individual associate physiological reactions combined with cognitive and behavioral strategies to gain improved control of these processes to help the individual cope more effectively
Supportive (6)	Formation of therapeutic relationship primarily for providing emotional support to prevent further deterioration in functioning during periods of particular stress Explanation: Often used in conjunction with other therapeutic approaches
Vocational (1)	Exploration of vocational interests, aptitudes and required adaptive behavior skills to develop and carry out a plan for achieving a successful vocational placement Includes/Examples: Includes enhancing work related adjustment and/or pursuing viable options in training education or preparation

Section H–Substance Abuse Treatment

ICD-10-PCS Value (Character 3)	Definition
Detoxification Services (2)	Detoxification from alcohol and/or drugs Explanation: Not a treatment modality, but helps the patient stabilize physically and psychologically until the body becomes free of drugs and the effects of alcohol
Family Counseling (6)	The application of psychological methods that includes one or more family members to treat an individual with addictive behavior Explanation: Provides support and education for family members of addicted individuals. Family member participation is seen as a critical area of substance abuse treatment.
Group Counseling (4)	The application of psychological methods to treat two or more individuals with addictive behavior Explanation: Provides structured group counseling sessions and healing power through the connection with others
Individual Counseling (3)	The application of psychological methods to treat an individual with addictive behavior Explanation: Comprised of several different techniques, which apply various strategies to address drug addiction
Individual Psychotherapy (5)	Treatment of an individual with addictive behavior by behavioral, cognitive, psychoanalytic, psychodynamic or psychophysiological means
Medication Management (8)	Monitoring and adjusting the use of replacement medications for the treatment of addiction
Pharmacotherapy (9)	The use of replacement medications for the treatment of addiction

Appendix K: Hospital Acquired Conditions

Hospital acquired conditions (HACs) are conditions considered reasonably preventable through the application of evidence-based guidelines. Although it is the ICD-10-CM diagnosis code that drives a HAC designation, in some cases a specific ICD-10-PCS procedure code must also be present before that diagnosis code can be considered a HAC. This resource provides only those HAC categories that require both an ICD-10-PCS code and an ICD-10-CM diagnosis code. The official descriptions for each code are also provided. To see all 14 HAC categories and their corresponding codes, refer to Optum's *ICD-10-CM Expert for Hospitals*.

Note: The resource used to compile this list is the proposed, version 40, MS-DRG Grouper software and Definitions Manual files published with the fiscal 2023 IPPS proposed rule. For the most current files, refer to the following: https://www.cms.gov/Medicare/Medicare-Fee-for-Service-Payment/AcuteInpatientPPS/MS-DRG-Classifications-and-Software.

HAC 08: Surgical Site Infection of Mediastinitis After Coronary Bypass Graft (CABG) Procedures

Secondary diagnosis not POA:

J98.51 Mediastinitis
J98.59 Other diseases of mediastinum, not elsewhere classified

AND

Any of the following procedures:

0210083 Bypass Coronary Artery, One Artery from Coronary Artery with Zooplastic Tissue, Open Approach
0210088 Bypass Coronary Artery, One Artery from Right Internal Mammary with Zooplastic Tissue, Open Approach
0210089 Bypass Coronary Artery, One Artery from Left Internal Mammary with Zooplastic Tissue, Open Approach
021008C Bypass Coronary Artery, One Artery from Thoracic Artery with Zooplastic Tissue, Open Approach
021008F Bypass Coronary Artery, One Artery from Abdominal Artery with Zooplastic Tissue, Open Approach
021008W Bypass Coronary Artery, One Artery from Aorta with Zooplastic Tissue, Open Approach
0210093 Bypass Coronary Artery, One Artery from Coronary Artery with Autologous Venous Tissue, Open Approach
0210098 Bypass Coronary Artery, One Artery from Right Internal Mammary with Autologous Venous Tissue, Open Approach
0210099 Bypass Coronary Artery, One Artery from Left Internal Mammary with Autologous Venous Tissue, Open Approach
021009C Bypass Coronary Artery, One Artery from Thoracic Artery with Autologous Venous Tissue, Open Approach
021009F Bypass Coronary Artery, One Artery from Abdominal Artery with Autologous Venous Tissue, Open Approach
021009W Bypass Coronary Artery, One Artery from Aorta with Autologous Venous Tissue, Open Approach
02100A3 Bypass Coronary Artery, One Artery from Coronary Artery with Autologous Arterial Tissue, Open Approach
02100A8 Bypass Coronary Artery, One Artery from Right Internal Mammary with Autologous Arterial Tissue, Open Approach
02100A9 Bypass Coronary Artery, One Artery from Left Internal Mammary with Autologous Arterial Tissue, Open Approach
02100AC Bypass Coronary Artery, One Artery from Thoracic Artery with Autologous Arterial Tissue, Open Approach
02100AF Bypass Coronary Artery, One Artery from Abdominal Artery with Autologous Arterial Tissue, Open Approach
02100AW Bypass Coronary Artery, One Artery from Aorta with Autologous Arterial Tissue, Open Approach

02100J3 Bypass Coronary Artery, One Artery from Coronary Artery with Synthetic Substitute, Open Approach
02100J8 Bypass Coronary Artery, One Artery from Right Internal Mammary with Synthetic Substitute, Open Approach
02100J9 Bypass Coronary Artery, One Artery from Left Internal Mammary with Synthetic Substitute, Open Approach
02100JC Bypass Coronary Artery, One Artery from Thoracic Artery with Synthetic Substitute, Open Approach
02100JF Bypass Coronary Artery, One Artery from Abdominal Artery with Synthetic Substitute, Open Approach
02100JW Bypass Coronary Artery, One Artery from Aorta with Synthetic Substitute, Open Approach
02100K3 Bypass Coronary Artery, One Artery from Coronary Artery with Nonautologous Tissue Substitute, Open Approach
02100K8 Bypass Coronary Artery, One Artery from Right Internal Mammary with Nonautologous Tissue Substitute, Open Approach
02100K9 Bypass Coronary Artery, One Artery from Left Internal Mammary with Nonautologous Tissue Substitute, Open Approach
02100KC Bypass Coronary Artery, One Artery from Thoracic Artery with Nonautologous Tissue Substitute, Open Approach
02100KF Bypass Coronary Artery, One Artery from Abdominal Artery with Nonautologous Tissue Substitute, Open Approach
02100KW Bypass Coronary Artery, One Artery from Aorta with Nonautologous Tissue Substitute, Open Approach
02100Z3 Bypass Coronary Artery, One Artery from Coronary Artery, Open Approach
02100Z8 Bypass Coronary Artery, One Artery from Right Internal Mammary, Open Approach
02100Z9 Bypass Coronary Artery, One Artery from Left Internal Mammary, Open Approach
02100ZC Bypass Coronary Artery, One Artery from Thoracic Artery, Open Approach
02100ZF Bypass Coronary Artery, One Artery from Abdominal Artery, Open Approach
0210483 Bypass Coronary Artery, One Artery from Coronary Artery with Zooplastic Tissue, Percutaneous Endoscopic Approach
0210488 Bypass Coronary Artery, One Artery from Right Internal Mammary with Zooplastic Tissue, Percutaneous Endoscopic Approach
0210489 Bypass Coronary Artery, One Artery from Left Internal Mammary with Zooplastic Tissue, Percutaneous Endoscopic Approach

021048C Bypass Coronary Artery, One Artery from Thoracic Artery with Zooplastic Tissue, Percutaneous Endoscopic Approach
021048F Bypass Coronary Artery, One Artery from Abdominal Artery with Zooplastic Tissue, Percutaneous Endoscopic Approach
021048W Bypass Coronary Artery, One Artery from Aorta with Zooplastic Tissue, Percutaneous Endoscopic Approach
0210493 Bypass Coronary Artery, One Artery from Coronary Artery with Autologous Venous Tissue, Percutaneous Endoscopic Approach
0210498 Bypass Coronary Artery, One Artery from Right Internal Mammary with Autologous Venous Tissue, Percutaneous Endoscopic Approach
0210499 Bypass Coronary Artery, One Artery from Left Internal Mammary with Autologous Venous Tissue, Percutaneous Endoscopic Approach
021049C Bypass Coronary Artery, One Artery from Thoracic Artery with Autologous Venous Tissue, Percutaneous Endoscopic Approach
021049F Bypass Coronary Artery, One Artery from Abdominal Artery with Autologous Venous Tissue, Percutaneous Endoscopic Approach
021049W Bypass Coronary Artery, One Artery from Aorta with Autologous Venous Tissue, Percutaneous Endoscopic Approach
02104A3 Bypass Coronary Artery, One Artery from Coronary Artery with Autologous Arterial Tissue, Percutaneous Endoscopic Approach
02104A8 Bypass Coronary Artery, One Artery from Right Internal Mammary with Autologous Arterial Tissue, Percutaneous Endoscopic Approach
02104A9 Bypass Coronary Artery, One Artery from Left Internal Mammary with Autologous Arterial Tissue, Percutaneous Endoscopic Approach
02104AC Bypass Coronary Artery, One Artery from Thoracic Artery with Autologous Arterial Tissue, Percutaneous Endoscopic Approach
02104AF Bypass Coronary Artery, One Artery from Abdominal Artery with Autologous Arterial Tissue, Percutaneous Endoscopic Approach
02104AW Bypass Coronary Artery, One Artery from Aorta with Autologous Arterial Tissue, Percutaneous Endoscopic Approach
02104J3 Bypass Coronary Artery, One Artery from Coronary Artery with Synthetic Substitute, Percutaneous Endoscopic Approach

HAC 08: Surgical Site Infection of Mediastinitis After Coronary Bypass Graft (CABG) Procedures (continued)

02104J8   Bypass Coronary Artery, One Artery from Right Internal Mammary with Synthetic Substitute, Percutaneous Endoscopic Approach

02104J9   Bypass Coronary Artery, One Artery from Left Internal Mammary with Synthetic Substitute, Percutaneous Endoscopic Approach

02104JC   Bypass Coronary Artery, One Artery from Thoracic Artery with Synthetic Substitute, Percutaneous Endoscopic Approach

02104JF   Bypass Coronary Artery, One Artery from Abdominal Artery with Synthetic Substitute, Percutaneous Endoscopic Approach

02104JW   Bypass Coronary Artery, One Artery from Aorta with Synthetic Substitute, Percutaneous Endoscopic Approach

02104K3   Bypass Coronary Artery, One Artery from Coronary Artery with Nonautologous Tissue Substitute, Percutaneous Endoscopic Approach

02104K8   Bypass Coronary Artery, One Artery from Right Internal Mammary with Nonautologous Tissue Substitute, Percutaneous Endoscopic Approach

02104K9   Bypass Coronary Artery, One Artery from Left Internal Mammary with Nonautologous Tissue Substitute, Percutaneous Endoscopic Approach

02104KC   Bypass Coronary Artery, One Artery from Thoracic Artery with Nonautologous Tissue Substitute, Percutaneous Endoscopic Approach

02104KF   Bypass Coronary Artery, One Artery from Abdominal Artery with Nonautologous Tissue Substitute, Percutaneous Endoscopic Approach

02104KW   Bypass Coronary Artery, One Artery from Aorta with Nonautologous Tissue Substitute, Percutaneous Endoscopic Approach

02104Z3   Bypass Coronary Artery, One Artery from Coronary Artery, Percutaneous Endoscopic Approach

02104Z8   Bypass Coronary Artery, One Artery from Right Internal Mammary, Percutaneous Endoscopic Approach

02104Z9   Bypass Coronary Artery, One Artery from Left Internal Mammary, Percutaneous Endoscopic Approach

02104ZC   Bypass Coronary Artery, One Artery from Thoracic Artery, Percutaneous Endoscopic Approach

02104ZF   Bypass Coronary Artery, One Artery from Abdominal Artery, Percutaneous Endoscopic Approach

0211083   Bypass Coronary Artery, Two Arteries from Coronary Artery with Zooplastic Tissue, Open Approach

0211088   Bypass Coronary Artery, Two Arteries from Right Internal Mammary with Zooplastic Tissue, Open Approach

0211089   Bypass Coronary Artery, Two Arteries from Left Internal Mammary with Zooplastic Tissue, Open Approach

021108C   Bypass Coronary Artery, Two Arteries from Thoracic Artery with Zooplastic Tissue, Open Approach

021108F   Bypass Coronary Artery, Two Arteries from Abdominal Artery with Zooplastic Tissue, Open Approach

021108W   Bypass Coronary Artery, Two Arteries from Aorta with Zooplastic Tissue, Open Approach

0211093   Bypass Coronary Artery, Two Arteries from Coronary Artery with Autologous Venous Tissue, Open Approach

0211098   Bypass Coronary Artery, Two Arteries from Right Internal Mammary with Autologous Venous Tissue, Open Approach

0211099   Bypass Coronary Artery, Two Arteries from Left Internal Mammary with Autologous Venous Tissue, Open Approach

021109C   Bypass Coronary Artery, Two Arteries from Thoracic Artery with Autologous Venous Tissue, Open Approach

021109F   Bypass Coronary Artery, Two Arteries from Abdominal Artery with Autologous Venous Tissue, Open Approach

021109W   Bypass Coronary Artery, Two Arteries from Aorta with Autologous Venous Tissue, Open Approach

02110A3   Bypass Coronary Artery, Two Arteries from Coronary Artery with Autologous Arterial Tissue, Open Approach

02110A8   Bypass Coronary Artery, Two Arteries from Right Internal Mammary with Autologous Arterial Tissue, Open Approach

02110A9   Bypass Coronary Artery, Two Arteries from Left Internal Mammary with Autologous Arterial Tissue, Open Approach

02110AC   Bypass Coronary Artery, Two Arteries from Thoracic Artery with Autologous Arterial Tissue, Open Approach

02110AF   Bypass Coronary Artery, Two Arteries from Abdominal Artery with Autologous Arterial Tissue, Open Approach

02110AW   Bypass Coronary Artery, Two Arteries from Aorta with Autologous Arterial Tissue, Open Approach

02110J3   Bypass Coronary Artery, Two Arteries from Coronary Artery with Synthetic Substitute, Open Approach

02110J8   Bypass Coronary Artery, Two Arteries from Right Internal Mammary with Synthetic Substitute, Open Approach

02110J9   Bypass Coronary Artery, Two Arteries from Left Internal Mammary with Synthetic Substitute, Open Approach

02110JC   Bypass Coronary Artery, Two Arteries from Thoracic Artery with Synthetic Substitute, Open Approach

02110JF   Bypass Coronary Artery, Two Arteries from Abdominal Artery with Synthetic Substitute, Open Approach

02110JW   Bypass Coronary Artery, Two Arteries from Aorta with Synthetic Substitute, Open Approach

02110K3   Bypass Coronary Artery, Two Arteries from Coronary Artery with Nonautologous Tissue Substitute, Open Approach

02110K8   Bypass Coronary Artery, Two Arteries from Right Internal Mammary with Nonautologous Tissue Substitute, Open Approach

02110K9   Bypass Coronary Artery, Two Arteries from Left Internal Mammary with Nonautologous Tissue Substitute, Open Approach

02110KC   Bypass Coronary Artery, Two Arteries from Thoracic Artery with Nonautologous Tissue Substitute, Open Approach

02110KF   Bypass Coronary Artery, Two Arteries from Abdominal Artery with Nonautologous Tissue Substitute, Open Approach

02110KW   Bypass Coronary Artery, Two Arteries from Aorta with Nonautologous Tissue Substitute, Open Approach

02110Z3   Bypass Coronary Artery, Two Arteries from Coronary Artery, Open Approach

02110Z8   Bypass Coronary Artery, Two Arteries from Right Internal Mammary, Open Approach

02110Z9   Bypass Coronary Artery, Two Arteries from Left Internal Mammary, Open Approach

02110ZC   Bypass Coronary Artery, Two Arteries from Thoracic Artery, Open Approach

02110ZF   Bypass Coronary Artery, Two Arteries from Abdominal Artery, Open Approach

0211483   Bypass Coronary Artery, Two Arteries from Coronary Artery with Zooplastic Tissue, Percutaneous Endoscopic Approach

0211488   Bypass Coronary Artery, Two Arteries from Right Internal Mammary with Zooplastic Tissue, Percutaneous Endoscopic Approach

0211489   Bypass Coronary Artery, Two Arteries from Left Internal Mammary with Zooplastic Tissue, Percutaneous Endoscopic Approach

021148C   Bypass Coronary Artery, Two Arteries from Thoracic Artery with Zooplastic Tissue, Percutaneous Endoscopic Approach

021148F   Bypass Coronary Artery, Two Arteries from Abdominal Artery with Zooplastic Tissue, Percutaneous Endoscopic Approach

021148W   Bypass Coronary Artery, Two Arteries from Aorta with Zooplastic Tissue, Percutaneous Endoscopic Approach

0211493   Bypass Coronary Artery, Two Arteries from Coronary Artery with Autologous Venous Tissue, Percutaneous Endoscopic Approach

0211498   Bypass Coronary Artery, Two Arteries from Right Internal Mammary with Autologous Venous Tissue, Percutaneous Endoscopic Approach

0211499   Bypass Coronary Artery, Two Arteries from Left Internal Mammary with Autologous Venous Tissue, Percutaneous Endoscopic Approach

021149C   Bypass Coronary Artery, Two Arteries from Thoracic Artery with Autologous Venous Tissue, Percutaneous Endoscopic Approach

021149F   Bypass Coronary Artery, Two Arteries from Abdominal Artery with Autologous Venous Tissue, Percutaneous Endoscopic Approach

021149W   Bypass Coronary Artery, Two Arteries from Aorta with Autologous Venous Tissue, Percutaneous Endoscopic Approach

02114A3   Bypass Coronary Artery, Two Arteries from Coronary Artery with Autologous Arterial Tissue, Percutaneous Endoscopic Approach

02114A8   Bypass Coronary Artery, Two Arteries from Right Internal Mammary with Autologous Arterial Tissue, Percutaneous Endoscopic Approach

02114A9   Bypass Coronary Artery, Two Arteries from Left Internal Mammary with Autologous Arterial Tissue, Percutaneous Endoscopic Approach

02114AC   Bypass Coronary Artery, Two Arteries from Thoracic Artery with Autologous Arterial Tissue, Percutaneous Endoscopic Approach

02114AF   Bypass Coronary Artery, Two Arteries from Abdominal Artery with Autologous Arterial Tissue, Percutaneous Endoscopic Approach

HAC 08: Surgical Site Infection of Mediastinitis After Coronary Bypass Graft (CABG) Procedures (continued)

02114AW Bypass Coronary Artery, Two Arteries from Aorta with Autologous Arterial Tissue, Percutaneous Endoscopic Approach

02114J3 Bypass Coronary Artery, Two Arteries from Coronary Artery with Synthetic Substitute, Percutaneous Endoscopic Approach

02114J8 Bypass Coronary Artery, Two Arteries from Right Internal Mammary with Synthetic Substitute, Percutaneous Endoscopic Approach

02114J9 Bypass Coronary Artery, Two Arteries from Left Internal Mammary with Synthetic Substitute, Percutaneous Endoscopic Approach

02114JC Bypass Coronary Artery, Two Arteries from Thoracic Artery with Synthetic Substitute, Percutaneous Endoscopic Approach

02114JF Bypass Coronary Artery, Two Arteries from Abdominal Artery with Synthetic Substitute, Percutaneous Endoscopic Approach

02114JW Bypass Coronary Artery, Two Arteries from Aorta with Synthetic Substitute, Percutaneous Endoscopic Approach

02114K3 Bypass Coronary Artery, Two Arteries from Coronary Artery with Nonautologous Tissue Substitute, Percutaneous Endoscopic Approach

02114K8 Bypass Coronary Artery, Two Arteries from Right Internal Mammary with Nonautologous Tissue Substitute, Percutaneous Endoscopic Approach

02114K9 Bypass Coronary Artery, Two Arteries from Left Internal Mammary with Nonautologous Tissue Substitute, Percutaneous Endoscopic Approach

02114KC Bypass Coronary Artery, Two Arteries from Thoracic Artery with Nonautologous Tissue Substitute, Percutaneous Endoscopic Approach

02114KF Bypass Coronary Artery, Two Arteries from Abdominal Artery with Nonautologous Tissue Substitute, Percutaneous Endoscopic Approach

02114KW Bypass Coronary Artery, Two Arteries from Aorta with Nonautologous Tissue Substitute, Percutaneous Endoscopic Approach

02114Z3 Bypass Coronary Artery, Two Arteries from Coronary Artery, Percutaneous Endoscopic Approach

02114Z8 Bypass Coronary Artery, Two Arteries from Right Internal Mammary, Percutaneous Endoscopic Approach

02114Z9 Bypass Coronary Artery, Two Arteries from Left Internal Mammary, Percutaneous Endoscopic Approach

02114ZC Bypass Coronary Artery, Two Arteries from Thoracic Artery, Percutaneous Endoscopic Approach

02114ZF Bypass Coronary Artery, Two Arteries from Abdominal Artery, Percutaneous Endoscopic Approach

0212083 Bypass Coronary Artery, Three Arteries from Coronary Artery with Zooplastic Tissue, Open Approach

0212088 Bypass Coronary Artery, Three Arteries from Right Internal Mammary with Zooplastic Tissue, Open Approach

0212089 Bypass Coronary Artery, Three Arteries from Left Internal Mammary with Zooplastic Tissue, Open Approach

021208C Bypass Coronary Artery, Three Arteries from Thoracic Artery with Zooplastic Tissue, Open Approach

021208F Bypass Coronary Artery, Three Arteries from Abdominal Artery with Zooplastic Tissue, Open Approach

021208W Bypass Coronary Artery, Three Arteries from Aorta with Zooplastic Tissue, Open Approach

0212093 Bypass Coronary Artery, Three Arteries from Coronary Artery with Autologous Venous Tissue, Open Approach

0212098 Bypass Coronary Artery, Three Arteries from Right Internal Mammary with Autologous Venous Tissue, Open Approach

0212099 Bypass Coronary Artery, Three Arteries from Left Internal Mammary with Autologous Venous Tissue, Open Approach

021209C Bypass Coronary Artery, Three Arteries from Thoracic Artery with Autologous Venous Tissue, Open Approach

021209F Bypass Coronary Artery, Three Arteries from Abdominal Artery with Autologous Venous Tissue, Open Approach

021209W Bypass Coronary Artery, Three Arteries from Aorta with Autologous Venous Tissue, Open Approach

02120A3 Bypass Coronary Artery, Three Arteries from Coronary Artery with Autologous Arterial Tissue, Open Approach

02120A8 Bypass Coronary Artery, Three Arteries from Right Internal Mammary with Autologous Arterial Tissue, Open Approach

02120A9 Bypass Coronary Artery, Three Arteries from Left Internal Mammary with Autologous Arterial Tissue, Open Approach

02120AC Bypass Coronary Artery, Three Arteries from Thoracic Artery with Autologous Arterial Tissue, Open Approach

02120AF Bypass Coronary Artery, Three Arteries from Abdominal Artery with Autologous Arterial Tissue, Open Approach

02120AW Bypass Coronary Artery, Three Arteries from Aorta with Autologous Arterial Tissue, Open Approach

02120J3 Bypass Coronary Artery, Three Arteries from Coronary Artery with Synthetic Substitute, Open Approach

02120J8 Bypass Coronary Artery, Three Arteries from Right Internal Mammary with Synthetic Substitute, Open Approach

02120J9 Bypass Coronary Artery, Three Arteries from Left Internal Mammary with Synthetic Substitute, Open Approach

02120JC Bypass Coronary Artery, Three Arteries from Thoracic Artery with Synthetic Substitute, Open Approach

02120JF Bypass Coronary Artery, Three Arteries from Abdominal Artery with Synthetic Substitute, Open Approach

02120JW Bypass Coronary Artery, Three Arteries from Aorta with Synthetic Substitute, Open Approach

02120K3 Bypass Coronary Artery, Three Arteries from Coronary Artery with Nonautologous Tissue Substitute, Open Approach

02120K8 Bypass Coronary Artery, Three Arteries from Right Internal Mammary with Nonautologous Tissue Substitute, Open Approach

02120K9 Bypass Coronary Artery, Three Arteries from Left Internal Mammary with Nonautologous Tissue Substitute, Open Approach

02120KC Bypass Coronary Artery, Three Arteries from Thoracic Artery with Nonautologous Tissue Substitute, Open Approach

02120KF Bypass Coronary Artery, Three Arteries from Abdominal Artery with Nonautologous Tissue Substitute, Open Approach

02120KW Bypass Coronary Artery, Three Arteries from Aorta with Nonautologous Tissue Substitute, Open Approach

02120Z3 Bypass Coronary Artery, Three Arteries from Coronary Artery, Open Approach

02120Z8 Bypass Coronary Artery, Three Arteries from Right Internal Mammary, Open Approach

02120Z9 Bypass Coronary Artery, Three Arteries from Left Internal Mammary, Open Approach

02120ZC Bypass Coronary Artery, Three Arteries from Thoracic Artery, Open Approach

02120ZF Bypass Coronary Artery, Three Arteries from Abdominal Artery, Open Approach

0212483 Bypass Coronary Artery, Three Arteries from Coronary Artery with Zooplastic Tissue, Percutaneous Endoscopic Approach

0212488 Bypass Coronary Artery, Three Arteries from Right Internal Mammary with Zooplastic Tissue, Percutaneous Endoscopic Approach

0212489 Bypass Coronary Artery, Three Arteries from Left Internal Mammary with Zooplastic Tissue, Percutaneous Endoscopic Approach

021248C Bypass Coronary Artery, Three Arteries from Thoracic Artery with Zooplastic Tissue, Percutaneous Endoscopic Approach

021248F Bypass Coronary Artery, Three Arteries from Abdominal Artery with Zooplastic Tissue, Percutaneous Endoscopic Approach

021248W Bypass Coronary Artery, Three Arteries from Aorta with Zooplastic Tissue, Percutaneous Endoscopic Approach

0212493 Bypass Coronary Artery, Three Arteries from Coronary Artery with Autologous Venous Tissue, Percutaneous Endoscopic Approach

0212498 Bypass Coronary Artery, Three Arteries from Right Internal Mammary with Autologous Venous Tissue, Percutaneous Endoscopic Approach

0212499 Bypass Coronary Artery, Three Arteries from Left Internal Mammary with Autologous Venous Tissue, Percutaneous Endoscopic Approach

021249C Bypass Coronary Artery, Three Arteries from Thoracic Artery with Autologous Venous Tissue, Percutaneous Endoscopic Approach

021249F Bypass Coronary Artery, Three Arteries from Abdominal Artery with Autologous Venous Tissue, Percutaneous Endoscopic Approach

021249W Bypass Coronary Artery, Three Arteries from Aorta with Autologous Venous Tissue, Percutaneous Endoscopic Approach

02124A3 Bypass Coronary Artery, Three Arteries from Coronary Artery with Autologous Arterial Tissue, Percutaneous Endoscopic Approach

HAC 08: Surgical Site Infection of Mediastinitis After Coronary Bypass Graft (CABG) Procedures (continued)

02124A8 Bypass Coronary Artery, Three Arteries from Right Internal Mammary with Autologous Arterial Tissue, Percutaneous Endoscopic Approach

02124A9 Bypass Coronary Artery, Three Arteries from Left Internal Mammary with Autologous Arterial Tissue, Percutaneous Endoscopic Approach

02124AC Bypass Coronary Artery, Three Arteries from Thoracic Artery with Autologous Arterial Tissue, Percutaneous Endoscopic Approach

02124AF Bypass Coronary Artery, Three Arteries from Abdominal Artery with Autologous Arterial Tissue, Percutaneous Endoscopic Approach

02124AW Bypass Coronary Artery, Three Arteries from Aorta with Autologous Arterial Tissue, Percutaneous Endoscopic Approach

02124J3 Bypass Coronary Artery, Three Arteries from Coronary Artery with Synthetic Substitute, Percutaneous Endoscopic Approach

02124J8 Bypass Coronary Artery, Three Arteries from Right Internal Mammary with Synthetic Substitute, Percutaneous Endoscopic Approach

02124J9 Bypass Coronary Artery, Three Arteries from Left Internal Mammary with Synthetic Substitute, Percutaneous Endoscopic Approach

02124JC Bypass Coronary Artery, Three Arteries from Thoracic Artery with Synthetic Substitute, Percutaneous Endoscopic Approach

02124JF Bypass Coronary Artery, Three Arteries from Abdominal Artery with Synthetic Substitute, Percutaneous Endoscopic Approach

02124JW Bypass Coronary Artery, Three Arteries from Aorta with Synthetic Substitute, Percutaneous Endoscopic Approach

02124K3 Bypass Coronary Artery, Three Arteries from Coronary Artery with Nonautologous Tissue Substitute, Percutaneous Endoscopic Approach

02124K8 Bypass Coronary Artery, Three Arteries from Right Internal Mammary with Nonautologous Tissue Substitute, Percutaneous Endoscopic Approach

02124K9 Bypass Coronary Artery, Three Arteries from Left Internal Mammary with Nonautologous Tissue Substitute, Percutaneous Endoscopic Approach

02124KC Bypass Coronary Artery, Three Arteries from Thoracic Artery with Nonautologous Tissue Substitute, Percutaneous Endoscopic Approach

02124KF Bypass Coronary Artery, Three Arteries from Abdominal Artery with Nonautologous Tissue Substitute, Percutaneous Endoscopic Approach

02124KW Bypass Coronary Artery, Three Arteries from Aorta with Nonautologous Tissue Substitute, Percutaneous Endoscopic Approach

02124Z3 Bypass Coronary Artery, Three Arteries from Coronary Artery, Percutaneous Endoscopic Approach

02124Z8 Bypass Coronary Artery, Three Arteries from Right Internal Mammary, Percutaneous Endoscopic Approach

02124Z9 Bypass Coronary Artery, Three Arteries from Left Internal Mammary, Percutaneous Endoscopic Approach

02124ZC Bypass Coronary Artery, Three Arteries from Thoracic Artery, Percutaneous Endoscopic Approach

02124ZF Bypass Coronary Artery, Three Arteries from Abdominal Artery, Percutaneous Endoscopic Approach

0213083 Bypass Coronary Artery, Four or More Arteries from Coronary Artery with Zooplastic Tissue, Open Approach

0213088 Bypass Coronary Artery, Four or More Arteries from Right Internal Mammary with Zooplastic Tissue, Open Approach

0213089 Bypass Coronary Artery, Four or More Arteries from Left Internal Mammary with Zooplastic Tissue, Open Approach

021308C Bypass Coronary Artery, Four or More Arteries from Thoracic Artery with Zooplastic Tissue, Open Approach

021308F Bypass Coronary Artery, Four or More Arteries from Abdominal Artery with Zooplastic Tissue, Open Approach

021308W Bypass Coronary Artery, Four or More Arteries from Aorta with Zooplastic Tissue, Open Approach

0213093 Bypass Coronary Artery, Four or More Arteries from Coronary Artery with Autologous Venous Tissue, Open Approach

0213098 Bypass Coronary Artery, Four or More Arteries from Right Internal Mammary with Autologous Venous Tissue, Open Approach

0213099 Bypass Coronary Artery, Four or More Arteries from Left Internal Mammary with Autologous Venous Tissue, Open Approach

021309C Bypass Coronary Artery, Four or More Arteries from Thoracic Artery with Autologous Venous Tissue, Open Approach

021309F Bypass Coronary Artery, Four or More Arteries from Abdominal Artery with Autologous Venous Tissue, Open Approach

021309W Bypass Coronary Artery, Four or More Arteries from Aorta with Autologous Venous Tissue, Open Approach

02130A3 Bypass Coronary Artery, Four or More Arteries from Coronary Artery with Autologous Arterial Tissue, Open Approach

02130A8 Bypass Coronary Artery, Four or More Arteries from Right Internal Mammary with Autologous Arterial Tissue, Open Approach

02130A9 Bypass Coronary Artery, Four or More Arteries from Left Internal Mammary with Autologous Arterial Tissue, Open Approach

02130AC Bypass Coronary Artery, Four or More Arteries from Thoracic Artery with Autologous Arterial Tissue, Open Approach

02130AF Bypass Coronary Artery, Four or More Arteries from Abdominal Artery with Autologous Arterial Tissue, Open Approach

02130AW Bypass Coronary Artery, Four or More Arteries from Aorta with Autologous Arterial Tissue, Open Approach

02130J3 Bypass Coronary Artery, Four or More Arteries from Coronary Artery with Synthetic Substitute, Open Approach

02130J8 Bypass Coronary Artery, Four or More Arteries from Right Internal Mammary with Synthetic Substitute, Open Approach

02130J9 Bypass Coronary Artery, Four or More Arteries from Left Internal Mammary with Synthetic Substitute, Open Approach

02130JC Bypass Coronary Artery, Four or More Arteries from Thoracic Artery with Synthetic Substitute, Open Approach

02130JF Bypass Coronary Artery, Four or More Arteries from Abdominal Artery with Synthetic Substitute, Open Approach

02130JW Bypass Coronary Artery, Four or More Arteries from Aorta with Synthetic Substitute, Open Approach

02130K3 Bypass Coronary Artery, Four or More Arteries from Coronary Artery with Nonautologous Tissue Substitute, Open Approach

02130K8 Bypass Coronary Artery, Four or More Arteries from Right Internal Mammary with Nonautologous Tissue Substitute, Open Approach

02130K9 Bypass Coronary Artery, Four or More Arteries from Left Internal Mammary with Nonautologous Tissue Substitute, Open Approach

02130KC Bypass Coronary Artery, Four or More Arteries from Thoracic Artery with Nonautologous Tissue Substitute, Open Approach

02130KF Bypass Coronary Artery, Four or More Arteries from Abdominal Artery with Nonautologous Tissue Substitute, Open Approach

02130KW Bypass Coronary Artery, Four or More Arteries from Aorta with Nonautologous Tissue Substitute, Open Approach

02130Z3 Bypass Coronary Artery, Four or More Arteries from Coronary Artery, Open Approach

02130Z8 Bypass Coronary Artery, Four or More Arteries from Right Internal Mammary, Open Approach

02130Z9 Bypass Coronary Artery, Four or More Arteries from Left Internal Mammary, Open Approach

02130ZC Bypass Coronary Artery, Four or More Arteries from Thoracic Artery, Open Approach

02130ZF Bypass Coronary Artery, Four or More Arteries from Abdominal Artery, Open Approach

0213483 Bypass Coronary Artery, Four or More Arteries from Coronary Artery with Zooplastic Tissue, Percutaneous Endoscopic Approach

0213488 Bypass Coronary Artery, Four or More Arteries from Right Internal Mammary with Zooplastic Tissue, Percutaneous Endoscopic Approach

0213489 Bypass Coronary Artery, Four or More Arteries from Left Internal Mammary with Zooplastic Tissue, Percutaneous Endoscopic Approach

021348C Bypass Coronary Artery, Four or More Arteries from Thoracic Artery with Zooplastic Tissue, Percutaneous Endoscopic Approach

021348F Bypass Coronary Artery, Four or More Arteries from Abdominal Artery with Zooplastic Tissue, Percutaneous Endoscopic Approach

021348W Bypass Coronary Artery, Four or More Arteries from Aorta with Zooplastic Tissue, Percutaneous Endoscopic Approach

HAC 08: Surgical Site Infection of Mediastinitis After Coronary Bypass Graft (CABG) Procedures (continued)

0213493	Bypass Coronary Artery, Four or More Arteries from Coronary Artery with Autologous Venous Tissue, Percutaneous Endoscopic Approach
0213498	Bypass Coronary Artery, Four or More Arteries from Right Internal Mammary with Autologous Venous Tissue, Percutaneous Endoscopic Approach
0213499	Bypass Coronary Artery, Four or More Arteries from Left Internal Mammary with Autologous Venous Tissue, Percutaneous Endoscopic Approach
021349C	Bypass Coronary Artery, Four or More Arteries from Thoracic Artery with Autologous Venous Tissue, Percutaneous Endoscopic Approach
021349F	Bypass Coronary Artery, Four or More Arteries from Abdominal Artery with Autologous Venous Tissue, Percutaneous Endoscopic Approach
021349W	Bypass Coronary Artery, Four or More Arteries from Aorta with Autologous Venous Tissue, Percutaneous Endoscopic Approach
02134A3	Bypass Coronary Artery, Four or More Arteries from Coronary Artery with Autologous Arterial Tissue, Percutaneous Endoscopic Approach
02134A8	Bypass Coronary Artery, Four or More Arteries from Right Internal Mammary with Autologous Arterial Tissue, Percutaneous Endoscopic Approach
02134A9	Bypass Coronary Artery, Four or More Arteries from Left Internal Mammary with Autologous Arterial Tissue, Percutaneous Endoscopic Approach
02134AC	Bypass Coronary Artery, Four or More Arteries from Thoracic Artery with Autologous Arterial Tissue, Percutaneous Endoscopic Approach
02134AF	Bypass Coronary Artery, Four or More Arteries from Abdominal Artery with Autologous Arterial Tissue, Percutaneous Endoscopic Approach
02134AW	Bypass Coronary Artery, Four or More Arteries from Aorta with Autologous Arterial Tissue, Percutaneous Endoscopic Approach
02134J3	Bypass Coronary Artery, Four or More Arteries from Coronary Artery with Synthetic Substitute, Percutaneous Endoscopic Approach
02134J8	Bypass Coronary Artery, Four or More Arteries from Right Internal Mammary with Synthetic Substitute, Percutaneous Endoscopic Approach
02134J9	Bypass Coronary Artery, Four or More Arteries from Left Internal Mammary with Synthetic Substitute, Percutaneous Endoscopic Approach
02134JC	Bypass Coronary Artery, Four or More Arteries from Thoracic Artery with Synthetic Substitute, Percutaneous Endoscopic Approach
02134JF	Bypass Coronary Artery, Four or More Arteries from Abdominal Artery with Synthetic Substitute, Percutaneous Endoscopic Approach
02134JW	Bypass Coronary Artery, Four or More Arteries from Aorta with Synthetic Substitute, Percutaneous Endoscopic Approach
02134K3	Bypass Coronary Artery, Four or More Arteries from Coronary Artery with Nonautologous Tissue Substitute, Percutaneous Endoscopic Approach
02134K8	Bypass Coronary Artery, Four or More Arteries from Right Internal Mammary with Nonautologous Tissue Substitute, Percutaneous Endoscopic Approach
02134K9	Bypass Coronary Artery, Four or More Arteries from Left Internal Mammary with Nonautologous Tissue Substitute, Percutaneous Endoscopic Approach
02134KC	Bypass Coronary Artery, Four or More Arteries from Thoracic Artery with Nonautologous Tissue Substitute, Percutaneous Endoscopic Approach
02134KF	Bypass Coronary Artery, Four or More Arteries from Abdominal Artery with Nonautologous Tissue Substitute, Percutaneous Endoscopic Approach
02134KW	Bypass Coronary Artery, Four or More Arteries from Aorta with Nonautologous Tissue Substitute, Percutaneous Endoscopic Approach
02134Z3	Bypass Coronary Artery, Four or More Arteries from Coronary Artery, Percutaneous Endoscopic Approach
02134Z8	Bypass Coronary Artery, Four or More Arteries from Right Internal Mammary, Percutaneous Endoscopic Approach
02134Z9	Bypass Coronary Artery, Four or More Arteries from Left Internal Mammary, Percutaneous Endoscopic Approach
02134ZC	Bypass Coronary Artery, Four or More Arteries from Thoracic Artery, Percutaneous Endoscopic Approach
02134ZF	Bypass Coronary Artery, Four or More Arteries from Abdominal Artery, Percutaneous Endoscopic Approach

HAC 10: Deep Vein Thrombosis (DVT) or Pulmonary Embolism (PE) with Total Knee or Hip Replacement

Secondary diagnosis not POA:

I26.02	Saddle embolus of pulmonary artery with acute cor pulmonale
I26.09	Other pulmonary embolism with acute cor pulmonale
I26.92	Saddle embolus of pulmonary artery without acute cor pulmonale
I26.93	Single subsegmental pulmonary embolism without acute cor pulmonale
I26.94	Multiple subsegmental pulmonary emboli without acute cor pulmonale
I26.99	Other pulmonary embolism without acute cor pulmonale
I82.401	Acute embolism and thrombosis of unspecified deep veins of right lower extremity
I82.402	Acute embolism and thrombosis of unspecified deep veins of left lower extremity
I82.403	Acute embolism and thrombosis of unspecified deep veins of lower extremity, bilateral
I82.409	Acute embolism and thrombosis of unspecified deep veins of unspecified lower extremity
I82.411	Acute embolism and thrombosis of right femoral vein
I82.412	Acute embolism and thrombosis of left femoral vein
I82.413	Acute embolism and thrombosis of femoral vein, bilateral
I82.419	Acute embolism and thrombosis of unspecified femoral vein
I82.421	Acute embolism and thrombosis of right iliac vein
I82.422	Acute embolism and thrombosis of left iliac vein
I82.423	Acute embolism and thrombosis of iliac vein, bilateral
I82.429	Acute embolism and thrombosis of unspecified iliac vein
I82.431	Acute embolism and thrombosis of right popliteal vein
I82.432	Acute embolism and thrombosis of left popliteal vein
I82.433	Acute embolism and thrombosis of popliteal vein, bilateral
I82.439	Acute embolism and thrombosis of unspecified popliteal vein
I82.441	Acute embolism and thrombosis of right tibial vein
I82.442	Acute embolism and thrombosis of left tibial vein
I82.443	Acute embolism and thrombosis of tibial vein, bilateral
I82.449	Acute embolism and thrombosis of unspecified tibial vein
I82.451	Acute embolism and thrombosis of right peroneal vein
I82.452	Acute embolism and thrombosis of left peroneal vein
I82.453	Acute embolism and thrombosis of peroneal vein, bilateral
I82.459	Acute embolism and thrombosis of unspecified peroneal vein
I82.491	Acute embolism and thrombosis of other specified deep vein of right lower extremity
I82.492	Acute embolism and thrombosis of other specified deep vein of left lower extremity
I82.493	Acute embolism and thrombosis of other specified deep vein of lower extremity, bilateral
I82.499	Acute embolism and thrombosis of other specified deep vein of unspecified lower extremity
I82.4Y1	Acute embolism and thrombosis of unspecified deep veins of right proximal lower extremity
I82.4Y2	Acute embolism and thrombosis of unspecified deep veins of left proximal lower extremity
I82.4Y3	Acute embolism and thrombosis of unspecified deep veins of proximal lower extremity, bilateral
I82.4Y9	Acute embolism and thrombosis of unspecified deep veins of unspecified proximal lower extremity
I82.4Z1	Acute embolism and thrombosis of unspecified deep veins of right distal lower extremity
I82.4Z2	Acute embolism and thrombosis of unspecified deep veins of left distal lower extremity
I82.4Z3	Acute embolism and thrombosis of unspecified deep veins of distal lower extremity, bilateral
I82.4Z9	Acute embolism and thrombosis of unspecified deep veins of unspecified distal lower extremity

AND

Any of the following procedures:

0SR9019	Replacement of Right Hip Joint with Metal Synthetic Substitute, Cemented, Open Approach
0SR901A	Replacement of Right Hip Joint with Metal Synthetic Substitute, Uncemented, Open Approach

HAC 10: Deep Vein Thrombosis (DVT) or Pulmonary Embolism (PE) with Total Knee or Hip Replacement (continued)

ØSR901Z   Replacement of Right Hip Joint with Metal Synthetic Substitute, Open Approach

ØSR9029   Replacement of Right Hip Joint with Metal on Polyethylene Synthetic Substitute, Cemented, Open Approach

ØSR902A   Replacement of Right Hip Joint with Metal on Polyethylene Synthetic Substitute, Uncemented, Open Approach

ØSR902Z   Replacement of Right Hip Joint with Metal on Polyethylene Synthetic Substitute, Open Approach

ØSR9039   Replacement of Right Hip Joint with Ceramic Synthetic Substitute, Cemented, Open Approach

ØSR903A   Replacement of Right Hip Joint with Ceramic Synthetic Substitute, Uncemented, Open Approach

ØSR903Z   Replacement of Right Hip Joint with Ceramic Synthetic Substitute, Open Approach

ØSR9049   Replacement of Right Hip Joint with Ceramic on Polyethylene Synthetic Substitute, Cemented, Open Approach

ØSR904A   Replacement of Right Hip Joint with Ceramic on Polyethylene Synthetic Substitute, Uncemented, Open Approach

ØSR904Z   Replacement of Right Hip Joint with Ceramic on Polyethylene Synthetic Substitute, Open Approach

ØSR9069   Replacement of Right Hip Joint with Oxidized Zirconium on Polyethylene Synthetic Substitute, Cemented, Open Approach

ØSR906A   Replacement of Right Hip Joint with Oxidized Zirconium on Polyethylene Synthetic Substitute, Uncemented, Open Approach

ØSR906Z   Replacement of Right Hip Joint with Oxidized Zirconium on Polyethylene Synthetic Substitute, Open Approach

ØSR907Z   Replacement of Right Hip Joint with Autologous Tissue Substitute, Open Approach

ØSR90EZ   Replacement of Right Hip Joint with Articulating Spacer, Open Approach

ØSR90J9   Replacement of Right Hip Joint with Synthetic Substitute, Cemented, Open Approach

ØSR90JA   Replacement of Right Hip Joint with Synthetic Substitute, Uncemented, Open Approach

ØSR90JZ   Replacement of Right Hip Joint with Synthetic Substitute, Open Approach

ØSR90KZ   Replacement of Right Hip Joint with Nonautologous Tissue Substitute, Open Approach

ØSRA009   Replacement of Right Hip Joint, Acetabular Surface with Polyethylene Synthetic Substitute, Cemented, Open Approach

ØSRA00A   Replacement of Right Hip Joint, Acetabular Surface with Polyethylene Synthetic Substitute, Uncemented, Open Approach

ØSRA00Z   Replacement of Right Hip Joint, Acetabular Surface with Polyethylene Synthetic Substitute, Open Approach

ØSRA019   Replacement of Right Hip Joint, Acetabular Surface with Metal Synthetic Substitute, Cemented, Open Approach

ØSRA01A   Replacement of Right Hip Joint, Acetabular Surface with Metal Synthetic Substitute, Uncemented, Open Approach

ØSRA01Z   Replacement of Right Hip Joint, Acetabular Surface with Metal Synthetic Substitute, Open Approach

ØSRA039   Replacement of Right Hip Joint, Acetabular Surface with Ceramic Synthetic Substitute, Cemented, Open Approach

ØSRA03A   Replacement of Right Hip Joint, Acetabular Surface with Ceramic Synthetic Substitute, Uncemented, Open Approach

ØSRA03Z   Replacement of Right Hip Joint, Acetabular Surface with Ceramic Synthetic Substitute, Open Approach

ØSRA07Z   Replacement of Right Hip Joint, Acetabular Surface with Autologous Tissue Substitute, Open Approach

ØSRA0J9   Replacement of Right Hip Joint, Acetabular Surface with Synthetic Substitute, Cemented, Open Approach

ØSRA0JA   Replacement of Right Hip Joint, Acetabular Surface with Synthetic Substitute, Uncemented, Open Approach

ØSRA0JZ   Replacement of Right Hip Joint, Acetabular Surface with Synthetic Substitute, Open Approach

ØSRA0KZ   Replacement of Right Hip Joint, Acetabular Surface with Nonautologous Tissue Substitute, Open Approach

ØSRB019   Replacement of Left Hip Joint with Metal Synthetic Substitute, Cemented, Open Approach

ØSRB01A   Replacement of Left Hip Joint with Metal Synthetic Substitute, Uncemented, Open Approach

ØSRB01Z   Replacement of Left Hip Joint with Metal Synthetic Substitute, Open Approach

ØSRB029   Replacement of Left Hip Joint with Metal on Polyethylene Synthetic Substitute, Cemented, Open Approach

ØSRB02A   Replacement of Left Hip Joint with Metal on Polyethylene Synthetic Substitute, Uncemented, Open Approach

ØSRB02Z   Replacement of Left Hip Joint with Metal on Polyethylene Synthetic Substitute, Open Approach

ØSRB039   Replacement of Left Hip Joint with Ceramic Synthetic Substitute, Cemented, Open Approach

ØSRB03A   Replacement of Left Hip Joint with Ceramic Synthetic Substitute, Uncemented, Open Approach

ØSRB03Z   Replacement of Left Hip Joint with Ceramic Synthetic Substitute, Open Approach

ØSRB049   Replacement of Left Hip Joint with Ceramic on Polyethylene Synthetic Substitute, Cemented, Open Approach

ØSRB04A   Replacement of Left Hip Joint with Ceramic on Polyethylene Synthetic Substitute, Uncemented, Open Approach

ØSRB04Z   Replacement of Left Hip Joint with Ceramic on Polyethylene Synthetic Substitute, Open Approach

ØSRB069   Replacement of Left Hip Joint with Oxidized Zirconium on Polyethylene Synthetic Substitute, Cemented, Open Approach

ØSRB06A   Replacement of Left Hip Joint with Oxidized Zirconium on Polyethylene Synthetic Substitute, Uncemented, Open Approach

ØSRB06Z   Replacement of Left Hip Joint with Oxidized Zirconium on Polyethylene Synthetic Substitute, Open Approach

ØSRB07Z   Replacement of Left Hip Joint with Autologous Tissue Substitute, Open Approach

ØSRB0EZ   Replacement of Left Hip Joint with Articulating Spacer, Open Approach

ØSRB0J9   Replacement of Left Hip Joint with Synthetic Substitute, Cemented, Open Approach

ØSRB0JA   Replacement of Left Hip Joint with Synthetic Substitute, Uncemented, Open Approach

ØSRB0JZ   Replacement of Left Hip Joint with Synthetic Substitute, Open Approach

ØSRB0KZ   Replacement of Left Hip Joint with Nonautologous Tissue Substitute, Open Approach

ØSRC069   Replacement of Right Knee Joint with Oxidized Zirconium on Polyethylene Synthetic Substitute, Cemented, Open Approach

ØSRC06A   Replacement of Right Knee Joint with Oxidized Zirconium on Polyethylene Synthetic Substitute, Uncemented, Open Approach

ØSRC06Z   Replacement of Right Knee Joint with Oxidized Zirconium on Polyethylene Synthetic Substitute, Open Approach

ØSRC07Z   Replacement of Right Knee Joint with Autologous Tissue Substitute, Open Approach

ØSRC0EZ   Replacement of Right Knee Joint with Articulating Spacer, Open Approach

ØSRC0J9   Replacement of Right Knee Joint with Synthetic Substitute, Cemented, Open Approach

ØSRC0JA   Replacement of Right Knee Joint with Synthetic Substitute, Uncemented, Open Approach

ØSRC0JZ   Replacement of Right Knee Joint with Synthetic Substitute, Open Approach

ØSRC0KZ   Replacement of Right Knee Joint with Nonautologous Tissue Substitute, Open Approach

ØSRC0L9   Replacement of Right Knee Joint with Medial Unicondylar Synthetic Substitute, Cemented, Open Approach

ØSRC0LA   Replacement of Right Knee Joint with Medial Unicondylar Synthetic Substitute, Uncemented, Open Approach

ØSRC0LZ   Replacement of Right Knee Joint with Medial Unicondylar Synthetic Substitute, Open Approach

ØSRC0M9   Replacement of Right Knee Joint with Lateral Unicondylar Synthetic Substitute, Cemented, Open Approach

ØSRC0MA   Replacement of Right Knee Joint with Lateral Unicondylar Synthetic Substitute, Uncemented, Open Approach

ØSRC0MZ   Replacement of Right Knee Joint with Lateral Unicondylar Synthetic Substitute, Open Approach

ØSRC0N9   Replacement of Right Knee Joint with Patellofemoral Synthetic Substitute, Cemented, Open Approach

ØSRC0NA   Replacement of Right Knee Joint with Patellofemoral Synthetic Substitute, Uncemented, Open Approach

ØSRC0NZ   Replacement of Right Knee Joint with Patellofemoral Synthetic Substitute, Open Approach

ØSRD069   Replacement of Left Knee Joint with Oxidized Zirconium on Polyethylene Synthetic Substitute, Cemented, Open Approach

ØSRD06A   Replacement of Left Knee Joint with Oxidized Zirconium on Polyethylene Synthetic Substitute, Uncemented, Open Approach

HAC 10: Deep Vein Thrombosis (DVT) or Pulmonary Embolism (PE) with Total Knee or Hip Replacement (continued)

ØSRDØ6Z Replacement of Left Knee Joint with Oxidized Zirconium on Polyethylene Synthetic Substitute, Open Approach

ØSRDØ7Z Replacement of Left Knee Joint with Autologous Tissue Substitute, Open Approach

ØSRDØEZ Replacement of Left Knee Joint with Articulating Spacer, Open Approach

ØSRDØJ9 Replacement of Left Knee Joint with Synthetic Substitute, Cemented, Open Approach

ØSRDØJA Replacement of Left Knee Joint with Synthetic Substitute, Uncemented, Open Approach

ØSRDØJZ Replacement of Left Knee Joint with Synthetic Substitute, Open Approach

ØSRDØKZ Replacement of Left Knee Joint with Nonautologous Tissue Substitute, Open Approach

ØSRDØL9 Replacement of Left Knee Joint with Medial Unicondylar Synthetic Substitute, Cemented, Open Approach

ØSRDØLA Replacement of Left Knee Joint with Medial Unicondylar Synthetic Substitute, Uncemented, Open Approach

ØSRDØLZ Replacement of Left Knee Joint with Medial Unicondylar Synthetic Substitute, Open Approach

ØSRDØM9 Replacement of Left Knee Joint with Lateral Unicondylar Synthetic Substitute, Cemented, Open Approach

ØSRDØMA Replacement of Left Knee Joint with Lateral Unicondylar Synthetic Substitute, Uncemented, Open Approach

ØSRDØMZ Replacement of Left Knee Joint with Lateral Unicondylar Synthetic Substitute, Open Approach

ØSRDØN9 Replacement of Left Knee Joint with Patellofemoral Synthetic Substitute, Cemented, Open Approach

ØSRDØNA Replacement of Left Knee Joint with Patellofemoral Synthetic Substitute, Uncemented, Open Approach

ØSRDØNZ Replacement of Left Knee Joint with Patellofemoral Synthetic Substitute, Open Approach

ØSRE009 Replacement of Left Hip Joint, Acetabular Surface with Polyethylene Synthetic Substitute, Cemented, Open Approach

ØSRE00A Replacement of Left Hip Joint, Acetabular Surface with Polyethylene Synthetic Substitute, Uncemented, Open Approach

ØSRE00Z Replacement of Left Hip Joint, Acetabular Surface with Polyethylene Synthetic Substitute, Open Approach

ØSRE019 Replacement of Left Hip Joint, Acetabular Surface with Metal Synthetic Substitute, Cemented, Open Approach

ØSRE01A Replacement of Left Hip Joint, Acetabular Surface with Metal Synthetic Substitute, Uncemented, Open Approach

ØSRE01Z Replacement of Left Hip Joint, Acetabular Surface with Metal Synthetic Substitute, Open Approach

ØSRE039 Replacement of Left Hip Joint, Acetabular Surface with Ceramic Synthetic Substitute, Cemented, Open Approach

ØSRE03A Replacement of Left Hip Joint, Acetabular Surface with Ceramic Synthetic Substitute, Uncemented, Open Approach

ØSRE03Z Replacement of Left Hip Joint, Acetabular Surface with Ceramic Synthetic Substitute, Open Approach

ØSRE07Z Replacement of Left Hip Joint, Acetabular Surface with Autologous Tissue Substitute, Open Approach

ØSRE0J9 Replacement of Left Hip Joint, Acetabular Surface with Synthetic Substitute, Cemented, Open Approach

ØSRE0JA Replacement of Left Hip Joint, Acetabular Surface with Synthetic Substitute, Uncemented, Open Approach

ØSRE0JZ Replacement of Left Hip Joint, Acetabular Surface with Synthetic Substitute, Open Approach

ØSRE0KZ Replacement of Left Hip Joint, Acetabular Surface with Nonautologous Tissue Substitute, Open Approach

ØSRR019 Replacement of Right Hip Joint, Femoral Surface with Metal Synthetic Substitute, Cemented, Open Approach

ØSRR01A Replacement of Right Hip Joint, Femoral Surface with Metal Synthetic Substitute, Uncemented, Open Approach

ØSRR01Z Replacement of Right Hip Joint, Femoral Surface with Metal Synthetic Substitute, Open Approach

ØSRR039 Replacement of Right Hip Joint, Femoral Surface with Ceramic Synthetic Substitute, Cemented, Open Approach

ØSRR03A Replacement of Right Hip Joint, Femoral Surface with Ceramic Synthetic Substitute, Uncemented, Open Approach

ØSRR03Z Replacement of Right Hip Joint, Femoral Surface with Ceramic Synthetic Substitute, Open Approach

ØSRR07Z Replacement of Right Hip Joint, Femoral Surface with Autologous Tissue Substitute, Open Approach

ØSRR0J9 Replacement of Right Hip Joint, Femoral Surface with Synthetic Substitute, Cemented, Open Approach

ØSRR0JA Replacement of Right Hip Joint, Femoral Surface with Synthetic Substitute, Uncemented, Open Approach

ØSRR0JZ Replacement of Right Hip Joint, Femoral Surface with Synthetic Substitute, Open Approach

ØSRR0KZ Replacement of Right Hip Joint, Femoral Surface with Nonautologous Tissue Substitute, Open Approach

ØSRS019 Replacement of Left Hip Joint, Femoral Surface with Metal Synthetic Substitute, Cemented, Open Approach

ØSRS01A Replacement of Left Hip Joint, Femoral Surface with Metal Synthetic Substitute, Uncemented, Open Approach

ØSRS01Z Replacement of Left Hip Joint, Femoral Surface with Metal Synthetic Substitute, Open Approach

ØSRS039 Replacement of Left Hip Joint, Femoral Surface with Ceramic Synthetic Substitute, Cemented, Open Approach

ØSRS03A Replacement of Left Hip Joint, Femoral Surface with Ceramic Synthetic Substitute, Uncemented, Open Approach

ØSRS03Z Replacement of Left Hip Joint, Femoral Surface with Ceramic Synthetic Substitute, Open Approach

ØSRS07Z Replacement of Left Hip Joint, Femoral Surface with Autologous Tissue Substitute, Open Approach

ØSRS0J9 Replacement of Left Hip Joint, Femoral Surface with Synthetic Substitute, Cemented, Open Approach

ØSRS0JA Replacement of Left Hip Joint, Femoral Surface with Synthetic Substitute, Uncemented, Open Approach

ØSRS0JZ Replacement of Left Hip Joint, Femoral Surface with Synthetic Substitute, Open Approach

ØSRS0KZ Replacement of Left Hip Joint, Femoral Surface with Nonautologous Tissue Substitute, Open Approach

ØSRT07Z Replacement of Right Knee Joint, Femoral Surface with Autologous Tissue Substitute, Open Approach

ØSRT0J9 Replacement of Right Knee Joint, Femoral Surface with Synthetic Substitute, Cemented, Open Approach

ØSRT0JA Replacement of Right Knee Joint, Femoral Surface with Synthetic Substitute, Uncemented, Open Approach

ØSRT0JZ Replacement of Right Knee Joint, Femoral Surface with Synthetic Substitute, Open Approach

ØSRT0KZ Replacement of Right Knee Joint, Femoral Surface with Nonautologous Tissue Substitute, Open Approach

ØSRU07Z Replacement of Left Knee Joint, Femoral Surface with Autologous Tissue Substitute, Open Approach

ØSRU0J9 Replacement of Left Knee Joint, Femoral Surface with Synthetic Substitute, Cemented, Open Approach

ØSRU0JA Replacement of Left Knee Joint, Femoral Surface with Synthetic Substitute, Uncemented, Open Approach

ØSRU0JZ Replacement of Left Knee Joint, Femoral Surface with Synthetic Substitute, Open Approach

ØSRU0KZ Replacement of Left Knee Joint, Femoral Surface with Nonautologous Tissue Substitute, Open Approach

ØSRV07Z Replacement of Right Knee Joint, Tibial Surface with Autologous Tissue Substitute, Open Approach

ØSRV0J9 Replacement of Right Knee Joint, Tibial Surface with Synthetic Substitute, Cemented, Open Approach

ØSRV0JA Replacement of Right Knee Joint, Tibial Surface with Synthetic Substitute, Uncemented, Open Approach

ØSRV0JZ Replacement of Right Knee Joint, Tibial Surface with Synthetic Substitute, Open Approach

ØSRV0KZ Replacement of Right Knee Joint, Tibial Surface with Nonautologous Tissue Substitute, Open Approach

ØSRW07Z Replacement of Left Knee Joint, Tibial Surface with Autologous Tissue Substitute, Open Approach

ØSRW0J9 Replacement of Left Knee Joint, Tibial Surface with Synthetic Substitute, Cemented, Open Approach

ØSRW0JA Replacement of Left Knee Joint, Tibial Surface with Synthetic Substitute, Uncemented, Open Approach

ØSRW0JZ Replacement of Left Knee Joint, Tibial Surface with Synthetic Substitute, Open Approach

ØSRW0KZ Replacement of Left Knee Joint, Tibial Surface with Nonautologous Tissue Substitute, Open Approach

ØSU90BZ Supplement Right Hip Joint with Resurfacing Device, Open Approach

ØSUA0BZ Supplement Right Hip Joint, Acetabular Surface with Resurfacing Device, Open Approach

ØSUB0BZ Supplement Left Hip Joint with Resurfacing Device, Open Approach

ØSUE0BZ Supplement Left Hip Joint, Acetabular Surface with Resurfacing Device, Open Approach

HAC 10: Deep Vein Thrombosis (DVT) or Pulmonary Embolism (PE) with Total Knee or Hip Replacement (continued)

ØSURØBZ Supplement Right Hip Joint, Femoral Surface with Resurfacing Device, Open Approach

ØSUSØBZ Supplement Left Hip Joint, Femoral Surface with Resurfacing Device, Open Approach

XRRGØL8 Replacement of Right Knee Joint with Synthetic Substitute, Lateral Meniscus, Open Approach, New Technology Group 8

XRRGØM8 Replacement of Right Knee Joint with Synthetic Substitute, Medial Meniscus, Open Approach, New Technology Group 8

XRRHØL8 Replacement of Left Knee Joint with Synthetic Substitute, Lateral Meniscus, Open Approach, New Technology Group 8

XRRHØM8 Replacement of Left Knee Joint with Synthetic Substitute, Medial Meniscus, Open Approach, New Technology Group 8

HAC 11: Surgical Site Infection-Bariatric Surgery

Principal diagnosis of:

E66.Ø1 Morbid (severe) obesity due to excess calories

AND

Secondary diagnosis not POA:

K68.11 Postprocedural retroperitoneal abscess
K95.Ø1 Infection due to gastric band procedure
K95.81 Infection due to other bariatric procedure
T81.4ØXA Infection following a procedure, unspecified, initial encounter
T81.41XA Infection following a procedure, superficial incisional surgical site, initial encounter
T81.42XA Infection following a procedure, deep incisional surgical site, initial encounter
T81.43XA Infection following a procedure, organ and space surgical site, initial encounter
T81.44XA Sepsis following a procedure, initial encounter
T81.49XA Infection following a procedure, other surgical site, initial encounter

AND

Any of the following procedures:

ØD16Ø79 Bypass Stomach to Duodenum with Autologous Tissue Substitute, Open Approach
ØD16Ø7A Bypass Stomach to Jejunum with Autologous Tissue Substitute, Open Approach
ØD16Ø7B Bypass Stomach to Ileum with Autologous Tissue Substitute, Open Approach
ØD16Ø7L Bypass Stomach to Transverse Colon with Autologous Tissue Substitute, Open Approach
ØD16ØJ9 Bypass Stomach to Duodenum with Synthetic Substitute, Open Approach
ØD16ØJA Bypass Stomach to Jejunum with Synthetic Substitute, Open Approach
ØD16ØJB Bypass Stomach to Ileum with Synthetic Substitute, Open Approach
ØD16ØJL Bypass Stomach to Transverse Colon with Synthetic Substitute, Open Approach
ØD16ØK9 Bypass Stomach to Duodenum with Nonautologous Tissue Substitute, Open Approach
ØD16ØKA Bypass Stomach to Jejunum with Nonautologous Tissue Substitute, Open Approach
ØD16ØKB Bypass Stomach to Ileum with Nonautologous Tissue Substitute, Open Approach
ØD16ØKL Bypass Stomach to Transverse Colon with Nonautologous Tissue Substitute, Open Approach

ØD16ØZ9 Bypass Stomach to Duodenum, Open Approach
ØD16ØZA Bypass Stomach to Jejunum, Open Approach
ØD16ØZB Bypass Stomach to Ileum, Open Approach
ØD16ØZL Bypass Stomach to Transverse Colon, Open Approach
ØD16479 Bypass Stomach to Duodenum with Autologous Tissue Substitute, Percutaneous Endoscopic Approach
ØD1647A Bypass Stomach to Jejunum with Autologous Tissue Substitute, Percutaneous Endoscopic Approach
ØD1647B Bypass Stomach to Ileum with Autologous Tissue Substitute, Percutaneous Endoscopic Approach
ØD1647L Bypass Stomach to Transverse Colon with Autologous Tissue Substitute, Percutaneous Endoscopic Approach
ØD164J9 Bypass Stomach to Duodenum with Synthetic Substitute, Percutaneous Endoscopic Approach
ØD164JA Bypass Stomach to Jejunum with Synthetic Substitute, Percutaneous Endoscopic Approach
ØD164JB Bypass Stomach to Ileum with Synthetic Substitute, Percutaneous Endoscopic Approach
ØD164JL Bypass Stomach to Transverse Colon with Synthetic Substitute, Percutaneous Endoscopic Approach
ØD164K9 Bypass Stomach to Duodenum with Nonautologous Tissue Substitute, Percutaneous Endoscopic Approach
ØD164KA Bypass Stomach to Jejunum with Nonautologous Tissue Substitute, Percutaneous Endoscopic Approach
ØD164KB Bypass Stomach to Ileum with Nonautologous Tissue Substitute, Percutaneous Endoscopic Approach
ØD164KL Bypass Stomach to Transverse Colon with Nonautologous Tissue Substitute, Percutaneous Endoscopic Approach
ØD164Z9 Bypass Stomach to Duodenum, Percutaneous Endoscopic Approach
ØD164ZA Bypass Stomach to Jejunum, Percutaneous Endoscopic Approach
ØD164ZB Bypass Stomach to Ileum, Percutaneous Endoscopic Approach
ØD164ZL Bypass Stomach to Transverse Colon, Percutaneous Endoscopic Approach
ØD16879 Bypass Stomach to Duodenum with Autologous Tissue Substitute, Via Natural or Artificial Opening Endoscopic
ØD1687A Bypass Stomach to Jejunum with Autologous Tissue Substitute, Via Natural or Artificial Opening Endoscopic
ØD1687B Bypass Stomach to Ileum with Autologous Tissue Substitute, Via Natural or Artificial Opening Endoscopic
ØD1687L Bypass Stomach to Transverse Colon with Autologous Tissue Substitute, Via Natural or Artificial Opening Endoscopic
ØD168J9 Bypass Stomach to Duodenum with Synthetic Substitute, Via Natural or Artificial Opening Endoscopic
ØD168JA Bypass Stomach to Jejunum with Synthetic Substitute, Via Natural or Artificial Opening Endoscopic
ØD168JB Bypass Stomach to Ileum with Synthetic Substitute, Via Natural or Artificial Opening Endoscopic
ØD168JL Bypass Stomach to Transverse Colon with Synthetic Substitute, Via Natural or Artificial Opening Endoscopic
ØD168K9 Bypass Stomach to Duodenum with Nonautologous Tissue Substitute, Via Natural or Artificial Opening Endoscopic

ØD168KA Bypass Stomach to Jejunum with Nonautologous Tissue Substitute, Via Natural or Artificial Opening Endoscopic
ØD168KB Bypass Stomach to Ileum with Nonautologous Tissue Substitute, Via Natural or Artificial Opening Endoscopic
ØD168KL Bypass Stomach to Transverse Colon with Nonautologous Tissue Substitute, Via Natural or Artificial Opening Endoscopic
ØD168Z9 Bypass Stomach to Duodenum, Via Natural or Artificial Opening Endoscopic
ØD168ZA Bypass Stomach to Jejunum, Via Natural or Artificial Opening Endoscopic
ØD168ZB Bypass Stomach to Ileum, Via Natural or Artificial Opening Endoscopic
ØD168ZL Bypass Stomach to Transverse Colon, Via Natural or Artificial Opening Endoscopic
ØDV64CZ Restriction of Stomach with Extraluminal Device, Percutaneous Endoscopic Approach

HAC 12: Surgical Site Infection-Certain Orthopedic Procedures of the Spine, Shoulder, and Elbow

Secondary diagnosis not POA:

K68.11 Postprocedural retroperitoneal abscess
T81.4ØXA Infection following a procedure, unspecified, initial encounter
T81.41XA Infection following a procedure, superficial incisional surgical site, initial encounter
T81.42XA Infection following a procedure, deep incisional surgical site, initial encounter
T81.43XA Infection following a procedure, organ and space surgical site, initial encounter
T81.44XA Sepsis following a procedure, initial encounter
T81.49XA Infection following a procedure, other surgical site, initial encounter
T84.6ØXA Infection and inflammatory reaction due to internal fixation device of unspecified site, initial encounter
T84.61ØA Infection and inflammatory reaction due to internal fixation device of right humerus, initial encounter
T84.611A Infection and inflammatory reaction due to internal fixation device of left humerus, initial encounter
T84.612A Infection and inflammatory reaction due to internal fixation device of right radius, initial encounter
T84.613A Infection and inflammatory reaction due to internal fixation device of left radius, initial encounter
T84.614A Infection and inflammatory reaction due to internal fixation device of right ulna, initial encounter
T84.615A Infection and inflammatory reaction due to internal fixation device of left ulna, initial encounter
T84.619A Infection and inflammatory reaction due to internal fixation device of unspecified bone of arm, initial encounter
T84.63XA Infection and inflammatory reaction due to internal fixation device of spine, initial encounter
T84.69XA Infection and inflammatory reaction due to internal fixation device of other site, initial encounter
T84.7XXA Infection and inflammatory reaction due to other internal orthopedic prosthetic devices, implants and grafts, initial encounter

AND

Any of the following procedures:

ØRG0070 Fusion of Occipital-cervical Joint with Autologous Tissue Substitute, Anterior Approach, Anterior Column, Open Approach

HAC 12: Surgical Site Infection-Certain Orthopedic Procedures of the Spine, Shoulder, and Elbow (continued)

ØRG0071 Fusion of Occipital-cervical Joint with Autologous Tissue Substitute, Posterior Approach, Posterior Column, Open Approach

ØRG007J Fusion of Occipital-cervical Joint with Autologous Tissue Substitute, Posterior Approach, Anterior Column, Open Approach

ØRG00A0 Fusion of Occipital-cervical Joint with Interbody Fusion Device, Anterior Approach, Anterior Column, Open Approach

ØRG00AJ Fusion of Occipital-cervical Joint with Interbody Fusion Device, Posterior Approach, Anterior Column, Open Approach

ØRG00J0 Fusion of Occipital-cervical Joint with Synthetic Substitute, Anterior Approach, Anterior Column, Open Approach

ØRG00J1 Fusion of Occipital-cervical Joint with Synthetic Substitute, Posterior Approach, Posterior Column, Open Approach

ØRG00JJ Fusion of Occipital-cervical Joint with Synthetic Substitute, Posterior Approach, Anterior Column, Open Approach

ØRG00K0 Fusion of Occipital-cervical Joint with Nonautologous Tissue Substitute, Anterior Approach, Anterior Column, Open Approach

ØRG00K1 Fusion of Occipital-cervical Joint with Nonautologous Tissue Substitute, Posterior Approach, Posterior Column, Open Approach

ØRG00KJ Fusion of Occipital-cervical Joint with Nonautologous Tissue Substitute, Posterior Approach, Anterior Column, Open Approach

ØRG0370 Fusion of Occipital-cervical Joint with Autologous Tissue Substitute, Anterior Approach, Anterior Column, Percutaneous Approach

ØRG0371 Fusion of Occipital-cervical Joint with Autologous Tissue Substitute, Posterior Approach, Posterior Column, Percutaneous Approach

ØRG037J Fusion of Occipital-cervical Joint with Autologous Tissue Substitute, Posterior Approach, Anterior Column, Percutaneous Approach

ØRG03A0 Fusion of Occipital-cervical Joint with Interbody Fusion Device, Anterior Approach, Anterior Column, Percutaneous Approach

ØRG03AJ Fusion of Occipital-cervical Joint with Interbody Fusion Device, Posterior Approach, Anterior Column, Percutaneous Approach

ØRG03J0 Fusion of Occipital-cervical Joint with Synthetic Substitute, Anterior Approach, Anterior Column, Percutaneous Approach

ØRG03J1 Fusion of Occipital-cervical Joint with Synthetic Substitute, Posterior Approach, Posterior Column, Percutaneous Approach

ØRG03JJ Fusion of Occipital-cervical Joint with Synthetic Substitute, Posterior Approach, Anterior Column, Percutaneous Approach

ØRG03K0 Fusion of Occipital-cervical Joint with Nonautologous Tissue Substitute, Anterior Approach, Anterior Column, Percutaneous Approach

ØRG03K1 Fusion of Occipital-cervical Joint with Nonautologous Tissue Substitute, Posterior Approach, Posterior Column, Percutaneous Approach

ØRG03KJ Fusion of Occipital-cervical Joint with Nonautologous Tissue Substitute, Posterior Approach, Anterior Column, Percutaneous Approach

ØRG0470 Fusion of Occipital-cervical Joint with Autologous Tissue Substitute, Anterior Approach, Anterior Column, Percutaneous Endoscopic Approach

ØRG0471 Fusion of Occipital-cervical Joint with Autologous Tissue Substitute, Posterior Approach, Posterior Column, Percutaneous Endoscopic Approach

ØRG047J Fusion of Occipital-cervical Joint with Autologous Tissue Substitute, Posterior Approach, Anterior Column, Percutaneous Endoscopic Approach

ØRG04A0 Fusion of Occipital-cervical Joint with Interbody Fusion Device, Anterior Approach, Anterior Column, Percutaneous Endoscopic Approach

ØRG04AJ Fusion of Occipital-cervical Joint with Interbody Fusion Device, Posterior Approach, Anterior Column, Percutaneous Endoscopic Approach

ØRG04J0 Fusion of Occipital-cervical Joint with Synthetic Substitute, Anterior Approach, Anterior Column, Percutaneous Endoscopic Approach

ØRG04J1 Fusion of Occipital-cervical Joint with Synthetic Substitute, Posterior Approach, Posterior Column, Percutaneous Endoscopic Approach

ØRG04JJ Fusion of Occipital-cervical Joint with Synthetic Substitute, Posterior Approach, Anterior Column, Percutaneous Endoscopic Approach

ØRG04K0 Fusion of Occipital-cervical Joint with Nonautologous Tissue Substitute, Anterior Approach, Anterior Column, Percutaneous Endoscopic Approach

ØRG04K1 Fusion of Occipital-cervical Joint with Nonautologous Tissue Substitute, Posterior Approach, Posterior Column, Percutaneous Endoscopic Approach

ØRG04KJ Fusion of Occipital-cervical Joint with Nonautologous Tissue Substitute, Posterior Approach, Anterior Column, Percutaneous Endoscopic Approach

ØRG1070 Fusion of Cervical Vertebral Joint with Autologous Tissue Substitute, Anterior Approach, Anterior Column, Open Approach

ØRG1071 Fusion of Cervical Vertebral Joint with Autologous Tissue Substitute, Posterior Approach, Posterior Column, Open Approach

ØRG107J Fusion of Cervical Vertebral Joint with Autologous Tissue Substitute, Posterior Approach, Anterior Column, Open Approach

ØRG10A0 Fusion of Cervical Vertebral Joint with Interbody Fusion Device, Anterior Approach, Anterior Column, Open Approach

ØRG10AJ Fusion of Cervical Vertebral Joint with Interbody Fusion Device, Posterior Approach, Anterior Column, Open Approach

ØRG10J0 Fusion of Cervical Vertebral Joint with Synthetic Substitute, Anterior Approach, Anterior Column, Open Approach

ØRG10J1 Fusion of Cervical Vertebral Joint with Synthetic Substitute, Posterior Approach, Posterior Column, Open Approach

ØRG10JJ Fusion of Cervical Vertebral Joint with Synthetic Substitute, Posterior Approach, Anterior Column, Open Approach

ØRG10K0 Fusion of Cervical Vertebral Joint with Nonautologous Tissue Substitute, Anterior Approach, Anterior Column, Open Approach

ØRG10K1 Fusion of Cervical Vertebral Joint with Nonautologous Tissue Substitute, Posterior Approach, Posterior Column, Open Approach

ØRG10KJ Fusion of Cervical Vertebral Joint with Nonautologous Tissue Substitute, Posterior Approach, Anterior Column, Open Approach

ØRG1370 Fusion of Cervical Vertebral Joint with Autologous Tissue Substitute, Anterior Approach, Anterior Column, Percutaneous Approach

ØRG1371 Fusion of Cervical Vertebral Joint with Autologous Tissue Substitute, Posterior Approach, Posterior Column, Percutaneous Approach

ØRG137J Fusion of Cervical Vertebral Joint with Autologous Tissue Substitute, Posterior Approach, Anterior Column, Percutaneous Approach

ØRG13A0 Fusion of Cervical Vertebral Joint with Interbody Fusion Device, Anterior Approach, Anterior Column, Percutaneous Approach

ØRG13AJ Fusion of Cervical Vertebral Joint with Interbody Fusion Device, Posterior Approach, Anterior Column, Percutaneous Approach

ØRG13J0 Fusion of Cervical Vertebral Joint with Synthetic Substitute, Anterior Approach, Anterior Column, Percutaneous Approach

ØRG13J1 Fusion of Cervical Vertebral Joint with Synthetic Substitute, Posterior Approach, Posterior Column, Percutaneous Approach

ØRG13JJ Fusion of Cervical Vertebral Joint with Synthetic Substitute, Posterior Approach, Anterior Column, Percutaneous Approach

ØRG13K0 Fusion of Cervical Vertebral Joint with Nonautologous Tissue Substitute, Anterior Approach, Anterior Column, Percutaneous Approach

ØRG13K1 Fusion of Cervical Vertebral Joint with Nonautologous Tissue Substitute, Posterior Approach, Posterior Column, Percutaneous Approach

ØRG13KJ Fusion of Cervical Vertebral Joint with Nonautologous Tissue Substitute, Posterior Approach, Anterior Column, Percutaneous Approach

ØRG1470 Fusion of Cervical Vertebral Joint with Autologous Tissue Substitute, Anterior Approach, Anterior Column, Percutaneous Endoscopic Approach

ØRG1471 Fusion of Cervical Vertebral Joint with Autologous Tissue Substitute, Posterior Approach, Posterior Column, Percutaneous Endoscopic Approach

ØRG147J Fusion of Cervical Vertebral Joint with Autologous Tissue Substitute, Posterior Approach, Anterior Column, Percutaneous Endoscopic Approach

ØRG14A0 Fusion of Cervical Vertebral Joint with Interbody Fusion Device, Anterior Approach, Anterior Column, Percutaneous Endoscopic Approach

HAC 12: Surgical Site Infection-Certain Orthopedic Procedures of the Spine, Shoulder, and Elbow (continued)

ØRG14AJ Fusion of Cervical Vertebral Joint with Interbody Fusion Device, Posterior Approach, Anterior Column, Percutaneous Endoscopic Approach

ØRG14JØ Fusion of Cervical Vertebral Joint with Synthetic Substitute, Anterior Approach, Anterior Column, Percutaneous Endoscopic Approach

ØRG14J1 Fusion of Cervical Vertebral Joint with Synthetic Substitute, Posterior Approach, Posterior Column, Percutaneous Endoscopic Approach

ØRG14JJ Fusion of Cervical Vertebral Joint with Synthetic Substitute, Posterior Approach, Anterior Column, Percutaneous Endoscopic Approach

ØRG14KØ Fusion of Cervical Vertebral Joint with Nonautologous Tissue Substitute, Anterior Approach, Anterior Column, Percutaneous Endoscopic Approach

ØRG14K1 Fusion of Cervical Vertebral Joint with Nonautologous Tissue Substitute, Posterior Approach, Posterior Column, Percutaneous Endoscopic Approach

ØRG14KJ Fusion of Cervical Vertebral Joint with Nonautologous Tissue Substitute, Posterior Approach, Anterior Column, Percutaneous Endoscopic Approach

ØRG2Ø7Ø Fusion of 2 or more Cervical Vertebral Joints with Autologous Tissue Substitute, Anterior Approach, Anterior Column, Open Approach

ØRG2Ø71 Fusion of 2 or more Cervical Vertebral Joints with Autologous Tissue Substitute, Posterior Approach, Posterior Column, Open Approach

ØRG2Ø7J Fusion of 2 or more Cervical Vertebral Joints with Autologous Tissue Substitute, Posterior Approach, Anterior Column, Open Approach

ØRG2ØAØ Fusion of 2 or more Cervical Vertebral Joints with Interbody Fusion Device, Anterior Approach, Anterior Column, Open Approach

ØRG2ØAJ Fusion of 2 or more Cervical Vertebral Joints with Interbody Fusion Device, Posterior Approach, Anterior Column, Open Approach

ØRG2ØJØ Fusion of 2 or more Cervical Vertebral Joints with Synthetic Substitute, Anterior Approach, Anterior Column, Open Approach

ØRG2ØJ1 Fusion of 2 or more Cervical Vertebral Joints with Synthetic Substitute, Posterior Approach, Posterior Column, Open Approach

ØRG2ØJJ Fusion of 2 or more Cervical Vertebral Joints with Synthetic Substitute, Posterior Approach, Anterior Column, Open Approach

ØRG2ØKØ Fusion of 2 or more Cervical Vertebral Joints with Nonautologous Tissue Substitute, Anterior Approach, Anterior Column, Open Approach

ØRG2ØK1 Fusion of 2 or more Cervical Vertebral Joints with Nonautologous Tissue Substitute, Posterior Approach, Posterior Column, Open Approach

ØRG2ØKJ Fusion of 2 or more Cervical Vertebral Joints with Nonautologous Tissue Substitute, Posterior Approach, Anterior Column, Open Approach

ØRG237Ø Fusion of 2 or more Cervical Vertebral Joints with Autologous Tissue Substitute, Anterior Approach, Anterior Column, Percutaneous Approach

ØRG2371 Fusion of 2 or more Cervical Vertebral Joints with Autologous Tissue Substitute, Posterior Approach, Posterior Column, Percutaneous Approach

ØRG237J Fusion of 2 or more Cervical Vertebral Joints with Autologous Tissue Substitute, Posterior Approach, Anterior Column, Percutaneous Approach

ØRG23AØ Fusion of 2 or more Cervical Vertebral Joints with Interbody Fusion Device, Anterior Approach, Anterior Column, Percutaneous Approach

ØRG23AJ Fusion of 2 or more Cervical Vertebral Joints with Interbody Fusion Device, Posterior Approach, Anterior Column, Percutaneous Approach

ØRG23JØ Fusion of 2 or more Cervical Vertebral Joints with Synthetic Substitute, Anterior Approach, Anterior Column, Percutaneous Approach

ØRG23J1 Fusion of 2 or more Cervical Vertebral Joints with Synthetic Substitute, Posterior Approach, Posterior Column, Percutaneous Approach

ØRG23JJ Fusion of 2 or more Cervical Vertebral Joints with Synthetic Substitute, Posterior Approach, Anterior Column, Percutaneous Approach

ØRG23KØ Fusion of 2 or more Cervical Vertebral Joints with Nonautologous Tissue Substitute, Anterior Approach, Anterior Column, Percutaneous Approach

ØRG23K1 Fusion of 2 or more Cervical Vertebral Joints with Nonautologous Tissue Substitute, Posterior Approach, Posterior Column, Percutaneous Approach

ØRG23KJ Fusion of 2 or more Cervical Vertebral Joints with Nonautologous Tissue Substitute, Posterior Approach, Anterior Column, Percutaneous Approach

ØRG247Ø Fusion of 2 or more Cervical Vertebral Joints with Autologous Tissue Substitute, Anterior Approach, Anterior Column, Percutaneous Endoscopic Approach

ØRG2471 Fusion of 2 or more Cervical Vertebral Joints with Autologous Tissue Substitute, Posterior Approach, Posterior Column, Percutaneous Endoscopic Approach

ØRG247J Fusion of 2 or more Cervical Vertebral Joints with Autologous Tissue Substitute, Posterior Approach, Anterior Column, Percutaneous Endoscopic Approach

ØRG24AØ Fusion of 2 or more Cervical Vertebral Joints with Interbody Fusion Device, Anterior Approach, Anterior Column, Percutaneous Endoscopic Approach

ØRG24AJ Fusion of 2 or more Cervical Vertebral Joints with Interbody Fusion Device, Posterior Approach, Anterior Column, Percutaneous Endoscopic Approach

ØRG24JØ Fusion of 2 or more Cervical Vertebral Joints with Synthetic Substitute, Anterior Approach, Anterior Column, Percutaneous Endoscopic Approach

ØRG24J1 Fusion of 2 or more Cervical Vertebral Joints with Synthetic Substitute, Posterior Approach, Posterior Column, Percutaneous Endoscopic Approach

ØRG24JJ Fusion of 2 or more Cervical Vertebral Joints with Synthetic Substitute, Posterior Approach, Anterior Column, Percutaneous Endoscopic Approach

ØRG24KØ Fusion of 2 or more Cervical Vertebral Joints with Nonautologous Tissue Substitute, Anterior Approach, Anterior Column, Percutaneous Endoscopic Approach

ØRG24K1 Fusion of 2 or more Cervical Vertebral Joints with Nonautologous Tissue Substitute, Posterior Approach, Posterior Column, Percutaneous Endoscopic Approach

ØRG24KJ Fusion of 2 or more Cervical Vertebral Joints with Nonautologous Tissue Substitute, Posterior Approach, Anterior Column, Percutaneous Endoscopic Approach

ØRG4Ø7Ø Fusion of Cervicothoracic Vertebral Joint with Autologous Tissue Substitute, Anterior Approach, Anterior Column, Open Approach

ØRG4Ø71 Fusion of Cervicothoracic Vertebral Joint with Autologous Tissue Substitute, Posterior Approach, Posterior Column, Open Approach

ØRG4Ø7J Fusion of Cervicothoracic Vertebral Joint with Autologous Tissue Substitute, Posterior Approach, Anterior Column, Open Approach

ØRG4ØAØ Fusion of Cervicothoracic Vertebral Joint with Interbody Fusion Device, Anterior Approach, Anterior Column, Open Approach

ØRG4ØAJ Fusion of Cervicothoracic Vertebral Joint with Interbody Fusion Device, Posterior Approach, Anterior Column, Open Approach

ØRG4ØJØ Fusion of Cervicothoracic Vertebral Joint with Synthetic Substitute, Anterior Approach, Anterior Column, Open Approach

ØRG4ØJ1 Fusion of Cervicothoracic Vertebral Joint with Synthetic Substitute, Posterior Approach, Posterior Column, Open Approach

ØRG4ØJJ Fusion of Cervicothoracic Vertebral Joint with Synthetic Substitute, Posterior Approach, Anterior Column, Open Approach

ØRG4ØKØ Fusion of Cervicothoracic Vertebral Joint with Nonautologous Tissue Substitute, Anterior Approach, Anterior Column, Open Approach

ØRG4ØK1 Fusion of Cervicothoracic Vertebral Joint with Nonautologous Tissue Substitute, Posterior Approach, Posterior Column, Open Approach

ØRG4ØKJ Fusion of Cervicothoracic Vertebral Joint with Nonautologous Tissue Substitute, Posterior Approach, Anterior Column, Open Approach

ØRG437Ø Fusion of Cervicothoracic Vertebral Joint with Autologous Tissue Substitute, Anterior Approach, Anterior Column, Percutaneous Approach

ØRG4371 Fusion of Cervicothoracic Vertebral Joint with Autologous Tissue Substitute, Posterior Approach, Posterior Column, Percutaneous Approach

ØRG437J Fusion of Cervicothoracic Vertebral Joint with Autologous Tissue Substitute, Posterior Approach, Anterior Column, Percutaneous Approach

ØRG43AØ Fusion of Cervicothoracic Vertebral Joint with Interbody Fusion Device, Anterior Approach, Anterior Column, Percutaneous Approach

HAC 12: Surgical Site Infection-Certain Orthopedic Procedures of the Spine, Shoulder, and Elbow (continued)

ØRG43AJ Fusion of Cervicothoracic Vertebral Joint with Interbody Fusion Device, Posterior Approach, Anterior Column, Percutaneous Approach

ØRG43JØ Fusion of Cervicothoracic Vertebral Joint with Synthetic Substitute, Anterior Approach, Anterior Column, Percutaneous Approach

ØRG43J1 Fusion of Cervicothoracic Vertebral Joint with Synthetic Substitute, Posterior Approach, Posterior Column, Percutaneous Approach

ØRG43JJ Fusion of Cervicothoracic Vertebral Joint with Synthetic Substitute, Posterior Approach, Anterior Column, Percutaneous Approach

ØRG43KØ Fusion of Cervicothoracic Vertebral Joint with Nonautologous Tissue Substitute, Anterior Approach, Anterior Column, Percutaneous Approach

ØRG43K1 Fusion of Cervicothoracic Vertebral Joint with Nonautologous Tissue Substitute, Posterior Approach, Posterior Column, Percutaneous Approach

ØRG43KJ Fusion of Cervicothoracic Vertebral Joint with Nonautologous Tissue Substitute, Posterior Approach, Anterior Column, Percutaneous Approach

ØRG447Ø Fusion of Cervicothoracic Vertebral Joint with Autologous Tissue Substitute, Anterior Approach, Anterior Column, Percutaneous Endoscopic Approach

ØRG4471 Fusion of Cervicothoracic Vertebral Joint with Autologous Tissue Substitute, Posterior Approach, Posterior Column, Percutaneous Endoscopic Approach

ØRG447J Fusion of Cervicothoracic Vertebral Joint with Autologous Tissue Substitute, Posterior Approach, Anterior Column, Percutaneous Endoscopic Approach

ØRG44AØ Fusion of Cervicothoracic Vertebral Joint with Interbody Fusion Device, Anterior Approach, Anterior Column, Percutaneous Endoscopic Approach

ØRG44AJ Fusion of Cervicothoracic Vertebral Joint with Interbody Fusion Device, Posterior Approach, Anterior Column, Percutaneous Endoscopic Approach

ØRG44JØ Fusion of Cervicothoracic Vertebral Joint with Synthetic Substitute, Anterior Approach, Anterior Column, Percutaneous Endoscopic Approach

ØRG44J1 Fusion of Cervicothoracic Vertebral Joint with Synthetic Substitute, Posterior Approach, Posterior Column, Percutaneous Endoscopic Approach

ØRG44JJ Fusion of Cervicothoracic Vertebral Joint with Synthetic Substitute, Posterior Approach, Anterior Column, Percutaneous Endoscopic Approach

ØRG44KØ Fusion of Cervicothoracic Vertebral Joint with Nonautologous Tissue Substitute, Anterior Approach, Anterior Column, Percutaneous Endoscopic Approach

ØRG44K1 Fusion of Cervicothoracic Vertebral Joint with Nonautologous Tissue Substitute, Posterior Approach, Posterior Column, Percutaneous Endoscopic Approach

ØRG44KJ Fusion of Cervicothoracic Vertebral Joint with Nonautologous Tissue Substitute, Posterior Approach, Anterior Column, Percutaneous Endoscopic Approach

ØRG6070 Fusion of Thoracic Vertebral Joint with Autologous Tissue Substitute, Anterior Approach, Anterior Column, Open Approach

ØRG6071 Fusion of Thoracic Vertebral Joint with Autologous Tissue Substitute, Posterior Approach, Posterior Column, Open Approach

ØRG607J Fusion of Thoracic Vertebral Joint with Autologous Tissue Substitute, Posterior Approach, Anterior Column, Open Approach

ØRG60AØ Fusion of Thoracic Vertebral Joint with Interbody Fusion Device, Anterior Approach, Anterior Column, Open Approach

ØRG60AJ Fusion of Thoracic Vertebral Joint with Interbody Fusion Device, Posterior Approach, Anterior Column, Open Approach

ØRG60JØ Fusion of Thoracic Vertebral Joint with Synthetic Substitute, Anterior Approach, Anterior Column, Open Approach

ØRG60J1 Fusion of Thoracic Vertebral Joint with Synthetic Substitute, Posterior Approach, Posterior Column, Open Approach

ØRG60JJ Fusion of Thoracic Vertebral Joint with Synthetic Substitute, Posterior Approach, Anterior Column, Open Approach

ØRG60KØ Fusion of Thoracic Vertebral Joint with Nonautologous Tissue Substitute, Anterior Approach, Anterior Column, Open Approach

ØRG60K1 Fusion of Thoracic Vertebral Joint with Nonautologous Tissue Substitute, Posterior Approach, Posterior Column, Open Approach

ØRG60KJ Fusion of Thoracic Vertebral Joint with Nonautologous Tissue Substitute, Posterior Approach, Anterior Column, Open Approach

ØRG6370 Fusion of Thoracic Vertebral Joint with Autologous Tissue Substitute, Anterior Approach, Anterior Column, Percutaneous Approach

ØRG6371 Fusion of Thoracic Vertebral Joint with Autologous Tissue Substitute, Posterior Approach, Posterior Column, Percutaneous Approach

ØRG637J Fusion of Thoracic Vertebral Joint with Autologous Tissue Substitute, Posterior Approach, Anterior Column, Percutaneous Approach

ØRG63AØ Fusion of Thoracic Vertebral Joint with Interbody Fusion Device, Anterior Approach, Anterior Column, Percutaneous Approach

ØRG63AJ Fusion of Thoracic Vertebral Joint with Interbody Fusion Device, Posterior Approach, Anterior Column, Percutaneous Approach

ØRG63JØ Fusion of Thoracic Vertebral Joint with Synthetic Substitute, Anterior Approach, Anterior Column, Percutaneous Approach

ØRG63J1 Fusion of Thoracic Vertebral Joint with Synthetic Substitute, Posterior Approach, Posterior Column, Percutaneous Approach

ØRG63JJ Fusion of Thoracic Vertebral Joint with Synthetic Substitute, Posterior Approach, Anterior Column, Percutaneous Approach

ØRG63KØ Fusion of Thoracic Vertebral Joint with Nonautologous Tissue Substitute, Anterior Approach, Anterior Column, Percutaneous Approach

ØRG63K1 Fusion of Thoracic Vertebral Joint with Nonautologous Tissue Substitute, Posterior Approach, Posterior Column, Percutaneous Approach

ØRG63KJ Fusion of Thoracic Vertebral Joint with Nonautologous Tissue Substitute, Posterior Approach, Anterior Column, Percutaneous Approach

ØRG6470 Fusion of Thoracic Vertebral Joint with Autologous Tissue Substitute, Anterior Approach, Anterior Column, Percutaneous Endoscopic Approach

ØRG6471 Fusion of Thoracic Vertebral Joint with Autologous Tissue Substitute, Posterior Approach, Posterior Column, Percutaneous Endoscopic Approach

ØRG647J Fusion of Thoracic Vertebral Joint with Autologous Tissue Substitute, Posterior Approach, Anterior Column, Percutaneous Endoscopic Approach

ØRG64AØ Fusion of Thoracic Vertebral Joint with Interbody Fusion Device, Anterior Approach, Anterior Column, Percutaneous Endoscopic Approach

ØRG64AJ Fusion of Thoracic Vertebral Joint with Interbody Fusion Device, Posterior Approach, Anterior Column, Percutaneous Endoscopic Approach

ØRG64JØ Fusion of Thoracic Vertebral Joint with Synthetic Substitute, Anterior Approach, Anterior Column, Percutaneous Endoscopic Approach

ØRG64J1 Fusion of Thoracic Vertebral Joint with Synthetic Substitute, Posterior Approach, Posterior Column, Percutaneous Endoscopic Approach

ØRG64JJ Fusion of Thoracic Vertebral Joint with Synthetic Substitute, Posterior Approach, Anterior Column, Percutaneous Endoscopic Approach

ØRG64KØ Fusion of Thoracic Vertebral Joint with Nonautologous Tissue Substitute, Anterior Approach, Anterior Column, Percutaneous Endoscopic Approach

ØRG64K1 Fusion of Thoracic Vertebral Joint with Nonautologous Tissue Substitute, Posterior Approach, Posterior Column, Percutaneous Endoscopic Approach

ØRG64KJ Fusion of Thoracic Vertebral Joint with Nonautologous Tissue Substitute, Posterior Approach, Anterior Column, Percutaneous Endoscopic Approach

ØRG7070 Fusion of 2 to 7 Thoracic Vertebral Joints with Autologous Tissue Substitute, Anterior Approach, Anterior Column, Open Approach

ØRG7071 Fusion of 2 to 7 Thoracic Vertebral Joints with Autologous Tissue Substitute, Posterior Approach, Posterior Column, Open Approach

ØRG707J Fusion of 2 to 7 Thoracic Vertebral Joints with Autologous Tissue Substitute, Posterior Approach, Anterior Column, Open Approach

ØRG70AØ Fusion of 2 to 7 Thoracic Vertebral Joints with Interbody Fusion Device, Anterior Approach, Anterior Column, Open Approach

ØRG70AJ Fusion of 2 to 7 Thoracic Vertebral Joints with Interbody Fusion Device, Posterior Approach, Anterior Column, Open Approach

ØRG70JØ Fusion of 2 to 7 Thoracic Vertebral Joints with Synthetic Substitute, Anterior Approach, Anterior Column, Open Approach

HAC 12: Surgical Site Infection-Certain Orthopedic Procedures of the Spine, Shoulder, and Elbow (continued)

ØRG7ØJ1 Fusion of 2 to 7 Thoracic Vertebral Joints with Synthetic Substitute, Posterior Approach, Posterior Column, Open Approach

ØRG7ØJJ Fusion of 2 to 7 Thoracic Vertebral Joints with Synthetic Substitute, Posterior Approach, Anterior Column, Open Approach

ØRG7ØKØ Fusion of 2 to 7 Thoracic Vertebral Joints with Nonautologous Tissue Substitute, Anterior Approach, Anterior Column, Open Approach

ØRG7ØK1 Fusion of 2 to 7 Thoracic Vertebral Joints with Nonautologous Tissue Substitute, Posterior Approach, Posterior Column, Open Approach

ØRG7ØKJ Fusion of 2 to 7 Thoracic Vertebral Joints with Nonautologous Tissue Substitute, Posterior Approach, Anterior Column, Open Approach

ØRG737Ø Fusion of 2 to 7 Thoracic Vertebral Joints with Autologous Tissue Substitute, Anterior Approach, Anterior Column, Percutaneous Approach

ØRG7371 Fusion of 2 to 7 Thoracic Vertebral Joints with Autologous Tissue Substitute, Posterior Approach, Posterior Column, Percutaneous Approach

ØRG737J Fusion of 2 to 7 Thoracic Vertebral Joints with Autologous Tissue Substitute, Posterior Approach, Anterior Column, Percutaneous Approach

ØRG73AØ Fusion of 2 to 7 Thoracic Vertebral Joints with Interbody Fusion Device, Anterior Approach, Anterior Column, Percutaneous Approach

ØRG73AJ Fusion of 2 to 7 Thoracic Vertebral Joints with Interbody Fusion Device, Posterior Approach, Anterior Column, Percutaneous Approach

ØRG73JØ Fusion of 2 to 7 Thoracic Vertebral Joints with Synthetic Substitute, Anterior Approach, Anterior Column, Percutaneous Approach

ØRG73J1 Fusion of 2 to 7 Thoracic Vertebral Joints with Synthetic Substitute, Posterior Approach, Posterior Column, Percutaneous Approach

ØRG73JJ Fusion of 2 to 7 Thoracic Vertebral Joints with Synthetic Substitute, Posterior Approach, Anterior Column, Percutaneous Approach

ØRG73KØ Fusion of 2 to 7 Thoracic Vertebral Joints with Nonautologous Tissue Substitute, Anterior Approach, Anterior Column, Percutaneous Approach

ØRG73K1 Fusion of 2 to 7 Thoracic Vertebral Joints with Nonautologous Tissue Substitute, Posterior Approach, Posterior Column, Percutaneous Approach

ØRG73KJ Fusion of 2 to 7 Thoracic Vertebral Joints with Nonautologous Tissue Substitute, Posterior Approach, Anterior Column, Percutaneous Approach

ØRG747Ø Fusion of 2 to 7 Thoracic Vertebral Joints with Autologous Tissue Substitute, Anterior Approach, Anterior Column, Percutaneous Endoscopic Approach

ØRG7471 Fusion of 2 to 7 Thoracic Vertebral Joints with Autologous Tissue Substitute, Posterior Approach, Posterior Column, Percutaneous Endoscopic Approach

ØRG747J Fusion of 2 to 7 Thoracic Vertebral Joints with Autologous Tissue Substitute, Posterior Approach, Anterior Column, Percutaneous Endoscopic Approach

ØRG74AØ Fusion of 2 to 7 Thoracic Vertebral Joints with Interbody Fusion Device, Anterior Approach, Anterior Column, Percutaneous Endoscopic Approach

ØRG74AJ Fusion of 2 to 7 Thoracic Vertebral Joints with Interbody Fusion Device, Posterior Approach, Anterior Column, Percutaneous Endoscopic Approach

ØRG74JØ Fusion of 2 to 7 Thoracic Vertebral Joints with Synthetic Substitute, Anterior Approach, Anterior Column, Percutaneous Endoscopic Approach

ØRG74J1 Fusion of 2 to 7 Thoracic Vertebral Joints with Synthetic Substitute, Posterior Approach, Posterior Column, Percutaneous Endoscopic Approach

ØRG74JJ Fusion of 2 to 7 Thoracic Vertebral Joints with Synthetic Substitute, Posterior Approach, Anterior Column, Percutaneous Endoscopic Approach

ØRG74KØ Fusion of 2 to 7 Thoracic Vertebral Joints with Nonautologous Tissue Substitute, Anterior Approach, Anterior Column, Percutaneous Endoscopic Approach

ØRG74K1 Fusion of 2 to 7 Thoracic Vertebral Joints with Nonautologous Tissue Substitute, Posterior Approach, Posterior Column, Percutaneous Endoscopic Approach

ØRG74KJ Fusion of 2 to 7 Thoracic Vertebral Joints with Nonautologous Tissue Substitute, Posterior Approach, Anterior Column, Percutaneous Endoscopic Approach

ØRG8Ø7Ø Fusion of 8 or More Thoracic Vertebral Joints with Autologous Tissue Substitute, Anterior Approach, Anterior Column, Open Approach

ØRG8Ø71 Fusion of 8 or More Thoracic Vertebral Joints with Autologous Tissue Substitute, Posterior Approach, Posterior Column, Open Approach

ØRG8Ø7J Fusion of 8 or More Thoracic Vertebral Joints with Autologous Tissue Substitute, Posterior Approach, Anterior Column, Open Approach

ØRG8ØAØ Fusion of 8 or More Thoracic Vertebral Joints with Interbody Fusion Device, Anterior Approach, Anterior Column, Open Approach

ØRG8ØAJ Fusion of 8 or More Thoracic Vertebral Joints with Interbody Fusion Device, Posterior Approach, Anterior Column, Open Approach

ØRG8ØJØ Fusion of 8 or More Thoracic Vertebral Joints with Synthetic Substitute, Anterior Approach, Anterior Column, Open Approach

ØRG8ØJ1 Fusion of 8 or More Thoracic Vertebral Joints with Synthetic Substitute, Posterior Approach, Posterior Column, Open Approach

ØRG8ØJJ Fusion of 8 or More Thoracic Vertebral Joints with Synthetic Substitute, Posterior Approach, Anterior Column, Open Approach

ØRG8ØKØ Fusion of 8 or More Thoracic Vertebral Joints with Nonautologous Tissue Substitute, Anterior Approach, Anterior Column, Open Approach

ØRG8ØK1 Fusion of 8 or More Thoracic Vertebral Joints with Nonautologous Tissue Substitute, Posterior Approach, Posterior Column, Open Approach

ØRG8ØKJ Fusion of 8 or More Thoracic Vertebral Joints with Nonautologous Tissue Substitute, Posterior Approach, Anterior Column, Open Approach

ØRG837Ø Fusion of 8 or More Thoracic Vertebral Joints with Autologous Tissue Substitute, Anterior Approach, Anterior Column, Percutaneous Approach

ØRG8371 Fusion of 8 or More Thoracic Vertebral Joints with Autologous Tissue Substitute, Posterior Approach, Posterior Column, Percutaneous Approach

ØRG837J Fusion of 8 or More Thoracic Vertebral Joints with Autologous Tissue Substitute, Posterior Approach, Anterior Column, Percutaneous Approach

ØRG83AØ Fusion of 8 or More Thoracic Vertebral Joints with Interbody Fusion Device, Anterior Approach, Anterior Column, Percutaneous Approach

ØRG83AJ Fusion of 8 or More Thoracic Vertebral Joints with Interbody Fusion Device, Posterior Approach, Anterior Column, Percutaneous Approach

ØRG83JØ Fusion of 8 or More Thoracic Vertebral Joints with Synthetic Substitute, Anterior Approach, Anterior Column, Percutaneous Approach

ØRG83J1 Fusion of 8 or More Thoracic Vertebral Joints with Synthetic Substitute, Posterior Approach, Posterior Column, Percutaneous Approach

ØRG83JJ Fusion of 8 or More Thoracic Vertebral Joints with Synthetic Substitute, Posterior Approach, Anterior Column, Percutaneous Approach

ØRG83KØ Fusion of 8 or More Thoracic Vertebral Joints with Nonautologous Tissue Substitute, Anterior Approach, Anterior Column, Percutaneous Approach

ØRG83K1 Fusion of 8 or More Thoracic Vertebral Joints with Nonautologous Tissue Substitute, Posterior Approach, Posterior Column, Percutaneous Approach

ØRG83KJ Fusion of 8 or More Thoracic Vertebral Joints with Nonautologous Tissue Substitute, Posterior Approach, Anterior Column, Percutaneous Approach

ØRG847Ø Fusion of 8 or More Thoracic Vertebral Joints with Autologous Tissue Substitute, Anterior Approach, Anterior Column, Percutaneous Endoscopic Approach

ØRG8471 Fusion of 8 or More Thoracic Vertebral Joints with Autologous Tissue Substitute, Posterior Approach, Posterior Column, Percutaneous Endoscopic Approach

ØRG847J Fusion of 8 or More Thoracic Vertebral Joints with Autologous Tissue Substitute, Posterior Approach, Anterior Column, Percutaneous Endoscopic Approach

ØRG84AØ Fusion of 8 or More Thoracic Vertebral Joints with Interbody Fusion Device, Anterior Approach, Anterior Column, Percutaneous Endoscopic Approach

ØRG84AJ Fusion of 8 or More Thoracic Vertebral Joints with Interbody Fusion Device, Posterior Approach, Anterior Column, Percutaneous Endoscopic Approach

ØRG84JØ Fusion of 8 or More Thoracic Vertebral Joints with Synthetic Substitute, Anterior Approach, Anterior Column, Percutaneous Endoscopic Approach

ØRG84J1 Fusion of 8 or More Thoracic Vertebral Joints with Synthetic Substitute, Posterior Approach, Posterior Column, Percutaneous Endoscopic Approach

HAC 12: Surgical Site Infection-Certain Orthopedic Procedures of the Spine, Shoulder, and Elbow (continued)

ØRG84JJ Fusion of 8 or More Thoracic Vertebral Joints with Synthetic Substitute, Posterior Approach, Anterior Column, Percutaneous Endoscopic Approach

ØRG84KØ Fusion of 8 or More Thoracic Vertebral Joints with Nonautologous Tissue Substitute, Anterior Approach, Anterior Column, Percutaneous Endoscopic Approach

ØRG84K1 Fusion of 8 or More Thoracic Vertebral Joints with Nonautologous Tissue Substitute, Posterior Approach, Posterior Column, Percutaneous Endoscopic Approach

ØRG84KJ Fusion of 8 or More Thoracic Vertebral Joints with Nonautologous Tissue Substitute, Posterior Approach, Anterior Column, Percutaneous Endoscopic Approach

ØRGAØ7Ø Fusion of Thoracolumbar Vertebral Joint with Autologous Tissue Substitute, Anterior Approach, Anterior Column, Open Approach

ØRGAØ71 Fusion of Thoracolumbar Vertebral Joint with Autologous Tissue Substitute, Posterior Approach, Posterior Column, Open Approach

ØRGAØ7J Fusion of Thoracolumbar Vertebral Joint with Autologous Tissue Substitute, Posterior Approach, Anterior Column, Open Approach

ØRGAØAØ Fusion of Thoracolumbar Vertebral Joint with Interbody Fusion Device, Anterior Approach, Anterior Column, Open Approach

ØRGAØAJ Fusion of Thoracolumbar Vertebral Joint with Interbody Fusion Device, Posterior Approach, Anterior Column, Open Approach

ØRGAØJØ Fusion of Thoracolumbar Vertebral Joint with Synthetic Substitute, Anterior Approach, Anterior Column, Open Approach

ØRGAØJ1 Fusion of Thoracolumbar Vertebral Joint with Synthetic Substitute, Posterior Approach, Posterior Column, Open Approach

ØRGAØJJ Fusion of Thoracolumbar Vertebral Joint with Synthetic Substitute, Posterior Approach, Anterior Column, Open Approach

ØRGAØKØ Fusion of Thoracolumbar Vertebral Joint with Nonautologous Tissue Substitute, Anterior Approach, Anterior Column, Open Approach

ØRGAØK1 Fusion of Thoracolumbar Vertebral Joint with Nonautologous Tissue Substitute, Posterior Approach, Posterior Column, Open Approach

ØRGAØKJ Fusion of Thoracolumbar Vertebral Joint with Nonautologous Tissue Substitute, Posterior Approach, Anterior Column, Open Approach

ØRGA37Ø Fusion of Thoracolumbar Vertebral Joint with Autologous Tissue Substitute, Anterior Approach, Anterior Column, Percutaneous Approach

ØRGA371 Fusion of Thoracolumbar Vertebral Joint with Autologous Tissue Substitute, Posterior Approach, Posterior Column, Percutaneous Approach

ØRGA37J Fusion of Thoracolumbar Vertebral Joint with Autologous Tissue Substitute, Posterior Approach, Anterior Column, Percutaneous Approach

ØRGA3AØ Fusion of Thoracolumbar Vertebral Joint with Interbody Fusion Device, Anterior Approach, Anterior Column, Percutaneous Approach

ØRGA3AJ Fusion of Thoracolumbar Vertebral Joint with Interbody Fusion Device, Posterior Approach, Anterior Column, Percutaneous Approach

ØRGA3JØ Fusion of Thoracolumbar Vertebral Joint with Synthetic Substitute, Anterior Approach, Anterior Column, Percutaneous Approach

ØRGA3J1 Fusion of Thoracolumbar Vertebral Joint with Synthetic Substitute, Posterior Approach, Posterior Column, Percutaneous Approach

ØRGA3JJ Fusion of Thoracolumbar Vertebral Joint with Synthetic Substitute, Posterior Approach, Anterior Column, Percutaneous Approach

ØRGA3KØ Fusion of Thoracolumbar Vertebral Joint with Nonautologous Tissue Substitute, Anterior Approach, Anterior Column, Percutaneous Approach

ØRGA3K1 Fusion of Thoracolumbar Vertebral Joint with Nonautologous Tissue Substitute, Posterior Approach, Posterior Column, Percutaneous Approach

ØRGA3KJ Fusion of Thoracolumbar Vertebral Joint with Nonautologous Tissue Substitute, Posterior Approach, Anterior Column, Percutaneous Approach

ØRGA47Ø Fusion of Thoracolumbar Vertebral Joint with Autologous Tissue Substitute, Anterior Approach, Anterior Column, Percutaneous Endoscopic Approach

ØRGA471 Fusion of Thoracolumbar Vertebral Joint with Autologous Tissue Substitute, Posterior Approach, Posterior Column, Percutaneous Endoscopic Approach

ØRGA47J Fusion of Thoracolumbar Vertebral Joint with Autologous Tissue Substitute, Posterior Approach, Anterior Column, Percutaneous Endoscopic Approach

ØRGA4AØ Fusion of Thoracolumbar Vertebral Joint with Interbody Fusion Device, Anterior Approach, Anterior Column, Percutaneous Endoscopic Approach

ØRGA4AJ Fusion of Thoracolumbar Vertebral Joint with Interbody Fusion Device, Posterior Approach, Anterior Column, Percutaneous Endoscopic Approach

ØRGA4JØ Fusion of Thoracolumbar Vertebral Joint with Synthetic Substitute, Anterior Approach, Anterior Column, Percutaneous Endoscopic Approach

ØRGA4J1 Fusion of Thoracolumbar Vertebral Joint with Synthetic Substitute, Posterior Approach, Posterior Column, Percutaneous Endoscopic Approach

ØRGA4JJ Fusion of Thoracolumbar Vertebral Joint with Synthetic Substitute, Posterior Approach, Anterior Column, Percutaneous Endoscopic Approach

ØRGA4KØ Fusion of Thoracolumbar Vertebral Joint with Nonautologous Tissue Substitute, Anterior Approach, Anterior Column, Percutaneous Endoscopic Approach

ØRGA4K1 Fusion of Thoracolumbar Vertebral Joint with Nonautologous Tissue Substitute, Posterior Approach, Posterior Column, Percutaneous Endoscopic Approach

ØRGA4KJ Fusion of Thoracolumbar Vertebral Joint with Nonautologous Tissue Substitute, Posterior Approach, Anterior Column, Percutaneous Endoscopic Approach

ØRGEØ4Z Fusion of Right Sternoclavicular Joint with Internal Fixation Device, Open Approach

ØRGEØ7Z Fusion of Right Sternoclavicular Joint with Autologous Tissue Substitute, Open Approach

ØRGEØJZ Fusion of Right Sternoclavicular Joint with Synthetic Substitute, Open Approach

ØRGEØKZ Fusion of Right Sternoclavicular Joint with Nonautologous Tissue Substitute, Open Approach

ØRGE34Z Fusion of Right Sternoclavicular Joint with Internal Fixation Device, Percutaneous Approach

ØRGE37Z Fusion of Right Sternoclavicular Joint with Autologous Tissue Substitute, Percutaneous Approach

ØRGE3JZ Fusion of Right Sternoclavicular Joint with Synthetic Substitute, Percutaneous Approach

ØRGE3KZ Fusion of Right Sternoclavicular Joint with Nonautologous Tissue Substitute, Percutaneous Approach

ØRGE44Z Fusion of Right Sternoclavicular Joint with Internal Fixation Device, Percutaneous Endoscopic Approach

ØRGE47Z Fusion of Right Sternoclavicular Joint with Autologous Tissue Substitute, Percutaneous Endoscopic Approach

ØRGE4JZ Fusion of Right Sternoclavicular Joint with Synthetic Substitute, Percutaneous Endoscopic Approach

ØRGE4KZ Fusion of Right Sternoclavicular Joint with Nonautologous Tissue Substitute, Percutaneous Endoscopic Approach

ØRGFØ4Z Fusion of Left Sternoclavicular Joint with Internal Fixation Device, Open Approach

ØRGFØ7Z Fusion of Left Sternoclavicular Joint with Autologous Tissue Substitute, Open Approach

ØRGFØJZ Fusion of Left Sternoclavicular Joint with Synthetic Substitute, Open Approach

ØRGFØKZ Fusion of Left Sternoclavicular Joint with Nonautologous Tissue Substitute, Open Approach

ØRGF34Z Fusion of Left Sternoclavicular Joint with Internal Fixation Device, Percutaneous Approach

ØRGF37Z Fusion of Left Sternoclavicular Joint with Autologous Tissue Substitute, Percutaneous Approach

ØRGF3JZ Fusion of Left Sternoclavicular Joint with Synthetic Substitute, Percutaneous Approach

ØRGF3KZ Fusion of Left Sternoclavicular Joint with Nonautologous Tissue Substitute, Percutaneous Approach

ØRGF44Z Fusion of Left Sternoclavicular Joint with Internal Fixation Device, Percutaneous Endoscopic Approach

ØRGF47Z Fusion of Left Sternoclavicular Joint with Autologous Tissue Substitute, Percutaneous Endoscopic Approach

ØRGF4JZ Fusion of Left Sternoclavicular Joint with Synthetic Substitute, Percutaneous Endoscopic Approach

ØRGF4KZ Fusion of Left Sternoclavicular Joint with Nonautologous Tissue Substitute, Percutaneous Endoscopic Approach

ØRGGØ4Z Fusion of Right Acromioclavicular Joint with Internal Fixation Device, Open Approach

HAC 12: Surgical Site Infection-Certain Orthopedic Procedures of the Spine, Shoulder, and Elbow (continued)

ØRGGØ7Z Fusion of Right Acromioclavicular Joint with Autologous Tissue Substitute, Open Approach

ØRGGØJZ Fusion of Right Acromioclavicular Joint with Synthetic Substitute, Open Approach

ØRGGØKZ Fusion of Right Acromioclavicular Joint with Nonautologous Tissue Substitute, Open Approach

ØRGG34Z Fusion of Right Acromioclavicular Joint with Internal Fixation Device, Percutaneous Approach

ØRGG37Z Fusion of Right Acromioclavicular Joint with Autologous Tissue Substitute, Percutaneous Approach

ØRGG3JZ Fusion of Right Acromioclavicular Joint with Synthetic Substitute, Percutaneous Approach

ØRGG3KZ Fusion of Right Acromioclavicular Joint with Nonautologous Tissue Substitute, Percutaneous Approach

ØRGG44Z Fusion of Right Acromioclavicular Joint with Internal Fixation Device, Percutaneous Endoscopic Approach

ØRGG47Z Fusion of Right Acromioclavicular Joint with Autologous Tissue Substitute, Percutaneous Endoscopic Approach

ØRGG4JZ Fusion of Right Acromioclavicular Joint with Synthetic Substitute, Percutaneous Endoscopic Approach

ØRGG4KZ Fusion of Right Acromioclavicular Joint with Nonautologous Tissue Substitute, Percutaneous Endoscopic Approach

ØRGHØ4Z Fusion of Left Acromioclavicular Joint with Internal Fixation Device, Open Approach

ØRGHØ7Z Fusion of Left Acromioclavicular Joint with Autologous Tissue Substitute, Open Approach

ØRGHØJZ Fusion of Left Acromioclavicular Joint with Synthetic Substitute, Open Approach

ØRGHØKZ Fusion of Left Acromioclavicular Joint with Nonautologous Tissue Substitute, Open Approach

ØRGH34Z Fusion of Left Acromioclavicular Joint with Internal Fixation Device, Percutaneous Approach

ØRGH37Z Fusion of Left Acromioclavicular Joint with Autologous Tissue Substitute, Percutaneous Approach

ØRGH3JZ Fusion of Left Acromioclavicular Joint with Synthetic Substitute, Percutaneous Approach

ØRGH3KZ Fusion of Left Acromioclavicular Joint with Nonautologous Tissue Substitute, Percutaneous Approach

ØRGH44Z Fusion of Left Acromioclavicular Joint with Internal Fixation Device, Percutaneous Endoscopic Approach

ØRGH47Z Fusion of Left Acromioclavicular Joint with Autologous Tissue Substitute, Percutaneous Endoscopic Approach

ØRGH4JZ Fusion of Left Acromioclavicular Joint with Synthetic Substitute, Percutaneous Endoscopic Approach

ØRGH4KZ Fusion of Left Acromioclavicular Joint with Nonautologous Tissue Substitute, Percutaneous Endoscopic Approach

ØRGJØ4Z Fusion of Right Shoulder Joint with Internal Fixation Device, Open Approach

ØRGJØ7Z Fusion of Right Shoulder Joint with Autologous Tissue Substitute, Open Approach

ØRGJØJZ Fusion of Right Shoulder Joint with Synthetic Substitute, Open Approach

ØRGJØKZ Fusion of Right Shoulder Joint with Nonautologous Tissue Substitute, Open Approach

ØRGJ34Z Fusion of Right Shoulder Joint with Internal Fixation Device, Percutaneous Approach

ØRGJ37Z Fusion of Right Shoulder Joint with Autologous Tissue Substitute, Percutaneous Approach

ØRGJ3JZ Fusion of Right Shoulder Joint with Synthetic Substitute, Percutaneous Approach

ØRGJ3KZ Fusion of Right Shoulder Joint with Nonautologous Tissue Substitute, Percutaneous Approach

ØRGJ44Z Fusion of Right Shoulder Joint with Internal Fixation Device, Percutaneous Endoscopic Approach

ØRGJ47Z Fusion of Right Shoulder Joint with Autologous Tissue Substitute, Percutaneous Endoscopic Approach

ØRGJ4JZ Fusion of Right Shoulder Joint with Synthetic Substitute, Percutaneous Endoscopic Approach

ØRGJ4KZ Fusion of Right Shoulder Joint with Nonautologous Tissue Substitute, Percutaneous Endoscopic Approach

ØRGKØ4Z Fusion of Left Shoulder Joint with Internal Fixation Device, Open Approach

ØRGKØ7Z Fusion of Left Shoulder Joint with Autologous Tissue Substitute, Open Approach

ØRGKØJZ Fusion of Left Shoulder Joint with Synthetic Substitute, Open Approach

ØRGKØKZ Fusion of Left Shoulder Joint with Nonautologous Tissue Substitute, Open Approach

ØRGK34Z Fusion of Left Shoulder Joint with Internal Fixation Device, Percutaneous Approach

ØRGK37Z Fusion of Left Shoulder Joint with Autologous Tissue Substitute, Percutaneous Approach

ØRGK3JZ Fusion of Left Shoulder Joint with Synthetic Substitute, Percutaneous Approach

ØRGK3KZ Fusion of Left Shoulder Joint with Nonautologous Tissue Substitute, Percutaneous Approach

ØRGK44Z Fusion of Left Shoulder Joint with Internal Fixation Device, Percutaneous Endoscopic Approach

ØRGK47Z Fusion of Left Shoulder Joint with Autologous Tissue Substitute, Percutaneous Endoscopic Approach

ØRGK4JZ Fusion of Left Shoulder Joint with Synthetic Substitute, Percutaneous Endoscopic Approach

ØRGK4KZ Fusion of Left Shoulder Joint with Nonautologous Tissue Substitute, Percutaneous Endoscopic Approach

ØRGLØ3Z Fusion of Right Elbow Joint with Sustained Compression Internal Fixation Device, Open Approach

ØRGLØ4Z Fusion of Right Elbow Joint with Internal Fixation Device, Open Approach

ØRGLØ5Z Fusion of Right Elbow Joint with External Fixation Device, Open Approach

ØRGLØ7Z Fusion of Right Elbow Joint with Autologous Tissue Substitute, Open Approach

ØRGLØJZ Fusion of Right Elbow Joint with Synthetic Substitute, Open Approach

ØRGLØKZ Fusion of Right Elbow Joint with Nonautologous Tissue Substitute, Open Approach

ØRGL33Z Fusion of Right Elbow Joint with Sustained Compression Internal Fixation Device, Percutaneous Approach

ØRGL34Z Fusion of Right Elbow Joint with Internal Fixation Device, Percutaneous Approach

ØRGL35Z Fusion of Right Elbow Joint with External Fixation Device, Percutaneous Approach

ØRGL37Z Fusion of Right Elbow Joint with Autologous Tissue Substitute, Percutaneous Approach

ØRGL3JZ Fusion of Right Elbow Joint with Synthetic Substitute, Percutaneous Approach

ØRGL3KZ Fusion of Right Elbow Joint with Nonautologous Tissue Substitute, Percutaneous Approach

ØRGL43Z Fusion of Right Elbow Joint with Sustained Compression Internal Fixation Device, Percutaneous Endoscopic Approach

ØRGL44Z Fusion of Right Elbow Joint with Internal Fixation Device, Percutaneous Endoscopic Approach

ØRGL45Z Fusion of Right Elbow Joint with External Fixation Device, Percutaneous Endoscopic Approach

ØRGL47Z Fusion of Right Elbow Joint with Autologous Tissue Substitute, Percutaneous Endoscopic Approach

ØRGL4JZ Fusion of Right Elbow Joint with Synthetic Substitute, Percutaneous Endoscopic Approach

ØRGL4KZ Fusion of Right Elbow Joint with Nonautologous Tissue Substitute, Percutaneous Endoscopic Approach

ØRGMØ3Z Fusion of Left Elbow Joint with Sustained Compression Internal Fixation Device, Open Approach

ØRGMØ4Z Fusion of Left Elbow Joint with Internal Fixation Device, Open Approach

ØRGMØ5Z Fusion of Left Elbow Joint with External Fixation Device, Open Approach

ØRGMØ7Z Fusion of Left Elbow Joint with Autologous Tissue Substitute, Open Approach

ØRGMØJZ Fusion of Left Elbow Joint with Synthetic Substitute, Open Approach

ØRGMØKZ Fusion of Left Elbow Joint with Nonautologous Tissue Substitute, Open Approach

ØRGM33Z Fusion of Left Elbow Joint with Sustained Compression Internal Fixation Device, Percutaneous Approach

ØRGM34Z Fusion of Left Elbow Joint with Internal Fixation Device, Percutaneous Approach

ØRGM35Z Fusion of Left Elbow Joint with External Fixation Device, Percutaneous Approach

ØRGM37Z Fusion of Left Elbow Joint with Autologous Tissue Substitute, Percutaneous Approach

ØRGM3JZ Fusion of Left Elbow Joint with Synthetic Substitute, Percutaneous Approach

ØRGM3KZ Fusion of Left Elbow Joint with Nonautologous Tissue Substitute, Percutaneous Approach

ØRGM43Z Fusion of Left Elbow Joint with Sustained Compression Internal Fixation Device, Percutaneous Endoscopic Approach

ØRGM44Z Fusion of Left Elbow Joint with Internal Fixation Device, Percutaneous Endoscopic Approach

ØRGM45Z Fusion of Left Elbow Joint with External Fixation Device, Percutaneous Endoscopic Approach

ØRGM47Z Fusion of Left Elbow Joint with Autologous Tissue Substitute, Percutaneous Endoscopic Approach

ØRGM4JZ Fusion of Left Elbow Joint with Synthetic Substitute, Percutaneous Endoscopic Approach

HAC 12: Surgical Site Infection-Certain Orthopedic Procedures of the Spine, Shoulder, and Elbow (continued)

ØRGM4KZ Fusion of Left Elbow Joint with Nonautologous Tissue Substitute, Percutaneous Endoscopic Approach

ØRQEØZZ Repair Right Sternoclavicular Joint, Open Approach

ØRQE3ZZ Repair Right Sternoclavicular Joint, Percutaneous Approach

ØRQE4ZZ Repair Right Sternoclavicular Joint, Percutaneous Endoscopic Approach

ØRQEXZZ Repair Right Sternoclavicular Joint, External Approach

ØRQFØZZ Repair Left Sternoclavicular Joint, Open Approach

ØRQF3ZZ Repair Left Sternoclavicular Joint, Percutaneous Approach

ØRQF4ZZ Repair Left Sternoclavicular Joint, Percutaneous Endoscopic Approach

ØRQFXZZ Repair Left Sternoclavicular Joint, External Approach

ØRQGØZZ Repair Right Acromioclavicular Joint, Open Approach

ØRQG3ZZ Repair Right Acromioclavicular Joint, Percutaneous Approach

ØRQG4ZZ Repair Right Acromioclavicular Joint, Percutaneous Endoscopic Approach

ØRQGXZZ Repair Right Acromioclavicular Joint, External Approach

ØRQHØZZ Repair Left Acromioclavicular Joint, Open Approach

ØRQH3ZZ Repair Left Acromioclavicular Joint, Percutaneous Approach

ØRQH4ZZ Repair Left Acromioclavicular Joint, Percutaneous Endoscopic Approach

ØRQHXZZ Repair Left Acromioclavicular Joint, External Approach

ØRQJØZZ Repair Right Shoulder Joint, Open Approach

ØRQJ3ZZ Repair Right Shoulder Joint, Percutaneous Approach

ØRQJ4ZZ Repair Right Shoulder Joint, Percutaneous Endoscopic Approach

ØRQJXZZ Repair Right Shoulder Joint, External Approach

ØRQKØZZ Repair Left Shoulder Joint, Open Approach

ØRQK3ZZ Repair Left Shoulder Joint, Percutaneous Approach

ØRQK4ZZ Repair Left Shoulder Joint, Percutaneous Endoscopic Approach

ØRQKXZZ Repair Left Shoulder Joint, External Approach

ØRQLØZZ Repair Right Elbow Joint, Open Approach

ØRQL3ZZ Repair Right Elbow Joint, Percutaneous Approach

ØRQL4ZZ Repair Right Elbow Joint, Percutaneous Endoscopic Approach

ØRQLXZZ Repair Right Elbow Joint, External Approach

ØRQMØZZ Repair Left Elbow Joint, Open Approach

ØRQM3ZZ Repair Left Elbow Joint, Percutaneous Approach

ØRQM4ZZ Repair Left Elbow Joint, Percutaneous Endoscopic Approach

ØRQMXZZ Repair Left Elbow Joint, External Approach

ØRUE07Z Supplement Right Sternoclavicular Joint with Autologous Tissue Substitute, Open Approach

ØRUEØJZ Supplement Right Sternoclavicular Joint with Synthetic Substitute, Open Approach

ØRUEØKZ Supplement Right Sternoclavicular Joint with Nonautologous Tissue Substitute, Open Approach

ØRUE37Z Supplement Right Sternoclavicular Joint with Autologous Tissue Substitute, Percutaneous Approach

ØRUE3JZ Supplement Right Sternoclavicular Joint with Synthetic Substitute, Percutaneous Approach

ØRUE3KZ Supplement Right Sternoclavicular Joint with Nonautologous Tissue Substitute, Percutaneous Approach

ØRUE47Z Supplement Right Sternoclavicular Joint with Autologous Tissue Substitute, Percutaneous Endoscopic Approach

ØRUE4JZ Supplement Right Sternoclavicular Joint with Synthetic Substitute, Percutaneous Endoscopic Approach

ØRUE4KZ Supplement Right Sternoclavicular Joint with Nonautologous Tissue Substitute, Percutaneous Endoscopic Approach

ØRUF07Z Supplement Left Sternoclavicular Joint with Autologous Tissue Substitute, Open Approach

ØRUFØJZ Supplement Left Sternoclavicular Joint with Synthetic Substitute, Open Approach

ØRUFØKZ Supplement Left Sternoclavicular Joint with Nonautologous Tissue Substitute, Open Approach

ØRUF37Z Supplement Left Sternoclavicular Joint with Autologous Tissue Substitute, Percutaneous Approach

ØRUF3JZ Supplement Left Sternoclavicular Joint with Synthetic Substitute, Percutaneous Approach

ØRUF3KZ Supplement Left Sternoclavicular Joint with Nonautologous Tissue Substitute, Percutaneous Approach

ØRUF47Z Supplement Left Sternoclavicular Joint with Autologous Tissue Substitute, Percutaneous Endoscopic Approach

ØRUF4JZ Supplement Left Sternoclavicular Joint with Synthetic Substitute, Percutaneous Endoscopic Approach

ØRUF4KZ Supplement Left Sternoclavicular Joint with Nonautologous Tissue Substitute, Percutaneous Endoscopic Approach

ØRUG07Z Supplement Right Acromioclavicular Joint with Autologous Tissue Substitute, Open Approach

ØRUGØJZ Supplement Right Acromioclavicular Joint with Synthetic Substitute, Open Approach

ØRUGØKZ Supplement Right Acromioclavicular Joint with Nonautologous Tissue Substitute, Open Approach

ØRUG37Z Supplement Right Acromioclavicular Joint with Autologous Tissue Substitute, Percutaneous Approach

ØRUG3JZ Supplement Right Acromioclavicular Joint with Synthetic Substitute, Percutaneous Approach

ØRUG3KZ Supplement Right Acromioclavicular Joint with Nonautologous Tissue Substitute, Percutaneous Approach

ØRUG47Z Supplement Right Acromioclavicular Joint with Autologous Tissue Substitute, Percutaneous Endoscopic Approach

ØRUG4JZ Supplement Right Acromioclavicular Joint with Synthetic Substitute, Percutaneous Endoscopic Approach

ØRUG4KZ Supplement Right Acromioclavicular Joint with Nonautologous Tissue Substitute, Percutaneous Endoscopic Approach

ØRUH07Z Supplement Left Acromioclavicular Joint with Autologous Tissue Substitute, Open Approach

ØRUHØJZ Supplement Left Acromioclavicular Joint with Synthetic Substitute, Open Approach

ØRUHØKZ Supplement Left Acromioclavicular Joint with Nonautologous Tissue Substitute, Open Approach

ØRUH37Z Supplement Left Acromioclavicular Joint with Autologous Tissue Substitute, Percutaneous Approach

ØRUH3JZ Supplement Left Acromioclavicular Joint with Synthetic Substitute, Percutaneous Approach

ØRUH3KZ Supplement Left Acromioclavicular Joint with Nonautologous Tissue Substitute, Percutaneous Approach

ØRUH47Z Supplement Left Acromioclavicular Joint with Autologous Tissue Substitute, Percutaneous Endoscopic Approach

ØRUH4JZ Supplement Left Acromioclavicular Joint with Synthetic Substitute, Percutaneous Endoscopic Approach

ØRUH4KZ Supplement Left Acromioclavicular Joint with Nonautologous Tissue Substitute, Percutaneous Endoscopic Approach

ØRUJ07Z Supplement Right Shoulder Joint with Autologous Tissue Substitute, Open Approach

ØRUJØJZ Supplement Right Shoulder Joint with Synthetic Substitute, Open Approach

ØRUJØKZ Supplement Right Shoulder Joint with Nonautologous Tissue Substitute, Open Approach

ØRUJ37Z Supplement Right Shoulder Joint with Autologous Tissue Substitute, Percutaneous Approach

ØRUJ3JZ Supplement Right Shoulder Joint with Synthetic Substitute, Percutaneous Approach

ØRUJ3KZ Supplement Right Shoulder Joint with Nonautologous Tissue Substitute, Percutaneous Approach

ØRUJ47Z Supplement Right Shoulder Joint with Autologous Tissue Substitute, Percutaneous Endoscopic Approach

ØRUJ4JZ Supplement Right Shoulder Joint with Synthetic Substitute, Percutaneous Endoscopic Approach

ØRUJ4KZ Supplement Right Shoulder Joint with Nonautologous Tissue Substitute, Percutaneous Endoscopic Approach

ØRUK07Z Supplement Left Shoulder Joint with Autologous Tissue Substitute, Open Approach

ØRUKØJZ Supplement Left Shoulder Joint with Synthetic Substitute, Open Approach

ØRUKØKZ Supplement Left Shoulder Joint with Nonautologous Tissue Substitute, Open Approach

ØRUK37Z Supplement Left Shoulder Joint with Autologous Tissue Substitute, Percutaneous Approach

ØRUK3JZ Supplement Left Shoulder Joint with Synthetic Substitute, Percutaneous Approach

ØRUK3KZ Supplement Left Shoulder Joint with Nonautologous Tissue Substitute, Percutaneous Approach

ØRUK47Z Supplement Left Shoulder Joint with Autologous Tissue Substitute, Percutaneous Endoscopic Approach

ØRUK4JZ Supplement Left Shoulder Joint with Synthetic Substitute, Percutaneous Endoscopic Approach

ØRUK4KZ Supplement Left Shoulder Joint with Nonautologous Tissue Substitute, Percutaneous Endoscopic Approach

ØRUL07Z Supplement Right Elbow Joint with Autologous Tissue Substitute, Open Approach

HAC 12: Surgical Site Infection-Certain Orthopedic Procedures of the Spine, Shoulder, and Elbow (continued)

ØRULØJZ Supplement Right Elbow Joint with Synthetic Substitute, Open Approach

ØRULØKZ Supplement Right Elbow Joint with Nonautologous Tissue Substitute, Open Approach

ØRUL37Z Supplement Right Elbow Joint with Autologous Tissue Substitute, Percutaneous Approach

ØRUL3JZ Supplement Right Elbow Joint with Synthetic Substitute, Percutaneous Approach

ØRUL3KZ Supplement Right Elbow Joint with Nonautologous Tissue Substitute, Percutaneous Approach

ØRUL47Z Supplement Right Elbow Joint with Autologous Tissue Substitute, Percutaneous Endoscopic Approach

ØRUL4JZ Supplement Right Elbow Joint with Synthetic Substitute, Percutaneous Endoscopic Approach

ØRUL4KZ Supplement Right Elbow Joint with Nonautologous Tissue Substitute, Percutaneous Endoscopic Approach

ØRUM07Z Supplement Left Elbow Joint with Autologous Tissue Substitute, Open Approach

ØRUMØJZ Supplement Left Elbow Joint with Synthetic Substitute, Open Approach

ØRUMØKZ Supplement Left Elbow Joint with Nonautologous Tissue Substitute, Open Approach

ØRUM37Z Supplement Left Elbow Joint with Autologous Tissue Substitute, Percutaneous Approach

ØRUM3JZ Supplement Left Elbow Joint with Synthetic Substitute, Percutaneous Approach

ØRUM3KZ Supplement Left Elbow Joint with Nonautologous Tissue Substitute, Percutaneous Approach

ØRUM47Z Supplement Left Elbow Joint with Autologous Tissue Substitute, Percutaneous Endoscopic Approach

ØRUM4JZ Supplement Left Elbow Joint with Synthetic Substitute, Percutaneous Endoscopic Approach

ØRUM4KZ Supplement Left Elbow Joint with Nonautologous Tissue Substitute, Percutaneous Endoscopic Approach

ØSG0070 Fusion of Lumbar Vertebral Joint with Autologous Tissue Substitute, Anterior Approach, Anterior Column, Open Approach

ØSG0071 Fusion of Lumbar Vertebral Joint with Autologous Tissue Substitute, Posterior Approach, Posterior Column, Open Approach

ØSG007J Fusion of Lumbar Vertebral Joint with Autologous Tissue Substitute, Posterior Approach, Anterior Column, Open Approach

ØSG00A0 Fusion of Lumbar Vertebral Joint with Interbody Fusion Device, Anterior Approach, Anterior Column, Open Approach

ØSG00AJ Fusion of Lumbar Vertebral Joint with Interbody Fusion Device, Posterior Approach, Anterior Column, Open Approach

ØSG00J0 Fusion of Lumbar Vertebral Joint with Synthetic Substitute, Anterior Approach, Anterior Column, Open Approach

ØSG00J1 Fusion of Lumbar Vertebral Joint with Synthetic Substitute, Posterior Approach, Posterior Column, Open Approach

ØSG00JJ Fusion of Lumbar Vertebral Joint with Synthetic Substitute, Posterior Approach, Anterior Column, Open Approach

ØSG00K0 Fusion of Lumbar Vertebral Joint with Nonautologous Tissue Substitute, Anterior Approach, Anterior Column, Open Approach

ØSG00K1 Fusion of Lumbar Vertebral Joint with Nonautologous Tissue Substitute, Posterior Approach, Posterior Column, Open Approach

ØSG00KJ Fusion of Lumbar Vertebral Joint with Nonautologous Tissue Substitute, Posterior Approach, Anterior Column, Open Approach

ØSG0370 Fusion of Lumbar Vertebral Joint with Autologous Tissue Substitute, Anterior Approach, Anterior Column, Percutaneous Approach

ØSG0371 Fusion of Lumbar Vertebral Joint with Autologous Tissue Substitute, Posterior Approach, Posterior Column, Percutaneous Approach

ØSG037J Fusion of Lumbar Vertebral Joint with Autologous Tissue Substitute, Posterior Approach, Anterior Column, Percutaneous Approach

ØSG03A0 Fusion of Lumbar Vertebral Joint with Interbody Fusion Device, Anterior Approach, Anterior Column, Percutaneous Approach

ØSG03AJ Fusion of Lumbar Vertebral Joint with Interbody Fusion Device, Posterior Approach, Anterior Column, Percutaneous Approach

ØSG03J0 Fusion of Lumbar Vertebral Joint with Synthetic Substitute, Anterior Approach, Anterior Column, Percutaneous Approach

ØSG03J1 Fusion of Lumbar Vertebral Joint with Synthetic Substitute, Posterior Approach, Posterior Column, Percutaneous Approach

ØSG03JJ Fusion of Lumbar Vertebral Joint with Synthetic Substitute, Posterior Approach, Anterior Column, Percutaneous Approach

ØSG03K0 Fusion of Lumbar Vertebral Joint with Nonautologous Tissue Substitute, Anterior Approach, Anterior Column, Percutaneous Approach

ØSG03K1 Fusion of Lumbar Vertebral Joint with Nonautologous Tissue Substitute, Posterior Approach, Posterior Column, Percutaneous Approach

ØSG03KJ Fusion of Lumbar Vertebral Joint with Nonautologous Tissue Substitute, Posterior Approach, Anterior Column, Percutaneous Approach

ØSG0470 Fusion of Lumbar Vertebral Joint with Autologous Tissue Substitute, Anterior Approach, Anterior Column, Percutaneous Endoscopic Approach

ØSG0471 Fusion of Lumbar Vertebral Joint with Autologous Tissue Substitute, Posterior Approach, Posterior Column, Percutaneous Endoscopic Approach

ØSG047J Fusion of Lumbar Vertebral Joint with Autologous Tissue Substitute, Posterior Approach, Anterior Column, Percutaneous Endoscopic Approach

ØSG04A0 Fusion of Lumbar Vertebral Joint with Interbody Fusion Device, Anterior Approach, Anterior Column, Percutaneous Endoscopic Approach

ØSG04AJ Fusion of Lumbar Vertebral Joint with Interbody Fusion Device, Posterior Approach, Anterior Column, Percutaneous Endoscopic Approach

ØSG04J0 Fusion of Lumbar Vertebral Joint with Synthetic Substitute, Anterior Approach, Anterior Column, Percutaneous Endoscopic Approach

ØSG04J1 Fusion of Lumbar Vertebral Joint with Synthetic Substitute, Posterior Approach, Posterior Column, Percutaneous Endoscopic Approach

ØSG04JJ Fusion of Lumbar Vertebral Joint with Synthetic Substitute, Posterior Approach, Anterior Column, Percutaneous Endoscopic Approach

ØSG04K0 Fusion of Lumbar Vertebral Joint with Nonautologous Tissue Substitute, Anterior Approach, Anterior Column, Percutaneous Endoscopic Approach

ØSG04K1 Fusion of Lumbar Vertebral Joint with Nonautologous Tissue Substitute, Posterior Approach, Posterior Column, Percutaneous Endoscopic Approach

ØSG04KJ Fusion of Lumbar Vertebral Joint with Nonautologous Tissue Substitute, Posterior Approach, Anterior Column, Percutaneous Endoscopic Approach

ØSG1070 Fusion of 2 or More Lumbar Vertebral Joints with Autologous Tissue Substitute, Anterior Approach, Anterior Column, Open Approach

ØSG1071 Fusion of 2 or More Lumbar Vertebral Joints with Autologous Tissue Substitute, Posterior Approach, Posterior Column, Open Approach

ØSG107J Fusion of 2 or More Lumbar Vertebral Joints with Autologous Tissue Substitute, Posterior Approach, Anterior Column, Open Approach

ØSG10A0 Fusion of 2 or More Lumbar Vertebral Joints with Interbody Fusion Device, Anterior Approach, Anterior Column, Open Approach

ØSG10AJ Fusion of 2 or More Lumbar Vertebral Joints with Interbody Fusion Device, Posterior Approach, Anterior Column, Open Approach

ØSG10J0 Fusion of 2 or More Lumbar Vertebral Joints with Synthetic Substitute, Anterior Approach, Anterior Column, Open Approach

ØSG10J1 Fusion of 2 or More Lumbar Vertebral Joints with Synthetic Substitute, Posterior Approach, Posterior Column, Open Approach

ØSG10JJ Fusion of 2 or More Lumbar Vertebral Joints with Synthetic Substitute, Posterior Approach, Anterior Column, Open Approach

ØSG10K0 Fusion of 2 or More Lumbar Vertebral Joints with Nonautologous Tissue Substitute, Anterior Approach, Anterior Column, Open Approach

ØSG10K1 Fusion of 2 or More Lumbar Vertebral Joints with Nonautologous Tissue Substitute, Posterior Approach, Posterior Column, Open Approach

ØSG10KJ Fusion of 2 or More Lumbar Vertebral Joints with Nonautologous Tissue Substitute, Posterior Approach, Anterior Column, Open Approach

ØSG1370 Fusion of 2 or More Lumbar Vertebral Joints with Autologous Tissue Substitute, Anterior Approach, Anterior Column, Percutaneous Approach

Appendix K: Hospital Acquired Conditions

HAC 12: Surgical Site Infection–Certain Orthopedic Procedures of the Spine, Shoulder, and Elbow (continued)

ØSG1371 Fusion of 2 or More Lumbar Vertebral Joints with Autologous Tissue Substitute, Posterior Approach, Posterior Column, Percutaneous Approach

ØSG137J Fusion of 2 or More Lumbar Vertebral Joints with Autologous Tissue Substitute, Posterior Approach, Anterior Column, Percutaneous Approach

ØSG13AØ Fusion of 2 or More Lumbar Vertebral Joints with Interbody Fusion Device, Anterior Approach, Anterior Column, Percutaneous Approach

ØSG13AJ Fusion of 2 or More Lumbar Vertebral Joints with Interbody Fusion Device, Posterior Approach, Anterior Column, Percutaneous Approach

ØSG13JØ Fusion of 2 or More Lumbar Vertebral Joints with Synthetic Substitute, Anterior Approach, Anterior Column, Percutaneous Approach

ØSG13J1 Fusion of 2 or More Lumbar Vertebral Joints with Synthetic Substitute, Posterior Approach, Posterior Column, Percutaneous Approach

ØSG13JJ Fusion of 2 or More Lumbar Vertebral Joints with Synthetic Substitute, Posterior Approach, Anterior Column, Percutaneous Approach

ØSG13KØ Fusion of 2 or More Lumbar Vertebral Joints with Nonautologous Tissue Substitute, Anterior Approach, Anterior Column, Percutaneous Approach

ØSG13K1 Fusion of 2 or More Lumbar Vertebral Joints with Nonautologous Tissue Substitute, Posterior Approach, Posterior Column, Percutaneous Approach

ØSG13KJ Fusion of 2 or More Lumbar Vertebral Joints with Nonautologous Tissue Substitute, Posterior Approach, Anterior Column, Percutaneous Approach

ØSG147Ø Fusion of 2 or More Lumbar Vertebral Joints with Autologous Tissue Substitute, Anterior Approach, Anterior Column, Percutaneous Endoscopic Approach

ØSG1471 Fusion of 2 or More Lumbar Vertebral Joints with Autologous Tissue Substitute, Posterior Approach, Posterior Column, Percutaneous Endoscopic Approach

ØSG147J Fusion of 2 or More Lumbar Vertebral Joints with Autologous Tissue Substitute, Posterior Approach, Anterior Column, Percutaneous Endoscopic Approach

ØSG14AØ Fusion of 2 or More Lumbar Vertebral Joints with Interbody Fusion Device, Anterior Approach, Anterior Column, Percutaneous Endoscopic Approach

ØSG14AJ Fusion of 2 or More Lumbar Vertebral Joints with Interbody Fusion Device, Posterior Approach, Anterior Column, Percutaneous Endoscopic Approach

ØSG14JØ Fusion of 2 or More Lumbar Vertebral Joints with Synthetic Substitute, Anterior Approach, Anterior Column, Percutaneous Endoscopic Approach

ØSG14J1 Fusion of 2 or More Lumbar Vertebral Joints with Synthetic Substitute, Posterior Approach, Posterior Column, Percutaneous Endoscopic Approach

ØSG14JJ Fusion of 2 or More Lumbar Vertebral Joints with Synthetic Substitute, Posterior Approach, Anterior Column, Percutaneous Endoscopic Approach

ØSG14KØ Fusion of 2 or More Lumbar Vertebral Joints with Nonautologous Tissue Substitute, Anterior Approach, Anterior Column, Percutaneous Endoscopic Approach

ØSG14K1 Fusion of 2 or More Lumbar Vertebral Joints with Nonautologous Tissue Substitute, Posterior Approach, Posterior Column, Percutaneous Endoscopic Approach

ØSG14KJ Fusion of 2 or More Lumbar Vertebral Joints with Nonautologous Tissue Substitute, Posterior Approach, Anterior Column, Percutaneous Endoscopic Approach

ØSG3070 Fusion of Lumbosacral Joint with Autologous Tissue Substitute, Anterior Approach, Anterior Column, Open Approach

ØSG3071 Fusion of Lumbosacral Joint with Autologous Tissue Substitute, Posterior Approach, Posterior Column, Open Approach

ØSG307J Fusion of Lumbosacral Joint with Autologous Tissue Substitute, Posterior Approach, Anterior Column, Open Approach

ØSG30AØ Fusion of Lumbosacral Joint with Interbody Fusion Device, Anterior Approach, Anterior Column, Open Approach

ØSG30AJ Fusion of Lumbosacral Joint with Interbody Fusion Device, Posterior Approach, Anterior Column, Open Approach

ØSG30JØ Fusion of Lumbosacral Joint with Synthetic Substitute, Anterior Approach, Anterior Column, Open Approach

ØSG30J1 Fusion of Lumbosacral Joint with Synthetic Substitute, Posterior Approach, Posterior Column, Open Approach

ØSG30JJ Fusion of Lumbosacral Joint with Synthetic Substitute, Posterior Approach, Anterior Column, Open Approach

ØSG30KØ Fusion of Lumbosacral Joint with Nonautologous Tissue Substitute, Anterior Approach, Anterior Column, Open Approach

ØSG30K1 Fusion of Lumbosacral Joint with Nonautologous Tissue Substitute, Posterior Approach, Posterior Column, Open Approach

ØSG30KJ Fusion of Lumbosacral Joint with Nonautologous Tissue Substitute, Posterior Approach, Anterior Column, Open Approach

ØSG3370 Fusion of Lumbosacral Joint with Autologous Tissue Substitute, Anterior Approach, Anterior Column, Percutaneous Approach

ØSG3371 Fusion of Lumbosacral Joint with Autologous Tissue Substitute, Posterior Approach, Posterior Column, Percutaneous Approach

ØSG337J Fusion of Lumbosacral Joint with Autologous Tissue Substitute, Posterior Approach, Anterior Column, Percutaneous Approach

ØSG33AØ Fusion of Lumbosacral Joint with Interbody Fusion Device, Anterior Approach, Anterior Column, Percutaneous Approach

ØSG33AJ Fusion of Lumbosacral Joint with Interbody Fusion Device, Posterior Approach, Anterior Column, Percutaneous Approach

ØSG33JØ Fusion of Lumbosacral Joint with Synthetic Substitute, Anterior Approach, Anterior Column, Percutaneous Approach

ØSG33J1 Fusion of Lumbosacral Joint with Synthetic Substitute, Posterior Approach, Posterior Column, Percutaneous Approach

ØSG33JJ Fusion of Lumbosacral Joint with Synthetic Substitute, Posterior Approach, Anterior Column, Percutaneous Approach

ØSG33KØ Fusion of Lumbosacral Joint with Nonautologous Tissue Substitute, Anterior Approach, Anterior Column, Percutaneous Approach

ØSG33K1 Fusion of Lumbosacral Joint with Nonautologous Tissue Substitute, Posterior Approach, Posterior Column, Percutaneous Approach

ØSG33KJ Fusion of Lumbosacral Joint with Nonautologous Tissue Substitute, Posterior Approach, Anterior Column, Percutaneous Approach

ØSG3470 Fusion of Lumbosacral Joint with Autologous Tissue Substitute, Anterior Approach, Anterior Column, Percutaneous Endoscopic Approach

ØSG3471 Fusion of Lumbosacral Joint with Autologous Tissue Substitute, Posterior Approach, Posterior Column, Percutaneous Endoscopic Approach

ØSG347J Fusion of Lumbosacral Joint with Autologous Tissue Substitute, Posterior Approach, Anterior Column, Percutaneous Endoscopic Approach

ØSG34AØ Fusion of Lumbosacral Joint with Interbody Fusion Device, Anterior Approach, Anterior Column, Percutaneous Endoscopic Approach

ØSG34AJ Fusion of Lumbosacral Joint with Interbody Fusion Device, Posterior Approach, Anterior Column, Percutaneous Endoscopic Approach

ØSG34JØ Fusion of Lumbosacral Joint with Synthetic Substitute, Anterior Approach, Anterior Column, Percutaneous Endoscopic Approach

ØSG34J1 Fusion of Lumbosacral Joint with Synthetic Substitute, Posterior Approach, Posterior Column, Percutaneous Endoscopic Approach

ØSG34JJ Fusion of Lumbosacral Joint with Synthetic Substitute, Posterior Approach, Anterior Column, Percutaneous Endoscopic Approach

ØSG34KØ Fusion of Lumbosacral Joint with Nonautologous Tissue Substitute, Anterior Approach, Anterior Column, Percutaneous Endoscopic Approach

ØSG34K1 Fusion of Lumbosacral Joint with Nonautologous Tissue Substitute, Posterior Approach, Posterior Column, Percutaneous Endoscopic Approach

ØSG34KJ Fusion of Lumbosacral Joint with Nonautologous Tissue Substitute, Posterior Approach, Anterior Column, Percutaneous Endoscopic Approach

ØSG7Ø4Z Fusion of Right Sacroiliac Joint with Internal Fixation Device, Open Approach

ØSG7Ø7Z Fusion of Right Sacroiliac Joint with Autologous Tissue Substitute, Open Approach

ØSG7ØJZ Fusion of Right Sacroiliac Joint with Synthetic Substitute, Open Approach

ØSG7ØKZ Fusion of Right Sacroiliac Joint with Nonautologous Tissue Substitute, Open Approach

HAC 12: Surgical Site Infection-Certain Orthopedic Procedures of the Spine, Shoulder, and Elbow (continued)

ØSG734Z Fusion of Right Sacroiliac Joint with Internal Fixation Device, Percutaneous Approach

ØSG737Z Fusion of Right Sacroiliac Joint with Autologous Tissue Substitute, Percutaneous Approach

ØSG73JZ Fusion of Right Sacroiliac Joint with Synthetic Substitute, Percutaneous Approach

ØSG73KZ Fusion of Right Sacroiliac Joint with Nonautologous Tissue Substitute, Percutaneous Approach

ØSG744Z Fusion of Right Sacroiliac Joint with Internal Fixation Device, Percutaneous Endoscopic Approach

ØSG747Z Fusion of Right Sacroiliac Joint with Autologous Tissue Substitute, Percutaneous Endoscopic Approach

ØSG74JZ Fusion of Right Sacroiliac Joint with Synthetic Substitute, Percutaneous Endoscopic Approach

ØSG74KZ Fusion of Right Sacroiliac Joint with Nonautologous Tissue Substitute, Percutaneous Endoscopic Approach

ØSG804Z Fusion of Left Sacroiliac Joint with Internal Fixation Device, Open Approach

ØSG807Z Fusion of Left Sacroiliac Joint with Autologous Tissue Substitute, Open Approach

ØSG80JZ Fusion of Left Sacroiliac Joint with Synthetic Substitute, Open Approach

ØSG80KZ Fusion of Left Sacroiliac Joint with Nonautologous Tissue Substitute, Open Approach

ØSG834Z Fusion of Left Sacroiliac Joint with Internal Fixation Device, Percutaneous Approach

ØSG837Z Fusion of Left Sacroiliac Joint with Autologous Tissue Substitute, Percutaneous Approach

ØSG83JZ Fusion of Left Sacroiliac Joint with Synthetic Substitute, Percutaneous Approach

ØSG83KZ Fusion of Left Sacroiliac Joint with Nonautologous Tissue Substitute, Percutaneous Approach

ØSG844Z Fusion of Left Sacroiliac Joint with Internal Fixation Device, Percutaneous Endoscopic Approach

ØSG847Z Fusion of Left Sacroiliac Joint with Autologous Tissue Substitute, Percutaneous Endoscopic Approach

ØSG84JZ Fusion of Left Sacroiliac Joint with Synthetic Substitute, Percutaneous Endoscopic Approach

ØSG84KZ Fusion of Left Sacroiliac Joint with Nonautologous Tissue Substitute, Percutaneous Endoscopic Approach

XRGAØR7 Fusion of Thoracolumbar Vertebral Joint using Customizable Interbody Fusion Device, Open Approach, New Technology Group 7

XRGA3R7 Fusion of Thoracolumbar Vertebral Joint using Customizable Interbody Fusion Device, Percutaneous Approach, New Technology Group 7

XRGA4R7 Fusion of Thoracolumbar Vertebral Joint using Customizable Interbody Fusion Device, Percutaneous Endoscopic Approach, New Technology Group 7

XRGBØR7 Fusion of Lumbar Vertebral Joint using Customizable Interbody Fusion Device, Open Approach, New Technology Group 7

XRGB3R7 Fusion of Lumbar Vertebral Joint using Customizable Interbody Fusion Device, Percutaneous Approach, New Technology Group 7

XRGB4R7 Fusion of Lumbar Vertebral Joint using Customizable Interbody Fusion Device, Percutaneous Endoscopic Approach, New Technology Group 7

XRGCØR7 Fusion of 2 or more Lumbar Vertebral Joints using Customizable Interbody Fusion Device, Open Approach, New Technology Group 7

XRGC3R7 Fusion of 2 or more Lumbar Vertebral Joints using Customizable Interbody Fusion Device, Percutaneous Approach, New Technology Group 7

XRGC4R7 Fusion of 2 or more Lumbar Vertebral Joints using Customizable Interbody Fusion Device, Percutaneous Endoscopic Approach, New Technology Group 7

XRGDØR7 Fusion of Lumbosacral Joint using Customizable Interbody Fusion Device, Open Approach, New Technology Group 7

XRGD3R7 Fusion of Lumbosacral Joint using Customizable Interbody Fusion Device, Percutaneous Approach, New Technology Group 7

XRGD4R7 Fusion of Lumbosacral Joint using Customizable Interbody Fusion Device, Percutaneous Endoscopic Approach, New Technology Group 7

HAC 13: Surgical Site Infection (SSI) Following Cardiac Implantable Electronic Device (CIED) Procedures

Secondary diagnosis not POA:

K68.11 Postprocedural retroperitoneal abscess

T81.40XA Infection following a procedure, unspecified, initial encounter

T81.41XA Infection following a procedure, superficial incisional surgical site, initial encounter

T81.42XA Infection following a procedure, deep incisional surgical site, initial encounter

T81.43XA Infection following a procedure, organ and space surgical site, initial encounter

T81.44XA Sepsis following a procedure, initial encounter

T81.49XA Infection following a procedure, other surgical site, initial encounter

T82.7XXA Infection and inflammatory reaction due to other internal orthopedic prosthetic devices, implants and grafts, initial encounter

AND

Any of the following procedures:

02H43JZ Insertion of Pacemaker Lead into Coronary Vein, Percutaneous Approach

02H43KZ Insertion of Defibrillator Lead into Coronary Vein, Percutaneous Approach

02H43MZ Insertion of Cardiac Lead into Coronary Vein, Percutaneous Approach

02H63JZ Insertion of Pacemaker Lead into Right Atrium, Percutaneous Approach

02H63MZ Insertion of Cardiac Lead into Right Atrium, Percutaneous Approach

02H73JZ Insertion of Pacemaker Lead into Left Atrium, Percutaneous Approach

02H73MZ Insertion of Cardiac Lead into Left Atrium, Percutaneous Approach

02HK3JZ Insertion of Pacemaker Lead into Right Ventricle, Percutaneous Approach

02HL3JZ Insertion of Pacemaker Lead into Left Ventricle, Percutaneous Approach

02HNØJZ Insertion of Pacemaker Lead into Pericardium, Open Approach

02HNØMZ Insertion of Cardiac Lead into Pericardium, Open Approach

02HN3JZ Insertion of Pacemaker Lead into Pericardium, Percutaneous Approach

02HN3MZ Insertion of Cardiac Lead into Pericardium, Percutaneous Approach

02HN4JZ Insertion of Pacemaker Lead into Pericardium, Percutaneous Endoscopic Approach

02HN4MZ Insertion of Cardiac Lead into Pericardium, Percutaneous Endoscopic Approach

02PAØMZ Removal of Cardiac Lead from Heart, Open Approach

02PA3MZ Removal of Cardiac Lead from Heart, Percutaneous Approach

02PA4MZ Removal of Cardiac Lead from Heart, Percutaneous Endoscopic Approach

02PAXMZ Removal of Cardiac Lead from Heart, External Approach

02WAØMZ Revision of Cardiac Lead in Heart, Open Approach

02WA3MZ Revision of Cardiac Lead in Heart, Percutaneous Approach

02WA4MZ Revision of Cardiac Lead in Heart, Percutaneous Endoscopic Approach

ØJH604Z Insertion of Pacemaker, Single Chamber into Chest Subcutaneous Tissue and Fascia, Open Approach

ØJH605Z Insertion of Pacemaker, Single Chamber Rate Responsive into Chest Subcutaneous Tissue and Fascia, Open Approach

ØJH606Z Insertion of Pacemaker, Dual Chamber into Chest Subcutaneous Tissue and Fascia, Open Approach

ØJH607Z Insertion of Cardiac Resynchronization Pacemaker Pulse Generator into Chest Subcutaneous Tissue and Fascia, Open Approach

ØJH608Z Insertion of Defibrillator Generator into Chest Subcutaneous Tissue and Fascia, Open Approach

ØJH609Z Insertion of Cardiac Resynchronization Defibrillator Pulse Generator into Chest Subcutaneous Tissue and Fascia, Open Approach

ØJH60PZ Insertion of Cardiac Rhythm Related Device into Chest Subcutaneous Tissue and Fascia, Open Approach

ØJH634Z Insertion of Pacemaker, Single Chamber into Chest Subcutaneous Tissue and Fascia, Percutaneous Approach

ØJH635Z Insertion of Pacemaker, Single Chamber Rate Responsive into Chest Subcutaneous Tissue and Fascia, Percutaneous Approach

ØJH636Z Insertion of Pacemaker, Dual Chamber into Chest Subcutaneous Tissue and Fascia, Percutaneous Approach

ØJH637Z Insertion of Cardiac Resynchronization Pacemaker Pulse Generator into Chest Subcutaneous Tissue and Fascia, Percutaneous Approach

ØJH638Z Insertion of Defibrillator Generator into Chest Subcutaneous Tissue and Fascia, Percutaneous Approach

ØJH639Z Insertion of Cardiac Resynchronization Defibrillator Pulse Generator into Chest Subcutaneous Tissue and Fascia, Percutaneous Approach

ØJH63PZ Insertion of Cardiac Rhythm Related Device into Chest Subcutaneous Tissue and Fascia, Percutaneous Approach

ØJH804Z Insertion of Pacemaker, Single Chamber into Abdomen Subcutaneous Tissue and Fascia, Open Approach

HAC 13: Surgical Site Infection (SSI) Following Cardiac Implantable Electronic Device (CIED) Procedures (continued)

ØJH805Z   Insertion of Pacemaker, Single Chamber Rate Responsive into Abdomen Subcutaneous Tissue and Fascia, Open Approach

ØJH806Z   Insertion of Pacemaker, Dual Chamber into Abdomen Subcutaneous Tissue and Fascia, Open Approach

ØJH807Z   Insertion of Cardiac Resynchronization Pacemaker Pulse Generator into Abdomen Subcutaneous Tissue and Fascia, Open Approach

ØJH808Z   Insertion of Defibrillator Generator into Abdomen Subcutaneous Tissue and Fascia, Open Approach

ØJH809Z   Insertion of Cardiac Resynchronization Defibrillator Pulse Generator into Abdomen Subcutaneous Tissue and Fascia, Open Approach

ØJH80PZ   Insertion of Cardiac Rhythm Related Device into Abdomen Subcutaneous Tissue and Fascia, Open Approach

ØJH834Z   Insertion of Pacemaker, Single Chamber into Abdomen Subcutaneous Tissue and Fascia, Percutaneous Approach

ØJH835Z   Insertion of Pacemaker, Single Chamber Rate Responsive into Abdomen Subcutaneous Tissue and Fascia, Percutaneous Approach

ØJH836Z   Insertion of Pacemaker, Dual Chamber into Abdomen Subcutaneous Tissue and Fascia, Percutaneous Approach

ØJH837Z   Insertion of Cardiac Resynchronization Pacemaker Pulse Generator into Abdomen Subcutaneous Tissue and Fascia, Percutaneous Approach

ØJH838Z   Insertion of Defibrillator Generator into Abdomen Subcutaneous Tissue and Fascia, Percutaneous Approach

ØJH839Z   Insertion of Cardiac Resynchronization Defibrillator Pulse Generator into Abdomen Subcutaneous Tissue and Fascia, Percutaneous Approach

ØJH83PZ   Insertion of Cardiac Rhythm Related Device into Abdomen Subcutaneous Tissue and Fascia, Percutaneous Approach

ØJPTØFZ   Removal of Subcutaneous Defibrillator Lead from Trunk Subcutaneous Tissue and Fascia, Open Approach

ØJPTØPZ   Removal of Cardiac Rhythm Related Device from Trunk Subcutaneous Tissue and Fascia, Open Approach

ØJPT3FZ   Removal of Subcutaneous Defibrillator Lead from Trunk Subcutaneous Tissue and Fascia, Percutaneous Approach

ØJPT3PZ   Removal of Cardiac Rhythm Related Device from Trunk Subcutaneous Tissue and Fascia, Percutaneous Approach

ØJWTØFZ   Revision of Subcutaneous Defibrillator Lead in Trunk Subcutaneous Tissue and Fascia, Open Approach

ØJWTØPZ   Revision of Cardiac Rhythm Related Device in Trunk Subcutaneous Tissue and Fascia, Open Approach

ØJWT3FZ   Revision of Subcutaneous Defibrillator Lead in Trunk Subcutaneous Tissue and Fascia, Percutaneous Approach

ØJWT3PZ   Revision of Cardiac Rhythm Related Device in Trunk Subcutaneous Tissue and Fascia, Percutaneous Approach

HAC 14: Iatrogenic Pneumothorax with Venous Catheterization

Secondary diagnosis not POA:

J95.811   Postprocedural pneumothorax

AND

Any of the following procedures:

02H633Z   Insertion of Infusion Device into Right Atrium, Percutaneous Approach

02HK33Z   Insertion of Infusion Device into Right Ventricle, Percutaneous Approach

02HS33Z   Insertion of Infusion Device into Right Pulmonary Vein, Percutaneous Approach

02HS43Z   Insertion of Infusion Device into Right Pulmonary Vein, Percutaneous Endoscopic Approach

02HT33Z   Insertion of Infusion Device into Left Pulmonary Vein, Percutaneous Approach

02HT43Z   Insertion of Infusion Device into Left Pulmonary Vein, Percutaneous Endoscopic Approach

02HV33Z   Insertion of Infusion Device into Superior Vena Cava, Percutaneous Approach

02HV43Z   Insertion of Infusion Device into Superior Vena Cava, Percutaneous Endoscopic Approach

05H033Z   Insertion of Infusion Device into Azygos Vein, Percutaneous Approach

05H043Z   Insertion of Infusion Device into Azygos Vein, Percutaneous Endoscopic Approach

05H133Z   Insertion of Infusion Device into Hemiazygos Vein, Percutaneous Approach

05H143Z   Insertion of Infusion Device into Hemiazygos Vein, Percutaneous Endoscopic Approach

05H333Z   Insertion of Infusion Device into Right Innominate Vein, Percutaneous Approach

05H343Z   Insertion of Infusion Device into Right Innominate Vein, Percutaneous Endoscopic Approach

05H433Z   Insertion of Infusion Device into Left Innominate Vein, Percutaneous Approach

05H443Z   Insertion of Infusion Device into Left Innominate Vein, Percutaneous Endoscopic Approach

05H533Z   Insertion of Infusion Device into Right Subclavian Vein, Percutaneous Approach

05H543Z   Insertion of Infusion Device into Right Subclavian Vein, Percutaneous Endoscopic Approach

05H633Z   Insertion of Infusion Device into Left Subclavian Vein, Percutaneous Approach

05H643Z   Insertion of Infusion Device into Left Subclavian Vein, Percutaneous Endoscopic Approach

05HM33Z   Insertion of Infusion Device into Right Internal Jugular Vein, Percutaneous Approach

05HN33Z   Insertion of Infusion Device into Left Internal Jugular Vein, Percutaneous Approach

05HP33Z   Insertion of Infusion Device into Right External Jugular Vein, Percutaneous Approach

05HQ33Z   Insertion of Infusion Device into Left External Jugular Vein, Percutaneous Approach

ØJH63XZ   Insertion of Vascular Access Device into Chest Subcutaneous Tissue and Fascia, Percutaneous Approach

Appendix L: Procedure Combination Tables

The tables below were developed to help simplify the relationship between ICD-10-PCS coding and MS-DRG assignment. The Centers for Medicare & Medicaid Services (CMS) has identified in the MS-DRG Definitions Manual certain procedure combinations that must occur in order to assign a specific MS-DRG. There are many factors influencing MS-DRG assignment, including principal and secondary diagnoses, MCC or CC use, sex of the patient, and discharge status. These tables should be used only as a guide. These tables were created based on the proposed, version 40, MS-DRG Grouper software and Definitions Manual files published with the fiscal 2023 IPPS proposed rule. To view the most current files, refer to the following: https://www.cms.gov/Medicare/Medicare-Fee-for-Service-Payment/AcuteInpatientPPS/MS-DRG-Classifications-and-Software.

DRG 001-002 Heart Transplant or Implant of Heart Assist System

Heart Transplant
Replacement of Right and Left Ventricle　02RK0JZ and 02RL0JZ

Insertion With Removal of Heart Assist System

Type of Heart Assist System	Code as appropriate Insertion by approach	Code also as appropriate Removal of Heart Assist System by approach
Biventricular External	02HA[0,3,4]RS	02PA[0,3,4]RZ
External	02HA[0,4]RZ	02PA[0,3,4]RZ

Revision With Removal of Heart Assist System

Type of Heart Assist System	Code as appropriate Revision by approach	Code also as appropriate Removal of Heart Assist System by approach
Implantable	02WA[0,3,4]QZ	02PA[0,3,4]RZ
External	02WA[0,3,4]RZ	02PA[0,3,4]RZ

DRG 008 Simultaneous Pancreas/Kidney Transplant

Transplanted Body Part	Code Transplant as appropriate by tissue type			Code also Pancreas Transplant as appropriate by tissue type		
	Allogeneic	Syngeneic	Zooplastic	Allogeneic	Syngeneic	Zooplastic
Kidney, Right	0TY00Z0	0TY00Z1	0TY00Z2	0FYG0Z0	0FYG0Z1	0FYG0Z2
Kidney, Left	0TY10Z0	0TY10Z1	0TY10Z2			

DRG 019 Simultaneous Pancreas/Kidney Transplant with Hemodialysis

Transplanted Body Part	Code Transplant as appropriate by tissue type			Code also Pancreas Transplant as appropriate by tissue type			Code also Hemodialysis		
	Allogeneic	Syngeneic	Zooplastic	Allogeneic	Syngeneic	Zooplastic	< 6 Hours	6-18 Hours	> 18 Hours
Kidney, Right	0TY00Z0	0TY00Z1	0TY00Z2	0FYG0Z0	0FYG0Z1	0FYG0Z2	5A1D07Z	5A1D80Z	5A1D90Z
Kidney, Left	0TY10Z0	0TY10Z1	0TY10Z2						

DRG 023-027 Craniotomy

Site of Neurostimulator Lead	Code as appropriate Insertion of Lead by approach	Code also as appropriate Insertion of Device by type and subcutaneous site						
		Neuro-stimulator Generator	Stimulator Multiple Array Code as appropriate by approach			Stimulator Multiple Array, Rechargeable Code as appropriate by approach		
		Skull	Chest	Back	Abdomen	Chest	Back	Abdomen
Brain	00H0[0,3,4]MZ	0NH00NZ	0JH6[0,3]DZ	0JH7[0,3]DZ	0JH8[0,3]DZ	0JH6[0,3]EZ	0JH7[0,3]EZ	0JH8[0,3]EZ
Cerebral Ventricle	00H6[0,3,4]MZ	0NH00NZ	0JH6[0,3]DZ	0JH7[0,3]DZ	0JH8[0,3]DZ	0JH6[0,3]EZ	0JH7[0,3]EZ	0JH8[0,3]EZ

DRG Ø28-Ø3Ø Spinal Procedures

Generator Type	Insertion of Generator by Site			Code also as appropriate Insertion of Neurostimulator Lead by approach	
	Chest	Abdomen	Back	Spinal Canal	Spinal Cord
Single Array	ØJH6[Ø,3]BZ	ØJH8[Ø,3]BZ	ØJH7[Ø,3]BZ	ØØHU[Ø,3,4]MZ	ØØHV[Ø,3,4]MZ
Single Array, Rechargeable	ØJH6[Ø,3]CZ	ØJH8[Ø,3]CZ	ØJH7[Ø,3]CZ	ØØHU[Ø,3,4]MZ	ØØHV[Ø,3,4]MZ
Multiple Array	ØJH6[Ø,3]DZ	ØJH8[Ø,3]DZ	ØJH7[Ø,3]DZ	ØØHU[Ø,3,4]MZ	ØØHV[Ø,3,4]MZ
Multiple Array, Rechargeable	ØJH6[Ø,3]EZ	—	ØJH7[Ø,3]EZ	ØØHU[Ø,3,4]MZ	ØØHV[Ø,3,4]MZ
Multiple Array, Rechargeable	—	ØJH8[Ø,3]EZ		ØØHU[Ø,3,4]MZ	ØØHV[Ø,3,4]MZ

DRG Ø4Ø-Ø42 Peripheral and Cranial Nerve and Other Nervous System Procedures

Insertion of Neurostimulator Generator and Lead

Insertion Single Array Generator, by Site		Code also Lead Insertion, by Site					
		Cranial Nerve	Peripheral Nerve	Azygos Vein	Innominate Vein, RT	Innominate Vein, LT	Stomach
Chest	ØJH6[Ø,3]BZ						
Back	ØJH7[Ø,3]BZ	ØØHE[Ø,3,4]MZ	Ø1HY[Ø,3,4]MZ	Ø5HØ[Ø,3,4]MZ	Ø5H3[Ø,3,4]MZ	Ø5H4[Ø,3,4]MZ	ØDH6[Ø,3,4]MZ
Abdomen	ØJH8[Ø,3]BZ						

Insertion Single Array, Rechargeable Generator, by Site		Code also Lead Insertion, by Site					
		Cranial Nerve	Peripheral Nerve	Azygos Vein	Innominate Vein, RT	Innominate Vein, LT	Stomach
Chest	ØJH6[Ø,3]CZ						
Back	ØJH7[Ø,3]CZ	ØØHE[Ø,3,4]MZ	Ø1HY[Ø,3,4]MZ	Ø5HØ[Ø,3,4]MZ	Ø5H3[Ø,3,4]MZ	Ø5H4[Ø,3,4]MZ	ØDH6[Ø,3,4]MZ
Abdomen	ØJH8[Ø,3]CZ						

Insertion Multiple Array Generator, by Site		Code also Lead Insertion, by Site					
		Cranial Nerve	Peripheral Nerve	Azygos Vein	Innominate Vein, RT	Innominate Vein, LT	Stomach
Chest	ØJH6[Ø,3]DZ						
Back	ØJH7[Ø,3]DZ	ØØHE[Ø,3,4]MZ	Ø1HY[Ø,3,4]MZ	Ø5HØ[Ø,3,4]MZ	Ø5H3[Ø,3,4]MZ	Ø5H4[Ø,3,4]MZ	ØDH6[Ø,3,4]MZ
Abdomen	ØJH8[Ø,3]DZ						

Insertion Multiple Array, Rechargeable Generator, by Site		Code also Lead Insertion, by Site					
		Cranial Nerve	Peripheral Nerve	Azygos Vein	Innominate Vein, RT	Innominate Vein, LT	Stomach
Chest	ØJH6[Ø,3]EZ						
Back	ØJH7[Ø,3]EZ	ØØHE[Ø,3,4]MZ	Ø1HY[Ø,3,4]MZ	Ø5HØ[Ø,3,4]MZ	Ø5H3[Ø,3,4]MZ	Ø5H4[Ø,3,4]MZ	ØDH6[Ø,3,4]MZ
Abdomen	ØJH8[Ø,3]EZ						

Insertion Stimulator Generator, by Site		Code also Lead Insertion, by Site					
		Cranial Nerve	Peripheral Nerve	Azygos Vein	Innominate Vein, RT	Innominate Vein, LT	Stomach
Chest	ØJH6[Ø,3]MZ						
Back	ØJH7[Ø,3]MZ	ØØHE[Ø,3,4]MZ	Ø1HY[Ø,3,4]MZ	Ø5HØ[Ø,3,4]MZ	Ø5H3[Ø,3,4]MZ	Ø5H4[Ø,3,4]MZ	ØDH6[Ø,3,4]MZ
Abdomen	ØJH8[Ø,3]MZ						

DRG 222-227 Cardiac Defibrillator Implant

Insertion of Generator With Insertion of Lead(s) into Coronary Vein, Atrium or Ventricle

Generator Type	Insertion of Generator by Site		Code also as appropriate Insertion of Leads by site				
	Chest	Abdomen	Coronary Vein	Atrium		Ventricle	
				Right	Left	Right	Left
Defibrillator	ØJH6[Ø,3]8Z	ØJH8[Ø,3]8Z	02H4[Ø,4]KZ	02H6[Ø,3,4]KZ	02H7[Ø,3,4]KZ	02HK[Ø,3,4]KZ	02HL[Ø,3,4]KZ
Cardiac Resynch Defibrillator Pulse Generator	ØJH6[Ø,3]9Z	ØJH8[Ø,3]9Z	02H4[Ø,3,4]KZ or 02H43[J,M]Z	02H6[Ø,3,4]KZ	02H7[Ø,3,4]KZ	02HK[Ø,3,4]KZ	02HL[Ø,3,4]KZ
Contractility Modulation Device	ØJH6[Ø,3]AZ	ØJH8[Ø,3]AZ	—	02H6[Ø,3,4]MZ	—	02HK[Ø,3,4]MZ	—

Insertion of Generator with Insertion of Lead(s) into Pericardium or Chest

Generator Type	Insertion of Generator by Site		Code also as appropriate Insertion of Leads by Site and Type			
	Chest	Abdomen	Pericardium			Chest
			Pacemaker	Defibrillator	Cardiac	Subcutaneous
Defibrillator	ØJH6[Ø,3]8Z	ØJH8[Ø,3]8Z	02HN[Ø,3,4]JZ	02HN[Ø,3,4]KZ	02HN[Ø,3,4]MZ	ØJH6[Ø,3]FZ
Cardiac Resynch Defibrillator Pulse Generator	ØJH6[Ø,3]9Z	ØJH8[Ø,3]9Z	02HN[Ø,3,4]JZ	02HN[Ø,3,4]KZ	02HN[Ø,3,4]MZ	ØJH6[Ø,3]FZ

DRG 242-244 Permanent Cardiac Pacemaker Implant

Insertion of Generator and Lead(s) Only

Generator Type	Insertion of Generator by Site		Code also Insertion of Lead, by Site			
	Chest	Abdomen	Coronary Vein	Right Atrium (6)/Left Atrium (7)	Right Ventricle (K)/ Left Ventricle (L)	Pericardium
Single Chamber	ØJH6[Ø,3]4Z	ØJH8[Ø,3]4Z	02H4[Ø,3,4][J,M]Z	02H[6,7][Ø,3,4][J,M]Z	02H[K,L][Ø,3,4][J,M]Z	02HN[Ø,3,4][J,M]Z
Single Chamber RR	ØJH6[Ø,3]5Z	ØJH8[Ø,3]5Z	02H4[Ø,3,4][J,M]Z	02H[6,7][Ø,3,4][J,M]Z	02H[K,L][Ø,3,4][J,M]Z	02HN[Ø,3,4][J,M]Z
Dual Chamber	ØJH6[Ø,3]6Z	ØJH8[Ø,3]6Z	02H4[Ø,3,4][J,M]Z	02H[6,7][Ø,3,4][J,M]Z	02H[K,L][Ø,3,4][J,M]Z	02HN[Ø,3,4][J,M]Z
Cardiac Resynch	ØJH6[Ø,3]7Z	ØJH8[Ø,3]7Z	02H4[Ø,3,4][J,M]Z	02H[6,7][Ø,3,4][J,M]Z	02H[K,L][Ø,3,4][J,M]Z	02HN[Ø,3,4][J,M]Z
Cardiac Rhythm Related	ØJH6[Ø,3]PZ	ØJH8[Ø,3]PZ	02H4[Ø,3,4][J,M]Z	02H[6,7][Ø,3,4][J,M]Z	02H[K,L][Ø,3,4][J,M]Z	02HN[Ø,3,4][J,M]Z

DRG 326-328 Stomach, Esophageal and Duodenal Procedures

Site	Resection by Open Approach	Code also as appropriate Resection of Pancreas by Open Approach
Duodenum	ØDT9ØZZ	ØFTGØZZ

DRG 344-346 Minor Small and Large Bowel Procedures

Site	Repair by Open Approach	Code also as appropriate Repair by external approach of Abdominal Wall Stoma
Small Intestine	ØDQ8ØZZ	ØWQFXZ2
Duodenum	ØDQ9ØZZ	ØWQFXZ2
Jejunum	ØDQAØZZ	ØWQFXZ2
Ileum	ØDQBØZZ	ØWQFXZ2
Large Intestine	ØDQEØZZ	ØWQFXZ2
Large Intestine, Right	ØDQFØZZ	ØWQFXZ2
Large Intestine, Left	ØDQGØZZ	ØWQFXZ2
Cecum	ØDQHØZZ	ØWQFXZ2
Ascending Colon	ØDQKØZZ	ØWQFXZ2
Transverse Colon	ØDQLØZZ	ØWQFXZ2
Descending Colon	ØDQMØZZ	ØWQFXZ2
Sigmoid Colon	ØDQNØZZ	ØWQFXZ2

DRG 456-458 Spinal Fusion Except Cervical with Spinal Curvature/Malignancy/ Infection or Extensive Fusions

Fusion of Thoracic and Lumbar Vertebra, Anterior Column

2 to 7 Thoracic Vertebra		Code also 2 or more Lumbar Vertebra	
ØRG[Ø,3,4][7,A,J,K]Ø	XRG7ØF3	ØSG1[Ø,3,4][7,A,J,K]Ø	XRGCØF3

Fusion of Thoracic and Lumbar Vertebra, Posterior Column

2 to 7 Thoracic Vertebra			Code also 2 or more Lumbar Vertebra		
Posterior Approach	Anterior Approach	New Technology	Posterior Approach	Anterior Approach	New Technology
ØRG7[Ø,3,4][7,J,K]1	ØRG7[Ø,3,4][7,A,J,K]J	XRG7Ø92 XRG7ØF3	ØSG1[Ø,3,4][7,J,K]1	ØSG1[Ø,3,4][7,A,J,K]J	XRGCØ92 XRGCØF3

DRG 461-462 Bilateral or Multiple Major Joint Procedures of Lower Extremity

For procedures to qualify as bilateral or multiple joint procedures, at least one replacement code or combination removal and replacement code from two different lower extremity sites from the following table(s) must be reported.

Examples: Left hip and right hip codes (bilateral); left hip and left knee codes (multiple); left hip and right ankle codes (multiple); left knee and right knee codes (bilateral); right hip removal and replacement, with right knee replacement

Hip, RT	Hip, LT	Knee, RT	Knee, LT	Ankle, RT	Ankle, LT		Hip, RT	Hip, LT	Knee, RT	Knee, LT	Ankle, RT	Ankle, LT
ØSR9Ø19	ØSRBØ19	ØSRCØ69	ØSRDØ69	ØSRFØ7Z	ØSRGØ7Z		ØSRAØ1Z	ØSREØ1Z	ØSRVØJZ	ØSRWØJZ		
ØSR9Ø1A	ØSRBØ1A	ØSRCØ6A	ØSRDØ6A	ØSRFØJ9	ØSRGØJ9		ØSRAØ39	ØSREØ39	ØSRVØKZ	ØSRWØKZ		
ØSR9Ø1Z	ØSRBØ1Z	ØSRCØ6Z	ØSRDØ6Z	ØSRFØJA	ØSRGØJA		ØSRAØ3A	ØSREØ3A	ØSPCØJZ	ØSPDØJZ		
ØSR9Ø29	ØSRBØ29	ØSRCØ7Z	ØSRDØ7Z	ØSRFØJZ	ØSRGØJZ		ØSRAØ3Z	ØSREØ3Z				
ØSR9Ø2A	ØSRBØ2A	ØSRCØJ9	ØSRDØJ9	ØSRFØKZ	ØSRGØKZ		ØSRAØ7Z	ØSREØ7Z				
ØSR9Ø2Z	ØSRBØ2Z	ØSRCØJA	ØSRDØJA				ØSRAØJ9	ØSREØJ9				
ØSR9Ø39	ØSRBØ39	ØSRCØJZ	ØSRDØJZ				ØSRAØJA	ØSREØJA				
ØSR9Ø3A	ØSRBØ3A	ØSRCØKZ	ØSRDØKZ				ØSRAØJZ	ØSREØJZ				
ØSR9Ø3Z	ØSRBØ3Z	ØSRCØL9	ØSRDØL9				ØSRAØKZ	ØSREØKZ				
ØSR9Ø49	ØSRBØ49	ØSRCØLA	ØSRDØLA				ØSRRØ19	ØSRSØ19				
ØSR9Ø4A	ØSRBØ4A	ØSRCØLZ	ØSRDØLZ				ØSRRØ1A	ØSRSØ1A				
ØSR9Ø4Z	ØSRBØ4Z	ØSRCØM9	ØSRDØM9				ØSRRØ1Z	ØSRSØ1Z				
ØSR9Ø69	ØSRBØ69	ØSRCØMA	ØSRDØMA				ØSRRØ39	ØSRSØ39				
ØSR9Ø6A	ØSRBØ6A	ØSRCØMZ	ØSRDØMZ				ØSRRØ3A	ØSRSØ3A				
ØSR9Ø6Z	ØSRBØ6Z	ØSRCØN9	ØSRDØN9				ØSRRØ3Z	ØSRSØ3Z				
ØSR9Ø7Z	ØSRBØ7Z	ØSRCØNA	ØSRDØNA				ØSRRØ7Z	ØSRSØ7Z				
ØSR9ØJ9	ØSRBØJ9	ØSRCØNZ	ØSRDØNZ				ØSRRØJ9	ØSRSØJ9				
ØSR9ØJA	ØSRBØJA	ØSRTØ7Z	ØSRUØ7Z				ØSRRØJA	ØSRSØJA				
ØSR9ØJZ	ØSRBØJZ	ØSRTØJ9	ØSRUØJ9				ØSRRØJZ	ØSRSØJZ				
ØSR9ØKZ	ØSRBØKZ	ØSRTØJA	ØSRUØJA				ØSRRØKZ	ØSRSØKZ				
ØSRAØØ9	ØSREØØ9	ØSRTØJZ	ØSRUØJZ				ØSU9ØBZ	ØSUBØBZ				
ØSRAØØA	ØSREØØA	ØSRTØKZ	ØSRUØKZ				ØSUAØBZ	ØSUEØBZ				
ØSRAØØZ	ØSREØØZ	ØSRVØ7Z	ØSRWØ7Z				ØSURØBZ	ØSUSØBZ				
ØSRAØ19	ØSREØ19	ØSRVØJ9	ØSRWØJ9				ØSP9ØJZ	ØSPBØJZ				
ØSRAØ1A	ØSREØ1A	ØSRVØJA	ØSRWØJA									

Hip Procedure Combinations

Open Removal of Hip Spacer with Replacement

Removal of Spacer		Code also as appropriate Replacement by Device Type					
		Metal	Metal on Poly	Ceramic	Ceramic on Poly	Oxidized Zirc on Poly	Synth Subst
Hip, RT	ØSP9Ø8Z	ØSR9Ø1[9,A,Z]	ØSR9Ø2[9,A,Z]	ØSR9Ø3[9,A,Z]	ØSR9Ø4[9,A,Z]	ØSR9Ø6[9,A,Z]	ØSR9ØJ[9,A,Z]
Hip, LT	ØSPBØ8Z	ØSRBØ1[9,A,Z]	ØSRBØ2[9,A,Z]	ØSRBØ3[9,A,Z]	ØSRBØ4[9,A,Z]	ØSRBØ6[9,A,Z]	ØSRBØJ[9,A,Z]

Open Removal of Hip Spacer with Replacement

Removal of Spacer		Code also as appropriate Replacement by Device Type						
		Acetabular Surface				Femoral Surface		
		Poly	Metal	Ceramic	Synthetic	Metal	Ceramic	Synth
Hip, RT	0SP908Z	0SRA00[9,A,Z]	0SRA01[9,A,Z]	0SRA03[9,A,Z]	0SRA0J[9,A,Z]	0SRR01[9,A,Z]	0SRR03[9,A,Z]	0SRR0J[9,A,Z]
Hip, LT	0SPB08Z	0SRE00[9,A,Z]	0SRE01[9,A,Z]	0SRE03[9,A,Z]	0SRE0J[9,A,Z]	0SRS01[9,A,Z]	0SRS03[9,A,Z]	0SRS0J[9,A,Z]

Open Removal of Hip Liner with Replacement

Removal of Liner		Code also as appropriate Replacement by Device Type					
		Metal	Metal on Poly	Ceramic	Ceramic on Poly	Oxidized Zirc on Poly	Synth Subst
Hip, RT	0SP909Z	0SR901[9,A,Z]	0SR902[9,A,Z]	0SR903[9,A,Z]	0SR904[9,A,Z]	0SR906[9,A,Z]	0SR90J[9,A,Z]
Hip, LT	0SPB09Z	0SRB01[9,A,Z]	0SRB02[9,A,Z]	0SRB03[9,A,Z]	0SRB04[9,A,Z]	0SRB06[9,A,Z]	0SRB0J[9,A,Z]

Open Removal of Hip Liner with Replacement

Removal of Liner		Code also as appropriate Replacement by Device Type						
		Acetabular Surface				Femoral Surface		
		Poly	Metal	Ceramic	Synthetic	Metal	Ceramic	Synth
Hip, RT	0SP909Z	0SRA00[9,A,Z]	0SRA01[9,A,Z]	0SRA03[9,A,Z]	0SRA0J[9,A,Z]	0SRR01[9,A,Z]	0SRR03[9,A,Z]	0SRR0J[9,A,Z]
Hip, LT	0SPB09Z	0SRE00[9,A,Z]	0SRE01[9,A,Z]	0SRE03[9,A,Z]	0SRE0J[9,A,Z]	0SRS01[9,A,Z]	0SRS03[9,A,Z]	0SRS0J[9,A,Z]

Open Removal of Hip Resurfacing Device with Replacement

Removal of Resurfacing Device		Code also as appropriate Replacement by Device Type					
		Metal	Metal on Poly	Ceramic	Ceramic on Poly	Oxidized Zirc on Poly	Synth Subst
Hip, RT	0SP90BZ	0SR901[9,A,Z]	0SR902[9,A,Z]	0SR903[9,A,Z]	0SR904[9,A,Z]	0SR906[9,A,Z]	0SR90J[9,A,Z]
Hip, LT	0SPB0BZ	0SRB01[9,A,Z]	0SRB02[9,A,Z]	0SRB03[9,A,Z]	0SRB04[9,A,Z]	0SRB06[9,A,Z]	0SRB0J[9,A,Z]

Open Removal of Hip Resurfacing Device with Replacement

Removal of Resurfacing Device		Code also as appropriate Replacement by Device Type						
		Acetabular Surface				Femoral Surface		
		Poly	Metal	Ceramic	Synthetic	Metal	Ceramic	Synth
Hip, RT	0SP90BZ	0SRA00[9,A,Z]	0SRA01[9,A,Z]	0SRA03[9,A,Z]	0SRA0J[9,A,Z]	0SRR01[9,A,Z]	0SRR03[9,A,Z]	0SRR0J[9,A,Z]
Hip, LT	0SPB0BZ	0SRE00[9,A,Z]	0SRE01[9,A,Z]	0SRE03[9,A,Z]	0SRE0J[9,A,Z]	0SRS01[9,A,Z]	0SRS03[9,A,Z]	0SRS0J[9,A,Z]

Open Removal of Hip Articulating Spacer with Replacement

Removal of Articulating Spacer		Code also as appropriate Replacement by Device Type					
		Metal	Metal on Poly	Ceramic	Ceramic on Poly	Oxidized Zirc on Poly	Synth Subst
Hip, RT	0SP90EZ	0SR901[9,A,Z]	0SR902[9,A,Z]	0SR903[9,A,Z]	0SR904[9,A,Z]	0SR906[9,A,Z]	0SR90J[9,A,Z]
Hip, LT	0SPB0EZ	0SRB01[9,A,Z]	0SRB02[9,A,Z]	0SRB03[9,A,Z]	0SRB04[9,A,Z]	0SRB06[9,A,Z]	0SRB0J[9,A,Z]

Open Removal of Hip Articulating Spacer with Replacement

Removal of Articulating Spacer		Code also as appropriate Replacement by Device Type						
		Acetabular Surface				Femoral Surface		
		Poly	Metal	Ceramic	Synthetic	Metal	Ceramic	Synth
Hip, RT	0SP90EZ	0SRA00[9,A,Z]	0SRA01[9,A,Z]	0SRA03[9,A,Z]	0SRA0J[9,A,Z]	0SRR01[9,A,Z]	0SRR03[9,A,Z]	0SRR0J[9,A,Z]
Hip, LT	0SPB0EZ	0SRE00[9,A,Z]	0SRE01[9,A,Z]	0SRE03[9,A,Z]	0SRE0J[9,A,Z]	0SRS01[9,A,Z]	0SRS03[9,A,Z]	0SRS0J[9,A,Z]

Open Removal of Hip Synthetic Substitute with Replacement

Removal of Synthetic Substitute		Code also as appropriate Replacement by Device Type					
		Metal	Metal on Poly	Ceramic	Ceramic on Poly	Oxidized Zirc on Poly	Synth Subst
Hip, RT	0SP[9,A,R]0JZ	0SR901[9,A,Z]	0SR902[9,A,Z]	0SR903[9,A,Z]	0SR904[9,A,Z]	0SR906[9,A,Z]	0SR90J[9,A,Z]
Hip, LT	0SP[B,E,S]0JZ	0SRB01[9,A,Z]	0SRB02[9,A,Z]	0SRB03[9,A,Z]	0SRB04[9,A,Z]	0SRB06[9,A,Z]	0SRB0J[9,A,Z]

Open Removal of Hip Synthetic Substitute with Replacement

Removal of Synthetic Substitute		Code also as appropriate Replacement by Device Type						
		Acetabular Surface				Femoral Surface		
		Poly	Metal	Ceramic	Synthetic	Metal	Ceramic	Synth
Hip, RT	ØSP[9,A,R]ØJZ	ØSRAØØ[9,A,Z]	ØSRAØ1[9,A,Z]	ØSRAØ3[9,A,Z]	ØSRAØJ[9,A,Z]	ØSRRØ1[9,A,Z]	ØSRRØ3[9,A,Z]	ØSRRØJ[9,A,Z]
Hip, LT	ØSP[B,E,S]ØJZ	ØSREØØ[9,A,Z]	ØSREØ1[9,A,Z]	ØSREØ3[9,A,Z]	ØSREØJ[9,A,Z]	ØSRSØ1[9,A,Z]	ØSRSØ3[9,A,Z]	ØSRSØJ[9,A,Z]

Percutaneous Endoscopic Removal of Hip Spacer with Open Replacement

Removal of Spacer		Code also as appropriate Replacement by Device Type					
		Metal	Metal on Poly	Ceramic	Ceramic on Poly	Oxidized Zirc on Poly	Synth Subst
Hip, RT	ØSP948Z	ØSR9Ø1[9,A,Z]	ØSR9Ø2[9,A,Z]	ØSR9Ø3[9,A,Z]	ØSR9Ø4[9,A,Z]	ØSR9Ø6[9,A,Z]	ØSR9ØJ[9,A,Z]
Hip, LT	ØSPB48Z	ØSRBØ1[9,A,Z]	ØSRBØ2[9,A,Z]	ØSRBØ3[9,A,Z]	ØSRBØ4[9,A,Z]	ØSRBØ6[9,A,Z]	ØSRBØJ[9,A,Z]

Percutaneous Endoscopic Removal of Hip Spacer with Open Replacement

Removal of Spacer		Code also as appropriate Replacement by Device Type						
		Acetabular Surface				Femoral Surface		
		Poly	Metal	Ceramic	Synthetic	Metal	Ceramic	Synth
Hip, RT	ØSP948Z	ØSRAØØ[9,A,Z]	ØSRAØ1[9,A,Z]	ØSRAØ3[9,A,Z]	ØSRAØJ[9,A,Z]	ØSRRØ1[9,A,Z]	ØSRRØ3[9,A,Z]	ØSRRØJ[9,A,Z]
Hip, LT	ØSPB48Z	ØSREØØ[9,A,Z]	ØSREØ1[9,A,Z]	ØSREØ3[9,A,Z]	ØSREØJ[9,A,Z]	ØSRSØ1[9,A,Z]	ØSRSØ3[9,A,Z]	ØSRSØJ[9,A,Z]

Percutaneous Endoscopic Removal of Hip Synthetic Substitute with Open Replacement

Removal of Synthetic Substitute		Code also as appropriate Replacement by Device Type					
		Metal	Metal on Poly	Ceramic	Ceramic on Poly	Oxidized Zirc on Poly	Synth Subst
Hip, RT	ØSP[9,A,R]4JZ	ØSR9Ø1[9,A,Z]	ØSR9Ø2[9,A,Z]	ØSR9Ø3[9,A,Z]	ØSR9Ø4[9,A,Z]	ØSR9Ø6[9,A,Z]	ØSR9ØJ[9,A,Z]
Hip, LT	ØSP[B,E,S]4JZ	ØSRBØ1[9,A,Z]	ØSRBØ2[9,A,Z]	ØSRBØ3[9,A,Z]	ØSRBØ4[9,A,Z]	ØSRBØ6[9,A,Z]	ØSRBØJ[9,A,Z]

Percutaneous Endoscopic Removal of Hip Synthetic Substitute with Open Replacement

Removal of Synthetic Substitute		Code also as appropriate Replacement by Device Type						
		Acetabular Surface				Femoral Surface		
		Poly	Metal	Ceramic	Synthetic	Metal	Ceramic	Synth
Hip, RT	ØSP[9,A,R]4JZ	ØSRAØØ[9,A,Z]	ØSRAØ1[9,A,Z]	ØSRAØ3[9,A,Z]	ØSRAØJ[9,A,Z]	ØSRRØ1[9,A,Z]	ØSRRØ3[9,A,Z]	ØSRRØJ[9,A,Z]
Hip, LT	ØSP[B,E,S]4JZ	ØSREØØ[9,A,Z]	ØSREØ1[9,A,Z]	ØSREØ3[9,A,Z]	ØSREØJ[9,A,Z]	ØSRSØ1[9,A,Z]	ØSRSØ3[9,A,Z]	ØSRSØJ[9,A,Z]

Knee Procedure Combinations

Removal of Knee Spacer with Replacement

Removal of Spacer		Code also Replacement by Type of Synthetic Substitute					
		Oxidized Zirc on Poly	Synthetic Substitute	Patello-femoral	Femoral Surface	Tibial Surface	Medial (L)/Lateral (M) Meniscus
Knee, RT	ØSPC[Ø,3,4]8Z	ØSRCØ6[9,A,Z]	ØSRCØJ[9,A,Z]	ØSRCØN[9,A,Z]	ØSRTØJ[9,A,Z]	ØSRVØJ[9,A,Z]	XRRGØ[L,M]8
Knee, LT	ØSPD[Ø,3,4]8Z	ØSRDØ6[9,A,Z]	ØSRDØJ[9,A,Z]	ØSRDØN[9,A,Z]	ØSRUØJ[9,A,Z]	ØSRWØJ[9,A,Z]	XRRHØ[L,M]8

Removal of Knee Liner with Replacement

Removal of Liner		Code also Replacement by Type of Synthetic Substitute						
		Oxidized Zirc on Poly	Synthetic Substitute	Medial (L)/Lateral (M) Unicondylar	Patello-femoral	Femoral Surface	Tibial Surface	Medial (L)/Lateral (M) Meniscus
Knee, RT	ØSPCØ9Z	ØSRCØ6[9,A,Z]	ØSRCØJ[9,A,Z]	ØSRCØ[L,M][9,A,Z]	ØSRCØN[9,A,Z]	ØSRTØJ[9,A,Z]	ØSRVØJ[9,A,Z]	XRRGØ[L,M]8
Knee, LT	ØSPDØ9Z	ØSRDØ6[9,A,Z]	ØSRDØJ[9,A,Z]	ØSRDØ[L,M][9,A,Z]	ØSRDØN[9,A,Z]	ØSRUØJ[9,A,Z]	ØSRWØJ[9,A,Z]	XRRHØ[L,M]8

Removal of Knee Articulating Spacer with Replacement

Removal of Articulating Spacer		Code also Replacement by Type of Synthetic Substitute				
		Oxidized Zirc on Poly	Synthetic Substitute	Femoral Surface	Tibial Surface	Medial (L)/ Lateral (M) Meniscus
Knee, RT	ØSPCØEZ	ØSRCØ6[9,A,Z]	ØSRCØJ[9,A,Z]	ØSRTØJ[9,A,Z]	ØSRVØJ[9,A,Z]	XRRGØ[L,M]8
Knee, LT	ØSPDØEZ	ØSRDØ6[9,A,Z]	ØSRDØJ[9,A,Z]	ØSRUØJ[9,A,Z]	ØSRWØJ[9,A,Z]	XRRHØ[L,M]8

Removal of Knee Patellar Surface with Replacement

Removal of Patellar Surface		Code also Replacement by Type of Synthetic Substitute					
		Oxidized Zirc on Poly	Synthetic Substitute	Patello-femoral	Femoral Surface	Tibial Surface	Medial (L)/Lateral (M) Meniscus
Knee, RT	ØSPC[Ø,4]JC	ØSRCØ6[9,A,Z]	ØSRCØJ[9,A,Z]	ØSRCØN[9,A,Z]	ØSRTØJ[9,A,Z]	ØSRVØJ[9,A,Z]	XRRGØ[L,M]8
Knee, LT	ØSPD[Ø,4]JC	ØSRDØ6[9,A,Z]	ØSRDØJ[9,A,7]	ØSRDØN[9,A,Z]	ØSRUØJ[9,A,Z]	ØSRWØJ[9,A,Z]	XRRHØ[L,M]8

Removal of Knee Synthetic Substitute with Replacement

Removal of Synthetic Substitute		Code also Replacement by Type of Synthetic Substitute						
		Oxidized Zirc on Poly	Synthetic Substitute	Medial (L)/ Lateral (M) Unicondylar	Patello-femoral	Femoral Surface	Tibial Surface	Medial (L)/ Lateral (M) Meniscus
Knee, RT	ØSPC[Ø,4]JZ	ØSRCØ6[9,A,Z]	ØSRCØJ[9,A,Z]	ØSRCØ[L,M][9,A,Z]	ØSRCØN[9,A,Z]	ØSRTØJ[9,A,Z]	ØSRVØJ[9,A,Z]	XRRGØ[L,M]8
Knee, LT	ØSPD[Ø,4]JZ	ØSRDØ6[9,A,Z]	ØSRDØJ[9,A,Z]	ØSRDØ[L,M][9,A,Z]	ØSRDØN[9,A,Z]	ØSRUØJ[9,A,Z]	ØSRWØJ[9,A,Z]	XRRHØ[L,M]8

Removal of Knee Unicondylar Device with Replacement

Removal of Medial (L)/ Lateral (M) Unicondylar Device		Code also Replacement by Type of Synthetic Substitute					
		Oxidized Zirc on Poly	Synthetic Substitute	Medial Unicondylar	Femoral Surface	Tibial Surface	Medial (L)/Lateral (M) Meniscus
Knee, RT	ØSPC[Ø,4][L,M]Z	ØSRCØ6[9,A,Z]	ØSRCØJ[9,A,Z]	ØSRCØL[9,A,Z]	ØSRTØJ[9,A,Z]	ØSRVØJ[9,A,Z]	XRRGØ[L,M]8
Knee, LT	ØSPD[Ø,4][L,M]Z	ØSRDØ6[9,A,Z]	ØSRDØJ[9,A,Z]	ØSRDØL[9,A,Z]	ØSRUØJ[9,A,Z]	ØSRWØJ[9,A,Z]	XRRHØ[L,M]8

Removal of Knee Patellofemoral Device with Replacement

Removal of Patellofemoral Device		Code also Replacement by Type of Synthetic Substitute					
		Oxidized Zirc on Poly	Synthetic Substitute	Medial Unicondylar	Femoral Surface	Tibial Surface	Medial (L)/Lateral (M) Meniscus
Knee, RT	ØSPC[Ø,4]NZ	ØSRCØ6[9,A,Z]	ØSRCØJ[9,A,Z]	ØSRCØL[9,A,Z]	ØSRTØJ[9,A,Z]	ØSRVØJ[9,A,Z]	XRRGØ[L,M]8
Knee, LT	ØSPD[Ø,4]NZ	ØSRDØ6[9,A,Z]	ØSRDØJ[9,A,Z]	ØSRDØL[9,A,Z]	ØSRUØJ[9,A,Z]	ØSRWØJ[9,A,Z]	XRRHØ[L,M]8

Removal of Knee Femoral/Tibial Surface Device with Replacement

Removal of Femoral (T,U)/ Tibial (V,W) Surface		Code also Replacement by Type of Synthetic Substitute					
		Oxidized Zirc on Poly	Synthetic Substitute	Articulating Spacer	Patello-femoral	Femoral Surface	Tibial Surface	Medial (L)/Lateral (M) Meniscus
Knee, RT	ØSP[T,V][Ø,4]JZ	ØSRCØ6[9,A,Z]	ØSRCØJ[9,A,Z]	ØSRCØEZ	ØSRCØN[9,A,Z]	ØSRTØJ[9,A,Z]	ØSRVØJ[9,A,Z]	XRRGØ[L,M]8
Knee, LT	ØSP[U,W][Ø,4]JZ	ØSRDØ6[9,A,Z]	ØSRDØJ[9,A,Z]	ØSRDØEZ	ØSRDØN[9,A,Z]	ØSRUØJ[9,A,Z]	ØSRWØJ[9,A,Z]	XRRHØ[L,M]8

466-468 Revision of Hip or Knee Replacement

Hip Procedure Combinations

Open Removal of Hip Spacer with Replacement

Removal of Spacer		Code also as appropriate Replacement by Device Type						
		Metal	Metal on Poly	Ceramic	Ceramic on Poly	Oxidized Zirc on Poly	Articulating Spacer	Synth Subst
Hip, RT	ØSP9Ø8Z	ØSR9Ø1[9,A,Z]	ØSR9Ø2[9,A,Z]	ØSR9Ø3[9,A,Z]	ØSR9Ø4[9,A,Z]	ØSR9Ø6[9,A,Z]	ØSR9ØEZ	ØSR9ØJ[9,A,Z]
Hip, LT	ØSPBØ8Z	ØSRBØ1[9,A,Z]	ØSRBØ2[9,A,Z]	ØSRBØ3[9,A,Z]	ØSRBØ4[9,A,Z]	ØSRBØ6[9,A,Z]	ØSRBØEZ	ØSRBØJ[9,A,Z]

Open Removal of Hip Spacer with Replacement

Removal of Spacer		Code also as appropriate Replacement by Device Type						
		Acetabular Surface				Femoral Surface		
		Poly	Metal	Ceramic	Synthetic	Metal	Ceramic	Synth
Hip, RT	ØSP9Ø8Z	ØSRAØØ[9,A,Z]	ØSRAØ1[9,A,Z]	ØSRAØ3[9,A,Z]	ØSRAØJ[9,A,Z]	ØSRRØ1[9,A,Z]	ØSRRØ3[9,A,Z]	ØSRRØJ[9,A,Z]
Hip, LT	ØSPBØ8Z	ØSREØØ[9,A,Z]	ØSREØ1[9,A,Z]	ØSREØ3[9,A,Z]	ØSREØJ[9,A,Z]	ØSRSØ1[9,A,Z]	ØSRSØ3[9,A,Z]	ØSRSØJ[9,A,Z]

Open Removal of Hip Spacer with Liner Insertion (supplement)

Removal of Spacer		Code also as appropriate Supplement of Body Part by Site		
		Joint	Acetabular Surface	Femoral Surface
Hip, RT	ØSP9Ø8Z	ØSU9Ø9Z	ØSUAØ9Z	ØSURØ9Z
Hip, LT	ØSPBØ8Z	ØSUBØ9Z	ØSUEØ9Z	ØSUSØ9Z

Open Removal of Hip Liner with Replacement

Removal of Liner		Code also as appropriate Replacement by Device Type						
		Metal	Metal on Poly	Ceramic	Ceramic on Poly	Oxidized Zirc on Poly	Articulating Spacer	Synth Subst
Hip, RT	ØSP9Ø9Z	ØSR9Ø1[9,A,Z]	ØSR9Ø2[9,A,Z]	ØSR9Ø3[9,A,Z]	ØSR9Ø4[9,A,Z]	ØSR9Ø6[9,A,Z]	ØSR9ØEZ	ØSR9ØJ[9,A,Z]
Hip, LT	ØSPBØ9Z	ØSRBØ1[9,A,Z]	ØSRBØ2[9,A,Z]	ØSRBØ3[9,A,Z]	ØSRBØ4[9,A,Z]	ØSRBØ6[9,A,Z]	ØSRBØEZ	ØSRBØJ[9,A,Z]

Open Removal of Hip Liner with Replacement

Removal of Liner		Code also as appropriate Replacement by Device Type						
		Acetabular Surface				Femoral Surface		
		Poly	Metal	Ceramic	Synthetic	Metal	Ceramic	Synth
Hip, RT	ØSP9Ø9Z	ØSRAØØ[9,A,Z]	ØSRAØ1[9,A,Z]	ØSRAØ3[9,A,Z]	ØSRAØJ[9,A,Z]	ØSRRØ1[9,A,Z]	ØSRRØ3[9,A,Z]	ØSRRØJ[9,A,Z]
Hip, LT	ØSPBØ9Z	ØSREØØ[9,A,Z]	ØSREØ1[9,A,Z]	ØSREØ3[9,A,Z]	ØSREØJ[9,A,Z]	ØSRSØ1[9,A,Z]	ØSRSØ3[9,A,Z]	ØSRSØJ[9,A,Z]

Open Removal of Hip Liner with Liner Insertion (supplement)

Removal of Liner		Code also as appropriate Supplement of Body Part by Site		
		Joint	Acetabular Surface	Femoral Surface
Hip, RT	ØSP9Ø9Z	ØSU9Ø9Z	ØSUAØ9Z	ØSURØ9Z
Hip, LT	ØSPBØ9Z	ØSUBØ9Z	ØSUEØ9Z	ØSUSØ9Z

Open Removal of Hip Resurfacing Device with Replacement

Removal of Resurfacing Device		Code also as appropriate Replacement by Device Type						
		Metal	Metal on Poly	Ceramic	Ceramic on Poly	Oxidized Zirc on Poly	Articulating Spacer	Synth Subst
Hip, RT	ØSP9ØBZ	ØSR9Ø1[9,A,Z]	ØSR9Ø2[9,A,Z]	ØSR9Ø3[9,A,Z]	ØSR9Ø4[9,A,Z]	ØSR9Ø6[9,A,Z]	ØSR9ØEZ	ØSR9ØJ[9,A,Z]
Hip, LT	ØSPBØBZ	ØSRBØ1[9,A,Z]	ØSRBØ2[9,A,Z]	ØSRBØ3[9,A,Z]	ØSRBØ4[9,A,Z]	ØSRBØ6[9,A,Z]	ØSRBØEZ	ØSRBØJ[9,A,Z]

Open Removal of Hip Resurfacing Device with Replacement

Removal of Resurfacing Device		Code also as appropriate Replacement by Device Type						
		Acetabular Surface				Femoral Surface		
		Poly	Metal	Ceramic	Synthetic	Metal	Ceramic	Synth
Hip, RT	ØSP9ØBZ	ØSRAØØ[9,A,Z]	ØSRAØ1[9,A,Z]	ØSRAØ3[9,A,Z]	ØSRAØJ[9,A,Z]	ØSRRØ1[9,A,Z]	ØSRRØ3[9,A,Z]	ØSRRØJ[9,A,Z]
Hip, LT	ØSPBØBZ	ØSREØØ[9,A,Z]	ØSREØ1[9,A,Z]	ØSREØ3[9,A,Z]	ØSREØJ[9,A,Z]	ØSRSØ1[9,A,Z]	ØSRSØ3[9,A,Z]	ØSRSØJ[9,A,Z]

Open Removal of Hip Resurfacing Device with Liner Insertion (supplement)

Removal of Resurfacing Device		Code also as appropriate Supplement of Body Part by Site		
		Joint	Acetabular Surface	Femoral Surface
Hip, RT	ØSP9ØBZ	ØSU9Ø9Z	ØSUAØ9Z	ØSURØ9Z
Hip, LT	ØSPBØBZ	ØSUBØ9Z	ØSUFØ9Z	ØSUSØ9Z

Open Removal of Hip Articulating Spacer with Replacement

Removal of Articulating Spacer		Code also as appropriate Replacement by Device Type					
		Metal	Metal on Poly	Ceramic	Ceramic on Poly	Oxidized Zirc on Poly	Synth Subst
Hip, RT	ØSP9ØEZ	ØSR9Ø1[9,A,Z]	ØSR9Ø2[9,A,Z]	ØSR9Ø3[9,A,Z]	ØSR9Ø4[9,A,Z]	ØSR9Ø6[9,A,Z]	ØSR9ØJ[9,A,Z]
Hip, LT	ØSPBØEZ	ØSRBØ1[9,A,Z]	ØSRBØ2[9,A,Z]	ØSRBØ3[9,A,Z]	ØSRBØ4[9,A,Z]	ØSRBØ6[9,A,Z]	ØSRBØJ[9,A,Z]

Open Removal of Hip Articulating Spacer with Replacement

Removal of Articulating Spacer		Code also as appropriate Replacement by Device Type						
		Acetabular Surface				Femoral Surface		
		Poly	Metal	Ceramic	Synthetic	Metal	Ceramic	Synth
Hip, RT	ØSP9ØEZ	ØSRAØØ[9,A,Z]	ØSRAØ1[9,A,Z]	ØSRAØ3[9,A,Z]	ØSRAØJ[9,A,Z]	ØSRRØ1[9,A,Z]	ØSRRØ3[9,A,Z]	ØSRRØJ[9,A,Z]
Hip, LT	ØSPBØEZ	ØSREØØ[9,A,Z]	ØSREØ1[9,A,Z]	ØSREØ3[9,A,Z]	ØSREØJ[9,A,Z]	ØSRSØ1[9,A,Z]	ØSRSØ3[9,A,Z]	ØSRSØJ[9,A,Z]

Open Removal of Hip Articulating Spacer with Liner Insertion (supplement)

Removal of Articulating Spacer		Code also as appropriate Supplement of Body Part by Site		
		Joint	Acetabular Surface	Femoral Surface
Hip, RT	ØSP9ØEZ	ØSU9Ø9Z	ØSUAØ9Z	ØSURØ9Z
Hip, LT	ØSPBØEZ	ØSUBØ9Z	ØSUEØ9Z	ØSUSØ9Z

Open Removal of Hip Synthetic Substitute with Replacement

Removal of Synthetic Substitute		Code also as appropriate Replacement by Device Type						
		Metal	Metal on Poly	Ceramic	Ceramic on Poly	Oxidized Zirc on Poly	Articulating Spacer	Synth Subst
Hip, RT	ØSP[9,A,R]ØJZ	ØSR9Ø1[9,A,Z]	ØSR9Ø2[9,A,Z]	ØSR9Ø3[9,A,Z]	ØSR9Ø4[9,A,Z]	ØSR9Ø6[9,A,Z]	ØSR9ØEZ	ØSR9ØJ[9,A,Z]
Hip, LT	ØSP[B,E,S]ØJZ	ØSRBØ1[9,A,Z]	ØSRBØ2[9,A,Z]	ØSRBØ3[9,A,Z]	ØSRBØ4[9,A,Z]	ØSRBØ6[9,A,Z]	ØSRBØEZ	ØSRBØJ[9,A,Z]

Open Removal of Hip Synthetic Substitute with Replacement

Removal of Synthetic Substitute		Code also as appropriate Replacement by Device Type						
		Acetabular Surface				Femoral Surface		
		Poly	Metal	Ceramic	Synthetic	Metal	Ceramic	Synth
Hip, RT	ØSP[9,A,R]ØJZ	ØSRAØØ[9,A,Z]	ØSRAØ1[9,A,Z]	ØSRAØ3[9,A,Z]	ØSRAØJ[9,A,Z]	ØSRRØ1[9,A,Z]	ØSRRØ3[9,A,Z]	ØSRRØJ[9,A,Z]
Hip, LT	ØSP[B,E,S]ØJZ	ØSREØØ[9,A,Z]	ØSREØ1[9,A,Z]	ØSREØ3[9,A,Z]	ØSREØJ[9,A,Z]	ØSRSØ1[9,A,Z]	ØSRSØ3[9,A,Z]	ØSRSØJ[9,A,Z]

Percutaneous Endoscopic Removal of Hip Spacer with Open Replacement

Removal of Spacer		Code also as appropriate Replacement by Device Type						
		Metal	Metal on Poly	Ceramic	Ceramic on Poly	Oxidized Zirc on Poly	Articulating Spacer	Synth Subst
Hip, RT	ØSP948Z	ØSR9Ø1[9,A,Z]	ØSR9Ø2[9,A,Z]	ØSR9Ø3[9,A,Z]	ØSR9Ø4[9,A,Z]	ØSR9Ø6[9,A,Z]	ØSR9ØEZ	ØSR9ØJ[9,A,Z]
Hip, LT	ØSPB48Z	ØSRBØ1[9,A,Z]	ØSRBØ2[9,A,Z]	ØSRBØ3[9,A,Z]	ØSRBØ4[9,A,Z]	ØSRBØ6[9,A,Z]	ØSRBØEZ	ØSRBØJ[9,A,Z]

Percutaneous Endoscopic Removal of Hip Spacer with Open Replacement

Removal of Spacer		Code also as appropriate Replacement by Device Type						
		Acetabular Surface				Femoral Surface		
		Poly	Metal	Ceramic	Synthetic	Metal	Ceramic	Synth
Hip, RT	0SP948Z	0SRA00[9,A,Z]	0SRA01[9,A,Z]	0SRA03[9,A,Z]	0SRA0J[9,A,Z]	0SRR01[9,A,Z]	0SRR03[9,A,Z]	0SRR0J[9,A,Z]
Hip, LT	0SPB48Z	0SRE00[9,A,Z]	0SRE01[9,A,Z]	0SRE03[9,A,Z]	0SRE0J[9,A,Z]	0SRS01[9,A,Z]	0SRS03[9,A,Z]	0SRS0J[9,A,Z]

Percutaneous Endoscopic Removal of Hip Spacer with Open Liner Insertion (supplement)

Removal of Spacer		Code also as appropriate Supplement of Body Part by Site		
		Joint	Acetabular Surface	Femoral Surface
Hip, RT	0SP948Z	0SU909Z	0SUA09Z	0SUR09Z
Hip, LT	0SPB48Z	0SUB09Z	0SUE09Z	0SUS09Z

Percutaneous Endoscopic Removal of Hip Synthetic Substitute with Open Replacement

Removal of Synthetic Substitute		Code also as appropriate Replacement by Device Type						
		Metal	Metal on Poly	Ceramic	Ceramic on Poly	Oxidized Zirc on Poly	Articulating Spacer	Synth Subst
Hip, RT	0SP[9,A,R]4JZ	0SR901[9,A,Z]	0SR902[9,A,Z]	0SR903[9,A,Z]	0SR904[9,A,Z]	0SR906[9,A,Z]	0SR90EZ	0SR90J[9,A,Z]
Hip, LT	0SP[B,E,S]4JZ	0SRB01[9,A,Z]	0SRB02[9,A,Z]	0SRB03[9,A,Z]	0SRB04[9,A,Z]	0SRB06[9,A,Z]	0SRB0EZ	0SRB0J[9,A,Z]

Percutaneous Endoscopic Removal of Hip Synthetic Substitute with Open Replacement

Removal of Synthetic Substitute		Code also as appropriate Replacement by Device Type						
		Acetabular Surface				Femoral Surface		
		Poly	Metal	Ceramic	Synthetic	Metal	Ceramic	Synth
Hip, RT	0SP[9,A,R]4JZ	0SRA00[9,A,Z]	0SRA01[9,A,Z]	0SRA03[9,A,Z]	0SRA0J[9,A,Z]	0SRR01[9,A,Z]	0SRR03[9,A,Z]	0SRR0J[9,A,Z]
Hip, LT	0SP[B,E,S]4JZ	0SRE00[9,A,Z]	0SRE01[9,A,Z]	0SRE03[9,A,Z]	0SRE0J[9,A,Z]	0SRS01[9,A,Z]	0SRS03[9,A,Z]	0SRS0J[9,A,Z]

Percutaneous Endoscopic Removal of Hip Synthetic Substitute with Open Liner Insertion (supplement)

Removal of Synthetic Substitute		Code also as appropriate Supplement of Body Part by Site		
		Joint	Acetabular Surface	Femoral Surface
Hip, RT	0SP[9,A,R]4JZ	0SU909Z	0SUA09Z	0SUR09Z
Hip, LT	0SP[B,E,S]4JZ	0SUB09Z	0SUE09Z	0SUS09Z

Knee Procedure Combinations

Removal of Knee Spacer with Replacement

Removal of Spacer		Code also Replacement by Type of Synthetic Substitute						
		Oxidized Zirc on Poly	Synthetic Substitute	Articulating Spacer	Patello-femoral	Femoral Surface	Tibial Surface	Medial (L)/ Lateral (M) Meniscus
Knee, RT	0SPC[0,3,4]8Z	0SRC06[9,A,Z]	0SRC0J[9,A,Z]	0SRC0EZ	0SRC0N[9,A,Z]	0SRT0J[9,A,Z]	0SRV0J[9,A,Z]	XRRG0[L,M]8
Knee, LT	0SPD[0,3,4]8Z	0SRD06[9,A,Z]	0SRD0J[9,A,Z]	0SRD0EZ	0SRD0N[9,A,Z]	0SRU0J[9,A,Z]	0SRW0J[9,A,Z]	XRRH0[L,M]8

Removal of Knee Liner with Replacement

Removal of Liner		Code also Replacement by Type of Synthetic Substitute							
		Oxidized Zirc on Poly	Synthetic Substitute	Articulating Spacer	Medial (L)/ Lateral (M) Unicondylar	Patello-femoral	Femoral Surface	Tibial Surface	Medial (L)/Lateral (M) Meniscus
Knee, RT	0SPC09Z	0SRC06[9,A,Z]	0SRC0J[9,A,Z]	0SRC0EZ	0SRC0[L,M][9,A,Z]	0SRC0N[9,A,Z]	0SRT0J[9,A,Z]	0SRV0J[9,A,Z]	XRRG0[L,M]8
Knee, LT	0SPD09Z	0SRD06[9,A,Z]	0SRD0J[9,A,Z]	0SRD0EZ	0SRD0[L,M][9,A,Z]	0SRD0N[9,A,Z]	0SRU0J[9,A,Z]	0SRW0J[9,A,Z]	XRRH0[L,M]8

Removal of Knee Articulating Spacer with Replacement

Removal of Articulating Spacer		Code also Replacement by Type of Synthetic Substitute				
		Oxidized Zirc on Poly	Synthetic Substitute	Femoral Surface	Tibial Surface	Medial (L)/Lateral (M) Meniscus
Knee, RT	ØSPCØEZ	ØSRC06[9,A,Z]	ØSRCØJ[9,A,Z]	ØSRTØJ[9,A,Z]	ØSRVØJ[9,A,Z]	XRRGØ[L,M]8
Knee, LT	ØSPDØEZ	ØSRD06[9,A,Z]	ØSRDØJ[9,A,Z]	ØSRUØJ[9,A,Z]	ØSRWØJ[9,A,Z]	XRRHØ[L,M]8

Removal of Knee Patellar Surface with Replacement

Removal of Patellar Surface		Code also Replacement by Type of Synthetic Substitute						
		Oxidized Zirc on Poly	Synthetic Substitute	Articulating Spacer	Patello-femoral	Femoral Surface	Tibial Surface	Medial (L)/Lateral (M) Meniscus
Knee, RT	ØSPC[Ø,4]JC	ØSRC06[9,A,Z]	ØSRCØJ[9,A,Z]	ØSRCØEZ	ØSRCØN[9,A,Z]	ØSRTØJ[9,A,Z]	ØSRVØJ[9,A,Z]	XRRGØ[L,M]8
Knee, LT	ØSPD[Ø,4]JC	ØSRD06[9,A,Z]	ØSRDØJ[9,A,Z]	ØSRDØEZ	ØSRDØN[9,A,Z]	ØSRUØJ[9,A,Z]	ØSRWØJ[9,A,Z]	XRRHØ[L,M]8

Removal of Knee Synthetic Substitute with Replacement

Removal of Synthetic Substitute		Code also Replacement by Type of Synthetic Substitute							
		Oxidized Zirc on Poly	Synthetic Substitute	Articulating Spacer	Medial (L)/Lateral (M) Unicondylar	Patello-femoral	Femoral Surface	Tibial Surface	Medial (L)/Lateral (M) Meniscus
Knee, RT	ØSPC[Ø,4]JZ	ØSRC06[9,A,Z]	ØSRCØJ[9,A,Z]	ØSRCØEZ	ØSRCØ[L,M][9,A,Z]	ØSRCØN[9,A,Z]	ØSRTØJ[9,A,Z]	ØSRVØJ[9,A,Z]	XRRGØ[L,M]8
Knee, LT	ØSPD[Ø,4]JZ	ØSRD06[9,A,Z]	ØSRDØJ[9,A,Z]	ØSRDØEZ	ØSRDØ[L,M][9,A,Z]	ØSRDØN[9,A,Z]	ØSRUØJ[9,A,Z]	ØSRWØJ[9,A,Z]	XRRHØ[L,M]8

Removal of Knee Unicondylar Device with Replacement

Removal of Medial (L)/Lateral (M) Unicondylar Device		Code also Replacement by Type of Synthetic Substitute					
		Oxidized Zirc on Poly	Synthetic Substitute	Medial Unicondylar	Femoral Surface	Tibial Surface	Medial (L)/Lateral (M) Meniscus
Knee, RT	ØSPC[Ø,4][L,M]Z	ØSRC06[9,A,Z]	ØSRCØJ[9,A,Z]	ØSRCØL[9,A,Z]	ØSRTØJ[9,A,Z]	ØSRVØJ[9,A,Z]	XRRGØ[L,M]8
Knee, LT	ØSPD[Ø,4][L,M]Z	ØSRD06[9,A,Z]	ØSRDØJ[9,A,Z]	ØSRDØL[9,A,Z]	ØSRUØJ[9,A,Z]	ØSRWØJ[9,A,Z]	XRRHØ[L,M]8

Removal of Knee Patellofemoral Device with Replacement

Removal of Patellofemoral Device		Code also Replacement by Type of Synthetic Substitute					
		Oxidized Zirc on Poly	Synthetic Substitute	Medial Unicondylar	Femoral Surface	Tibial Surface	Medial (L)/Lateral (M) Meniscus
Knee, RT	ØSPC[Ø,4]NZ	ØSRC06[9,A,Z]	ØSRCØJ[9,A,Z]	ØSRCØL[9,A,Z]	ØSRTØJ[9,A,Z]	ØSRVØJ[9,A,Z]	XRRGØ[L,M]8
Knee, LT	ØSPD[Ø,4]NZ	ØSRD06[9,A,Z]	ØSRDØJ[9,A,Z]	ØSRDØL[9,A,Z]	ØSRUØJ[9,A,Z]	ØSRWØJ[9,A,Z]	XRRHØ[L,M]8

Removal of Knee Femoral/Tibial Surface Device with Replacement

Removal of Femoral (T,U)/Tibial (V,W) Surface		Code also Replacement by Type of Synthetic Substitute						
		Oxidized Zirc on Poly	Synthetic Substitute	Articulating Spacer	Patello-femoral	Femoral Surface	Tibial Surface	Medial (L)/Lateral (M) Meniscus
Knee, RT	ØSP[T,V][Ø,4]JZ	ØSRC06[9,A,Z]	ØSRCØJ[9,A,Z]	ØSRCØEZ	ØSRCØN[9,A,Z]	ØSRTØJ[9,A,Z]	ØSRVØJ[9,A,Z]	XRRGØ[L,M]8
Knee, LT	ØSP[U,W][Ø,4]JZ	ØSRD06[9,A,Z]	ØSRDØJ[9,A,Z]	ØSRDØEZ	ØSRDØN[9,A,Z]	ØSRUØJ[9,A,Z]	ØSRWØJ[9,A,Z]	XRRHØ[L,M]8

DRG 485-489 Knee Procedures

Joint	Removal of Liner by open approach	Code also as appropriate Supplement of Tibial Surface by Site
Knee, RT	ØSPCØ9Z	ØSUVØ9Z
Knee, LT	ØSPDØ9Z	ØSUWØ9Z

DRG 515-517 Other Musculoskeletal System and Connective Tissue Procedures

Site	Reposition of Vertebra by percutaneous approach	Code also as appropriate Supplement With Synthetic Substitute by Percutaneous Approach at site of Repositioned Vertebra
Cervical	ØPS33ZZ	ØPU33JZ
Coccyx	ØQSS3ZZ	ØQUS3JZ
Lumbar	ØQS03ZZ	ØQU03JZ
Sacrum	ØQS13ZZ	ØQU13JZ
Thoracic	ØPS43ZZ	ØPU43JZ

DRG 518-52Ø Back and Neck Procedures, Except Spinal Fusion, or Disc Devices/Neurostimulators

Generator Type	Insertion of Generator by Site			Code also as appropriate Insertion Neurostimulator Lead by approach and Site	
	Chest	Abdomen	Back	Spinal Canal	Spinal Cord
Single Array	ØJH6[Ø,3]BZ	ØJH8[Ø,3]BZ	ØJH7[Ø,3]BZ	00HU[Ø,3,4]MZ	00HV[Ø,3,4]MZ
Single Array, Rechargeable	ØJH6[Ø,3]CZ	ØJH8[Ø,3]CZ	ØJH7[Ø,3]CZ	00HU[Ø,3,4]MZ	00HV[Ø,3,4]MZ
Multiple Array	ØJH6[Ø,3]DZ	ØJH8[Ø,3]DZ	ØJH7[Ø,3]DZ	00HU[Ø,3,4]MZ	00HV[Ø,3,4]MZ
Multiple Array, Rechargeable	ØJH6[Ø,3]EZ	—	ØJH7[Ø,3]EZ	00HU[Ø,3,4]MZ	00HV[Ø,3,4]MZ
Multiple Array, Rechargeable	—	ØJH8[Ø,3]EZ	—	00HU[Ø,3,4]MZ	00HV[Ø,3,4]MZ

DRG 582-583 Mastectomy for Malignancy

Site	Resection by Open approach	Code also as appropriate Resection of Lymph Nodes by Open approach by site			Code also as appropriate Resection of Thorax Muscle by Open approach	
		Axillary	Internal Mammary	Thorax	Right	Left
Breast, Right	ØHTTØZZ	07T5ØZZ	07T8ØZZ	07T7ØZZ	ØKTHØZZ	—
Breast, Left	ØHTUØZZ	07T6ØZZ	07T9ØZZ	07T7ØZZ	—	ØKTJØZZ
Breast, Bilateral	ØHTVØZZ	07T5ØZZ and 07T6ØZZ	07T8ØZZ and 07T9ØZZ	07T7ØZZ	ØKTHØZZ	ØKTJØZZ

DRG 584-585 Breast Biopsy, Local Excision and Other Breast Procedures

Resection of Breast With Resection of Lymph Nodes and Thorax Muscle

Site	Resection by Open approach	Code also as appropriate Resection of Lymph Nodes by Open approach by site			Code also as appropriate Resection of Thorax Muscle by Open approach	
		Axillary	Internal Mammary	Thorax	Right	Left
Breast, Right	ØHTTØZZ	07T5ØZZ	07T8ØZZ	07T7ØZZ	ØKTHØZZ	—
Breast, Left	ØHTUØZZ	07T6ØZZ	07T9ØZZ	07T7ØZZ	—	ØKTJØZZ
Breast, Bilateral	ØHTVØZZ	07T5ØZZ and 07T6ØZZ	07T8ØZZ and 07T9ØZZ	07T7ØZZ	ØKTHØZZ	ØKTJØZZ

Replacement of Breast Tissue

Site	Replacement by Percutaneous approach with Autologous Tissue	Code also as appropriate Extraction of Subcutaneous Tissue by Percutaneous approach					
		Abdomen	Back	Buttock	Chest	Leg, Upper, Right	Leg, Upper, Left
Breast, Right	ØHRT37Z	ØJD83ZZ	ØJD73ZZ	ØJD93ZZ	ØJD63ZZ	ØJDL3ZZ	ØJDM3ZZ
Breast, Left	ØHRU37Z	ØJD83ZZ	ØJD73ZZ	ØJD93ZZ	ØJD63ZZ	ØJDL3ZZ	ØJDM3ZZ
Breast, Bilateral	ØHRV37Z	ØJD83ZZ	ØJD73ZZ	ØJD93ZZ	ØJD63ZZ	ØJDL3ZZ	ØJDM3ZZ

DRG 628-63Ø Other Endocrine, Nutritional and Metabolic Procedures

Hip Procedure Combinations

Open Removal of Hip Spacer with Replacement

Removal of Spacer		Code also as appropriate Replacement by Device Type					
		Metal	Metal on Poly	Ceramic	Ceramic on Poly	Oxidized Zirc on Poly	Synthetic Substitute
Hip, RT	ØSP9Ø8Z	ØSR9Ø1[9,A,Z]	ØSR9Ø2[9,A,Z]	ØSR9Ø3[9,A,Z]	ØSR9Ø4[9,A,Z]	ØSR9Ø6[9,A,Z]	ØSR9ØJ[9,A,Z]
Hip, LT	ØSPBØ8Z	ØSRBØ1[9,A,Z]	ØSRBØ2[9,A,Z]	ØSRBØ3[9,A,Z]	ØSRBØ4[9,A,Z]	ØSRBØ6[9,A,Z]	ØSRBØJ[9,A,Z]

Open Removal of Hip Spacer with Replacement

Removal of Spacer		Code also as appropriate Replacement by Device Type						
		Acetabular Surface				Femoral Surface		
		Poly	Metal	Ceramic	Synthetic	Metal	Ceramic	Synthetic
Hip, RT	ØSP908Z	ØSRAØØ[9,A,Z]	ØSRAØ1[9,A,Z]	ØSRAØ3[9,A,Z]	ØSRAØJ[9,A,Z]	ØSRRØ1[9,A,Z]	ØSRRØ3[9,A,Z]	ØSRRØJ[9,A,Z]
Hip, LT	ØSPBØ8Z	ØSREØØ[9,A,Z]	ØSREØ1[9,A,Z]	ØSREØ3[9,A,Z]	ØSREØJ[9,A,Z]	ØSRSØ1[9,A,Z]	ØSRSØ3[9,A,Z]	ØSRSØJ[9,A,Z]

Open Removal of Hip Spacer with Liner Insertion (supplement)

Removal of Spacer		Code also as appropriate Supplement of Body Part by Site		
		Joint	Acetabular Surface	Femoral Surface
Hip, RT	ØSP908Z	ØSU9Ø9Z	ØSUAØ9Z	ØSURØ9Z
Hip, LT	ØSPBØ8Z	ØSUBØ9Z	ØSUEØ9Z	ØSUSØ9Z

Open Removal of Hip Liner with Replacement

Removal of Liner		Code also as appropriate Replacement by Device Type					
		Metal	Metal on Poly	Ceramic	Ceramic on Poly	Oxidized Zirc on Poly	Synthetic Substitute
Hip, RT	ØSP9Ø9Z	ØSR9Ø1[9,A,Z]	ØSR9Ø2[9,A,Z]	ØSR9Ø3[9,A,Z]	ØSR9Ø4[9,A,Z]	ØSR9Ø6[9,A,Z]	ØSR9ØJ[9,A,Z]
Hip, LT	ØSPBØ9Z	ØSRBØ1[9,A,Z]	ØSRBØ2[9,A,Z]	ØSRBØ3[9,A,Z]	ØSRBØ4[9,A,Z]	ØSRBØ6[9,A,Z]	ØSRBØJ[9,A,Z]

Open Removal of Hip Liner with Replacement

Removal of Liner		Code also as appropriate Replacement by Device Type						
		Acetabular Surface				Femoral Surface		
		Poly	Metal	Ceramic	Synthetic	Metal	Ceramic	Synthetic
Hip, RT	ØSP9Ø9Z	ØSRAØØ[9,A,Z]	ØSRAØ1[9,A,Z]	ØSRAØ3[9,A,Z]	ØSRAØJ[9,A,Z]	ØSRRØ1[9,A,Z]	ØSRRØ3[9,A,Z]	ØSRRØJ[9,A,Z]
Hip, LT	ØSPBØ9Z	ØSREØØ[9,A,Z]	ØSREØ1[9,A,Z]	ØSREØ3[9,A,Z]	ØSREØJ[9,A,Z]	ØSRSØ1[9,A,Z]	ØSRSØ3[9,A,Z]	ØSRSØJ[9,A,Z]

Open Removal of Hip Liner with Liner Insertion (supplement)

Removal of Liner		Code also as appropriate Supplement of Body Part by Site		
		Joint	Acetabular Surface	Femoral Surface
Hip, RT	ØSP9Ø9Z	ØSU9Ø9Z	ØSUAØ9Z	ØSURØ9Z
Hip, LT	ØSPBØ9Z	ØSUBØ9Z	ØSUEØ9Z	ØSUSØ9Z

Open Removal of Hip Resurfacing Device with Replacement

Removal of Resurfacing Device		Code also as appropriate Replacement by Device Type					
		Metal	Metal on Poly	Ceramic	Ceramic on Poly	Oxidized Zirc on Poly	Synthetic Substitute
Hip, RT	ØSP9ØBZ	ØSR9Ø1[9,A,Z]	ØSR9Ø2[9,A,Z]	ØSR9Ø3[9,A,Z]	ØSR9Ø4[9,A,Z]	ØSR9Ø6[9,A,Z]	ØSR9ØJ[9,A,Z]
Hip, LT	ØSPBØBZ	ØSRBØ1[9,A,Z]	ØSRBØ2[9,A,Z]	ØSRBØ3[9,A,Z]	ØSRBØ4[9,A,Z]	ØSRBØ6[9,A,Z]	ØSRBØJ[9,A,Z]

Open Removal of Hip Resurfacing Device with Replacement

Removal of Resurfacing Device		Code also as appropriate Replacement by Device Type						
		Acetabular Surface				Femoral Surface		
		Poly	Metal	Ceramic	Synthetic	Metal	Ceramic	Synthetic
Hip, RT	ØSP9ØBZ	ØSRAØØ[9,A,Z]	ØSRAØ1[9,A,Z]	ØSRAØ3[9,A,Z]	ØSRAØJ[9,A,Z]	ØSRRØ1[9,A,Z]	ØSRRØ3[9,A,Z]	ØSRRØJ[9,A,Z]
Hip, LT	ØSPBØBZ	ØSREØØ[9,A,Z]	ØSREØ1[9,A,Z]	ØSREØ3[9,A,Z]	ØSREØJ[9,A,Z]	ØSRSØ1[9,A,Z]	ØSRSØ3[9,A,Z]	ØSRSØJ[9,A,Z]

Open Removal of Hip Resurfacing Device with Liner Insertion (supplement)

Removal of Resurfacing Device		Code also as appropriate Supplement of Body Part by Site		
		Joint	Acetabular Surface	Femoral Surface
Hip, RT	ØSP9ØBZ	ØSU9Ø9Z	ØSUAØ9Z	ØSURØ9Z
Hip, LT	ØSPBØBZ	ØSUBØ9Z	ØSUEØ9Z	ØSUSØ9Z

Open Removal of Hip Synthetic Substitute with Replacement

Removal of Synthetic Substitute		Code also as appropriate Replacement by Device Type					
		Metal	Metal on Poly	Ceramic	Ceramic on Poly	Oxidized Zirc on Poly	Synthetic Substitute
Hip, RT	ØSP9ØJZ	ØSR9Ø1[9,A,Z]	ØSR9Ø2[9,A,Z]	ØSR9Ø3[9,A,Z]	ØSR9Ø4[9,A,Z]	ØSR9Ø6[9,A,Z]	ØSR9ØJ[9,A,Z]
Hip, LT	ØSPBØJZ	ØSRBØ1[9,A,Z]	ØSRBØ2[9,A,Z]	ØSRBØ3[9,A,Z]	ØSRBØ4[9,A,Z]	ØSRBØ6[9,A,Z]	ØSRBØJ[9,A,Z]

Open Removal of Hip Synthetic Substitute with Replacement

Removal of Synthetic Substitute		Code also as appropriate Replacement by Device Type						
		Acetabular Surface				Femoral Surface		
		Poly	Metal	Ceramic	Synthetic	Metal	Ceramic	Synthetic
Hip, RT	ØSP9ØJZ	ØSRAØØ[9,A,Z]	ØSRAØ1[9,A,Z]	ØSRAØ3[9,A,Z]	ØSRAØJ[9,A,Z]	ØSRRØ1[9,A,Z]	ØSRRØ3[9,A,Z]	ØSRRØJ[9,A,Z]
Hip, LT	ØSPBØJZ	ØSREØØ[9,A,Z]	ØSREØ1[9,A,Z]	ØSREØ3[9,A,Z]	ØSREØJ[9,A,Z]	ØSRSØ1[9,A,Z]	ØSRSØ3[9,A,Z]	ØSRSØJ[9,A,Z]

Open Removal of Hip Acetabular/Femoral Surface with Replacement

Removal of Acetabular/Femoral Surface		Code also as appropriate Replacement by Device Type					
		Metal	Metal on Poly	Ceramic	Ceramic on Poly	Oxidized Zirc on Poly	Synthetic Substitute
Hip, RT	ØSP[A,R]ØJZ	ØSR9Ø1[9,A,Z]	ØSR9Ø2[9,A,Z]	ØSR9Ø3[9,A,Z]	ØSR9Ø4[9,A,Z]	ØSR9Ø6[9,A,Z]	ØSR9ØJ[9,A,Z]
Hip, LT	ØSP[E,S]ØJZ	ØSRBØ1[9,A,Z]	ØSRBØ2[9,A,Z]	ØSRBØ3[9,A,Z]	ØSRBØ4[9,A,Z]	ØSRBØ6[9,A,Z]	ØSRBØJ[9,A,Z]

Open Removal of Hip Acetabular/Femoral Surface with Replacement

Removal of Acetabular/Femoral Surface		Code also as appropriate Replacement by Device Type						
		Acetabular Surface				Femoral Surface		
		Poly	Metal	Ceramic	Synthetic	Metal	Ceramic	Synthetic
Hip, RT	ØSP[A,R]ØJZ	ØSRAØØ[9,A,Z]	ØSRAØ1[9,A,Z]	ØSRAØ3[9,A,Z]	ØSRAØJ[9,A,Z]	ØSRRØ1[9,A,Z]	ØSRRØ3[9,A,Z]	ØSRRØJ[9,A,Z]
Hip, LT	ØSP[E,S]ØJZ	ØSREØØ[9,A,Z]	ØSREØ1[9,A,Z]	ØSREØ3[9,A,Z]	ØSREØJ[9,A,Z]	ØSRSØ1[9,A,Z]	ØSRSØ3[9,A,Z]	ØSRSØJ[9,A,Z]

Percutaneous Endoscopic Removal of Hip Spacer with Replacement

Removal of Spacer		Code also as appropriate Replacement by Device Type					
		Metal	Metal on Poly	Ceramic	Ceramic on Poly	Oxidized Zirc on Poly	Synthetic Substitute
Hip, RT	ØSP948Z	ØSR9Ø1[9,A,Z]	ØSR9Ø2[9,A,Z]	ØSR9Ø3[9,A,Z]	ØSR9Ø4[9,A,Z]	ØSR9Ø6[9,A,Z]	ØSR9ØJ[9,A,Z]
Hip, LT	ØSPB48Z	ØSRBØ1[9,A,Z]	ØSRBØ2[9,A,Z]	ØSRBØ3[9,A,Z]	ØSRBØ4[9,A,Z]	ØSRBØ6[9,A,Z]	ØSRBØJ[9,A,Z]

Percutaneous Endoscopic Removal of Hip Spacer with Replacement

Removal of Spacer		Code also as appropriate Replacement by Device Type						
		Acetabular Surface				Femoral Surface		
		Poly	Metal	Ceramic	Synthetic	Metal	Ceramic	Synthetic
Hip, RT	ØSP948Z	ØSRAØØ[9,A,Z]	ØSRAØ1[9,A,Z]	ØSRAØ3[9,A,Z]	ØSRAØJ[9,A,Z]	ØSRRØ1[9,A,Z]	ØSRRØ3[9,A,Z]	ØSRRØJ[9,A,Z]
Hip, LT	ØSPB48Z	ØSREØØ[9,A,Z]	ØSREØ1[9,A,Z]	ØSREØ3[9,A,Z]	ØSREØJ[9,A,Z]	ØSRSØ1[9,A,Z]	ØSRSØ3[9,A,Z]	ØSRSØJ[9,A,Z]

Percutaneous Endoscopic Removal of Hip Spacer with Liner Insertion (supplement)

Removal of Spacer		Code also as appropriate Supplement of Body Part by Site		
		Joint	Acetabular Surface	Femoral Surface
Hip, RT	ØSP948Z	ØSU9Ø9Z	ØSUAØ9Z	ØSURØ9Z
Hip, LT	ØSPB48Z	ØSUBØ9Z	ØSUEØ9Z	ØSUSØ9Z

Percutaneous Endoscopic Removal of Hip Synthetic Substitute with Replacement

Removal of Synthetic Substitute		Code also as appropriate Replacement by Device Type					
		Metal	Metal on Poly	Ceramic	Ceramic on Poly	Oxidized Zirc on Poly	Synthetic Substitute
Hip, RT	ØSP94JZ	ØSR9Ø1[9,A,Z]	ØSR9Ø2[9,A,Z]	ØSR9Ø3[9,A,Z]	ØSR9Ø4[9,A,Z]	ØSR9Ø6[9,A,Z]	ØSR9ØJ[9,A,Z]
Hip, LT	ØSPB4JZ	ØSRBØ1[9,A,Z]	ØSRBØ2[9,A,Z]	ØSRBØ3[9,A,Z]	ØSRBØ4[9,A,Z]	ØSRBØ6[9,A,Z]	ØSRBØJ[9,A,Z]

Percutaneous Endoscopic of Hip Synthetic Substitute with Replacement

Removal of Synthetic Substitute		Code also as appropriate Replacement by Device Type						
		Acetabular Surface				Femoral Surface		
		Poly	Metal	Ceramic	Synthetic	Metal	Ceramic	Synthetic
Hip, RT	ØSP94JZ	ØSRA00[9,A,Z]	ØSRA01[9,A,Z]	ØSRA03[9,A,Z]	ØSRA0J[9,A,Z]	ØSRR01[9,A,Z]	ØSRR03[9,A,Z]	ØSRR0J[9,A,Z]
Hip, LT	ØSPB4JZ	ØSRE00[9,A,Z]	ØSRE01[9,A,Z]	ØSRE03[9,A,Z]	ØSRE0J[9,A,Z]	ØSRS01[9,A,Z]	ØSRS03[9,A,Z]	ØSRS0J[9,A,Z]

Percutaneous Endoscopic Removal of Hip Synthetic Substitute with Liner Insertion (supplement)

Removal of Synthetic Substitute		Code also as appropriate Supplement of Body Part by Site		
		Joint	Acetabular Surface	Femoral Surface
Hip, RT	ØSP94JZ	ØSU909Z	ØSUA09Z	ØSUR09Z
Hip, LT	ØSPB4JZ	ØSUB09Z	ØSUE09Z	ØSUS09Z

Percutaneous Endoscopic Removal of Hip Acetabular/Femoral Surface with Replacement

Removal of Acetabular/Femoral Surface		Code also as appropriate Replacement by Device Type					
		Metal	Metal on Poly	Ceramic	Ceramic on Poly	Oxidized Zirc on Poly	Synthetic Substitute
Hip, RT	ØSP[A,R]4JZ	ØSR901[9,A,Z]	ØSR902[9,A,Z]	ØSR903[9,A,Z]	ØSR904[9,A,Z]	ØSR906[9,A,Z]	ØSR90J[9,A,Z]
Hip, LT	ØSP[E,S]4JZ	ØSRB01[9,A,Z]	ØSRB02[9,A,Z]	ØSRB03[9,A,Z]	ØSRB04[9,A,Z]	ØSRB06[9,A,Z]	ØSRB0J[9,A,Z]

Percutaneous Endoscopic of Hip Acetabular/Femoral Surface with Replacement

Removal of Acetabular/Femoral Surface		Code also as appropriate Replacement by Device Type						
		Acetabular Surface				Femoral Surface		
		Poly	Metal	Ceramic	Synthetic	Metal	Ceramic	Synthetic
Hip, RT	ØSP[A,R]4JZ	ØSRA00[9,A,Z]	ØSRA01[9,A,Z]	ØSRA03[9,A,Z]	ØSRA0J[9,A,Z]	ØSRR01[9,A,Z]	ØSRR03[9,A,Z]	ØSRR0J[9,A,Z]
Hip, LT	ØSP[E,S]4JZ	ØSRE00[9,A,Z]	ØSRE01[9,A,Z]	ØSRE03[9,A,Z]	ØSRE0J[9,A,Z]	ØSRS01[9,A,Z]	ØSRS03[9,A,Z]	ØSRS0J[9,A,Z]

Percutaneous Endoscopic Removal of Hip Acetabular/Femoral Surface with Liner Insertion (supplement)

Removal of Acetabular/Femoral Surface		Code also as appropriate Supplement of Body Part by Site		
		Joint	Acetabular Surface	Femoral Surface
Hip, RT	ØSP[A,R]4JZ	ØSU909Z	ØSUA09Z	ØSUR09Z
Hip, LT	ØSP[E,S]4JZ	ØSUB09Z	ØSUE09Z	ØSUS09Z

Knee Procedure Combinations

Removal of Knee Liner with Replacement

Removal of Liner		Code also Replacement by Device Type						
		Oxidized Zirc on Poly	Synthetic Substitute	Medial (L)/ Lateral (M) Unicondylar	Patello-femoral	Femoral Surface	Tibial Surface	Medial (L)/ Lateral (M) Meniscus
Knee, RT	ØSPC09Z	ØSRC06[9,A,Z]	ØSRC0J[9,A,Z]	ØSRC0[L,M][9,A,Z]	ØSRC0N[9,A,Z]	ØSRT0J[9,A,Z]	ØSRV0J[9,A,Z]	XRRG0[L,M]8
Knee, LT	ØSPD09Z	ØSRD06[9,A,Z]	ØSRD0J[9,A,Z]	ØSRD0[L,M][9,A,Z]	ØSRD0N[9,A,Z]	ØSRU0J[9,A,Z]	ØSRW0J[9,A,Z]	XRRH0[L,M]8

Removal of Knee Patellar Surface with Replacement

Removal of Patellar Surface		Code also Replacement by Device Type	
		Femoral Surface	Tibial Surface
Knee, RT	ØSPC[0,4]JC	ØSRT0J[9,A,Z]	ØSRV0J[9,A,Z]
Knee, LT	ØSPD[0,4]JC	ØSRU0J[9,A,Z]	ØSRW0J[9,A,Z]

Removal of Knee Synthetic Substitute with Replacement

Removal of Synthetic Substitute		Code also Replacement by Device Type	
		Femoral Surface	Tibial Surface
Knee, RT	ØSPC[0,4]JZ	ØSRT0J[9,A,Z]	ØSRV0J[9,A,Z]
Knee, LT	ØSPD[0,4]JZ	ØSRU0J[9,A,Z]	ØSRW0J[9,A,Z]

Removal of Knee Unicondylar Device with Replacement

Removal of Medial (L)/ Lateral (M) Unicondylar Device		Code also Replacement by Device Type	
		Femoral Surface	**Tibial Surface**
Knee, RT	ØSPC[Ø,4][L,M]Z	ØSRTØJ[9,A,Z]	ØSRVØJ[9,A,Z]
Knee, LT	ØSPD[Ø,4][L,M]Z	ØSRUØJ[9,A,Z]	ØSRWØJ[9,A,Z]

Removal of Knee Patellofemoral Device with Replacement

Removal of Patellofemoral Device		Code also Replacement by Device Type	
		Femoral Surface	**Tibial Surface**
Knee, RT	ØSPC[Ø,4]NZ	ØSRTØJ[9,A,Z]	ØSRVØJ[9,A,Z]
Knee, LT	ØSPD[Ø,4]NZ	ØSRUØJ[9,A,Z]	ØSRWØJ[9,A,Z]

Removal of Knee Femoral/Tibial Surface Device with Replacement

Removal of Femoral (T,U)/Tibial (V,W) Surface		Code also Replacement by Device Type	
		Femoral Surface	**Tibial Surface**
Knee, RT	ØSP[T,V][Ø,4]JZ	ØSRTØJ[9,A,Z]	ØSRVØJ[9,A,Z]
Knee, LT	ØSP[U,W][Ø,4]JZ	ØSRUØJ[9,A,Z]	ØSRWØJ[9,A,Z]

DRG 662-664 Minor Bladder Procedure

Repair of Bladder	Code also as appropriate Repair of Abdominal Wall	
	with Stoma	**without Stoma**
ØTQB[Ø,3,4]ZZ	ØWQFXZ2	ØWQFXZZ

DRG 665-667 Prostatectomy

Site	Resection by approach				Code also as appropriate Resection of Seminal Vesicles, Bilateral by approach	
	Open	**Percutaneous Endoscopic**	**Via Natural or Artificial Opening**	**Via Natural or Artificial Opening Endoscopic**	**Open**	**Percutaneous Endoscopic**
Prostate	ØVTØØZZ	ØVTØ4ZZ	ØVTØ7ZZ	ØVTØ8ZZ	ØVT3ØZZ	ØVT34ZZ

DRG 7Ø7-7Ø8 Major Male Pelvic Procedures

Site	Resection by approach				Code also as appropriate Resection of Seminal Vesicles, Bilateral by approach	
	Open	**Percutaneous Endoscopic**	**Via Natural or Artificial Opening**	**Via Natural or Artificial Opening Endoscopic**	**Open**	**Percutaneous Endoscopic**
Prostate	ØVTØØZZ	ØVTØ4ZZ	ØVTØ7ZZ	ØVTØ8ZZ	ØVT3ØZZ	ØVT34ZZ

DRG 734-735 Pelvic Evisceration, Radical Hysterectomy and Radical Vulvectomy

Pelvic Evisceration

Resection by Site						
Bladder	**Cervix**	**Fallopian Tubes, Bilateral**	**Ovaries, Bilateral**	**Urethra**	**Uterus**	**Vagina**
ØTTBØZZ	ØUTCØZZ	ØUT7ØZZ	ØUT2ØZZ	ØTTDØZZ	ØUT9ØZZ	ØUTGØZZ

Radical Hysterectomy

Approach	Resection by Site		
	Cervix	**Uterus**	**Uterine Support Structure**
Vaginal	ØUTC[7,8]ZZ	ØUT9[7,8]ZZ	ØUT4[7,8]ZZ
Abdominal, Endoscopic	ØUTC4ZZ	ØUT9[4,F]ZZ	ØUT44ZZ
Abdominal, Open	ØUTCØZZ	ØUT9ØZZ	ØUT4ØZZ

Radical Vulvectomy

Resection by Site	Code also as appropriate Excision of Inguinal Lymph Nodes by Approach	
Vulva	Right	Left
ØUTM[Ø,X]ZZ	Ø7BH[Ø,4]ZZ	Ø7BJ[Ø,4]ZZ

Non-OR procedure combinations

Note: The following table identifies procedure combinations that are considered Non-OR even though one or more procedures of the combination are considered valid DRG OR procedures

Insertion With Removal of Intraluminal Device

Code as appropriate Insertion of Intraluminal Device into Hepatobiliary Duct	Code also as appropriate Removal of Intraluminal Device by Approach and Site			
	Via Natural or Artificial Opening		External	
	Hepatobiliary Duct	Pancreatic Duct	Hepatobiliary Duct	Pancreatic Duct
ØFHB7DZ	ØFPB[7,8]DZ	ØFPD[7,8]DZ	ØFPBXDZ	ØFPDXDZ

Appendix M: Coding Exercises and Answers

Using the ICD-10-PCS tables construct the code that accurately represents the procedure performed.

Medical Surgical Section

Procedure	Code
1. Excision of malignant melanoma from skin of right ear	
2. Laparoscopy with excision of endometrial implant from left ovary	
3. Percutaneous needle core biopsy of right kidney	
4. EGD with excisional gastric biopsy	
5. Open endarterectomy of left common carotid artery	
6. Excision of basal cell carcinoma of lower lip	
7. Open excision of tail of pancreas	
8. Percutaneous biopsy of right gastrocnemius muscle	
9. Sigmoidoscopy with sigmoid polypectomy	
10. Open excision of lesion from right Achilles tendon	
11. Open resection of cecum	
12. Total excision of pituitary gland, open	
13. Explantation of left failed kidney, open	
14. Open left axillary total lymphadenectomy	
15. Laparoscopic-assisted vaginal hysterectomy	
16. Right total mastectomy, open	
17. Open resection of papillary muscle	
18. Total retropubic prostatectomy, open	
19. Laparoscopic cholecystectomy	
20. Endoscopic bilateral total maxillary sinusectomy	
21. Amputation at right elbow level	
22. Right below-knee amputation, proximal tibia/fibula	
23. Fifth ray carpometacarpal joint amputation, left hand	
24. Right leg and hip amputation through ischium	
25. DIP joint amputation of right thumb	
26. Right wrist joint amputation	
27. Trans-metatarsal amputation of foot at left big toe	
28. Mid-shaft amputation, right humerus	
29. Left fourth toe amputation, mid-proximal phalanx	
30. Right above-knee amputation, distal femur	
31. Cryotherapy of wart on left hand	
32. Percutaneous radiofrequency ablation of right vocal cord lesion	
33. Left heart catheterization with laser destruction of arrhythmogenic focus, A-V node	
34. Cautery of nosebleed	
35. Transurethral endoscopic laser ablation of prostate	
36. Percutaneous cautery of oozing varicose vein, left calf	
37. Laparoscopy with destruction of endometriosis, bilateral ovaries	
38. Laser coagulation of right retinal vessel, percutaneous	
39. Thoracoscopic pleurodesis, left side	
40. Percutaneous insertion of Greenfield IVC filter	
41. Forceps total mouth extraction, upper and lower teeth	

Procedure	Code
42. Removal of left thumbnail	
43. Extraction of right intraocular lens without replacement, percutaneous	
44. Laparoscopy with needle aspiration of ova for in vitro fertilization	
45. Nonexcisional debridement of skin ulcer, right foot	
46. Open stripping of abdominal fascia, right side	
47. Hysteroscopy with D&C, diagnostic	
48. Liposuction for medical purposes, left upper arm	
49. Removal of tattered right ear drum fragments with tweezers	
50. Microincisional phlebectomy of spider veins, right lower leg	
51. Routine Foley catheter placement	
52. Incision and drainage of external anal abscess	
53. Percutaneous drainage of ascites	
54. Laparoscopy with left ovarian cystotomy and drainage	
55. Laparotomy and drain placement for liver abscess, right lobe	
56. Right knee arthrotomy with drain placement	
57. Thoracentesis of left pleural effusion	
58. Phlebotomy of left median cubital vein for polycythemia vera	
59. Percutaneous chest tube placement for right pneumothorax	
60. Endoscopic drainage of left ethmoid sinus	
61. External ventricular CSF drainage catheter placement via burr hole	
62. Removal of foreign body, right cornea	
63. Percutaneous mechanical thrombectomy, left brachial artery	
64. Esophagogastroscopy with removal of bezoar from stomach	
65. Foreign body removal, skin of left thumb	
66. Transurethral cystoscopy with removal of bladder stone	
67. Forceps removal of foreign body in right nostril	
68. Laparoscopy with excision of old suture from mesentery	
69. Incision and removal of right lacrimal duct stone	
70. Nonincisional removal of intraluminal foreign body from vagina	
71. Right common carotid endarterectomy, open	
72. Open excision of retained sliver, subcutaneous tissue of left foot	
73. Extracorporeal shockwave lithotripsy (ESWL), bilateral ureters	
74. Endoscopic retrograde cholangiopancreatography (ERCP) with lithotripsy of common bile duct stone	
75. Thoracotomy with crushing of pericardial calcifications	
76. Transurethral cystoscopy with fragmentation of bladder calculus	
77. Hysteroscopy with intraluminal lithotripsy of left fallopian tube calcification	
78. Division of right foot tendon, percutaneous	

Procedure	Code
79. Left heart catheterization with division of bundle of HIS	
80. Open osteotomy of capitate, left hand	
81. EGD with esophagotomy of esophagogastric junction	
82. Sacral rhizotomy for pain control, percutaneous	
83. Laparotomy with exploration and adhesiolysis of right ureter	
84. Incision of scar contracture, right elbow	
85. Frenulotomy for treatment of tongue-tie syndrome	
86. Right shoulder arthroscopy with coracoacromial ligament release	
87. Mitral valvulotomy for release of fused leaflets, open approach	
88. Percutaneous left Achilles tendon release	
89. Laparoscopy with lysis of peritoneal adhesions	
90. Manual rupture of right shoulder joint adhesions under general anesthesia	
91. Open posterior tarsal tunnel release	
92. Laparoscopy with freeing of left ovary and fallopian tube	
93. Liver transplant with donor matched liver	
94. Orthotopic heart transplant using porcine heart	
95. Right lung transplant, open, using organ donor match	
96. Transplant of large intestine, organ donor match	
97. Left kidney/pancreas organ bank transplant	
98. Replantation of avulsed scalp	
99. Reattachment of severed right ear	
100. Reattachment of traumatic left gastrocnemius avulsion, open	
101. Closed replantation of three avulsed teeth, lower jaw	
102. Reattachment of severed left hand	
103. Right open palmaris longus tendon transfer	
104. Endoscopic radial to median nerve transfer	
105. Fasciocutaneous flap closure of left thigh, open	
106. Transfer left index finger to left thumb position, open	
107. Percutaneous fascia transfer to fill defect, right neck	
108. Trigeminal to facial nerve transfer, percutaneous endoscopic	
109. Endoscopic left leg flexor hallucis longus tendon transfer	
110. Right scalp advancement flap to right temple	
111. Resection right breast with TRAM flap reconstruction, open	
112. Skin transfer flap closure of complex open wound, left lower back	
113. Open fracture reduction, right tibia	
114. Laparoscopy with gastropexy for malrotation	
115. Left knee arthroscopy with reposition of anterior cruciate ligament	
116. Open transposition of ulnar nerve	
117. Closed reduction with percutaneous internal fixation of right femoral neck fracture	
118. Trans-vaginal intraluminal cervical cerclage	
119. Cervical cerclage using Shirodkar technique	
120. Thoracotomy with banding of left pulmonary artery using extraluminal device	
121. Restriction of thoracic duct with intraluminal stent, percutaneous	

Procedure	Code
122. Craniotomy with clipping of cerebral aneurysm	
123. Nonincisional, transnasal placement of restrictive stent in right lacrimal duct	
124. Catheter-based temporary restriction of blood flow in abdominal aorta for treatment of cerebral ischemia	
125. Percutaneous ligation of esophageal vein	
126. Percutaneous embolization of left internal carotid-cavernous fistula	
127. Laparoscopy with bilateral occlusion of fallopian tubes using Hulka extraluminal clips	
128. Open suture ligation of failed AV graft, left brachial artery	
129. Percutaneous embolization of vascular supply, intracranial meningioma	
130. Percutaneous embolization of right uterine artery, using coils	
131. Open occlusion of left atrial appendage, using extraluminal pressure clips	
132. Percutaneous suture exclusion of left atrial appendage, via femoral artery access	
133. ERCP with balloon dilation of common bile duct	
134. PTCA of two coronary arteries, LAD with stent placement, RCA with no stent	
135. Cystoscopy with intraluminal dilation of bladder neck stricture	
136. Open dilation of old anastomosis, left femoral artery	
137. Dilation of upper esophageal stricture, direct visualization, with Bougie sound	
138. PTA of right brachial artery stenosis	
139. Transnasal dilation and stent placement in right lacrimal duct	
140. Hysteroscopy with balloon dilation of bilateral fallopian tubes	
141. Tracheoscopy with intraluminal dilation of tracheal stenosis	
142. Cystoscopy with dilation of left ureteral stricture, with stent placement	
143. Open gastric bypass with Roux-en-Y limb to jejunum	
144. Right temporal artery to intracranial artery bypass using Gore-Tex graft, open	
145. Tracheostomy formation with tracheostomy tube placement, percutaneous	
146. PICVA (percutaneous in situ coronary venous arterialization) of single coronary artery	
147. Open left femoral-popliteal artery bypass using cadaver vein graft	
148. Shunting of intrathecal cerebrospinal fluid to peritoneal cavity using synthetic shunt	
149. Colostomy formation, open, transverse colon to abdominal wall	
150. Open urinary diversion, left ureter, using ileal conduit to skin	
151. CABG of LAD using pedicled left internal mammary artery, open off-bypass	
152. Open pleuroperitoneal shunt, right pleural cavity, using synthetic device	
153. Percutaneous placement of ventriculoperitoneal shunt for treatment of hydrocephalus	
154. End-of-life replacement of spinal neurostimulator generator, multiple array, in lower abdomen	
155. Percutaneous insertion of spinal neurostimulator lead, lumbar spinal cord	

Procedure	Code
156. Percutaneous replacement of broken pacemaker lead in left atrium	
157. Open placement of dual chamber pacemaker generator in chest wall	
158. Percutaneous placement of venous central line in right internal jugular, with tip in superior vena cava	
159. Open insertion of multiple channel cochlear implant, left ear	
160. Percutaneous placement of Swan-Ganz catheter in pulmonary trunk	
161. Bronchoscopy with insertion of Low Dose, Pd-103 brachytherapy seeds, right lung	
162. Open insertion of interspinous process device into lumbar vertebral joint	
163. Open placement of bone growth stimulator, left femoral shaft	
164. Cystoscopy with placement of brachytherapy seeds in prostate gland	
165. Percutaneous insertion of Greenfield IVC filter	
166. Full-thickness skin graft to right lower arm, autograft (do not code graft harvest for this exercise)	
167. Excision of necrosed left femoral head with bone bank bone graft to fill the defect, open	
168. Penetrating keratoplasty of right cornea with donor matched cornea, percutaneous approach	
169. Excision of abdominal aorta with Gore-Tex graft replacement, open	
170. Total right knee arthroplasty with insertion of total knee prosthesis	
171. Tenonectomy with graft to right ankle using cadaver graft, open	
172. Mitral valve replacement using porcine valve, open	
173. Percutaneous phacoemulsification of right eye cataract with prosthetic lens insertion	
174. Transcatheter replacement of pulmonary valve using of bovine jugular vein valve	
175. Total left hip replacement using ceramic on ceramic prosthesis, without bone cement	
176. Aortic valve annuloplasty using ring, open	
177. Laparoscopic repair of left inguinal hernia with marlex plug	
178. Autograft nerve graft to right median nerve, percutaneous endoscopic (do not code graft harvest for this exercise)	
179. Exchange of liner in femoral component of previous left hip replacement, open approach	
180. Anterior colporrhaphy with polypropylene mesh reinforcement, open approach	
181. Implantation of CorCap cardiac support device, open approach	
182. Abdominal wall herniorrhaphy, open, using synthetic mesh	
183. Tendon graft to strengthen injured left shoulder using autograft, open (do not code graft harvest for this exercise)	
184. Onlay lamellar keratoplasty of left cornea using autograft, external approach	
185. Resurfacing procedure on right femoral head, open approach	
186. Exchange of drainage tube from right hip joint	
187. Tracheostomy tube exchange	
188. Change chest tube for left pneumothorax	
189. Exchange of cerebral ventriculostomy drainage tube	

Procedure	Code
190. Foley urinary catheter exchange	
191. Open removal of lumbar sympathetic neurostimulator lead	
192. Nonincisional removal of Swan-Ganz catheter from right pulmonary artery	
193. Laparotomy with removal of pancreatic drain	
194. Extubation, endotracheal tube	
195. Nonincisional PEG tube removal	
196. Transvaginal removal of brachytherapy seeds	
197. Transvaginal removal of extraluminal cervical cerclage	
198. Incision with removal of K-wire fixation, right first metatarsal	
199. Cystoscopy with retrieval of left ureteral stent	
200. Removal of nasogastric drainage tube for decompression	
201. Removal of external fixator, left radial fracture	
202. Trimming and reanastomosis of stenosed femorofemoral synthetic bypass graft, open	
203. Open revision of right hip replacement, with readjustment of prosthesis	
204. Adjustment of position, pacemaker lead in left ventricle, percutaneous	
205. External repositioning of Foley catheter to bladder	
206. Taking out loose screw and putting larger screw in fracture repair plate, left tibia	
207. Revision of totally implantable VAD port placement in chest wall, causing patient discomfort, open	
208. Thoracotomy with exploration of right pleural cavity	
209. Diagnostic laryngoscopy	
210. Exploratory arthrotomy of left knee	
211. Colposcopy with diagnostic hysteroscopy	
212. Digital rectal exam	
213. Diagnostic arthroscopy of right shoulder	
214. Endoscopy of maxillary sinus	
215. Laparotomy with palpation of liver	
216. Transurethral diagnostic cystoscopy	
217. Colonoscopy, discontinued at sigmoid colon	
218. Percutaneous mapping of basal ganglia	
219. Heart catheterization with cardiac mapping	
220. Intraoperative whole brain mapping via craniotomy	
221. Mapping of left cerebral hemisphere, percutaneous endoscopic	
222. Intraoperative cardiac mapping during open heart surgery	
223. Hysteroscopy with cautery of post-hysterectomy oozing and evacuation of clot	
224. Open exploration and ligation of post-op arterial bleeder, left forearm	
225. Control of post-operative retroperitoneal bleeding via laparotomy	
226. Reopening of thoracotomy site with drainage and control of post-op hemopericardium	
227. Arthroscopy with drainage of hemarthrosis at previous operative site, right knee	
228. Radiocarpal fusion of left hand with internal fixation, open	
229. Posterior approach spinal fusion at L1-L3 level with BAK cage interbody fusion device, open	
230. Intercarpal fusion of right hand with bone bank bone graft, open	

Procedure	Code
231. Sacrococcygeal fusion with bone graft from same operative site, open	
232. Interphalangeal fusion of left great toe, percutaneous pin fixation	
233. Suture repair of left radial nerve laceration	
234. Laparotomy with suture repair of blunt force duodenal laceration	
235. Perineoplasty with repair of old obstetric laceration, open	
236. Suture repair of right biceps tendon (upper arm) laceration, open	
237. Closure of abdominal wall stab wound	
238. Cosmetic face lift, open, no other information available	
239. Bilateral breast augmentation with silicone implants, open	
240. Cosmetic rhinoplasty with septal reduction and tip elevation using local tissue graft, open	
241. Abdominoplasty (tummy tuck), open	
242. Liposuction of bilateral thighs	
243. Creation of penis in female patient using tissue bank donor graft	
244. Creation of vagina in male patient using synthetic material	
245. Laparoscopic vertical (sleeve) gastrectomy	
246. Left uterine artery embolization with intraluminal biosphere injection	

Obstetrics

Procedure	Code
1. Abortion by dilation and evacuation following laminaria insertion	
2. Manually assisted spontaneous abortion	
3. Abortion by abortifacient insertion	
4. Bimanual pregnancy examination	
5. Extraperitoneal C-section, low transverse incision	
6. Fetal spinal tap, percutaneous	
7. Fetal kidney transplant, laparoscopic	
8. Open in utero repair of congenital diaphragmatic hernia	
9. Laparoscopy with total excision of tubal pregnancy	
10. Transvaginal removal of fetal monitoring electrode	

Placement

Procedure	Code
1. Placement of packing material, right ear	
2. Mechanical traction of entire left leg	
3. Removal of splint, right shoulder	
4. Placement of neck brace	
5. Change of vaginal packing	
6. Packing of wound, chest wall	
7. Sterile dressing placement to left groin region	
8. Removal of packing material from pharynx	
9. Placement of intermittent pneumatic compression device, covering entire right arm	
10. Exchange of pressure dressing to left thigh	

Administration

Procedure	Code
1. Peritoneal dialysis via indwelling catheter	
2. Transvaginal artificial insemination	
3. Infusion of total parenteral nutrition via central venous catheter	
4. Esophagogastroscopy with Botox injection into esophageal sphincter	
5. Percutaneous irrigation of knee joint	
6. Systemic infusion of recombinant tissue plasminogen activator (r-tPA) via peripheral venous catheter	
7. Transabdominal in vitro fertilization, implantation of donor ovum	
8. Autologous bone marrow transplant via central venous line	
9. Implantation of anti-microbial envelope with cardiac defibrillator placement, open	
10. Sclerotherapy of brachial plexus lesion, alcohol injection	
11. Percutaneous peripheral vein injection, glucarpidase	
12. Introduction of anti-infective envelope into subcutaneous tissue, open	

Measurement and Monitoring

Procedure	Code
1. Cardiac stress test, single measurement	
2. EGD with biliary flow measurement	
3. Right and left heart cardiac catheterization with bilateral sampling and pressure measurements	
4. Temperature monitoring, rectal	
5. Peripheral venous pulse, external, single measurement	
6. Holter monitoring	
7. Respiratory rate, external, single measurement	
8. Fetal heart rate monitoring, transvaginal	
9. Visual mobility test, single measurement	
10. Left ventricular cardiac output monitoring from pulmonary artery wedge (Swan-Ganz) catheter	
11. Olfactory acuity test, single measurement	

Extracorporeal or Systemic Assistance and Performance

Procedure	Code
1. Intermittent mechanical ventilation, 16 hours	
2. Liver dialysis, single encounter	
3. Cardiac countershock with successful conversion to sinus rhythm	
4. IPPB (intermittent positive pressure breathing) for mobilization of secretions, 22 hours	
5. Renal dialysis, 12 hours	
6. IABP (intra-aortic balloon pump) continuous	
7. Intraoperative cardiac pacing, continuous	
8. Intraoperative ECMO (extracorporeal membrane oxygenation), central	
9. Controlled mechanical ventilation (CMV), 45 hours	
10. Pulsatile compression boot with intermittent inflation	

Extracorporeal or Systemic Therapies

Procedure	Code
1. Donor thrombocytapheresis, single encounter	
2. Bili-lite phototherapy, series treatment	
3. Whole body hypothermia, single treatment	
4. Circulatory phototherapy, single encounter	
5. Shock wave therapy of plantar fascia, single treatment	
6. Antigen-free air conditioning, series treatment	
7. TMS (transcranial magnetic stimulation), series treatment	
8. Therapeutic ultrasound of peripheral vessels, single treatment	
9. Plasmapheresis, series treatment	
10. Extracorporeal electromagnetic stimulation (EMS) for urinary incontinence, single treatment	

Osteopathic

Procedure	Code
1. Isotonic muscle energy treatment of right leg	
2. Low velocity-high amplitude osteopathic treatment of head	
3. Lymphatic pump osteopathic treatment of left axilla	
4. Indirect osteopathic treatment of sacrum	
5. Articulatory osteopathic treatment of cervical region	

Other Procedures

Procedure	Code
1. Near infrared spectroscopy of leg vessels	
2. CT computer assisted sinus surgery	
3. Suture removal, abdominal wall	
4. Isolation after infectious disease exposure	
5. Robotic assisted open prostatectomy	
6. In vitro fertilization	

Chiropractic

Procedure	Code
1. Chiropractic treatment of lumbar region using long lever specific contact	
2. Chiropractic manipulation of abdominal region, indirect visceral	
3. Chiropractic extra-articular treatment of hip region	
4. Chiropractic treatment of sacrum using long and short lever specific contact	
5. Mechanically-assisted chiropractic manipulation of head	

Imaging

Procedure	Code
1. Noncontrast CT of abdomen and pelvis	
2. Intravascular ultrasound, left subclavian artery	
3. Fluoroscopic guidance for insertion of central venous catheter in SVC, low osmolar contrast	
4. Chest x-ray, AP/PA and lateral views	
5. Endoluminal ultrasound of gallbladder and bile ducts	
6. MRI of thyroid gland, contrast unspecified	
7. Esophageal videofluoroscopy study with oral barium contrast	

Procedure	Code
8. Portable x-ray study of right radius/ulna shaft, standard series	
9. Routine fetal ultrasound, second trimester twin gestation	
10. CT scan of bilateral lungs, high osmolar contrast with densitometry	
11. Fluoroscopic guidance for percutaneous transluminal angioplasty (PTA) of left common femoral artery, low osmolar contrast	

Nuclear Medicine

Procedure	Code
1. Tomo scan of right and left heart, unspecified radiopharmaceutical, qualitative gated rest	
2. Technetium pentetate assay of kidneys, ureters, and bladder	
3. Uniplanar scan of spine using technetium oxidronate, with first-pass study	
4. Thallous chloride tomographic scan of bilateral breasts	
5. PET scan of myocardium using rubidium	
6. Gallium citrate scan of head and neck, single plane imaging	
7. Xenon gas nonimaging probe of brain	
8. Upper GI scan, radiopharmaceutical unspecified, for gastric emptying	
9. Carbon 11 PET scan of brain with quantification	
10. Iodinated albumin nuclear medicine assay, blood plasma volume study	

Radiation Therapy

Procedure	Code
1. Plaque radiation of left eye, single port	
2. 8 MeV photon beam radiation to brain	
3. IORT of colon, 3 ports	
4. HDR brachytherapy of prostate using low dose palladium-103, unidirectional source	
5. Electron radiation treatment of right breast, with custom device	
6. Hyperthermia oncology treatment of pelvic region	
7. Contact radiation of tongue	
8. Heavy particle radiation treatment of pancreas, four risk sites	
9. LDR brachytherapy to spinal cord using iodine	
10. Whole body Phosphorus 32 administration with risk to hematopoietic system	

Physical Rehabilitation and Diagnostic Audiology

Procedure	Code
1. Bekesy assessment using audiometer	
2. Individual fitting of left eye prosthesis	
3. Physical therapy for range of motion and mobility, patient right hip, no special equipment	
4. Bedside swallow assessment using assessment kit	
5. Caregiver training in airway clearance techniques	
6. Application of short arm cast in rehabilitation setting	
7. Verbal assessment of patient's pain level	
8. Caregiver training in communication skills using manual communication board	

Procedure	Code
9. Group musculoskeletal balance training exercises, whole body, no special equipment	
10. Individual therapy for auditory processing using tape recorder	

Mental Health

Procedure	Code
1. Cognitive-behavioral psychotherapy, individual	
2. Narcosynthesis	
3. Light therapy	
4. ECT (electroconvulsive therapy), unilateral, multiple seizure	
5. Crisis intervention	
6. Neuropsychological testing	
7. Hypnosis	
8. Developmental testing	
9. Vocational counseling	
10. Family psychotherapy	

Substance Abuse Treatment

Procedure	Code
1. Naltrexone treatment for drug dependency	
2. Substance abuse treatment family counseling	
3. Medication monitoring of patient on methadone maintenance	
4. Individual interpersonal psychotherapy for drug abuse	
5. Patient in for alcohol detoxification treatment	
6. Group motivational counseling	
7. Individual 12-step psychotherapy for substance abuse	
8. Post-test infectious disease counseling for IV drug abuser	
9. Psychodynamic psychotherapy for drug dependent patient	
10. Group cognitive-behavioral counseling for substance abuse	

New Technology

Procedure	Code
1. Infusion of terlipressin via peripheral venous catheter	
2. Transcatheter dilation of left peroneal artery with 2 SAVAL stents	

Answers to Coding Exercises

Medical Surgical Section

Procedure	Code
1. Excision of malignant melanoma from skin of right ear	ØHB2XZZ
2. Laparoscopy with excision of endometrial implant from left ovary	ØUB14ZZ
3. Percutaneous needle core biopsy of right kidney	ØTBØ3ZX
4. EGD with excisional gastric biopsy	ØDB68ZX
5. Open endarterectomy of left common carotid artery	Ø3CJØZZ
6. Excision of basal cell carcinoma of lower lip	ØCB1XZZ
7. Open excision of tail of pancreas	ØFBGØZZ
8. Percutaneous biopsy of right gastrocnemius muscle	ØKBS3ZX
9. Sigmoidoscopy with sigmoid polypectomy	ØDBN8ZZ
10. Open excision of lesion from right Achilles tendon	ØLBNØZZ
11. Open resection of cecum	ØDTHØZZ
12. Total excision of pituitary gland, open	ØGTØØZZ
13. Explantation of left failed kidney, open	ØTT1ØZZ
14. Open left axillary total lymphadenectomy	Ø7T6ØZZ (RESECTION is coded for cutting out a chain of lymph nodes.)
15. Laparoscopic-assisted vaginal hysterectomy	ØUT9FZZ
16. Right total mastectomy, open	ØHTTØZZ
17. Open resection of papillary muscle	Ø2TDØZZ (The papillary muscle refers to the heart and is found in the *Heart and Great Vessels* body system.)
18. Total retropubic prostatectomy, open	ØVTØØZZ
19. Laparoscopic cholecystectomy	ØFT44ZZ
20. Endoscopic bilateral total maxillary sinusectomy	Ø9TQ8ZZ, Ø9TR8ZZ
21. Amputation at right elbow level	ØX6BØZZ
22. Right below-knee amputation, proximal tibia/fibula	ØY6HØZ1 (The qualifier *High* here means the portion of the tib/fib closest to the knee.)
23. Fifth ray carpometacarpal joint amputation, left hand	ØX6KØZ8 (A *complete* ray amputation is through the carpometacarpal joint.)
24. Right leg and hip amputation through ischium	ØY62ØZZ (The *Hindquarter* body part includes amputation along any part of the hip bone.)
25. DIP joint amputation of right thumb	ØX6LØZ3 (The qualifier *low* here means through the distal interphalangeal joint.)
26. Right wrist joint amputation	ØX6JØZØ (Amputation at the wrist joint is actually complete amputation of the hand.)
27. Trans-metatarsal amputation of foot at left big toe	ØY6NØZ9 (A *partial* amputation is through the shaft of the metatarsal bone.)
28. Mid-shaft amputation, right humerus	ØX68ØZ2
29. Left fourth toe amputation, mid-proximal phalanx	ØY6WØZ1 (The qualifier *High* here means anywhere along the proximal phalanx.)
30. Right above-knee amputation, distal femur	ØY6CØZ3
31. Cryotherapy of wart on left hand	ØH5GXZZ
32. Percutaneous radiofrequency ablation of right vocal cord lesion	ØC5T3ZZ
33. Left heart catheterization with laser destruction of arrhythmogenic focus, A-V node	Ø2583ZZ
34. Cautery of nosebleed	Ø93K7ZZ
35. Transurethral endoscopic laser ablation of prostate	ØV5Ø8ZZ
36. Percutaneous cautery of oozing varicose vein, left calf	ØY3J3ZZ
37. Laparoscopy with destruction of endometriosis, bilateral ovaries	ØU524ZZ
38. Laser coagulation of right retinal vessel, percutaneous	Ø85G3ZZ (The *Retinal Vessel* body-part values are in the *Eye* body system.)
39. Thoracoscopic pleurodesis, left side	ØB5P4ZZ
40. Percutaneous insertion of Greenfield IVC filter	Ø6HØ3DZ
41. Forceps total mouth extraction, upper and lower teeth	ØCDWXZ2, ØCDXXZ2
42. Removal of left thumbnail	ØHDQXZZ (No separate body-part value is given for thumbnail, so this is coded to *Fingernail*.)
43. Extraction of right intraocular lens without replacement, percutaneous	Ø8DJ3ZZ
44. Laparoscopy with needle aspiration of ova for in vitro fertilization	ØUDN4ZZ
45. Nonexcisional debridement of skin ulcer, right foot	ØHDMXZZ
46. Open stripping of abdominal fascia, right side	ØJD8ØZZ
47. Hysteroscopy with D&C, diagnostic	ØUDB8ZX
48. Liposuction for medical purposes, left upper arm	ØJDF3ZZ (The *Percutaneous* approach is inherent in the liposuction technique.)
49. Removal of tattered right ear drum fragments with tweezers	Ø9D77ZZ
50. Microincisional phlebectomy of spider veins, right lower leg	Ø6DY3ZZ
51. Routine Foley catheter placement	ØT9B7ØZ
52. Incision and drainage of external anal abscess	ØD9QXZZ
53. Percutaneous drainage of ascites	ØW9G3ZZ (This is drainage of the cavity and not the peritoneal membrane itself.)
54. Laparoscopy with left ovarian cystotomy and drainage	ØU914ZZ
55. Laparotomy and drain placement for liver abscess, right lobe	ØF91ØØZ
56. Right knee arthrotomy with drain placement	ØS9CØØZ
57. Thoracentesis of left pleural effusion	ØW9B3ZZ (This is drainage of the pleural cavity)
58. Phlebotomy of left median cubital vein for polycythemia vera	Ø59C3ZZ (The median cubital vein is a branch of the basilic vein)
59. Percutaneous chest tube placement for right pneumothorax	ØW993ØZ
60. Endoscopic drainage of left ethmoid sinus	Ø99V4ZZ
61. External ventricular CSF drainage catheter placement via burr hole	ØØ963ØZ
62. Removal of foreign body, right cornea	Ø8C8XZZ

Procedure	Code
63. Percutaneous mechanical thrombectomy, left brachial artery	03C83ZZ
64. Esophagogastroscopy with removal of bezoar from stomach	0DC68ZZ
65. Foreign body removal, skin of left thumb	0HCGXZZ (There is no specific value for thumb skin, so the procedure is coded to *Hand*.)
66. Transurethral cystoscopy with removal of bladder stone	0TCB8ZZ
67. Forceps removal of foreign body in right nostril	09CKXZZ (Nostril is coded to the *Nasal mucosa and soft tissue* body-part value.)
68. Laparoscopy with excision of old suture from mesentery	0DCV4ZZ
69. Incision and removal of right lacrimal duct stone	08CX0ZZ
70. Nonincisional removal of intraluminal foreign body from vagina	0UCG7ZZ (The approach *External* is also a possibility. It is assumed here that since the patient went to the doctor to have the object removed, that it was not in the vaginal orifice.)
71. Right common carotid endarterectomy, open	03CH0ZZ
72. Open excision of retained sliver, subcutaneous tissue of left foot	0JCR0ZZ
73. Extracorporeal shockwave lithotripsy (ESWL), bilateral ureters	0TF6XZZ, 0TF7XZZ (The *Bilateral Ureter* body-part value is not available for the root operation FRAGMENTATION, so the procedures are coded separately.)
74. Endoscopic retrograde cholangiopancreatography (ERCP) with lithotripsy of common bile duct stone	0FF98ZZ (ERCP is performed through the mouth to the biliary system via the duodenum, so the approach value is *Via Natural or Artificial Opening Endoscopic*.)
75. Thoracotomy with crushing of pericardial calcifications	02FN0ZZ
76. Transurethral cystoscopy with fragmentation of bladder calculus	0TFB8ZZ
77. Hysteroscopy with intraluminal lithotripsy of left fallopian tube calcification	0UF68ZZ
78. Division of right foot tendon, percutaneous	0L8V3ZZ
79. Left heart catheterization with division of bundle of HIS	02883ZZ
80. Open osteotomy of capitate, left hand	0P8N0ZZ (The capitate is one of the carpal bones of the hand.)
81. EGD with esophagotomy of esophagogastric junction	0D948ZZ
82. Sacral rhizotomy for pain control, percutaneous	018R3ZZ
83. Laparotomy with exploration and adhesiolysis of right ureter	0TN60ZZ
84. Incision of scar contracture, right elbow	0HNDXZZ (The skin of the elbow region is coded to *Lower Arm*.)
85. Frenulotomy for treatment of tongue-tie syndrome	0CN7XZZ (The frenulum is coded to the body-part value *Tongue*.)
86. Right shoulder arthroscopy with coracoacromial ligament release	0MN14ZZ

Procedure	Code
87. Mitral valvulotomy for release of fused leaflets, open approach	02NG0ZZ
88. Percutaneous left Achilles tendon release	0LNP3ZZ
89. Laparoscopy with lysis of peritoneal adhesions	0DNW4ZZ
90. Manual rupture of right shoulder joint adhesions under general anesthesia	0RNJXZZ
91. Open posterior tarsal tunnel release	01NG0ZZ (The nerve released in the posterior tarsal tunnel is the tibial nerve.)
92. Laparoscopy with freeing of left ovary and fallopian tube	0UN14ZZ, 0UN64ZZ
93. Liver transplant with donor matched liver	0FY00Z0
94. Orthotopic heart transplant using porcine heart	02YA0Z2 (The donor heart comes from an animal [pig], so the qualifier value is *Zooplastic*.)
95. Right lung transplant, open, using organ donor match	0BYK0Z0
96. Transplant of large intestine, organ donor match	0DYE0Z0
97. Left kidney/pancreas organ bank transplant	0FYG0Z0, 0TY10Z0
98. Replantation of avulsed scalp	0HM0XZZ
99. Reattachment of severed right ear	09M0XZZ
100. Reattachment of traumatic left gastrocnemius avulsion, open	0KMT0ZZ
101. Closed replantation of three avulsed teeth, lower jaw	0CMXXZ1
102. Reattachment of severed left hand	0XMK0ZZ
103. Right open palmaris longus tendon transfer	0LX50ZZ
104. Endoscopic radial to median nerve transfer	01X64Z5
105. Fasciocutaneous flap closure of left thigh, open	0JXM0ZC (The qualifier identifies the body layers in addition to fascia included in the procedure.)
106. Transfer left index finger to left thumb position, open	0XXP0ZM
107. Percutaneous fascia transfer to fill defect, right neck	0JX43ZZ
108. Trigeminal to facial nerve transfer, percutaneous endoscopic	00XK4ZM
109. Endoscopic left leg flexor hallucis longus tendon transfer	0LXP4ZZ
110. Right scalp advancement flap to right temple	0HX0XZZ
111. Resection right breast with TRAM flap reconstruction, open	0HTT0ZZ, 0HRT076 (Code both the resection and the replacement per guideline B3.18)
112. Skin transfer flap closure of complex open wound, left lower back	0HX6XZZ
113. Open fracture reduction, right tibia	0QSG0ZZ
114. Laparoscopy with gastropexy for malrotation	0DS64ZZ
115. Left knee arthroscopy with reposition of anterior cruciate ligament	0MSP4ZZ
116. Open transposition of ulnar nerve	01S40ZZ
117. Closed reduction with percutaneous internal fixation of right femoral neck fracture	0QS634Z
118. Trans-vaginal intraluminal cervical cerclage	0UVC7DZ
119. Cervical cerclage using Shirodkar technique	0UVC7ZZ
120. Thoracotomy with banding of left pulmonary artery using extraluminal device	02VR0CZ
121. Restriction of thoracic duct with intraluminal stent, percutaneous	07VK3DZ

Procedure	Code
122. Craniotomy with clipping of cerebral aneurysm	03VG0CZ (The clip is placed lengthwise on the outside wall of the widened portion of the vessel.)
123. Nonincisional, transnasal placement of restrictive stent in right lacrimal duct	08VX7DZ
124. Catheter-based temporary restriction of blood flow in abdominal aorta for treatment of cerebral ischemia	04V03DJ
125. Percutaneous ligation of esophageal vein	06L33ZZ
126. Percutaneous embolization of left internal carotid-cavernous fistula	03LL3DZ
127. Laparoscopy with bilateral occlusion of fallopian tubes using Hulka extraluminal clips	0UL74CZ
128. Open suture ligation of failed AV graft, left brachial artery	03L80ZZ
129. Percutaneous embolization of vascular supply, intracranial meningioma	03LG3DZ
130. Percutaneous embolization of right uterine artery, using coils	04LE3DT
131. Open occlusion of left atrial appendage, using extraluminal pressure clips	02L70CK
132. Percutaneous suture exclusion of left atrial appendage, via femoral artery access	02L73ZK
133. ERCP with balloon dilation of common bile duct	0F798ZZ
134. PTCA of two coronary arteries, LAD with stent placement, RCA with no stent	02703DZ, 02703ZZ (A separate procedure is coded for each artery dilated, since the device value differs for each artery.)
135. Cystoscopy with intraluminal dilation of bladder neck stricture	0T7C8ZZ
136. Open dilation of old anastomosis, left femoral artery	047L0ZZ
137. Dilation of upper esophageal stricture, direct visualization, with Bougie sound	0D717ZZ
138. PTA of right brachial artery stenosis	03773ZZ
139. Transnasal dilation and stent placement in right lacrimal duct	087X7DZ
140. Hysteroscopy with balloon dilation of bilateral fallopian tubes	0U778ZZ
141. Tracheoscopy with intraluminal dilation of tracheal stenosis	0B718ZZ
142. Cystoscopy with dilation of left ureteral stricture, with stent placement	0T778DZ
143. Open gastric bypass with Roux-en-Y limb to jejunum	0D160ZA
144. Right temporal artery to intracranial artery bypass using Gore-Tex graft, open	031S0JG
145. Tracheostomy formation with tracheostomy tube placement, percutaneous	0B113F4
146. PICVA (percutaneous in situ coronary venous arterialization) of single coronary artery	02103D4
147. Open left femoral-popliteal artery bypass using cadaver vein graft	041L0KL
148. Shunting of intrathecal cerebrospinal fluid to peritoneal cavity using synthetic shunt	00160J6
149. Colostomy formation, open, transverse colon to abdominal wall	0D1L0Z4
150. Open urinary diversion, left ureter, using ileal conduit to skin	0T170ZC
151. CABG of LAD using pedicled left internal mammary artery, open off-bypass	02100Z9

Procedure	Code
152. Open pleuroperitoneal shunt, right pleural cavity, using synthetic device	0W190JG
153. Percutaneous placement of ventriculoperitoneal shunt for treatment of hydrocephalus	00163J6
154. End-of-life replacement of spinal neurostimulator generator, multiple array, in lower abdomen	0JH80DZ (Taking out of the old generator is coded separately to the root operation Removal)
155. Percutaneous insertion of spinal neurostimulator lead, lumbar spinal cord	00HV3MZ
156. Percutaneous replacement of broken pacemaker lead in left atrium	02H73JZ (Taking out the broken pacemaker lead is coded separately to the root operation Removal.)
157. Open placement of dual chamber pacemaker generator in chest wall	0JH606Z
158. Percutaneous placement of venous central line in right internal jugular, with tip in superior vena cava	02HV33Z
159. Open insertion of multiple channel cochlear implant, left ear	09HE06Z
160. Percutaneous placement of Swan-Ganz catheter in pulmonary trunk	02HP32Z (The Swan-Ganz catheter is coded to the device value Monitoring Device because it monitors pulmonary artery output.)
161. Bronchoscopy with insertion of Low Dose Pd-103 brachytherapy seeds, right lung	0BHK81Z, DB11BBZ
162. Open insertion of interspinous process device into lumbar vertebral joint	0SH00BZ
163. Open placement of bone growth stimulator, left femoral shaft	0QHY0MZ
164. Cystoscopy with placement of brachytherapy seeds in prostate gland	0VH081Z
165. Percutaneous insertion of Greenfield IVC filter	06H03DZ
166. Full-thickness skin graft to right lower arm, autograft (do not code graft harvest for this exercise)	0HRDX73
167. Excision of necrosed left femoral head with bone bank bone graft to fill the defect, open	0QR70KZ
168. Penetrating keratoplasty of right cornea with donor matched cornea, percutaneous approach	08R83KZ
169. Excision of abdominal aorta with Gore-Tex graft replacement, open	04R00JZ
170. Total right knee arthroplasty with insertion of total knee prosthesis	0SRC0JZ
171. Tenonectomy with graft to right ankle using cadaver graft, open	0LRS0KZ
172. Mitral valve replacement using porcine valve, open	02RG08Z
173. Percutaneous phacoemulsification of right eye cataract with prosthetic lens insertion	08RJ3JZ
174. Transcatheter replacement of pulmonary valve using of bovine jugular vein valve	02RH38Z
175. Total left hip replacement using ceramic on ceramic prosthesis, without bone cement	0SRB03A
176. Aortic valve annuloplasty using ring, open	02UF0JZ
177. Laparoscopic repair of left inguinal hernia with marlex plug	0YU64JZ
178. Autograft nerve graft to right median nerve, percutaneous endoscopic (do not code graft harvest for this exercise)	01U547Z
179. Exchange of liner in femoral component of previous left hip replacement, open approach	0SUS09Z (Taking out of the old liner is coded separately to the root operation Removal)

Procedure	Code
180. Anterior colporrhaphy with polypropylene mesh reinforcement, open approach	0JUC0JZ
181. Implantation of CorCap cardiac support device, open approach	02UA0JZ
182. Abdominal wall herniorrhaphy, open, using synthetic mesh	0WUF0JZ
183. Tendon graft to strengthen injured left shoulder using autograft, open (do not code graft harvest for this exercise)	0LU207Z
184. Onlay lamellar keratoplasty of left cornea using autograft, external approach	08U9X7Z
185. Resurfacing procedure on right femoral head, open approach	0SUR0BZ
186. Exchange of drainage tube from right hip joint	0S2YX0Z
187. Tracheostomy tube exchange	0B21XFZ
188. Change chest tube for left pneumothorax	0W2BX0Z
189. Exchange of cerebral ventriculostomy drainage tube	0020X0Z
190. Foley urinary catheter exchange	0T2BX0Z (This is coded to *Drainage Device* because urine is being drained.)
191. Open removal of lumbar sympathetic neurostimulator lead	01PY0MZ
192. Nonincisional removal of Swan-Ganz catheter from right pulmonary artery	02PYX2Z
193. Laparotomy with removal of pancreatic drain	0FPG00Z
194. Extubation, endotracheal tube	0BP1XDZ
195. Nonincisional PEG tube removal	0DP6XUZ
196. Transvaginal removal of brachytherapy seeds	0UPH71Z
197. Transvaginal removal of extraluminal cervical cerclage	0UPD7CZ
198. Incision with removal of K-wire fixation, right first metatarsal	0QPN04Z
199. Cystoscopy with retrieval of left ureteral stent	0TP98DZ
200. Removal of nasogastric drainage tube for decompression	0DP6X0Z
201. Removal of external fixator, left radial fracture	0PPJX5Z
202. Trimming and reanastomosis of stenosed femorofemoral synthetic bypass graft, open	04WY0JZ
203. Open revision of right hip replacement, with readjustment of prosthesis	0SW90JZ
204. Adjustment of position, pacemaker lead in left ventricle, percutaneous	02WA3MZ
205. External repositioning of Foley catheter to bladder	0TWBX0Z
206. Taking out loose screw and putting larger screw in fracture repair plate, left tibia	0QWH04Z
207. Revision of totally implantable VAD port placement in chest wall, causing patient discomfort, open	0JWT0WZ
208. Thoracotomy with exploration of right pleural cavity	0WJ90ZZ
209. Diagnostic laryngoscopy	0CJS8ZZ
210. Exploratory arthrotomy of left knee	0SJD0ZZ
211. Colposcopy with diagnostic hysteroscopy	0UJD8ZZ
212. Digital rectal exam	0DJD7ZZ
213. Diagnostic arthroscopy of right shoulder	0RJJ4ZZ
214. Endoscopy of maxillary sinus	09JY4ZZ
215. Laparotomy with palpation of liver	0FJ00ZZ
216. Transurethral diagnostic cystoscopy	0TJB8ZZ
217. Colonoscopy, discontinued at sigmoid colon	0DJD8ZZ
218. Percutaneous mapping of basal ganglia	00K83ZZ
219. Heart catheterization with cardiac mapping	02K83ZZ
220. Intraoperative whole brain mapping via craniotomy	00K00ZZ

Procedure	Code
221. Mapping of left cerebral hemisphere, percutaneous endoscopic	00K74ZZ
222. Intraoperative cardiac mapping during open heart surgery	02K80ZZ
223. Hysteroscopy with cautery of post-hysterectomy oozing and evacuation of clot	0W3R8ZZ
224. Open exploration and ligation of post-op arterial bleeder, left forearm	0X3F0ZZ
225. Control of post-operative retroperitoneal bleeding via laparotomy	0W3H0ZZ
226. Reopening of thoracotomy site with drainage and control of post-op hemopericardium	0W3D0ZZ
227. Arthroscopy with drainage of hemarthrosis at previous operative site, right knee	0Y3F4ZZ
228. Radiocarpal fusion of left hand with internal fixation, open	0RGP04Z
229. Posterior approach spinal fusion at L1-L3 level with BAK cage interbody fusion device, open	0SG10AJ
230. Intercarpal fusion of right hand with bone bank bone graft, open	0RGQ0KZ
231. Sacrococcygeal fusion with bone graft from same operative site, open	0SG507Z
232. Interphalangeal fusion of left great toe, percutaneous pin fixation	0SGQ34Z
233. Suture repair of left radial nerve laceration	01Q60ZZ (The approach value is *Open*, though the surgical exposure may have been created by the wound itself.)
234. Laparotomy with suture repair of blunt force duodenal laceration	0DQ90ZZ
235. Perineoplasty with repair of old obstetric laceration, open	0WQN0ZZ
236. Suture repair of right biceps tendon (upper arm) laceration, open	0LQ30ZZ
237. Closure of abdominal wall stab wound	0WQF0ZZ
238. Cosmetic face lift, open, no other information available	0W020ZZ
239. Bilateral breast augmentation with silicone implants, open	0H0V0JZ
240. Cosmetic rhinoplasty with septal reduction and tip elevation using local tissue graft, open	090K07Z
241. Abdominoplasty (tummy tuck), open	0W0F0ZZ
242. Liposuction of bilateral thighs	0J0L3ZZ, 0J0M3ZZ
243. Creation of penis in female patient using tissue bank donor graft	0W4N0K1
244. Creation of vagina in male patient using synthetic material	0W4M0J0
245. Laparoscopic vertical (sleeve) gastrectomy	0DB64Z3
246. Left uterine artery embolization with intraluminal biosphere injection	04LF3DU

Appendix M: Coding Exercises and Answers

Obstetrics

Procedure	Code
1. Abortion by dilation and evacuation following laminaria insertion	10A07ZW
2. Manually assisted spontaneous abortion	10E0XZZ (Since the pregnancy was not artificially terminated, this is coded to *Delivery* because it captures the procedure objective. The fact that it was an abortion will be identified in the diagnosis code.)
3. Abortion by abortifacient insertion	10A07ZX
4. Bimanual pregnancy examination	10J07ZZ
5. Extraperitoneal C-section, low transverse incision	10D00Z1
6. Fetal spinal tap, percutaneous	10903ZA
7. Fetal kidney transplant, laparoscopic	10Y04ZS
8. Open in utero repair of congenital diaphragmatic hernia	10Q00ZK (Diaphragm is classified to the *Respiratory* body system in the *Medical and Surgical* section.)
9. Laparoscopy with total excision of tubal pregnancy	10T24ZZ
10. Transvaginal removal of fetal monitoring electrode	10P073Z

Placement

Procedure	Code
1. Placement of packing material, right ear	2Y42X5Z
2. Mechanical traction of entire left leg	2W6MX0Z
3. Removal of splint, right shoulder	2W5AX1Z
4. Placement of neck brace	2W32X3Z
5. Change of vaginal packing	2Y04X5Z
6. Packing of wound, chest wall	2W44X5Z
7. Sterile dressing placement to left groin region	2W27X4Z
8. Removal of packing material from pharynx	2Y50X5Z
9. Placement of intermittent pneumatic compression device, covering entire right arm	2W18X7Z
10. Exchange of pressure dressing to left thigh	2W0PX6Z

Administration

Procedure	Code
1. Peritoneal dialysis via indwelling catheter	3E1M39Z
2. Transvaginal artificial insemination	3E0P7LZ
3. Infusion of total parenteral nutrition via central venous catheter	3E0436Z
4. Esophagogastroscopy with Botox injection into esophageal sphincter	3E0G8GC (Botulinum toxin is a paralyzing agent with temporary effects; it does not sclerose or destroy the nerve.)
5. Percutaneous irrigation of knee joint	3E1U38Z
6. Systemic infusion of recombinant tissue plasminogen activator (r-tPA) via peripheral venous catheter	3E03317
7. Transabdominal in vitro fertilization, implantation of donor ovum	3E0P3Q1
8. Autologous bone marrow transplant via central venous line	30243G0
9. Implantation of anti-microbial envelope with cardiac defibrillator placement, open	3E0102A
10. Sclerotherapy of brachial plexus lesion, alcohol injection	3E0T3TZ

Procedure	Code
11. Percutaneous peripheral vein injection, glucarpidase	3E033GQ
12. Introduction of anti-infective envelope into subcutaneous tissue, open	3E0102A

Measurement and Monitoring

Procedure	Code
1. Cardiac stress test, single measurement	4A02XM4
2. EGD with biliary flow measurement	4A0C85Z
3. Right and left heart cardiac catheterization with bilateral sampling and pressure measurements	4A023N8
4. Temperature monitoring, rectal	4A1Z7KZ
5. Peripheral venous pulse, external, single measurement	4A04XJ1
6. Holter monitoring	4A12X45
7. Respiratory rate, external, single measurement	4A09XCZ
8. Fetal heart rate monitoring, transvaginal	4A1H7CZ
9. Visual mobility test, single measurement	4A07X7Z
10. Left ventricular cardiac output monitoring from pulmonary artery wedge (Swan-Ganz) catheter	4A1239Z
11. Olfactory acuity test, single measurement	4A08X0Z

Extracorporeal or Systemic Assistance and Performance

Procedure	Code
1. Intermittent mechanical ventilation, 16 hours	5A1935Z
2. Liver dialysis, single encounter	5A1C00Z
3. Cardiac countershock with successful conversion to sinus rhythm	5A2204Z
4. IPPB (intermittent positive pressure breathing) for mobilization of secretions, 22 hours	5A09358
5. Renal dialysis, 12 hours	5A1D80Z
6. IABP (intra-aortic balloon pump) continuous	5A02210
7. Intra-operative cardiac pacing, continuous	5A1223Z
8. Intraoperative ECMO (extracorporeal membrane oxygenation), central	5A15A2F
9. Controlled mechanical ventilation (CMV), 45 hours	5A1945Z
10. Pulsatile compression boot with intermittent inflation	5A02115 (This is coded to the function value *Cardiac Output*, because the purpose of such compression devices is to return blood to the heart faster.)

Extracorporeal or Systemic Therapies

Procedure	Code
1. Donor thrombocytapheresis, single encounter	6A550Z2
2. Bili-lite phototherapy, series treatment	6A601ZZ
3. Whole body hypothermia, single treatment	6A4Z0ZZ
4. Circulatory phototherapy, single encounter	6A650ZZ
5. Shock wave therapy of plantar fascia, single treatment	6A930ZZ
6. Antigen-free air conditioning, series treatment	6A0Z1ZZ
7. TMS (transcranial magnetic stimulation), series treatment	6A221ZZ

Procedure	Code
8. Therapeutic ultrasound of peripheral vessels, single treatment	6A750Z6
9. Plasmapheresis, series treatment	6A551Z3
10. Extracorporeal electromagnetic stimulation (EMS) for urinary incontinence, single treatment	6A210ZZ

Osteopathic

Procedure	Code
1. Isotonic muscle energy treatment of right leg	7W06X8Z
2. Low velocity-high amplitude osteopathic treatment of head	7W00X5Z
3. Lymphatic pump osteopathic treatment of left axilla	7W07X6Z
4. Indirect osteopathic treatment of sacrum	7W04X4Z
5. Articulatory osteopathic treatment of cervical region	7W01X0Z

Other Procedures

Procedure	Code
1. Near infrared spectroscopy of leg vessels	8E023DZ
2. CT computer assisted sinus surgery	8E09XBG (The primary procedure is coded separately.)
3. Suture removal, abdominal wall	8E0WXY8
4. Isolation after infectious disease exposure	8E0ZXY6
5. Robotic assisted open prostatectomy	8E0W0CZ (The primary procedure is coded separately.)
6. In vitro fertilization	8E0ZXY1

Chiropractic

Procedure	Code
1. Chiropractic treatment of lumbar region using long lever specific contact	9WB3XGZ
2. Chiropractic manipulation of abdominal region, indirect visceral	9WB9XCZ
3. Chiropractic extra-articular treatment of hip region	9WB6XDZ
4. Chiropractic treatment of sacrum using long and short lever specific contact	9WB4XJZ
5. Mechanically-assisted chiropractic manipulation of head	9WB0XKZ

Imaging

Procedure	Code
1. Noncontrast CT of abdomen and pelvis	BW21ZZZ
2. Intravascular ultrasound, left subclavian artery	B342ZZ3
3. Fluoroscopic guidance for insertion of central venous catheter in SVC, low osmolar contrast	B5181ZA
4. Chest x-ray, AP/PA and lateral views	BW03ZZZ
5. Endoluminal ultrasound of gallbladder and bile ducts	BF43ZZZ
6. MRI of thyroid gland, contrast unspecified	BG34YZZ
7. Esophageal videofluoroscopy study with oral barium contrast	BD11YZZ
8. Portable x-ray study of right radius/ulna shaft, standard series	BP0JZZZ
9. Routine fetal ultrasound, second trimester twin gestation	BY4DZZZ

Procedure	Code
10. CT scan of bilateral lungs, high osmolar contrast with densitometry	BB240ZZ
11. Fluoroscopic guidance for percutaneous transluminal angioplasty (PTA) of left common femoral artery, low osmolar contrast	B41G1ZZ

Nuclear Medicine

Procedure	Code
1. Tomo scan of right and left heart, unspecified radiopharmaceutical, qualitative gated rest	C226YZZ
2. Technetium pentetate assay of kidneys, ureters, and bladder	CT631ZZ
3. Uniplanar scan of spine using technetium oxidronate, with first-pass study	CP151ZZ
4. Thallous chloride tomographic scan of bilateral breasts	CH22SZZ
5. PET scan of myocardium using rubidium	C23GQZZ
6. Gallium citrate scan of head and neck, single plane imaging	CW1BLZZ
7. Xenon gas nonimaging probe of brain	C050VZZ
8. Upper GI scan, radiopharmaceutical unspecified, for gastric emptying	CD15YZZ
9. Carbon 11 PET scan of brain with quantification	C030BZZ
10. Iodinated albumin nuclear medicine assay, blood plasma volume study	C763HZZ

Radiation Therapy

Procedure	Code
1. Plaque radiation of left eye, single port	D8Y0FZZ
2. 8 MeV photon beam radiation to brain	D0011ZZ
3. IORT of colon, 3 ports	DDY5CZZ
4. HDR brachytherapy of prostate using low dose palladium-103, unidirectional source	DV10BB1
5. Electron radiation treatment of right breast, with custom device	DM013ZZ
6. Hyperthermia oncology treatment of pelvic region	DWY68ZZ
7. Contact radiation of tongue	D9Y57ZZ
8. Heavy particle radiation treatment of pancreas, four risk sites	DF034ZZ
9. LDR brachytherapy to spinal cord using iodine	D016B9Z
10. Whole body Phosphorus 32 administration with risk to hematopoietic system	DWY5GFZ

Physical Rehabilitation and Diagnostic Audiology

Procedure	Code
1. Bekesy assessment using audiometer	F13Z31Z
2. Individual fitting of left eye prosthesis	F0DZ8UZ
3. Physical therapy for range of motion and mobility, patient right hip, no special equipment	F07L0ZZ
4. Bedside swallow assessment using assessment kit	F00ZHYZ
5. Caregiver training in airway clearance techniques	F0FZ8ZZ
6. Application of short arm cast in rehabilitation setting	F0DZ7EZ (Inhibitory cast is listed in the equipment reference table under E, *Orthosis*.)
7. Verbal assessment of patient's pain level	F02ZFZZ

Procedure	Code
8. Caregiver training in communication skills using manual communication board	F0FZJMZ (Manual communication board is listed in the equipment reference table under M, *Augmentative/ Alternative Communication*.)
9. Group musculoskeletal balance training exercises, whole body, no special equipment	F07M6ZZ (Balance training is included in the motor treatment reference table under *Therapeutic Exercise*.)
10. Individual therapy for auditory processing using tape recorder	F09Z2KZ (Tape recorder is listed in the equipment reference table under *Audiovisual Equipment*.)

Mental Health

Procedure	Code
1. Cognitive-behavioral psychotherapy, individual	GZ58ZZZ
2. Narcosynthesis	GZGZZZZ
3. Light therapy	GZJZZZZ
4. ECT (electroconvulsive therapy), unilateral, multiple seizure	GZB1ZZZ
5. Crisis intervention	GZ2ZZZZ
6. Neuropsychological testing	GZ13ZZZ
7. Hypnosis	GZFZZZZ
8. Developmental testing	GZ10ZZZ
9. Vocational counseling	GZ61ZZZ
10. Family psychotherapy	GZ72ZZZ

Substance Abuse Treatment

Procedure	Code
1. Naltrexone treatment for drug dependency	HZ94ZZZ
2. Substance abuse treatment family counseling	HZ63ZZZ
3. Medication monitoring of patient on methadone maintenance	HZ81ZZZ
4. Individual interpersonal psychotherapy for drug abuse	HZ54ZZZ
5. Patient in for alcohol detoxification treatment	HZ2ZZZZ
6. Group motivational counseling	HZ47ZZZ
7. Individual 12-step psychotherapy for substance abuse	HZ53ZZZ
8. Post-test infectious disease counseling for IV drug abuser	HZ3CZZZ
9. Psychodynamic psychotherapy for drug dependent patient	HZ5CZZZ
10. Group cognitive-behavioral counseling for substance abuse	HZ42ZZZ

New Technology

Procedure	Code
1. Infusion of terlipressin via peripheral venous catheter	XW03367
2. Transcatheter dilation of left peroneal artery with 2 SAVAL stents	X27U395